# Oral and Maxillofacial Surgery for the Clinician

Krishnamurthy Bonanthaya
Elavenil Panneerselvam • Suvy Manuel
Vinay V. Kumar • Anshul Rai
Editors

# Oral and Maxillofacial Surgery for the Clinician

Volume I

Springer

*Editors*
Krishnamurthy Bonanthaya
Bhagwan Mahaveer Jain hospital
Bangalore
India

Suvy Manuel
Ananthapuri Hospitals & Research Institute
Kerala Institute of Medical Sciences
Trivandrum, Kerala
India

Anshul Rai
Associate Professor
Department of Dentistry
All India Institute of Medical Sciences
Bhopal, Madhya Pradesh
India

Elavenil Panneerselvam
Associate Professor
SRM Dental College, Ramapuram
Chennai, Tamil Nadu
India

Vinay V. Kumar
Department of Maxillofacial Plastic Surgery
Uppsala University Hospital
Uppsala
Sweden

*Video Editors*
Jimson Samson
Vice Principal
Prof & Head of Department
Department of Oral & Maxillofacial Surgery
Tagore Dental College & Hospital
Chennai, India

Nehal Patel
Director, DCKH Cleft Center
K. P. Sanghvi Hospital
Surat, India

*Illustrator*
Mr Brishank Pratap
Goa, India

*Voice-over for Videos*
Madhulaxmi Marimuthu
Professor
Saveetha Dental College
Chennai, India

Vivek Narayanan
Dean, SRM Dental College
Kaatangulathur
Chennai, India

This book is an open access publication.
ISBN 978-981-15-1345-9 ISBN 978-981-15-1346-6 (eBook)
https://doi.org/10.1007/978-981-15-1346-6



This Springer imprint is published by the registered company Springer Nature Singapore Pte Ltd.
The registered company address is: 152 Beach Road, #21-01/04 Gateway East, Singapore 189721, Singapore

# Preface

An important question that always comes up when a book of this scope and extent is written is: why do we need one more?

This deserves a thoughtful answer and we shall try to do that while tracing the origin and evolution of this book from an idea. Since its inception in 1969, the *Association of Oral and Maxillofacial Surgeons of India* (AOMSI) has made steady and significant progress in terms of its vision and commitment to promote the field. The members of AOMSI have also evolved into a vibrant, multidimensional, passionate, and committed community of oral and maxillofacial surgeons who are making substantial contribution to the field in India and around the world. So it was only natural that the association decided to express its commitment to academic medicine coinciding with its 50th year in existence.

And what better way to express it than publishing an open source comprehensive textbook on oral and maxillofacial surgery. This book showcases the experts and expertise of AOMSI and has been made freely available to surgeons worldwide through generous funding from the association. We are delighted to see this open access book published for free use by worldwide community of MaxFac surgeons, especially the young surgeons and trainees in the field. This book is published with a CCBY license and we encourage associations and institutes to widely distribute the link to this book for maximum possible usage.

The AOMSI was very conscious that the development of our speciality was not an insular one. As we evolved, we looked for guidance and training from colleagues around the world, and in return, we provided our bit of experience and insights. This exchange of knowledge is extremely important for ultimately improving patient treatment methods, techniques, and outcomes. The same spirit was applied in producing this book as well' as we requested eminent clinicians and researchers from around the world along with our members to contribute to this book.

The book has contributions by society's members within India as well as 41 international authors from various countries. Thus, the extent of this makes it one of the most comprehensive textbooks on the topic. The contributors were invited by the AOMSI keeping in mind their scholastic profile while ensuring diversity and inclusiveness as well as a mix of young and experienced surgeons. All the contributors have a track record of being high-volume clinicians and educators in their field of expertise and are generally working at prestigious teaching institutions. This textbook as a scholarly venture condenses and amalgamates both the authors' personal experience as well as being in line with the current evidence-based treatment principles in the field of maxillofacial surgery. In the beginning, the heterogeneous source of knowledge did pose editorial challenges in standardization of the chapter structuring and scope. However, the final outcome has achieved a blend of evidence-based, diverse surgical practices along with cutting-edge technology for the practice of maxillofacial surgery in a fairly uniform format.

As the title suggests, this is meant to be a comprehensive resource for all clinicians, postgraduate trainees, and young surgeons in their day-to-day clinical work. Graduate students and surgeons will find this book useful in preparing for their university exams as well as board-certified exams from professional organizations. The book will help in decision-making, implementing treatment plans, and managing problems that may arise while executing these plans. Overall, the key objective is to help crystallize current evidence and provide protocols, guidelines, and recommendations to assist dealing with most clinical scenarios. Keeping this objective in mind, we have included components like case scenarios and video recordings of surgical procedures in the book.

*Oral and Maxillofacial Surgery for the Clinician* is a compilation of 22 sections incorporating 88 chapters dealing with the nuances in the principles and practice of cranio-maxillofacial and head and neck surgery. An important value addition is the library of 68 demonstrational videos that have been compiled to give the readers a more interactive feel with audiovisual inputs.

The book is structured in a step-ladder fashion to guide the reader through the basic principles of surgery before exposing to the full spectrum of specialty cranio-maxillofacial work. The first section is devoted to the origin and scope of oral and maxillofacial surgery as a specialty and a description of the training standards practiced globally. The next four sections are tailored to discuss the prospective patient, investigations, patient preparation, and anesthesia techniques. Subsequent sections focus on minor surgical procedures involving the practice of dento-alveolar surgery, implantology, and orofacial infections. With the above as the basis, the textbook progresses to complex surgical procedures including facial trauma, orthognathic surgery, TMJ, surgical pathology, and craniofacial and reconstructive surgery. The book also features two exclusive sections which provide the readers a perspective on practice management and research and publication.

The editors of the book would like to thank the office bearers of the AOMSI, in particular, the dynamic and effervescent secretary, Pritham Shetty, for the constant support he gave while undertaking this project.

Brishank Pratap, our tireless and innovative illustrator, needs a special mention for his superb rendition of medical and technical illustrations throughout this book.

Our publisher Springer, particularly, Naren Aggarwal and Jagjeet Kaur, deserves our gratitude for constant support and advice throughout the preparation of this book.

Last but not least, we would like to express our deep appreciation for the authors for their time, efforts, and priceless contributions.

We hope this book will be read worldwide, and we look forward to hear its critical reviews.

Bangalore, India — Krishnamurthy Bonanthaya
Chennai, India — Elavenil Panneerselvam
Trivandrum, India — Suvy Manuel
Uppsala, Sweden — Vinay V. Kumar
Bhopal, India — Anshul Rai
Chennai, India — Jimson Samson
Surat, India — Nehal Patel

# Contents

# List of Videos

# Chapter Contributors and Video Contributors

## Contributors

**Avni Pandey Acharya** GSR Institute of Cranio-maxillofacial & Facial Plastic Surgery, Hyderabad, Telangana, India

**H. S. Adenwalla** Department of Plastic Surgery, Burns and the Charles Pinto Centre for Cleft Lip, Palate and Craniofacial Anomalies, Jubilee Mission Medical College and Research Institute, Thrissur, Kerala, India

**Neha Aggarwal** Nair Hospital Dental College, Mumbai, Maharashtra, India

Meenakshi Cleft and Craniofacial Centre, Chennai, Tamil Nadu, India

**Nisheet Anant Agni** Department of Oral and Maxillofacial Surgery, SMBT Institute of Dental Sciences and Research, Nashik, India

**Suman Ananathanarayana** Department of Anesthesiology, Columbia Asia Referral Hospital, Yeshwantpur, Bangalore, Karnataka, India

**Sonal Anchlia** Department of Oral & Maxillofacial Surgery, Government Dental College & Hospital, Ahmedabad, Gujarat, India

**Neelam N. Andrade** Department of Oral and Maxillofacial Surgery, Nair Hospital Dental College, Mumbai, Maharashtra, India

**Yashoda Ashok** Department of Oral and Maxillofacial Surgery, Meenakshi Ammal Dental College and Hospitals, Chennai, Tamil Nadu, India

**Prithvi S. Bachalli** Department of Oral and Maxillofacial Surgery, Rangadore Memorial Hospital, Apollo Hospitals, Bangalore, Karnataka, India

**Mirza Farhatullah Baig** Department of Oral and Maxillofacial Surgery, Saveetha Dental College, Chennai, Tamil Nadu, India

**Kannan Balaraman** Department of Oral and Maxillofacial Surgery, Ganga Medical Centre and Hospitals, Coimbatore, Tamil Nadu, India

**Rishi Kumar Bali** Postgraduate Department of OMFS, DAV Dental College Hospital, Yamunanagar, Haryana, India

**Peter A. Brennan** Maxillofacial Unit, Queen Alexandria Hospital, Portsmouth, UK

**Srinivasa R. Chandra** Department of Head and Neck Oncology and Reconstructive Microvascular and Oral and Maxillofacial Surgery, Fred and Pamela Buffett Cancer Center, UNMC, Omaha, NE, USA

**Jaideep Singh Chauhan** Department of Maxillofacial Surgery, the Smile Train CHL Hospital, Indore, Madhya Pradesh, India

**Aarti Chowdhary** Department of Periodontology, SD Dental College and Hospital, Parbhani, Maharashtra, India

**John Collin** Department of Oral and Maxillofacial Surgery, University of Florida, Jacksonville, FL, USA

**Ashok Dabir** D. Y. Patil University School of Dentistry, Nerul, Navi Mumbai, India

Breach Candy Hospital, Mumbai, India

**Abhay Datarkar** Department of Oral and Maxillofacial Surgery, Government Dental College and Hospital, Medical College Premises, Nagpur, Maharashtra, India

**Vijay Deshmukh** Deshmukh Institute of Maxillofacial Surgery and Research Centre, Aurangabad, Maharashtra, India

JIIU'S Indian Institute of Medical Sciences, Jalna, Maharashtra, India

**Amit Dhawan** Department of Oral and Maxillofacial Surgery, SGRD Dental Institute, Amritsar, India

**George Dimitroulis** Maxillofacial Unit, St. Vincent's Hospital—University of Melbourne, Melbourne, Australia

**Vikas Dhupar** Department of Oral and Maxillofacial Surgery, Goa Dental College and Hospital, Bambolim, Goa, India

**Supriya Ebenezer** Department of Oral Surgery and Stomatology, University of Bern, Bern, Switzerland

**El Mustafa** Department of Oral and Maxillofacial Surgery, Queen Elizabeth Hospital, Birmingham, UK

**Madan G. Ethunandan** Consultant Oral and Maxillofacial/Skull Base Surgeon, Honorary Senior Clinical Lecturer, Lead, Head and Neck Cancer, University Hospital Southampton, Southampton, UK

**Carlo Ferretti** , Johannesburg, South Africa

Department of Maxillofacial and Oral Surgery, University of Pretoria, Pretoria, South Africa

**Rui Fernandes** Department of Oral and Maxillofacial Surgery, Head and Neck Oncologic Surgery and Microvascular Fellowship, University of Florida, Jacksonville, FL, USA

**Rajasekhar Gaddipati** Department of Oral and Maxillofacial Surgery, Mamata Dental College, Khammam, Telangana, India

**Divya P. Gadre** Gadre Clinic, Pune, Maharashtra, India

**Kiran S. Gadre** Gadre Clinic, Pune, Maharashtra, India

Department of Oral and Maxillofacial Surgery, Bharati Vidyapeeth Dental College and Hospital, Pune, Maharashtra, India

**Raja Sekhar Gali** Department of Oral and Maxillofacial Surgery, Narayana Dental College and Hospital, Nellore, Andhra Pradesh, India

Medicover Hospital, Nellore, Andhra Pradesh, India

**Kandasamy Ganesan** Department of Oral and Maxillofacial Surgery, Southend University Hospitals NHS Trust, Southend-on-Sea, UK

University of Leeds, Leeds, UK

**Jaime Grant** Birmingham Children's Hospital, Birmingham, UK

**Beat Hammer** CFC Hirslanden Kopf Zentrum, Aarau, Switzerland

**Kalarikkal Mukundan Harish** Department of Oral & Maxillofacial Surgery, Ragas Dental College, Chennai, Tamil Nadu, India

**Velupillai Ilankovan** Oral and Maxillofacial Surgery, Poole Hospital NHS Foundation Trust, Poole, UK

**D' Souza Jacob** Maxillofacial Unit, Royal Surrey County Hospital, Guilford, UK

**Oommen Aju Jacob** Department of Oral and Maxillofacial Surgery, Ananthapuri Hospitals and Research Institute, Trivandrum, Kerala, India

Kerala Institute of Medical Sciences, Trivandrum, Kerala, India

**Rebecca Jacob** Department of Anesthesiology, Columbia Asia Referral Hospital, Yeshwantpur, Bangalore, Karnataka, India

**Anuj Jain** Oral and Maxillofacial Surgeon, Department of Trauma and Emergency Medicine, All India Institute of Medical Sciences, Bhopal, Madhya Pradesh, India

**B. S. Jayanth** Oral and Maxillofacial Surgeon, ABMSS, Bengaluru, Karnataka, India

**Samson Jimson** Department of Oral and Maxillofacial Surgery, Tagore Dental College and Hospital, Chennai, Tamil Nadu, India

**Bobby John** Department of Oral and Maxillofacial Surgery, Government Dental College, Kottayam, Kerala, India

Kerala University of Health Sciences, Thrissur, Kerala, India

**Reena Rachel John** Department of Oral and Maxillofacial Surgery, Vinayaka Mission's Sankarachariar Dental College and Hospital, VMRF, DU, Salem, India

**Maj Anson Jose** Oral and Maxillofacial Surgery, ADC R&R, New Delhi, India

**Shyamsundar K. Joshi** Department of Radiology, SDM College of Medical Sciences and Hospital, Shri Dharmasthala Manjunatheshwara University, Dharwad, India

**Takahiro Kanno** Department of Oral and Maxillofacial Surgery, Shimane University, Faculty of Medicine, Izumo, Shimane, Japan

**Taranjit Kaur** Department of Oral and Maxillofacial Surgery, Government Dental College and Hospital, Jamnagar, Gujarat, India

**Manal M. Khan** Department of Burns and Plastic Surgery, AIIMS Bhopal, Bhopal, Madhya Pradesh, India

**Rakshit Vijay Sinai Khandeparker** Department of Oral and Maxillofacial Surgery, Goa Dental College and Hospital, Bambolim, Goa, India

**Annie I. Kochuveettil** Department of Radiology, SDM College of Medical Sciences and Hospital, Shri Dharmasthala Manjunatheshwara University, Dharwad, India

**David Koppel** Scottish National Craniofacial Service for Children and Young People, Royal Hospital for Children, Glasgow, UK

**Shreya Krishna** Oral and Maxillofacial Surgery, Rangadore Memorial Hospital, Apollo Hospitals, Bangalore, India

**V. B. Krishnakumar Raja** Department of Oral & Maxillofacial Surgery, SRM Dental College & Hospital, Ramapuram, Chennai, Tamil Nadu, India

**B. Krishnan** Department of Dentistry, Jawaharlal Institute of Postgraduate Medical Education and Research (JIPMER), Puducherry, India

**Deepak G. Krishnan** Oral and Maxillofacial Surgery, University of Cincinnati Medical Center, Cincinnati, OH, USA

Cincinnati Children's Hospital and Medical Center, Cincinnati, OH, USA

**Balasubramanya Kumar** Department of Oral and Maxillofacial Surgery, St. Marthas's Hospital, Bangalore, Karnataka, India

Bhagwan Mahaveer Jain Hospital, Vikram Hospital, Bangalore, Karnataka, India

**Vinay V. Kumar** Department of Maxillofacial and Plastic Surgery, Uppsala University Hospital, Uppsala, Sweden

**Moni Abraham Kuriakose** Cochin Cancer Research Centre, Kochi, Kerala, India

**Paritkumar Ladani** Swiss Cleft and Craniofacial Centre, BSES MG Hospital, Mumbai, India

**Subramanyam S. Mahankali** Department of Anesthesiology, Columbia Asia Referral Hospital, Yeshwantpur, Bangalore, Karnataka, India

**Neelima Malik** Department of Oral and Maxillofacial Surgery, Krishna Institute of Medical Sciences "Deemed to be University", Karad, Maharashtra, India

**Varghese Mani** Department of Oral and Maxillofacial Surgery, Mar Baselios Dental College, Kothamangalam, Kerala, India

**Suvy Manuel** Department of Oral and Maxillofacial Surgery, Ananthapuri Hospitals and Research Institute, Trivandrum, Kerala, India

Kerala Institute of Medical Sciences, Trivandrum, Kerala, India

**Renita Maria** Department of Anesthesiology, Columbia Asia Referral Hospital, Yeshwantpur, Bangalore, Karnataka, India

**Madhulaxmi Marimuthu** Department of Oral & Maxillofacial Surgery, Saveetha Dental College & Hospital, Chennai, Tamil Nadu, India

**Paul Mathai** Nair Hospital Dental College, Mumbai, Maharashtra, India

Department of Oral and Maxillofacial Surgery, Jubilee Mission Medical College & Research Institute, Thrissur, Kerala, India

**Philip Mathew** Department of Oral and Maxillofacial Surgery, Jubilee Mission Medical College & Research Institute, Thrissur, Kerala, India

**Sainath Matsa** Praseedha Clinic for Maxillofacial Cosmetic Surgery, Chennai, Tamil Nadu, India

**Divya Mehrotra** Department of Oral and Maxillofacial Surgery, King George's Medical University, Lucknow, India

**Sushma Mehta** Mazumdar Shaw Cancer Center, Bengaluru, Karnataka, India

**Suresh Menon** Department of Oral and Maxillofacial Surgery, Vydehi Institute of Dental Sciences and Research Centre, Bangalore, Karnataka, India

**Aditya Moorthy** Department of Oral and Maxillofacial Surgery, Rangadore Memorial Hospital, Apollo Hospitals, Bangalore, Karnataka, India

**Mustafa. K** Department of Craniofacial Surgery, Kanachur Institute of Medical Sciences, Mangalore, Karnataka, India

**Veerabahu Muthusubramanian** Department of Oral & Maxillofacial Surgery, Ragas Dental College, Chennai, Tamil Nadu, India

**Sowjanya Nagamalla** Department of Oral and Maxillofacial Surgery, Virginia Commonwealth University Medical Center, Richmond, VA, USA

**Sanjiv Nair** Department of Oral and Maxillofacial Surgery, Bhagwan Mahaveer Jain Hospital, Bengaluru, Karnataka, India

**P. V. Narayanan** Consultant Plastic Surgeon, Jubilee Mission Medical College & Research Institute, Thrissur, Kerala, India

**Nasir A. Nasser** Barts & London NHS Trust, Whipps Cross University Hospital, London, UK

University Hospital, Berne, Switzerland

**J. Naveen Kumar** Oral and Maxillofacial Surgery, Sri Ramachandra Institute of Higher Education and Research, Chennai, India

**Kishore Nayak** Bhagvan Jain Mahaveer Hospital, Bangalore, India

**R. S. Neelakandan** Department of Oral and Maxillofacial Surgery, Meenakshi Ammal Dental College and Hospital, MAHER, Chennai, Tamil Nadu, India

**Rachel S. Oeppen** Consultant Radiologist, University Hospital Southampton, Southampton, UK

**Arun Kumar Panda** Department of Oral & Maxillofacial Surgery, SD Dental College and Hospital, Parbhani, Maharashtra, India

**Elavenil Panneerselvam** Department of Oral and Maxillofacial Surgery, SRM Dental College, Ramapuram, Chennai, Tamil Nadu, India

Department of Orbit & Oculoplasty, Aravind Eye Hospital, Chennai, Tamil Nadu, India

**Shreya Panwar** Department of Oral & Maxillofacial Surgery, Meenakshi Ammal Dental College & Hospital, Chennai, Tamil Nadu, India

**Ananthanarayanan Parameswaran** Department of Oral and Maxillofacial Surgery, Meenakshiammal Dental College & Hospital, Chennai, Tamil Nadu, India

Department of Orbit, Oculoplasty, Reconstructive & Aesthetic Surgery, Shankara Nethralaya, Chennai, Tamil Nadu, India

Department of Orbit & Oculoplasty, Aravind Eye Hospital, Chennai, Tamil Nadu, India

**Satyen Parida** Department of Anesthesiology and Critical Care, Jawaharlal Institute of Postgraduate Medical Education and Research (JIPMER), Puducherry, India

**Sat Parmar** Department of Oral and Maxillofacial Surgery, Queen Elizabeth Hospital, Birmingham, UK

**Mamatha Patil** Department of Oral and Maxillofacial Surgery, Sparsh Hospital, Bangalore, Karnataka, India

**George Paul** Kerala University of Health Sciences, Thrissur, Kerala, India

Dr MGR Medical University, Chennai, Tamil Nadu, India

**Vijay Pillai** Department of Head and Neck Surgical Oncology, Mazumdar Shaw Cancer Center, Narayana Health, Bangalore, Karnataka, India

**Sreedhar Reddy Pothula** Oral and Maxillofacial Surgery, Pioneer advanced Hair Transplant Centre, Bengaluru, Karnataka, India

**Abhinand Potturi** SVS Institute of Dental Sciences, Mahabubnagar, Telangana State, India

**Akhilesh Prathap** Department of Oral and Maxillofacial Surgery, Pushpagiri College of Dental Sciences, Thiruvalla, Kerala, India

**Prav Praveen** Department of Oral and Maxillofacial Surgery, Queen Elizabeth Hospital, Birmingham NHS Foundation Trust, Birmingham, UK

**Boyapati Raghu** Maxillofacial Unit, Royal Surrey County Hospital, Guilford, UK

**Anshul Rai** Department of Dentistry, All India Institute of Medical Sciences, Bhopal, Madhya Pradesh, India

**Manjunath Rai** Department of OMFS, A. J. Institute of Dental Sciences, Mangalore, Karnataka, India

Faculty of Dentistry, RGUHS, Bangalore, India

**Manikandhan Ramanathan** Department of Oral and Maxillofacial surgery, Meenakshi Ammal Dental College and Hospital, MAHER University, Chennai, Tamil Nadu, India

Meenakshi Cleft and Craniofacial Centre, Chennai, Tamil Nadu, India

**Dipesh Rao** Bhagwan Mahaveer Jain Hospital, Bangalore, Karnataka, India

**Latha P. Rao** Department of Craniomaxillofacial Surgery, Aster Medcity, Kochi, Kerala, India

**Neelam Rathod** Department of Oral and Maxillofacial Surgery, Southend University Hospitals NHS trust, Southend-on-Sea, UK

**Poornima Ravi** Department of Oral and Maxillofacial Surgery, SRM Dental College, Ramapuram, Chennai, Tamil Nadu, India

**Srinivas Gosla Reddy** GSR Institute of Cranio-maxillofacial & Facial Plastic Surgery, Hyderabad, Telangana, India

**N. Viveka Vardhan Reddy** Oral and Maxillofacial Surgery, SVS Institute of Dental Sciences, Mahabubnagar, Telangana, India

**Shravan Renapurkar** Department of Oral and Maxillofacial Surgery, Virginia Commonwealth University Medical Center, Richmond, VA, USA

**Christoph Renné** Group Practice for Pathology Wiesbaden, Wiesbaden, Germany

**Tara Renton** Oral Surgery, Kings College, London, UK

**Johan P. Reyneke** Center for Orthognathic Surgery, Mediclinic, Cape Town, South Africa

Department of Oral and Maxillofacial Surgery, Faculty of Health Sciences, University of the Western Cape, Cape Town, South Africa

Department of Oral and Maxillofacial Surgery, University of Oklahoma, Oklahoma City, OK, USA

**Sunil Richardson** Richardson's Dental and Craniofacial Hospital, Nagercoil, Tamil Nadu, India

**Saurabh Saigal** Department of Anaesthesiology, AIIMS Bhopal, Bhopal, Madhya Pradesh, India

**B. Sasikala** Department of Oral and Maxillofacial Surgery, SRM Dental College, Ramapuram, Chennai, Tamil Nadu, India

**Anna Sayan** Poole Hospital NHS Foundation Trust, Poole, UK

**Tian Ee Seah** TES Clinic for Face and Jaw, Singapore, Singapore

**Nallamilli V. S. Sekhar Reddy** Panineeya Institute of Dental Sciences and Research Centre, Hyderabad, Telangana, India

**Anjan Kumar Shah** Department of Oral and Maxillofacial Surgery, Rajarajeswari Dental College, Bangalore, India

Bhagwan Mahaveer Jain Hospital, Bangalore, India

**Garima Sharma** Department of Anesthesiology, Columbia Asia Referral Hospital, Yeshwantpur, Bangalore, Karnataka, India

**Lt Col Rohit Sharma** Oral and Maxillofacial Surgery, 11 Corps Dental Unit, Jalandhar Cantt, India

**Kishore Shekar** Head and Neck Surgeon (OMFS), Ninewells Hospital and Dundee, University Medical School, Dundee, UK

**Pritham N. Shetty** Department of Oral and maxillofacial surgery, Bangalore Institute of Dental Science, Bangalore, Karnataka, India

**Omkar Anand Shetye** Department of Oral and Maxillofacial Surgery, Goa Dental College and Hospital, Bambolim, Goa, India

**Sunil S. Shroff** Department of Oral and Maxillofacial Surgery, Bhagwan Mahaveer Jain Hospital, Bengaluru, Karnataka, India

**Anand Shukla** Department of Oral and Maxillofacial Surgery, King George's Medical University, Lucknow, India

**Deepti Simon** Department of Oral and Maxillofacial Surgery, Government Dental College, Trivandrum, Kerala, India

Kerala University of Health Sciences, Thrissur, Kerala, India

**Robert A. Strauss** Department of Oral and Maxillofacial Surgery, Virginia Commonwealth University Medical Center, Richmond, VA, USA

**Shintaro Sukegawa** Division of Oral and Maxillofacial Surgery, Kagawa Prefectural Central Hospital, Takamatsu, Kagawa, Japan

**Shikha Tayal** Department of Oral and Maxillofacial Surgery, Government Dental College and Hospital, Medical College Premises, Nagpur, Maharashtra, India

**Mary Thomas** Department of Anesthesiology, Regional Cancer Centre, Medical College Campus, Thiruvananthapuram, Kerala, India

**Andreas Thor** Department of Maxillofacial and Plastic Surgery, Uppsala University Hospital, Uppsala, Sweden

**Asha Thomson** Norfolk and Norwich University Hospitals, Norfolk, UK

**Benjamin Turner** Department of Oral and Maxillofacial Surgery, University of Florida, Jacksonville, FL, USA

**Jayesh Vahanwala** Department of Oral and Maxillofacial Surgery, Vaidik Dental College & Research Centre, Nani Daman, India

Breach Candy Hospital, Mumbai, India

**George Varghese** Principal, Professor and Head, Department of Oral and Maxillofacial Surgery, Pushpagiri College of Dental Sciences, Tiruvalla, Kerala, India

**Ravi Veeraraghavan** Department of Oral and Maxillofacial Surgery, Amrita School of Dentistry, Ernakulam, India

**Payal Verma** Oral and Maxillofacial Surgery, University of Cincinnati Medical Center, OH, Cincinnati, USA

**Christian Walter** Oral and Maxillofacial Surgery—Plastic Surgery, Mediplus Clinic Mainz, Mainz, Germany

**Gary Warburton** Department of Oral and Maxillofacial Surgery, University of Maryland School of Dentistry, Baltimore, MD, USA

**Frank Wilde** Department of Oral and Plastic Maxillofacial Surgery, Armed Forces Hospital, Ulm, Germany

Department of Oral and Maxillofacial Surgery, University Hospital, Ulm, Germany

**Abhilasha Yadav** Department of Oral and Maxillofacial Surgery, Awadh Dental College & Hospital, Jamshedpur, Jharkhand, India

## Video Contributors

**Prithvi S. Bachalli** Department of Oral and Maxillofacial Surgery, Rangadore Memorial Hospital, Apollo Hospitals, Bangalore, Karnataka, India

**Ramdas Balakrishna** Department of Oral and Maxillofacial Surgery, KLE's Institute of Dental Science and Research, Bangalore, India

**Anandh Balasubramanian** Department of Oral and Maxillofacial Surgery, Tagore Dental College and Hospital, Chennai, Tamil Nadu, India

**Mohan Baliga** Department of Oral and Maxillofacial Surgery, Manipal College of Dental Sciences, MAHE, Mangalore, Karnataka, India

**Biswajit Kumar Biswas** Avinash Institute of craniofacial and Reconstructive Surgery, Kolkata, India

**Lokesh Bhanumurthy** Department of Oral and Maxillofacial Surgery, Tagore Dental College and Hospital, Chennai, Tamil Nadu, India

**Rohit Chandra** Oral and Maxillofacial Surgeon, Department of Plastic Surgery, Max Hospitals, Vaishali and Noida, India

**Jaideep Singh Chauhan** Department of Oral and Maxillofacial Surgery, CHL Hospitals, Indore, Madhya Pradesh, India

**Anil Kumar Desai** Craniofacial Unit, SDM College of Dental Sciences & Hospital, Dharwad, India

**Anjaneya Dube** Department of Oral and Maxillofacial Surgery, Saptarshi Hospital and Cancer Centre, Jabalpur National Hospital, Jabalpur, India

**Gunjan Dube** Dube Surgical and Dental Hospital, Jabalpur, Madhya Pradesh, India

**Shehzana Fatima** Oral and Maxillofacial Surgeon, Dubai Health Authority, Dubai, UAE

**S. Girish Rao** Oral and Maxillofacial Surgeon, Shri Shankara Cancer Hospital and Research Center, Apollo Hospitals, Sagar Hospitals, Trustwell Hospital, NIMHANS, Bangalore, India

**Charu Girotra** Department of OMFS, School of Dentistry, D. Y. Patil Deemed to be University, Navi Mumbai, Maharashtra, India

**Gaurav Mahesh Gupta** Centre for Craniomaxillo Facial and Facial Plastic Surgery, Pushpanjali Hospital & Research Centre, Agra, Uttar Pradesh, India

**Rebecca Jacob** Department of Anesthesiology, Columbia Asia Referral Hospital, Yeshwantpur, Bangalore, India

**Jagadish Chandra** Department of OMFS, Yenepoya Dental College, Yenepoya Deemed to be University, Mangalore, India

**Samson Jimson** Department of Oral & Maxillofacial Surgery, Tagore Dental College & Hospital, Chennai, India

**Adarsh Kudva** Department of Oral and Maxillofacial Surgery, Manipal College of Dental Sciences, Mahe University, Manipal, India

**Deepak Kulkarni** Department of Oral and Maxillofacial Surgery, Dr D Y Patil Dental College, Pune, India

**Balasubramanya Kumar** Department of Oral and Maxillofacial Surgery, Bhagwan Mahaveer Jain Hospital, Vikram Hospital, Bangalore, India

**Paritkumar Ladani** Swiss Cleft and Craniofacial Centre, BSES MG Hospital, Mumbai, India

**Ummar Mangalath** Department of Oral and Maxillofacial Surgery, MES Dental College, Perinthalmanna, Kerala, India

**Philip Mathew** Department of Oral and Maxillofacial Surgery, Jubilee Mission Medical College and Hospital, Thrissur, Kerala, India

**Sainath Matsa** Praseedha Clinic for Maxillofacial Cosmetic Surgery, Chennai, Tamil Nadu, India

**Aditya Moorthy** Department of Oral and Maxillofacial Surgery, Rangadore Memorial Hospital, Apollo Hospitals, Bangalore, Karnataka, India

**Ravindran Nair** Department of Oral and Maxillofacial Surgery, Government Medical College, Manjeri, Kerala, India

**Anuradha Navaneetham** Department of Oral and Maxillofacial Surgery, M R Ambedkar Dental College, Rajiv Gandhi University, Bangalore, India

**Nilesh Pagaria** Oral and Maxillofacial Surgeon, Shrikrishna Hospital, Raipur, Chhattisgarh, India

**Arun Kumar Panda** Department of Oral & Maxillofacial Surgery, SD Dental College and Hospital, Parbhani, Maharashtra, India

**Ananthanarayanan Parameswaran** Department of Oral and Maxillofacial Surgery, Meenakshi Ammal Dental College & Hospital, Chennai, Tamil Nadu, India

**Nehal Patel** NuFace Maxillofacial Hospital, Surat, Gujarat, India

**Kavitha Prasad** Faculty of Dental Sciences, Ramaiah University of Applied Sciences, Bengaluru, India

**Satish Kumaran Pugazhendi** Department of Oral and Maxillofacial Surgery, M. R. Ambedkar Dental College, Bangalore, India

**Gunaseelan Rajan** Oral and Maxillofacial Surgeon, Rajan Dental Hospital, Chennai, Tamil Nadu, India

**Rajasekhar Gaddipati** Department of Oral and Maxillofacial Surgery, Mamata Dental College, Khammam, Telangana, India

**Sushmitha Rajmohan** Department of Dentistry & Maxillofacial Surgery, ESIC Model Hospital, Indore, India

Aasya the Clinic for Face Jaws & Teeth, Vijaynagar, Indore, MP, India

**Vidya Rattan** Unit of Oral & Maxillofacial Surgery, Oral Health Sciences Centre, Postgraduate Institute of Medical Education & Research, Chandigarh, India

**Pothula Sreedhar Reddy** Oral and Maxillofacial Surgeon, Pioneer Advanced Hair Transplant Center, Bangalore, India

**Sunil Richardson** Richardson's Dental and Craniofacial Hospital, Nagercoil, Tamil Nadu, India

**Senthil Murugan** Department of Oncology & Reconstructive Microsurgery, Saveetha Dental College, Saveetha University, Chennai, Tamil Nadu, India

DWIJAN Microsurgery Research & Training Centre, Chennai, India

**Navin Shah Sunderlal** Department of Oral and Maxillofacial Surgery, KM Shah Dental College, Sumandeep Vidyapeeth, A Central deemed to be University, Vadodara, Gujarat, India

**Yeshaswini Thelekkat** Department of Oral & Maxillofacial Surgery, Azeezia College of Dental Sciences and Research Kollam, Kollam, Kerala, India

**Joji Thomas** Department of Oral and Maxillofacial Surgery, Cosmopolitan Hospital Pvt Ltd, Trivandrum, Kerala, India

**P. Varun Menon** The Charles Pinto Centre for Cleft Lip, Palate and Craniofacial Anomalies, Jubilee Mission, Medical College & Research Institute, Thrissur, Kerala, India

**Sankar Vinod Vichattu** Department of OMFS, Mar Baselious Dental College, Kotamangalam, Kerala, India

**B. Vikraman** Department of Oral and Maxillofacial Surgery, Ragas Dental College & Hospital, Chennai, Tamil Nadu, India

**Gary Warburton** Department of Oral & Maxillofacial Surgery, University of Maryland Dental School, Baltimore, MD, USA

# About the Editors

**Krishnamurthy Bonanthaya** did his postgraduate dental studies from Mangalore University, and then he obtained his MBBS from Kasturba Medical College, Manipal. He is also a fellow of the Royal College of Surgeons of England and Royal College of Surgeons of Ireland. He is currently the project director of Smile Train Project treating cleft lip and palate deformities at Bhagwan Mahaveer Jain Hospital, Bangalore. He also holds the position of professor of oral and maxillofacial surgery, Bangalore Institute of Dental Sciences, which involves undergraduate and postgraduate training and the routine mix of maxillofacial surgical management. He is the editor in chief emeritus of the *Journal of Maxillofacial and Oral Surgery* and has numerous publications to his credit.

**Elavenil Panneerselvam** completed her postgraduation in oral and maxillofacial surgery from the Tamil Nadu Dr. M.G.R. Government Medical University, Chennai, India. She also has a master's degree in business administration, specializing in hospital management, fellowship in Aesthetic Medicine and has been awarded Fellowship in Dental Surgery by the Royal College of Physicians & Surgeons of Glasgow. She has contributed to textbooks on oral anatomy, local anesthesia, plastic surgery, and pediatric TMJ surgery. Presently, she holds a faculty position at the SRM Dental College (Ramapuram), Chennai, as associate professor in oral and axillofacial surgery. She is a recipient of the MM Cooper Memorial Research Award from the Indian Society for Anatomists and the Ginwalla Trophy from the Association of Oral & Maxillofacial Surgeons of India.

**Suvy Manuel** after his postgraduation from Government Dental College, Trivandrum, University of Kerala, in 2002, gained the Diplomate of National Board in Oral & Maxillofacial Surgery, Membership from the National Academy of Medical Sciences, New Delhi, India; and Diploma of Membership in Oral surgery, Royal College of Surgeons, Edinburgh.

During his tenure in the UK, he attained the Membership of the Faculty of Dental Surgery, Royal College of Surgeons, England. Subsequently, he attained the Fellowship in Dental Surgery, Royal College of Surgeons, Edinburgh. He is the MOMS RCSEd (Diploma of Membership in Oral Surgery) Examiner for the Royal College of Surgeons of Edinburgh in the Faculty of Dental Examiners, as appointed by the Dental Examinations Committee, RCS Edinburgh.

He is former professor and postgraduate guide at the Kerala University of Health Sciences and is a reviewer for the *Journal of Maxillofacial and Oral Surgery*.

Currently, he is attached to the maxillofacial units at Ananthapuri and KIMS Hospitals, Trivandrum, India.

**Vinay V. Kumar** completed his master's in oral and maxillofacial surgery from Nair Hospital Dental College, Mumbai, India, in 2008. He was an ITI Scholar in the Department of Maxillofacial and Plastic Surgery in Johannes Gutenberg University (JGU) Mainz, Germany, in 2010, where he went on to complete his Doctorate of Medicine in Dentistry (2013), obtain a practicing license, and served as a visiting faculty. He completed the MD and PhD program at the University of Medicine, Rostock, Germany in 2018. He is currently a Specialist Oral and Maxillofacial Surgeon in the Department of Maxillofacial and Plastic Surgery, Uppsala University Hospital, Sweden in the Department of Maxillofacial Surgery, Uppsala University, Sweden.

**Anshul Rai** is an Associate Professor in Department of Dentistry at All India Institute of Medical Sciences Bhopal, MP. He has 54 publications to his credit out of which 24 belong to prestigious international journals. He has contributed as a coauthor to *Textbook of Oral and Maxillofacial Surgery* by Dr. Borle. He is a Fellow of Indian Board of Oral and Maxillofacial Surgery (FIBOMS) and a fellow of the International Board for the Certification of Specialists in Oral and Maxillofacial Surgery (FIBCSOMS). He is a reviewer for *Journal of Maxillofacial and oral surgery and Indian Journal of Dental Research.*

**Jimson Samson** completed his postgraduate studies at the prestigious the Tamil Nadu Dr. M.G.R. Medical University, Chennai. Since completing his MDS, he has been in academics. He is a journal reviewer and also a section editor. He has lectured at various national and international conferences. He was also a faculty at OMFS workshops.

His special interest in research has made him Vice-Principal—Research at Tagore Dental College & Hospital, Chennai. In addition, he also heads the Department of Oral and Maxillofacial Surgery. He has published in indexed journals. He is now the Hon. State Secretary of the Association of Oral and Maxillofacial Surgeons of India, Tamil Nadu and Puducherry Branch. He is also an elected member of the Executive Committee of the National Association.

He is a member of the Board of Studies for Postgraduate Studies of Oral and Maxillofacial Surgery at the Tamil Nadu Dr. M.G.R. Medical University, Chennai.

**Nehal Patel** completed his master's in oral and maxillofacial surgery from A.B. Shetty Institute of Dental Sciences, Mangalore. He did his fellowship in Cleft and Craniofacial Surgery from Mangalore. He did his mini residency in TMJ Arthroscopy and Total Joint replacement from the USA. He worked as consultant cleft and craniofacial surgeon in BSES MG Hospital. He is currently working as Director, ABMSS CLEFT PROJECT in Surat, Gujarat.

# Part I

# Introduction

# 1 Oral and Maxillofacial Surgery in India: How Did We Get Here and Where Are We Going?

Kishore Nayak

## 1.1 History of Our Missions and Our Challenges

Any discussion about the history of surgery inevitably begins with an invariable reference to *Suśruta* and his contributions to facial surgery, in particular. While the contributions of the sixth-century sage surgeon may somewhat be nebulous in a foggy poorly documented history, they are inevitably (and arguably) numerous but need not be elaborated here in any manner. What is lesser known and not often spoken about is that Suśruta considered surgery the first and foremost branch of medicine and stated, "Surgery has the superior advantage of producing instantaneous effects by means of surgical instruments and appliances. Hence, it is the highest in value of all the medical tantras. It is eternal and a source of infinite piety, imports fame and opens the gates of Heaven to its votaries. It prolongs the duration of human existence on earth and helps men in successfully fulfilling their missions and earning a decent competence in life." [1, 2]

When applied specifically to the context of the specialty of Oral and Maxillofacial surgery (OMS) emerging in India, it raises many important questions on how we have emerged and more importantly what we see ourselves evolving into in the years to come. Perhaps all those debates that we labored along numerous times were all a part of our coming of age!

Like elsewhere in the world, in the mid-twentieth century, we were probably practitioners of dentoalveolar surgery working under very trying circumstances moving on to where we are today. The specialty in India today, is truly all encompassing in its scope. It embraces the entire and extended spectrum of the practice of oral and maxillofacial surgery, and as the Association of Oral and Maxillofacial Surgeons of India (AOMSI) approaches its 50th year in 2019, there is no better time to look back and reflect on the past and contemplate where we are heading. The changes that we have witnessed have been rapid and hopefully progressive. From being oral surgeons, we transitioned and added maxillofacial surgery and to our quiver and perhaps to the chagrin competing specialties treaded into areas, once considered "gray" and broadened the scope of our practices.

Mino S Ginwalla is regarded as the pioneer of oral and maxillofacial surgery in India. In the 1950s, Dr. Ginwalla arrived in Mumbai following surgical training in Montreal, Canada, and set up his practice at Nair Hospital. He was a part of the founding group of surgeons of the AOMSI in 1969. By the mid-70s, training programs were established in most of the major dental colleges throughout India. Today, there are numerous OMS training programs in India.

The dental qualified persons are governed by the statutes of the Dental Council of India [3]. Currently, the Dental Council of India provides for a comprehensive 3-year program that includes a syllabus and curriculum that exposes trainees to standard procedures covering the full spectrum of oral and maxillofacial surgery [4]. This provides a legal framework for the OMS to function. This qualification itself is only permission to practice the specialty. In today's system, competence and eventual ownership of key surgical domains often only come from structured post-qualification training.

Thus, traditionally, the specialty in India continues to be predominately a dental subspecialty that leans toward the idea of a surgical branch of dentistry. While many arguments have been made for and against the need for a medical degree to augment the specialty, it is safe to postulate that for the near future, we will remain a dental specialty for a variety of reasons. North Americans seem to have found a middle ground and of the 101 OMS training programs in the US, 55 are single-degree programs (dental degree only) and 43 are dual-degree (dental and medical) programs, and three offer both options.

Drawing comparisons to the international scenario, the specialty has always been on a pendulous path remaining undecided on the idea of whether it wants to stay a dental

K. Nayak (✉)
Bhagwan Mahaveer Jain Hospital, Bangalore, India


K. Bonanthaya et al. (eds.), *Oral and Maxillofacial Surgery for the Clinician*, https://doi.org/10.1007/978-981-15-1346-6_1

specialty or whether it wants to incorporate the medical degree. In the USA where this trend initially started, the practice of the specialty is protected by national, regional, and local legislature as a dental specialty. In reality, there is no perceivable practical difference in the scope of practice between single- or double-degree practitioners in the States. In the UK and many parts of Europe, the specialty has taken leaps and bounds toward the medical path of training and it could very well be only a matter of time before the Specialty remains only remotely associated with Dentistry. The primary challenge was a lack of understanding, which centered on the debate of whether a medical as well as a dental qualification was required prior to surgical training [5].

Oral and maxillofacial surgery remains a specialty of dentistry in India and most training programs involve a graduate study and thesis to obtain the Masters in Dental Surgery (MDS) degree. The dental practice act allows all qualified dentally trained oral and maxillofacial surgeons to practice the unrestricted and full scope of the specialty, similar to what occurs in the European nations that require a medical degree. In most of Europe, OMS has become a medical subspecialty.

Public perception of the scope of practice of the specialty remains below par. The specialty gets confused with other surgical domains within both dentistry and medicine that we share a scope.

## 1.2 Expertise, Familiarity, and Competence

"Innovation is the combination of different ideas and contribution of the different minds."

Laskin [6] attempts to address this problem by dividing the scope of oral and maxillofacial surgery into three parts: areas of expertise, competence, and familiarity.

- Areas of expertise include oral pathology/oral medicine, dentoalveolar surgery, preprosthetic surgery (including implantology), and maxillofacial traumatology.
- Areas of competence involve orthognathic surgery, temporomandibular joint surgery, and local reconstructive surgery.
- Areas of familiarity are cleft lip and palate surgery, regional reconstructive surgery, oncologic surgery, craniofacial surgery, and cosmetic surgery.

Laskin's system of classification, while seemingly appearing comprehensive, opens itself to a lot of debate and question. While there is no doubt that the areas of "expertise" are unique to our specialty, it is our foray into those areas of competence and familiarity that has led to the expansion of the scope of our specialty. This expansion and contraction of our scope may also be fundamental to continual evolution. A large majority of our colleagues in India and worldwide operate within the boundaries of that scope of practice defined as "expertise." However, to turn areas of familiarity into competence and expertise will require that the training units and staff have the required skills and volume of cases to ensure hands-on experience and documentation. Only under these circumstances can we be assured that the skill sets and competencies will be transferred and become enduring.

It is ideal that all trainees are trained to achieve competence in craniomaxillofacial trauma, orthognathic surgery, and TMJ surgery (i.e., maxillofacial surgery). This and only this can provide the transition from Oral to Maxillofacial surgery. There, however, is a clear and present reality that not all training programs are equipped to achieve this goal. Even though training standards and syllabi exist, these standards are so broad that even programs with a very limited scope of training will meet accreditation standards by reporting a narrow set of hospital-based procedures that are not representative of the scope of practice required of modern OMS. Further, the interest of the trainee in training in the full scope of surgery is a factor that leads to mediocre training. The system of choosing a postgraduate training in OMS in India is severely handicapped and primitive. The factors that decide a trainee's choice of an advanced training program have nothing to do with their aptitude or interest in a specialty. It is purely based on their standing in a national entrance examination or their affordability of a position in a private institution. This leads to complete neglect of the student's natural aptitudes leading to prosthodontists becoming orthodontists and endodontists doomed into the world of oral and maxillofacial surgery. A disinterested trainee will be barely motivated to improve the scope of their practice following completion of their training, often limiting their practice to general dentistry and minimal indulgence in areas of "expertise."

Bell [7], when contemplating the future of education and training in the specialty, raises some very valid concerns, which seem to reflect the issues that affect the specialty and its future worldwide. Many reasons for the training disparities exist today—including training program location, the presence or absence of a trauma center, limited head and neck surgery experience, and local politics—but regardless, the goal should be the same: to train oral and maxillofacial surgeons to competence in the core areas of the specialty that they will eventually practice.

The key point is that we, as a specialty, should ensure that we train to competence and expertise based on geographic location, years in practice, fellowship training, and academic involvement. In years past, if an OMS graduate wished to obtain training in any areas beyond basics, then he or she often sought it outside of the specialty, in either otolaryngology or plastic surgery. With the emergence of several teaching hospitals and colleges as well as standalone independent centers of excellence, this scenario has drastically transformed in India. Further, the development of a number of fellowships that have been facilitated by the AOMSI has resulted in a robust system within the specialty that caters to the trainee's desire, merit, and quite often desire to embrace technique and technology. The rapid and natural advent of OMS into areas of oncology and reconstruction, cleft lip and palate, craniofacial surgery, and aesthetic surgery has been unprecedented and the critical mass of those who now fit in comfortably with these are their areas of expertise is on the rise.

This has been a radical transformation. A few decades ago, wandering beyond the realms of dentoalveolar surgery and facial trauma inevitably encountered a glass ceiling. Today this has been most certainly breached. Moreover, while the majority of the specialty holds itself within the original areas of expertise, there is no doubt that the Big Bang Moment for OMS in India has happened and it is a great time to contemplate where we are heading. What does the future hold for the specialty as we drift on our very own Starship Enterprise?

## 1.3 Predicting the Future

"Look back over the past, with its changing empires that rose and fell, and you can foresee the future, too." Marcus Aurelius

Are we truly at a threshold or are we pieces in some continuum? What factors will drive our evolution as a specialty in India and our extended regions? What trends can we predictably follow to predict our future? Can we perhaps take a page from other fields in medicine to learn about ourselves? Will changing attitudes and aptitude of a new generation have a powerful impact on our profession or will we forever remain loyal to the vestiges of the legacy left behind for us?

Technology will undoubtedly play an important role in our future. Not just technology in patient care, but technology in our lives. Telemedicine and teleconsults will become a part of our everyday practice allowing us to practice beyond geographic limitations. Teleconferencing will make biannual AOMSI face-to-face conferences obsolete. In 2018, the American Association of Oral and Maxillofacial Surgeons (AAOMS) simulcasted their Dental Implant Conference, as did the American Society of Anesthesiologists. Their experience is that the while their total registration at these meetings went up, the number of in-person registrants did not dissipate. Consultant oral and maxillofacial surgeons all over the world have embraced telemedicine naturally, whether they realized it or not. Mobile technology allows the transfer of patient images and radiographs easily both for opinions and treatment planning. Such ease of access to patient images and documents has become a routine tool in emergency room triages of patients in the evaluation of the priority of care.

While technology in its current form is often perceived, as interruptive to one's lifestyle choices, the advent and immersion of artificial intelligence (AI) will make today's technology ubiquitous without being intrusive. Operating theaters of the future are likely to be guarded by artificial intelligence. Imagine an operating theater that prepares itself based on the radiofrequency identification (RFID) of the surgeon who swipes her/his badge at the door—that surgeon's preference cards get read by the system and a central core will prepare the instruments and supplies based on that surgeon's choices for that particular case booked for him.

Anesthesiology, radiology, and pathology are low-hanging fruits in the AI world. Radiologists in large tertiary-care centers in China, today, do not read radiographs anymore; they simply look at false positives read the previous night by their AI system. The system then learns from such mistakes and makes corrections forever. Computer systems today have the capacity of a thousand human brains to process data. The more data we feed these AI systems, the smarter they get. Google's AI product called LYNA or LymphNode Assistant is a trained algorithm that is capable of spotting the features of tumors that have metastasized, which are notoriously difficult to detect. Self-teaching algorithm systems will likely replace monitoring duties of the anesthesiologists and critical care nurses in the hospital.

Surgical robots are also constantly evolving incorporating precision haptics and AI. Robotic arms can already perform tasks independent of a surgeon yielding it. Imperfections and errors that a surgeon may cause in an operation are avoided in robotic surgery by consistent movements, angles, and access that can only be achieved by that robot. Imagine a robotic arm that can be programed to remove a mesioangular impacted mandibular third molar? The robot surgeon can assess the angulation of the impacted tooth based on the patient's radiograph, adjust its angulation and access, make a buccal trough, and split the tooth precisely. Less error and more precision, perhaps?

The day is not far before a robotic arm can obtain a tissue sample from our patients at a mall kiosk. Algorithms can then diagnose that tissue and their radiographs distancing the patient further away from the conventional practice of medicine. What is the future of our practices and our education in these scenarios? A well-informed patient with access to information and technology may surpass the traditional medicine man for their healthcare. Direct to consumer marketing of healthcare tools such as genetic testing is already prevalent in many countries. Several patients are aware of which chemotherapy may be best effective for the management of their cancers even before they see their doctor, today. Where does that place a specialist in the future?

In a keynote address at the Royal College of Surgeons in London at the 50th anniversary of the IAOMS, Brian Schmidt DDS, MD, PhD, Director, Bluestone Center for Clinical Research, and Professor of Oral and Maxillofacial Surgery at New York University pondered about the future of OMS internationally. He emphasized three units of care that oral and maxillofacial surgeons provide universally—

1. Management of maxillofacial trauma.
2. Management of oral cancer.
3. Management of craniofacial anomalies.

His views suggested that the advent of seatbelts, airbags, and safer road conditions in most countries is diminishing our total volume of trauma. Further, patterns of wars have changed from the bayonets of World War I to drone-controlled annihilation that ensures death! While bar fights and interpersonal violence continue to create left-sided ZMC and mandibular fractures, the world of facial trauma is most certainly changing.

He recognized examples of how personalized medicine is influencing the care of cancer patients. With our ability to map genomes and mutations, our ability to interpret cancer biology has had a meteoric rise even in the last decade. This leads to personalizing management via either chemotherapy or radiotherapy with predictable success making most cancers chronically manageable diseases rather than a death sentence. The future of personalized medicine will most likely put the cancer surgeon out of an occupation.

He introduced a study that demonstrated how a serendipitous finding in mice with Treacher-Collin's syndrome treated for endometrial cancer with a chemotherapeutic agent knocked out the gene causing the craniofacial anomaly in the following generation. This suggested that we could potentially be looking at gene therapy for craniofacial anomalies, including cleft lip and palate.

Schmidt's observations and predictions suggest that the diseases and conditions that are the mainstay to our profession will alter significantly in the future. Laboratories in Boston are very close to creating a template stem cells construct that will replace dental implants with naturally grown teeth. A dental caries vaccine is pending worldwide use.

How will these fundamental changes alter the practice of our specialty in the future?

Super specialization within the specialty is bound to happen. Attendees of the annual sessions of the British Association of Oral and Maxillofacial Surgeons will be struck by the design of the sessions. There are sessions designed for oral surgeons, implantologists, educators, deformities surgeons, ablative surgeons, and separately for reconstructive surgeons, as there are for minimally invasive surgery, aesthetic surgeons, and lab research. Larger sister specialties like ENT-Otolaryngology have also separated themselves into subspecialties. In the US, Pediatric otolaryngology, head and neck Surgery, facial plastic surgery, otology, skull-based surgery and surgery for sleep disorders are all recognized subspecialties within ENT in the US, for which fellowship training is offered. The pediatric otolaryngologist who specializes in airway surgery is unlikely to attend a conference organized for the otologists.

Similarly, domains within oral and maxillofacial surgery are already starting to branch out into subspecialty pods and practices are being limited to the practice of such subspecialties. That focus on a specific area within the specialty is also likely to be influenced by reimbursement for services. The subspecialties that rake in more money for the provider will thrive quicker and heftier than the latter. Changes in reimbursement strategies by hospitals will also evolve in this equation. For instance, in the US, where a large third-party payer system exists, clinical production for a practitioner is often not measured in actual dollars, but in revenue value units (RVUs). Complex longer cases like a head and neck disease ablation and reconstruction may not be related to a large reimbursement of dollars for the surgery alone; but the fact that the operating facility was used for several hours with the utilization of other resources such as nursing care, critical care, specialists like physical therapists, speech therapists, nutritionists, and a follow-up rehabilitation facility, all add up value to the health system ensuring reimbursement.

While this model seems to be working for now, the practice of medicine in the future unfortunately will be largely devised by the market and economics. The educational debt for training our future generation is getting out of hand. In a world where access to information is undoubtedly easier, the cost of a formal education is skyrocketing. Alternate models of education may arise disrupting this traditional model. Apprenticeships of the Osler era may be aft. Centers of excellence are likely to develop that allows a pathway of nontraditional training to an interested and talented trainee. Validation agencies like the International Board of Certification of Oral and Maxillofacial Surgeons (IBSCOMS) will have a bigger role in providing bonafide certification outside of the current commercialized and often-diluted education system.

The millennial and the gen Z student will also play a large role in the evolution of the specialty. Today's trainee learns differently, synthesizes information differently. They grew up on smartphones and Google searches and not in libraries or poring over Encyclopedia Britannica. They are visual learners with a panache for hand-eye coordination. They are multitaskers. No doubt that there will exist friction between a generation of older teachers and this generation of learners. And, that too will only be momentary. The new trainee is focused on lifestyle choices and is not unabatingly focused on education and patient care. The new trainee values life outside of work just as much as work. This will bring a new kind of diversity to the workplace. To make things worse, they will be treating a generation of aging patients who are used to a different kind of doctor from their times. The average patient is older and healthier and has demands that may have been considered unreasonable at one time. They are likely to be tech-savvy themselves. They will seek many opinions before they commit to the recommendations of their provider. They are likely to choose a surgeon based on the reviews on social media and the internet. Globalization of the medical industry and technology means that they might be willing to travel to have the same procedure and product used elsewhere than their hometown hospital.

Surgeons are working longer than they ever did as well. What impact does that have in a crowded marketplace? Will aging populations of patients and surgeons see an impact on the way we work? Will longevity and increased career years keep the younger ambitious surgeon from getting to the top? The retirement age of surgeons differs all over the world. Surgery is mentally and physically demanding. What effects does that chronic stress have on both the cognitive and physical decline in surgeons? Bhatt et al. did a narrative review on the topics of "ageing" and "surgeon" in Medline in 2016 [8]. They could not find any common ground in these studies. A surgeon who has to hang up his knife at 40 because of severe carpal tunnel in his hands is very different from one that has excellent physical health but severe cognitive decline. The variables were too many for them to consider any consensus on their research question—"when should surgeons retire?" They concluded that," Competence should be assessed at an individual level, focusing on functional ability over chronological age; this should inform retirement policies for surgeons."

OMS is like no other branch of medicine or dentistry. It has innovated, expanded, and usurped. It has replicated the old kingdoms, which created vast expanses as it rolled along. Eventually though, experience tells us that it can collapse under its own weight and might. As we look into the future, we must not ignore our past. Empires end for two reasons… problems from within and failure to protect their borders. As for empires, so for OMS. Our mistakes and pettiness must be acknowledged, accounted for, and learned so as not to repeat them.

We might have the ability as a specialty to control most of our destiny, but some of it may be adapted based on our environments. At the end of it all, if the specialty takes heed of three fundamental principles—patient care, education, and meaningful research, we will continue to justify our existence in the future.

## References

1. Suśruta Samhita. English translation by Kaviraj Kunja Lal Bhishagratna, Calcutta, 1907, Chapter 16, 152–154.
2. Raju VK. Suśruta of ancient India. Indian J Ophthalmol. 2003;51:119–22.
3. Paul G. The future of maxillofacial surgery as a specialty of dentistry. J Maxillofac Oral Surg. 2017;16(1):1–2. Published online 2017 Jan 16.
4. Revised 2007 regulation of the Dental Council of India, Gazette of India Extraordinary No DE 22–2007, Government of India, dated 20th November 2007, pp 56–68.
5. Nayak K. Oral and maxillofacial surgery: It's future as a specialty. J Maxillofac Oral Surg. 2011;10(4):281–2.
6. Laskin M. The past, present, and future of oral and maxillofacial surgery. J Oral Maxillofac Surg. 2008;66:1037–40.
7. Bryan Bell R. Infinite cornucopia: the future of education and training in oral and maxillofacial surgery. Oral Surg Oral Med Oral Pathol Oral Radiol. 2016;121(5):447–9.
8. Bhatt NR, Morris M, O'Neil A, Gillis A, Ridgway PF. When should surgeons retire? Br J Surg. 2016;103(1):35–42.

# Part II

# Preoperative Assessment and Patient Preparation/Optimization

# Preoperative Evaluation and Investigations for Maxillofacial Surgery

2

B. Krishnan and Satyen Parida

## 2.1 Introduction

A meticulous preoperative evaluation with the intention of identifying modifiable clinical conditions and understanding the risk stratification is imperative for all patients being subjected to any invasive procedure, inclusive of oral and maxillofacial surgery. Preoperative evaluation of such patients would of course differ, often dictated by age and the overall health condition that they present with. The choice of anesthesia may vary depending on the surgical procedure intended: general anesthesia, conscious sedation, regional blocks, local anesthesia, or various combinations of all of these. The current chapter focuses on the preoperative evaluation of patients posted for maxillofacial surgery under a general anesthetic in a formal operating room setting. Nevertheless, it is essential to realize that a preoperative evaluation is more or less standardized, irrespective of the type of surgery and practice (office-based dentoalveolar surgery, trauma, orthognathic surgery, elective esthetic surgery, craniofacial surgery, etc.) and anesthesia being planned. The goals of preoperative evaluation are summarized in Fig. 2.1 [1]. The intention is to minimize perioperative morbidity and mortality, to the best possible extent. The major step toward this goal requires the surgeon to be conscientiously aware of the general condition and clinical state of the patient so that in the eventuality of a critical event, he can intervene effectively and pertinently. This would involve modifying and customization of the patient's overall management to ensure that perioperative adverse events are avoided.

B. Krishnan (✉)
Department of Dentistry, Jawaharlal Institute of Postgraduate Medical Education and Research (JIPMER), Puducherry, India

S. Parida
Department of Anesthesiology and Critical Care, Jawaharlal Institute of Postgraduate Medical Education and Research (JIPMER), Puducherry, India

## 2.2 Preoperative Evaluation

The process of preoperative evaluation often begins with a standard history-taking and physical examination for the particular patient. A detailed history of prior medical problems, any previous surgical procedures, family, personal, and social history, any chronic medications and allergies or addictions needs to be obtained. In addition, it is worthwhile obtaining details about the patient's family physician if any, whether he has health insurance, the employer's details if the patient is employed, contact details of relatives, and any other information that may be deemed appropriate. The maxillofacial surgeon has to judge how the medical problems of the patient will affect perioperative care, and conversely, how perioperative events would influence the management of the patient's medical conditions. The patient's comorbidities could result in a significant physiologic decompensation due to myriad factors such as stress of the surgical procedure, original goals of the surgical intervention not being adequately met, and potential interactions between the regular medications that a patient may be on or with drugs that may be required to be instituted as part of the perioperative protocol. The maxillofacial surgeon should, therefore, be cognizant of what could possibly go wrong, and how those situations could be remedied. Also, it is critical that the surgeon be aware of all the medications (antidiabetic drugs, anticoagulants, antiplatelets, etc.) and medical comorbidities (cardiopulmonary, central nervous system, hepatic and renal disease, etc.) that the patient may be exposed to that could threaten the safe performance of the surgical procedure and have an adverse impact during the postoperative period. It is essential that every member of the perioperative team must be able to perform an independent assessment of the patient. This does not imply being ignorant of the other person's assessment since information needs to be shared by all components of the team, but each member should have his own way of assimilating such information by adding to it by his own independent assessment. This is important because


K. Bonanthaya et al. (eds.), *Oral and Maxillofacial Surgery for the Clinician*, https://doi.org/10.1007/978-981-15-1346-6_2

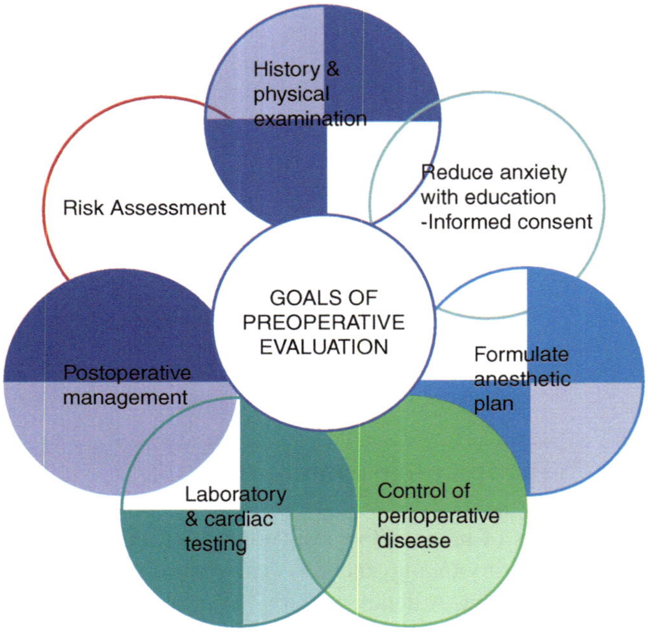


**Fig. 2.1** Goals of preoperative evaluation

**Table 2.1** Preoperative medical evaluation questions for a healthy patient

| Questions |
|---|
| 1. Do you usually get chest pain or breathlessness when you climb up two flights of stairs at normal speed? |
| 2. Do you have kidney disease? |
| 3. Has anyone in your family (blood relatives) had a problem following an anesthetic? |
| 4. Have you ever had a heart attack? |
| 5. Have you ever been diagnosed with an irregular heartbeat? |
| 6. Have you ever had a stroke? |
| 7. If you have been put to sleep for an operation, were there any anesthetic problems? |
| 8. Do you suffer from epilepsy or seizures? |
| 9. Do you have any problems with pain, stiffness, or arthritis in your neck or jaw? |
| 10. Do you have thyroid disease? |
| 11. Do you suffer from angina? |
| 12. Do you have liver disease? |
| 13. Have you ever been diagnosed with heart failure? |
| 14. Do you suffer from asthma? |
| 15. Do you have diabetes that requires insulin? |
| 16. Do you have diabetes that requires tablets only? |
| 17. Do you take any regular medications like antiplatelet or anticoagulants? |
| 18. Are you taking any over-the-counter medications, psychiatric medications, natural remedies? |
| 19. Do you have habits like smoking, alcohol, or use of recreational drugs? |

every specialty would have its independent perspective, about the patient, although they would all be in the latter's best interests. For example, the surgeon might look upon older age in terms of postoperative functional recovery, while the anesthesiologist would be contemplating the various comorbidities that could be associated. Accordingly, each specialist would have his own concerns regarding the state of the patient, and therefore, the preoperative assessment provides a meeting ground for all these concerns after everyone has performed his own independent assessment. The use of a medical history questionnaire provides the maxillofacial surgeon with valuable information about the physical and psychological condition of the patient. Any medical history questionnaire can either be extremely useful or totally worthless and its ultimate value depends upon the ability of the surgeon to interpret the significance of the answers and to elicit additional information through physical examination and dialogue history. A prototype of a health history questionnaire is seen in Table 2.1 [2].

A preoperative physical examination begins with a recording of the patient's vital signs. The oral and maxillofacial system, by virtue, of the proposed surgical site, receives close attention by the surgeon. Of particular interest for the surgeon would be recognizing potential difficulties in surgical access and the need for alternative strategies and additional surgeries (e.g., bone grafting/skin grating). The cardiopulmonary examination assesses the rate and rhythm, murmurs, wheezing, rhonchi, and stridor. The musculoskeletal examination will include a range of neck motion and potential donor site evaluation. Finally, a neurological examination would assess the patient's mental status and any signs of pre-existing nerve or head injuries. A detailed description of the examination of all systems is beyond the scope of this chapter and the reader is advised to consult the references at the end of this chapter [1, 3–5].

Once the history and physical examination are complete, the clinician would be in a situation to risk stratifying the patient according to the American Society of Anesthesiologists' (ASA) classification system (please see chapter on Ambulatory anesthesia for ASA table). Further investigations or specialist consultation is determined by the ASA status. This is especially imperative in patients with ASA Class III or IV who need to be further evaluated for their ability to withstand the proposed surgical procedure. Such patients, almost always, require inpatient admission due to a higher risk of perioperative adverse events. Patients of ASA Class V are extremely moribund and would therefore invariably require admission irrespective of the surgical procedure involved. It is extremely uncommon for a patient in this category to undergo any maxillofacial surgical procedure.

Preoperative risk stratification can also include a surgical classification system [6] (Table 2.2). This classification is quite useful for healthy patients undergoing a surgical procedure, as risk assessment in these patients is now determined solely by the nature of the procedure rather than the ASA

**Table 2.2** Cardiac Risk Stratification for Noncardiac Surgical procedures

| Cardiac risk stratification | Procedure examples |
|---|---|
| High Risk (>5%) | Aortic, Major vascular Surgery, Peripheral vascular Surgery |
| Intermediate Risk (1–5%) | Intraperitoneal and Intrathoracic Surgery, Carotid endarterectomy, Head and neck surgery, Orthopedic Surgery, Prostate Surgery. |
| Low Risk (<1%) | Endoscopic procedures, Superficial procedures, Cataract surgery, Breast surgery, Ambulatory surgery |

classification [7]. A similar surgical severity classification for oral and maxillofacial procedures has also been offered [8].

The preoperative assessment for oral and maxillofacial surgery will also require appropriate radiologic imaging for diagnostic information and treatment planning. These include panoramic, periapical, and occlusal radiographs, ultrasound, CT and MRI imaging. The clinical evaluation and imaging studies should help in the formation of a surgical plan, as to whether the surgery is going to be a simple or a complex one, what kind of instrumentation will be required for the same, or whether it would require the expertise of other surgical specialties such as Ophthalmology, ENT, and Plastic Surgery. The anesthesia team can also examine these imaging modalities to identify potential difficulties that may be encountered while intubating and securing the airway.

## 2.3 Laboratory Investigations

Preoperative patient assessment, ASA physical status, and severity of the proposed oral and maxillofacial surgical procedure guide the clinician to select the appropriate adjunctive studies for treatment planning. The ordering of adjunctive laboratory and radiological investigations is often determined by a complex interplay of pre-existing attitudes, practice patterns learnt during training, ease of ordering, fear of medicolegal consequences, and patient requests. When ordering a test, clinicians are attempting to discriminate between patients who have normal values and those who have abnormal ones. This is used to determine the possibility of the existence of a pathological condition that could impact the proposed surgical and anesthetic plan. The "normal" reference range for many clinical lab tests excludes the upper and lower 2.5% of results, and therefore 5% of normal individuals will obtain an "abnormal" result. While these "abnormal results" can be ignored, sometimes they are not and the result is an additional unnecessary investigation. Clinicians must be confident that there is a clinical justification for the actual need for the test. Studies indicate that less than 0.25% of all "abnormal" results of preoperative tests before an elective surgery influences the perioperative management [9]. "Routine" investigations, viz., those carried out preoperatively on all patients, and not directly related to the planned surgical procedure or the patient's physical condition, are not recommended [10, 11]. Age-based criteria are controversial as test abnormalities are common in older patients but are not as predictive of complications as information gained from a detailed history and physical examination. "Cost consciousness" and "stewardship of resources" also have to be considered by the clinician as the commonly ordered "battery of tests," though relatively inexpensive by themselves, can contribute to a significant proportion of healthcare expenditure as a result of the frequency with which they are ordered [12]. Beyond economics, the costs borne by patients include discomfort of needle sticks and blood loss with repeated phlebotomy, exposure to radiation, and additional unnecessary workup of spurious results. Good communication between the surgeon, medical consultant, anesthesia team, and the patient is essential when considering preoperative testing that may affect the timing of the surgery. Fit, young patients who are scheduled for outpatient surgery or low-risk surgery generally do not require any routine preoperative testing and, in the pediatric age group, a thorough clinical examination has been found to be of greater value [13, 14]. Routine urine or blood testing of the pediatric patient is not clinically warranted without a specific indication [15]. In general, test results within the past 6 months are acceptable if the patient's history has not changed. If the patient's condition has changed in the interim, adjunctive tests within the past 2 weeks are more favored [1].

The American Association of Oral and Maxillofacial Surgeons (AAOMS) recommendations on adjunctive studies prior to oral and maxillofacial surgery include, but are not limited to, both laboratory and imaging investigations [16] (Table 2.3). Similarly, algorithms based on the ASA classification, surgical procedure, and age of the patient are also available to assist the clinician to choose the appropriate adjunctive preoperative tests [17, 18].

While most standard texts would lead one to believe that extensive investigations in patients who are supposedly normal on history and clinical appraisal are not instrumental in improving outcomes or economically justified, it must be remembered that these perceptions are built upon data accumulated from the West, where regular health checkups and assessments are the norms. In contrast, in countries like India, a patient's first visit to a hospital may be for the surgery he is being posted for. Patients may also not be aware of existing comorbidities or details of any earlier interventions. This often leaves the clinician with no other option than to do order a "battery" of the so-called routine investigations to screen out potential pathological conditions. Ultimately, the choice of what laboratory investigations a patient may be subjected to is decided by the particular operating unit. It is important that such practices be customized to the population that the hospital caters to, and must be based on reasonable risk-benefit and cost analysis.

Table 2.3 Indications for commonly ordered preoperative laboratory tests based on specific findings during history and physical examination (independent of patient age, American Society of Anesthesiologists' classification, or surgical procedure)

| Investigations | Indications |
|---|---|
| *Laboratory investigations* | |
| 1. Complete Blood Counts: | |
| WBC count | Patients with infection/fever<br>On chemotherapy<br>Myeloproliferative disorders<br>Immune-compromised states (HIV)<br>History of cancer, chemotherapy, or radiation treatment |
| Platelet count | History of low platelets<br>Bleeding history<br>Thrombopathy<br>Pregnancy<br>Autoimmune disease<br>Splenectomy<br>Liver disease |
| Hemoglobin/Hematocrit | Anticipated blood loss greater than 500 ml<br>Suspicion of anemia<br>Recent chemotherapy/Radiotherapy (within 2 months)<br>Renal disease<br>Active cardiac symptoms<br>Recent blood loss<br>Sickle cell anemia/thalassemia<br>Recent autologous blood transfusion<br>Older patients undergoing major surgery |
| 2. Chemistry: | |
| Electrolytes/BUN/Creatinine | Chronic Kidney Disease<br>Liver cirrhosis<br>Medications (diuretics, ACE inhibitor, digoxin)<br>Diabetes mellitus<br>Malnutrition<br>Dehydration<br>Infections<br>On renal dialysis—$K^+$ tested immediately prior to surgery |
| Creatinine | Older patients undergoing intermediate-or-high-risk surgery<br>Patient for whom nephrotoxins will be used<br>When large fluid shifts or hypotension is likely |
| Glucose-(Fasting/Random/ Postprandial/Glucose Tolerance Test (GTT) /HbA1C) | Diabetes mellitus<br>Long-term steroid medications<br>Liver cirrhosis<br>Pregnancy<br>Infections<br>Pancreatic disease<br>Adrenal disease<br>Pituitary disease<br>>45 Years of age with no prior history of diabetes mellitus |
| 3. Coagulation profile | |
| Prothrombin Time (PT)<br>International Normalized Ration (INR)<br>Partial Thromboplastin Time (PTT) | Personal/ family history of bleeding diathesis or clotting disorders<br>Evidence of purpura or petechiae<br>On current or recent anticoagulation medications (warfarin/heparin)<br>Liver disease<br>Abnormal liver function (jaundice)<br>Alcoholism<br>Severe malnutrition<br>Chronic renal failure<br>History of stroke<br>Autoimmune disorders |
| PT (for warfarin)<br>PTT (for heparin) | Repeated on the evening before/morning of the surgery to document normal coagulation parameters after stopping these medications, if indicated. |
| Bleeding Time (BT) | Not a reliable preoperative indicator of platelet function. Not recommended for presurgical workup |
| Clotting Time (CT) | Time consuming, poor reproducibility, insensitive to high doses of heparin, and sensitive in only extreme factor deficiencies<br>Not of much value in modern laboratory settings |

**Table 2.3** (continued)

| Investigations | Indications |
|---|---|
| 4. Liver function tests | Cirrhosis<br>Hepatitis<br>Jaundice<br>Hepatomegaly<br>Alcohol abuse<br>Pancreatic disease<br>History of cancer<br>Easy bleeding and bruising<br>Malnutrition |
| 5. Type, screen, and cross-sensitivity | Patients with bleeding or coagulation disorders<br>Surgeries with a potential for blood loss (>500 ml) even if transfusion is not expected.<br>*This may help minimize the risk of later transfusion reaction.* |
| 6. Pregnancy testing (Serum/Urine) | Premenopausal women of child-bearing age who have not had tubal ligation or hysterectomy (Urine Human Chorionic Gonadotropin—HCG).<br>*History and physical examination are insufficient to determine early pregnancy, and patients are often unreliable in suspecting that they may be pregnant. Management protocols often change if it is discovered that the patient is pregnant.* |
| 7. Arterial blood gases (ABG) | Only if suspicion for hypoxemia or $CO_2$ retention that would affect postoperative management. |
| 8. Pulmonary function tests | Previously unknown obstructive lung disease<br>Severe asthma<br>Symptomatic COPD<br>Scoliosis |
| 9. Urinalysis | Active symptoms of Urinary tract infection (UTI), dysuria<br>*No good evidence that preoperative abnormal urinalysis is associated with any postoperative complication in nonurinary tract surgery.* |
| 10. Blood cultures | Only if clinical suspicion of septicemia. |
| *Imaging* | |
| 1. Chest X Ray | Significant risk factors for postoperative pulmonary complications (severe/uncontrolled COPD, active pulmonary disease/symptoms, abnormal lung sounds on physical examination, recent pneumonia) with no previous chest X-ray for past 1 year may warrant preoperative chest X-ray irrespective of age.<br>Asymptomatic patients older than 50 years with no risk factors—insufficient evidence for ordering a chest X-ray.<br>Should not be considered as an unequivocal indication for extremes of age, smoking, COPD, stable cardiac disease, and recent resolved upper Respiratory Tract Infection (RTI).<br>*Without symptoms or pertinent medical history, abnormal chest X rays do not predict a worse clinical outcome.* |
| 2. 12 Lead ECG | History of cardiac disease (coronary artery disease, significant arrhythmia, structural heart disease, compensated or prior heart failure)<br>Peripheral artery disease<br>Chest pains<br>Lung disease<br>Morbid obesity<br>History of stroke/cerebrovascular disease<br>Diabetes mellitus<br>Renal insufficiency<br>Patient is having an intermediate- or high-risk surgery<br>*Consider in high-risk group based on epidemiology (males >40 years and females >50 years of age)* |
| 3. Echocardiogram | Recent myocardial infarction<br>Congestive heart failure<br>Abnormal ECG<br>Unstable angina<br>Significant arrhythmias<br>Severe valvular heart disease<br>Previous history of coronary artery disease<br>Dyspnea of unknown origin<br>History of heart failure with progressive symptoms<br>Unstable cardiomyopathy |

## 2.4 Preanesthetic Evaluation

The preanesthetic evaluation aims at getting a favorable outcome, from the points of view of both the surgeon and the anesthesiologist by focusing on risk stratification and modification, and by developing a plan that appropriately addresses the risk-benefit ratio from the procedure, and also explores the other options available. It involves putting together all the elements of the patient's history, physical examination, medications, allergies, laboratory studies, and certain examinations of interest to the anesthesiologist (e.g., airway). This information is assimilated, and decisions are made regarding the plan for anesthetizing the patient once the full picture emerges. This, however, is a dynamic process, and hence accommodates changes in the plan, if new information surfaces, in the best interests of the patient and surgeon. It is also important to be aware of the strengths and limitations of the set-up in which the particular surgical intervention is being undertaken. Further, the preanesthetic evaluation also attempts to allay patient anxiety regarding the procedure, takes necessary steps for risk reduction and to get informed consent. Finally, it leads to the choice of the anesthetic plan to be followed, guided by the risk factors uncovered by the medical history, which covers the entire perioperative period, inclusive of a plan as to where the patient will be cared for postoperatively, and what kind of pain relief he/she should receive after surgery.

## 2.5 Aspects of Evaluation Unique to Anesthesia

The perspective of each specialty also drives the way physical examination is conducted by each of them. All clinicians learn early as part of their training that relevant positive and negative points not only direct the elicitation of history but also examination. Airway examination is something that is uniquely specific to anesthesiologists with the intention of predicting a difficult airway, that is, one that might result in difficulty in ventilating or intubating the patient, or both. The ASA task force on the management of the difficult airway stresses importance on the physical examination of the airway [19]. While no single method can be deemed to be foolproof in this regard, the anesthesiologist is trained to examine different aspects as well as scoring systems to be able to make the assessment of a difficult airway [20–22]. The mnemonic **LEMON** is a helpful tool for assessing the potential for difficult intubation [23, 24] (Fig. 2.2). The Mallampati classification, which relates tongue size to pharyngeal size, is a common component of a thorough airway examination [25]. The examination is performed with the patient in the sitting position, the head held in a neutral position, the mouth wide open, and the tongue protruding to the maximum. The subsequent classification is assigned according to the pharyngeal structures that are visible: (Fig. 2.3).

Class I: visualization of the soft palate, fauces, uvula, and anterior and posterior pillars.
Class II: visualization of the soft palate, fauces, and uvula.
Class III: visualization of the soft palate and the base of the uvula.
Class IV: soft palate not visible at all.

The important aspects of the airway, which can affect intubation, include the degree of mouth opening, the size of the tongue in relation to other oral structures, and the capability to align the oral, pharyngeal, and laryngeal axes in more or less one straight line, with the patient's head and neck in the sniffing position. While the Mallampati classification relates to soft-tissue sizes and their relationships with each other, apart from mouth opening, there are several other anatomical features that need to be considered in the evaluation of the airway (Table 2.4). Examination of systems, other than the cardiopulmonary system, is dependent upon the proposed surgical procedure and planned anesthesia, along with the clinical features of the patient. For example, a patient with a Le Fort II or III fracture may require a careful neurological and ophthalmological examination. Documentation of the findings of history and physical examination must focus on the positive and negative findings after integrating information from the surgeon, patient, and other sources.

## 2.6 Assessment of the Pediatric Patient

The objective of preoperative assessment in the apparently healthy child is to discover medical or anatomic issues, hitherto not acknowledged, that will escalate the risk of surgery and anesthesia. Special attention is warranted by virtue of specific anatomical and physiological differences from the adult patient. Additional risk factors in pediatric patients, apart from the surgery-specific and patient-specific risks,

**Fig. 2.2** LEMON Assessmer.t for difficult intubation

| Physical Signs | Less difficult airway | More difficult airway |
|---|---|---|
| Look externally | Normalface and neck<br>No face or neck pathology | Abnormally face shape<br>Sunken cheeks<br>Edentulous<br>Buck teeth<br>Receding mandible<br>Narrow mouth<br>Obesity<br>Face or neck pathology |
| Evaluate 3-3-2 rule | Mouth opening> 3 fingers<br>Hyoid-chin distance > 3 fingers<br>Thyroid cartilage to mouth floor distance> 2 fingers | Mouth opening < 3 fingers<br>Hyoid-chin distance < 3 fingers<br>Thyroid cartilage to mouth floor distance < 2 fingers |
| Mallampatti scale | Class I and II (Can see the soft palate, uvula, fauces, ± facial pillars) | Class III and IV (Can only see the hard palate ± soft palate ± base of uvula) |
| Obstruction | None | Pathology within or surrounding the upper airway (e.g., peritonsillar adscess, epiglottis, retropharyngeal abscess) |
| Neck mobility | Can flex and extend the neck normally | Limited range of motion of the neck |



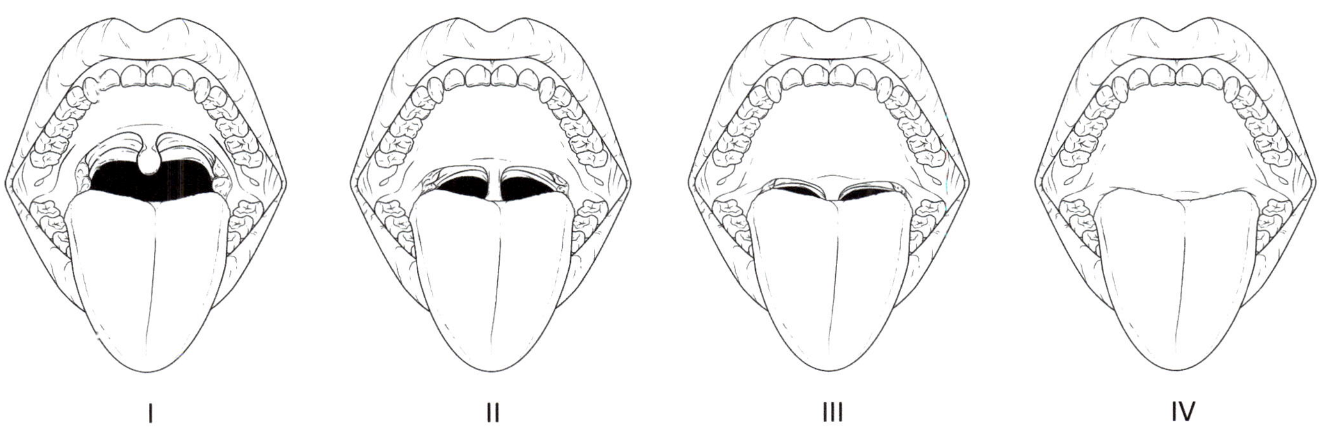


**Fig. 2.3** Mallampati Classification for assessment for intubation. Class I: Cmplete visualization of the soft palate. No additional difficulty. Class II: Complete visualizatin of the uvula. No additional difficulty. Class III: Visualization f only the base of the uvula. Moderate difficulty. Class IV: Soft palate is not visible at all. Severe difficulty

**Table 2.4** Airway compromising conditions

- *Congenital*
  - Pierre-Robin syndrome: micrognathia, macroglossia, cleft soft palate
  - Treacher-Collins syndrome: auricular and ocular defects, malar and mandibular hypoplasia
  - Goldenhar's syndrome: auricular and ocular defects, malar and mandibular hypolasia
  - Down's syndrome: poorly developed or absent bridge of the nose, macroglossia
  - Kippel-Feil syndrome: congenital fusion of a variable number of cervical vertebrae, restriction of neck movement
  - Goiter: compression of trachea, deviation of larynx/trachea
- *Infections*
  - Supraglottis: laryngeal edema
  - Croup: laryngeal edema
  - Abscess (intraoral, retropharygeal): distortion of the airway and trismus
  - Ludwig's angina: distortion of the airway and trismus
- *Arthritis*
  - Rheumatoid arthritis: temporomandibular joint ankylosis, cricoarytenoid arthritis, deviation of laynrx, restricted mobility of cervical spine
  - Ankylosing spondylitis: ankylosis of cervical spine, less commonly ankylosis of temporomandibular joints, lack of mobility of cervical spine
- *Benign tumors*
  - Cystic hygroma, lipoma, adenoma, goiter: stenosis or distortion of the airway, fixation of larynx or adjacent tissues secondary to infiltration or fibrosis from irradiation
- *Malignant tumor, facial injury, cervical spine injury, laryngeal or tracheal trauma*: edema of the airway, hematoma, unstable fracture(s) of the maxillae, mandible and cervical vertebrae
- *Obesity*: short thick neck, redundant tissue in the oropharynx, sleep apnea
- *Acromegaly*: macroglossia, prognathism
- *Acute burns*: edema of airway

include the clinician-related risks; an acknowledgment that superior skills are called for in managing this extremely vulnerable patient population. Children with chronic medical problems require appropriate management and prediction of possible difficulties in management, which the preoperative assessment needs to focus on. Especially for infants, enquiries about prematurity, developmental milestones, and medical background check probing for possible congenital diseases of the cardiac and respiratory systems need to be made. Congenital cardiovascular malformations are frequently associated with many facial malformations, which require a thorough preoperative assessment. Another challenge that pediatric patients present, especially for the anesthesiologist, is the pediatric airway management due to a difference in the airway anatomy vis-a-vis adults. The relatively larger soft tissues in the oropharynx, a more cephalad and anterior position of the vocal cords and the larynx, and a shorter length of the trachea are among the few differences between an adult and pediatric airway anatomy [26]. These unique variations can result in airway management issues, including difficulties in sustaining a patent airway, mask ventilation, insertion of supraglottic airway devices, and endotracheal intubation.

## 2.7 Assessment of the Elderly Patient

Another vulnerable population is the geriatric age group. This is because older age is associated not only with dwindling functions of almost all organ systems but also an increase in the incidence of comorbidities. Further, as life expectancy increases, clinicians are likely to encounter a substantial number of elderly people in their practice, and it is conceivable that a large proportion of these may present for surgery. It is therefore vital that clinicians dealing with patients of this age group should be able to comprehend the alterations in physiology and pathophysiology that occur with aging. A diminished cardiopulmonary reserve puts this patient population under a higher risk of perioperative adverse events. Incidence of coronary artery disease is also prevalent in the geriatric population. Further, there is an increased risk of cognitive dysfunction such as dementia, delirium, and depression, which may be exacerbated in the acute postoperative phase. Elderly patients have impaired hepatic and renal metabolism and delayed clearance of drugs in the systemic circulation, which can cause increased sensitivity to intravenous anesthetics. Also important in relation to the elderly patient are several anatomical alterations, which can affect management. Predominant among these are changes in airway anatomy, such as nasopharyngeal fragility, macroglossia, microstomia, etc. [27]. These can result in difficulty in mask ventilation and placement of supraglottic airway devices and endotracheal tube.

## 2.8 Specialist Consultation and Work-up

The initial evaluation of the patient then leads to subsequent work-up, including obtaining consultations from other specialties if deemed necessary, re-evaluating the need for any additional investigations, taking steps to limit perioperative risks as deemed necessary, evolving an anesthetic plan, and getting informed consent from the patient. As more and more areas of concern may develop, further testing, specialist consultation, and varied approaches to risk management strategies may become imperative. As this dynamic process of comprehensive patient assessment evolves, revision of the anesthetic plan and eliciting additional specific terms of consent from the patient may also become inevitable.

Specialist consultations are needed when the particular condition being evaluated does not come under the purview of the training of the anesthesiologist or surgeon. Such consultations must be specific and try to elicit whether the patient is in the best possible condition with regard to his particular comorbidity to undergo the proposed intervention, or whether the malady for which consultation is being sought, can be further optimized and at what stage of the particular ailment the patient is at. When consultations are merely sent without stating specific objectives of such request, they might meet with a similarly nonspecific response from the consultant that the referral is being sent to, and hence proving to be of not much help for the clarification sought for. Thus, referrals to other disciplines need to be very specific, as to the expectations that the referring unit has of the evaluation and the advice that they should receive. The consultant to whom the referral goes now becomes an important component of the perioperative team. It is essential that this consultant must also appreciate his role in the assessment of the patient, and this would be possible by building support networks among disciplines. This will also save time in the perioperative period, since a few investigations that the consultant being referred to would advise, may be carried out prior to the referral itself. An example would be getting an ECG and echocardiogram done prior to referring a patient with significant coronary artery disease to the cardiologist. Thus, the requirement for circulation of information, among disciplines, is vital and is especially true with regard to communication between consultants. Often, communicating personally with the consultant to whom the patient is being referred to, can expedite the evaluation to a very great extent.

## 2.9 The Process of Risk Assessment

Following a thorough evaluation and perusal of the results of the investigations, the patient-specific risks are evident, while the surgery-specific risks need to be considered upon, the summation of both of which contribute to the overall risk to the patient. Technical factors such as fluid shifts, total blood loss, as well as the site of the surgical intervention, are components of the surgery-specific factors that contribute to the total risk assessment [28]. Oral and maxillofacial surgery being classified as head and neck surgery, would normally be considered as an intermediate risk surgery, unless undertaken as emergency or anticipated to have a risk of excessive blood loss, wherein it would be classified as a high-risk procedure. The correlation between expected blood loss and specific maxillofacial surgeries has been demonstrated [29]. With improving the safety of anesthesia equipment and medications, the historical dangers of anesthesia administration are quite low, and patient- and surgery-specific risk factors almost completely determine the overall risk to the patient [30, 31].

Once the overall risk of the patient is known and calculated, the next step would be to devise a strategy for risk management.

## 2.10 Risk Reduction Strategies

Risk reduction blueprints must be assessed and a risk-benefit ratio evaluated in performing any elective oral or maxillofacial surgical procedure. Alternative procedures and occasionally even avoiding any intervention could be considered when the overall risks in terms of morbidity and mortality to the patient are substantial. Obviously, the most critical step in risk reduction would be to get the patient in the best physical condition to undergo an interventional procedure. To this effect, modifiable risk factors should be addressed (e.g., anemia, hyperglycemia, hypertension) always ensuring that the risk-benefit ratio stays in the patient's favor. As an example, in a smoker who is to undergo an intermediate- or high-risk surgery, the obvious risk reduction strategy would be to quit smoking [32, 33].

This then allows the patient's body to reap the benefits of a simple risk reduction maneuver with the risk now decreasing to a degree that might cause a favorable impact on the morbidity and mortality otherwise expected. Appropriate medical management of the comorbidities might be successful in optimizing patients to a state where they can withstand the rigors of the surgical procedure. The particular anesthetic technique apart, there are at least five other areas that may be targeted as part of overall risk reduction strategies, namely: (a) premedication, (b) antiaspiration prophylaxis, (c) perioperative beta-blockade, (d) postoperative nausea and vomiting (PONV) prophylaxis and (e) effective postoperative pain management.

### 2.10.1 Premedication [4]

An increase in heart rate is the major factor increasing myocardial oxygen demand in the perioperative period. This makes appropriate anxiolysis and management of postoperative pain absolute vital cogs in the overall care of the patient undergoing surgery since anxiety and/or pain can set off a noxious cycle of events starting with tachycardia and hypertension, which could, in turn, result in perioperative myocardial infarction, the incidence of which is highest in the first 72 h. Benzodiazepines induce anterograde amnesia, anxiolysis with mild sedation. Opiates were previously believed to be a vital part of preemptive analgesia, but later they were found to sensitize patients to pain. Clonidine may also be considered preemptive analgesia, especially when administered epidurally. However, the entire concept of pre-emptive analgesia, or antinociceptive treatment prior to initiation of the pain stimulus that prevents the establishment of altered processing of afferent input, that amplifies postoperative pain, is currently mired in controversy. Clonidine has a cardioprotective effect and also decreases the minimum alveolar concentration (MAC). Antihistamines may be used for their sedative and antiemetic properties. However, the clinician needs to know that promethazine, the most commonly prescribed antihistaminic, now carries an FDA warning for apnea and death in children. Anticholinergics are no longer used routinely, but rather to produce an antisialagogue effect when desirable (endoscopic procedures), sedation/amnesia, or to prevent reflex bradycardia.

### 2.10.2 Fasting Guidelines

Patients with a full stomach at the time of induction of anesthesia are perceived to be at high risk of aspiration of gastric contents into their respiratory tract, and also present difficulty with intubation if gastric contents are regurgitated at the time of airway manipulation. This may lead to acute lung injury manifested as pneumonitis, aspiration pneumonia, respiratory failure, or acute respiratory distress syndrome [34]. Following administration of a general anesthetic, patients can no longer have the ability to maintain a patent airway, respiration, or protective reflexes like gagging or coughing. The driving force for inducing aspiration is the barrier pressure, which is the difference between the gastroesophageal sphincter tone that opposes aspiration and the hydrostatic pressure within the stomach. In the presence of a negative barrier pressure, the possibility of regurgitation, vomiting, and aspiration is increased. One of the ways to maintain the barrier pressure positive during the vulnerable period of anesthesia is to instruct the patient to be "nil per oral" prior to surgery, such that the gastric hydrostatic pressure is kept low. What constitutes an appropriate period of fasting before anesthesia has been the subject of substantial research over several years, and current guidelines are based both on the nature of oral intake and the age of the patient [35, 36, 37] (Table 2.5). These recommendations, however, need to be viewed as guidelines, rather than a set of inviolable instructions. The reason why these rules should not be looked upon as impregnable is because these were intended for normal patients. Individual situations may sometimes prevent these nil-per-oral guidelines from providing foolproof safety from aspiration. Conditions that inhibit gastric emptying, including diabetes, morbid obesity (body mass index [BMI] >35), pregnancy, bowel obstruction, previous upper gastrointestinal surgery, and gastrointestinal disease such as gastric ulcer, scleroderma, etc. will all escalate the risk of aspiration and deserve as much attention that a full stomach does [38–40]. Another group of patients who are believed to be at high risk for aspiration comprises those with difficult airways, as these patients will require more prolonged airway manipulation and thus a greater time to intubation [41]. The airway remains unprotected and unsecured for a longer time and hence these patients may benefit from prophylaxis against aspiration. The preanesthetic evaluation needs to identify this special category of patients who appear to be at higher risk of aspiration, despite adhering faithfully to standard nil per oral guidelines and premedicate them for elective surgery. A prokinetic drug and an alkalinizing agent could reduce the complications from gastric aspiration by combating the corrosive acidic nature of gastric juice, even if aspiration does occur [3].

**Table 2.5** Preoperative fasting recommendations for healthy patients undergoing elective surgery

| Liquid and food intake | Minimum fasting period |
|---|---|
| Clear liquids (Water, tea, black coffee, fruit juice without pulp, carbonated beverages) | 2 h |
| Breast milk | 4 h |
| Nonhuman milk, including infant milk formula | 6 h |
| Light meal (e.g., toast and clear liquids) | 6 h |
| Regular or heavy meal (may include fried or fatty food, meat) | 8 h |

The most widely prescribed prokinetic in this regard is the dopamine-antagonist metoclopramide (10 mg orally/IV). However, this drug has the potential to cause extrapyramidal symptoms and should be used cautiously. The other pharmacological agent that increases the pH of gastric juice and makes it less acidic is a Histamine 2 (H2) receptor blocker, viz., ranitidine (150 mg orally; 50 mg IV) or famotidine (20 mg IV). Cimetidine is no longer used due to its ability to induce hepatic enzymes and influence the metabolism of several anesthetic agents. Usually, the prokinetic along with the H2 blocker is administered both on the night before and on the morning of the surgery. Administration of two doses each of both the medications guarantees adequate plasma levels required for an effective action. Lastly, the use of particulate antacids such as citric acid/sodium citrate (30 ml) typically within 2 h prior to the anticipated induction of anesthesia also can neutralize the gastric acid, and reduce the incidence of chemical pneumonitis even if the aspiration occurs. However, its bitter taste and propensity to induce emesis necessitates that it be administered a substantial period prior to intubation.

### 2.10.3 Perioperative Beta-Blocker Therapy

Organ ischemia is a result of an imbalance between the oxygen supply and demand. The heart is especially vulnerable since myocardial work and oxygen demand are very tightly coupled. However, the precise level of myocardial demand at which it outstrips the supply is unclear. Hence, a patient who is susceptible to the development of myocardial ischemia needs to be managed perioperatively in a manner that keeps the demand lowest, while at the same time maximizing supply. Pharmacological manipulation of the myocardial demand is probably effected easier than a significant manipulation of the supply. Physiologically, tachycardia is the most important parameter that increases myocardial demand, with increases in systemic vascular resistance being the second most important [42–44]. Patients having a significant cardiovascular risk need a cardiologist's opinion for an evaluation of the extent of risk and preoperative optimization [6] (Table 2.6). Obviously, modifiable risk factors and reversible disorders need to be addressed and managed. The ACC recommends perioperative beta-blocker therapy for patients with two or more intermediate risk factors or a single major risk factor, especially if being posted for an intermediate-to-high-risk surgical procedure [6]. The evaluating physician can be requested to assess the benefits of beta-blockade in the patient scheduled for maxillofacial surgery. The commonest way of introducing beta-blockade is with the drug metoprolol for a target basal heart rate of 60–65 beats per minute (bpm), and to sustain the rates at no more than 85 bpm during the perioperative period. Beta-blockade should, however, be started well before the surgery so that ample time is available to adjust the dose to the target heart rate and address any side effects that may develop. The administration of a beta-blocker just prior to an emergency surgery is controversial as this has been observed to be associated with a greater risk of perioperative strokes [45, 46]. More research is needed to clearly identify which patient subsets might benefit most from the beta-blockade, and in whom the side effects may be substantial.

**Table 2.6** Clinical predictors of increased perioperative cardiovascular risk

*Major clinical predictors (markers of unstable coronary artery disease)*
- Myocardial infarction <6 weeks: Delay elective surgery, consultation with cardiologist
- Unstable or severe angina (Canadian Cardiovascular Society class III or IV)
- Decompensated heart failure
- Significant arrhythmias (e.g., causing hemodynamic instability)
- Severe valvular heart disease (e.g., aortic or mitral valve stenosis with valve area < 1 cm$^2$)
- CABG or PTCA <6 weeks

*Intermediate clinical predictors (markers of stable coronary artery disease)*
- Previous Myocardial infarction >6 weeks but <3 months (> 3 months if complicated) based on the history or presence of pathologic Q waves on the Electrocardiogram
- Mild angina (Canadian Cardiovascular Society class I to II)
- Silent ischemia (Holter monitoring)
- Compensated heart failure, ejection fraction <0.35
- Post CABG or PTCA >6 weeks and < 3 months, or > 6 years, or on antianginal therapy
- Diabetes mellitus
- Renal insufficiency

*Mild clinical predictors (increased probability of coronary artery disease)*
- Familial history of coronary artery disease
- Age > 70 years
- ECG abnormalities (arrhythmias, LVH, Left bundle branch block)
- Low functional capacity
- History of stroke
- Uncontrolled systemic hypertension
- Hypercholesterolemia
- Smoking
- Post infarction (> 3 months, asymptomatic without treatment
- Post CABG or PTCA (> 3 months and < 6 years, and no symptoms of angina nor on antianginal therapy)

*Major clinical predictors*: All elective operations should be postponed and the patients properly investigated and treated.
*Intermediate clinical predictors*: Proof of well-established but controlled coronary artery disease. Further risk stratification and optimization in consultation with cardiologist.
*Minor clinical predictors*: Increased probability of coronary artery disease, but not of an increased perioperative risk. Further risk stratification and optimization in consultation with cardiologist.
*Emergency procedures*: Proceed for surgery with perioperative surveillance and postoperative risk stratification and risk factor management.

*CABG* Coronary Artery Bypass Grafting, *PTCA* Percutaneous Transluminal Coronary Angioplasty, *LVH* Left Ventricular Hypertrophy

### 2.10.4 PONV Prophylaxis [47]

Oral and Maxillofacial surgeries are generally not considered as high risk for the incidence of postoperative nausea and vomiting (PONV) [48]. Risk factors, including female gender, previous history of PONV or motion sickness, non-smoking status, and younger age patients, have been associated with an increased incidence and severity of PONV [49]. Therefore, the preoperative assessment should be sensitive to the presence of these indicators and must devise a plan for offering pharmacological prophylaxis to this patient population. The plan for anesthesia devised preoperatively should also take into consideration that use of volatile anesthetics, opioids, and nitrous oxide may be associated with higher PONV incidence, and thus influence the choice of anesthetic agents used. The choices for PONV prophylaxis are between 5HT3 antagonists (ondansetron, granisetron, palonosetron, etc.), dexamethasone, subanesthetic doses of propofol, scopolamine patches, etc. [50]. Generally, a combination of agents seems to work much better than a single agent.

### 2.10.5 Plan for Postoperative Analgesia [51]

Regional anesthesia techniques, including peripheral nerve blocks, are excellent in terms of providing quality analgesia postoperatively, but they do have their own set of risks and may cause discomfort from the ensuing numbness. Hence, it is important that the patient is taken into confidence about the risks and benefits of this modality of pain relief, while also offering alternative approaches that could be opted for. Local anesthesia in adequate concentrations and volume is essential for a pain-free postoperative period. Contrary to earlier practices, the mixing of local anesthetic solutions to apparently harness the best pharmacological effects of both is an approach, which is currently being discouraged. In fact, a successful preoperative nerve block may also be used so as to minimize the incidence of tachycardia during the intraoperative noxious stimuli, and then repeated at the culmination of the procedure, so that the effect can extend into the postprocedure period. This option can be employed by the maxillofacial surgeon resultant to their expertise in regional nerve blocks of the orofacial region. Opioids have traditionally been the workhorse for postoperative analgesia. Intravenous patient-controlled analgesia is an attractive option for the postoperative pain control for the inpatient in whom the effects of the nerve blocks are expected to wane after a few hours. However, there is accumulating evidence that a multimodal approach to pain management works best, with the intent of reducing the side effects of opioids and improving pain scores. Enhanced recovery after surgery (ERAS) protocols to minimize postsurgery hospital stay are gaining wider acceptance, and an important part of such protocols is the inclusion of multimodal opioid-sparing pain management protocols [52].

## 2.11 Preoperative Decision Making and Obtaining Informed Consent: The Team Concept [53]

The preoperative plan blends the patient's requirements, the competence of the perioperative team, and the infrastructure provided by the hospital to get the particular intervention done. This, it is expected, would help achieve the favorable outcome of the intervention. Quite often, the optimization of all of these conditions may not always be possible. The onus then is upon both the patient and the operating team to take a decision on what may be the acceptable course of action. Whether to pursue the performance of a particular intervention or not is, therefore, also an integral part of the preoperative decision-making process.

The final element of a comprehensive preoperative assessment is the process of obtaining a valid, written, and informed consent. Obviously, this process can be initiated, only after a thorough risk estimation has been made, based on the preceding evaluation of the patient, and a tentative anesthetic and surgical plan have been evolved, including strategies for management of postoperative pain. For all practical purposes, an informed consent necessitates presentation of the final residual risk that the patient has, which cannot be further optimized, and its expected interaction with the proposed surgical intervention. The main players in the process of obtaining informed are obviously the surgeon, anesthesiologist, and the patient. Typically, any of them has the autonomy to reject or to suggest modifications to the proposed sequence for the intervention. It is important to note that informed consent is a process of ensuring the patient understands the risks and benefits of the available surgical and anesthetic options. It is not merely signing a consent form. The capacity of a patient refers to the ability to make decisions about their care, and to decide whether to agree to, or refuse, an examination, investigation, or treatment. To have the capacity, a patient must be able to understand and retain information regarding the treatment, evaluate the risks and benefits of treatment, reach a decision regarding their course of treatment, and communicate their decision to the clinician [54]. A patient undergoing surgery is understandably apprehensive, and hence the process of imparting information to him while taking consent must be handled professionally, yet with the utmost sensitivity [55]. It is important that the anesthesiologist and the surgeon should have thrashed out issues relating to perioperative care and broken common ground on all aspects before involving the patient (Table 2.7).

Following discussion and concordance between the surgeon and the anesthesiologist on the course of action, the patient is taken into confidence, informed about the procedure, and his/her consent for the same, sought. The information provided to the patient includes the nature of the risk involved, the benefits, and the alternatives to the proposed plan. If the proposal or any particular element of it is unacceptable to the patient, the operating team must be ready for course correction and should be able to come up with alternatives, which would be acceptable to the patient. However, if no substitute plan can be offered, and the patient is resolute in not accepting the proposed one, there is no option than to abort the proposed surgery. Options, such as referrals to other surgical teams, with different expertise or set-ups that may address the patient's concerns better and satisfy his expectations can be considered. Consequently, acquiring informed consent is a highly interactive process, with the patient being the pivot, to whom the risk-benefit ratio is projected taking into consideration his/her wishes and needs. The Association of Oral and Maxillofacial Surgeons of India consent forms can serve as a useful template for consent taking in one's clinical practice [56].

**Table 2.7** Points of concurrence between surgeon and anesthesiologist before seeking informed consent from the patient

- Diagnosis
- Nature and purpose of the proposed treatment or procedure
- Risks, complications, and consequences of the proposed treatment or procedure
- Alternatives to proposed treatment or procedure
- The consequences if the proposed treatment or procedure is refused
- Benefits and expected results if the proposed treatment or procedure is accepted
- Conflicts of interest
- Who will be providing the treatment or procedure

## 2.12 Conclusion

"Do not operate on a stranger" is the most important mantra to be followed by any surgeon. The preoperative evaluation of oral and maxillofacial surgery patient comprises a critical part of the perioperative period and hence requires a watchful and staged outlook to risk identification and management, putting in place a plan for anesthesia, surgery, and postsurgical pain management. There is no substitute for a properly performed and detailed history and physical examination. Literature suggests that most clinically relevant conditions are recognized during the history and physical examination without the need for further laboratory testing. The surgical team needs to ascertain the risks involved with the comorbidities that the patient may be suffering from, and be able to juxtapose this against the procedure-specific risks to identify the overall risk of the procedure in that particular patient. Risk management and optimization strategies involve the rational use of adjunctive laboratory and imaging studies and professional opinions of consultants of other specialties. This helps evaluate the degree of physiological decompensation a patient might be having due to his comorbidities, and whether this could be either reversed or ameliorated. Acquiring informed consent from the patient involves the development of consensus between the surgeon and anesthesiologist first, with regard to the perioperative plan, irrespective of whether the consent forms for anesthesia and surgery are the same or different documents. This proposed plan, which has the concurrence of both the surgeon and the anesthesiologist, is then presented to the patient along with clear information about the risks and benefits of different clinical strategies, such that the patient can make his up his/her mind, or else request refinement of the proposed plan. This thorough process of preoperative evaluation, it is expected, would be able to keep morbidity and mortality related to the maxillofacial surgery, to an absolute minimum.

## References


1. Galway UA. Preoperative evaluation. In: Sikka PK, Beaman ST, Street JA, editors. Basic clinical anesthesia. New York: Springer; 2015. p. 7–15.
2. Hilditch WG, Asbury AJ, Jack E, McGrane S. Validation of a pre-anaesthetic screening questionnaire. Anaesthesia. 2003;58:874.
3. Wijeysundera DN, Sweitzer BJ. Preoperative evaluation. In: Miller RD, editor. Miller's anesthesia. 8th ed. Philadelphia: Elsevier Saunders; 2015. p. 1085–155.
4. Hata TM, Hata JS. Preoperative patient assessment and management. In: Barash PG, Cullen BF, Stoelting RK, Cahalan MK, Stock MC, Ortega R, Sharar SR, Holt NF, editors. Clinical anesthesia. 8th ed. Philadelphia: Wolters Kluwer; 2017. p. 1479–544.
5. Gupta A, Shiveley T. The preoperative patient evaluation. In: Ehrenfeld JM, Urman RD, Segal S, editors. Anesthesia student survival guide-a case based approach. 2nd ed. New York: Springer; 2016. p. 89–106.
6. Fleisher LA, Beckman JA, Brown KA, Calkins H, Chaikpf E, Fleischmann K, et al. ACC/AHA 2007 Guidelines on Perioperative Cardiovascular Evaluation and Care for Noncardiac Surgery: a Report of the American College of Cardiology/American Heart Association Task Force on Practice Guidelines (Writing Committee to Revise the 2002 Guidelines on Perioperative Cardiovascular Evaluation for Noncardiac Surgery). Circulation. 2007;116:e418–99.
7. Owens WD. American Society of Anesthesiologist physical classification system is not a risk classification system. Anesthesiology. 2001;94:378.
8. Henry A, Dewi F, Atan R, Patel N, Bhatia S. Pre-operative investigations in patients undergoing oral and maxillofacial procedures. Oral Surg. 2016;9:155–9.
9. Tasse JL, Janzen ML, Ahmed NA, Chung RS. Screening laboratory and radiology panels for trauma patients have low utility and arenot cost effective. J Trauma. 2008;65:1114–6.
10. Bryson GL, Wyand A, Bragg PR. Preoperative testing is inconsistent with published guidelines and rarely changes management. Can J Anaesth. 2006;53:236–41.
11. Smetana GW, Macpherson DS. The case against routine preoperative laboratory testing. Med Clin North Am. 2003;87:7–40.
12. Weinberger SE. Providing high-value, cost-conscious care: a critical seventh general competency for physicians. Ann Intern Med. 2011;155:386–8.
13. Benarroch-Gampel J, Riall TS. What laboratory tests are required for ambulatory surgery? Adv Surg. 2013;47:81–98.
14. Feely MA, Collins CS, Daniels PR, Kebede EB, Jatoi A, Mauck KF. Preoperative testing before noncardiac surgery: guidelines and recommendations. Am Fam Physician. 2013;87(6):414–8.
15. Czoski-Murray C, Lloyd Jones M, McCabe C, Claxton K, Oluboyede Y, Roberts J, et al. What is the value of routinely testing full blood count, electrolytes and urea, and pulmonary function tests before elective surgery in patients with no apparent clinical indication and in subgroups of patients with common comorbidities: a systematic review of the clinical and cost-effective literature? Health Technol Assess. 2012;16(i–xvi):1–159.
16. Parameters of Care; AAOMS clinical practice guidelines for oral and maxillofacial surgery (AAOMS ParCare), 6th ed; 2017; J Oral Maxillofac Surg 75:Suppl 1e12-1e33.
17. Fattahi T. Perioperative laboratory and diagnostic testing-what is needed and when? Oral Maxillofac Surg Clins North Am. 2006;18:1–6.
18. National Institute for Health and Care Excellence (NICE) guidelines. Routine pre-operative tests for elective surgery 2016. www.nice.org.uk/guidance/ng45.
19. Apfelbaum JL, Hagberg CA, Caplan RA, Blitt CD, Connis RT, Nickinovich DG, et al. Practice guidelines for management of the difficult airway: an updated report by the American Society of Anesthesiologists Task Force on Management of the Difficult Airway. Anesthesiology. 2013;118:251–70.
20. Prakash S, Mullick P, Bhandari S, Kumar A, Gogia AR, Singh R. Sternomental distance and sternomental displacement as predictors of difficult laryngoscopy and intubation in adult patients. Saudi J Anaesth. 2017;11:273–8.
21. O'Dell K. Predictors of difficult intubation and the otolaryngology perioperative consult. Anesthesiol Clin. 2015;33:279–90.
22. Reed MJ, Dunn MJG, McKeown DW. Can an airway assessment score predict difficulty at intubation in the emergency department? Emerg Med. 2005;22:99–102.
23. Murphy Michael F, Walls RM. Identification of the difficult and failed airway. In: Walls RM, Michael F, editors. Emergency airway management. 3rd ed. Philadelphia: Lippincott Williams & Wilkins; 2008. p. 82–93.
24. Advanced Trauma Life Support (ATLS) Student course manual. Airway and ventilatory management. 9th ed. Chicago IL, 2012. American College of Surgeons Committee on Trauma: 36.

25. Mallampati SR, Gatt SP, Gugino LD, Desai SP, Waraksa B, Freiberger D, et al. A clinical sign to predict difficult tracheal intubation: a prospective study. Can Anaesth Soc J. 1985;32:429–34.
26. Advanced Trauma Life Support (ATLS) student course manual. Pediatric trauma. 9th ed. Chicago IL, 2012. American College of Surgeons Committee on Trauma: 251.
27. Advanced Trauma Life Support (ATLS) student course manual. Geriatric trauma. 9th ed. Chicago IL, 2012. American College of Surgeons Committee on Trauma: 275.
28. Glance LG, Lustik SJ, Hannan EL, Osler TM, Mukamel DB, Qian F, et al. The Surgical Mortality Probability Model: derivation and validation of a simple risk prediction rule for noncardiac surgery. Ann Surg. 2012;255:696–702.
29. Akinbami BO, Onajin-Obembe B. Assessment of intraoperative blood loss during oral and maxillofacial surgical procedures in a Nigerian tertiary health care center. J Blood Transfus. 2014;2014:301467.
30. Lanier WL. A three-decade perspective on anesthesia safety. Am Surg. 2006;72:985–9.
31. Botney R. Improving patient safety in anesthesia: a success story? Int J Radiat Oncol Biol Phys. 2008;71:S182–6.
32. Rodrigo C. The effects of cigarette smoking on anesthesia. Anesth Prog. 2000;47:143–50.
33. Warner DO. Perioperative abstinence from cigarettes: physiologic and clinical consequences. Anesthesiology. 2006;104:356–67.
34. Warner MA, Warner ME, Weber JG. Clinical significance of pulmonary aspiration during the perioperative period. Anesthesiology. 1993;78:56–62.
35. Apfelbaum JL, Caplan RA, Connis RT, Epstein BS, Nickinovich DG, Warner MA. American Society of Anesthesiologists Committee. Practice guidelines for preoperative fasting and the use of pharmacologic agents to reduce the risk of pulmonary aspiration: application to healthy patients undergoing elective procedures: an updated report by the American Society of Anesthesiologists Committee on Standards and Practice Parameters. Anesthesiology. 2011;114:495–511.
36. Brady M, Kinn S, Stuart P. Preoperative fasting for adults to prevent perioperative complications. Cochrane Database Syst Rev. 2003;4:CD004423.
37. Stuart PC. The evidence base behind modern fasting guidelines. Best Pract Res Clin Anaesthesiol. 2006;20:457–69.
38. Fleisher LA, Mythen M. Anesthetic implications of concurrent diseases. In: Miller RD, editor. Miller's anesthesia. 8th ed. Philadelphia: Elsevier Saunders; 2015. p. 1156–225.
39. Krishnan B. Obese oral and maxillofacial surgical patient. J Craniofac Surg. 2009;20:53–7.
40. Hoefnagel A, Yu A, Kaminski A. Anesthetic complications in pregnancy. Crit Care Clin. 2016;32:1–28.
41. Neuman MD, Fleisher LA. Risk of anesthesia. In: Miller RD, editor. Miller's anesthesia. 8th ed. Philadelphia: Elsevier Saunders; 2015. p. 1056–84.
42. Fox KM, Ferrari R. Heart rate: a forgotten link in coronary artery disease? Nat Rev Cardiol. 2011;8:369–79.
43. Tardif JC. Heart rate as a treatable cardiovascular risk factor. Br Med Bull. 2009;90:71–84.
44. Braunwald E. Control of myocardial oxygen consumption: physiologic and clinical considerations. Am J Cardiol. 1971;27:416–32.
45. Lindholm LH, Carlberg B, Samuelsson O. Should beta blockers remain first choice in the treatment of primary hypertension? A meta-analysis. Lancet. 2005;366:1545–53.
46. Bangalore S, Messerli FH, Kostis JB, Pepine CJ. Cardiovascular protection using betablockers: a critical review of the evidence. J Am Coll Cardiol. 2007;50:563–72.
47. Fowler MA, Spiess BD. Postanesthesia recovery. In: Barash PG, Cullen BF, Stoelting RK, Cahalan MK, Stock MC, Ortega R, Sharar SR, Holt NF, editors. Clinical anesthesia. 8th ed. Philadelphia: Wolters Kluwer; 2017. p. 3854–918.
48. Alexander M, Krishnan B, Yuvraj V. Prophylactic antiemetics in oral and maxillofacial surgery: a requiem? J Oral Maxillofac Surg. 2009;67:1873–7.
49. Habib AS, Gan TJ. Evidence-based management of postoperative nausea and vomiting: a review. Can J Anaesth. 2004;51:326–41.
50. Cao X, White PF, Ma H. An update on the management of postoperative nausea and vomiting. J Anesth. 2017;31:617–26.
51. White PF, Kehlet H, Neal JM, Schricker T, Carr DB, Carli F, et al. The role of the anesthesiologist in fast-track surgery: from multimodal analgesia to perioperative medical care. Anesth Analg. 2007;104:1380–96.
52. Misiołek H, Cettler M, Woroń J, Wordliczek J, Dobrogowski J, Mayzner-Zawadzka E. The 2014 guidelines for post-operative pain management. Anaesthesiol Intensive Ther. 2014;46:221–44.
53. Barry MJ, Edgman-Levitan S. Shared decision making–pinnacle of patient-centered care. N Engl J Med. 2012;366:780–1.
54. General Medical Council (GMC). Consent: patients and doctors making decisions together [online]. GMC, 2008. Available: http://www.gmc-uk.org/static/documents/content/Consent-English0414.pdf
55. Sjöling M, Nordahl G, Olofsson N, Asplund K. The impact of preoperative information on state anxiety, postoperative pain and satisfaction with pain management. Patient Educ Couns. 2003;51:169–76.
56. Association of Oral and Maxillofacial Surgeons of India (AOMSI): https://www.aomsi.com/WebPages/downloads.aspx

# Management of Medical Comorbidities in Maxillofacial Surgery

# 3

Aditya Moorthy and Shreya Krishna

## 3.1 Introduction

The management of the medically compromised patient is a topic that has received a great deal of attention in recent times. Unfortunately, most of the literature available discusses this topic from a western context. While the human species and the physiology remains unchanged, challenges in South Asia, especially India, stem from a vastly different social structure, a massive urban-rural socioeconomic divide, and social variables that have a major impact on the practice of medicine. In addition, a mixture of patient ignorance, poor training in soft skills of doctors, and an irresponsible fourth estate has vitiated a hitherto-friendly doctor-patient relationship.

While this chapter is not designed to provide a comprehensive guide to the medical management of a maxillofacial patient (which deserves a textbook in its own right), it attempts to provide an insight into the management of medically compromised patients requiring maxillofacial surgery.

## 3.2 Changing Demographics in India

India encompasses almost a fifth of the world's population with a population estimate of about 1.34 billion [1]. The life expectancy at birth in India has improved from 59.7 years in 1990 to 70.3 years in 2016 for females, and from 58.3 years to 66.9 years for males [1]. In short, the average life span of an Indian has increased by 11 years in the last decade leading to an increase in the geriatric population of the country. The crude death rate has also steadily declined in the last decade from 7.5 to 6.4 per 1000 population [2]. The population continues to grow, as the birth rate has superseded the death rate. This change, while an indicator of improved healthcare delivery, adds to the health burden of the country, and creates a different spectrum of diseases—particularly lifestyle diseases.

There has also been a shift in the societal patterns. We see an increase in urban nuclear families resulting in unattended elderly parents whose medical conditions stay undiagnosed and uncontrolled.

## 3.3 Lifestyle Changes in India

There has been a sea of change in the lifestyle of today's population compared to a couple of decades ago. Sedentary lifestyle, processed food, industrialization, occupational hazards, etc. have led India to a "dual disease burden" scenario. So, even as the incidence of lifestyle diseases is steadily on the rise, a vast majority of rural and poor patients still suffer from infectious and acute diseases.

As recently as 2016, cardiovascular diseases like Ischaemic Heart Disease (IHD) and stroke contributed 28.1% toward mortality in India. This was a 34.3% increase over 16 years, suggesting the impact of lifestyle disease on society. The major contributors for this change are rapidly aging population, pollution, high blood pressure, dyslipidemia, high fasting plasma glucose, and an increased BMI (body-mass index) [3]. Respiratory diseases like chronic obstructive pulmonary disease (COPD) and bronchial asthma—are the second-largest contributors to the total mortality burden of India—at 10.9%. Diabetes analysis shows that it contributes 3.1% toward the total mortality burden.

Air pollution is a major risk factor for both cardiovascular and respiratory illness and increases the risks for acute respiratory infections and exacerbates asthma [4]. Such unique challenges raise questions of following treatment protocols based on western studies. A preoperative chest X-Ray may

A. Moorthy (✉)
Rangadore Memorial Hospital, Apollo Hospitals, Bangalore, Karnataka, India

S. Krishna
Oral and Maxillofacial Surgery, Rangadore Memorial Hospital, Bangalore, India


K. Bonanthaya et al. (eds.), *Oral and Maxillofacial Surgery for the Clinician*, https://doi.org/10.1007/978-981-15-1346-6_3

find an indication in an apparently fit and healthy 28-year-old living in New Delhi (with record levels of pollution) when it would be considered unnecessary for a similar patient from rural Yorkshire.

With the rise of urbanization and urban migration, the problems of air pollution, inadequate sanitation, and an unhealthy diet are accentuated. Population residing in urban areas in India, according to 1901 census, was 11.4%. This count increased to 28.53% by 2001, and the numbers increased to 34% in 2017 [5].

"Cyberchondria" has become a challenge with patients tending to diagnose and treat their problems themselves, and unsurprisingly getting it wrong. India is also among one of the most depressed countries in the world. A World Health Organization (WHO) study states that at least 6.5% of the Indian population suffers from some form of serious mental disorder. The average suicide rate in India is 10.9 for every hundred thousand people with the majority of victims being less than 44 years of age [6]. Diminished mental health is associated with a host of consequences like lack of participation in social activities, odd eating habits, and withdrawal from income generation and employment opportunities—all of which can cascade onto other serious illnesses and even death.

## 3.4 The Changing Face of Oral and Maxillofacial Surgery

As always, training is struggling to keep up with the changing trends in medicine. Trainees are often unaware of new protocols and the changed scenario of medical comorbidities of the population. Surgery has become heavily technology oriented, sometimes at the cost of clinical expertise. Furthermore, there is improved awareness among medical professionals for crossreferral to review dentition, seen mostly by maxillofacial surgeons rather than general dentists. Referrals are required now before radiotherapy, chemotherapy, cardiac surgery, transplants, etc.

Furthermore, maxillofacial surgery as a specialty has blazed a trail hitherto unimagined with successful foray into head and neck surgery, craniofacial reconstruction, and microvascular surgery. This now has put the onus on the surgeon to educate himself enough to be able to manage a sick patient on the ward to the extent of preventing complications and making appropriate referrals. Gone are the days when a physician could be asked to do the job for us and we could enjoy the comfort of being surgical technicians!

### 3.4.1 Medical History and India

While veritable treatises about the science and art of history taking, this part of clinical medicine is a unique investigative effort in the Indian context. The challenges to the maxillofacial surgeon are multifold. The first difficulty is encountered with the patient who may deny illness (often hypertension or diabetes) because he/she is adequately treated and all parameters are within normal limits. The next hurdle is when the patient decides to withhold information wantonly due to social taboos or plain ignorance of its importance to the treating doctor. Dentists and maxillofacial surgeons who question their patients seated on dental chairs in an outpatient setting often experience the latter. This stems from the patients' assumption that the information is inconsequential to their treatment. The last situation is the uneducated patient who is truly unaware of his medical condition.

With these intricacies, the oral surgeon needs to employ several out-of-the-box techniques to extract the history. This includes the much-derided leading questions, questioning relatives, sometimes in private, and playing Sherlock by asking them to bring in their medication and working backwards. But this effort is still of paramount importance in this technology-driven age and the modern oral and maxillofacial surgeon will do well to assimilate all the conventional history-taking skills and learn a few new ones as well.

## 3.5 Cardiovascular System

### 3.5.1 Hypertension

Hypertension is an extremely common condition and often undiagnosed. Since it is mostly asymptomatic, the oral surgeon has the unique opportunity to be the first healthcare professional to identify the condition. Hence, it is imperative that every procedure should begin with recording the patients' vital signs. The following table offers a guideline for the diagnosis and risk stratification of hypertension (Table 3.1).

The authors stress that aneroid manometers are more accurate than digital ones. Like any delicate instrument, these too need frequent calibration [8].

The long-term effects of hypertension have far-reaching implications on maxillofacial surgery, especially under general anesthesia (Fig. 3.1).

**Table 3.1** Guidelines for diagnosis of hypertension [7]

| Category | Systolic (mmHg) | Diastolic (mmHg) |
|---|---|---|
| Optimal | <120 | <80 |
| Normal | 120–129 | And/or 80–84 |
| High normal | 130–139 | And/or 85–89 |
| Grade 1 hypertension | 140–159 | And/or 90–99 |
| Grade 2 hypertension | 160–179 | And/or 100–109 |
| Grade 3 hypertension | >180 | And/or >110 |
| Isolated systolic hypertension | >140 | And <90 |

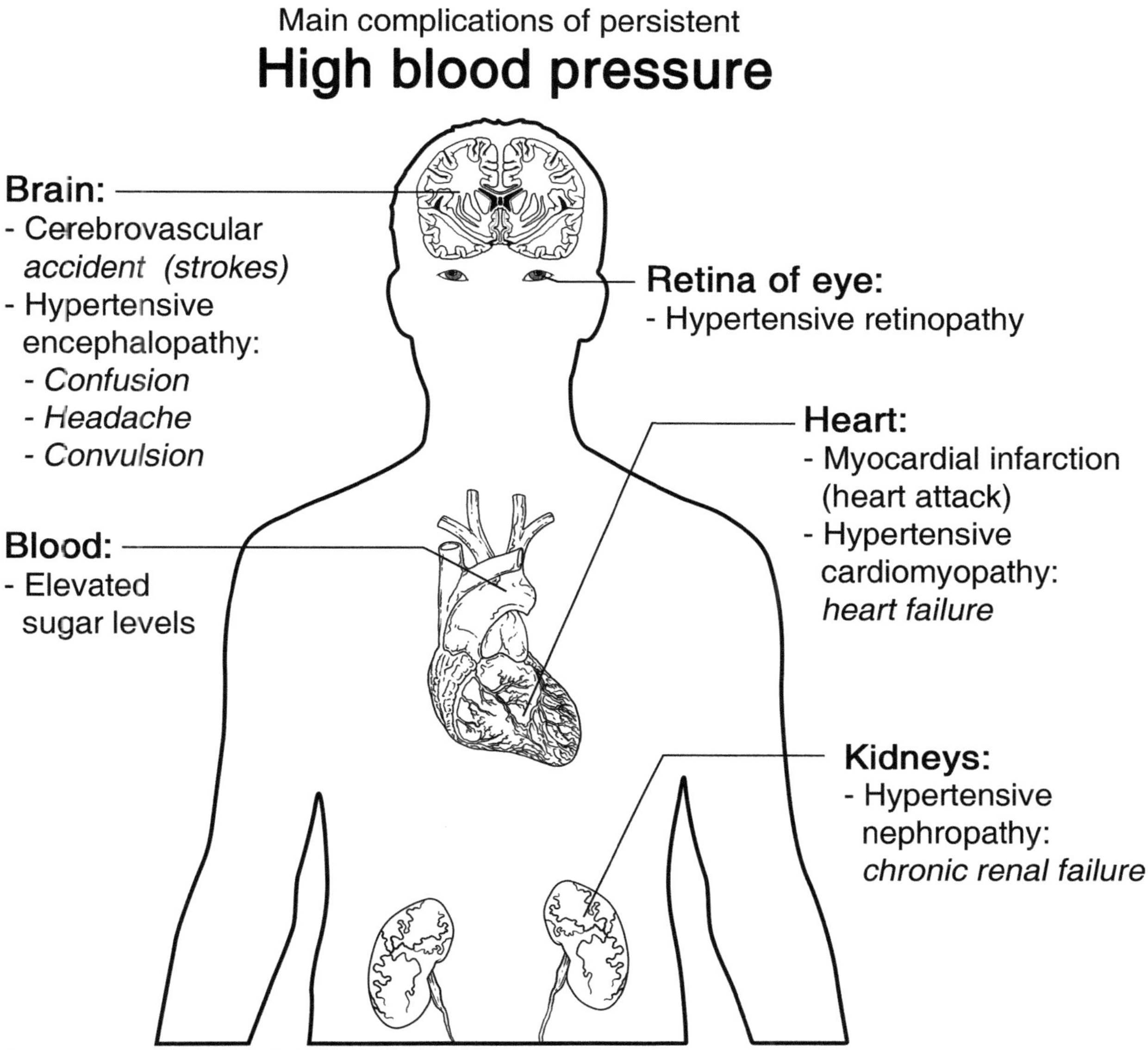


**Fig. 3.1** Long-term effects of hypertension

#### 3.5.1.1 Minor Oral Surgery

A thorough history will elicit symptoms of poor blood pressure control and symptoms of end-organ damage in a known hypertensive.

Conversely, end-organ damage points to poor blood pressure control. If such symptoms exist, elective procedures are to be deferred until good control is achieved. The absolute cut off of blood pressure is supposed to be 180/110 mmHg [9]. However, it is the author's experience that this is too high a cut off in the Indian context with social and logistic challenges. This is especially true for an out-of-hospital standalone dental clinic where the average oral surgeon performs his outpatient procedures. This is because there is a lack of clarity on the effect of stress-induced hypertension (white coat hypertension) and the effect it can have in an already-hypertensive patient. Hence, it is advisable to limit elective extractions to stage 2 hypertension [10] (SBP < 160 mmHg and DBP < 100 mmHg). When minor oral surgery is performed within these parameters, excessive bleeding is an unlikely complication.

#### 3.5.1.2 Major Maxillofacial Surgery

Major surgery introduces two important variables into the mix. First is the procedure itself with surgical trauma and the attendant physiologic response (Table 3.2). The second is the requirement of a general anesthetic. While the anesthesiologist takes the final call on the safety of administering general anesthesia, the surgeon is the one who needs to provide the input regarding the intensity of the surgery. For example, fixing a fractured zygomatic bone can wait while operating on a patient with stridor from Ludwig's angina cannot.

Additionally, perioperative hypotension can also be of significant concern, both systemically and surgically (microvascular flaps need excellent perfusion and hypotension with peripheral vasoconstriction can lead to a flap loss). The surgeon and the anesthetist need to walk a tightrope, especially in a hypertensive patient.

**Table 3.2** Causes of hemodynamic changes [7]

| Hemodynamic changes | Causes |
|---|---|
| Hypotension | Systemic vasodilatation (GA) |
| | Sympathetic blockade (spinal/epidural anesthesia) |
| | Hypovolemia |
| | Blood loss |
| | Mechanical ventilation |
| | Drugs (angiotensin receptor blockers) |
| | Arrhythmias |
| | Acute coronary events |
| | Pulmonary thromboembolism (high-risk surgery for pulmonary thromboembolism and/or patient predisposing factors) |
| Hypertension | Laryngoscopy and intubation |
| | Surgical stimulus |
| | Inadequate plane of anesthesia/analgesia |
| | Hypothermia |
| | Hypervolemia |
| | Reversal and recovery |
| | Hypoxia (post-op) |
| | Inadequate analgesia (post-op) |
| | Full bladder (post-op) |

#### 3.5.1.3 Vasoconstrictors and Hypertension

Vasoconstrictors are routinely used in conjunction with a local anesthetic to reduce bleeding, increase the duration of action, and reduce the requirement of the total volume of the anesthetic. The most commonly used vasoconstrictor is adrenaline. Felypressin (Octapressin) is also available as a vasoconstrictor with Prilocaine—but only in a cartridge. The concentration of adrenaline as a vasoconstrictor ranges from 1:80,000 to 1:200,000.

Physiologic effects of adrenaline in varying concentration [11]:

- 1:80,000 significantly increase in systolic blood pressure (SBP), diastolic blood pressure (DBP), and heart rate;
- 1:100,000 concentrations can increase SBP and heart rate; and
- 1:200,000 is limited to an increase in heart rate, but less significant

Pain itself has a significant effect on SBP, DBP on heart rate and adrenaline, even in the concentration of 1:200,000 significantly increases the duration and depth of local anesthetic. Adrenalin has a beneficial effect in this concentration without negative cardiovascular implications [11].

### 3.5.2 Ischemic Heart Disease (IHD)

Atherosclerosis is a progressive disease involving medium-to-large caliber arteries. It may result in ischemic lesions of the brain, heart or extremities leading to thrombosis, infarction of affected vessels, and end-organ damage.

Ischemic heart disease could present as angina or myocardial infarction (Figs. 3.2 and 3.3). Both conditions are caused

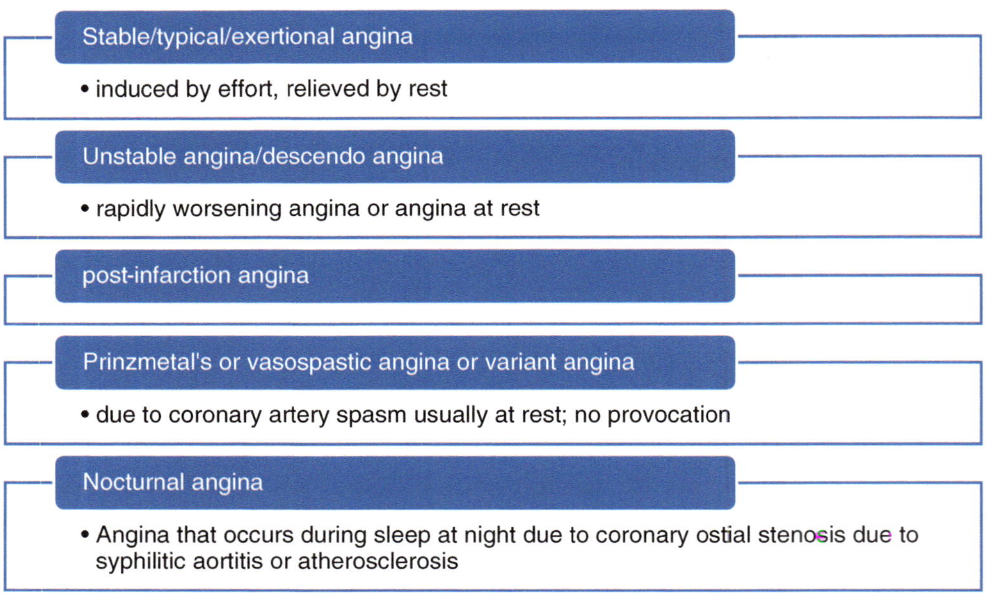

**Fig. 3.2** Types of Angina

©Association of Oral and Maxillofacial Surgeons of India

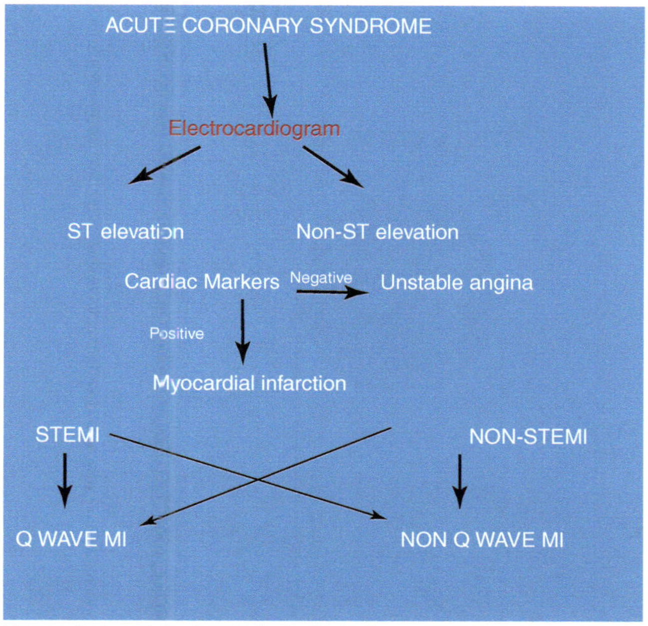


©Association of Oral and Maxillofacial Surgeons of India

**Fig. 3.3** Types of Acute Coronary Syndrome

by decreased coronary blood flow, increased myocardial oxygen demand, and form two ends of a spectrum with several subclassifications.

Oral surgical procedures cause significant surgical, physiological, and psychological stress. It is imperative that the patient is assessed thoroughly prior to any intervention. Patients with IHD are susceptible for another cardiac event within 6 months [12]. With changing management strategies in cardiac patients and medicolegal aspects in mind, it is prudent to liaise with the cardiologist for all but the most straightforward of situations.

#### 3.5.2.1 Minor Oral Surgery

Previous myocardial infarction or unstable angina does not form a contraindication for dental extractions. However, timing and planning are of paramount importance. In the quoted study, about 10% of patients have reported postoperative chest pain [12]. While the sample size of the quoted article is small, it underscores the importance of risk-benefit analysis before undertaking these procedures. The treatment planning may need further input from a cardiologist.

If such patients are on antiplatelet medication, it is of extreme importance to note that single antiplatelet agents do not constitute a contraindication for most minor oral surgery [13]. *Refer to the section on antiplatelet and anticoagulant drugs and surgery.*

#### 3.5.2.2 Major Surgery

Since most surgery considered in this context is emergent or urgent in nature (trauma, oncosurgery, space infections), the benefit of the life-saving procedure by far outweighs the risk of a further cardiac episode. Such procedures are ideally done in a center equipped to deal with any adverse cardiac event. In a country like India, the onus of keeping the appropriate specialty appraised of the situation before starting the procedure is on the operating surgeon.

### 3.5.3 Postintervention Cardiac Patients

#### 3.5.3.1 Percutaneous Coronary Angioplasty (PTCA) and Coronary Artery Bypass Graft (CABG) and Valve Replacement Procedures

With access to healthcare improving, it is becoming more common for the surgeon to encounter patients with IHD who have had interventions. These range from conventional CABG to Percutaneous angioplasties with stents in place and minimal access CABGs. In our context, the clinician needs to know what these are not only to analyze the impact these procedures have on the maxillofacial procedure but also to tease the information out of the reluctant historian.

**PTCA/PCA**

Percutaneous transluminal coronary angioplasty has become the intervention of choice for coronary artery disease. This procedure involves the insertion of a stent in the narrowed portion of the artery (Fig. 3.4). This stent intimately hugs the endothelium of the vessel and is reliably and completely endothilized in 6 months to a year. The patient is susceptible to stent thrombosis in this period and hence the antiplatelets. There are many varieties of stents and the design and features are always in a state of flux. Therefore, any changes to antiplatelet therapy are to be made in consultation with the treating cardiologist [14].

Types of coronary stents:

- Bare metal stents
- Drug-eluting stents
- Bioresorbable scaffold system
- Drug-eluting balloons

Following successful revascularization procedures, the patient is expected to be in a far better hemodynamic state than before. If the patient remains symptomatic, then he/she requires to be seen by the cardiothoracic surgery team. The only challenge in these patients is the antiplatelet/anticoagulant medication. In the case of patients with prosthetic cardiac valves, it is vital to provide endocarditis prophylaxis (read following content).

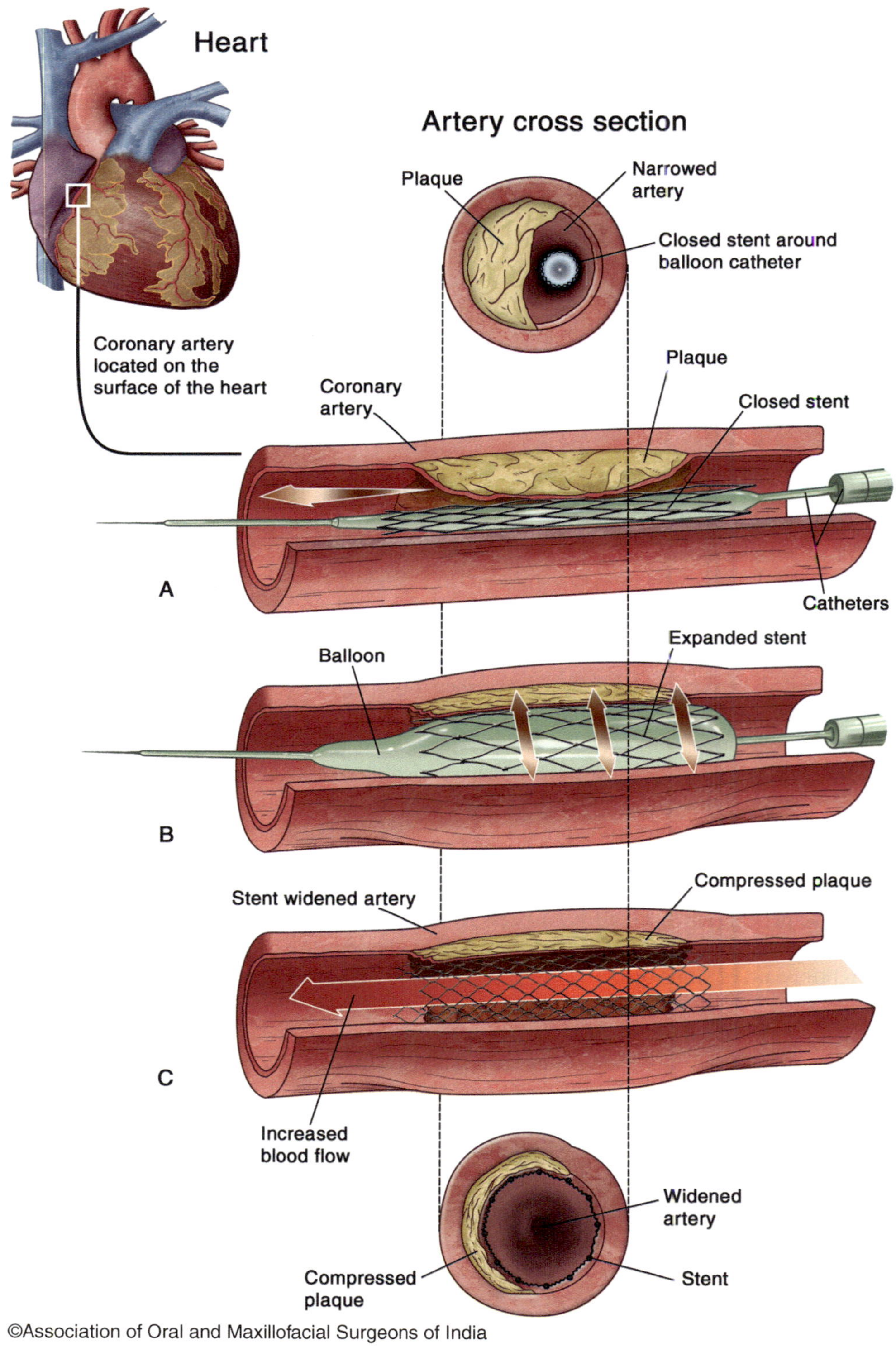


**Fig. 3.4** Mechanism of PTCA

### 3.5.4 Conventional Antiplatelets, Anticoagulants, and Novel Oral Anticoagulants (NOAC)

#### 3.5.4.1 Minor Dentoalveolar Surgery: Antiplatelets

There are several concerns regarding the risk of excessive bleeding following minor oral surgery in anticoagulated patients and those on antiplatelet medication. Most of these are unfounded for dentoalveolar procedures. In most dentoalveolar procedures, we have the advantage of a bony cavity where physical pressure can be effectively applied to obtain hemostasis. This can be further augmented with other local hemostatic measures (sutures, surgical R, AbgelR, etc.). This obviates the need to stop antiplatelet drugs (read following content). However, in patients on dual antiplatelet therapy, the authors suggest caution when operating in critical areas like the floor of the mouth as hematomas can cause airway embarrassment.

Conventional antiplatelets bind irreversibly to platelets and the normal clotting process is restored only with the production of new, unaffected platelets (Fig. 3.5, Table 3.3). It takes 5–10 days for platelets to be produced in the quantity required to produce a clinically normal platelet action. In the interim, if a procedure causes excessive bleeding, the only reliable way to ensure hemostasis is platelet transfusion. However, the newer ones are reversible and can be stopped for 24 h prior to the procedure as a “switch on-switch off”

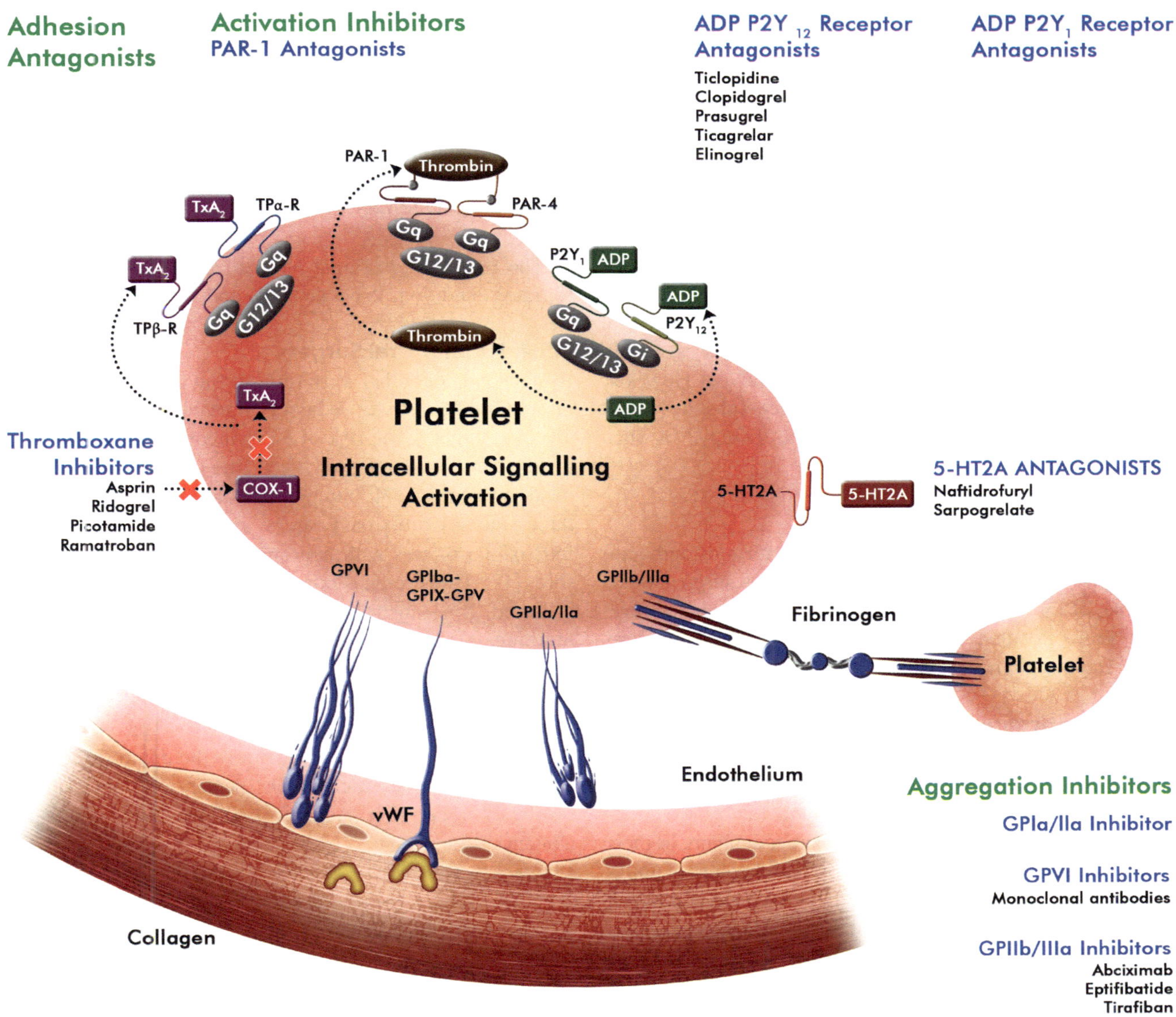


**Fig. 3.5** Mechanism of action of commonly used antiplatelet drugs

**Table 3.3** Commonly used antiplatelet agents and their characteristics [15]

| Drug | Mechanism of action | Loading dose | Maintenance dose | Half-life | Time to recover platelet function after drug withdrawal | Platelet inhibition | Administration route |
|---|---|---|---|---|---|---|---|
| Aspirin | COX-1 inhibition | 325 mg | 75–325 mg daily | 15–20 min | 30% at 48 h | Irreversible inhibition | Oral |
| Clopidogrel | P2Y12 receptor inhibition | 30–600 mg | 75 mg daily | 7–9 h | 40% at 3 days | Irreversible inhibition | Oral |
| Prasugrel | P2Y12 receptor inhibition | 60 mg | 10 mg daily | 7 h | 2–3 days | Irreversible inhibition | Oral |
| Ticagrelor | P2Y12 and Partly P2Y1 receptor inhibition | 180 mg | 90 mg twice a day | 7–9 h | 57% at 24 h | Reversible inhibition | Oral |
| Cangrelor | Adenosine triphosphate analogue with a high affinity for the P2Y12 receptor | 30 μg/kg | 2–4 μg/kg/min | 3–6 min | Rapid (mins–hours) | Reversible inhibition | i.v |
| Abciximab | Glycoprotein IIb/IIIa receptor inhibitor | 0.25 μg/kg | 0.125 μg/kg/min | 10–15 min | 12 h | Reversible inhibition | i.v |
| Eptifibatide | Glycoprotein IIb/IIIa receptor inhibitor | 180 μg/kg | 2 μg/kg/min | 2.5 h | 2–4 h | Reversible inhibition | i.v |
| Tirofiban | Glycoprotein IIb/IIIa receptor inhibitor | 0.4 μg/kg | 0.1 μg/kg/min | 2 h | 2–4 h | Reversible inhibition | i.v |

drug. But these are very expensive and most of the below-poverty-line patients are likely to be on older antiplatelets for some time to come.

#### 3.5.4.2 Maxillofacial Surgery

Patients who need procedures with low risk of bleeding (e.g., fixation of fracture of the parasymphysis) may continue oral antiplatelet/anticoagulation therapy. This applies especially to high-risk patients (e.g., mechanical heart valves). However, when the risk of bleeding is obvious, it outweighs the benefit of continuing antiplatelet/anticoagulant therapy. In such cases, heparin is used as bridge therapy.

#### 3.5.4.3 Bridging with Heparin

In cases where the patient is at high risk for a thromboembolic episode, a "bridge"—a balance between surgical bleed and risk of thrombosis may be achieved either with intravenous unfractionated heparin or with subcutaneous low-molecular-weight heparin [16].

#### 3.5.4.4 Anticoagulants and Oral/Maxillofacial Surgery

While several indications exist for the use of anticoagulants, the authors have noted that there is significant resistance in the medical community to prescribe anticoagulants in these cases and they are often replaced by antiplatelets in India. This is especially true for the rural patient who may not have regular access to monitor his anticoagulation status. However, in urban centers, NOAC are in regular use.

Common indications for anticoagulation—prevention of thrombotic events in:

Mechanical Heart Valves.
Atrial Fibrillation.
Deep Vein Thrombosis and Pulmonary Embolism.
Myocardial infarction.
Acute Ischemic Stroke

The target International Normalized Ratio (INR) range for most conditions is between 2.5 and 3.5.

#### 3.5.4.5 Minor Oral Surgery

It is beyond doubt that warfarin/acetrom therapy need not be discontinued and INR need not be normalized prior to dento-alveolar surgery. The risk of a thrombotic episode does not justify the risk of a minor bleed that can be controlled by local measures [17]. Simple dentoalveolar surgery (e.g., three simple extractions) can be safely performed with an INR of 3.5 or less with appropriate local hemostatic measures [18]. However, it is imperative that the patient is closely followed. It is sensible to schedule these procedures in the morning.

#### 3.5.4.6 Major Maxillofacial Surgery

Depending on the indication for anticoagulant therapy and the drug used, the decision regarding the control of anticoagulation is made. Ideally the prescribing physician is involved in decision making (Fig. 3.6) (read following content).

### 3.5.5 Infective Endocarditis Prophylaxis

Much has changed over the years with regard to infective endocarditis (IE) and antibiotic prophylaxis. Since the guidelines change by the year, the authors strongly recommend that the surgeon takes recourse to his smartphone to keep abreast of the changing scenery (Tables 3.4 and 3.5).

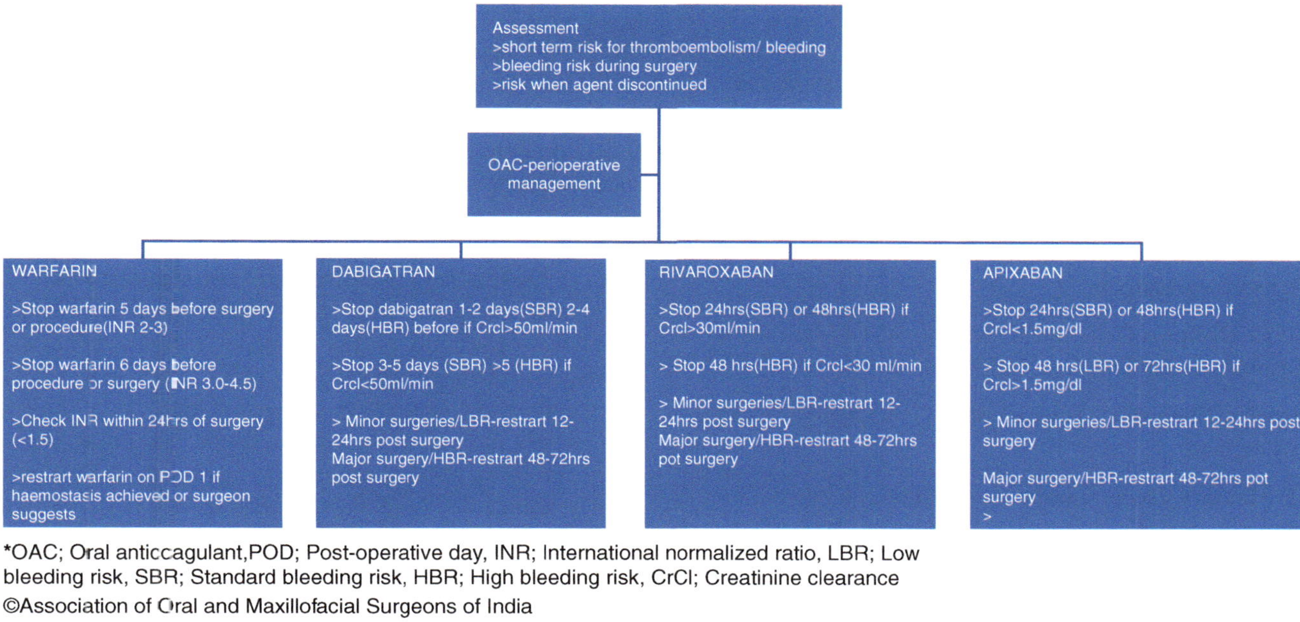


**Fig. 3.6** Perioperative management of oral anticoagulants [19]

### 3.5.6 Implantable Cardioverter Defibrillators (ICD)

An ICD is a battery-powered device implanted in a patient that generates a small electrical impulse. Indications are patients at risk of sudden cardiac death—ventricular fibrillation/ventricular tachycardia, malignant ventricular tachyarrhythmias. ICDs are also used to treat Brugada syndrome [21].

#### 3.5.6.1 Implications

Bleeding: patients may either be on antiplatelets or anticoagulated. (read earlier content).

Devices: Electrocautery, especially monopolar diathermy, may interfere with the device and this may have to be turned to a "safe mode" by the electrophysiology technician. The concerned cardiologist should be able to assist with the technical details.

Infective endocarditis prophylaxis: Risk being low, current guidelines DO NOT recommend prophylaxis for these patients.

## 3.6 Impact of Central Nervous System Disorders in Maxillofacial Surgery

Of the many conditions which affect this system, the effects of epilepsy and stroke are most commonly encountered in maxillofacial surgical practice.

**Table 3.4** AHA, ESC, and NICE guidelines for infective endocarditis prophylaxis

| 2007 AHA guidelines | 2015 ESC guidelines | 2016 NICE guidelines |
|---|---|---|
| Highest risk of adverse outcomes:<br>• Previous IE<br>• Prosthetic valve<br>• Unrepaired cyanotic congenital heart disease (CHD)<br>• 6-month period postprosthetic repair of CHD<br>• Repaired CHD with residual defects<br>• Cardiac transplant with valvulopathy | Highest risk of IE:<br>• Previous IE<br>• Prosthetic valve/ Prosthetic material for valve repair<br>• Any cyanotic CHD<br>• 6-month period postprosthetic repair of CHD<br>Intermediate risk of IE:<br>• History of rheumatic fever<br>• Any form of native valve disease<br>• Unrepaired noncyanotic CHD | Risk of developing IE:<br>• Previous IE<br>• Valve replacement<br>• Acquired valvular heart disease<br>• Structural Congenital heart disease<br>• Hypertrophic cardiomyopathy |
| Antibiotic prophylaxis:<br>• All dental procedures involving gingival tissue manipulation or periapical region of teeth or oral mucosa perforation<br>• Procedures on respiratory tract or infected skin/ musculoskeletal tissue. | Antibiotic prophylaxis: Considered for dental procedures involving gingival tissue manipulation or periapical region of teeth or oral mucosa perforation | Antibiotic prophylaxis: Not routinely recommended |

**Table 3.5** Revised AHA guidelines for infective endocarditis prophylaxis [20]

| Patient group | Antibiotic | Dose (30–60 min before procedure) Adults | Children |
|---|---|---|---|
| Able to take oral medicine | Amoxicillin | 2 g | 50 mg/kg |
| Unable to take oral medication | Ampicillin | 2 g i.m/i.v | 50 mg/kg i.m/i.v |
| | or | | |
| | Cefazolin/ ceftriaxone | 1 g i.m/i.v | 50 mg/kg i.m/i.v |
| Allergic to penicillin or ampicillin and able to take oral medication | Cephalexin[a,b] | 2 g | 50 mg/kg |
| | or | | |
| | Clindamycin | 600 mg | 20 mg/kg |
| | or | | |
| | Azithromycin/ clarithromycin | 500 mg | 15 mg/kg |
| Allergic to penicillins or ampicillin and unable to take oral medication | Cefazolin/ ceftriaxone[b] | 1 g i.m/i.v | 50 mg/kg i.m/i.v |
| | or | | |
| | Clindamycin | 600 mg | 20 mg/kg |

Note: *i.m* intramuscular; *i.v* intravenous

[a]Or other first- or second-generation cephalosporins at equivalent adult and pediatric dose

[b]Cephalosporins should not be given to a patient with a history of anaphylaxis, angioedema, or urticaria with penicillin or ampicillin

## 3.6.1 Epilepsy

A seizure is a result of excessive electrical discharges in a group of brain cells, whereas epilepsy is described as a disease characterized by recurrent seizures. A single seizure does not constitute epilepsy, which is defined as having at least two or more unprovoked seizures. The incidence worldwide is approximately 0.5–0.9%, affecting over 50 million individuals [22].

Etiology of epilepsy can be divided as primary or idiopathic, where the cause is unknown and this constitutes the vast majority of cases. In secondary or acquired epilepsy, the cause can be determined and these include metabolic, genetic, structural, and functional abnormalities.

An increase in the incidence in the elderly can be attributed to conditions such as stroke, tumors, trauma, and Alzheimer's disease. Systemic conditions include diabetes, hypertension, infections, electrolyte imbalances and dehydration, or lack of oxygen. Withdrawal from high-dose, long-term use of drugs such as cocaine, heroin, barbiturates, amphetamines, and alcohol can also precipitate seizures [23]. Seizures generally last for a few seconds to minutes. Although many types exist, they are broadly divided into two groups (Fig. 3.7).

Primary generalized seizures—which begin with involvement both sides of the cerebral hemispheres.

Partial seizures—start in a localized area [25].

### 3.6.1.1 Basic considerations

While recording history, the duration, type, frequency of the seizure as well as the most recent episode must be recorded as well as the type of medication taken, if any. If the patient is aware of how the seizure starts, if there is any warning or "aura," this too must be noted [23].

Several factors are capable of provoking seizures. These include improper use of medication, lack of sleep, drug abuse, drug interactions, hypoglycemia, electrolyte imbalance among others. Antiepileptic drugs should generally be continued without alteration.

### 3.6.1.2 Outpatient maxillofacial considerations

If seizures are predictable, then appointments should be scheduled accordingly. Frequency of seizures determines the urgency of treatment. Procedures, unless emergent, should be postponed if frequency of seizures is high. The clinician must reduce anxiety to the patient. Short morning appointments are ideal. Sudden bright lights, noise, or movements must be avoided as these may trigger a seizure [23].

### 3.6.1.3 Major Surgical Considerations

Trauma is a common consequence of seizures and may result in lacerations of the face or oral cavity and fractures of the maxillofacial skeleton. Other injuries include hematomas, dislocation of temporomandibular joint (TMJ) fracture/loss of teeth. An electroencephalogram (EEG) along with imaging such as CT/MRI is recommended if there is no previous seizure history. Open reduction should be preferred over closed for treatment of facial fractures, as further episodes of seizures might lead to aspiration if intermaxillary fixation (IMF) is attempted [25].

Local anesthetic is considered safe in well-controlled epileptics, as is sedation. General anesthesia is preferred in uncontrolled epileptics, especially if coupled with a mental deficit, as a seizure might be triggered due to stress from difficulties in communication. One drawback of general anesthetic is temporary anoxia to the brain, which itself might trigger a seizure [26].

### 3.6.1.4 Precautions, complications, & management

As mentioned earlier, appropriate recording of history gives an insight into planning the procedure, particularly for elective surgeries. Objects with the potential to cause harm must be kept away from the vicinity of the patient. Antiepileptics such as phenytoin have been known to cause gingival enlargement, which can be managed either by surgery or by a change in medication. Aspirin, antifungal azoles, metronidazole can interfere with phenytoin. Propoxyphene and erythromycin can interfere with carbemezepine. Contraindicated drugs are chlorpromazine, flumazenil, ketamine, lignocaine in large doses and quinolones, tramadol, and tricyclic antidepressants [25].

### 3.6.1.5 Management of an acute episode on the dental chair

If possible, all foreign body/material should be removed from the oral cavity. The chair should be reclined to a supine position with the patient turned onto their side to minimize the

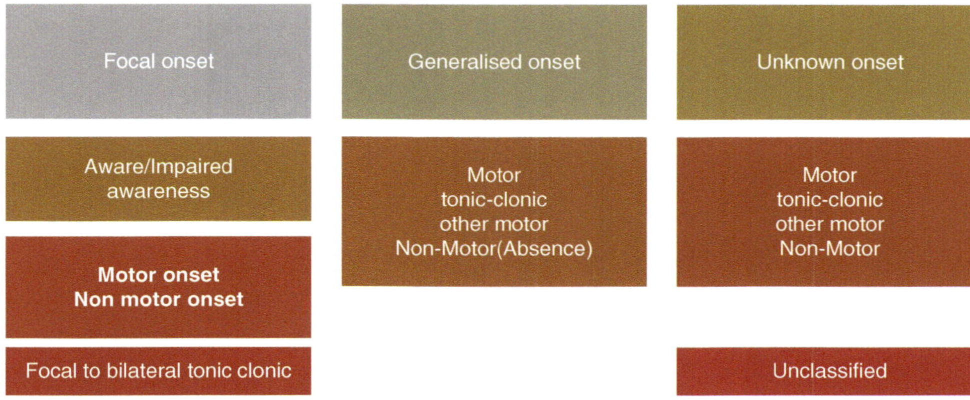


©Association of Oral and Maxillofacial Surgeons of India

**Fig. 3.7** ILAE 2017 classifications of seizure types basic version [24]

risk of aspiration. Passive restraint is used only to prevent them from falling out of the chair. A recurrent seizure or a seizure of more than 3 min requires drug administration. The patient should be monitored to prevent airway obstruction. After the patient recovers, appropriate medical consults should be arranged. Elective treatment should be postponed [23]. However, prolonged seizures, which continue in spite of medication, may lead to status epilepticus, which may be fatal if untreated. Airway patency and peripheral venous access are first line of management. If seizures persist even after administration of drugs such as lorazepam or diazepam, the patient must be shifted to the hospital for further management.

## 3.6.2 Stroke

Stroke (cerebrovascular accident) is a serious, occasionally fatal neurologic event characterized by the rapid appearance of a focal deficit of brain function. It is estimated that 85% of patients presenting with stroke would have sustained a cerebral infarction because of inadequate blood flow to a part of the brain, with the remainder suffering from an intracerebral hemorrhage. Often, survivors of cerebrovascular accidents are left debilitated in motor function and/or speech [27].

A stroke may be a result of hemorrhage or ischemia as given later (Fig. 3.8).

The initial presentation of stroke includes loss of combination of sensory and motor functions with occasional loss of consciousness. The presenting features include hemiparesis or paraparesis, dysphagia, ataxia, aphasia, dysarthria, loss of vision. Early detection is by assessing facial and arm weakness and any slurring of speech. Mechanism of stroke may be ischemic, primary intracerebral hemorrhage, and subarachnoid hemorrhage. The oral impact of stroke includes facial weakness, dysphagia, and speech impairment [29].

### 3.6.2.1 Basic Considerations

At the outset, it is paramount to assess the extent of disability of the patient—both physical and mental, as this is vital in determining whether performing the procedure is safe in the outpatient setting. There may be a dependence on others for basic needs. History of past strokes needs to be elicited: including dates, severity and current neurological deficit. Treatment is performed in consultation with the neurologist and precautions according to the specific characteristics of the stroke.

### 3.6.2.2 Maxillofacial considerations

Outpatient appointments must be ideally scheduled in the morning and must be of short duration. Patients must be treated in an upright position as much as possible, as they are more prone to aspiration due to impaired protective reflexes. Another important consideration is difficulty in oral hygiene maintenance due to facial weakness and xerostomia, which may be observed as a side effect of medications prescribed [24]. Although procedures must be deferred for as long as possible, in unavoidable circumstances such as trauma or progressing head and neck cancers, general anesthesia is reasonably safe. Shorter duration surgery, intraoperative monitoring and maintaining cerebral perfusion, anticoagulation status, and precaution all aid in reducing the incidence of a further episode.

Antiplatelets and anticoagulation: Ref previous section.

### 3.6.2.3 Precautions

Monitoring of Blood pressure pre- and postprocedure is vital, procedures should be deferred if systolic is >180 mmHg or diastolic is >110 mmHg. Poststroke patients are usually on antiplatelet or anticoagulant medications; hence, coagulation status must be ascertained prior to any procedure. Vasoconstrictors are to be used cautiously as they can increase the risk of adverse outcomes like cerebral hemorrhage due to acute hypertension [29].

Opiods are best avoided as they may result in severe hypotension and benzodiazepines may cause respiratory depression. The practitioner must be mindful that sudden loss of consciousness could result from stroke, and emergency management is the protection of airway and shift to hospital [24].

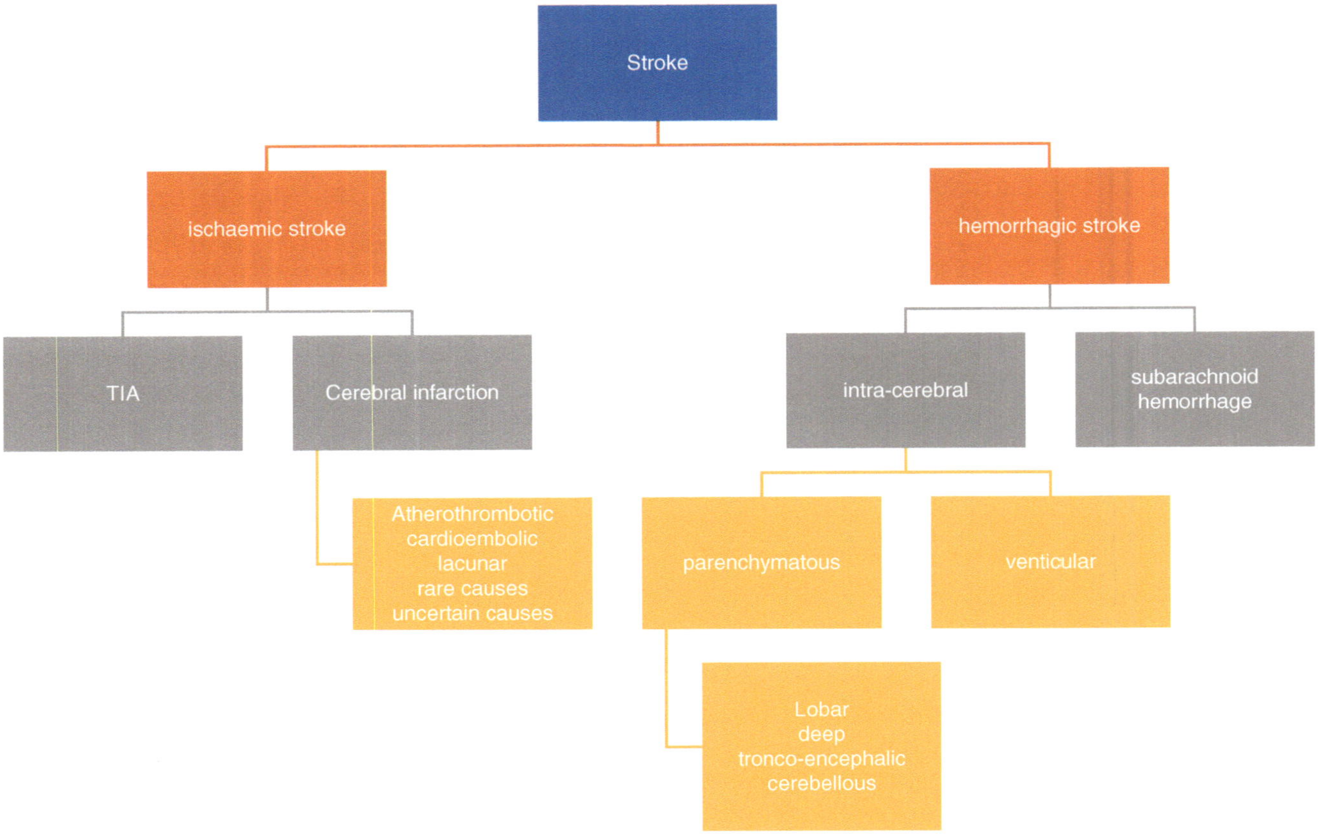




**Fig. 3.8** Common causes of stroke [28]

## 3.7 Impact of Psychiatric Disorders in Maxillofacial Surgery

Psychiatric and psychological disorders are of rising concern in modern society, affecting all aspects of a patient's life, including oral health. Poor oral hygiene is usually due to a combination of lethargy, side effect of medications, and possibly fear of treatment [30]. Common disorders encountered in practice are related to mood, anxiety, substance dependence, eating, or somatoform in nature [31].

Occasionally, oral symptoms may be the initial or single manifestations of the underlying issue. Patients who present with atypical facial pain with vague symptoms, oral dysesthesia, abnormal sensation or movement, salivation often with no identifiable physical cause could be suffering from undiagnosed underlying emotional disturbances. Early detection in such cases benefits both the patient and the practitioner [32, 33].

### 3.7.1 Maxillofacial Considerations

Pain related to the TMJ and associated structures seems to be another condition, which fits into the previous category, commonly seen and treated by the maxillofacial surgeon. In the absence of an identifiable organic cause, there must be a low threshold for considering an underlying emotional disturbance.

Patients with diagnosed psychiatric conditions and on medication present with obvious oral symptoms. Most common among these are dental caries and periodontal disease. The primary cause of these is due to decreased salivary flow or xerostomia, which is a side effect of medications, including tricyclic antidepressants, lithium carbonate, phenothiazines, and benzodiazepines. Sialorrhea or excessive salivation is a well-known side effect of clozapine and reduction in dose may be of use [32]. Candidiasis is another condition, which may manifest due to xerostomia, especially in denture wearers. Fear of dental treatment is well known. However, recognition of the nature and extent of this fear is important to prevent noncompliance. Anxiety disorders and phobia often stem from two types of experiences, a painful or traumatic procedure, usually at a young age, or a negative interaction with healthcare professional [32]. A specific maxillofacial consideration in this respect is suturing of facial wounds under local anesthetic, in young children. The authors recommend sedation if not a general anesthetic, particularly in extremely young children, where such procedures are required.

Alcohol, tobacco, and drug abusers are particularly tricky to treat, be it minor or major maxillofacial surgery. The amount of local anesthetic required to produce adequate analgesia tends to be higher in such patients. These groups of patients are at a higher risk of developing oral cancer. Effects of withdrawal can be significant and this must be kept in mind preoperatively, intraoperatively, and postoperatively—especially where procedures of long duration and extended stay are planned. Use of drugs like chlordiazepoxide might be required to offset delirium tremens, particularly in the postoperative period. Head and neck cancer particularly affects the psyche, making a psychologist a very important member of the multidisciplinary team.

Patients suffering from clefts of the orofacial region require multiple surgeries at various stages of their life and the effects of surgery and rehabilitation can be debilitating on both the child and the parents. Timing of surgeries is vital as they disrupt the life of the entire family of the child and for this parental counselling is extremely important [33].

While management of trauma might be comparatively straightforward, one must not underestimate the effect on the psyche in the recovery phase, especially if this is coupled with post-traumatic stress disorder (PTSD). Although these injuries are among the most common treated, these can lead to depression, drug abuse, antisocial behavior, especially in those with a post-traumatic residual defect [34].

Orthognathic surgery, while primarily carried out for cosmetic reasons, occasionally may be performed for functional reasons, as in obstructive sleep apnea. Counselling prior to surgery is useful and the entire process can take up to 3 years. Serious psychological and psychosocial problems have been reported [33].

While awareness of maxillofacial surgery and its benefits is gradually growing in our country, with most centers providing information about technical aspects of surgery, the psychological aspect is often ignored. Communication needs to improve and an assessment of patients' emotional state before and after surgery could help in improving patient satisfaction [33].

## 3.8 Dental and Maxillofacial Implications in Liver Disease

### 3.8.1 Introduction

At approximate of 1.4 kg, this reddish, rubbery structure forms an important organ system. Along with the Gall Bladder and Pancreas, the liver works to digest, process, and absorb food. Liver aids in detoxification in the body and is the primary organ of drug metabolism. It also helps in the production and transport of bile [35].

#### 3.8.1.1 The Function of the Liver [36]

Detoxification—Removal of ammonia, exogenous hormones

(a) Alcohol metabolism
(b) Synthesis of essential Serum Proteins (Albumin)
(c) Synthesis—coagulation Factors (V, VII, IX, X), prothrombin, fibrinogen.
(d) Production of Bile and its transporters
(e) Regulation of nutrients
(f) Conjugation of lipophilic compounds

Liver dysfunction hence alters all of these functions, thereby disrupting the homeostasis in the body, which has to be taken into consideration when providing dental and maxillofacial therapy.

Vitamin K levels are significantly lowered in advanced liver disease hampering the production of coagulation factors. This, along with portal hypertension, results in thrombocytopenia, thus resulting in excessive bleeding, which is of consideration during dental and maxillofacial management [37].

### 3.8.2 Classification of Liver Dysfunctions [35]

Acute or Chronic

(a) Infective (Hepatitis) & Noninfective (Substance abuse)
(b) Extent of damage—steatosis (fatty liver), fibrosis, cirrhosis, hepatocellular carcinoma

#### 3.8.2.1 Viral Hepatitis

Hepatitis A—caused due to Hepatitis A virus, spreads via the orofecal route. It is endemic in nature and is self-limiting.

Hepatitis B—caused by (HBV) that replicates within the hepatocyte; it is a dangerous form of viral disease with high risk to healthcare workers. The surface antigen is routinely detected in the saliva of infected individuals, and hence transmission through the saliva is of concern to the Oral Surgeon [38]. Prevalence of HBV infection is three to five times more in dentists than the general population. Younger individuals with chronic HBV infections have a greater prevalence of developing hepatocellular carcinoma.

Hepatitis C—Caused by a bloodborne virus, it is the most common cause for chronic hepatitis, which over long term could lead to cirrhosis or hepatocellular carcinoma.

#### 3.8.2.2 Autoimmune Hepatitis

It is a chronic liver inflammatory disease as a result of IgG Hypergammaglobinemia as a result of environmental or viral factors inciting an autoimmune response leading to cirrhosis [39].

#### 3.8.2.3 Fulminant Hepatitis

A sudden acute and severe dysfunction of the liver with resulting hepatocellular necrosis and encephalopathy with a very poor prognosis. These patients require liver transplant.

#### 3.8.2.4 Cirrhosis

It is the irreversible damage to the hepatic architecture due to long-term fibrous scarring. A rise in the production of total liver collagen and matrix protein that is troublesome to the function and form of the liver [40].

#### 3.8.2.5 Hepatocellular Carcinoma

It is the fifth most common cancer and a life-threatening malignancy with poor survival rates. HBV and HCV are the most common causes of it.

#### 3.8.2.6 Alcoholic Liver Disease

It is the 10th most common cause of death with 3% of fatalities in the industrialized world [35]. Alcoholism results in varied disruption of the hepatic system ranging from simple fatty liver to complicated life-threatening cirrhosis.

### 3.8.3 Oral Manifestations of Liver Disease

Foetor hepaticus (Breath of the dead odor of rotten eggs with garlic) is a characteristic late feature of liver dysfunction [36]. Evidence of liver diseases has been noted in the oral cavity as icteric mucosal alteration with gingival bleeding and also associated hemorrhagic changes like hematoma, petechiae [37]. HCV-associated hepatitis is noted as a common cause for Sjogren's syndrome and lichen planus in the oral cavity [41]. Alcoholic hepatitis in association with nutritional deficiencies could cause glossitis along with delayed healing post surgery [37]. Occasionally, parotid enlargement is also noted. These oral manifestations are associated with concomitant general symptoms of liver disease such as hepatomegaly, malaise, confusion, fatigue, weight loss, nausea, and altering the well being of the person [37].

### 3.8.4 Implications of Liver Disease

1. Hepatic metabolism of drugs is Unpredictable
2. Defective hemostatic cascade and poor coagulation
3. Increased risk of infection

#### 3.8.4.1 Liver Disease and Maxillofacial Surgery

Risk of viral contagion and crossinfection is one of the implications of viral hepatic disease. Hep C viruses are found to be stable at room temperatures for approximately 5 days. The virus is also detected at different surfaces in the clinic after the patient is treated. It is vital to maintain adequate sterilization and observe strict universal protection when treating such patients. Needlestick injury precautions must be adhered to.

Detailed history taking is important to identify any indications of liver disease, including that of hepatitis, jaundice, alcohol intake, recreational drugs, or rank abuse. Abnormal bleeding patterns are elicited in history [42]. Past surgical history provides a valuable indicator for any doubts regarding the adequate functioning of the liver system. Additional information of identifying the etiology for cirrhosis and any continued risk factors like alcohol consumption should be noted [35]. Review of blood investigations such as serum bilirubin, albumin, alanine aminotransferase (ALT), Aspartate aminotransferase (AST), complete blood counts, and coagulation profile must be performed prior to any surgical planning [43].

Elective surgery is contraindicated in acute phases of viral hepatitis and acute liver failure. Patients who present with hepatitis due to alcohol/drug abuse are poor candidates for elective surgery due to liver dysfunction and psychological impact of withdrawal during their hospital stay.

Plasma level of coagulation factors is depressed in liver disease and can potentially alter the hemostasis. Complete blood counts, PT, PTT, INR, and liver functions tests are mandatory in all patients with any signs/symptoms of liver dysfunctions. The goal of surgical therapy is to minimize trauma to the tissues. It is also advisable to involve the hematologist if required. Any dental or minor oral surgical procedure must terminate with the use of local hemostatic agents or antifibrinolytic agents to aid in hemostasis. Maxillofacial surgical work and major invasive oral surgery are ideally performed in the hospital. Fresh Frozen Plasma and Vitamin K infusions to optimize the coagulating process might be required to offset intraoperative bleeding.

Patients with liver disease are more susceptible to infection with a greater risk post invasive dental or maxillofacial procedure. Antibiotic prophylaxis is recommended.

Drug metabolism is altered in these patients (Table 3.6). Unlike serum creatinine, which is an indicator of renal function, the liver function test is more of an indicator for liver damage. Hence, it is difficult to obtain exact dose modification formulae when medicating patients with liver disease. Drug usage, dosage, and interactions must be consulted with the specialist prior to their usage.

The metabolism of these drugs is well tolerated in mild liver dysfunctions but is impaired in severe dysfunction and hence requires modifications and contraindications. The beta lactams mainly utilized in maxillofacial surgery are quite safe. NSAIDS are to be used with caution to avoid gastric bleedings [35]. Hepatotoxic drugs should be avoided eg. erythromycin, ketoconazole, halothane, phenytoin etc. Prilocaine or articaine is preferred over lidocaine. Sedatives,

Table 3.6 Drugs metabolized in the liver [37]

| | |
|---|---|
| Local anesthetics | Lidocaide, Bupivacaine, Prilocaine, |
| Sedatives | Barbiturates, Diazepam |
| Analgesics | Paracetamol, Aspirin, Ibuprofen, Codiene |
| Antibiotics | Erythromycin, Clindamycin, Tetracyclin |
| Antifungal | Ketaconozol, Fluconozol |

hypnotics or opiods should be used with caution. A balance has to be struck constantly to maintain the anesthesia and concern is of the depressive action of alcohol and central nervous system depressors. Postoperative care in view of alcohol withdrawal must be noted. Ensure alcohol-based mouth rinses are avoided.

## 3.9 Maxillofacial Implications in GI Disorders

### 3.9.1 Perioperative Maxillofacial Implications

#### 3.9.1.1 GERD

Extraesophageal symptoms of GERD must be identified to prevent any airway issues primarily. Due to delayed gastric emptying, preoperative fasting hours must be prolonged. In high-risk patients, Proton pump inhibitors and H2 receptor antagonists are potent drugs to increase gastric pH and reduce secretions. Nasogastric suctioning through nasogastric tube aids in protecting the airway from gastric secretions during surgery. It is important to manage nausea and vomiting postoperatively effectively.

#### 3.9.1.2 Peptic Ulcers

Stress reduction protocol is vital. GI symptoms from NSAIDS are delayed and identified when the ulcers are in an advanced stage with a greater risk of bleeding. Corticosteroids must be avoided in these patients along with NSAIDS. GI bleeding due to ulceration could cause anemia and has to be managed prior to any surgery. Surgery is contraindicated in active peptic ulcers. Ranitidine, when used over a long phase for management, could cause thrombocytopenia [44].

#### 3.9.1.3 Ulcerative Colitis

One must rule out anemia in these patients and assess the effect of long-term steroid therapy. Antibiotics such as clindamycin, ampicillin, and cephalosporins are implicated in aggravation of colitis and are hence avoided. If the patient has undergone Vitamin K malabsorption, its effects are considered.

Postoperative nausea and vomiting, though not a complication, is still detrimental in patient management perioperatively. Volatile inhalation anesthetic agents and opiod analgesics are emetogenic and need to be used with caution. Postoperative anxiety, dehydration, and pain could result in nausea and vomiting. Scarred ulcers in the duodenum delay gastric emptying resulting in vomitus. Antiemetics in these patients must be prescribed at the end of the surgery and dexamethasone 1 h prior to the surgery is helpful if not contraindicated. In high-risk patients, antiemetics must be administered prior to anesthesia itself [45]. Postoperative ileus could occur due to prolonged opiate use during anesthesia, decreased potassium levels, trauma or due to iliac bone harvesting as a complication or resultant severe pain.

## 3.10 Pregnancy

Pregnancy is often associated with changes in cardiovascular, endocrine, hematological, respiratory, gastrointestinal, and genitourinary system. These alterations may occasionally be subtle and can lead to disastrous complications if not identified [46].

### 3.10.1 Physiologic Changes

There will be increase in the heart rate leading to an increase in cardiac output. Cardiac output increases mostly in the first trimester and remains fairly unchanged with minimal increase in the final trimester.

During the second and final trimesters, a decrease in blood pressure and cardiac output may occur while the patient is in a supine position. This is caused by the gravid uterus compressing the inferior vena cava leading to a decreased venous return to the heart leading to hypotension, bradycardia, and syncope. This phenomenon is called *supine hypotension syndrome* [47].

The concentration of all coagulation factors, other than factors XI and XIII, is increased. As Thrombin-mediated fibrin generation increases during pregnancy, this combines with an increase in the aforementioned clotting factors and hematocrit, leading to the hypercoagulable state of pregnancy. This leads to a higher risk of deep vein thrombosis (DVT) and pulmonary embolism (PE).

In the abdomen, the enlarging uterus displaces the stomach onto the spleen and liver leading to high intragastric pressure. This and the delayed gastric emptying leads to regurgitation and gastric reflux. Hyperventilation that begins in the first trimester might increase throughout pregnancy. This has obvious implications on drug dosage, route and timing of administration.

In the first trimester, glomerular filtration rate increases 30–50%, which results in an increase in clearance of creatinine, uric acid, and urea. This leads to a decrease in levels of the same. While prescribing drugs, doses may need to be increased to account for this rapid clearance [48].

### 3.10.2 Treatment Protocol

#### 3.10.2.1 Minor Surgery

While minor oral surgery is not a contraindication in the pregnant patient, it is advised that the oral surgeon should consult with the patient's obstetrician to address specific concerns should dental emergencies arise during the first trimester.

Unless emergency treatment is required, it is advisable to defer treatment during the first trimester because of the potential vulnerability of the fetus. The second trimester is the safest time to perform the routine dental treatment. No elective treatment is advisable late in the third trimester.

#### 3.10.2.2 Dental Radiology

Two important factors to be considered are the dose of radiation to be given and the time of gestation. Animal and human data clearly support the conclusion that no increase in congenital anomalies due to exposures totaling less than 0.05–0.1 Gy during pregnancy. The amount of radiation used in dental radiographs is well below the threshold dose [47]. With modern features such as high-speed film, filtration, collimation, and use of lead aprons, dental radiography is deemed quite safe.

#### 3.10.2.3 Major Surgery

Elective surgery should be postponed until after delivery. If possible, nonurgent surgery should be performed in the second trimester when preterm contractions and spontaneous abortion are least likely. Fetal safety requires that potentially dangerous drugs are avoided and adequate uteroplacental perfusion is ensured. No anesthetic drugs have been proven to be clearly hazardous to the human fetus. However, teratogenic effects of nitrous oxide have been demonstrated in animal models following prolonged administration in high concentration [49].

Anxiety in itself leads to decrease in uteroplacental perfusion secondary to increase in circulating catecholamines. Appropriate timing of surgery and anxiolysis is of paramount importance.

### 3.10.3 Drug Usage in Pregnancy

Most drugs cross the placental barrier by simple diffusion. Hence, the major concern of drug administration during pregnancy is the potential of teratogenic adverse effects. The period of maximum risk for teratogenicity is during organogenesis. This occurs from the end of the predifferentiation period until the end of the 10th week after the last menstrual period (Table 3.7).

**Table 3.7** Commonly used safe and unsafe drugs during pregnancy [46]

| Drug | Safe | Unsafe |
|---|---|---|
| Local anesthetics | Articaine<br>Lignocaine<br>Prilocaine | Bupivacaine |
| Analgesics | Paracetamol<br>Ibuprofen (first and second trimesters) | Aspirin<br>Diclofenac<br>Ibuprofen (third trimester)<br>Naproxen |
| Antibacterials | Amoxicillin<br>Azithromycin<br>Cephalosporins<br>Erythromycin | Aminoglycosides<br>Metronidazole<br>Sulfonamides<br>Tetracyclines |
| Antifungals | Fluconazole<br>Nystatin | Ketoconazole |
| Anxiolytics | None | Alprazolam<br>Diazepam |

## 3.11 Endocrine Disorders

### 3.11.1 Diabetes

Diabetes is an endocrine disease manifesting as hyperglycemia, leading to microvascular and cardiovascular complications. Type 1 diabetes mellitus is an autoimmune pancreatic beta cell destruction leading to inadequate production of insulin. In type 2 diabetes mellitus, there is a condition of insulin resistance in addition to defects in insulin secretion by the pancreatic beta cells, and increased endogenous glucose production, primarily by the liver [50].

The current recommendation for diagnosis of diabetes stands at >126 mg/dl of fasting plasma glucose levels or a 2-h plasma glucose level of 200 mg/dl [51]. The Endocrine Society guidelines indicate that patients with hyperglycemia and glycated haemoglobin (HbA1c) of 6.5% or higher can be identified as having diabetes [52].

Optimal glycemic control is advised in each patient to avoid hyperglycemia or hypoglycemia. The surgical patient with diabetes is at higher risk of perioperative morbidity and mortality and subsequently longer length of hospital stays. This is mainly due to increased chances of surgical site infections and systemic infections, other complications like acute kidney injury, acute coronary syndromes, acute cerebrovascular accidents, hospital-acquired diabetic ketoacidosis, etc [53].

The stress of surgery and anesthesia derails the glycemic control of the patient due to the metabolic response to surgery. Nondiabetic patients evoke a catabolic response with a release of cortisol, glucagon, catecholamines, etc., promoting hepatic glycogenolysis and gluconeogenesis causing hyperglycemia. There is a catecholamine-induced inhibition of insulin production as well as insulin resistance. The type of anesthesia and the length of the procedure are also said to influence the amount of catabolism [54].

The preoperative preparation for a diabetic patient begins with a thorough history, including the type and dosing of medications, any history of cardiac events, or diabetic ketoacidosis. ECG is mandated as these patients have a higher occurrence of hypercholesterolemia, hypertension, macrovascular disease, autonomic neuropathy, and hence silent ischemia. If the ECG does suggest so, further investigation is indicated [55].

Renal function tests should include serum urea and creatinine. Hypertension should be ruled out or treated if present. Diabetic neuropathy should be evaluated as it may cause aspiration, silent myocardial ischemia, or even sudden death. It may manifest as postural hypotension, heartburn, or resting tachycardia [56].

HbA1c is usually advised in diabetic patients undergoing treatment as it reflects mean control over the previous 3 months. This allows one to estimate the quality of glycemic control before the consultation and adaptation of treatment to fixed objectives. It is also important to know the duration of the diabetes, dependence on insulin, and whether the glycemic control is achieved by oral hypoglycemics and lifestyle modification.

#### 3.11.1.1 Management of Patients Undergoing Procedures

The recommendations for target glycemic control vary. The Endocrine Society and the American Diabetes Association/AACE Practice Guidelines recommend that patients on insulin maintain a target preprandial glucose of less than 140 mg/dl and a random Blood Glucose (BG) of less than 180 mg/dl for patients treated [52]. The Joint British Diabetes Societies guideline, however, recommends that insulin therapy be commenced when random blood glucose levels exceed 180 mg/dl [53].

#### 3.11.1.2 Preoperative Glycemic Control in patients on Oral Hypoglycemic Agents

##### 3.11.1.2.1 Minor surgery

Patient should adhere to his daily oral diabetic medication and follow his usual diet [50].

##### 3.11.1.2.2 Major surgery

- Most oral hypoglycemics can be continued till the day before surgery. Sulfonylureas and insulin secretagogues should be stopped on the day of surgery to reduce the chances of hypoglycemia [52].
- If normal oral intake is expected to resume on the day of surgery, metformin may be given on the day of surgery [53].
- Metformin is discontinued if there is either prolonged state of fasting or use of i.v contrast dyes or reduced renal function
- (Dipeptyl Peptidase-4) DPP-4 inhibitors are not contraindicated throughout the perioperative period [54].

#### 3.11.1.3 Preoperative Glycemic Control in Type 2 Diabetics on Insulin

Patients on basal insulin: If they are on twice daily dosing then morning dose to be reduced to 80% of normal dose; whereas if those on single dose then evening dose to be reduced to 80% [57].

If the morning glucose levels are above 120 mg/dl, Neutral protamine Hagedorn (NPH) insulin and premixed formulations are reduced by 20% the evening before surgery and by 50% the morning of surgery. If not, morning insulin dose is withheld [58].

Naturally, these are guidelines and the diabetologist will tailor the doses to the individual requirement of the patient.

#### 3.11.1.4 Preoperative Glycemic Control in Type 1 Diabetics on Insulin

##### 3.11.1.4.1 Minor surgery:

- Well-controlled patients should halve their daily dose of insulin the morning of surgery and also eat their normal breakfast.
- Morning appointments are preferred. If preoperative glucose is between 100 and 200 mg/dl, surgery can be performed.
- If blood glucose is >200 mg/dl, an intravenous infusion of 10% dextrose in half-normal saline is initiated. 10-mEq potassium chloride should be added to each 500 ml of dextrose/saline infusion.
- Rapid-acting insulin is administered subcutaneously.
- Blood glucose should be monitored hourly if the surgery lasts beyond 1 h [50].

##### 3.11.1.4.2 Major surgery:

These patients are at risk of developing stress-induced hyperglycemia and ketoacidosis and hence need insulin coverage during perioperative period. These patients should receive 80% of basal insulin dose the evening before surgery and on the morning of surgery in order to prevent hypoglycemia [54].

##### 3.11.1.4.3 Intraoperative glycemic control:

The endocrine society recommends an intraoperative BG level within 180 mg/dl [52].

Levels above that are treated either with subcutaneous rapid-acting insulin analogs or with an IV infusion of regular insulin. In patients undergoing short surgeries (under 4-h operative time), ambulatory surgeries, expected hemodynamic stability and those expected to resume oral diet soon can be managed with subcutaneous rapid-acting insulin correction scales [3]. When it is used, the BG should be checked every 2 h [52].

An IV insulin infusion is preferred where there is anticipated hemodynamic disturbance, significant fluid shifts, expected changes in temperature, inotropic support, or lengthy operative times (greater than 4 h). In this situation, hourly insulin monitoring is needed.

#### 3.11.1.4.4 Postoperative glycemic control:

For noncritical and non-ICU patients, the subcutaneous sliding scale insulin is used with BG being checked every 2 h. If BG drops below 70 mg/dl, insulin is stopped and oral dextrose or iv dextrose is given. For patients in the ICU, continuous iv insulin infusion is given instead of the subcutaneous sliding scale for BG > 180 mg/dl. Oral antidiabetic agents are best avoided in hospitalized patients due to the limited data available on their safety and efficacy. DPP-4 has shown promising results for in-patient hyperglycemia control [54].

## 3.11.2 Hypo/Hyperthyroidism

The thyroid gland releases the hormone thyroxine (T4) and its active form T3. The thyroid hormones are released upon stimulation by the thyroid-stimulating hormone (TSH) released from the pituitary gland. This is, in turn, stimulated by thyrotropin release hormone (TRH). Secretion of T3 and T4 is regulated by the negative feedback loop modulating release of TSH [59].

Thyroid hormones play a critical role in maintaining metabolic homeostasis in the adult. Thyroid-related disorders are due to either overproduction of thyroid hormones (thyrotoxicosis) or hormone deficiency (hypothyroidism). These situations may arise due to infectious, autoimmune, proliferative, or tumorous pathologies [60].

Most patients with well-compensated thyroid disease do not need special consideration prior to surgery. Patients with a newly diagnosed thyroid disorder around the time of surgery will need to undergo risk assessment and optimization before surgery.

Routine thyroid screening is not done for asymptomatic patients unless there is a reason to suspect thyroid dysfunction. Thyroid disease present with a myriad of symptoms clinically. These include-unexplained weight changes, and fine tremor or changes in bowel habits, skin, hair, exophthalmos, goiter, abnormal reflexes. Palpitations, tachycardia, or bradycardia are common cardiovascular manifestations. In such situations as well as in patients with a known thyroid disorder, a TSH test should be included in the preoperative analysis [61].

### 3.11.2.1 Hypothyroidism

Hypothyroidism may be primary (due to thyroid disease) or secondary due to hypothalamo-pituitary disorders. Commonly, it is due to thyroid loss from surgery, irradiation, autoimmune diseases, or drug induced [59]. The diagnosis is confirmed by blood tests revealing low T3 and T4 levels and high TSH in primary and decreased TSH in secondary hypothyroidism. These patients pose challenges during perioperative period due to their effects on various organ systems.

#### 3.11.2.1.1 Physiologic Challenges

Cardiac disturbances like increased peripheral vascular resistance, decreased cardiac output; Respiratory implications like increased incidence of pneumonia, impaired respiratory drive, respiratory muscle weakness. Decreased renal perfusion, decreased gastric motility, and slower drug metabolism need to be considered.

One of the most serious complications of surgery in hypothyroid patients is myxedema coma. It is associated with a mortality rate as high as 80%. It is characterized by altered mental status, which may manifest as coma or seizure, and hypothermia, bradycardia, hyponatremia, heart failure, and hypopnea. It is precipitated by surgery, infection, cold exposure, and administration of sedatives [61].

#### 3.11.2.1.2 Management

A condition of euthyroidism is usually targeted preoperatively and elective surgery is usually postponed. Once TSH values normalize, surgery can be performed. Use of sedatives, benzodiazepenes and Opiods should be avoided [59].

For urgent and emergent procedures, surgery may be performed in mild-to-moderate hypothyroidism with levothyroxine cover preoperatively. Surgery should be postponed in patients with severe hypothyroidism in case of nonemergent surgery. In an emergency, thyroid hormone levels should be normalized as rapidly as possible, using IV levothyroxine in a loading dose of 200–500 μg followed by 50–100 μg IV daily [62].

### 3.11.2.2 Hyperthyroidism

It is commonly due to autoimmune disease (e.g., Graves' disease), multinodular goiter, or adenoma presenting as thyroid nodule. The diagnosis is confirmed by elevated serum T3 and T4. It usually causes exopthalmos, heat intolerance, anxiety, sweating, diarrhea, and weight loss [59]. It has a positive ionotropic and chronotropic effect on the heart coupled with decreased vascular resistance [61]. Hence, these patients manifest tachycardia, arrhythmias, or cardiac failure frequently.

Thyroid storm is a severe manifestation of uncontrolled hyperthyroidism and is characterized by tachycardia, confusion, fever, gastrointestinal complaints, and potentially leading to cardiovascular collapse. It is precipitated by pain, anxiety, trauma, or GA. Hence, elective surgery should always be postponed in patients with overt untreated hyperthyroidism. Hyperthyroidism is usually treated by β-blockers like atenolol or metoprolol as they decrease the sympathetic overactivity. When there is no time to render a patient euthyroid as in emergency cases, cardiac monitoring and adequate β-blockers with antithyroid medication should be given [61]. While epinephrine with lidocaine is not contraindicated, caution should be exercised. Benzodiapines should be avoided. Carbamizole causes agranulocytosis and this can manifest as oral ulcers.

### 3.11.3 Adrenal Gland Disorders

#### 3.11.3.1 Primary Adrenocortical Hypofunction

Addison's disease occurs due to autoantibody-mediated destruction of the adrenal cortex leading to failed cortisol and aldosterone secretion. It may also occur due to tuberculosis, histoplasmosis, sarcoidosis, etc [59]. Due to lack of adequate corticosteroid production, these patients are prone to hypotensive collapse, hypoglycemia, profound weakness, and dehydration (Adrenal crisis).

Adrenal crisis is rare in outpatient oral surgery. However, patients with Addison's disease who need surgery should be covered with supplemental steroids. Drugs like barbiturates, azole antifungals, etomidates, phenytoin, and rifampins should be avoided as they accelerate cortisol metabolism.

#### 3.11.3.2 Secondary Adrenocortical Insufficiency

Corticosteroids are prescribed as long-term treatment for various ailments such as inflammatory bowel disease, blood dyscrasias like idiopathic thrombocytopenia, rheumatologic disease, reactive airway disease, and immunosuppression for transplant recipients, etc. due to their immunosuppressive, anti-inflammatory, metabolic, and hemodynamic properties. This external source of long-term steroid can lead to secondary adrenal insufficiency that may manifest in the perioperative period [63].

In a healthy individual, corticotrophin-releasing hormone (CRH) has a diurnal pattern of release from the hypothalamus. This in turn acts on the anterior pituitary to release the Adrenocorticotrophic hormone (ACTH). ACTH acts on the adrenal cortex to release cortisol (hydrocortisone), corticosterone, and mineralocorticoids. Circulating corticosteroids have a subsequent negative feedback effect on CRH and ACTH release. This constitutes the hypothalamic-pituitary adrenocortical (HPA) axis [59].

Normally, an unstressed adrenal gland secretes approximately 8–10 mg of cortisol per day (Table 3.8). Stress, such as illness or surgery, is the stimulus for raised production of cortisol. During surgical stress, the rate varies between individuals and also upon the type of surgery. It is usually up to 50 mg/day for minor procedures and up to 75–150 mg/day for more complex procedures, rarely exceeding 200 mg/day. However, patients on exogenous corticosteroids aren't able to secrete adequate amounts of corticosteroids in response to stress due to HPA axis suppression and a resulting low level of ACTH and CRH leading to atrophy of the zona fasciculate of adrenal cortex [63].This may predispose them to develop adrenal crisis, with rapidly developing hypotension, hypoglycemia, collapse, and even death [59].

Even though there is no consensus on the exact dosage of corticosteroids that leads to hypofunction of the adrenal cortex, doses greater than physiologic doses of cortisol lead to suppression [59]. HPAA suppression does not extend beyond 1 year after exogenous steroid therapy is stopped [64]. Hence, those at risk are:

- Patients currently taking >5 mg of systemic prednisolone
- Corticosteroids been taken in the past 30 days
- Corticosteroids taken for more than a month during the past 1 year.

These patients require steroid cover/supplementation when undertaken for surgeries. Most dentoalveolar and maxillofacial surgeries result in stress and hence require steroid supplements, but most other dental procedures do not require any additional steroid supplements [59].

Following table shows the normal corticosteroid response to the particular level of stress and the appropriate steroid cover needed in cases of adrenal suppression (Table 3.9):

During the procedure, blood pressure and blood sugar levels should be monitored. NSAIDs should be avoided to avoid increasing risk of peptic ulceration. Prophylactic antibiotics should be given in such patients to avoid postoperative infections.

### 3.11.4 Renal Disorders

The kidneys are responsible for eliminating metabolic waste; fluid and electrolyte homeostasis; and to maintain acid and base balance. The kidneys also affect the cardiovascular and hematologic systems.

**Table 3.8** Approximate potencies of systemic corticosteroids relative to cortisol [59]

| Steroid | Glucocorticoid activity | Mineralocorticoid activity | Equivalent dose (IV/PO) |
|---|---|---|---|
| Cortisol (hydrocortisone) | 1 | 1 | 20 |
| Cortisone | 0.8 | 0.8 | 25 |
| Prednisone | 4 | 0.8 | 5 |
| Prednisolone | 4 | 0.8 | 5 |
| Methylprednisolone | 5 | 0.5 | 4 |
| Dexamethasone | 30–40 | 0 | 0.5–0.75 |

**Table 3.9** Normal corticosteroid response to the particular level of stress and the appropriate steroid cover needed in cases of adrenal suppression [63]

| Surgery type | Endogenous cortisol secretion rate | Examples | Recommended steroid dosing |
|---|---|---|---|
| Superficial | 8–10 mg/day (baseline) | Dental surgery<br>Biopsy | Usual daily dose |
| Minor | 50 mg/day | Multiple extractions LA, Dental implant surgery<br>Inguinal hernia repair<br>Colonoscopy<br>Uterine curettage<br>Hand surgery | Usual daily dose<br>plus<br>Hydrocortisone: 50 mg IV before incision<br>Hydrocortisone: 25 mg IV every 8 h × 24 h<br>Then usual daily dose |
| Moderate | 75–150 mg/day | Minor maxillofacial trauma,<br>Orthognathic surgery<br>Lower-extremity revascularization<br>Total joint replacement<br>Cholecystectomy<br>Colon resection<br>Abdominal hysterectomy | Usual daily dose<br>plus<br>Hydrocortisone: 50 mg IV before incision<br>Hydrocortisone: 25 mg IV every 8 h × 24 h<br>Then usual daily dose |
| Major esophagectomy | 75–150 mg/day | Total proctocolectomy<br>Major cardiac/vascular<br>Hepaticojejunostomy<br>Delivery<br>Trauma | Usual daily dose<br>plus<br>Hydrocortisone: 100 mg IV before incision<br>Followed by continuous IV infusion of 200 mg of hydrocortisone<br>more than 24 h<br>or<br>Hydrocortisone: 50 mg IV every 8 h × 24<br>Taper dose by half per day until usual daily dose reached<br>plus<br>Continuous IV fluids with 5% dextrose and 0.2–0.45% NaCl<br>(based on degree of hypoglycemia) |

The best parameter to assess the function of the kidneys is the glomerular filtration rate (GFR). It is measured by calculating the creatinine clearance based on serum creatinine (SC). The normal value of GFR for an adult male is 130 ml/1.73 m$^2$ and is 120 ml/1.73 m$^2$ for an adult female. Chronic kidney disease occurs when the GFR is reduced by at least 50 ml/min [65].

Patients with chronic kidney disease who are either on dialysis, dialysis naive, or renal transplant recipients or post-transplant patients require modification of treatment plan from a surgical point of view. These patients always have a risk of developing acute renal failure in the postoperative period either due to pre-existing renal dysfunction or solely due to the effects of surgery.

#### 3.11.4.1 Acute Renal Failure (ARF)

ARF is the rapid loss of renal function over the course of days to weeks, resulting in the patient's inability to clear nitrogenous waste, including creatinine and urea, from the body [66]. The term Acute Kidney Injury (AKI) has replaced acute renal failure in current literature. Perioperative AKI is a leading cause of morbidity and mortality due to increased risk of sepsis, anemia, coagulopathy, and mechanical ventilation.

There are three types of ARF based on etiology: prerenal, renal, and postrenal causes. The most common cause of AKI in perioperative period is the prerenal cause and the ischemic acute tubular necrosis (renal AKI) due to hypoxic damage to medullary region secondary to hypovolemia, hypotension, and dehydration [67]. Prerenal AKI and ischemic ATN are a part of a spectrum of manifestations of renal hypoperfusion. Hypotension or hypovolemia may be due to preoperative factors like hemorrhage, diarrhea, fasting, use of diuretics, due to intraoperative factors like ongoing blood loss, activation of sympathetic reflexes, and due to postoperative factors like intravascular volume depletion, myocardial infarction, etc [68]. Hypotension and hypovolemia result in activation of the sympathetic nervous system and the renin–angiotensin–aldosterone axis, which compromises GFR by inducing afferent arteriolar renal vasoconstriction. Other common causes of AKI are the use of NSAIDs, ACE inhibitors, nephrotoxic drugs like aminoglycosides, radiocontrast materials, myoglobin, hemoglobin, and amphotericin B. Pre-existing diseases like diabetes, hypertension, and obstructions of the urinary system also lead to perioperative AKI [68].

The strategy around perioperative AKI is ideally prevention. Preoperatively potential risk factors such as volume depletion, hypotension, sepsis, nephrotoxin exposure, and pre-existing chronic kidney disease should be identified and elective surgery should be postponed till optimization is complete. Anemia should be corrected before surgery. The choice of fluid in intraoperative resuscitation is usually a balanced crystalloid solution like Ringer's lactate and not a chloride-rich crystalloid. Hydroxyethyl starch is best avoided. Mean arterial pressure should be maintained and hemodynamic stability is of utmost importance. Diuretics should be only given in cases of volume overload and not for increasing GFR. Norepinephrine is preferred over dopamine as it maintains renal perfusion pressure, but the role is still not very clear [67].

#### 3.11.4.2 Chronic Renal Failure (CRF)

CRF is permanent renal insufficiency that develops over months or years caused by the structural and intrinsic damage of the glomerulus or tubulointerstitial system. This usually occurs when GFR is reduced by 50 ml/min. If necessary treatment is not started, most cases of CRF would lead to End Stage Renal Disease (ESRD). ESRD is maintained by regular dialysis or by transplant, in the absence of which, death may occur [68].

Preoperative assessment:

Detailed history and physical examination;
Cardiac work up as dictated by clinical symptoms. ECG and Echocardiogram
Complete blood count
Metabolic panel, serum magnesium, and phosphorus levels
Coagulation profile.

Coronary artery disease and congestive heart failure are commonly found in patients with ESRD and those on dialysis. Hence, cardiac workup and monitoring is required in the perioperative period. Maintaining euvolemia perioperatively in ESRD patients is mandatory. For patients not undergoing dialysis, euvolemia can be achieved with appropriate hydration or diuresis. Dialysis is usually performed a day before surgery to prevent fluid overload and to reduce uremic complications (bleeding). Postoperative dialysis helps to achieve euvolemia if large amounts of fluids were given during surgery. Heparin is withheld if dialysis is performed on the day of surgery.

Anemia complicates CKD due to the decreased production of erythropoietin. Transfusion should be considered in the perioperative period when hemoglobin levels fall below 8–10 g/dl due to surgical blood loss in patients with ESRD. If anemia has been detected, erythropoietin should be initiated several weeks before the elective surgery with iron supplementation to raise hemoglobin to the desired level. Patients who have ESRD may be susceptible to more intraoperative and postoperative bleeding due to platelet dysfunction caused by uremia. Hence, NSAIDs and dipyridamole should not be given within 72 h before surgery to patients who have ESRD due to their effects on platelet function. Hypertension and glycemic control should be tightly monitored in such patients as well.

These patients have inefficient mechanisms of drug clearance that inherently predispose them to adverse drug responses. Hence, NSAIDs, aminoglycosides, benzodiazipines, morphine, and radiocontrast media are avoided. Drugs like propofol, fentanyl, and inhalational anesthetics are usually the preferred drugs of choice.

## 3.12 Patients with Non-head and Neck Malignancies

### 3.12.1 Introduction

The most common cancers in India in women are Breast, Oral, Cervical, ovary, and esophagus. Men tend to be afflicted with head and neck cancers, lung, esophagus, stomach, and colorectal cancer [69]. The cancers that most commonly metastatize to the jaws and oral soft tissues are breast, lung, prostrate, thyroid, kidney, stomach, and colon [70]. Another group of malignancies that receive chemoradiotherapy are the lymphoproliferative and hematologic malignancies [70].

*Chemotherapy* is often employed either with an intent of palliation or for cure. It may be administered as adjuvant therapy or as neoadjuvant therapy. Cytotoxic chemotherapeutic agents have hematologic effects (myelosuppression) as well as nonhematologic effects. The effects of myelosuppression, i.e., leukopenia, thrombocytopenia, and anemia start after 5–7 days with the nadir occurring at 10–14 days. It is usually followed by bone marrow recovery [71]. Hence, the oral surgical treatment should be planned in a manner that it doesn't coincide with the nadir of the myelosuppression where the neutropenia can be as low as 500.

*Radiotherapy* is a part of treatment for a variety of Head and neck cancers either as primary treatment modality or as adjuvant therapy to the primary tumor or to the associated lymphatic structures. Unlike the effects of chemotherapy, effects of radiotherapy are more long lasting. These include mucositis, xerostomia, trismus, radiation-induced fibrosis, and dysguesia.

### 3.12.2 Treatment Protocol

#### 3.12.2.1 Chemotherapy

It is best to undertake a dental screening before the start of the chemotherapy so that the hopeless teeth can be extracted, be restored, periodontal therapy, alveoloplasty be performed, and primary closure be done. After extraction, it takes approximately 10 days to 6 weeks for healing to be enough for chemotherapy to start [72]. Ill-fitting and loose dentures should be discontinued and replaced ideally with implants especially in patients scheduled to take systemic bisphosphonates or RANK-L therapy as it might lead to osteonecrosis of the jaws [73]. Fluoride treatment can also be done.

However, patients suffering from leukemia, lymphomas have a state of myelosuppression even before the start of the

**Table 3.10** Modification of invasive dental treatment according to hematologic indices [75]

| Platelet count | Treatment modification | Neutrophil count | Treatment modification |
|---|---|---|---|
| >75,000 cells/mm³ | No modification | >1000 cell/mm³ | No need for antibiotic prophylaxis. |
| 40,000–75,000 cell/mm³ | Platelet transfusion may be considered in the preoperative and postoperative (24 h). | <1000 cell/mm³ | Postpone the dental treatment. In cases of emergency, discuss antibiotic coverage and endocarditis prophylaxis before treatment with the medical team. Hospitalization may be required |
| <40,000 cell/mm³ | Postpone the dental treatment. In the case of dental emergency, contact the patient's physician before dental treatment to discuss supportive measures, such as platelet transfusion, control of bleeding, and need for hospitalization. Other coagulation tests may be necessary in some cases. | | |

chemotherapy. Only acute situations need to be dealt with. Elective treatments can wait till the time the patient is in optimal clinical and hematological parameters, which is usually until after chemotherapy is over. Hence, extractions of grossly carious and severely periodontally compromised teeth, ill-fitting denture, etc. should be addressed. For extractions to be done, or other invasive dental procedures, hematologic indices should be evaluated and antibiotic prophylaxis should be considered [74] (Table 3.10).

Once the chemotherapy starts, a gap of 1 week before the next cycle is essential before any dental intervention. For surgical procedures that cannot wait, like facial trauma or infection, the complete blood counts should be assessed and consultation should be sought with the medical oncologist to determine the nadir in blood counts, the timing of the chemotherapy cycle, and duration [72]. For platelet levels below 40,000/mm$^3$, platelet transfusions are usually needed [76].

Opportunistic infections may complicate mucositis and may be of viral, fungal, or bacterial origins. Treatment should be guided by culture and sensitivity. Febrile neutropenia needs to be treated usually by intravenous antibiotics like amoxicillin and clavulanic acid with a fluoroquinolone or clindamycin with fluoroquinolone. Hematopoeitic growth factors like granulocyte colony-stimulating factors or granulocyte-macrophage colony-stimulating factors are effective drugs for prophylaxis and treatment of febrile neutropenia. Mucositis occurs in almost all patients and causes great difficulty in feeding, hydrating, and causes pain. It is preferable to manage it with saline mouth rinses rather than with chlorhexidine mouthwashes. Some chemotherapeutic agents are also neurotoxic and cause a deep mandibular pain as well as altered taste sensation and dysguesia. Most of these symptoms subside after cessation of treatment [72].

#### 3.12.2.2 Radiotherapy

The same prophylactic measures of extraction, restoration, alveoloplasty, etc. have to be taken before radiotherapy as for chemotherapy. Additionally, jaw-opening exercises should be initiated and coronoidectomy should be considered as a part of the ablative procedure [72].

### 3.12.3 Prevention and Treatment of Osteonecrosis After Chemotherapy and Radiation

Osteonecrosis of the jaws occurring in an irradiated bone is called osteoradionecrosis (ORN). Those occurring in a patient on antiresorptive therapy like bisphosphonates or monoclonal antibodies to RANK-L is termed Antiresorptive osteonecrosis of jaws (AONJ) [72]. The incidence of ORN in areas of jaws that have received greater than 60 Gy of radiation is 5–15%. Incidence of AONJ in patients who have received denosumab is 1.3% and is 1.8% in patients treated with nitrogen-containing bisphosphonates [77, 78].

**Acknowledgments** Dr Prithvi Bachalli, Consultant Oral and Maxillofacial Surgeon
Rangadore Memorial Hospital, Bangalore
Dr. Prashanth Bhat, Consultant Oral and Maxillofacial Surgeon
Rangadore Memorial Hospital, Bangalore
Dr Shobha Hegde, Registrar Oral and Maxillofacial Surgeon
Rangadore Memorial Hospital, Bangalore

## References

1. 'Indians have gained 10 years of life expectancy since 1990'. The Business Line [Document on internet]. Updated on 09 Jan 2018. https://www.thehindubusinessline.com/news/science/indians-have-gained-10-years-of-life-expectancy-since-1990/article9958774.ece. Accessed 14 Nov 2017.
2. Central Bureau of Health intelligence. National Health profile 2018 [Document on internet]. New Delhi: India Offset Press. https://cdn.downtoearth.org.in/pdf/NHP-2018.pdf. Accessed 27 Apr 2018.
3. Arokiasamy P. India's escalating burden of non-communicable diseases. The Lancet; Global Health. 2018;6(12):1262–3.
4. Indian council of medical research, Public health foundation of India, and Institute for health metrics and evaluation. India: Health

of the Nation's states-The India state-level disease burden initiative. New Delhi: ICMR, PHFI and IHME; 2017. https://www.healthdata.org/sites/default/files/files/policy_report/2017/India_Health_of_the_Nation%27s_States_Report_2017.pdf
5. Government of India: Ministry of Housing and Urban Affairs. Urban Growth [document on the internet]. New Delhi; 2019. Last updated 9 May 2019. http://mohua.gov.in/cms/urban-growth.php#skip
6. India is the most depressed country in the world: Mental Health Day 2018. India Today Web Desk, 2018 [Document on the internet]. New Delhi; 2018. Updated: 10 Oct 2018. https://www.indiatoday.in/education-today/gk-current-affairs/story/india-is-the-most-depressed-country-in-the-world-mental-health-day-2018-1360096-2018-10-10. Accessed 10 Oct 2018.
7. Misra S. Systemic hypertension and noncardiac surgery. Indian J Anaesth. 2017;61:697–704.
8. Shahbabu B, Dasgupta A, Sarkar K, Sahoo SK. Which is more accurate in measuring the blood pressure? A digital or an aneroid sphygmomanometer. J Clin Diagn Res. 2016;10(3)
9. Hogan J, Radhakrishnan J. The assessment and importance of hypertension in the dental setting. J Dent Clin N Am. 2012 Oct;56(4):731–45.
10. Foëx P, Sear JW. The surgical hypertensive patient. Continuing Education in Anaesthesia Critical Care & Pain. 2004 Oct;4(5):139–14.
11. Southerland JH, Gill DG, Gangula PR, Halpern LR, Cardona CY, Mouton CP. Dental management in patients with hypertension: challenges and solutions. Clin Cosmet Investig Dent. 2016;8:111–20.
12. Niwa H, Sato Y, Matsuura H. Safety of dental treatment in patients with previously diagnosed acute myocardial infarction or unstable angina pectoris. Oral Surg Oral Med Oral Pathol Oral Radiol Endod. 2000;89(1):35–41.
13. Ferrari E, Benhamou M, Cerboni P, Marcel B. Coronary syndromes following aspirin withdrawal. J Am Coll Cardiol. 2005;45(3):456–9.
14. Zain MA, Siddiqui WJ. Coronary stents. [Updated 24 Jan 2019]. In: StatPearls [Internet]. Treasure Island (FL): StatPearls Publishing; 2019. https://www.ncbi.nlm.nih.gov/books/NBK507804
15. Oprea AD, Popescu WM. Perioperative management of antiplatelet therapy. Br J Anaes. 2013;111(Suppl 1):i3–i17.
16. Yeung LYY, Sarani B, Weinberg JA, McBeth PB, May AK. Surgeon's guide to anticoagulant and antiplatelet medications. Part Two: Antiplatelet agents and perioperative management of long-term anticoagulation. Trauma Surg Acute Care Open. 2016;1:1–7.
17. León AMD, López BC, Esteve CG. Dental management of patients receiving anticoagulant and/or antiplatelet treatment. J Clin Exp Dent. 2014 Apr;5(2):e155–61.
18. Abdullah WA, Khalil H. Dental extraction in patients on warfarin treatment. Clin Cosmet Investig Dent. 2014;6:65–9.
19. Shah SN. Oral anticoagulation in special population and conditions. J Assoc Phy Ind. 2014;62. http://www.japi.org/june_2014_special_issue/07_oral_anticoagulation_in.htm
20. Lam DK, Jan A, Sándor GK, Clokie CM. Prevention of infective endocarditis: Revised guidelines from the American Heart Association and the implications for dentists. J Can Dent Assoc. 2008;74(5):449–53.
21. Shah AH, Khalil HS, Kola MZ. Dental management of a patient fitted with subcutaneous Implantable Cardioverter Defibrillator device and concomitant warfarin treatment. Saudi Dent J. 2015;27(3):165–70.
22. Turner MD, Glickman RS. Epilepsy in the oral and maxillofacial patient: current therapy. J Oral Maxillofac Surg. 2005;63:996–1005.
23. Jacobsen PL, Eden O. Epilepsy and the dental management of the epileptic patient. J Contemp Dent Pract. 2008;9(1):1–13.
24. Scheffer IE, Berkovic S, Capovilla G, Connolly MB, French J, Guilhoto L, et al. ILAE classification of the epilepsies: position paper of the ILAE Commission for Classification and Terminology. Epilepsia. 2017;58(4):512–21.
25. Scully C. Neurology. In: Scully's medical problems in dentistry. 7th ed. Haryana: Churchill Livingstone, Elsevier; 2014. p. 345–93.
26. Mehmet Y, Senem O, Sülün T, Hümeyra K. Management of epileptic patients in dentistry. Surg Sci. 2012;3:47–52.
27. Bodnar DC, Varlan CM, Varlan V, Vaideanu T, Popa MB. Dental management in Stroke patients. TMJ. 2008;58(3–4):228–35.
28. Arboix A, Pérez Sempere A, Alvarez SJ. Ictus: etiological types and diagnostic criteria. In: Díez Tejedor E, editor. Guide for the diagnosis and treatment of stroke. Barcelona: Prous Science; 2006. p. 1–23.
29. British Society of Gerodontology. Guidelines for the oral healthcare of stroke survivors. June 2010. p. 4–10.
30. MBA A, Abbas G, Latifeh Y, Hamadah O. The oral manifestations of psychiatric disorders. Oral Health Dent Manag. 2018;17(4):1–6.
31. Al-Atram Majmaah AA. The ability of dentists to identify psychiatric symptoms in their patients. J Health Sci. 2017;5(2)
32. Tomar B, Bhati NK, Kumar P, Bhatia MS, Shah RJ. The psychiatric and dental inter-relationship. Delhi Psychiatry Journal. 2011;14(1)
33. Sousa AD. Psychological issues in oral and maxillofacial reconstructive surgery. Br J Oral Maxillofac Surg. 2008;46(8):661–4.
34. Nassab ISAHG, Samieirad S, Zadeh MV, Aghahi RK, Hashemipour MA. Depression and anxiety disorders in a sample of facial trauma: a study. Med Oral Patol Oral Cir Bucal. 2016 Jul 1;21(4):e477–82.
35. Pamplona MC, Muñoz MM, Pérez MGS. Dental considerations in patients with liver disease. J Clin Exp Dent. 2011;3(2):127–34.
36. Grau-García-Moreno DM. Dental management of patients with liver disease. Med Oral. 2003;8:231.
37. Golla K, Epstein JB, Cabay RJ. Liver disease: current perspectives on medical and dental management. Oral Surg Oral Med Oral Pathol Oral Radiol Endod. 2004;98:516–21.
38. Dienstag JL, Isselbacher KJ. Acute viral hepatitis [Internet]. Columbus, OH: The McGraw-Hill. http://harrisons.accessmedicine.com.proxy.cc.uic.edu. Accessed 12 Sep 2004.
39. Al-Khalidi JA, Czaja AJ. Current concepts in the diagnosis, pathogenesis, and treatment of autoimmune hepatitis. Mayo Clin Proc. 2001;76:1237–52.
40. Iredale JP. Cirrhosis: new research provides a basis for rational and targeted treatments. Br Med J. 2003;327:143–7.
41. Haddad J, Deny P, Munz-Gotheil C, Ambrosini JC, Trinchet JC, et al. Lymphocyte sialadenitis of Sjogren's syndrome associated with chronic Hepatitis C virus liver disease. Lancet. 1992;339:1425–6.
42. Greenwood M, Meecham JG. General medicine and surgery for dental practitioners. Part 5: Liver disease. Br Dent J. 2003;195:71–3.
43. John Firriolo F. Dental management of patients with end stage liver disease. Dent Clin N Am. 2006;50:563–90.
44. Edwards CR, Boucher IA. Davidson's principles and practice of medicine. 17th ed. London: Churchill Livingston; 1996. p. 405–82.
45. Gan TJ. Postoperative nausea and vomiting-can it be eliminated? JAMA. 2002;287:1233–6.
46. Scully C. Age and gender issues. In: Scully's medical problems in dentistry. 7th ed. Haryana: Churchill Livingstone, Elsevier; 2014. p. 642–6.
47. Cengiz SB. The pregnant patent: consideration for dental management and drug use. Quintessence Int. 2007;38:777e733-742.

48. Turner M, Aziz SR. Management of the pregnant oral and maxillofacial surgery patient. J Oral Maxillofoc Surg. 2002;60:1479–88.
49. Upadya M, Saneesh PJ. Anaesthesia for non-obstetric surgery during pregnancy. Indian J Anaesth. 2016 Apr;60(4):234–41.
50. Bergman SA. Perioperative management of the diabetic patient. Oral Surg Oral Med Oral Pathol Oral Radiol Endod. 2007;103:731–7.
51. Definition and diagnosis of diabetes mellitus and intermediate hyperglycemia: Report of a WHO/IDF consultation (Document on the internet). WHO Document Production Services, Geneva. 2006. https://www.who.int/diabetes/publications/Definition%20and%20diagnosis%20of%20diabetes_new.pdf
52. Umpierrez GE, Hellman R, Korytkowski MT, Kosiborod M, Maynard GA, Montori VM, Seley JJ, Van den Berghe G. Endocrine Society: Management of hyperglycemia in hospitalized patients in non-critical care setting: an endocrine society clinical practice guideline. J Clin Endocrinol Metab. 2012;97:16–38.
53. Dhatariya K, Levy N, Kilvert A, et al. NHS Diabetes guideline for the perioperative management of the adult patient with diabetes. Diabetic Med. 2012;29:420–33.
54. Duggan EW, Carlson K, Umpierrez GE. Perioperative hyperglycaemia management: an Update. Anesthesiology. 2017;126:547–60.
55. Plodkowski RA, Edelman SV. Pre-surgical evaluation of diabetic patients. Clin Diabetes. 2001;19:92–5.
56. Yoo HK, Serafin BL. Perioperative management of the diabetic patient. Oral Maxillofacial Surg Clin N Am. 2006;18:255–60.
57. Rosenblatt SI, Dukatz T, Jahn R, Ramsdell C, Sakharova A, Henry M, et al. Insulin glargine dosing before next-day surgery: comparing three strategies. J Clin Anesth. 2012;24:610–7.
58. Likavec A, Moitra V, Greenberg J, Drum M, Sweitzer BJ. Comparison of preoperative blood glucose levels in patients receiving different insulin regimens. Anesthesiology. 2006;105:A567.
59. Scully C. Endocrinology. In: Scully's medical problems in dentistry. 7th ed. Haryana: Churchill Livingstone, Elsevier; 2014. p. 171–99.
60. Fauci AS, Kasper DL, Longo DL, Braunwald E, Hauser SL, Jameson JL, Loscalzo J. Harrison's internal medicine. 17th ed. https://doi.org/10.1111/j.1445-5994.2008.01837.
61. Palace MR. Perioperative management of thyroid dysfunction. Health Serv Insights. 2017; https://doi.org/10.1177/1178632916689677.
62. Bennet Guerrero E, Kramer DC, Schwinn DA. Effect of chronic and acute thyroid hormone reduction on perioperative outcome. Anesth Analg. 1997;85:30–6.
63. Liu MM, Reidy AB, Saatee S, et al. Perioperative steroid management: approaches based on current evidence. Anesthesiology. 2017;127:166–72.
64. Axelrod L. Perioperative management of patients treated with glucocorticoids. Endocrinol Metab Clin N Am. 2003;32:367–83.
65. Horio M, Orita Y, Fukunaga M. Assessment of renal function. In: Johnson RJ, Feehally J, editors. Comprehensive clinical nephrology. Philadelphia: Mosby; 2000. p. 3.1–6.
66. Anderson RJ, Schrier RW. Clinical spectrum of oliguric and nonoliguric acute renal failure. Contemporary issues in nephrology, Vol. 6. New York: Churchill Livingstone; 1980. p. 1–16.
67. Goren O, Matot I. Perioperative acute kidney injury. Br J Anaesth. 2015;115(Suppl 2):ii3–14.
68. Carrasco LR, Chou JC. Perioperative management of patients with renal disease. Oral Maxillofacial Surg Clin N Am. 2006;18:203–12.
69. India: Globocan 2018. International Agency for research on cancer. 2019. http://gco.iarc.fr/today/data/factsheets/populations/356-india-fact-sheets.pdf
70. Scully C. Malignant disease. In: Scully's medical problems in dentistry. 7th ed. Haryana: Churchill Livingstone, Elsevier; 2014. p. 576–93.
71. Motzer RJ, Geller NL, Bosl GJ. The effect of a 7-day delay in chemotherapy cycles on complete response and event-free survival in good-risk disseminated germ cell tumor patients. Cancer. 1990;66(5):857–61.
72. Demian NM, Shun JW, Kessel IL, Eid A. Oral surgery in patients undergoing chemoradiation therapy. Oral Maxillofacial Surg Clin N Am. 2014;26:193–207.
73. Yamashita J, Mc Cauley LK. Antiresorptives and osteonecrosis of the jaw. J Evid Based Dent Pract. 2012;12(Suppl 3):233–47.
74. Zimmermann C, Meurer MI, Grando LJ, et al. Dental treatment in patients with leukemia. J Oral Oncol. 2015;2015:Article ID 571739, 14 pages. https://doi.org/10.1155/2015/571739.
75. American Academy of Pediatric Dentistry. Guideline on dental management of pediatric patients receiving chemotherapy, hematopoietic cell transplantation, and/or radiation. J Pediat Dentistry. 2013;35(5):E185–93. http://www.ncbi.nlm.nih.gov/pubmed/24290549.
76. Lopez BC, Esteve CG, Perez MG. Dental treatment considerations in the chemotherapy patient. J Clin Exp Dent. 2011;3(1):e31–2.
77. Jacobson AS, Buchbinder D, Hu K, et al. Paradigm shifts in the management of osteoradionecrosis of the mandible. Oral Oncol. 2010;46(11):795–801.
78. Saad F, Brown J, Van Poznack C, et al. Incidence, risk factors and outcomes of osteonecrosis of the jaws: integrated analysis from three blinded active controlled phase III trials in cancer patients with bone metastasis. Ann Oncol. 2012;23(5):1341–7.

# Medical Emergencies in Oral and Maxillofacial Surgical Practice

4

Nallamilli V. S. Sekhar Reddy

## 4.1 Introduction

Oral and Maxillofacial Surgery has evolved over the last few decades. Although it is now practiced as a full-fledged hospital-based specialty, a significant amount of work is still carried out under local anesthesia; predisposing toward a medical emergency precipitated particularly by stress. Oral and Maxillofacial surgeons thus deal with the medical emergencies in an office or hospital setting on a regular basis.

Emergency team response in most countries is prompt. The published guidelines from these countries reflect this in the advice for the general practitioner; doing the essential minimum toward the sustenance of life in case of a medical emergency and to prioritize escalation of call for help to the emergency team. However, in some parts of the world, the response time of the emergency team is expected to be comparatively longer, due to various policy issues. The chapter considers these special circumstances, to suggest some additional measures toward the management of the emergency, while waiting for the arrival of the emergency team.

Also, the general advice in the management of a medical emergency during an outpatient procedure in a clinic is aimed at general practitioners, who may not necessarily be exposed to training in clinical skills like the placement of an intravenous cannula. Oral and Maxillofacial surgeons are expected to be well versed with this life-saving simple clinical skill and the protocols discussed here take this into consideration.

The management of emergency should follow the universally accepted ABCDE approach [1], which helps the clinician to follow a systematic approach in an emergency situation where the most life-threatening condition is assessed and is given the top priority. Lack of airway kills the patient first, then the lack of ability to breathe followed by the absence of circulation. ABCDE approach incorporates:

A: Airway
B: Breathing
C: Circulation
D: Disability (refers to neurological function)
E: Exposure

Medical Emergencies that are life threatening and need immediate remedial measures on an emergency basis are discussed here:

1. Acute Asthmatic Attack
2. Adrenal Crisis
3. Airway Obstruction
4. Anaphylaxis
5. Chest Pain
6. Cardiac Arrest
7. Hypoglycemia
8. Tonic-Clonic Seizure
9. Syncope.

## 4.2 Acute Asthmatic Attack

Stress, Anxiety, and Infection can precipitate an asthmatic attack in individuals who are prone. Unfortunately, all three of them can be part of OMFS practice.

**Box 4.1**
Note: Asthma that is part of a generalized anaphylactic reaction needs Adrenaline via intramuscular route.

**Signs and Symptoms:**
- Difficulty in breathing
- Cough
- Wheezing
- Use of accessory muscles of respiration
- Tightness of chest

N. V. S. Sekhar Reddy (✉)
Panineeya Institute of Dental Sciences and Research Centre, Hyderabad, Telangana, India


K. Bonanthaya et al. (eds.), *Oral and Maxillofacial Surgery for the Clinician*, https://doi.org/10.1007/978-981-15-1346-6_4

- Rapid breathing and Tachycardia
- Pale and anxious-looking face

**Management:**

- Keep the patient in a sitting position.
- Give two puffs of Salbutamol (100 μg/puff) inhaler [2, 3].
- If no rapid response, give further puffs through a spacer device.
- Consider oxygen supplementation.
- If no improvement, consider urgent transfer to a medical center.

### 4.2.1 Life-Threatening Acute Asthma

Asthmatic attack can sometimes be severe and may fail to respond to standard bronchodilator therapy. This can be fatal if no proper treatment is given. When an asthmatic attack failed to respond to the treatment and getting worse, the patient will need urgent transfer to appropriate medical center.

**Signs and symptoms of severe life-threatening asthma:**

- Silent chest, poor respiratory effort, cyanosis
- $SPO_2 < 92\%$
- Exhaustion
- Altered consciousness
- Weak or irregular pulse

**Treatment:**

- Urgent transfer to hospital is needed.
- Oxygen supplementation.
- Salbutamol 100 μg/puff; give four puffs through spacer device, followed by two puffs every 2 min according to response, up to a maximum of ten puffs or if there is nebulizer available, give salbutamol 5 mg [4].
- Hydrocortisone: 100 mg IV, or Prednisolone: 40–50 mg Orally [4].
- For children 5 years and above, use Oral Prednisolone 30–40 mg.
- For children less than 5 years, give salbutamol inhalation up to a maximum of ten puffs while awaiting transfer to an appropriate medical facility [2].

## 4.3 Acute Adrenal Insufficiency/Adrenal Crisis/Steroid Crisis/Addisonian Crisis

Sudden and severe hypotension in patients who cannot mount a normal stress-induced cortisol response. The stress can be physiological or psychological. Adrenal crisis can be seen in patients who were taking glucocorticoids regularly or who have taken glucocorticoids for a considerable period of time in the past, patients with Addison's disease, hypopituitarism, or in other conditions associated with decreased adrenocorticotropic hormone (ACTH) production.

**Box 4.2**

*Oxygen—Supports Combustion*

*Keep cylinders away from open flames and heat sources*

*Oxygen cylinder should be stored in a well-ventilated area*

*Do not oil, grease, or lubricate cylinder controls.*

**Signs and Symptoms:**

- Severe hypotension, which can manifest as weakness, confusion, dizziness, drowsiness, loss of consciousness.
- Nausea, vomiting.
- Seizure may occur following deep faint.

**Treatment:**

- Lay patient flat.
- Give high flow oxygen.
- Arrange for urgent transfer to a medical center.
- Establish Intravenous access.
- Administer Hydrocortisone sodium succinate by IV. Dosage given below [5, 6]:
  - Children from age 2 to 11 years, 2–4 mg/kg body weight.
  - Above 11 years: give adult dose.
  - Adult dose: 100 mg by IV.
  - If unable to secure IV access, give the same dose by IM route.
- Start IV infusion of 0.9% Normal Saline.

## 4.4 Airway Obstruction

As the mouth is the primary area of our specialty, clinicians may have to deal with acute airway obstruction. As with everything else, prevention is the most important thing.

**Signs and Symptoms:**

- Distressed patient.
- Abnormal noises like gurgling, crowing, snoring.
- Forced inspiratory efforts.
- No sounds at all in complete airway obstruction
- Various degrees of cyanosis leading to loss of consciousness.

**Treatment** [7]:

- Encourage the patient to cough.
- If an object could be visualized, retrieve it with an appropriate instrument.
- If obstruction is caused by fluids, use high-volume suction.
- Back slaps: up to five back blows between the scapulae while the patient is supported leaning forward.
- Abdominal thrusts: (Heimlich maneuver) up to five abdominal thrusts by standing behind the patient.

- If obstruction fails to relieve, continue with five back blows alternating with abdominal thrusts.
- If these measures fail, the patient will lose consciousness. Lay the patient down on floor and start with CPR.
  - Start with chest compressions even if there is pulse, as chest compressions can help relieving the obstruction.
- If there is partial obstruction, which could not be relieved by the foregoing means, arrange for emergency transfer to appropriate medical care.
  - Patient may need oxygen supplementation.
- In patients with a completely obstructed airway, where the obstruction could not be relieved with these measures, where there are no facilities or skill to use a laryngoscope, emergency invasive procedures like jet insufflation or cricothyroidotomy may be needed as life-saving measures.
- Jet Insufflation involves placing a wide bore cannula (12–14 gauge) through cricothyroid membrane and connect this to a high flow oxygen source.
- It is advised to read further about Jet insufflation and Cricothyroidotomy as the full detailed description is beyond the scope of this textbook.

**Box 4.3**

Aspiration of small objects like burs, endodontic files, and reamers may not cause immediate life-threatening airway obstruction, but retrieval of these rather small and prickly instruments from lungs is a very difficult task needing bronchoscopy and can result in serious lung infections and damage. Prevention takes priority.

## 4.5 Anaphylaxis

Sudden onset, severe form of life-threatening allergic reaction, which can be seen following exposure to an allergen. Remember topical anesthetic gels, chlorhexidine mouth wash, and even contact with latex gloves can trigger anaphylaxis in individuals who are sensitive [8].

Prompt recognition and immediate response are key to success.

**Signs and Symptoms:**

- Face—red and hot.
- Generalized skin rash with itching.
- Various degrees of breathing difficulties manifested as stridor, wheezing, or hoarseness.
- Pulse may initially be rapid but can gradually become weak or impalpable.
- Hypotension can progress to cardiac arrest.

**Treatment:**

- Make sure airway is clear.
- Administer Adrenaline [9].
- Position the patient in supine position unless the patient prefers to sit up due to breathing difficulties.
- Make arrangements for emergency transfer to appropriate medical center.
- While waiting for transfer [10],
  - Oxygen supplementation at 15 L/min.
  - Keep assessing the airway and provide necessary support.
  - Chlorpheniramine maleate IM or IV.
  - Hydrocortisone sodium succinate IM or IV.
  - Establish Intravenous access.
  - Ringer's lactate solution or 0.9% Normal saline to support circulation.
  - Reassess the need for further adrenaline.
- Start CPR in case of cardiac arrest.

**Box 4.4**

Adrenaline is to be administered if there is severe respiratory distress or when there are signs of shock.

**Box 4.5**

Adrenaline—Life-saving drug for Anaphylaxis
Repeat after 5 min if not getting better
Supply: 1 mL ampoule containing 1 mg adrenaline in 1:1000 concentration
Site: I.M Anterolateral thigh
Dosage:
Adult: 500 μg IM 0.5 mL
Child More than 12 years: 500 μg IM 0.5 mL
Child 6–12 years: 300 μg IM 0.3 mL
Less than 6 years: 150 μg IM 0.15 mL

**Box 4.6**

**Second-line drugs:**
Hydrocortisone sodium succinate: 100 mg
Route: IM or Slow IV
12 years and adults: 200 mg IM/IV
6–12 years: 100 mg IM/IV
6 months to 6 years: 50 mg IM/IV
Chlorpheniramine Maleate
Supply: Chlorpheniramine Maleate 10 mg/1 mL Ampoule
Route: IM or IV
12 years and adults: 10 mg IM/IV
6–12 years: 5 mg IM/IV
6 months to 6 years: 2.5 mg IM/IV

## 4.6 Chest Pain

Experiencing chest pain in an outpatient office can be a frightening experience for both the patient and to the attending clinician. Thorough understanding of the pathophysiology of these acute cardiac events is very important for the clinician to stay composed and initiate appropriate measures to prevent mortality. Myocardial infarction may not always have the typical features of chest pain and especially diabetic patients may not have pain. Hence, a high index of suspicion is what is required.

Causes of chest pain:

- Angina
- Myocardial Infarction
- Hyperventilation

Hyperventilation is associated with anxiety and often a young person who is quite frightened of the intended treatment, the breathing gets very heavy resulting in decreased carbon dioxide levels in the blood.

### 4.6.1 Angina

Transient decrease of oxygen supply to cardiac muscle precipitates pain.

Precipitating factors:

Anxiety, stress, exertion, strong emotions, heavy meal, and extreme weather conditions.

**Signs and Symptoms:**

If you are looking for typical symptoms of chest pain, you may miss some cases. List of all possible presentations being:

- Pain, heaviness, or tightness in the chest.
- Pain in the neck, throat, arms, stomach, and back.
- Pain can be associated with light-headedness, nausea, shortness of breath, and sweating.

**Management:**

- Stop the procedure and reassure the patient.
- Clear the mouth from any foreign bodies.
- Let the patient attain a comfortable position (may not like to lie flat).
- Administer Glyceryl trinitrate sublingual spray or Glyceryl trinitrate sublingual tablets [11].
- Oxygen supplementation.
- Check for any irregularities of pulse.

Simple angina should resolve very quickly with rest alone or with sublingual glyceryl trinitrate spray or tablets. In simple angina, the cardiac output is not impaired, and pulse should be regular. In a patient with chest pain, having an irregular pulse, suspect MI.

### 4.6.2 Myocardial Infarction (Heart Attack)

Progressive/Sudden ischemia of the cardiac muscle leads to necrosis of cardiac muscle. This can cause cardiac arrest.

**Signs and Symptoms:**

- Same as angina but can be more severe in intensity and lasts long.
- Pain in the center of the chest.
- Pain radiates to neck, arms, jaw, back, or stomach.
- Pain associated with sweating, vomiting, shortness of breath, lightheadedness, or dizziness.
- Chest discomfort associated with a feeling of weakness and unwell.
- Chest pain associated with an irregular pulse.
- Chest pain fails to relieve with two doses of Nitroglycerin sublingual Spray.
- Chest pain getting progressively worse.
- Patient with previous experience of angina, now experiencing an unusual type of chest discomfort.
- Weak pulse.
- Falling Blood pressure.
- Skin—pale and clammy.

**Management:**

- The moment MI is suspected, arrange for an emergency transfer of the patient to an appropriate medical facility.
- Let the patient attain the most comfortable position. The patient may like to sit up to avoid venous congestion on the heart and lungs.
- Administer soluble Aspirin, 300 mg [12]. Chew and swallow for rapid action.
- By this time, the patient should have received at least two doses of sublingual Glyceryl trinitrate spray or tablets [12], this may need a repeating.
- While waiting for transfer, the following measures can be done, but do not delay transfer, early expert care improves outcome.
  - Establish IV access.
  - Give antiemetic Metoclopramide hydrochloride by IV [13].

    Adult > 60 kg, dose 10 mg

    Small-sized Adult <60 kg, dose 5 mg
  - Administer analgesia - Paracetamol by slow IV (Morphine, diamorphine 7 fentanyl, are not easily available in India) [13].

Adult >50 kg, dose 1000 mg in 100 mL
Small-sized Adult <50 kg, dose 750 mg in 75 mL
When no IV access, alternatively, give Oral Paracetamol 650 mg

- Do not routinely administer oxygen. Supplemental oxygen only when hypoxic.
- Patients where consciousness level deteriorates.
  - Watch for signs of cardiac arrest.
  - Start CPR, if cardiac arrest occurs.

**Box 4.7**
Drugs for MI:
Glyceryl Trinitrate Aerosol Spray: 400 μg/metered dose
Glyceryl Trinitrate: 300-μg tablets
Soluble Aspirin: 300-mg tablets
Metoclopromide: 10-mg solution for IV
Paracetamol: 1000-mg/100-mL solution for IV
Paracetamol: 500-mg tablets
Paracetamol 650 mg tablets

## 4.7 Cardiac Arrest

Cardiac arrest is a sudden loss of heart function resulting in hypoxic damage to body organs. Lack of oxygen to the brain causes loss of consciousness, victim falls to the ground and stops breathing. Cardiac arrest can occur suddenly with or without any symptoms.

Following cardiac arrest neurons start to die within 4–6 min without oxygen. Chances of survival can be increased by early defibrillation (where indicated) and good-quality Cardiopulmonary Resuscitation, that's instituted quickly and performed with minimal interruptions. Automated External Defibrillators (AED) are increasingly available and these can analyze the rhythm, whether it's shockable or not and can suggest you through the process of CPR by voice commands. In centers where AEDs are not available, CPR is continued until appropriate help arrives. Often, in busy countries like India, this can take quite a considerable amount of time, so hospitals and healthcare establishments should be encouraged to buy AEDs.

Recognition of cardiac arrest:

- Unconscious
- Unresponsive
- Not breathing normally (agonal breathing/gasping) or absent breathing
  - Some people may have a seizure when cardiac arrest occurs as a result of severe cerebral hypoxia.

**Box 4.8**
Chest pain in a patient with previous history of stable angina: Urgent transfer to appropriate medical facility is to be done, if the patient feels the pain is unusual or if the pain doesn't resolve with rest and Sublingual Glyceryl Trinitrate.

**Box 4.9**
Do not waste time, for example, trying to find a vein while the ambulance is waiting! Antiplatelet medication (aspirin) within few minutes of suspecting MI and early thrombolysis by the Physicians can significantly reduce the mortality associated.

**Management:**

- Call for help and ask to bring defibrillator and emergency drug kit.
- Second person can call for ambulance.
- Start CPR [14]
  - CPR can be executed in the dental chair.
- Start with chest compressions.
  - Second person checks airway, gets ready for ventilations, preferably using a bag valve mask.
- Give 30 chest compressions.
- Give two ventilations.
- Carry on CPR at 30:2 until expert help or AED arrives.
- Stop CPR when patient shows signs of life.

CPR with AED:

- Continue with CPR while the pads of AED are being attached.
- Stop CPR and do not touch victim while the AED starts analyzing the rhythm [15].
  - Nonshockable rhythm observed by AED—continue CPR until signs of life or AED starts analyzing rhythm again [16].
  - Shock advised by AED—Make sure no one touches the patient directly or indirectly—Deliver the shock.
- Continue CPR at 30:2 while the pads remain attached.
- After 2 min, AED will start reanalyzing the rhythm and the cycle to be continued until the patient shows signs of life.

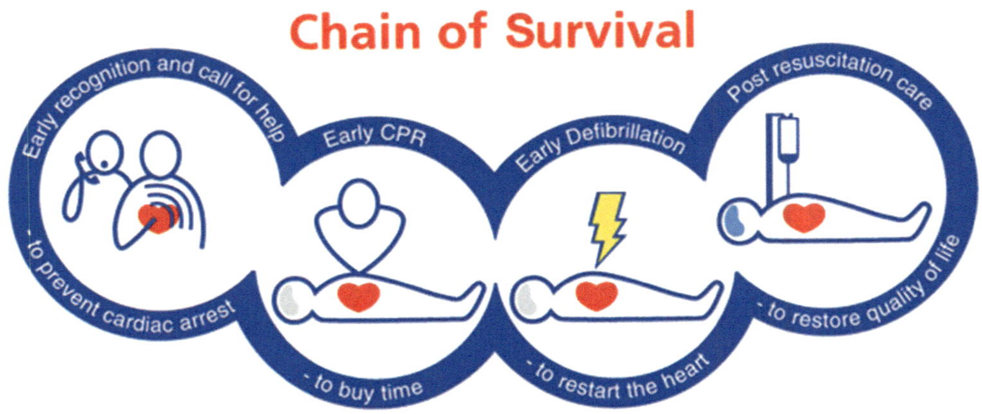


**Fig. 4.1** Chain of survival

- Once the patient regains consciousness, put the patient in recovery position and maintain saturations above 94%, supplemental oxygen may be needed.
- The patient should receive appropriate post-resuscitation care and keep monitoring as chances of a second cardiac arrest is high in the immediate post-resuscitation period.

To improve overall outcome in cardiac arrest patients, it is necessary to follow these four important aspects of care:

1. *Early recognition and call for help*—do not waste time trying to ascertain if pulse is there or not. A patient who is unresponsive and not breathing should be considered in cardiac arrest unless until proven otherwise.
2. *Early CPR*—the victim soon after cardiac arrest will have some oxygen in the blood and starting with chest compressions early will be extremely beneficial to the cells starved of oxygen.
3. *Early Defibrillation*: The chances of reversing a shockable rhythm diminish with the passage of time.
4. *Post resuscitation care:* All patients who have been successfully reversed from cardiac arrest should be transferred to an appropriate center with cardiac care facilities.

The four points are incorporated into this internationally recognized "chain of survival," which is given here (adapted from the Resuscitation Council UK; website: https://www.resus.org.uk/EasysiteWeb/getresource.axd?AssetID=3907&type=Full&servicetype=Attachment) (Fig. 4.1):

**Box 4.10**

All healthcare workers should undergo proper training in CPR. Healthcare organizations throughout the world are now insisting on a CPR certificate. Such a training has to be done on a periodic basis so that the skills are retained. The reader is strongly advised to undergo training periodically and a valid certificate will prevent you from future litigation if an unfortunate event occurs to one of your patients.

## 4.8 Hypoglycemia

Glucose is essential for the effective functioning of neurons. When the glucose levels in blood drop to a very low level, brain function will get affected and if the glucose levels are not restored quickly, permanent neurologic damage can occur within 4–6 min. Hypoglycemia can occur in diabetic patients taking Insulin, who skipped meal, and is also the leading cause of loss of consciousness in children. Hypoglycemia occurs when blood glucose level falls below 70 mg/dL.

**Signs and Symptoms:**

- Anxious, confused, irritable, or aggressive behavior.
- Sweating
- Nausea and vomiting
- Hungry
- Visual disturbances
- Convulsions
- Loss of consciousness.

**Management** [17]:

Management depends on consciousness level and the ability of the patient to take food orally without the risk of aspiration.

- Conscious patient:
  - 10–20 g of glucose
    10 g of glucose in two teaspoons of granulated sugar
    Two teaspoons of Glucon-D powder contain 15 g of Glucose
  - Can be repeated in 10–15 min
  - Once the patient's condition improves, provide a carbohydrate snack or meal as appropriate to raise blood glucose level.
- Unconscious patient:
  - Check if airway is clear—ABCDE approach
  - Put patient in recovery position
  - Oxygen supplementation at 15 L/min

- Give Glucagon by IM route into the anterolateral thigh
- If Glucagon is not available
  - Arrange for emergency transfer of patient
  - Give 100 mL of 10% dextrose by IV route
  - Severe cases of hypoglycemia need 50 mL of 50% Dextrose
  - Higher concentrations of dextrose are thicker solutions, need a larger bore cannula.
  - Once the patient regains consciousness, give oral glucose and carbohydrate as earlier.

**Box 4.11**
Glucagon either by IM or SC route
Dose: Adult—1 mg
Child under 8 years or less than 25 kg should be given 500 μg (0.5 mg)
Keep patient in lateral position to prevent risk of aspiration

## 4.9 Grand Mal Seizures

Enquire with patients about how frequently they get seizures and their compliance with medication. Patients with frequent seizure history or patients who are irregular with their medications are more likely to have a seizure while having dental procedures. Provide the treatment in a calm, stress-free environment, avoid any seizure-triggering factors.

**Signs and Symptoms:**

- Seizure activity may have a brief period of aura, where the patient can behave indifferently, spaced out, and detached.
- The patient will go rigid, lose consciousness, lose balance, and may cry-tonic (rigidity) phase.
- After a few seconds, sudden rhythmic jerking movements of the body lasting for up to 2 min.
- Mouth goes rigid. Frothy saliva can be noticed.
- Cyanosis around the mouth can be noticed as breathing stops.
- Possible urination.
- Following the seizure, patient can go into varying periods of confused state and may fall asleep.

**Treatment** [18]:

- Prevent injury to patient
  - Remove all the sharps away
  - Create safe space around a fitting patient
  - Provide cushions like a pillow or blanket
  - Pay particular attention to head
- Do not restrain
- Do not attempt to insert any object between teeth
- Supplemental oxygen at 15 L/min
- Have a suction readily available, with a yankauer suction tube clear oral cavity of any fluids after seizure stops [19].
- Ascertain hypoglycemia as a possible cause by checking blood glucose level by a finger prick test. This should be done in a patient with no previous history of epilepsy. Hypoglycemia is common in children and in diabetic patients [19].
- Once the convulsions are stopped:
  - Provide reassurance and empathy to the patient
  - Explain what had happened
  - Examine the mouth for any fluids and use suction
  - Examine for any bleeding, lacerations of tongue secondary to biting
  - Place the patient in a recovery position
  - Examine for any other injuries
  - Provide oxygen as required
  - Stay with the patient until the patient is fully recovered
  - Do not give anything orally until the patient is fully conscious, to avoid the risk of aspiration
  - Do not attempt to arouse a patient who is sleeping after a convulsive episode
- Prolonged Convulsions beyond 5 min or repeated seizure activity without proper recovery constitutes—status epilepticus [20], which can be fatal and needs to be managed as:
  - Make arrangements for urgent transfer to appropriate medical center
  - Administer midazolam intravenously [21]
  - Where IV access is not possible:
    - Rectal route can be used effectively, especially in children.
    - Buccal midazolam gel can be instilled into buccal vestibule with the help of a syringe with no needle.
    - Midazolam sprays, which can be used via nasal route, are slowly being available in India.
    - Buccal and nasal routes are increasingly being used and the reader is advised to look up for more up-to-date information as suitable formulations are not routinely available in India.

**Box 4.12**
Midazolam Dosage:
I.V route: Above 12 years, 5 mg slowly—patient may need encouragement to breathe after IV midazolam.
I.M route: Adult: 0.2 mg/kg, Not to exceed 10 mg in total.
Child: 0.1–0.2 mg/kg, not to exceed 10 mg in total
Nasal Spray: Child: 0.2 mg/kg body weight (Max: 5 mg/nares)
Rectal: Adult and children above 12 years: 10–20 mg, can be repeated once after 10–15 min if needed
Child 2–11 years: 5–10 mg, can be repeated once after 10–15 min

**Box 4.13**
Remember generalized tonic-clonic seizures can be seen in:

- Epilepsy
- Head injury
- Hypoglycemia
- Hypoxia
- Alcohol withdrawal
- Drugs
- Local anesthesia overdose or Intravascular injection
- Febrile convulsions

**Box 4.14**
Midazolam is a benzodiazepine that carries the risk of respiratory depression. Patients need close monitoring after drug administration and may need respiratory support.

**Box 4.15**
Typical grand mal seizure, in a known epileptic patient, where the seizure has subsided within a couple of minutes, patient can be discharged with the carer, provided all the vital signs are with in normal range. Urgent hospital transfer is indicated in all other epileptic seizures.

## 4.10 Syncope

Energy demands of the brain are met primarily by oxidation of glucose. A regular and constant supply of glucose and oxygen is essential for brain function. Supply of both glucose and oxygen depends on effective perfusion of the brain. When brain perfusion decreases beyond a critical level, the patient loses consciousness and the balance gets affected and the patient falls.

**Signs and Symptoms:**

- Feeling unwell
- Nausea, Lightheadedness
- Blurred vision
- Pallor
- Sweaty, especially forehead
- Sudden loss of consciousness and collapse
- Seizure, if the patient is not positioned in a horizontal position quickly.

**Management** [22]:

- Clear airway and reassure
- Change position to a flat or legs elevated
- Let fresh air by opening a window or a fan
- Do not let people to crowd around
- Place cold towel on forehead
- Supplemental Oxygen can be given, but usually, if it's simple faint consciousness should recover very quickly.
- Once recovered, encourage the patient to have a sugary drink.
- Examine for injuries secondary to fall.

## 4.11 Other Causes of Loss of Consciousness

Although syncope is the most common cause of loss of consciousness, the other causes should also be borne in mind, as some of them can be quite serious, such as:

- Postural Hypotension
- Hyperventilation
- Epilepsy
- Adrenaline crisis
- Hypoglycemia
- Stroke
- Cardiac Arrest

**Postural Hypotension:**

- Loss of consciousness following a sudden change of posture from supine or sitting to standing upright.
- Usually in patients who are taking antihypertensives or elderly.
- Place them in a supine position and bring them to the upright position slowly.

**Hyperventilation:**

Excessive breathing in an anxiety state or excessive crying resulting in drop of blood $CO_2$ level.

- Feeling lightheaded, dizzy
- Chest discomfort to chest pain
- Muscle spasms, especially in hands and feet
- Tingling or numbness in the arms and in the perioral region
- Control the crying/breathing through suggestion
- Use a paper bag to rebreath exhaled air to build up $CO_2$ levels

## 4.12 Conclusion

Preparedness for emergency is the key and when you are prepared, emergencies are easier to manage. The maxillofacial surgeon should be able to recognize these conditions and initiate appropriate management before professional emergency help is available. More often, maxillofacial surgeon is the lone clinician and is the sole responder in an emergency. It is prudent for the surgeon to know what to do and what not to do to get the best out of the worst scenario or situation.

It is imperative that the maxillofacial surgeons thoroughly understand the pathophysiology and extend their skills to recognize and manage expeditiously and effectively the emergencies that may arise. It is advisable that the contemporary clinicians update their knowledge and skills periodically with proper training courses.

Protocols given here are based on the currently available evidence, keeping in view of the local healthcare systems and access. As protocols are only suggestive, the clinician is strongly advised to use his or her own discretion when dealing with medical emergencies (Table 4.1; Flowchart 4.1).

Table 4.1 Causes of loss of consciousness and its age distribution

| Causes of unconsciousness | | |
|---|---|---|
| Child | Teen-mid 30 | Above 40 |
| Hypoglycemia | Syncope | Cardiovascular causes |
| Epilepsy | Hypoglycemia | |
| Congenital heart disease | Epilepsy | |

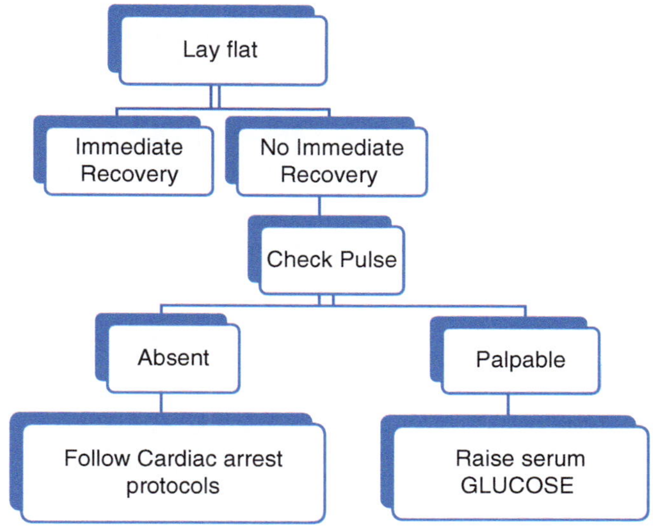


Flowchart 4.1 Management algorithm for a collapsed patient where the cause of collapse is not known

## References

1. Thim T, Krarup NHV, et al. Initial asseement and treatment with the Airway, Breathing, Circulation, Disability, Exposure (ABCDE) approach. Int J Gen Med. 2012;5:117–21.
2. Saglani S, Fleming L, Sonnappa S, et al. Advances in the aetiology, management, and prevention of acute asthmatic attack in children. Lancet Child Adolesc Health. 2019;3(5):354–64.
3. Fergeson JE, Patel SS, Lockey RF. Acute asthma, prognosis, and treatment. J Allergy Clin Immunol. 2017;139(2):438–47.
4. Marsh B, Drake MG. Outpatient management of acute exacerbations of obstructive lung diseases. Med Clin N Am. 2017;101(3):537–51.
5. Hahner S. Acute adrenal crisis and mortality in adrenal insufficiency. Ann Endocrinol. 2018;79(3):164–6.
6. Paur THK, Stikkelbroeck NMMI, et al. Adrenal crisis: still a deadly event in the 21st century. Am J Med. 2016;129(3):339.
7. Schwartz A. Airway mangement for the oral surgery patient. Oral Maxillofac Surg Clin N Am. 2018;30(2):207–26.
8. Chapman J, Lalkhen AG. Anaphylaxis. Anaesth Intensive Care Med. 2017;18(1):16–21.
9. Young NH, Nimmo GR. Anaphylaxis. Medicine. 2017;45(3):157–62.
10. Moore LE, Kemp AM, Kemp SF. Recognition, treatment, and prevention of Anaphylaxis. Immunol Allergy Clin N Am. 2015;35(2):363–74.
11. Waller JR, Waller DG. Drugs for systemic hypertension and angina. Medicine. 2018;46(9):566–72.
12. Dym H, Barzani G, et al. Emergency drugs for the dental office. Dent Clin N Am. 2016;60(2):287–94.

13. Herman WW, Ferguson HW. Dental care for patients with heart failure: an update. J Am Dent Assoc. 2010;141(7):845–53.
14. Yates EJ, Schmidbauer S, et al. Out of hospital cardiac arrest termination of resuscitation with ongoing CPR: an observational study. Resuscitation. 2018;130:21–7.
15. Fernando SM, Vaillancourt C, et al. Analysis of bystander CPR quality out of hospital cardiac arrest using data derived from AED. Resuscitation. 2018;18:138–43.
16. Pollack RA, Brown SP, et al. Bystander automated external defibrillator application in non-shockable out of patient cardiac arrest. Resuscitation. 2019;137:168–74.
17. Bansal N, Dhaliwal R, et al. Management of diabetes in elderly. Med Clin N Am. 2015;99(2):351–77.
18. Johnson EI. Seizures & epilepsy. Med Clin N Am. 2019;103(2):309–24.
19. Thijs RD, Surges R, et al. Epilepsy in adults. Lancet. 2019;393(10172):689–701.
20. Paris M, Reddy U. Update on the management of status epilepticus. Anaesth Intensive Care Med. 2018;19(3):83–6.
21. Papavasiliou AS, Kotsalis C, et al. Intravenous midazolam in convulsive status epilepticus in children with pharmacoresistant epilepsy. Epilepsy Behav. 2009;14(4):661–4.
22. Numeroso F, Mossini G, et al. Emergency department management of patients with syncope according to the 2018 ESC guidelines. Int J Cardiol. 2019;283:119–21.

# Part III

# Anesthesia for Oral and Maxillofacial Surgery

# Local Anesthesia in Oral and Maxillofacial Surgery

# 5

Reena Rachel John

## 5.1 Introduction

Pain, the dreaded symptom, is an unpleasant sensation that draws the attention of the individual as a whole. Its management has greatly evolved in the field of dentistry, starting from the leaves of a coca tree to articaine, Comfort Control Syringe (CCS) system, Transcutaneous Electrical Nerve Stimulation (TENS), Computer-Controlled Local Anesthetic Delivery System as well as oral and intravenous sedatives. Apart from all these, local anesthesia (LA) is the favored mode of pain control in the profession. The painless surgery under LA is must; otherwise, endogenous catecholamines are released if there is excessive pain during dental treatment, which can alter the hemodynamic status such as an increase in blood pressure and heart rate and even dysrhythmias [1].

### 5.1.1 Historical Background

The first local anesthetic isolated from the leaves of a coca tree in 1860 by Neiman was cocaine, and it was Karl Koller in 1884 who showed the anesthetic effect of Cocaine. In 1905, Einhorn popularized Procaine as an effective local anesthetic. It was derived from benzoic acid and diethyl amino ethanol. In 1948, the anesthetic property of lignocaine was discovered by Lofgren, and T. Gordh applied it in dental surgery [2].

### 5.1.2 Definition

Local anesthesia is defined as a reversible loss of sensation in the circumscribed area of the body caused by depression of excitation in the nerve endings or inhibition of the conduction process in peripheral nerves [2].

### 5.1.3 Ideal Characteristic of Local Anesthesia

An ideal local anesthetic must have the following characteristics:

- It should be nonirritating and nonallergic.
- It should not cause structural changes to nerve and have low systemic toxicity.
- Its onset of action should be short and should be stable in solution.
- It should be effective as both injectable and topical application.
- Its action should be long enough to allow the procedure to be completed.

## 5.2 Classification (Tables 5.1 and 5.2)

**Table 5.1** Classification of local anesthetic agents: based on chemical structure

| Chemical structure | Example |
|---|---|
| Esters of benzoic acid | Cocaine, Benzocaine, Butacaine, Piperocaine, Tetracaine |
| Esters of para amino benzoic acid | Procaine, Chloroprocaine, Propoxycaine |
| Amides | Articaine, Bupivicaine, Lidocaine, Dibucaine, Mepivacaine, Prilocaine |
| Quinolone derivatives | Centbucridine |

R. R. John (✉)
Department of Oral and Maxillofacial Surgery,
Vinayaka Mission's Sankarachariar Dental College and Hospital,
VMRF DU, Salem, India



K. Bonanthaya et al. (eds.), *Oral and Maxillofacial Surgery for the Clinician*, https://doi.org/10.1007/978-981-15-1346-6_5

Table 5.2 Classification of local anesthetic agents: based on duration of action

| Duration of action | Example |
|---|---|
| Ultra short acting<br>Pulpal anesthesia: less than 10 min<br>Soft-tissue anesthesia: 30–45 min | Chloroprocaine, Procaine |
| Short acting<br>Pulpal anesthesia: 5–10 min<br>Soft-tissue anesthesia: 60–120 min | Lidocaine, Prilocaine |
| Medium acting<br>Pulpal anesthesia: 45–90 min<br>Soft-tissue anesthesia: 120–240 min | Mepivacine, Articaine |
| Long acting<br>Pulpal anesthesia: 90–180 min<br>Soft-tissue anesthesia: 240–540 min | Bupivicaine, Etidocaine |

## 5.3 Local Anesthetic Agents

The LA agents have been divided into Esters and Amides groups. The commonly used Amides are Lidocaine, Articaine, and Bupivacain [2].

### 5.3.1 Lidocaine (Lignocaine)

Lofgren in 1943 introduced the prototype amide local anesthetic [2], i.e., Lidocaine.

The other similar names are xylocaine, octocaine, dentocaine. Chemically, it is Diethyl 2, 6 dimethyl acetanilide. The maximum recommended dosage for Lignocaine with vasoconstrictor is 7 mg/kg not exceeding 500 mg and without vasoconstrictor is 4.4 mg/kg not exceeding 300 mg. Its onset of action is 2–3 min and duration of action with vasoconstrictor is 45–75 min, without vasoconstrictor is less than 30 min. Its contraindications include Ehlers Danlos syndrome and Attention-deficit hyperactive syndrome. Lignocaine is available in the form of jelly, spray, patches, and ointments. The toxicity arises from inadvertent intravascular administration or from overdose.

Recently, Howlader et al. [3] suggested open reduction and internal fixation (ORIF) of isolated subcondylar fractures under local anesthesia by using 2% lidocaine with 1:200,000 epinephrine for mandibular nerve block and superior cervical plexus blocks (SCPB).

To anesthetize the cutaneous branches of SCP (lesser occipital, greater auricular, transverse cervical, and supraclavicular nerve), the solution is deposited at the midpoint of the posterior border of sternocleidomastoid muscle border, as well as inferior and superior to that point subcutaneously creating a field block.

The anesthetic agent selection should be based on three main clinical considerations: anesthetic potency and latency, onset, and duration. The composition of the local anesthetic solution is shown in Table 5.3.

Table 5.3 Composition of local anaesthetic solution (Lignocaine with Adrenaline)

| Ingredients | Functions |
|---|---|
| Lignocaine HCl 2% (21.3 mg) | Anesthetic agent |
| Adrenaline 1:80,000 (0.0125 mg) | Vasoconstrictor, decreased absorption of LA in blood |
| Sodium Metabisulfite (0.5 mg) | Preservative |
| Methyl Paraben (1.0 mg) | Preservative to increase shelf life |
| Sodium Chloride (0.6 mg) | Isotonicity of solution to the tissues |
| Sodium Hydroxide | To maintain and adjust pH |
| Thymol | Fungicidal |
| Distilled water | Dilution |
| Nitrogen Bubble | 1–2 mm in diameter, present to prevent oxygen from being trapped in cartridge and potentially destroying vasopressor or vasoconstrictor. |

### 5.3.2 Bupivacaine

Its chemical name is 1 butyl-2,6piperoloxylidine hydrochloride.

It is four times more potent than prilocaine, lidocaine, and mepivacaine. It is less toxic than lidocaine and mepivacaine and it is metabolized in the liver by amidases and excretion via kidney 16% unchanged. Its onset of action is similar to lidocaine, mepivacaine, and prilocaine. Effective dental concentration is 0.5% and anesthetic half-life is 2.5 h.

Maximum recommended dose is 1.3 mg/kg body wt to a maximum of 90 mg. Because of its long duration of action, it is advisable for use in lengthy surgical procedure and the management of postoperative pain. Hence, the patient's requirement for postoperative opioid analgesics is lessened when bupivacaine is used. Bupivacaine is not recommended in young patients as the risk of self-mutilation is increased.

The duration of soft-tissue anesthesia has been consistently shown to be longer than with lidocaine [4] and thereby reducing postoperative pain experience [5].

### 5.3.3 Articaine

Its chemical structure is 3-N Propylaminoproprionylamino 2-Carbomethoxy 4-Methylthiophene hydrochloride.

The potency of Articaine is 1.5 times more than lignocaine and 1.9 times than procaine. Its onset of action when used with vasoconstrictor is 1–2 min. Half-life is approximately 21 min and it is metabolized to pharmacologically inactive metabolite called articaine acid glucoronide. Since it is rapidly biotransformed to its inactive metabolite, it is a safe local anesthetic agent. It is excreted via kidney

**Table 5.4** Maximum recommended dose of common Local Anesthetic used

| Local Anesthetic | mg/kg | mg/lb | MRD (mg) |
|---|---|---|---|
| *Articaine* | | | |
| With vasoconstrictor | 7.0 | 3.2 | 500 |
| *Bupivacaine* | | | |
| With vasoconstrictor | 1.3 | 0.6 | 90 |
| *Lidocaine* | | | |
| No vasoconstrictor | 4.4 | 2.0 | 300 |
| With vasoconstrictor | 6.6 | 3.0 | 500 |

unchanged (5–10%) and as metabolite (90%). The maximum recommended dosage for articaine is 0.8 mg/kg body weight.

Contraindications for the use of articaine are Idiopathic or congenital methemoglobinuria, hemoglobinopathies, hypoxia, and in patients with cardio-respiratory failures. Prolonged paraesthesia has been reported as a complication following inferior alveolar nerve block (IANB) [6].

Articaine with epinephrine is the best choice to improve anesthesia in both inflamed and in uninflamed tissues with good results, and more effective anesthesia for longer duration can be achieved [7]. Table 5.4 shows maximum recommended dose of commonly used LA.

## 5.4 Vasoconstrictors

Importance of vasoconstrictors in local anesthetic solution include

1. To decrease the tissue perfusion and therefore to decrease the blood flow at the site of drug administration, which further decreases the absorption of local anesthetics into the circulatory system. Therefore, the blood levels of the anesthetic agents remain low, thereby decreasing the risk of toxicity [2].
2. It also increases the time taken by the local anesthetic to be absorbed from the site of administration and therefore increases the duration of action of the local anesthetic.

Most commonly used vasoconstrictors are epinephrine, norepinephrine, levonordefrin hydrochloride, phenylephrine hydrochloride.

### 5.4.1 Dilution of Vasoconstrictor

The explanation of 1:1000 vasoconstrictor concentration is that 1 g/1000 mg of solute is present in 1000 ml of the solution, which means 1 mg of solute in 1 ml of solution. In the local anesthetic solution, the concentration of vasoconstrictor is less. The concentrations used are 1:80,000 or 1:100,000 or 1:200,000. The concentration of 1:100,000 of the vasoconstrictor would contain 1000 mg in 100,000 ml of the solution. Therefore, 1 ml of 1:100,000 concentration would contain 0.01 mg in 1 ml.

**Table 5.5** Quantity of vasoconstrictor with varying dilutions

| Concentration (dilution) | Milligrams per milliliter (mg/ml) | Micrograms per milliliter (μg/ml) | Microgram per cartridge (1.8 ml) |
|---|---|---|---|
| 1:1000 | 1.0 | 1000 | |
| 1:2500 | 0.4 | 400 | |
| 1:10,000 | 0.1 | 100 | |
| 1:20,000 | 0.05 | 50 | 90 |
| 1:30,000 | 0.033 | 33.3 | 73 |
| 1:50,000 | 0.02 | 20 | 36 |
| 1:80,000 | 0.0125 | 12.5 | 27.5 |
| 1:100,000 | 0.01 | 10 | 18 |
| 1:200,000 | 0.05 | 5 | 9 |

The absorption of vasoconstrictors is dose dependent and may last from minutes to half an hour. The patients with cardiovascular compromise are at increased risk with endogenously released epinephrine in response to stress rather than the epinephrine, which is injected with the local anesthetic (Table 5.5).

## 5.5 Causes of Failure of LA

1. Anatomic variation
2. Bifid or double nerve supply
3. Secondary supply by a soft-tissue nerve
4. Inadequate dose
5. Injection into the blood vessel
6. Degradation of vasoconstrictor
7. Patient having sepsis

## 5.6 LA Toxicity and Antidote for Toxicity

Symptoms, which reflect toxicity from the administration of local anesthetic solution, may range from mild cutaneous reactions to severe life-threatening anaphylactic reactions. There are a variety of methods and drugs to treat these reactions symptomatically. However, the reversal of toxicity, including damage to vital organs such as the heart and brain, is still less understood. A clinically efficient antidote for a complete reversal of toxicity is still beyond our grasp currently.

### 5.6.1 Reversal of Cardiomyotoxicity

Intravenous lipid emulsion (IVLE) is being reported as a rescue measure for LA toxicity. This has been studied and proven in both animal models and in limited human trials with successful resuscitation outcomes. The lipid emulsion acts on the plasma and tissue and extracts the lipophilic anesthetic molecules, thereby reversing their inhibitory myocardial effects. Bolus doses of 1.2–2 ml/kg followed by continuous infusion of 0.25–0.5 ml/kg/min are currently advocated for adequate efficacy. This drug needs to be used judiciously as optimal dosages have not been established and the risks of overdosage are not clearly understood.

## 5.7 Reversal of Soft-Tissue Anesthesia

The duration of soft-tissue anesthesia often exceeds that of pulpal or bony anesthesia. This is an important reason for the occurrence of undesirable events like accidental lip or tongue biting, difficulties in speaking, eating, or drinking liquids, etc. Various drugs have been studied to decrease the postoperative duration of anesthesia. Of the various drugs tried clinically, phentolamine is one drug, which has demonstrated appreciable clinical efficacy.

Phentolamine is a nonselective alpha-adrenergic antagonist that is reversible. Its main action is vasodilatation. It has been used effectively for controlling hypertensive emergencies, especially in pheochromocytomas. In dental practice, Phentolamine in the form of phentolamine mesylate injections has been used as a reversal agent against LA by reversing the action of vasoconstrictors in the LA solution and expedites the metabolism of the LA molecules. The recommended dose for phentolamine is the administration of 1.8 ml of the solution containing 0.4 mg of phentolamine mesylate immediately after treatment.

## 5.8 Plain Local Anesthetic (Without Epinephrine)

It is preferred for patients having comorbidities such as circulatory disorder to avoid complications and adverse systemic effects of vasoconstrictors [8]. Lip laceration is one of the common cases, which are attended to by a maxillofacial surgeon in the emergency department for suturing. Localized blanching caused by the use of local anesthetic with adrenalin at the lacerated wound causes difficulty in locating the exact demarcation between skin, white roll, and lip. Therefore, LA without epinephrine is preferred in such cases before suturing [9].

## 5.9 Topical Local Anesthetic Agent

The solution used for this purpose is 5% Lignocaine, 10% Lignocaine, combination of 2.5% lignocaine and 2.5% prilocaine [10]. They are indicated in patients [11, 12]

- For removal of maxillary and mandibular arch bars
- Gingival probing
- Deep Scaling
- Closure of facial lacerations in younger children
- Before LA injections in small patients

In suture and staple removal

## 5.10 Surface Anesthesia

The form of drug used to obtain this includes ointment, gel, viscous, cream, spray, etc. Topical application of these forms can produce anesthesia on the surface, particularly of the oral mucosa.

This is used often, before an actual injection for L.A, at the site of injection, in order to reduce the pain of the needle prick itself. It can also be used to obtund pain in situations where the oral mucosa is breached, as in an ulcer in the oral mucosa. The gel may also be used to anesthetize the surface mucosa, e.g., nasal, pharyngeal, etc., before a diagnostic endoscopy.

The concentration of a local anesthetic applied topically is typically greater than the same drug administered by injection. Drugs that are commonly employed in topical L.A formulations are Benzocaine and Lidocaine.

EMLA, which is a eutectic mixture of local anesthetic agents, lignocaine, & prilocaine in the ratio 1:1 by weight, has been found to be a very useful topical agent to be applied on the skin, before painful procedures like injection, venipuncture, etc. and is used extensively in children. This particular cream, which is oil-in-water emulsion, may also be used for surface anesthesia of the oral mucosa for purposes listed earlier.

## 5.11 Methods of Local Anesthetic Administration

There are major three different types of methods:

- Local infiltration
- Field block
- Nerve block

In local infiltration, deposition of the local anesthetic solution in the area of the surgery to anesthetize small terminal nerve endings. Field block involves the deposition of anesthetic solution near the large terminal nerve branches to prevent the passage of impulses from teeth to the central nervous system. In nerve block, local anesthesia is deposited away from the site of surgery, but close to the main nerve trunk.

Different techniques for mandibular nerve block anesthesia have been published, including the mental/incisive nerve block [13–15].

1. The standard (Halsted) technique
2. The standard indirect technique
3. Mental nerve (incisive nerve) block
   - standard approach for mandibular anteriors and soft tissue
   - anterior approach
   - extraoral approach
4. Clarke-Holmes technique (1959)

5. Vazirani technique (1960)
6. Akinosi technique (1977) closed-mouth technique
7. Wolfe technique (1992)
8. Sargenti technique (1966)
9. Gow-Gates technique (1973)
10. Ipsilateral open-mouth technique (2007)
11. Morishita (positive aspiration) technique (2007)
12. Extraoral submandibular approach
13. Lateral extraoral approach
14. Anterior extraoral approach. (1969)

Different maxillary nerve block techniques have been described.

1. Anterior-superior alveolar nerve and infraorbital nerve blocks,
   - intraoral approach (bicuspid approach)
   - Bisecting approach (central incisor)
   - extraoral approach
   - nasal approach (1969)
2. Posterior-superior alveolar nerve block (tuberosity block)
3. Middle-superior alveolar nerve block (buccal approach)
4. Middle and anterior-superior alveolar nerve block (palatal approach)
5. Sphenopalatine (incisive) nerve block
6. Greater palatine nerve and lesser palatine nerves block
7. Maxillary nerve blocks,
   - High tuberosity approach
   - Greater palatine canal approach
   - nasal approach
   - lateral extraoral approach
   - suprazygomatic extraoral approach extraoral approach
   - anterior-lateral extraoral approach.

### 5.11.1 Percentage of Blood Vessel Penetration During IANB

During IANB, the intravenous injection of local anesthetic is very common. Frangiskos F et al. [16], in their study, found positive aspiration (the tip of the needle is in the blood vessel) 20% times. The positive aspiration was more commonly seen in young patient's age ranging from 9 to 19 years. To avoid systemic complications while giving local anesthesia, aspiration is must in each and every case.

### 5.11.2 Controversy in the Use of Bilateral IANB and Lingual Nerve Block [17]

Has bilateral IAN and Lingual nerve block been given? Some surgeons recommend, while some do not, but there are no published data available regarding its contraindications. The common complications associated with its use are

- Collection of fluid in the oral cavity
- Injury to tongue
- Loss of control of tongue, which can lead to respiratory embarrassment
- Unpleasant effects of bilateral anesthesia [18].

Many authors advocated the use of sodium bicarbonate in addition to the lignocaine solution to reduce the duration of onset of anesthesia, and it is very effective in reducing pain during the injection. Sodium bicarbonate ions also nonspecifically reduce the safety margin for nerve conduction and it has a direct action on the binding of Local anesthetic to the sodium channel [19–21].

## 5.12 Techniques

### 5.12.1 Inferior Alveolar Nerve Block (*Also Known as* Mandibular Nerve Block) [Along with Lingual & Long Buccal Nerve Blocks]

This is the single most important nerve block, whose technique needs to be mastered. With this, we can anesthetize the whole of the mandibular soft and hard tissues, including the cheek, and many procedures in this region can be carried out.

Secondly unlike in the maxilla, infiltration techniques do not provide adequate anesthesia to the hard tissue in the mandible, particularly the teeth. This is due to the dense cortical bone in the mandible, in contrast to the porous maxillary bone, where a paraperiosteal deposition of the solution can allow the solution to diffuse through the bone to the periapical region easily and cause anesthesia of the teeth and their supporting structures.

### 5.12.2 Technique

This description is for injection on the right side of the patient and for a right-handed operator. The surgeon is on the right side of the patient, in front of the patient. The patient is asked to open the mouth wide.

With the left hand, the operator palpates the posterior buccal sulcus, runs the index finger posteriorly to feel the external oblique ridge and the anterior border of the coronoid process. As the finger proceeds upwards, palpate the coronoid process up and down to determine the deepest point on its anterior border. This is the coronoid notch. [This is a very important landmark because this determines the vertical height at which the needle should be inserted, the reason being the Mandibular foramen on the medial aspect of the ramus where we want the needle to reach is in direct line with the coronoid notch] Fig. 5.1.

Once the coronoid notch is palpated with the pulp of the index finger, the finger is rotated such that the nail faces medially. At the same time, the finger retracts the soft tissue

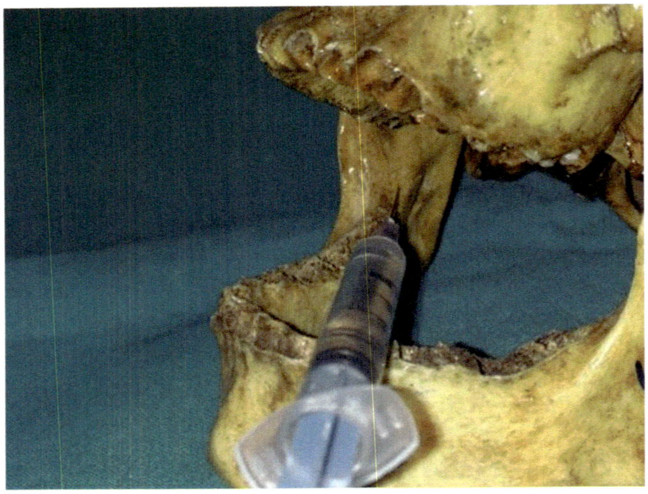



**Fig. 5.1** Dry mandible showing the position of needle and the coronoid notch

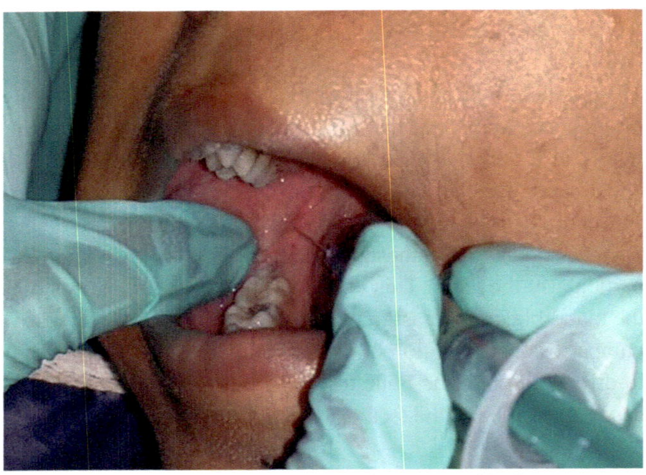



**Fig. 5.2** Picture showing needle insertion position from the soft tissue for IAN block

to reveal a depression called the pterygo mandibular depression, which is medial to the finger between the finger and the pterygo Mandibular raphe (Fig. 5.2).

Now the needle with solution in the syringe is taken in the right hand and is introduced into the mouth from the opposite side (i.e., left side) corner of the mouth/premolar area.

The syringe and needle are kept parallel to the Mandibular occlusal plane and are introduced into the pterygo temporal depression at the same height as the nail of the index finger (on the coronoid notch). The needle is advanced slowly in the soft tissue till the needle strikes the bone and resistance is felt. Now the needle is in the pterygo mandibular space bounded laterally by the medial surface of the ramus of the mandible and it is just above the lingula in the area of the opening of the mandibular foramen.

The syringe is aspirated and 1 ml of the solution is deposited. This will anesthetize the inferior alveolar nerve as it enters the mandible. Now, the needle with the syringe is swung on to the corner of the mouth on the same side, i.e., right, and is slowly withdrawn after about half the length is inserted and 0.5–0.8 ml of the solution is deposited here. This will take care of the lingual nerve, which is anteromedial to the inferior alveolar nerve.

Now the needle is withdrawn completely out of the soft tissue and is reinserted into the cheek, posterior to the last molar teeth at the level of the occlusal plane of the mandibular teeth for a short distance. After aspiration, the remaining 0.5 ml of the solution is deposited. This anesthetizes the long buccal nerve [for the left-sided block, the surgeon is slightly behind the patient on the right side with the left hand coming around].

This classical Mandibular Nerve block of inferior alveolar nerve with lingual & long buccal is done together if the mandibular molars and their adjoining soft tissues need to be anaesthetized. The reason being the pulp and the periodontium of these teeth are supplied by the inferior alveolar nerve. The lingual gingiva is supplied by the lingual nerve and the buccal gingiva by the long buccal nerve.

### 5.12.3 Areas Anesthetized by This Block

1. *Inferior Alveolar Nerve Block*
   (a) All mandibular teeth and the bone surrounding them.
   (b) The buccal gingiva in relation to the Mandibular anterior and premolar teeth.
   (c) Lower lip on the same half up to the midline.
2. *Lingual Nerve Block*
   (a) The lingual gingiva of the Mandibular teeth along with the lingual Mandibular mucosa.
   (b) The Anterior 2/3rd of the tongue on the same side.
3. *Long buccal nerve Block*
   (a) The cheek mucosa.
   (b) Buccal gingiva and mandibular mucosa in relation to the molar teeth.

### 5.12.4 Signs and Symptoms of Anesthesia

It usually takes about 3–5 min before adequate depth of anesthesia is obtained after any injection. In other words, although symptoms of anesthesia may be felt almost instantly after the injection, for the patient to feel no pain during the procedure a wait of at least 5 min is needed.

It has been conventional to confirm the anesthesia obtained with two parameters:

1. Subjective symptoms of anesthesia as experienced by the patient.
2. Objective signs elicited by the surgeon.

Subjective symptoms may or may not be present with certain nerve blocks, e.g., nasopalatine block. However with the classical inferior alveolar/mental nerve block, a *tingling and numbness* on one half of the lip (same side) will be felt. There will be an area of sharp demarcation between the numb side of the lip and the normal side at the midline. The tingling or numbness will start instantly to become heavy in about 3–5 min. Similar sensation of numbness will be felt on the same side of the tongue particularly the tip as a result of the lingual nerve block. There may be no symptoms of numbness felt by the patients in the other anaesthetized areas, e.g., the gingiva, teeth, or the cheek.

The objective sign as elicited by the surgeon is more reliable and may be the only means of ascertaining anesthesia in the absence of subjective symptoms. The objective sign of anesthesia is *lack of pain in the area anesthetized when stimulus is applied* with a blunt instrument, e.g., the end of a periosteal elevator. [It should be noted from the earlier discussion that the patient might feel the pressure of the instrument and an apprehensive patient might occasionally interpret this as pain.]

In checking for anesthesia of the inferior alveolar nerve, the blunt instrument must be applied on the buccal gingiva anterior to the mental foramen, because the lack of sensation in the posterior buccal soft tissue indicates a successful long buccal nerve and not inferior alveolar nerve block. The same blunt instrument must be applied in the gingival sulcus on the lingual side of the tooth to be extracted for lingual nerve anesthesia. The same can be done to check the buccal nerve anesthesia.

### 5.12.5 **Complications** (Table 5.6)

These were discussed very briefly as local complications of L.A in the earlier section. Specific complications after an Inferior Alveolar Nerve block include:

1. Failure to obtain anesthesia
2. Hematoma formation
3. Transient facial nerve palsy/weakness
4. Trismus
5. Breakage of the needle.

**Table 5.6** Complications with local anesthetics

| Local | Systemic |
|---|---|
| Needle breakage | Syncope |
| Paresthesia | Adverse drug reactions |
| Facial nerve paralysis | Overdose drug reactions |
| Trismus | Psychogenic reactions |
| Soft-tissue injury | |
| Hematoma | |
| Pain on injection | |
| Burning on injection | |
| Infection | |
| Edema | |
| Sloughing postanesthetic intraoral lesion | |

#### 5.12.5.1 Failure to Obtain Anesthesia

It is the most common problem and usually due to the wrong technique. Repeating the block employing the right technique is usually the solution. However, this might be encountered in two other situations.

1. Failure to anesthetize the myolohyoid branch, which might occasionally innervate the site of the procedure.
2. Also as already mentioned, in an apprehensive patient, the symptoms of pressure may be interpreted as pain. In this situation, anxiety reduction techniques may be needed or alternately some other form of anesthesia, e.g., conscious sedation or General Anesthesia may have to be employed. The subjective symptom of numbness in the lower lip (same side) and tip of the tongue will be the distinguishing feature between a faulty technique and an apprehensive patient. In the former, it will be absent, and in the latter very much present.

#### 5.12.5.2 Hematoma Formation

This may occur within the pterygo mandibular space as a result of bleeding induced by the needle prick. It may be a rare problem. The patient might have pain, swelling, & difficulty in opening the mouth. The treatment is symptomatic and possibly prophylactic antibiotic cover. It will resolve spontaneously.

#### 5.12.5.3 Transient Facial Nerve Palsy

May occasionally occur as a result of a faulty technique where the needle is inserted farther posteriorly into the substance of the parotid gland (in this situation, the needle would have failed to encounter bony resistance) and paralyzes the facial nerve.

The patient will have typical signs of ipsilateral facial nerve palsy/weakness, which includes difficulty in closing the eye, absence of wrinkles on the forehead, and drooping of the corner of the mouth ipsilaterally with a possible asymmetry. This effect will be transient, till such time the local anesthetic effect persists (about 1–1½ h) and the patient needs to be reassured.

#### 5.12.5.4 Trismus

Is a relatively more common complication and will be seen usually postoperatively. It could be due to a variety of causes, including:

1. Muscle spasm due to injury
2. Infection
3. Necrosis of tissue due to contact with contaminants, etc.

Most of the time it resolves spontaneously. But on occasion, this will require anti-inflammatory analgesics, muscle relaxants, and vigorous physiotherapy to overcome the problem. Wherever an infection is suspected, a suitable antibiotic cover may also be needed.

#### 5.12.5.5 Accidental Breakage of the Needle

Occurring within the tissues of the pterygo mandibular space, this is a very rare complication today where we use disposable needles for one use only. But when this happens, a radiographic guided exploration and removal of the broken piece may be needed. Gerbino G et al. [22] advocated use of brain LAB vector vision neuronavigation system for the retrieval of broken needle. This Intraoperative navigation system is very helpful in locating the broken needle fragment.

## 5.13 Vazirani–Akinosi (VA) Versus Inferior Alveolar Nerve Block

The closed mouth VA technique to anesthetize the IAN, lingual, and long buccal nerve simultaneously was described in 1977 [23]. VA is used only secondarily to conventional IAN block.

### 5.13.1 Indications for VA [24]

1. In patients with restricted mouth opening
2. In cases of failure of IAN blocks
3. Difficult-to-locate landmarks for IAN block

The percentage of Positive aspiration is much higher with IAN block in comparison to VA. This is because of the close proximity of the inferior alveolar artery, which enters the mandibular foramen just behind the nerve [25]. To avoid frequent aspiration, many surgeons prefer VA technique in normal patients also.

### 5.13.2 Akinosi–Vazirani Technique (Closed-Mouth Technique)

A 25-gauge long needle is used. The operator is in front of the patient on the right side (right-handed operator) for both sides on the patient.

With the left index finger or thumb, the coronoid notch is palpated and the soft tissues on the medial aspect of the ramus are pushed laterally. The needle is held parallel to the maxillary occlusal plane on the same side of the injection and is inserted adjacent to the maxillary third molar into the soft tissue overlying the medial border of the ramus, just adjacent to the maxillary tuberosity. This is now advanced posteriorly & slightly laterally. The bevel of the needle is away from the mandibular ramus and in an average-sized adult the needle is inserted about 25 mm into the tissue. At this point, the tip of the needle will be in the middle of the pterygo mandibular space close to the branches of the mandibular nerve. After aspiration, the LA solution is injected.

The areas anesthetized, signs and symptoms of anesthesia are similar to the open-mouth technique of mandibular nerve block.

Another viable alternative to the VA block is the technique of Gow-Gates described in 1973. In the Gow-Gates technique, anesthesia is administered more proximally, at the neck of the condyle and relies on extraoral landmark [26].

### 5.13.3 Technique

A 25-gauge long needle is used. The operator stands in front of the patient. It is very essential for the patient to extend his neck & open the mouth as wide as possible. Here the needle is inserted into the mucosa medial to the mandibular ramus on a line parallel to a line drawn from the intertragic notch to the corner of the mouth—just distal to the maxillary second molar. The needle is inserted from the corner of the mouth on the opposite side. The height of insertion is just at the level of the mesiolingual cusp of the maxillary second molar. Slowly advance the needle till the bone is contacted. (The needle here is in contact with the neck of the condyle. The position the patient is asked to assume, i.e., extend neck & open mouth wide, is to facilitate a more frontal position of the condyle closer to the mandibular nerve trunk). The average depth of insertion is about 25 mm. Aspirate & inject 2 ml of the solution slowly. Unlike with the classical method, injection is at one site only in this technique. This anesthetizes the inferior alveolar, lingual, long buccal branches of the mandibular here with similar effect as the classical block (Fig. 5.3a, b).

## 5.14 Mental/Incisive Nerve Block

These are two very similar blocks except that in a mental block the solution is deposited around the mental nerve as it exits the mandible at the mental foramen, whereas for an incisive nerve block, the solution is injected into the mandible through the mental foramen. This blocks the incisive nerve, which is the continuation of the inferior alveolar nerve anteriorly, up to the midline.

### 5.14.1 Technique

This may be carried out with the operator standing in front of the patient (can also be done easily with the operator standing behind).

With the left-hand thumb or index finger, palpate the mucobuccal fold on the mandible starting in the molar region moving anteriorly when depression will be felt. This is usually in relation to the apex of the premolar teeth where the mental foramen is present. The needle is now directed vertically to be inserted into this area with the bevel facing the bone. With the mental nerve block, the solution is deposited in the soft tissues, whereas for the incisive the needle is inserted into the foramen for a short distance before injection.

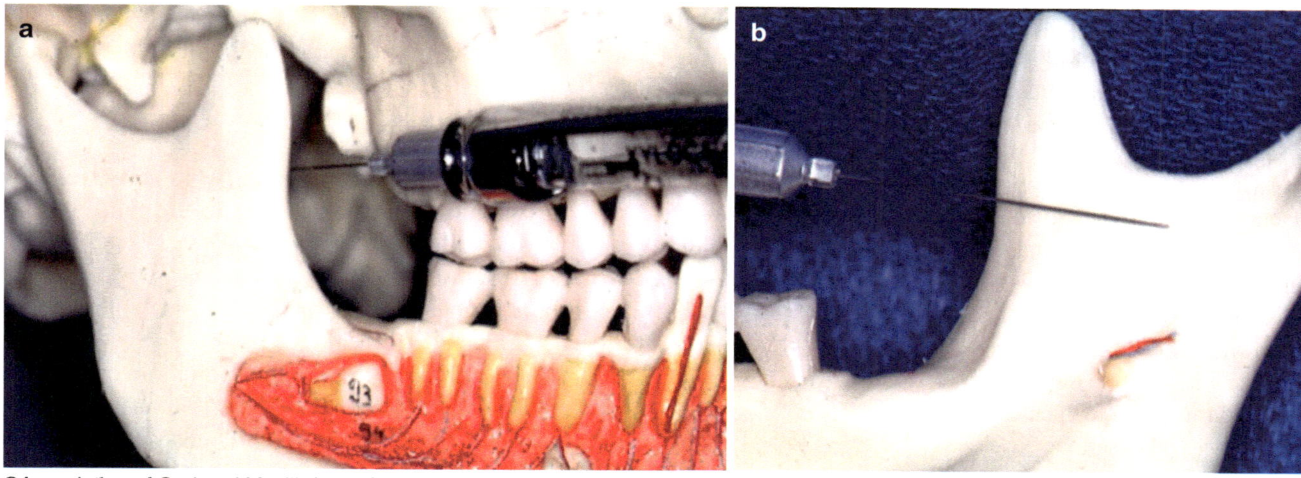



**Fig. 5.3** (**a**, **b**) Position of needle from medial and lateral aspect in case of closed-mouth technique

### 5.14.2 Areas Anesthetized

*Mental Nerve Block*: Buccal mucosa and gingiva in the mandible anterior to the premolar area, lower lip mucosa, and skin on the same side.

*Incisive Nerve Block*: In addition to the aforementioned structures, mandibular teeth anterior to the mental foramen, i.e., incisors, canine, and the premolars (which are anterior to the mental foramen).

### 5.14.3 Signs and Symptoms

*Subjective:* Tingling and numbness in the lower lip on the same side for both blocks as it is for the inferior alveolar block.

*Objective*: Lack of pain on probing with a blunt instrument over the buccal gingival/mucosa in the anterior Mandibular region.

*Complications:* Hematoma formation: If there is bleeding submucosally or subcutaneously, pressure application to stem the flow is all that is needed, with reassurance to the patient that it will resolve spontaneously in a short period of days.

## 5.15 Nerve Blocks in the Maxilla

As already mentioned, in maxilla buccal & palatal infiltration techniques are often followed because they are effective, particularly if the surgical area is limited, e.g., extraction of a single tooth. However nerve blocks are useful at times, particularly when anesthesia of a larger area is sought.

### 5.15.1 Posterior Superior Alveolar Nerve Block Technique

The position of the operator is on the front of the patient for both sides, on the right side, for a right-handed operator.

Palpate the maxillary mucobuccal fold after asking the patient to open mouth partially and retracting the buccal soft tissue with the index finger of the left hand. Insert the needle (25/27 gauge—20-mm length) into the height of the mucobuccal fold opposite the upper second (second) molar tooth. Advance the needle in inward, upward, backward direction with the needle at 45° angle to the maxillary plane for about 10–15 mm. The tip of the needle will now be close to the entry of the posterior superior alveolar nerve into the maxilla on its posterior surface. Inject 1–1.5 ml of the solution after aspiration (Fig. 5.4).

#### 5.15.1.1 Areas Anesthetized

1. Buccal alveolar mucosa and gingiva in relation to the maxillary molar teeth.
2. All the three maxillary molar teeth except the mesiobuccal root of the first molar in some instances. (This may be supplied by the middle superior alveolar nerve occasionally. In this case, to anesthetize the first molar tooth completely, a buccal infiltration has to be given in addition to the posterior superior alveolar nerve block if employed.)

Hence, this is a nerve block, which may be used if multiple extractions of molar teeth have to be done in the maxilla or any other procedure in this area.

#### 5.15.1.2 Signs and Symptoms

*Subjective*: The patient usually will not feel any tingling or numbness in this case.

*Objective*: Lack of pain on probing with the blunt instrument as with any other local anesthetic injection.

*Complications*: Most common problem is a swiftly developing hematoma particularly if the needle goes too far distally into the area of the pterygoid venous plexus.

As in earlier instances, pressure needs to be applied in this case, on the face above the area where the swelling is developing. The sudden swelling can be alarming but is of little consequence once the application of pressure stops flows. Once again, reassurance to the patient is needed. Prophylactic antibiotics to prevent secondary infection of the hematoma may be considered.

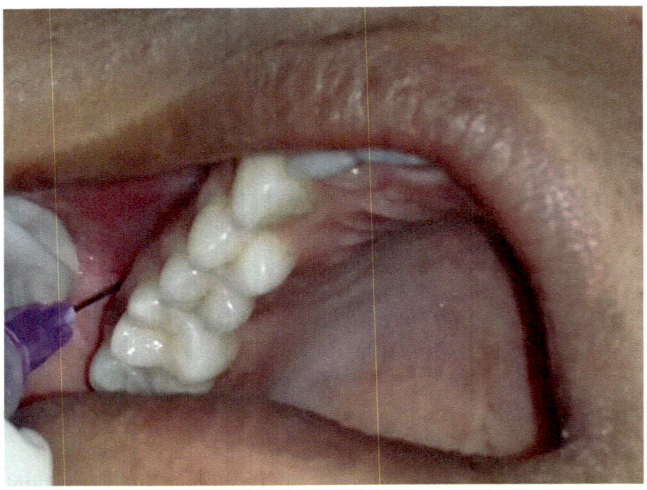



**Fig. 5.4** Needle insertion position in posterior superior alveolar nerve block

### 5.15.2 Infraorbital Nerve Block [Also Anterior and Middle Superior Nerve Blocks]

#### 5.15.2.1 Technique

The operator (right handed) is on the right side of the patient for both sides, i.e., left & right.

With the left index finger, the infraorbital rim on the face is palpated. A notch is felt on the medial third of this region, the finger is now slid down to feel for depression below this notch on the anterior surface of the maxilla. This is the position of the infraorbital foramen. With the left index finger over the infraorbital foramen, the cheek is retracted with the thumb and a 25-gauge needle is inserted intraorally into the height of the mucobuccal fold opposite the first premolar with the bevel of the needle directed toward the bone and the needle being parallel to the long axis of the tooth. The needle is advanced until gentle bone contact is made, and this will be the upper rim of the infraorbital foramen.

Aspirate and inject about 1–1.5 ml of the solution. As the solution is deposited, firm pressure is applied over the infraorbital foramen by the left-hand index finger so as to facilitate entry of the solution into the infraorbital canal through the foramen (Fig. 5.5a, b).

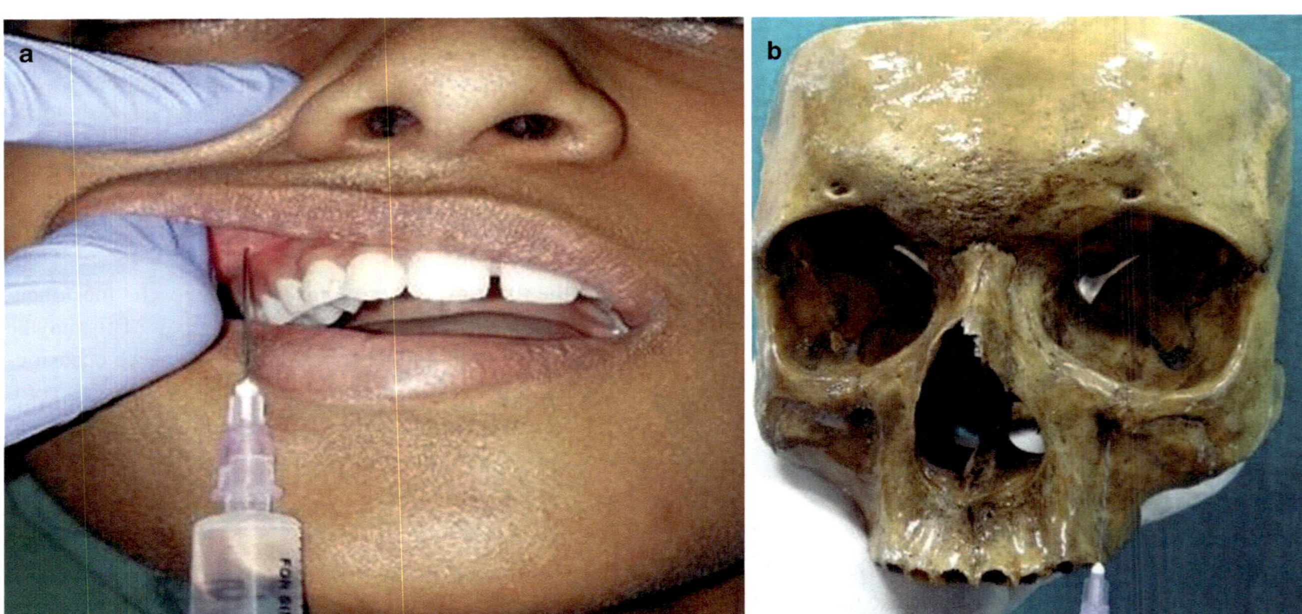



**Fig. 5.5** (**a**, **b**) Position of needle insertion and target point in dry skull in Infraorbital nerve block

#### 5.15.2.2 Areas Anesthetized

1. The lower eyelid, lateral side of the nose, and the upper lip on the same side (This is due to blockade of the terminal branches of the infraorbital nerve after it exits the foramen and will happen irrespective of whether the solution has entered into the foramen)
2. The buccal gingiva & mucosa, as well as the upper anterior and premolar teeth on the same side as well as the mesiobuccal root of the first molar if it is supplied by the middle superior alveolar nerve. (For this to happen, the anesthetic solution injected should diffuse into the infraorbital canal in the floor of the orbit from where the branches, anterior, & middle superior alveolar nerve are given off.)

#### 5.15.2.3 Signs and Symptoms of Anesthesia

*Subjective:* Tingling & numbness in the areas supplied by the terminal branches of the infraorbital nerve, i.e., the lower eyelid, lateral side of the nose, and the upper lip on the same side. (This symptom does not necessarily mean that the anterior & middle superior alveolar nerves have been anesthetized. This can be confirmed only objectively.)

*Objective*: Like always, lack of pain on probing with a blunt instrument in the area anesthetized.

*Complication*: Are few. Rarely a hematoma may develop.

### 5.15.3 Palatal Anesthesia

Injection into the palatal tissues, whether an infiltration or a nerve block, is the most painful. The reason is the palatal mucoperiostem is tightly adherent to the bone and there is no easy space for the solution to flow. This also makes the process of injection difficult as often there is backflow due to the resistance offered.

Most often, particularly when a single tooth is involved, infiltration anesthesia is preferred in the palate. However, two nerve blocks are often used particularly when a larger area is involved

1. Greater palatine nerve block
2. Nasopalatine or Anterior Palatine Nerve block.

#### 5.15.3.1 Greater Palatine Nerve Block

*Technique*: The greater palatine foramen in the adult is usually present on the palatal side of the second molar tooth at the junction of the alveolus and the horizontal palatine bone. (This may be palpated as a depression in this area but need not be done for the purpose of the nerve block.)

A 25/27-gauge short needle is inserted from the opposite side with the operator standing in front (for both sides of the patient) into the area palatal to the second molar at the junction of the alveolus & the palatine bone (Fig. 5.6a, b). A little solution is deposited (0.1–0.2 ml) at the point of entry and

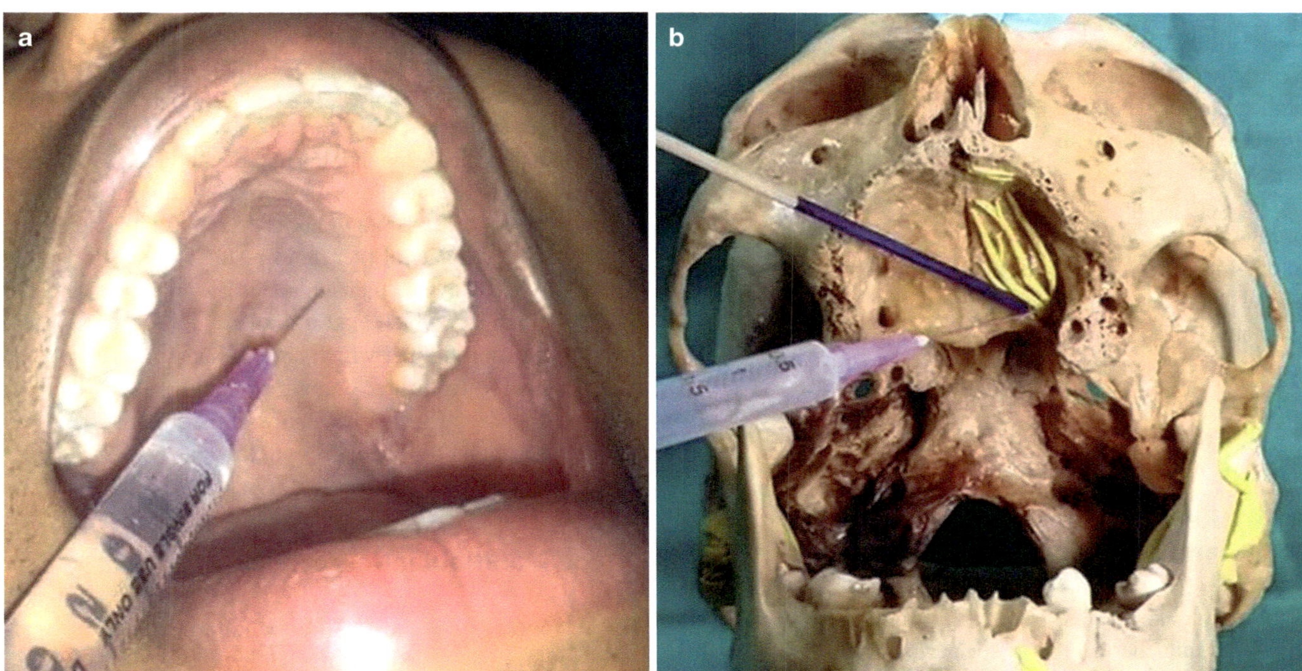




**Fig. 5.6** (**a**, **b**) Intraoral and in dry skull showing insertion of needle in greater palatine nerve block

the needle is advanced into the foramen for a variable distance (0.5–0.7 cm) and the rest, about 0.8 ml is deposited. As *usual, always aspirate* before depositing any solution.

*Areas Anesthetized*: The palatal gingiva of the maxillary teeth till the second premolar on the same side as well as the palatal mucosa & bone on the same side till the premolar region.

**Signs and Symptoms of Anesthesia**

*Subjective*: May not always be there. However, numbness in the posterior hard palate mucosa may be present.

*Objective*: Confirmation of anesthesia is always by lack of pain in the area and tested by probing with a blunt instrument.

#### 5.15.3.2 Nasopalatine Nerve Block

*Technique*: Operator in front with the patient mouth wide open, a 25/27 gauge needle is inserted into the palate just lateral to the incisive papilla. A small amount 0.1–0.2 ml of the solution is injected after aspiration. Now the needle is advanced further into the incisive foramen for a distance of about 0.5–0.75 cm and 1 ml of the solution is deposited as always after aspiration.

*Areas Anesthetized*: Probably the only nerve block, which anesthetizes bilaterally symmetrical areas and hence there is no separate right- & left-sided blocks. The palatal gingiva of the anterior teeth up to the first premolar on either side as well as the palatal mucosa and bone in the same anterior region.

**Signs and Symptoms**

*Subjective*: May be variable if present there is numbness of the anterior palate.

*Objective*: lack of pain in the anesthetized area on blunt probing.

The various nerve blocks discussed so far are the commonly used techniques. Usually this set of techniques is sufficient for all requirements of local anesthesia in the oral cavity. There are a number of alternative techniques, intraoral and extraoral, which are described in literature and may be popular in some parts of the world. However, a couple of them will be discussed here because they may have a specific indication or may be a popular technique.

## 5.16 Regional Blocks in Oral and Maxillofacial Surgery

Regional blocks are fast becoming popular in providing not only local anesthetic support for performing surgical procedures of the head and neck, but also as a method for perioperative pain control in the form of pre-emptive anesthetic techniques.

This section focuses on a few regional blocks, which can be added to the armamentarium of today's maxillofacial surgeon.

1. Maxillary nerve block
2. Mandibular nerve block
3. Greater auricular nerve block
4. Glossopharyngeal nerve block &
5. Sphenopalatine ganglion nerve block

### 5.16.1 Maxillary Nerve Block

There are numerous techniques for achieving total maxillary nerve anesthesia for dental and maxillofacial surgical procedures. These may be divided into intraoral and extraoral methods [27].

The intraoral techniques include:

1. *The "Greater Palatine Canal" Approach* where a 25-gauge needle is passed and manipulated through the greater palatine canal to reach the maxillary nerve trunk at the pterygopalatine fissure (PTM fissure) and
2. *The "High Tuberosity" Block Technique* where the maxillary nerve is anesthetized as it traverses the pterygomaxillary fissure. The technique involves the insertion of a 1.5-in. 25-gauge needle through the depth of the mucobuccal fold lateral to the maxillary tuberosity in a fashion similar to the posterior superior alveolar nerve block. The depth of penetration is about 30 mm and the target area is the pterygomaxillary (ptm) fissure posterolateral to the maxillary tuberosity.

*The extraoral technique* [28, 29]:

It involves a subzygomatic, technique. The clinical landmarks include the area below the zygomatic arch anterior to the articular eminence. This corresponds to the region above the midpoint of the sigmoid notch of the mandible. A 25-gauge 90-mm-long spinal needle is preferred for this method; the needle is inserted to a depth of about 45 mm till it contacts the lateral side of the lateral pterygoid plate. The needle is then withdrawn half-way and then angulated 15° in the forward and upward directions, which lead it to the region of the superior aspect of the ptm fissure, which corresponds to the exit of the maxillary nerve from the foramen rotundum across the ptm fissure. After negative aspiration, a volume of 2 ml is injected into the space, and the needle is withdrawn (Fig. 5.7).

### 5.16.2 Mandibular Nerve Block

The extraoral technique for the mandibular nerve block is very similar to the maxillary nerve block [30].

*Technique*—The surface landmarks and point of penetration for the block are the same and so is the armamentarium. The needle after penetrating the skin is advanced to

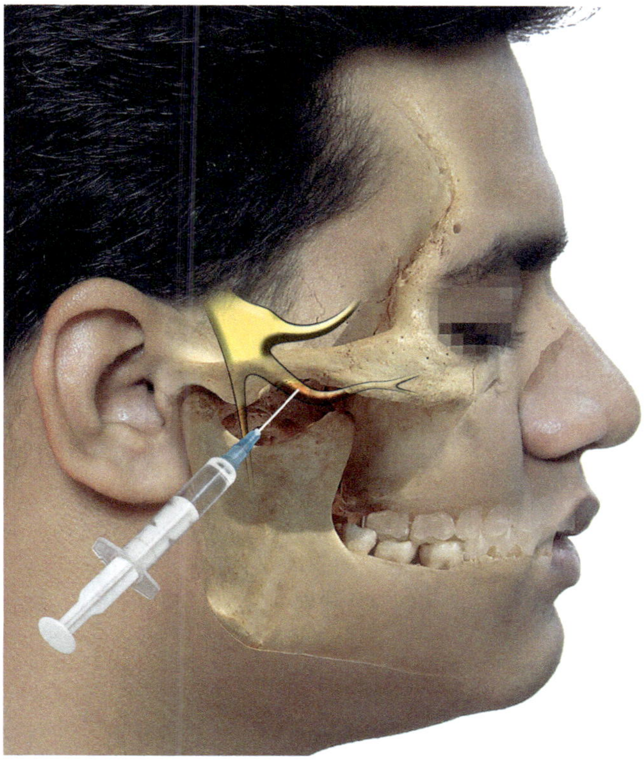



**Fig. 5.7** Representing pathway of needle in extraoral maxillary nerve block

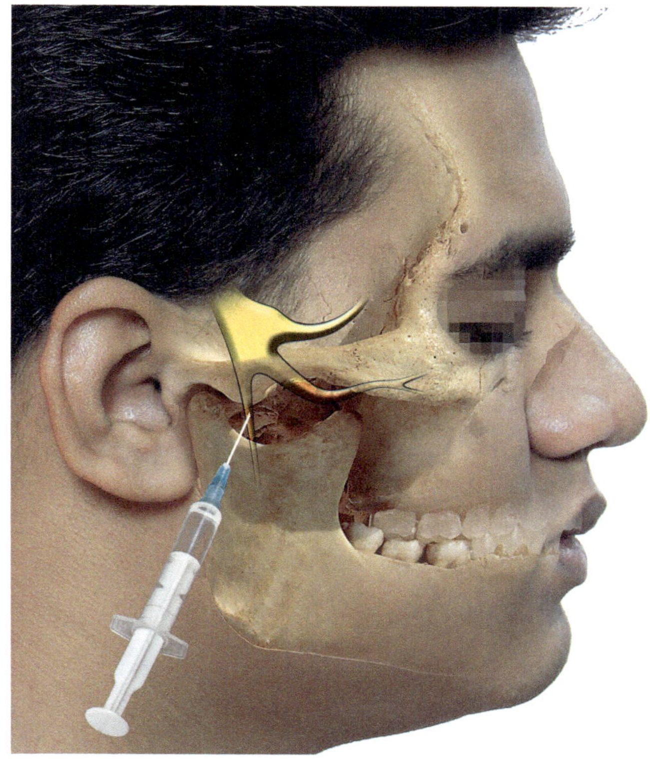



**Fig. 5.8** Showing position of needle insertion in extraoral mandibular nerve block

contact the lateral pterygoid plate as described earlier, following which the needle is withdrawn half way and turned posteriorly by 15° to the same depth of 45 mm. This area corresponds to the region just caudal to the foramen ovale through which the mandibular nerve trunk exits the skull base. After negative aspiration, a volume of 2.5–3 ml is injected to anesthetize the mandibular nerve.

The extraoral mandibular nerve block with suprazygomatic access can be safely and efficiently used with this unique approach for the mandibular nerve block to get relief in pain and Trismus. After local infiltration, an 18-gauge insulated and stimulating cannula is inserted into the retrozygomatic space just above the zygomatic arch and directed to the angle of mandible with medial and posterior inclination (Fig. 5.8) [31].

### 5.16.3 Greater Auricular Nerve Block

This nerve block is performed as an extraoral technique and provides good surface anesthesia to the periauricular skin and skin over the angle of the mandible [32].

*Technique*—The landmarks used for this technique include the cricoid cartilage and the posterior border of the sternocleidomastoid muscle. With the patient supine or semisupine, a line is drawn from the cricoid cartilage to intersect the posterior border of the sternomastoid muscle. This corresponds to the area where the superficial branches of the cervical plexus emerge from under the sternomastoid muscle, wrapping around the posterior border. A small subcutaneous injection of local anesthetic solution (around 2 ml) will anesthetize the greater auricular nerve and its area of distribution (Fig. 5.9).

### 5.16.4 Glossopharyngeal Nerve Block

The utility of the glossopharyngeal block has been studied in indications such as:

1. Excessive gag reflex during oral procedures
2. Excellent adjuvant for oropharyngeal anesthesia during awake endotracheal intubations (blind nasal or fibro-optic)
3. Management of pain due to glossopharyngeal neuralgias and atypical facial pain secondary to Eagle's syndrome [33–35]. The block can be administered both via an intraoral and an extraoral method. The intraoral technique is a relatively easy and simple technique to administer producing good outcomes.

*Technique*—A 25-gauge, 1 inch needle is chosen. The landmark for penetration is the base of the anterior tonsillar

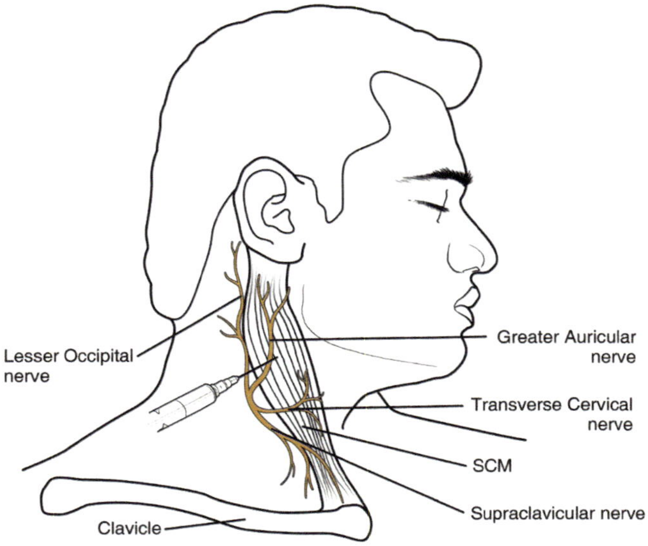




**Fig. 5.9** Showing position of needle for greater auricular nerve block

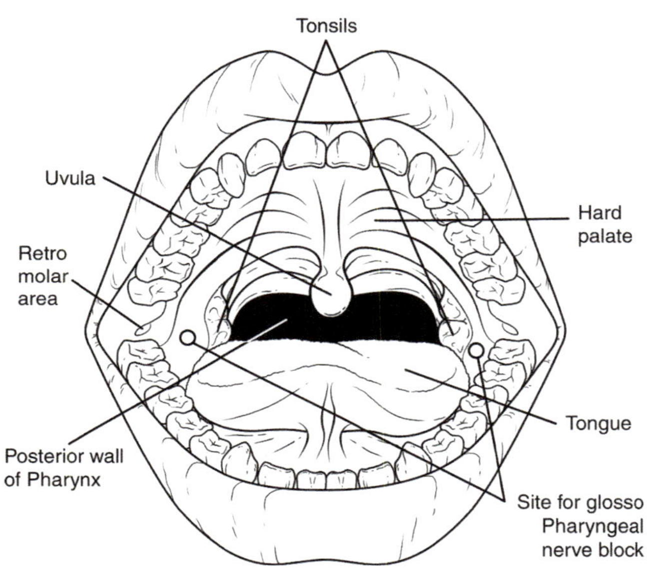




**Fig. 5.10** Target area for glossopharyngeal nerve block

pillar lateral to the base of the tongue. The syringe is positioned with the barrel near the maxillary premolar of the contralateral side with the needle facing the base of the anterior tonsillar pillar. The tongue is retracted medially to provide good visualization of the involved site. The needle is then made to pierce the mucosa and advance by 5 mm. This corresponds to the target site for the glossopharyngeal nerve in the submucosal space. After judicious aspiration, if found negative, a volume of 3 ml of anesthetic solution (2% lignocaine) is administered to block the nerve trunk (Fig. 5.10).

### 5.16.5 Sphenopalatine Ganglion Block

Indications for sphenopalatine ganglion block include:

1. Management of cluster headaches and migraine
2. Treatment for atypical facial pain
3. Palliative pain control for patients with maxillary malignancies and
4. Pre-Emptive nerve blockade for perioperative pain control in surgical procedures of the maxilla and palate [36, 37]

*Technique*—There are numerous techniques for the administration of sphenopalatine block, but the most commonly followed methods are the greater palatine approach and the transmucosal approach in the posterior aspect of the middle meatus. The greater palatine approach is the same as the maxillary nerve block via the greater palatine canal, which simultaneously blocks the sphenopalatine ganglion as well. The transmucosal method, which is most commonly followed, maybe done blind or using endoscopic guidance. A cotton pledget on a long application stick is dipped in anesthetic solution or gel and is advanced transnasally to the posterior aspect of the middle turbinate to reach the end of the middle meatus. This corresponds to the level of the sphenopalatine ganglion, which is a very superficial structure. The local anesthetic gel is then deposited, which produces anesthesia through transmucosal perfusion. Another recent technique involves the submucosal injection of the anesthetic solution into the posterior aspect of the middle meatus for achieving the block (Fig. 5.11) [37].

## 5.17 Recent Advances in Local Anesthesia

Research is ongoing to find newer modalities of pain management. In order to administer local anesthesia with less pain and adverse effects, newer technologies have been developed. Some of them are:

### 5.17.1 Vibrotactile Devices

This device is based on the Gate Control theory, which proposes that pain during injection can be decreased by simultaneous stimulation of nerve fibers by vibration.

#### 5.17.1.1 Vibraject [38]

An attachment, which is battery operated, is snapped on to the barrel to deliver strong vibrations, which is felt by the patient and therefore reducing the perception of pain.

#### 5.17.1.2 Dental Vibe [39]

It is a handheld device, which delivers pulsed percussive oscillations to the site of injection, thereby closing the pain

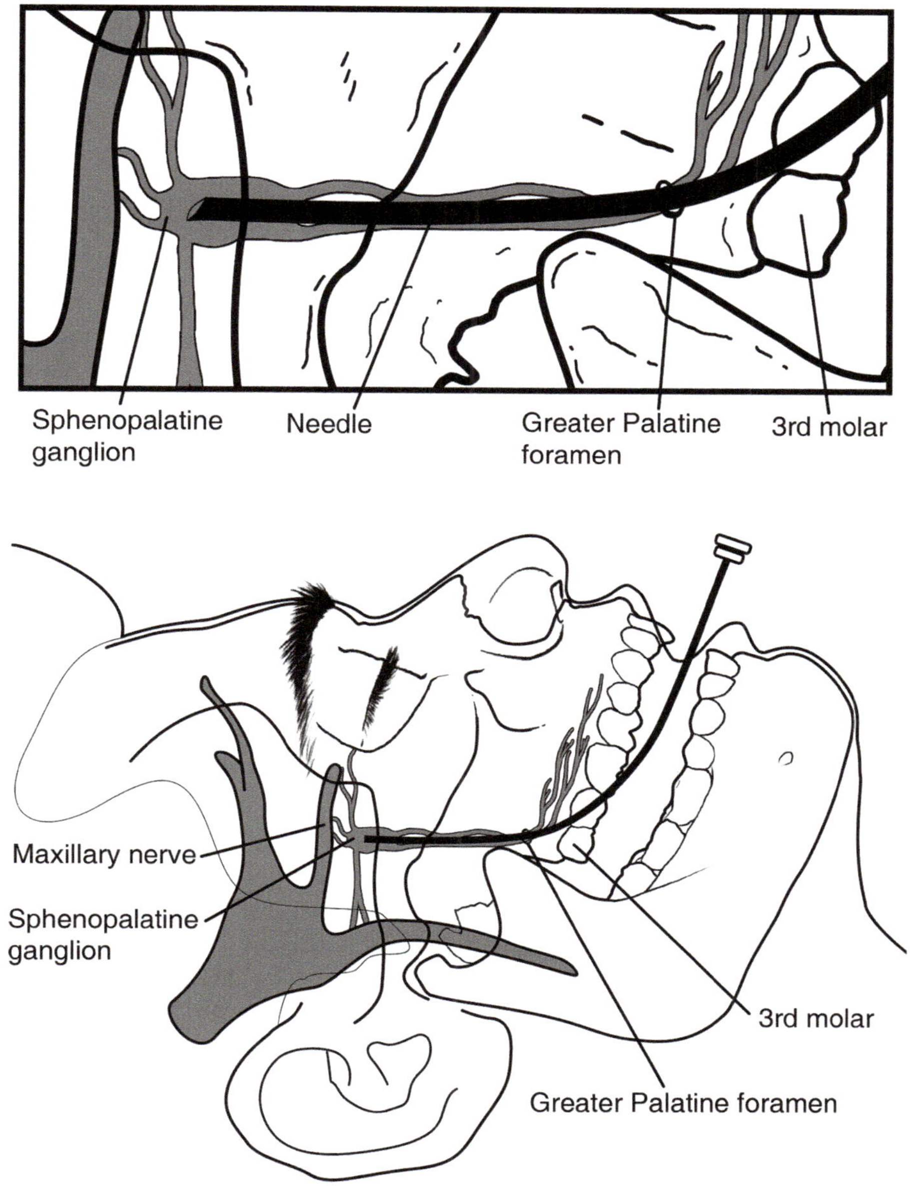


©Association of Oral and Maxillofacial Surgeons of India

**Fig. 5.11** Showing technique of sphenopalatine ganglion block

gate. It does not have a cord and it can be recharged. Dental vibe significantly lowered the self-reported pain during local anesthesia injections compared to a conventional approach.

#### 5.17.1.3 Accupal

It is a cordless device, which shuts the pain gate by preconditioning the site of injection by pressure and vibration. To energize the dental tissue in and around the site to be punctured by the needle, Accupal incorporates the "Pain Gate theory" [40].

### 5.17.2 C-CLAD (Computer-Controlled Local Anesthetic Delivery)

With this device, there is a controlled delivery of the anesthetic and hence reduction of pain during injection. With this device, we can slowly administer anesthesia and control the injection speed [41].

**Advantages of C-CLAD device**

Higher success rates for single tooth anesthesia. The absence of pain especially in pediatric patient with disruptive behavior. More effective than a traditional syringe.

**Disadvantage**—Difficulty in locating the precise site for needle placement.
*C-CLAD* technology led to the development of an instrument for medical and dental injections capable of controlling all variables of subcutaneous injection event.

### 5.17.3 Compu-Flo

Allows instantaneous real-time measurement of fluid exit pressure at the tip of the needle. This approach to fluid exit pressure at the tip of the needle is called dynamic pressure-sensing technology (DPS) technology.

### 5.17.4 STA—single tooth anesthesia

More predictable, reliable, comfortable anesthesia than high-pressure mechanical syringe. The system incorporates the safety of using dynamic pressure-sensing technology allowing low-pressure administration of local anesthetic drugs. All patients receiving PDL with STA device reported subjective pain responses of minimal or no pain.

### 5.17.5 Jet Injection

The principle of Jet injection is that the mechanical energy is used to force a thin column of the local anesthetic solution through a small opening into the soft tissue under pressure without causing tissue damage. There is less or no pain during this procedure [42].

### 5.17.6 MED-JET H III

Local anesthetic solution in extremely small amount is administered under pressure through an orifice seven times smaller than the smallest available.

### 5.17.7 Safety Dental Syringes [43]

The protective sheath over the needle prevents accidental needle stick injury.

**Ultrasafety Plus XL Syringe**
The plunger, which is autoclavable and reusable, has a sterile disposable protective shield. It does not have to be disassembled prior to disposal.

**Ultrasafe Syringe**
Transparent disposable syringe with retractable needle sheath is helpful in aspiration and helps in seeing the aspirated contents in the syringe barrel.

**Hyposafety Syringe**
Disposable syringe and needle, which is translucent with a retractable needle into the barrel. Hence, less chance of needle stick injury. The main disadvantage is that the needle cannot be re-exposed to readminister the remaining solution.

**REV VAC Safety Syringe**
It is similar to the standard conventional syringe, the difference being that when the plunger reaches the bottom after all the medicine has been administered, further push on the plunger will cause breakage of the needle, which retracts into the plunger. It can be used only once.

### 5.17.8 Devices for Intraosseous Anesthesia [44]

**Stabident**
This device can be used with the armamentarium that is available in the clinic to administer the anesthetic solution. The main disadvantage is that inaccessible areas cannot be anesthetized with this equipment.

**X-Tip**
It is a single-step method. An initial drill is placed, which allows entry and withdrawal in one step during administration.

## 5.18 Conclusion

Pain is always a deterrent to seek treatment and hence local anesthesia is a boon to all clinicians and patients alike. Although the medication provides pain relief, its administration has always instilled fear in one and all. The advances in equipment and techniques of local anesthesia administration have undergone continuous research and development to make it as painless as possible.

## References

1. Ouchi K, Koga Y, Nakao S, Sugiyama K. Dexmedetomidine dose dependently enhances local anesthetic action of lidocaine. J Oral Maxillofac Surg. 2014;72:474.
2. Holmdahl MH. Xylocain (lidocaine, lignocaine), its discovery and Gordh's contribution to its clinical use. Acta Anaesthesiol Scand Suppl. 1998;113:8–12.
3. Howlader D, et al. Surgical management of mandibular subcondylar fractures under local anesthesia: a proposed protocol. J Oral Maxillofac Surg. 2019;77:1040.e1–9.
4. Burm AG, Van der Meer AD, Van Kleef JW. Pharmacokinetics of the enantiomers of bupivacaine following intravenous administration of the racemate. Br J Clin Pharmacol. 1994;38:125.
5. Chapman P. A controlled comparison of the effectiveness of bupivacaine for post-operative pain control. Aust Dent J. 1988;33:288.
6. Van Eeden SP, Patel MF. Prolonged paraesthesia following inferior alveolar nerve block using articaine. Br Oral Maxillofac Surg. 2002;40:519–20.

7. Da Silva CB, et al. Anaesthetic efficacy of unilamellar and multilamellar liposomal formulations of articaine in inflamed and uninflamed tissue. Br Oral Maxillofac Surg. 2016;54:295–300.
8. Neal JM. Effects of epinephrine in local anesthetics on the central and peripheral nervous systems: Neurotoxicity and neural blood flow. Reg Anesth Pain Med. 2003;28:124.
9. Vempaty S, et al. Is lignocaine with out adrenaline a better choice for lip wounds crossing vermillion border? Int J Oral Maxillofac Surg. 2017;46:90–1.
10. Haasio J, Jokinen T, Numminen M, Rosenberg PH. Topical anaesthesia of gingival mucosa by 5% eutectic mixture of lignocaine and prilocaine or by 10% lignocaine spray. Br J Oral Maxillofac Surg. 1990;28:99–101.
11. Pere P, Iizuka T, Rosenberg PH, Lindqvist C. Topical application of 5% eutectic mixture of lignocaine and prilocaine (Emla) before removal of arch bars. Br J Oral Maxillofac Surg. 1992;30:153–6.
12. Svensson P, Kolsen Petersen J, Svensson H. Efficacy of a topical anesthetic on pain and unpleasantness during scaling of gingival pockets. Anesth Prog. 1994;41:35–9.
13. Gow-Gates G, Watson JE. Gow-Gates mandibular block: applied anatomy and histology. Anesth Prog. 1989;36:193–5.
14. Gaum LI, Moon AC. The ART mandibular block. Can J Dent Assoc. 1997;63:454–9.
15. Aggarwal V, Singla M, Kabi D. Comparative evaluation of anesthetic efficacy of GowGates mandibular conduction anesthesia, Vazirani-Akinosi technique, buccal-plus-lingual infiltrations, and conventional inferior alveolar nerve anesthesia in patients with irreversible pulpitis. Oral Surg Oral Med Oral Pathol Oral Radiol Endod. 2010;109:303–8.
16. Frangiskos F, et al. Incidence of penetration of a blood vessel during inferior alveolar nerve block. Br Oral Maxillofac Surg. 2003;41:188–9.
17. Jabar J. Should we be giving bilateral inferior alveolar and lingual nerve blocks for third molar surgery? Br Oral Maxillofac Surg. 2014;52:16–7.
18. Singh B. Mandibular nerve block for the removal of dentures during trismus caused by tetanus. Anesth Analg. 2006;103:252–3.
19. Kashyap VM, et al. Effect of alkalinisation of lignocaine for intraoral nerve block on pain during injection, and speed of onset of anaesthesia. Br Oral Maxillofac Surg. 2011;49:e72–5.
20. Vinay M. Int J Oral Maxillofac Surg. 2007;36:1031.
21. Milner QJ, Guard BC, Allen JG. Alkalinization of amide local anaesthetics by addition of 1% sodium bicarbonate solution. Eur J Anaesthesiol. 2000;17:38–42.
22. Gerbino G, et al. Management of needle breakage using intraoperative navigation following inferior alveolar nerve block. J Oral Maxillofac Surg. 2013;71:1819–24.
23. Akinosi JO. A new approach to the mandibular nerve block. Br J Oral Surg Oral Med Oral Pathol Oral Radiol Endod. 1977;15:83.
24. Haas D. Alternative mandibular nerve block techniques. JAMA. 2011;142:8S.
25. Martinez Gonzalez J, Benito BP, Fernandez FC, et al. A comparative study of direct mandibular nerve block and the Akinosi technique. Med Oral. 2003;8:143.
26. Gow-Gates GA. Mandibular conduction anesthesia: a new technique using extraoral landmarks. Oral Surg Oral Med Oral Pathol. 1973;36:321.
27. Malamed SF. Techniques of regional anaesthesia in dentistry. Handbook of local anesthesia. St. Louis, MO: Elsevier; 2013.
28. Stojcev Stajcić L, Gacić B, Popović N, Stajcić Z. Anatomical study of the pterygopalatine fossa pertinent tothe maxillary nerve block at the foramen rotundum. Int J Oral Maxillofac Surg. 2010;39(5):493–6.
29. Stajcić Z, Todorović L. Blocks of the foramen rotundum and the oval foramen: a reappraisal of extraoralmaxillary and mandibular nerve injections. Br J Oral Maxillofac Surg. 1997;35:328–33.
30. Kampitak W, Tansatit T, Shibata Y. A novel technique of ultrasound-guided selective mandibular nerve block with a lateral pterygoid plate approach: a cadaveric study. Reg Anesth Pain Med. 2018;43:763–7.
31. Dziadzko MA, Heritier F. Suprazygomatic access for continuous bilateral mandibular nerve block for pain and trismus relief in the tetraplegic patient. J Oral Maxillofac Surg. 2016;74:1947.e1–5.
32. Suresh S, Barcelona SL, Young NM, Heffner CL, Coté CJ. Does a pre-emptive block ofthe great auricular nerve improve postoperativeanalgesia in children undergoing tympanomastoid surgery? Anesth Analg. 2004 Feb;98(2):330–3.
33. Garg R, Singhal A, Agrawal K, Agrawal N. Managing endodontic patients with severe gag reflex by glossopharyngeal nerveblock technique. J Endod. 2014 Sep;40(9):1498–500.
34. Rao S, Rao S. Glossopharyngeal nerve block: the premolar approach. Craniomaxillofac Trauma Reconstr. 2018 Dec;11(4):331–2.
35. Henthorn RW, et al. Which method for intraoral glossopharyngeal nerve block is better? Anesth Analg. 1995 Nov;81(5):1113–4.
36. Parameswaran A, Ganeshmurthy MV, Ashok Y, Ramanathan M, Markus AF, Sailer HF. Does sphenopalatine ganglion block improve pain control and intraoperative hemodynamics in children undergoing palatoplasty? A randomized controlled trial. J Oral Maxillofac Surg. 2018 Sep;76(9):1873–81.
37. Binfalah M, Alghawi E, Shosha E, Alhilly A, Bakhiet M. Sphenopalatine ganglion block for the treatment of acute migraine headache. Pain Res Treat. 2018;2018:2516953.
38. Roeber B, et al. Evaluation of the effects of the VibraJect attachment on pain in children receiving local anesthesia. Pediatr Dent. 2011;33(1):46–50.
39. Ching D, et al. Effect of the Dental Vibe injection system on pain during local anesthesia injections in adolescent patients. Pediatr Dent. 2014;36(1):51–5.
40. Melzack R, Wall PD. Pain mechanisms: a new theory. Science. 1965 Nov 19;150(699):971–9.
41. Kwak EJ, et al. Computer-controlled local anesthetic delivery for painless anesthesia: a literature review. J Dent Anesth Pain Med. 2016;16:81–8.
42. Lambrianidis T, et al. Dental analgesia by jet injection. Br J Oral Surg. 1979–80;17:227–31.
43. Zakrzewska JM, Boon EC. Use of safety dental syringes in British and Irish dental schools. Br Dent J. 2003;195:207–9.
44. Feridoz J, Raj JD. Intraosseous anesthesia in dentistry – a review. Drug Invention Today. 2018;10:3035–40.

# 6 Office-Based Anesthesia in Oral and Maxillofacial Surgery-The American Model and Training

Payal Verma and Deepak G. Krishnan

## 6.1 Introduction

Anxiety and pain control has been the center of dental health provision from its inception. Dentists continue to practice some form of pain and anxiety control throughout the world. In the United States (US), Oral and maxillofacial surgery (OMS) has maintained a unique privilege where the surgeon is able to provide both anesthetic and surgical treatment for most of the procedures that are completed in a setting outside of the operation theater. The extensive, focused training received during OMS residency in the delivery of anesthesia, as well as continued education in anesthesia is central to this privilege. The art and science of alleviating pain and anxiety by providing office-based surgical treatment using various anesthetic techniques is associated with tremendous responsibility. Therefore, appropriate training along with local licensure, credentialing, and continuous education is of paramount importance.

While the Commission on Dental Accreditation (CODA) of the American Dental Association (ADA) stipulates standards in training OMS residents in anesthesia, American Association of Oral and Maxillofacial Surgeons (AAOMS) and state dental societies have developed parameters and protocols that are enforced among practicing OMSs, ensuring patient safety.

For the remainder of this chapter, the term ambulatory anesthesia would refer to the provision of anesthesia outside of a hospital operatory, such as a dental or an OMS office. Generally, this would entail provision of "open-airway" deep sedation with drugs delivered through an intra-venous (IV), intra-muscular (IM) or inhalational routes.

The American Society of Anesthesiology (ASA) recognizes four stages of anesthesia (Table 6.1) [1]. The most common forms of anesthesia used in an ambulatory office setting are mild-to-moderate sedation as well as deep sedation/general anesthesia with the use of inhalational and intravenous agents. As defined by ASA, moderate sedation/analgesia (replacing the term "Conscious Sedation," which has been condoned) is a medication-induced depression of consciousness during which patients respond purposefully to verbal commands, either alone or often accompanied by light tactile stimulation. Other interventions are not required to maintain a patent airway, while spontaneous ventilation is adequate, and cardiovascular function is usually maintained. Whereas deep sedation/analgesia is a drug-induced depression of consciousness during which patients cannot be easily aroused but respond purposefully following repeated or painful stimulation. The ability to independently maintain ventilatory function may be impaired and may require assistance in maintaining a patent airway. However, it is important that the cardiovascular function is maintained.

Given that the process of sedation is a continuum, the patient's response is unpredictable. Hence, practitioners should be able to rescue the patients whose level of sedation becomes deeper than initially intended. An oral and maxillofacial surgeon is well trained in airway management and advanced life support.

## 6.2 Brief History of Anesthesia in OMS

Over several decades, Oral and maxillofacial surgeons have been at the forefront of anesthesia and pain control among all dental specialties and have been providing safe outpatient anesthesia.

Nitrous oxide was produced by Joseph Priestly and was termed as "laughing gas" by Humphrey Davy in eighteenth

P. Verma (✉)
Oral & Maxillofacial Surgery, University of Cincinnati Medical Center, OH, Cincinnati, USA
e-mail: vermapl@ucmail.uc.edu

D. G. Krishnan
Oral & Maxillofacial Surgery, University of Cincinnati Medical Center, OH, Cincinnati, USA

Oral & Maxillofacial Surgery, Cincinnati Children's Hospital and Medical Center, OH, Cincinnati, USA


K. Bonanthaya et al. (eds.), *Oral and Maxillofacial Surgery for the Clinician*, https://doi.org/10.1007/978-981-15-1346-6_6

**Table 6.1** Continuum of depth of sedation: definition of general anesthesia and levels of sedation/analgesia

| | Minimal Sedation Anxiolysis | Moderate Sedation/ Analgesia ("Conscious Sedation") | Deep Sedation/ Analgesia | General Anesthesia |
|---|---|---|---|---|
| *Responsiveness* | Normal response to verbal stimulation | Purposeful response to verbal or tactile stimulation | Purposeful response following repeated or painful stimulation | Unarousable even with painful stimulus |
| *Airway* | Unaffected | No intervention required | Intervention may be required | Intervention often required |
| *Spontaneous ventilation* | Unaffected | Adequate | May be inadequate | Frequently inadequate |
| *Cardiovascular function* | Unaffected | Usually maintained | Usually maintained | May be impaired |

century [2, 3]. It was first used as an anesthetic agent in dental practice by Dr. Horace Wells [4] of Connecticut. He demonstrated the use of nitrous oxide for dental extractions that was aimed at the prevention of pain during surgery. Unfortunately, he was dismissed due to lack of medical background. His friend, William T G Morton [4], later demonstrated the use of ether vapors as anesthetic for the removal of a jaw tumor. Morton was therefore credited for the first anesthetic (October 16, 1846; also known as Ether Day). This solidified the foundation for the use of anesthetics in dental practice.

A prominent step forward in the provision of safe ambulatory anesthesia was the development and further refinement of the intravenous route of administration. It provided a safe route for rapid delivery and titration of medications along with giving the surgeon the ability to provide emergency medications. The practice of intravenous techniques allowed fast onset and recovery.

Adrian O. Hubbell [5] was critical in popularizing outpatient general anesthesia among OMS. He completed his training at Mayo Clinic and later demonstrated the safety of administering barbiturate anesthesia in an outpatient setting. He also advocated the utility and safety of recovering patients on their side or abdomen postoperatively to prevent aspiration of vomitus. Sylvan Shane [6] later reported on the use of intravenous drugs (benzodiazepines) for inducing sedation known as a "balanced" anesthetic. It was rapidly accepted due to its property of anxiolysis as a sole agent.

Another drug that became popular was methohexital [7] but was quickly overtaken by the introduction of Propofol [8], which is currently the most favored primary agent. In 1989, Propofol was officially approved for use, and its benefits related to the faster onset, improved recovery, and inherent antiemetic activity were soon recognized.

It became evident soon that to continue the privilege of administering outpatient anesthesia, it was important to receive adequate formal general anesthesia training and to maintain the highest standard of care. Today, Intravenous drug anesthesia is the mainstay of providing sedation in the outpatient setting of oral and maxillofacial surgery and has a history of safety [9].

## 6.3 The Anesthesia Team

A majority of the OMSs in the US work in private practice settings where ambulatory anesthesia is the mainstay of practice. This has led to the development of a unique office anesthesia model known as the Anesthesia Team model for OMS practice [10]. This was originally described as the operator-anesthetist model. That was a misnomer because in reality the entire team involved in patient care is trained to monitor and manage the patient under anesthesia in various capacities.

In a typical setting, it is the surgeon who performs the surgery and administers anesthesia. Apart from the surgeon, two or more other team members are present in the room (Fig. 6.1). At least one of these team members is required to be BLS (Basic life support) trained. Most commonly, one trained staff member observes the monitors, records drugs and vitals, and helps with i.v. drug administration, while another member acts as a surgical assistant. Assistant's job is to retract, suction, and irrigate during the surgery along with helping in supporting the airway (Fig. 6.2). Often surgeons employ a registered nurse with advanced cardiac life support (ACLS) training in their offices as well. The entire team is well versed with emergency equipment and is well trained to handle an airway emergency by providing positive pressure oxygen.

## 6.4 AAOMS Office Anesthesia Guidelines

AAOMS strives to ensure that its members throughout the country are in compliance with strict and mandated guidelines. It provides these guidelines through often-updated Office Anesthesia Evaluation document made available through the association. These guidelines are created by the Committee on Anesthesia (CAN) of the AAOMS. This committee uses the latest evidence-based recommendations and guidelines to make this document. This document is then vetted by the ASA to ensure that it gets the highest level of scrutiny and approval by that organization. This multilevel peer-review process of the guidelines is important for ensur-

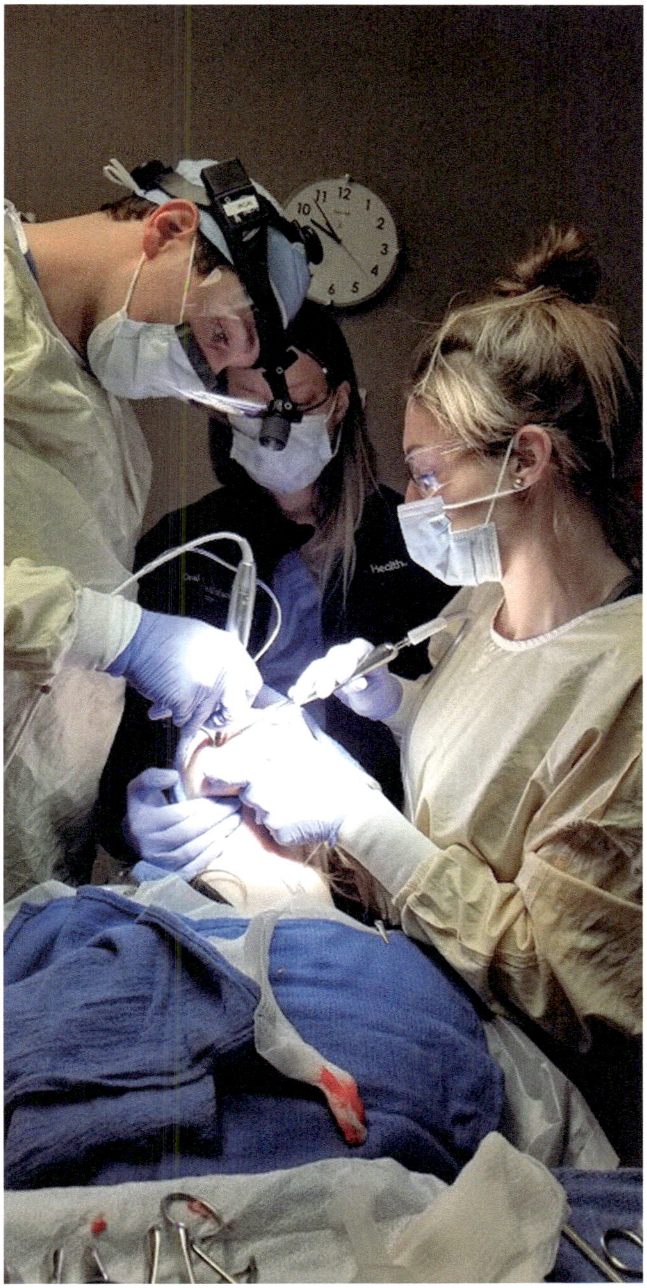



**Fig. 6.1** Example of the office anesthesia team. The surgeon provides the anesthesia and performs the procedure, one trained staff member supports the airway, and a second staff member is the surgical assistant

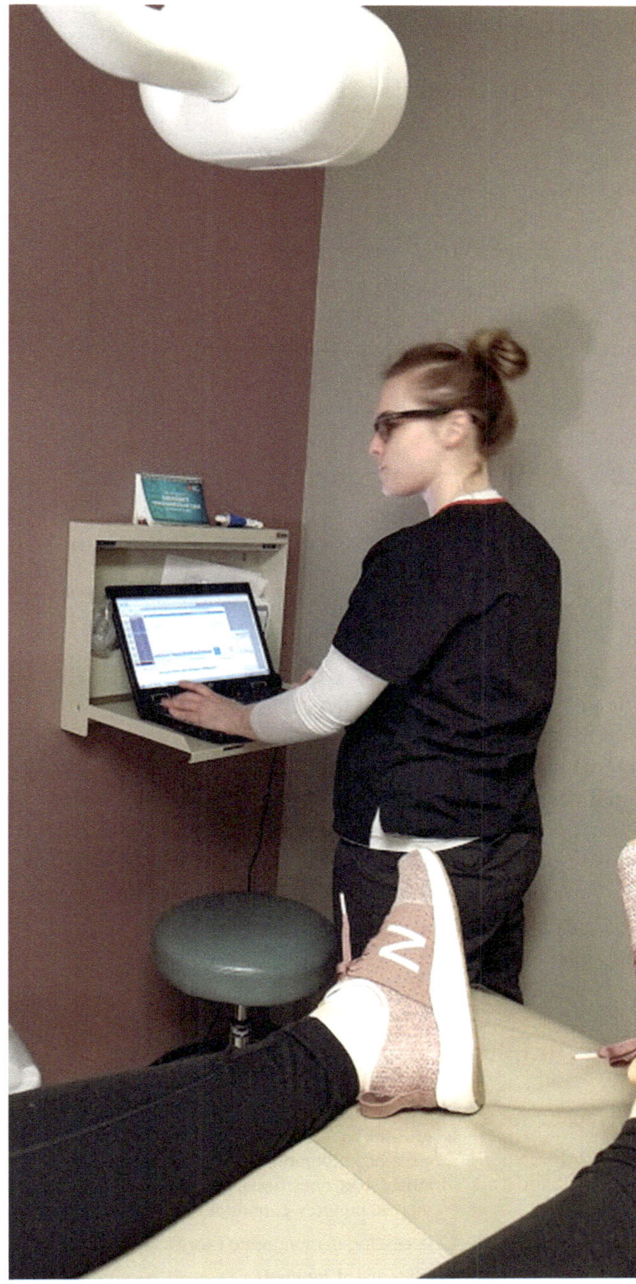



**Fig. 6.2** A dedicated registered nurse with ACLS training is often in charge of monitoring the patient under sedation

ing the safe delivery of anesthesia in the ambulatory OMS setting.

Every AAOMS member (close to 10,000 members) goes through a periodic office anesthesia evaluation process by peers to ensure that each office and team is current and well equipped to perform safe anesthetic practice in their setting (Fig. 6.3). Failure to pass such an evaluation leads to punitive action and inability to perform anesthesia in the office setting until corrective actions are taken. AAOMS, state dental societies, and third-party insurance carriers take this process seriously. Public safety cannot be compromised.

## Sample Anesthesia On-site Inspection and Evaluation Form

Date Sent to Society ______________________________

Name of Practitioner Evaluated ______________________________ General Anesthesia Permit Number (if applicable) ______________________________

Location(s) Inspected ______________________________ Telephone Number ______________________________

Date(s) of Evaluation ______________________________ Time of Evaluation ______________________________

Names of Evaluators ______________________________

______________________________

### A. Personnel

1. ACLS Certificate (Please have doctor's ACLS Certification available)
2. PALS Certificate (if appropriate)
3. Evidence of: one year advanced training in anesthesiology, Fellow of the American Dental Society of Anesthesiology, Diplomate of the American Board of Oral and Maxillofacial Surgery, eligible for examination by American Board of Oral and Maxillofacial Surgery, or Fellow of the American Association of Oral and Maxillofacial Surgeons
4. List of assisting staff's credentials/CV/training:
   a. ______________________________
   b. ______________________________
   c. ______________________________

### B. Records

Have available three charts of patients who have been treated in your office with intravenous sedation or general anesthesia.

1. An adequate medical history of the patient.
2. An adequate physical evaluation of the patient.
3. Anesthesia records showing: continuous monitoring of heart rate, blood pressure, and respiration using electrocardiographic monitoring and pulse oximetry, and ventilation by capnography. In patients undergoing inhalational anesthesia, preoperative and postoperative temperature monitoring, and if the procedure is longer than 30 minutes, continuous temperature monitoring.
4. Recording of monitoring every five minutes.
5. Evidence of continuous recovery monitoring, with notation of patient's condition upon discharge and person to whom the patient was discharged.
6. Accurate recording of medications administered, including amounts and time administered.
7. Records illustrating length of procedure.
8. Records reflecting any complications of anesthesia.

### C. Office Facility and Equipment

1. ***Noninvasive Blood Pressure Monitor***
2. ***Electrocardiograph***



**Fig. 6.3** Sample on site form for periodic office anesthesia evaluation. Available at www.aaoms.org

3. ***Defibrillator/Automated External Defibrillator***
4. ***Pulse Oximeter***
5. ***Capnography equipment***
6. ***Operating Theater***
   a. Is the operating theater large enough to accommodate the patient on a table or in an operating chair adequately?
   b. Does the operating theater permit an operating team consisting of at least three individuals to move freely about the patient?
   c. Does the operating theater allow easy access for emergency personnel and transportation equipment?
7. ***Operating Chair or Table***
   a. Does the operating chair or table permit the patient to be positioned so the operating team can maintain the airway?
   b. Does the operating chair or table permit the team to alter the patient's position quickly in an emergency?
   c. Does the operating chair or table provide a firm platform for the management of cardiopulmonary resuscitation?
8. ***Lighting System***
   a. Does the lighting system permit evaluation of the patient's skin and mucosal color?
   b. Is there a battery-powered backup lighting system?
   c. Is the backup lighting system of sufficient intensity and power for an adequate period of time to permit completion of any operation underway at the time of general power failure?
9. ***Suction Equipment***
   a. Does the suction equipment permit aspiration of the oral and pharyngeal cavities?
   b. Is there a backup suction device available?
10. ***Oxygen Delivery System***
   a. Does the oxygen delivery system have adequate full-face masks and appropriate connectors, and is it capable of delivering oxygen to the patient under positive pressure?
   b. Is there an adequate backup oxygen delivery system?
11. ***Recovery Area (recovery area can be the operating theater)***
   a. Does the recovery area have available oxygen?
   b. Does the recovery area have available adequate suction?
   c. Does the recovery area have adequate lighting?
   d. Does the recovery area have adequate electrical outlets?
   e. Can the patient be observed by a member of the staff at all times during the recovery period?
12. ***Ancillary Equipment***
   a. Is there a working laryngoscope complete with an adequate selection of blades, spare batteries and bulbs?
   b. Are there endotracheal tubes and appropriate connectors?
   c. Are there oral airways?
   d. Are there any supraglottic airway devices?
   e. Is there a tonsillar or pharyngeal type suction tip adaptable to all office outlets?
   f. Are there endotracheal tube forceps?
   g. Is there a sphygmomanometer and stethoscope?
   h. Are there an electrocardioscope and defibrillator/automated external defibrillator?



**Fig. 6.3** (continued)

*Office Anesthesia Evaluation Manual: 9th Edition*

i. Is there a pulse oximeter?

j. Is there a capnography monitor?

k. Is there adequate equipment for the establishment of an intravenous infusion?

### D. Drugs

1. Vasopressor drug available?
2. Corticosteroid drug available?
3. Bronchodilator drug available?
4. Muscle-relaxant drug available?
5. Intravenous medication for treatment of cardiopulmonary arrest available?
6. Narcotic antagonist drug available?
7. Benzodiazepine antagonist drug available?
8. Antihistamine drug available?
9. Antiarrhythmic drug available?
10. Anticholinergic drug available?
11. Coronary artery vasodilator drug available?
12. Antihypertensive drug available?
13. Mechanism of response for dantrolene (Dantrium)?

**Overall Equipment – Facility** ________ **Adequate** ________ **Inadequate**

Comments ______________________________

______________________________

______________________________

______________________________

Recommendations ______________________________

______________________________

______________________________

______________________________

Signature(s) of Evaluators ______________________________

______________________________

**Printed Name(s) of Evaluators** ______________________________

______________________________

10

**Fig. 6.3** (continued)

## 6.5 Office Requirements

The facilities where ambulatory anesthesia is provided in OMS practices are subject to stringent guidelines [11]. Specific building codes and local fire department regulations have to be followed for installation of remote gases. Proximity to a larger healthcare facility and access to emergency personnel are of paramount importance. Recommendations per Centers for Disease Control (CDC) and prevention on controls for exposure to anesthetic gases and other potential chemical hazards, as well as sterilization of the instruments and facilities are enforced. Office's fire safety and emergency protocols should be known by all staff and easily accessible for reference. Telephone numbers of the local ambulance service and nearest hospital should be clearly displayed and their location known to all office staff.

## 6.6 Record Keeping

Medical record keeping is paramount in current OMS practice. For the purpose of OMS procedures, proper electronic records have to be maintained. This includes preanesthesia assessment forms, i.e., history and physical evaluation, consent forms, intraoperative anesthesia records, operative notes as well as recovery records (Fig. 6.4). Anesthesia records typically consist of vital signs (recorded every 5 min), type and amount of drugs administered with time of administration, start and end times of anesthesia and surgery, surgeon and other team members' names, and details of complications and management, if any.

## 6.7 Office Anesthesia Evaluation Program and Parameters of Care

Every practicing AAOMS member agrees to a uniform peer inspection of their properly equipped office and their techniques and preparation for managing emergencies and complications of anesthesia in the treatment of the OMS patient in their office or outpatient setting.

In 1975, the AAOMS established the Office Anesthesia Evaluation Program. This program was conceived, developed, and implemented by the AAOMS through its component state societies to benefit the public, whom its members serve. This ensures a level of safety to the practice of anesthesia in the OMS office, which is often outside a hospital or other healthcare facility. Since 1990, AAOMS Bylaws require official component societies' constitutions and bylaws to include provision for the fulfillment of an onsite office evaluation based on the AAOMS Office Anesthesia Evaluation Program as a prerequisite for active membership. The office anesthesia evaluation is now required every 5–6 years for every AAOMS member.

AAOMS periodically offers an Office Anesthesia Evaluation Manual [12] with the following intent—"AAOMS Committee on Anesthesia developed the Office Anesthesia Evaluation Manual to provide information that could aid oral and maxillofacial surgeons in preparing themselves and their offices for the management of anesthetic complications. It presents scientific and clinical information and can serve as a reference for the practitioner." The most recent evaluation manual is available for purchase by the members in 2019.

In addition, a separate document called "AAOMS Parameters of Care" [13, 14] is intended to reflect practice considerations for 11 designated areas of oral and maxillofacial surgery and is an additional guide for AAOMS members to establish parameters of care for anesthesia in outpatient facilities. The most recent version of this document was published in 2017. The document provides complementary recommendations for the provision of safe sedation and anesthesia in the office. Members are encouraged to review both documents, which provide essential information on contemporary OMS office anesthesia practice and practice accordingly.

## 6.8 AAOMS National Simulation Program

AAOMS recognizes that the provision of anesthesia at an OMS office is a team effort. It expects each member of the team—from the surgeon to the assistants—to be highly trained and qualified to address every anesthesia-related situation that may occur during a surgical procedure. This training is initiated in OMS residencies but is continuous throughout the surgeon's career, mandated by continuing education and team exercised. Similar to professional sports teams, successful oral and maxillofacial surgery teams train as a unit to ensure they can seamlessly and quickly manage an unexpected airway emergency. The most recent AAOMS offering to help the office anesthesia team partners with advanced simulation technology making it possible to train surgeons and staff by simulating a full range of real-life emergency airway situations [15]. This program allows participants to practice and master critical techniques for administering and monitoring office-based anesthesia; a standardized approach that ensures that every participant experiences the same simulated events. The program allows for evaluation of each participant's performance and can pinpoint those areas that may benefit from additional training. The three-module program offers oral and maxillofacial surgeons and their staff an effective method of assessing their readiness to meet an office anesthesia emergency situation by practicing these in a low-risk, high-stake simulation scenario.

# Sedation and Anesthesia Record

Patient ______________________________

ID # ______________________________

☐ Premed ______________________________

☐ Equipment Check Dx: ______________

☐ Time Out Tx: ______________

Preoperative start time: ______________

| Date | Age | NPO | ASA | Surgeon | Anesthetist |
|---|---|---|---|---|---|
| | | | 1 2 3 | | |
| **Weight** | **Height** | **BMI** | **Airway** | **Surgeon Asst.** | **Anesthetist Asst.** |
| | | | Mallampati 1 2 3 4 | | |

| Agents/Drugs | 0 | 5 | 10 | 15 | 20 | 25 | 30 | 35 | 40 | 45 | 50 | 55 | 60 | 65 | 70 | 75 | TOTAL |
|---|---|---|---|---|---|---|---|---|---|---|---|---|---|---|---|---|---|
| Midazolam | | | | | | | | | | | | | | | | | |
| Fentanyl 50 mcg/ml | | | | | | | | | | | | | | | | | |
| Propofol 10 mg/ml | | | | | | | | | | | | | | | | | |
| Methohexital 10 mg/mL | | | | | | | | | | | | | | | | | |
| Ketamine | | | | | | | | | | | | | | | | | |
| Dexamethasone 4 mg/mL | | | | | | | | | | | | | | | | | |
| Remifentanil mcg/cc | | | | | | | | | | | | | | | | | |
| Zofran mg | | | | | | | | | | | | | | | | | |
| Exparel mg | | | | | | | | | | | | | | | | | |
| Sevoflurane % | | | | | | | | | | | | | | | | | |
| Lidocaine 2% 1:100 k epi | | | | | | | | | | | | | | | | | |
| Articaine 4% 1:100 200k epi | | | | | | | | | | | | | | | | | |
| Mepivacaine 3% | | | | | | | | | | | | | | | | | |
| Fluids NS RL | | | | | | | | | | | | | | | | | |
| Nitrous Oxide L/min | | | | | | | | | | | | | | | | | |
| Oxygen L/min % | | | | | | | | | | | | | | | | | |

| MONITORS |
|---|
| ☐ Auto BP R L |
| ☐ ECG (Lead II) |
| ☐ Pulse Oximeter |
| ☐ Stethoscope |
| ☐ Capnograph |
| ☐ BIS |
| ☐ Temp |
| **SYMBOLS** |
| SBP v |
| DBP ʌ |
| Pulse • |
| Resp ❍ |
| Anes x |
| Anes x̲ |
| Surg ⊙ |
| Surg ⊙̲ |
| **POSITION** |
| ☐ Reclined |
| ☐ Supine |

| | 0 | 5 | 10 | 15 | 20 | 25 | 30 | 35 | 40 | 45 | 50 | 55 | 60 | 65 | 70 | 75 |
|---|---|---|---|---|---|---|---|---|---|---|---|---|---|---|---|---|
| ECG | | | | | | | | | | | | | | | | |
| $SpO_2$ | | | | | | | | | | | | | | | | |
| mmHg | | | | | | | | | | | | | | | | |
| Temp | | | | | | | | | | | | | | | | |
| 200 | | | | | | | | | | | | | | | | |
| | | | | | | | | | | | | | | | | |
| 180 | | | | | | | | | | | | | | | | |
| | | | | | | | | | | | | | | | | |
| 160 | | | | | | | | | | | | | | | | |
| | | | | | | | | | | | | | | | | |
| 140 | | | | | | | | | | | | | | | | |
| | | | | | | | | | | | | | | | | |
| 120 | | | | | | | | | | | | | | | | |
| | | | | | | | | | | | | | | | | |
| 100 | | | | | | | | | | | | | | | | |
| | | | | | | | | | | | | | | | | |
| 80 | | | | | | | | | | | | | | | | |
| | | | | | | | | | | | | | | | | |
| 60 | | | | | | | | | | | | | | | | |
| | | | | | | | | | | | | | | | | |
| 40 | | | | | | | | | | | | | | | | |
| | | | | | | | | | | | | | | | | |
| 20 | | | | | | | | | | | | | | | | |
| | | | | | | | | | | | | | | | | |
| 0 | | | | | | | | | | | | | | | | |

| IV | |
|---|---|
| ☐ 22G Catheter | x___ |
| ☐ 20G Catheter | x___ |
| ☐ __________ | x___ |
| R ☐ Antecubital | x___ |
| ☐ Radial | x___ |
| L ☐ Dorsum hand | x___ |
| ☐ __________ | x___ |
| **AIRWAY** | |
| ☐ Nasal Cannula | |
| ☐ Nasal Mask | |
| ☐ Mask | |
| ☐ Nasopharyngeal | |
| ☐ Oral | |
| ☐ LMA | |
| ☐ ET Tube | |

Comments ______________________________ Dr. Signature ______________________________

______________________________

17

**Fig. 6.4** Sample sedation and anesthesia record form. Available at www.aaoms.org

## 6.9 Dental Anesthesia Assistant National Certification Examination (DAANCE)

The practice of office-based anesthesia depends largely on the skillset of the assistants in the office as much as it does on the surgeon leading the team. In an effort to elevate the education and knowledge base of the other team members, a program called the Dental Anesthesia Assistant National Certification Examination (DAANCE) was implemented nationwide. This is a continuing education program that comprises 36 h of self-education and a computerized exam to be completed in 6 months. This course is designed primarily for OMS assistants. Upon successful completion of the final examination, certification is provided.

The course is designed to cover important topics, including general review of basic sciences, patient's medical history evaluation, basic knowledge on anesthetic drugs and techniques, role of anesthesia equipment and monitoring, and covers basic maneuvers to handle office anesthesia emergencies.

This course is available to allied staff all year round to register and complete. More and more states in the US are now mandating courses like DAANCE or others to all team members in an effort to keep the practice of ambulatory anesthesia team model safe and viable in the OMS office.

## 6.10 Anesthesia Training during OMS Residency

OMS trainees in the US have a rigorous curriculum in anesthesia. The Commission on Dental Accreditation (CODA) of the American Dental Association (ADA) is the independent body that accredits all residency training programs. This accreditation is based on a peer-review process that enforces adherence to training standards created and vetted by the CODA. The educational standards for anesthesia read as follows:

> 4-3.1... Anesthesia Service: The assignment must be for a minimum of 5 months, should be consecutive, and one of these months should be dedicated to pediatric anesthesia. The resident must function as an anesthesia resident with commensurate level of responsibility.
> *Intent: The pediatric portion could include Pediatric intensive care unit (PICU), Neonatal intensive care unit (NICU), pediatric anesthesia service, or ambulatory pediatric anesthesia. Oral and maxillofacial surgery residents rotating on the anesthesia service have levels of responsibility identical to those of the anesthesia residents, and abide by the anesthesia department's assignments and schedules. Part of this time can be during medical school as long as oral and maxillofacial surgery trainee functions at the anesthesia resident level.*
>
> 4-9... The off-service rotation in anesthesia must be supplemented by longitudinal and progressive experience throughout the training program in all aspects of pain and anxiety control. The ambulatory oral and maxillofacial anesthetic experience must include the administration of general anesthesia/deep sedation for oral and maxillofacial surgery procedures to pediatric, adult, and geriatric populations, including the demonstration of competency in airway management. Examples of evidence to demonstrate compliance may include:
> - Resident's anesthetic log.
> - Clinical tracking system.
> - Anesthesia records.
> - Oral and Maxillofacial Surgery Benchmarks.
>
> 4-9.1... The cumulative anesthetic experience of each graduating resident must include administration of general anesthesia/deep sedation for a minimum of 300 cases. This experience must involve care for 50 patients younger than 13. A minimum of 150 of the 300 cases must be ambulatory anesthetics for oral and maxillofacial surgery outside of the operating room. Intent: The cumulative experience includes time on the anesthesia rotation as well as anesthetics administered while on the oral and maxillofacial surgery service. Locations for ambulatory anesthesia may include dental school clinics, hospital clinics, emergency rooms, and oral and maxillofacial surgery offices.
> Examples of evidence to demonstrate compliance may include:
> - Resident's anesthetic log.
> - Clinical tracking system.
> - Anesthesia records.
> - Oral and Maxillofacial Surgery Benchmarks.
>
> 4-9.2 ...In addition to general anesthesia/deep sedation, the residents must obtain extensive training and experience in all sedation techniques.
> Examples of evidence to demonstrate compliance may include:
> - Detailed curriculum plans
> - Patient charts
> - Simulation experience
>
> 4-9.3 ...The clinical program must be supported in part by a core comprehensive didactic program on general anesthesia, deep sedation, and other methods of pain and anxiety control. The didactic program must include lectures and seminars emphasizing:
> - Patient evaluation
> - Risk assessment
> - Anesthesia and sedation techniques
> - Monitoring and
> - The diagnosis and management of complications
>
> 4-9.4 ...Advanced Cardiac Life Support (ACLS) must be obtained in the first year of residency and must be maintained throughout residency training and thereafter.

Examples of evidence to demonstrate compliance may include:

- ACLS certification records and cards

4-9.5... Each resident must be certified in Pediatric Advanced Life Support (PALS) prior to completion of training.
Examples of evidence to demonstrate compliance may include:

- PALS certification records and cards

Adherence to these standards is strictly enforced ensuring a standardized education in anesthesia to each OMS resident in training in the US.

## 6.11 Preanesthetic Evaluation of the Patient

The OMS planning an office-based anesthetic is trained to do a thorough preoperative evaluation of the patient to deem them fit for office anesthesia. Just as an anesthesiologist would evaluate the patient for systemic disease, functional capacity and medications along with a detailed anesthetic history and physical examination to classify every patient into an American Society of Anesthesiologists (ASA) status (Table 6.2) [16], every OMS would do the same for formulating an anesthetic plan for the patient.

Ideally, ASA I and II patients are best suited for office-based anesthetics. Careful preanesthetic patient evaluation is critical in choosing the type and venue for the anesthetic. This evaluation has the following essential steps:

- Reviewing and understanding patient's medical, family, social, surgical, and anesthetic history through questionnaire and interview.
- Full physical examination of all systems.

This detailed preop evaluation gives the OMS the knowledge to classify all according to the ASA classification and adequately plan for an appropriate anesthesia technique.

## 6.12 Monitoring

Provision of anesthesia in the OMS office requires that monitoring is done according to the ASA standards and more.

This includes the following minimal time-stamped monitoring and documentation [17].

1. Noninvasive monitoring of blood pressure every 5 min
2. Continuous ECG monitoring
3. Continuous pulse oximetry
4. Continuous end-tidal CO2 monitoring of ventilatory effort

**Table 6.2** ASA physical status classification system.

| | | |
|---|---|---|
| *ASA I* | A normal healthy patient | Healthy, nonsmoking, no or minimal alcohol use |
| *ASA II* | A patient with mild systemic disease | Mild diseases only without substantive functional limitations. Examples include (but not limited to): Current smoker, social alcohol drinker, pregnancy, obesity (30 < BMI < 40), well-controlled DM/HTN, mild lung disease |
| *ASA III* | A patient with severe systemic disease | Substantive functional limitations; one or more moderate-to-severe diseases. Examples include (but not limited to): Poorly controlled DM or HTN, COPD, morbid obesity (BMI ≥40), active hepatitis, alcohol dependence or abuse, implanted pacemaker, moderate reduction of ejection fraction, ESRD undergoing regularly scheduled dialysis, premature infant PCA < 60 weeks, history (>3 months) of MI, CVA, TIA, or CAD/stents. |
| *ASA IV* | A patient with severe systemic disease that is a constant threat to life | Examples include (but not limited to): Recent (< 3 months) MI, CVA, TIA, or CAD/stents, ongoing cardiac ischemia or severe valve dysfunction, severe reduction of ejection fraction, sepsis, DIC, ARD or ESRD not undergoing regularly scheduled dialysis |
| *ASA V* | A moribund patient who is not expected to survive without the operation | Examples include (but not limited to): Ruptured abdominal/thoracic aneurysm, massive trauma, intracranial bleed with mass effect, ischemic bowel in the face of significant cardiac pathology or multiple organ/system dysfunction |
| *ASA VI* | A declared brain-dead patient whose organs are being removed for donor purposes | |

Developed By: ASA House of Delegates/Executive Committee

5. Ability to measure temperature, i.e., very essential in a setting where Malignant Hyperthermia (MH) triggering agents are in use.

Majority of OMS offices now use monitor units (Fig. 6.5) that interface directly with an electronic health record. The entire team is clued into monitoring with a staff member often dedicated to only monitoring the patient.

All patients receive supplemental oxygen before, during, and after the procedure. Most facilities have a separate recovery area with the same monitors, although there are several offices that recover in the operatory. The goal is the improvement of efficacious monitoring to establish the safe performance of anesthetic without the need for a separate anesthesia provider. It is imperative to have a meticulously trained team to allow for continuous monitoring, thus facilitating immediate recognition of changes in patient's vital signs. A properly evaluated and selected patient is unlikely to have a catastrophe in the OMS anesthetic, but when an untoward event does occur, it is often a respiratory event.

### 6.12.1 Methods for Monitoring Ventilation

Data available from closed claims cases from the OMS National Insurance Corporation (OMSNIC) allow us as a specialty to audit the near-misses and tragic outcomes from our offices. The data suggest a strong correlation between airway-related failure and adverse events in the open-airway anesthetic techniques. The emphasis is on monitoring of both ventilation and oxygenation to allow adequate monitoring of the respiratory system during anesthesia. This can be achieved by using a pulse oximeter, which is a device that measures oxygen saturation and provides an indirect indication of oxygenation. Recently, AAOMS recommended a newer ASA standard monitoring of ventilation with continuous capnography. Although chest movements are a reliable method but are least exact, hence the addition of capnography. Most OMSs use a pretracheal/precordial stethoscope (Fig. 6.6) to auscultate while the patient is sedated.

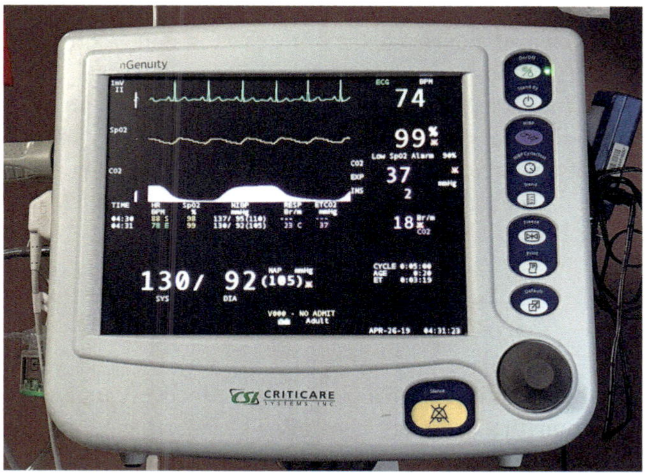



**Fig. 6.5** Example of monitor commonly used in oral and maxillofacial surgery anesthetic administration. The single unit clearly displays the electrocardiogram, noninvasive blood pressure monitor, oxygen saturation, and end-tidal carbon dioxide

Historically, pulse oximetry has been used for respiratory monitoring. But due to its limitation in lacking real-time responsiveness to major respiratory events like airway obstruction or respiratory depression, there was an imminent need to incorporate a different parameter to provide a real-time assessment. Thus was developed capnography [18], which is the noninvasive measurement of the partial pressure of carbon dioxide ($CO_2$) from the airway during inspiration and expiration. It can provide real-time sensitivity to early changes in ventilation and is reliable even in low-perfusion states.

Although, in the nonintubated sedated patient, there is loss of $CO_2$ through the nose and mouth, and thus requires modification of the collection cannula, it still provides valuable clinical information on patient's ventilation during sedation.

It cannot be stressed enough how critical it is to manage intraoperative airway and monitor respiratory status. Ventilation is monitored by inspection of chest movement by the assistants, monitoring of capnography as well as auscul-

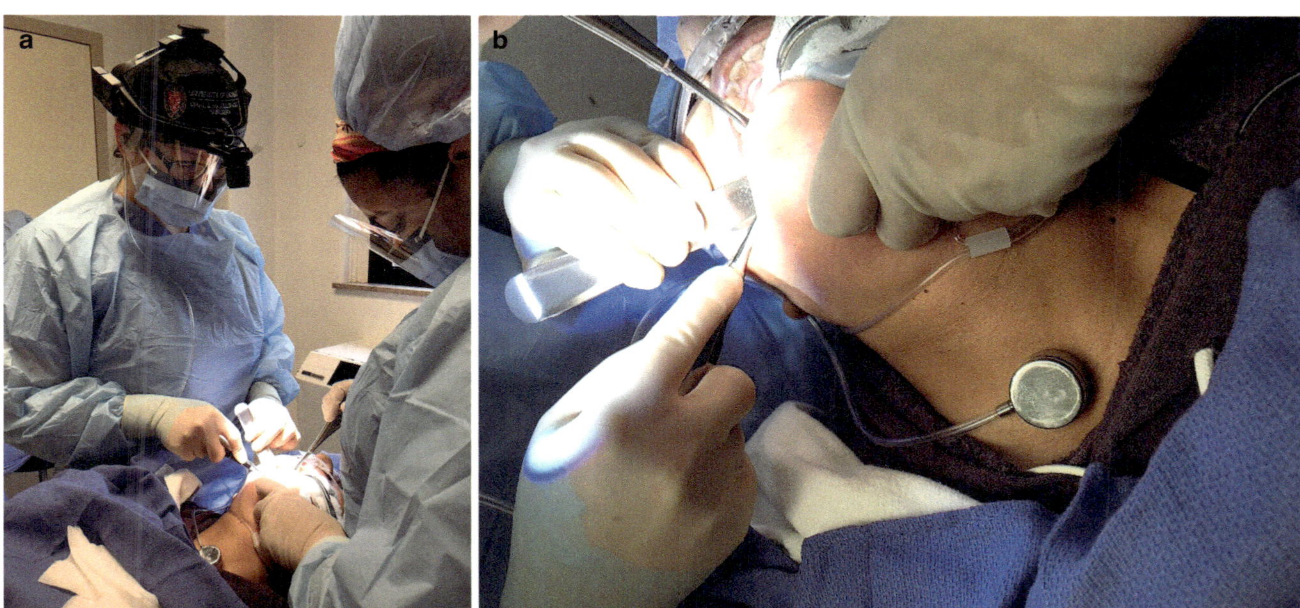



**Fig. 6.6** (**a**, **b**) Pretracheal/precordial stethoscope used by the surgeon to auscultate while the patient is sedated

tation with a precordial stethoscope. The newer Bluetooth models of the precordial stethoscope allow wireless speakers that allow the entire team to listen to the patient's respiratory patterns.

Now with multiple modalities such as a real-time capnography tracing, listening to breath sounds with high fidelity, OMS team has an opportunity to assess and act promptly on potential airway threats even before the adverse respiratory event comes to light. With these available modalities, along with surgeon's experience and developed senses, anticipation and prediction of an impending laryngospasm or bronchospasm prompts the team to act preemptively. Even before a drop in oxygen saturation or loss of waveform on capnography becomes apparent, both the depth and rate of breathing as well as the cessation of breathing can be promptly recognized.

## 6.13 Airway Armamentarium

Despite several preventive modalities available to the OMS performing anesthesia, emergencies are bound to happen. The unit must be prepared to handle airway and other emergencies. All the anesthesia providers should be exceptionally familiar with emergency airway equipment that must be readily accessible in both the operating suites and the recovery area [11].

Emergency airway equipment must include full face mask, bag-valve-mask device capable of providing positive pressure ventilation, oral and nasopharyngeal airways, supraglottic airway devices, endotracheal tubes, and laryngoscope and cricothyrotomy kit. All these equipment should be available in both pediatric and adult sizes. The entire staff should have periodic in-office training to familiarize themselves with the equipment and their use. Apart from emergency airway instruments, all offices are required to have either a basic monophasic defibrillator or automated external defibrillator.

## 6.14 Oxygen and Supplemental Gas Delivery System

In addition to oxygen, most OMS offices utilize other gases such as nitrous oxide and inhalational anesthetics as well as air. The oxygen delivery system should be able to deliver metered oxygen to the patient under positive pressure. A standard fail-safe mechanism along with scavenging system should be part of all gas delivery machines installed in the office. This prevents delivery of any hypoxic amount of gases. To prevent the accidental administration of an incorrect gas, the gas outlets used should be pin-indexed. The gas delivery machines also are mandated to have periodic calibration records, which should be maintained with proper documentation stored at a known location. Anesthesia equipment, including ventilators, are similarly required to have a periodic inspection by biomedical engineers. The OMS office is responsible for ensuring this happens and the office anesthesia evaluation is a mechanism to keep a check on this.

## 6.15 Suction Equipment

As trivial as it may seem, the office suction unit (central and portable) is an integral part of both the normal and emergency functions of that office. A portable suction unit must be readily accessible in the operatory and recovery area in case of unanticipated power failure or central suction pump failure. Again, routine maintenance of the suction system and its documentation is required.

## 6.16 Recovery Room

Most OMS offices have a postoperative recovery unit separate from the operatory that allows unobstructed patient observation. The design of this area must allow resuscitation and management of the patient during an emergency. The recovery area should have a suction system, oxygen delivery system, all appropriate monitors and emergency equipment as detailed earlier. It is also the responsibility of the recovery nurse to document the patient's recovery from anesthetic to deem their fitness to leave the office. A recovery checklist such as the Modified Aldrete Scale is useful in making this determination.

## 6.17 Techniques in Anesthesia

Training in anesthesia exposes the oral and maxillofacial surgeon to the different modalities of anesthesia from light to deep sedation. As described before, levels of anesthesia are a continuum (Table 6.1). The effects of different drugs and techniques may vary between individuals. Patients may achieve deeper or lighter levels of anesthesia than anticipated based on their unique metabolic responses to the different anesthetics administration. The OMS team is prepared to anticipate these differences in responses and intervene accordingly.

The techniques utilized to get to different levels of anesthesia include inhalational anesthesia, oral anesthetic technique, parenteral anesthesia, and local anesthesia. Regardless of the technique employed, the goals of each of these techniques are to reduce anxiety, establish cooperation, amnesia and analgesia, ensuring comfort and hemodynamic stability. In order to choose the level of anesthesia, one should consider the age of the patient, level of anxiety and ability to cooperate, detailed medical history, and prior anesthesia experience.

### 6.17.1 Enteral Anesthesia

Oral or nasal route of delivery of drugs is the least threatening route of administration of anesthesia. While some anxiolysis is achieved via this modality, it is rarely used to achieve deeper levels of anesthesia. Often the oral route of sedation is used as a premedication prior to IV access in an uncooperative patient. Various ingestives such as syrups, popsicles, needleless syringes, other creative methods are employed to get the patient to consume the medication. Dosing is adjusted in such a way that a higher dose of the drug may be administered in a limited volume to prevent the likelihood of aspiration. Despite that, a crying child or a coughing adult may end up aspirating the medication. The other disadvantages of this technique include a slow onset and variable response to the action of the drug as well as an unpredictable recovery pattern. In an uncooperative patient, patient compliance will limit oral or nasal administration of any drug. Additionally, oral dosing is often empiric with almost predictable erratic absorption. Titration of the drug is difficult via this route.

Yet, it remains a convenient mode of administration, requiring very little training to deliver, and any adverse reactions are slow to the onset and usually less severe and manageable. In the US, a medical provider providing oral sedation in the office does not have an increase in their malpractice premiums because of this practice. In contrast, practitioners of general anesthesia have higher malpractice coverage due to the inherent risks of that practice.

An ideal oral medication must be able to provide rapid absorption, must have a rapid onset, and must have a high therapeutic index allowing rapid and predictable recovery.

The following are the drugs most commonly used in oral sedation techniques:

- Benzodiazepines
- Histamine blockers
- Opioids
- Scopolamine
- Chloral hydrate
- Barbiturates
- Alpha agonists—Dexmedetomadine, Clonidine

Oral sedation techniques are primarily useful in the OMS as a premedication tool. An orally sedated patient is likely to accept a mask or an IV for further induction of anesthesia. Several minor procedures, however, can be performed with oral sedation and good local anesthesia alone.

### 6.17.2 Parenteral Anesthesia: Intravenous Anesthesia and Inhalational Anesthesia

Hubbell [5] was known to promote the use of intravenous thiopental anesthesia. It was eventually replaced by the shorter-acting barbiturate methohexital. This became the primary agent used for office-based anesthesia for multiple decades. A shortage in supply of methohexital and an increased use of Propofol [8] in the operating theater setting prompted an adaptation of the use of that drug in the office-based anesthetic technique. The basic technique for deep sedation and general anesthetic in the nonintubated patient in the OMS office typically employs a cocktail of medications under strict ASA-mandated guidelines for monitoring with the personnel as described earlier.

These medications include, but are not limited to, the following:

- A benzodiazepine such as Midazolam for anxiolysis, amnesia, sedation, and hypnosis
- A potent narcotic analgesic such as Fentanyl or Remifentanil
- A potent non-narcotic analgesic such as Ketamine
- A sedative hypnotic such as Propofol. It also acts as an adjunct antiemetic agent.
- Adjuvant drugs such as dexamethasone for prevention of postoperative edema and nausea and vomiting.
- Toradol or i.v. Tylenol for adjunct pain control

Most of these medications are characterized by their ability to have a rapid onset and offset. Medications such as Propofol rapidly redistribute and metabolize and are eliminated from the system. The combination of these medications often results in a cumulative effect of sedation and hypnosis in addition to central analgesia. Discomfort from the administration of local anesthesia is often obtunded by this level of sedation. Patients maintain their ventilation and careful monitoring of their vital signs and protection of their airway allows for smooth sedation. The surgeon who is performing the procedure is in close proximity to the patient's airway understanding its minute undulations and sensing the level of the patient's sedation and acting preemptively to either prolong or discontinue the sedation. It is an art and science that is built on years of training and experience.

The dosing of these medications is based on the patient's ideal body weight. The administration of these medications is through a continuous intravenous catheter infusion with an appropriate IV fluid. Typically, a 20- or a 22-gauge catheter is inserted into a peripheral vein in the upper extremity. Most OMSs practice the bolus technique, which introduces incremental doses of each medication, titrated to effect. Infusion pumps are often utilized in longer cases, while shorter cases of sedation seldom require infusion.

Using a continuous infusion has the following tangible advantages:

- Minimize fluctuations in drug serum concentration
- Smoother intraoperative course
- Enhanced cardiovascular stability
- Enhanced respiratory stability
- Less patient movement
- More rapid recovery
- Minimal drug utilization

## 6.18 Emergency Drugs

The ninth edition of the AAOMS Office Anesthesia Evaluation Manual [12] provides a detailed list of medications that can be used during anesthetic emergency. OMS offices are recommended to have a refrigerator designated for medications requiring cold storage. Pharmacy boards of different states control the storage and distribution of these drugs.

Listed are suggested drugs used in the event of anesthetic emergencies:

- Intravenous fluids: normal saline, lactated Ringer, etc.
- Cardiovascular medications: Oxygen, Atropine, Nitroglycerin, Dopamine, Epinephrine, Dobutamine, Ephedrine, Phenylephrine, Lidocaine, Propranolol, Procainamide, Verapamil, Amiodarone, Adenosine
- Antihypertensive medications: Diazoxide, Hydralazine, Esmolol, Labetalol
- Diuretics: Furosemide (Lasix)
- Antiemetics: Prochlorperazine, Ondansetron
- Reversal agents: Naloxone (Narcan), Flumazenil (Romazicon)

**Additional Drugs**

- Dextrose 50%, Dexamethasone (Decadron), Hydrocortisone sodium succinate or Methyl prednisolone sodium succinate (Solu-Medrol), Glycopyrolate (Robinul), Diazepam (Valium), Midazolam (Versed), Albuterol inhaler, Succinylcholine (Anectine), Morphine sulfate, Dantrolene (Dantrium), Lidocaine, Nonenteric-coated aspirin, Famotidine (Pepcid), Diphenhydramine (Benadryl)

## 6.19 Activism and Leadership in Office-Based Anesthesia

Dental anesthesia is an ADA-recognized specialty in the US as of 2019. Several dental practitioners, including OMSs, practice anxiolysis and sedation in their offices, outside a hospital operating suite and without a separate anesthesia provider. The concerted efforts by various interested parties to politically organize and better protect our intellectual and political interests in the discipline make this practice a reality in the US.

To ensure the commitment to patient safety, the AAOMS and its Board of Trustees have embraced a multipronged approach:

- undiluted enforcement of educational standards that requires resident rotation on the medical anesthesia service
- a self-imposed mandatory AAOMS Office Anesthesia Evaluation Program
- a devotion to the anesthesia team approach and development of the DAANCE program for the assistants
- the development of anesthesia and emergency management simulation programs such as Basic Emergency Airway Management [BEAM] and Office-Based Crisis Management [OBCM] are some examples of some of this commitment.

The AAOMS developed an Anesthesia Safety Conference for our own specialty that was held on April 27, 2017, at the American Society of Anesthesiologists headquarters in Schaumburg, Illinois. Representatives of the ASA as well as representatives of the appropriate disciplines of dentistry attended this meeting. In April 2019, a second patient safety conference focusing on pediatric sedation was organized at the AAOMS headquarters in Rosemont, Illinois.

By staying on the forefront of office-based anesthesia and by enforcing the highest standards of safety in patient care, OMS as a specialty has become stalwart in this arena. Continued positive momentum with nationwide simulation workshops and a mobile application supporting the office anesthesia evaluation will enhance our role as leaders in ambulatory anesthesia in our offices. The rapid response and emergency system and the healthcare infrastructure in the US allows for OMSs in this country to adapt this technique and methodology into their practices almost effortlessly. In other parts of the world, this may not be a model that is easy to replicate.

## Video Links

https://myoms.org/procedures/anesthesia

## References

1. American Society of Anesthesiologists (ASA). Continuum of depth of sedation: definition of general anesthesia and levels of sedation/analgesia. (Approved by the ASA House of Delegates on October 13, 1999 and last amended on October 15, 2014). Available at: https://www.asahq.org/standards-and-guidelines/continuum-of-

depth-of-sedation-definition-of-general-anesthesia-and-levels-of-sedationanalgesia
2. Bicentenary of nitrous oxide. Br Med J. 1972 May 13;2(5810):367-368. PubMed PMID: 4554156; PubMed Central PMCID: PMC1788276.
3. West JB. Humphry Davy, nitrous oxide, the pneumatic institution, and the royal institution. Am J Physiol Lung Cell Mol Physiol 2014 Nov 1;307(9):L661-L667.
4. Desai MS, Desai SP. Discovery of modern anesthesia: a counterfactual narrative about Crawford W. long, Horace Wells, Charles T. Jackson, and William T. G. Morton. AANA J 2015 Dec;83(6):410-415. PubMed PMID: 26742335.
5. Hubbell AO, Adams CR. Intravenous anesthesia for dental surgery with sodium ethyl (1-Methylbutyl) Thiobarbituric acid. J ADA. 1940;27(8):1186–91.
6. Shane SM. Intravenous amnesia for total dentistry in one sitting. J Oral Surg 1966 Jan;24(1):27-32. PubMed PMID: 5214559.
7. Lieblich SE. Methohexital versus propofol for outpatient anesthesia. Part I: Methohexital is superior. J Oral Maxillofac Surg 1995 Jul;53(7):811-815. Review. PubMed PMID: 7595796.
8. Dembo JB. Methohexital versus propofol for outpatient anesthesia. Part II: Propofol is superior. J Oral Maxillofac Surg 1995 Jul;53(7):816-820. Review. PubMed PMID: 7595797.
9. Lieblich S. Providing anesthesia in the Oral and maxillofacial surgery office: a look Back, where we are now and a look ahead. J Oral Maxillofac Surg 2018 May;76(5):917-925. Review.
10. Drew SJ. Oral and maxillofacial surgery team anesthesia model and anesthesia assistant training. Oral Maxillofac Surg Clin North Am 2018 May;30(2):145-153. Review.
11. Chung WL. Anesthesia equipment for the oral and maxillofacial surgery practice. Oral Maxillofac Surg Clin North Am 2013 Aug;25(3):373-383.
12. American Association of Oral and Maxillofacial Surgeons (AAOMS). Office anesthesia evaluation manual. 9th edition. 2018. Available at: http://www.aaoms.org.
13. American Association of Oral and Maxillofacial Surgeons (AAOMS). Parameters of Care: AAOMS Clinical Practice Guidelines for Oral and Maxillofacial Surgery (AAOMS ParCare) Sixth Edition 2017. Patient assessment. Available at: https://www.aaoms.org/images/uploads/pdfs/parcare_assessment.pdf
14. American Association of Oral and Maxillofacial Surgeons (AAOMS). Parameters of Care: AAOMS Clinical Practice Guidelines for Oral and Maxillofacial Surgery (AAOMS ParCare) Sixth Edition 2017. Anesthesia in outpatient facilities. Available at: https://www.joms.org/article/S0278-2391(17)30488-3/pdf
15. Todd DW, Schaefer JJ 3rd. The American Association of Oral and Maxillofacial Surgeons Simulation Program. Oral Maxillofac Surg Clin North Am 2018 May;30(2):195-206. Review.
16. ASA Physical Status Classification System. Developed By: ASA House of Delegates/Executive Committee, Last Amended: October 15, 2014 (original approval: October 15, 2014). Available at: https://www.asahq.org/standards-and-guidelines/asa-physical-status-classification-system.
17. American Society of Anesthesiologists (ASA). Standards for basic anesthetic monitoring. Developed By: Committee on Standards and Practice Parameters (CSPP) Last Amended: October 28, 2015 (original approval: October 21, 1986). Available at: https://www.asahq.org/standards-and-guidelines/standards-for-basic-anesthetic-monitoring.
18. Farish SE, Garcia PS. Capnography primer for Oral and maxillofacial surgery: review and technical considerations. J Anesth Clin Res 2013 Mar 18;4(3):295. PubMed PMID: 24459603; PubMed Central PMCID: PMC3897173.

## Additional Reading

White Paper by American Association of Oral and Maxillofacial Surgeons (AAOMS). Office-Based Anesthesia Provided by the Oral and Maxillofacial Surgeon. 2016. Available at: https://www.aaoms.org/docs/govt_affairs/advocacy_white_papers/advocacy_office_based_anesthesia_whitepaper.pdf

# Anaesthesia for Maxillo Facial Surgery

7

Rebecca Jacob, Subramanyam S. Mahankali, Renita Maria, Suman Ananathanarayana, Garima Sharma, and Mary Thomas

## 7.1 Introduction

Maxillofacial surgery encompasses a wide range of procedures on the head and neck, combining oral and facial procedures with the ear, nose and throat (ENT), plastic surgery, neurosurgery and base of skull specialities. It ranges from simple dental extractions to complex reconstructive and free flap surgery.

Patients of all age groups may present for maxillofacial surgery. The main issues involve managing a shared airway; providing good access to head, neck and oral cavity. The management of difficult airways and measures to reduce tissue bleeding and oedema, both intra- and post-operatively pose a unique challenge to the anaesthetist. Good communication between all members of the team is essential [1].

## 7.2 Preoperative Assessment

All patients should be assessed preoperatively and an anaesthetic plan should be formulated as these patients may have a suspected or a known difficult airway or are undergoing complex or prolonged surgery. Patients may give the history of poor oral intake and nutritional state due to pain, dysphagia and odynophagia. If dyspnoea is present, it should be evaluated as to whether it is cardiac or respiratory in origin.

Previous surgeries, medication history and comorbidities diagnosed earlier should be noted. Medication history is important in all patients, especially elderly patients with cardiac, respiratory or renal involvement. It is also important to ascertain whether the patients have any comorbid ailments like hypertension, diabetes, thyrotoxicosis or myxoedema, a history of epistaxis or bleeding tendency and use of anticoagulants [2, 3].

### 7.2.1 Patients on anticoagulants

Patients on anticoagulants may present for emergency or elective surgery. The type of anticoagulant the patient is on should be noted during pre-operative assessment. Risk of peri-operative bleeding versus thrombosis on discontinuation of anticoagulants should be stratified and accordingly discontinued or bridged with preferably unfractionated heparin or low-molecular-weight heparin prior to elective surgery. Usually, three half-lives ($T_{1/2}$) discontinuation of anticoagulants prior to surgery is considered optimal to prevent blood loss (Table 7.1) [3].

In emergency situations, the main goals are discontinuation of anticoagulation, delaying semi-urgent procedures as appropriate and employment of reversal strategies like plate-

**Table 7.1** Recommendations for discontinuation of anticoagulation prior to elective surgery

| Drug | Time of discontinuation |
|---|---|
| Warfarin | 5 days |
| Factor Xa inhibitors | > 24 h |
| Rivaroxaban | ROCKET AF ≥ 3 days |
| Apixaban | Low bleed risk ≥24 h<br>High bleed risk ≥48 h |
| Low-molecular-weight heparin | 12 h |
| Prophylactic | 24 h |
| Therapeutic dose | |

American College of Chest Physician 2012 Guidelines published in Chest, the RE-LY trial published in Circulation 2014, the ROCKET AF trial, and the manufacturer's recommendations

**Electronic Supplementary Material** The online version of this chapter (https://doi.org/10.1007/978-981-15-1346-6_7) contains supplementary material, which is available to authorized users.

R. Jacob (✉) · S. S. Mahankali · R. Maria · S. Ananathanarayana · G. Sharma
Department of Anesthesiology, Columbia Asia Referral Hospital, Yeshwantpur, Bangalore, Karnataka, India

M. Thomas
Department of Anesthesiology, Regional Cancer Centre, Medical College Campus, Thiruvananthapuram, Kerala, India



K. Bonanthaya et al. (eds.), *Oral and Maxillofacial Surgery for the Clinician*, https://doi.org/10.1007/978-981-15-1346-6_7

let transfusions, fresh frozen plasma, vitamin K antagonists, and prothrombin complex concentrates.

The previous anaesthetic charts should be reviewed for the techniques used, ease of mask ventilation, best direct laryngoscopy grade, Endotracheal tube (ETT) size used, and any difficulties encountered and should be noted. The airway of previously operated patients may be altered due to previous surgeries and/or oedema, so this should be taken into account while reviewing the anaesthetic and follow-up records of the patient. If nasal intubation is required, one should enquire about nostril patency (history of nasal polyps or deviated septum). Contraindications to the use of controlled hypotension, e.g. cerebrovascular, reno-vascular and moderate-to-severe coronary artery disease should also be assessed. Specific attention should be given to the needs of each class of patient.

### 7.2.2 Oncology Patients

Patients with head and neck cancer sometimes constitute the most challenging patients. Their upper airway may be seriously distorted, and they may have tracheal stenosis or hardening and fixation of the soft tissues due to radiotherapy.

In these patients, documents concerning previous surgeries, radiation and chemotherapy should be studied. The difficult airway may have been encountered, tracheostomy and residual tracheal stenosis, limited mouth opening, and neck extension may have been recorded [4].

Symptoms such as hoarse voice, stridor, and dyspnoea will indicate whether there is airway compromise due to stenosis, tumour, nerve damage or oedema. Post radiation, the patients may have tissue fibrosis with limited mouth opening or neck extension. Make a note of chemotherapy drugs, duration and interval since the last cycle of chemotherapy.

### 7.2.3 Trauma Patients

Trauma patients require a thorough history of the mechanism of injury, which would indicate intracerebral or spinal injury. Drug and/or alcohol ingestion is often a contributory factor, and 15% have other injuries. There is also potential for injuries to other organs and massive blood loss. Cervical spine injury occurs in 5–10% of patients with blunt trauma to the head and face. Therefore, the patient should be evaluated from 'head to toe' [5].

### 7.2.4 Paediatric Patients

Consider age, weight, prematurity, feeding, nutritional status and position during sleep. In patients with craniofacial abnormalities, look for associated syndromes such as Pierre Robin sequence or Treacher Collins syndrome as in addition to a difficult airway these patients may have involvement of other systems, such as cardiac, as a part of the syndrome, which will require specialist consultation [6].

### 7.2.5 Toxic Airway/Infections

Infection of dental and facial structures commonly leads to erythema and swelling of tissues. This can result in obstruction of airway and difficulty in airway management. Toxic airways (e.g. Ludwig's angina, dental cysts and osteomyelitis) with spreading infection often present as acute emergencies and may pose an extreme airway maintenance challenge. Direct laryngoscopy due to trismus, tissue distortion, oedema or abscess cavity and pus may not be possible and other means of securing the airway must be considered [4] (Fig. 7.1a, b).

**Examination Table 7.2**

## 7.3 Airway Assessment

A detailed airway assessment based on criteria in the 'L-E-M-O-N' method would help to stratify the risk of difficult intubation. The 'LEMON Law' can be used to quickly assess for potentially difficult airways [7]. A total score of 10 can be given as per the criteria and higher scores are associated with poor glottic visualization and difficult intubation.

Please refer the Fig. 2.2 on LEMON in Chap. 2 on preoperative evaluation and investigations.

In paediatric patients, the Mallampati score does not accurately predict a poor view of the glottis and there are no standard values for the thyromental and horizontal length of the mandible. Thus, an adaptation is required, and this is found in the 'COPUR SCALE' (Table 7.3) [7, 8].

Once the airway assessment is done, check

- Whether mask ventilation would be possible after induction of General Anaesthesia (GA).
- Anticipated view during direct laryngoscopy.
- Whether it would be possible to use a supraglottic airway as a rescue device.
- Possibility and accessibility of a surgical airway in case of a dire emergency.

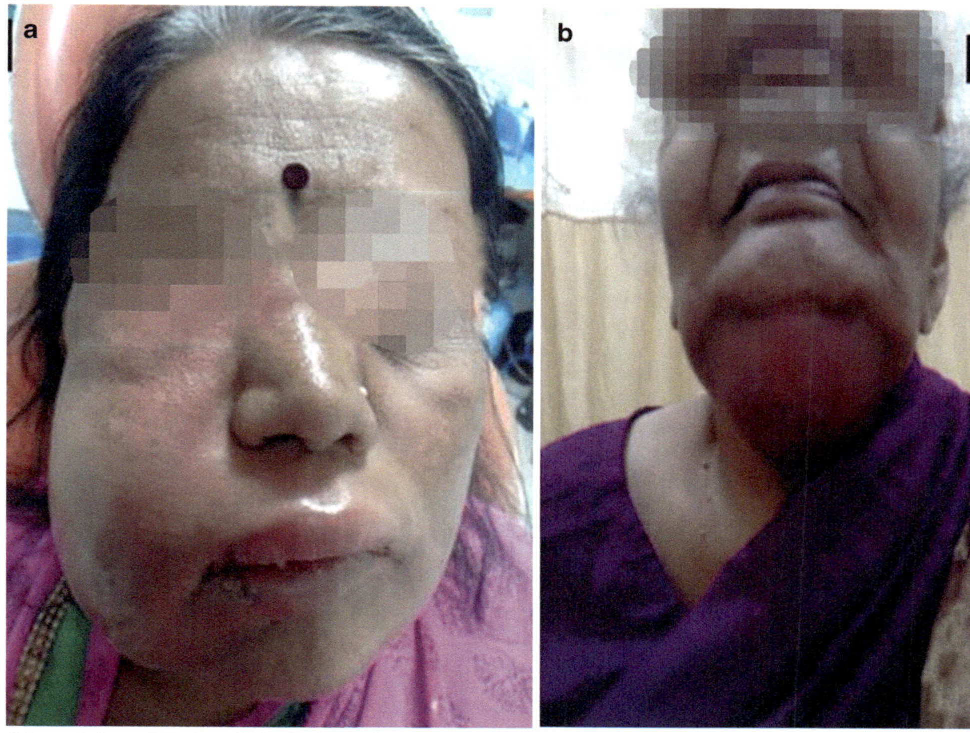


Fig. 7.1 (a) Buccal abscess (b) ludwigs angina



Table 7.2 Checklist of things for a safe surgery

| Pre-Anaesthesia Checklist |
|---|
| • Age and weight of the patient |
| • Type of maxillofacial surgery |
| • Previous surgeries/ associated complications |
| • Comorbidities and detailed medication list |
| • Known drug allergies |
| • CVS, RS, abdomen examination |
| • Detailed airway examination |
| • Venous access |
| • Adequate blood and blood products |

## 7.4 General Physical Examination

Look for pallor, icterus, cyanosis, clubbing, lymphadenopathy and oedema as well as the general nutritional status. Follow this up with pulse rate, blood pressure, respiratory rate, oxygen saturation, signs of dehydration, and responses denoted as AVPU–Alert, Verbal, Pain, Unresponsive.

AVPU is a simplified version of the Glasgow Coma Scale (GCS), which is easy to remember and apply to patients (Table 7.4) [9, 10]. It consists of four possible stages. When recording AVPU, it is important to document the time the observation was taken and to track any changes over time as this will help monitor the progress of the patient (Table 7.4).

Apart from these, specific systemic examination, including cardiovascular, respiratory, per-abdomen and central nervous system, should be done and if in any doubt a specialist should be consulted.

There are various scales used to record a patient's level of consciousness. One of the most detailed is the GCS, which is used worldwide (Table 7.5) [9, 10]. The GCS is a reasonably complicated system, which, unless you use regularly, can be difficult to remember and apply correctly.

### 7.4.1 Investigations

In addition to routine blood tests like complete blood counts, kidney function tests, blood sugars, coagulation profile, serology, blood grouping and cross-matching is required for major surgery.

Chest X-ray helps in visualising any pathology in the lungs. It may also reveal tracheal deviation. X-ray soft-tissue neck, airway ultrasound, computerized tomography (CT), and magnetic resonance imaging (MRI) scans may be helpful in cancer, infections, abscesses or trauma cases.

For cancer surgery, a nasoendoscopy & indirect laryngoscopy provides valuable information about the upper airway anatomy.

Electrocardiogram (ECG), echocardiogram, cardiopulmonary exercise testing or pulmonary function tests are required if there are symptoms or signs of cardiorespiratory disease.

**Table 7.3** Description of COPUR scale

| COPUR SCALE | |
|---|---|
| *C = Chin* | Normal –1<br>Small, moderately hypoplastic - 2<br>Markedly recessive – 3<br>Extremely hypoplastic – 4 |
| *O – Opening*<br>Interdental space between front teeth | > 40 mm – 1<br>20-40 mm – 2<br>10-20 mm – 3<br>< 10 mm – 4 |
| *P – Previous intubation or OSA* | Previous easy – 1<br>No attempt/no h/o OSA – 2<br>OSA, previous difficult intubation – 3<br>Extremely difficult intubation/ tracheostomy/can't lie down supine – 4 |
| *U – Uvula*<br>Mouth open tongue out | Tip of uvula visible – 1<br>Uvula partially visible – 2<br>Uvula concealed/soft palate visible – 3<br>Soft palate not visible – 4 |
| *R – Range*<br>Line from eye to orbit, range of motion looking up & down | >120°– 1<br>60–120° –2<br>30–60°–3<br>< 30°– 4 |
| *Prediction points for ease of intubation*<br>5–7: Easy normal intubation<br>8–10: Laryngeal help may be required<br>12: More difficult, may be less traumatic<br>14: Difficult intubation, fibre optic or other advanced technique may be required<br>16: Dangerous airway, consider awake intubation/potential tracheostomy | |

**Table 7.4** AVPU scale described with examples

| | Adult Behaviour | Paediatric Behaviour |
|---|---|---|
| A ALERT | Eyes open spontaneously.<br>Appears aware of and responsive to the environment.<br>Follows commands, eyes track people and objects | Child is active and responds appropriately to parents and other external stimuli |
| V VOICE | Eyes do not open spontaneously but open to verbal stimuli.<br>Able to respond in some meaningful way when spoken to | Responds only when his or her name is called |
| P PAIN | Does not respond to questions but moves or cries out in response to painful stimuli such as pinching the skin or earlobe | Responds only when painful stimuli are received such as pinching the nail bed |
| U UNRESPONSIVE | Patient does not respond to any stimuli | No response at all |

**Table 7.5** Glasgow Coma Scale described in detail

| Glasgow Coma Scale | | |
|---|---|---|
| Behaviour | Response | Score |
| Eye opening (E) | Spontaneous | 4 |
| | To speech | 3 |
| | To pressure | 2 |
| | None | 1 |
| Verbal response (V) | Orientated | 5 |
| | Confused | 4 |
| | Words, but not coherent | 3 |
| | Sounds, but no words | 2 |
| | None | 1 |
| Motor response (M) | Obeys command | 6 |
| | Moves to localised pain | 5 |
| | Flexion withdrawal to pain | 4 |
| | Abnormal flexion (decorticate) | 3 |
| | Abnormal extension (Decerebrate) | 2 |
| | No response | 1 |
| Total score | Best response | 15 |
| | Comatose | </=6 |
| | Totally unresponsive | 3 |

### 7.4.2 Counselling and Reassurance

This is essential in all cases but especially so in patients who may have dramatic cosmetic changes or are undergoing cancer surgery like hemi-mandibulectomy. The possibility of tracheostomy and loss of voice must also be discussed with empathy. Video counselling may be resorted to in case of need.

### 7.4.3 Informed Consent

Any patient above the age of 18 years may give consent for surgery and anaesthesia. In the case of patients younger than 18 years, consent must be obtained from a parent or guardian after full explanation of procedures. The consent must be documented and signed by both the person taking the consent and the person giving the consent.

### 7.4.4 Transport to Operation Theatre (OT)

Should be with a trained health care worker especially if the patient has been given a sedative premedication. It is advisable for a parent or guardian to accompany younger children to the OT.

### 7.4.5 Handover Documents

All documents pertaining to the case must be handed over to the OT personnel and the handover documented.

## 7.5 Intraoperative Considerations

### 7.5.1 Before Induction (Figs. 7.2, 7.3, 7.4, 7.5, 7.6, 7.7, and 7.8) [6]

- Discuss the procedure and options with the lead surgeon
- Ensure patients vitals are stable
- Check anaesthetic machine and all equipment, including the 'Difficult Airway' cart and 'rescue devices' like Laryngeal Mask Airway (LMA) and tracheostomy tubes.
- If an 'uncommon' ETT like a flexometallic or (RAE) Ring-Adair-Elwyn tube is to be used, ensure that a regular tube of the appropriate size and one size smaller are available
- Ensure you have adequate help and each one knows what is expected of him/her
- Check intravenous (IV) access and all drugs available in the CT—drawn up and labelled.
- Check that blood is available if deemed necessary
- If intubation is difficult do not try more than 2–3 times with any one method (you will precipitate oedema and make matters worse)
- *CALL FOR HELP EARLY*

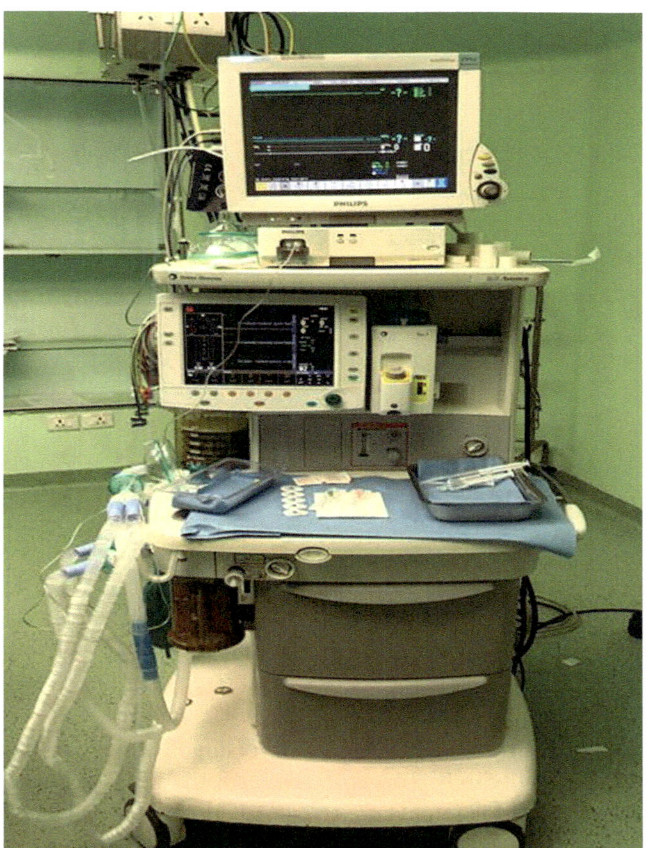



**Fig. 7.2** Anaesthetic apparatus

- Continue oxygenation with spontaneous respiration and wake up the patient if intubation is unsuccessful

*More patients have died from lack of oxygen than from lack of an endotracheal tube!*

*Please see Chap. 42 in this book to read about avoidable human errors for a safer patient care. (A case of loss of airway is discussed in Chap. 42).*

### 7.5.2 Induction

Anaesthesia may be induced either intravenously or with an inhalational agent. The choice of technique depends on:

- *Airway factors:* For example, an anticipated 'difficult airway' or limited mouth opening
- *Patient factors:*
  Paediatrics
  Post radiation
  Trauma
- *Associated comorbidities:* e.g. ischemic heart disease or emphysema.
  Nil-per-oral status
- *Surgical factors:*
  Trauma
  Cancer surgery
  Cosmetic
  Infective
  Vascular malformation

### 7.5.3 Monitoring

In young patients belonging to ASA (American Society of Anesthesiologists) Grade I and II, standard monitoring will suffice. Invasive arterial blood pressure monitoring may be required if controlled hypotension is planned or if comorbidities warrant. Monitoring of temperature is required in children and those undergoing prolonged surgeries like corrective LeFort osteotomies. Urinary catheterization may be required during prolonged surgeries.

### 7.5.4 *Airway management:* (Flow Chart 1)

The method of securing the airway should be discussed with the surgeon. This depends on:

- Patient factors, such as age, obesity, pan-facial trauma or anticipated difficult airway
- Site of operation may require oral or nasal intubation with specially configured tubes.
- Anaesthetists'/surgeons' preferences.

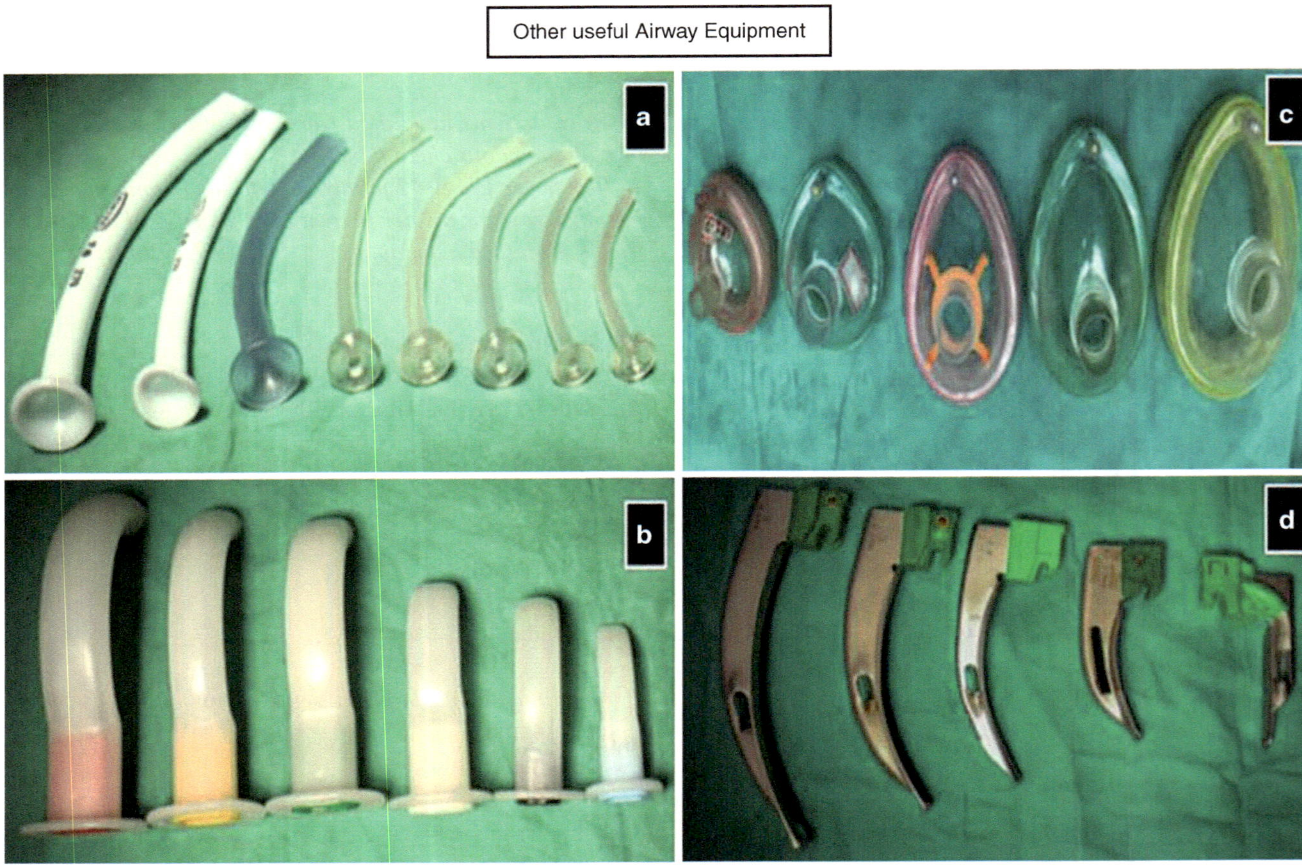




**Fig. 7.3** (**a**) Nasal airway, (**b**) Oral airway, (**c**) Ventilation mask and (**d**) Laryngoscope blades

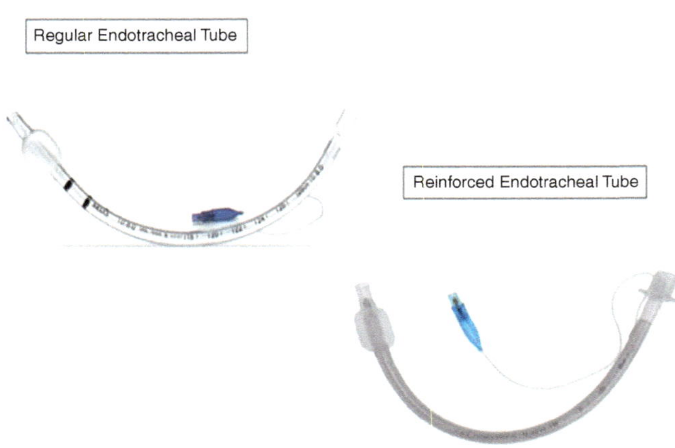


**Fig. 7.4** Endotracheal tubes

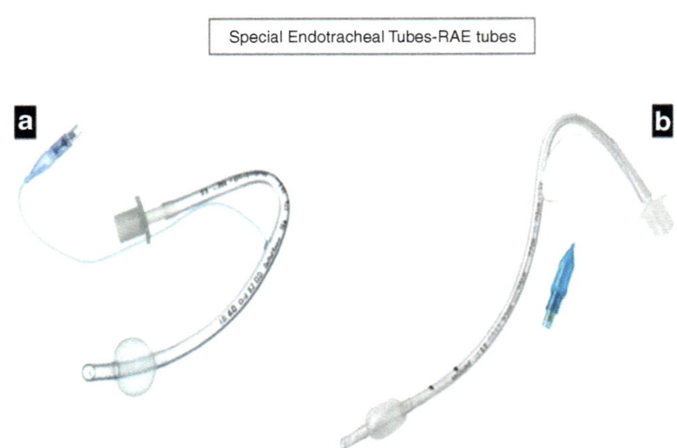


**Fig. 7.5** RAE tubes

Simple intraoral operations with no anticipated difficult airways can be done with standard nasal intubation or oral intubation under general anaesthesia with endotracheal tube pushed to the side opposite of surgery. Use of specially preformed tubes like RAE tubes and Reinforced/Armoured tube can be used to give good access to the surgical area (Figs. 7.4 and 7.5). However, major corrective surgeries will require the oral cavity to be empty and hence warrant nasal intubation, submental intubation or a tracheostomy. Anticipated non-obstructed difficult airway as assessed by history and/or examination or suspected (cervical) C-spine injury should be managed with awake fibre optic bronchoscopy or blind nasal

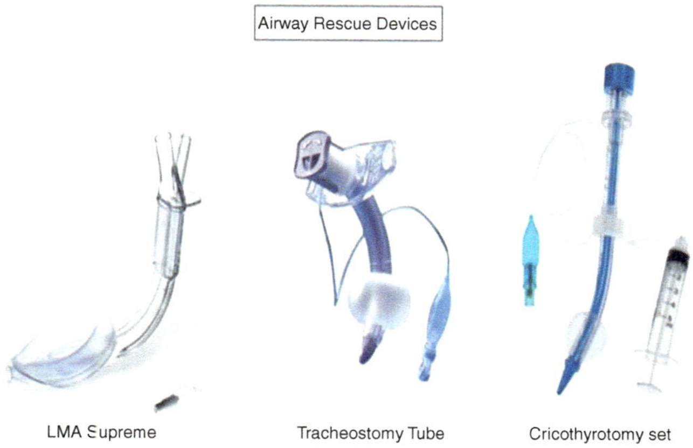


**Fig. 7.6** Airway rescue devices

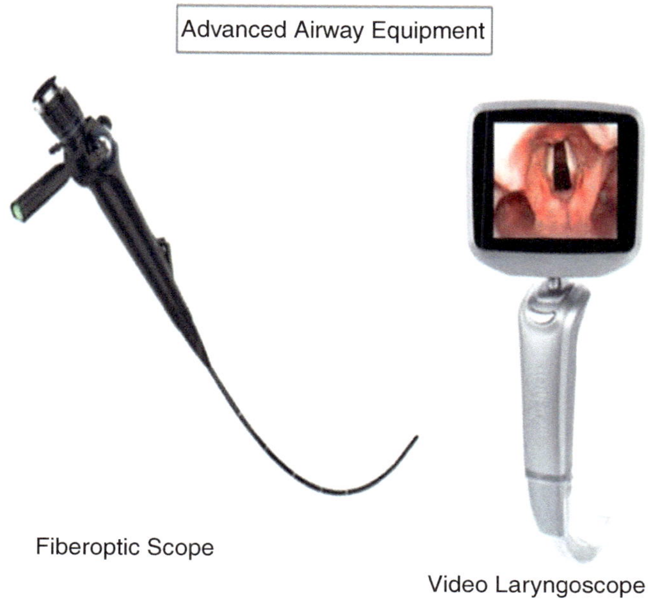


**Fig. 7.8** Advanced airway equipment

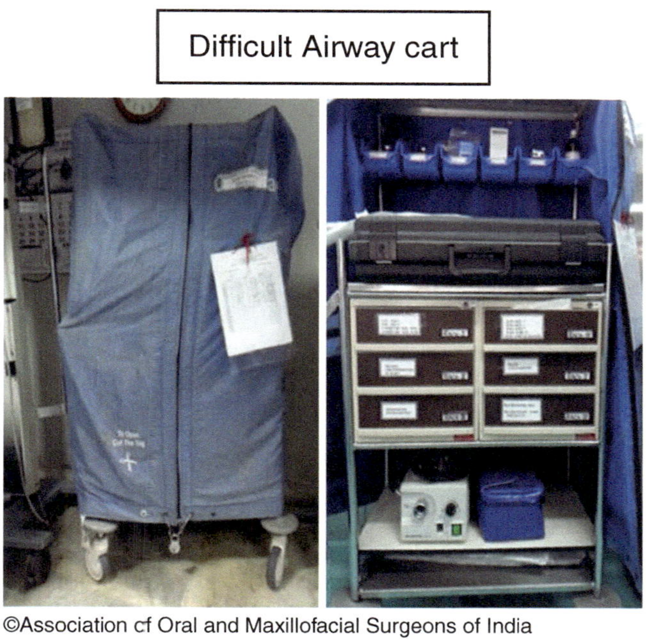


**Fig. 7.7** Difficult airway cart

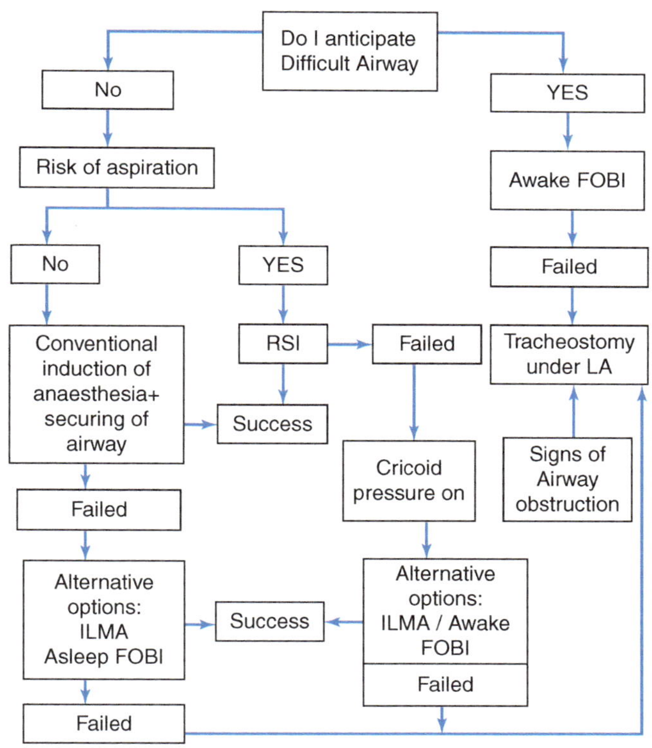


**Flow Chart 1** Airway management in oro-maxillo-facial surgery

intubation. The safety of awake intubation relies on the maintenance of spontaneous breathing, and the ability to stop and perform a different technique, such as awake tracheostomy, if intubation is unsuccessful. Most anaesthesiologists prefer the nasal route for fibre optic intubation, as it is technically easier. For this, the patency of the nostril should be assessed preoperatively, and roomier nostril should be chosen and prepared with vasoconstrictor drops like oxymetazoline hydrochloride.

Sedation may enhance the acceptability of awake fibre optic intubation. Dexmedetomidine infusion [11] serves this purpose very well. Airway instrumentation can be facilitated by local anaesthetic topicalisation of airway either by means of lignocaine nebulisation or 'spray as you go' technique and/airway blocks (glossopharyngeal, superior laryngeal and recurrent laryngeal nerve blocks) [12]. An antisialogoguelike glycopyrrolate administered 30–45 min prior will reduce the secretions and will facili-

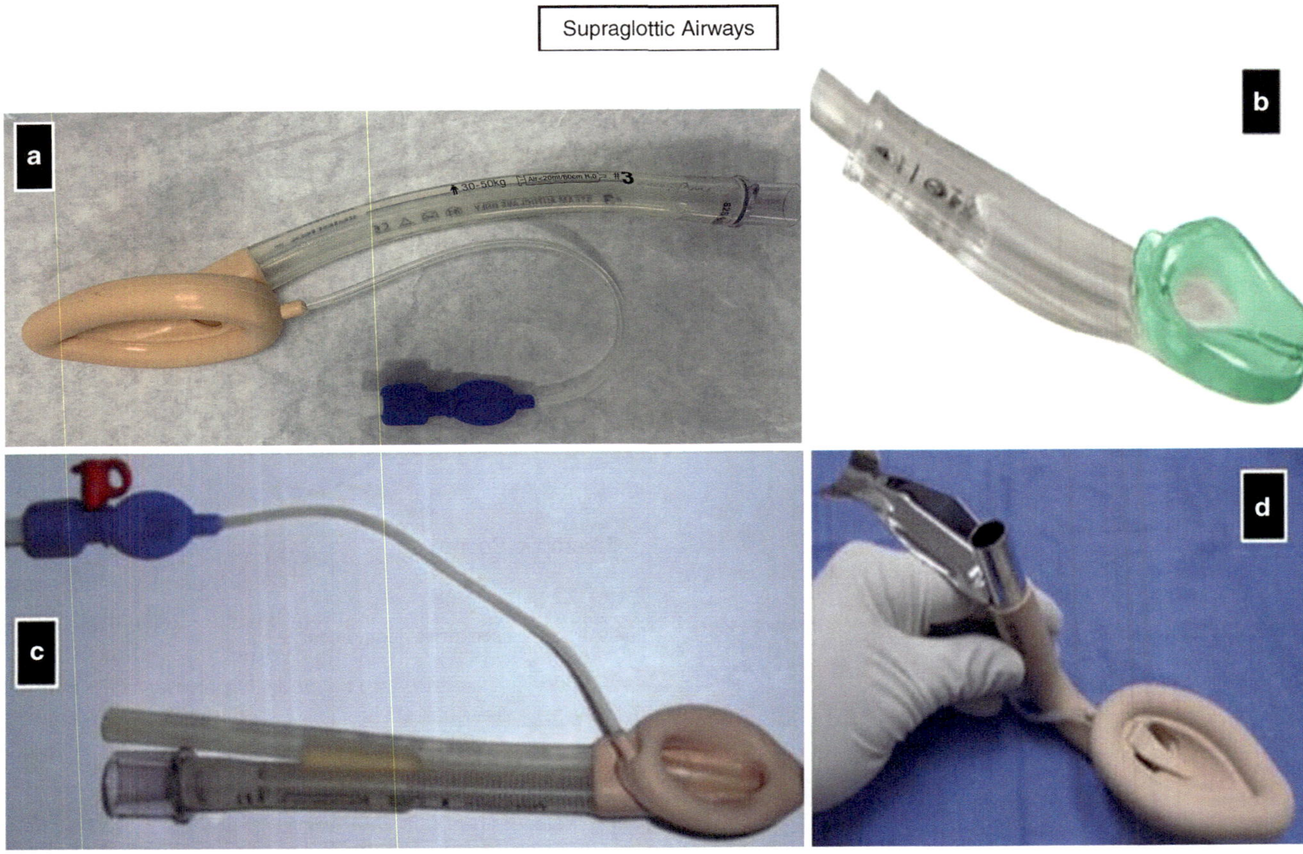


©Association of Oral and Maxillofacial Surgeons of India

**Fig. 7.9** (**a**,**b**,**c**,**d**) Supraglottic airways

tate awake fibre optic intubation. Airway blocks may not be an option to facilitate awake intubation in cases such as extensive pan-facial fractures or post-radiation fibrosis of the neck. Fibre optic intubation may be impractical in case of oro-maxillofacial trauma if associated with severe airway bleeding that can obscure visibility and other options such as tracheostomy under local anaesthesia (LA) should be considered.

The traditional 'blind nasal intubation' is rarely employed these days but may be used if a fibre optic scope is not available or not possible (Video 7.1).

A 'plan B' should always be present if intubation by one method is unsuccessful.

During long surgery and if ventilated in the post-operative period, the Endotracheal (or tracheostomy) cuff pressure should be measured using an aneroid manometer. A pressure of 20–30 cm of $H_2O$ is considered as standard in adults.

In supraglottic obstruction—associated with stridor and respiratory distress, as in case of upper airway trauma, rapidly expanding infections like epiglottitis, Ludwig's angina, etc. awake fibre optic bronchoscopy and intubation may not be the right choice. In such a situation, an awake tracheostomy under local anaesthesia must be considered.

### 7.5.5 Supraglottic Airway Devices

Several varieties of supraglottic airway devices are available (Fig. 7.9). However, these are not ideal devices for oro-maxillofacial surgeries requiring the oral cavity to be empty, but can be lifesaving as rescue devices in 'cannot ventilate, cannot intubate' situations to ventilate a patient until the definitive airway is secured. However, a flexible reinforced LMA can be used for simple dental extractions and nasal, zygomatic and superficial facial surgery. However, obstruction and dislodgement can occur, especially when the mandible is moved.

## 7.6 Special Considerations

*Paediatrics:* [6] Children will not co-operate for awake fibre optic intubation. Hence, in such cases, the airway can be secured after inhalational induction without relaxation after establishing IV access. A nasopharyngeal airway may be passed gently into one nostril and connected to a breathing circuit while monitoring the end-tidal carbon dioxide ($EtCO_2$) and continuing the anaesthetic and oxygenation via the airway. The other nostril may now be prepared with a vasoconstrictor and local anaesthetic and used for fibre optic intubation (Fig. 7.10).

### 7.6.1 Retromolar and Submental Intubation

These techniques were developed as alternatives to tracheostomy in maxillofacial surgeries requiring intra-operative inter-dental fixation for malocclusion correction like comminuted fracture of the mid-face or the nose, where nasal intubation is contraindicated.

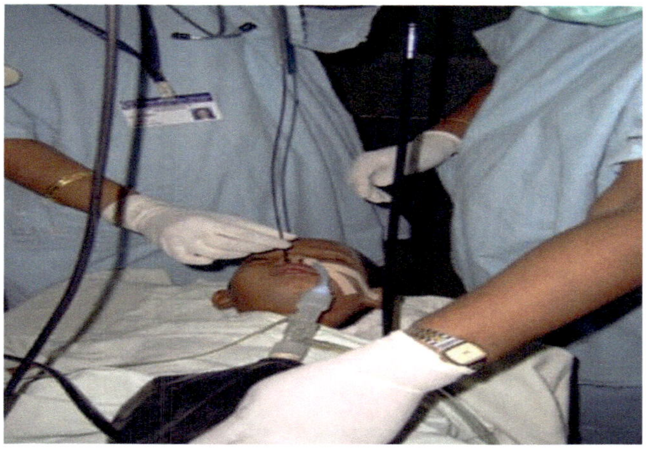



**Fig. 7.10** Fibre optic intubation in children

#### 7.6.1.1 Retromolar Intubation

Pre-operatively check the adequacy of the retromolar space. This is done to prevent kinking of the endotracheal tube in retromolar space by insinuating the index finger behind the third molar and asking the patient to clench his teeth. The patients' airway is then intubated by the conventional method and the ETT is pushed in the retromolar space and brought out from the angle of the mouth and connected to the ventilator. The spiral reinforced/armoured ETT is preferred as it is kink resistant (Fig. 7.11).

#### 7.6.1.2 Submental Orotracheal Intubation: [13] (Fig. 7.12a–f)

(See additional reading material on submental intubation given at the end of the chapter).

Just like retromolar intubation, it also requires the use of a spiral reinforced/armoured ETT in order to prevent the tube from kinking during its usage. Following conventional orotracheal intubation, a 2-cm incision is made lateral to the midline between the chin and the angle of the mandible and an opening is made in the floor of the mouth by the surgeon, avoiding the submandibular salivary glands. The machine end of the ETT without the connector is pulled through the tunnel, using gentle rotational movements. Following this manoeuvre, the tube is connected to the ventilating machine and sutures are used to fix the tube in position. If the procedure of disconnecting the ETT is long and pulling it out is prolonged, there is a possibility of hypoxia. So monitor oximetry closely and use high oxygen concentrations immediately before and after the placement of the submental tube (Video 7.2).

**Fig. 7.11** Retromolar intubation

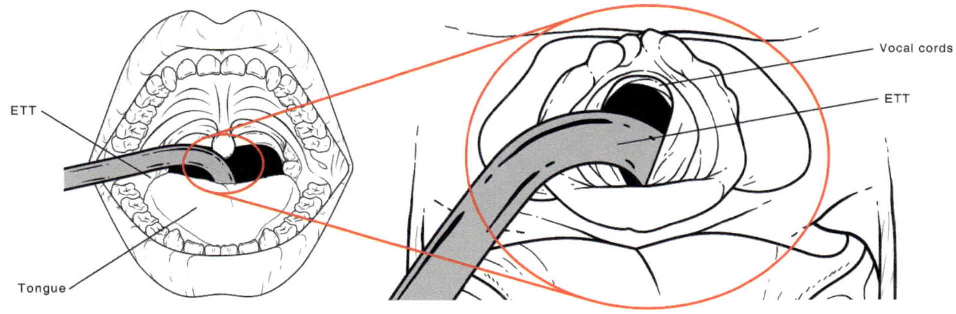

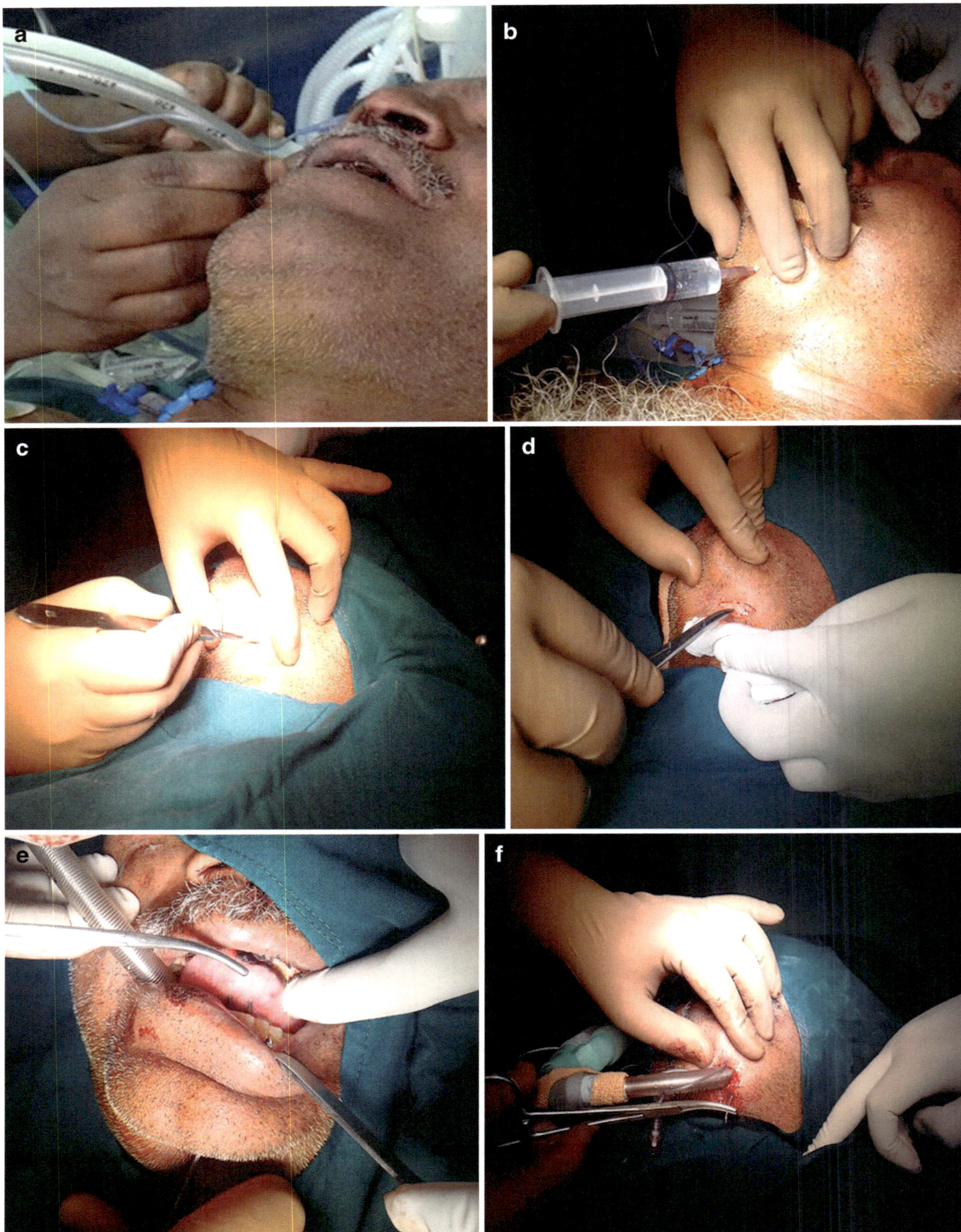




**Fig. 7.12** (**a**–**f**) Various steps in submental intubation

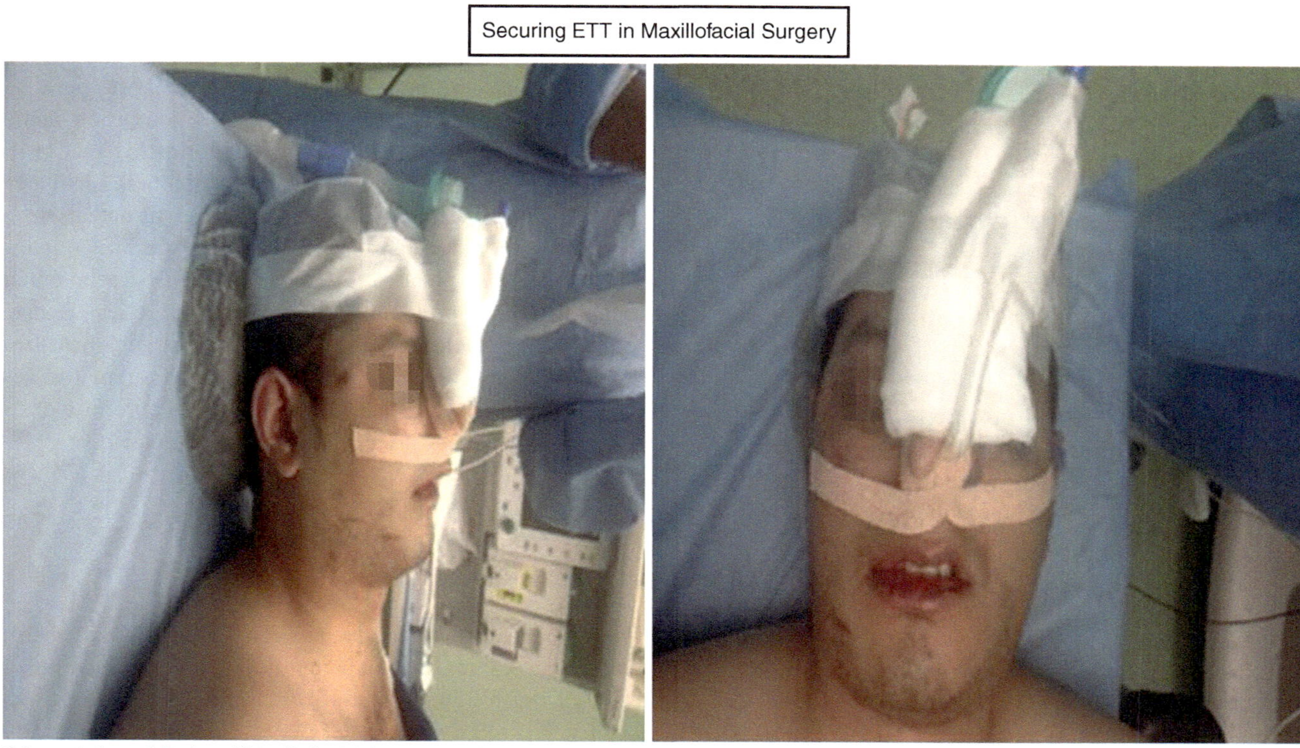




**Fig. 7.13** Securing ETT in maxillofacial surgery

**Securing the Endotracheal Tube**

The ETT may dislodge intra-operatively as the airway is shared between the surgeon and anaesthetist; hence, special attention should be paid to securing the ETT. Preformed nasal RAE tubes, if used, should be supported on the nasal bridge and forehead with the help of preformed supports or pads and secured on the forehead with tapes in addition to securing at the nostril (Fig. 7.13). Submental tubes can be secured with sutures (Fig. 7.14) South Pole oral RAE tubes are usually fixed in the middle of the lower jaw with tapes (Fig. 7.15).

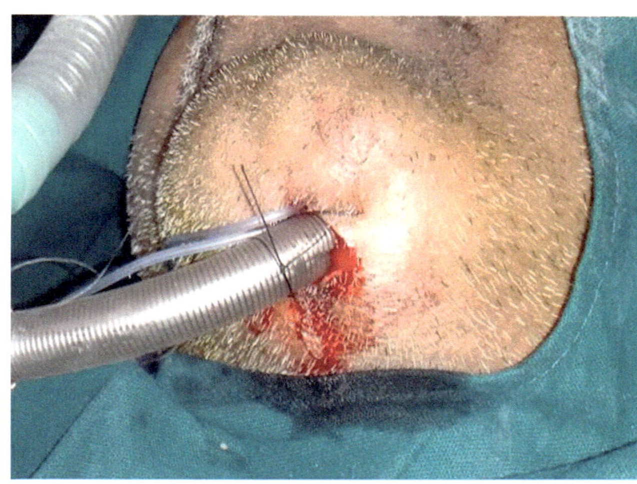



**Fig. 7.14** Securing submental tube with sutures

### 7.6.2 Eyes

Preferably taped with transparent dressing or specialized eye pads to capture moisture and prevent drying especially during prolonged surgeries (Fig. 7.15).

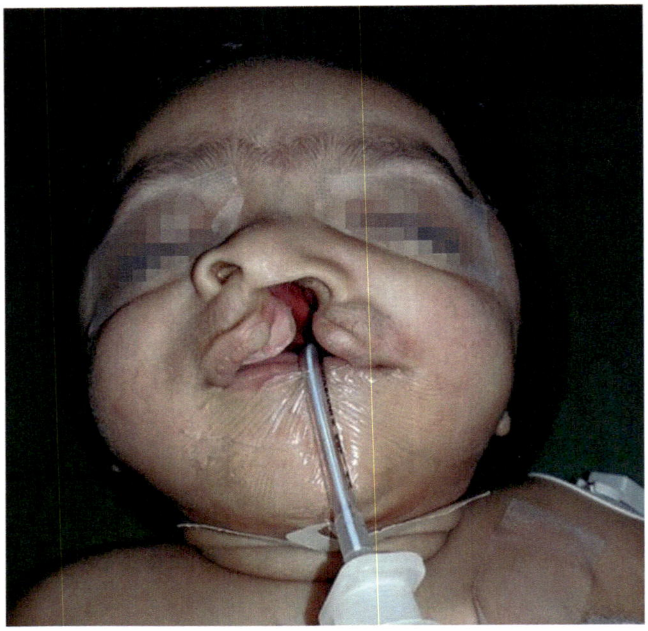



**Fig. 7.15** Securing oral south pole tubes/protection of the eyes with tapes

### 7.6.3 Positioning

Reverse Trendelenburg (anti-gravity) position with shoulder roll for adequate surgical exposure is preferred. Further, the operation table may be turned away from the anaesthetist and the anaesthesia machine by 90° or 180°. Hence, long breathing circuits, IV extensions and long cables for monitoring will be required.

### 7.6.4 Throat Pack

Saline-soaked throat packs will be required to protect the airway from blood, debris and saliva. It is advised to fix the tail end of the throat pack to the oral endotracheal tube whenever feasible to prevent accidental leaving behind of the throat pack at the end of surgery. Time of insertion and removal of the throat pack should be documented and carefully checked before extubation. If interdental wiring is planned at the end of surgery, then prior to doing so all throat packs should be removed and gauze counts should be confirmed.

## 7.7 Maintenance of Anaesthesia

Once the airway is secured, anaesthesia can be maintained with total intravenous anaesthesia (TIVA) or with volatile anaesthetics or combination of both as described earlier. Controlled ventilation with an intermediate-acting muscle relaxant such as atracurium or vecuronium is used.

Intra-operative analgesia is preferably provided with short-acting opioids such as fentanyl. Dexamethasone can be administered intra-operatively to reduce post-operative swelling, for its analgesic properties and as a prophylactic against post-operative nausea and vomiting (PONV) [14]. Orthognathic surgeries are associated with a high incidence of PONV; hence, additional antiemetics such as ondansetron should be administered prior to extubation especially if interdental wires are planned. Hypothermia can be a potential complication of prolonged orthognathic surgeries. Hence, temperature should be monitored and warming measures like intra-operative warm I.V fluids, forced air mattresses should be used. If there is a fear of airway compromise post-extubation, a tracheostomy should be done electively.

### 7.7.1 Deep Vein Thrombosis (DVT) Prophylaxis

Cancer patients and patients undergoing long surgery are at risk of developing thromboembolic complications. One or more of the following methods may be used to reduce its incidence.

Mechanical—Thromboembolic deterrent/Compression stockings (TEDS), pneumatic calf compression boots.

Pharmacological—Low-molecular-weight heparin such as Clexane could be used in patients at high risk for venous thromboembolism (VTE).

### 7.7.2 Control of Bleeding

The head and neck region receives rich blood supply from the branches of the carotid artery, and hence there is a tendency to bleed profusely during maxillofacial surgeries. Major bleeding can occur from branches of the maxillary artery or from pterygoid venous plexuses, leading to significant blood loss, warranting blood transfusion. Further, some of these procedures especially corrective osteotomies are extensive and time consuming. Surgical haemostasis is hampered by limited access. Risks involved in allogeneic blood transfusion have also been well documented and hence it is important to institute measures to reduce intra-operative blood loss and blood transfusion.

**Methods to control intra-operative blood loss include:**
Reverse Trendelenburg (anti-gravity) positioning.
Ensuring adequate venous drainage.
Antifibrinolytics, e.g. Tranexamic acid.
Infiltration of the tissues with vasoconstrictors like adrenaline.
Controlled hypotension.
Intermittent positive pressure ventilation and maintenance of mild hypocarbia.

1&2. *Positioning and venous drainage*: Reverse Trendelenburg (anti-gravity) positioning by 30° is recommended as it decreases bleeding by causing mild postural hypotension. Neck should be preferably positioned in the neutral position or turned slightly towards the surgeon. Extreme flexion or rotation of the neck to one side should be avoided to prevent venous engorgement. A minimum of 2-finger breadth space is recommended between chin and chest if flexion of neck is required.

3. *Antifibrinolytics:* A number of clinical trials have shown that the use of antifibrinolytics like tranexamic acid (TXA) reduces the peri-operative blood loss and the need for blood transfusion significantly. In 2011 World Health Organization added tranexamic acid (TXA) to its list of essential drugs [15]. The European guidelines on management of major bleeding and coagulopathy following trauma suggests a 1A recommendation for the use of TXA in the case of traumatic and perioperative bleeding [16]. Dose reduction is required in renal impairment. Also, caution should be exercised while administering to patients with history of seizures.
4. *Infiltration of the tissues with lignocaine + adrenaline:* Usually the surgeons infiltrate the tissues with lignocaine, a local anaesthetic (LA), and adrenaline, a vasoconstrictor, prior to incision so as to reduce bleeding. Before doing so, the maximum allowable dose of local anaesthetic and adrenaline must be calculated and not exceeded to avoid toxicity and arrhythmias. A dilution of 1:200000 adrenaline is considered safe. If a local anaesthetic drug has been used for securing the airway, the dose of LA used must be considered in total calculation. ECG should always be monitored during and after infiltration.
5. *Controlled hypotension:* is defined as iatrogenic reversible reduction of the patients mean arterial blood pressure. Controlled hypotension can be achieved either by decreasing peripheral vascular resistance and/or cardiac output [17]. However, hypotension induced by decreasing cardiac output may not be ideal as it decreases tissue perfusion. A reduction by 30% from the baseline mean arterial pressure (MAP) level is generally considered to be safe. But it may be unsafe in some patients such as those with chronic kidney disease, ischemic heart disease and carotid artery disease [17]. Therefore, their suitability for controlled hypotension should be assessed and recorded during the pre-anaesthetic workup.

Over the years, several protocols have been developed. The main strategies are

- Standard anaesthesia with non-pharmacological measures.
- Deep anaesthesia with analgesia.
- Standard anaesthesia with hypotensive drugs.

Standard anaesthesia with Non-pharmacological measures: This relies on

- Optimal anti-Trendelenburg positioning to achieve postural hypotension.
- Intermittent positive pressure ventilation with mild hypocarbia.

*Pharmacological measures:* It relies on drugs used to either deepen the plane of anaesthesia and/or produce vasodilatation.

The ideal drug used for controlled hypotension should be easy to administer, quick in onset and recovery with predictable effect, no toxic metabolites and should preserve organ perfusion [17]. At present, no such drug is available and hence a combination of drugs is often used.

Deep anaesthesia can be achieved either with volatile anaesthetics or with intravenous agents.

Most volatile anaesthetic agents are potent vasodilators. This property can be exploited to reduce blood pressure. However, when used alone, the minimum alveolar concentration (MAC) values required to achieve this are high and can result in hepatic and renal injury and also delay awakening. They are therefore used at lower concentrations with other pharmacological agents. Most commonly used volatile agents include isoflurane, sevoflurane and desflurane. Halothane is preferably avoided due to its arrhythmogenic potential with adrenaline.

*Propofol Infusions:* This has been extensively used in neuro anaesthesia for controlled hypotension as part of total intravenous anaesthesia (TIVA). It can be used either as part of TIVA or combined with volatile anaesthetics.

*Opioids:* Opioids decrease the doses of agents required to produce anaesthesia and hypotension by decreasing pain. Most commonly used short-acting opioids include fentanyl and remifentanil.

#### 7.7.2.1 Hypotensive Drugs: (Appendix II)

Hypotension should be carried out only to that level needed to reduce bleeding and only for that time of the surgery where it is of benefit in reducing significant blood loss. A number of drugs have been tried either alone or in combination to reduce blood pressure. While using them, one needs to be aware of their potential complications and contraindications. Drugs commonly used are beta-blockers, glyceryl trinitrate and sodium nitroprusside. Newer drugs like dexmedetomidine along with a propofol/remifentanil combination are gaining popularity [18, 19].

Invasive arterial blood pressure monitoring is recommended if infusions of hypotensive drugs are used for controlled hypotension. Intra-op serial monitoring of ABG (arterial blood gases), acid–base balance and lactate levels

**Table 7.6** Potential complications in specific maxillofacial procedures

| Complications | Surgery | Pathogenesis | Management |
|---|---|---|---|
| Bradycardia [21] | Levering of zygomatic fractures.<br>Manipulation of midface | Oculocardiac reflex | 1. Cessation of stimulus.<br>2. Anticholinergics: Atropine/ glycopyrrolate |
| Intra-operative bleeding:<br>Occurs due to high vascularity of the area not amenable to cauterization. | Maxillary osteotomies.<br>LeFort-I osteotomies | Bleeding from Pterygoid venous plexuses.<br>Sphenopalatine artery<br>Descending palatine artery<br>Internal maxillary artery | 1. Large bore I.V. cannula.<br>2. Intraoperative tranexamic acid.<br>3. Controlled hypotension.<br>4. Autologous blood donation.<br>5. Blood transfusion may be needed. |
| Tracheal tube damage | Lateral nasal osteotomies [20]<br>Le fort surgeries | Direct damage.<br>Bubbling of gas from the nose-Anaesthesia circuit leak with inability to ventilate. | 1. Immediate tube change.<br>2. Laryngeal packing may be attempted.<br>3. Precautions – Careful surgery<br>4. Unilateral: Intubate via contralateral nare. |
| Wiring of tracheal tube to maxilla | | | |
| Wide haemodynamic swings – Bradyarrythmias/ asystole | Radical neck dissections | Carotid sinus stimulation/ stellate ganglion stimulation. | 1. Cessation of stimulus<br>2. Carotid sinus block with LA<br>3. Stellate ganglion block.<br>4. Vagolysis. |

with hourly urine-output measurement should help to prevent organ dysfunction.

*Isovolaemic haemodilution* was once considered an adjunct in orthognathic surgeries to induce hypotension to reduce blood transfusion. It has become less common these days. The technique involves preoperative blood donation with IV fluids replacement of circulating volume followed by autologous whole blood transfusion as needed in the intra- or post-operative period.

*Intra-op Analgesia* can be achieved with NSAIDs, Paracetamol, opioids, intraoral LA infiltration and by mandibular or maxillary nerve blocks performed intra-op by the surgeon.

*Intra-operative complications:* The anaesthetist must be aware of and prepared for potential intra-operative complications [20, 21] (Table 7.6).

### 7.7.3 Elective Tracheostomy

Indications for elective tracheostomy are:

- Airway obstruction above the glottis - consider tracheostomy under LA.
- After extubation, Known or anticipated presence of an obstructed airway.
- Other general conditions requiring tracheostomy:
  - Certain head injuries
  - Massive chest injuries
  - Incidental pre-existing disease

  Inadequate postoperative nursing care.

## 7.8 Post-Operative

*Emergence and extubation* [22] Flow Chart 2—AIDAA (All India Difficult Airway Association) Guidelines for the management of anticipated difficult extubation and Table 7.7.

(flow chart 2 re-used with permission from IJA and AIDAA)

- After discussion with the surgeon, the decision of extubation post-surgery should be taken on a case-by-case basis.
- Before completion of the surgery, the induced hypotension should be ceased and time should be given to the surgeon to check for haemostasis. To check haemostasis, few surgeons prefer to increase mean blood pressure by 20–30% above pre-op level.
- At the end of the surgery, throat packs should be removed and clots or debris should be suctioned from the oropharynx.
- Prior to extubation cuff leak test may be performed to check for no airway oedema.
- A smooth emergence and extubation with less coughing and bucking is desirable. With the risk of the possibility of ongoing bleeding in the upper airway it is usual for patients to be extubated awake. Confirm that the patient is awake and breathing spontaneously.
- The Endotracheal tube should be left in situ, until the patient is fully conscious when the jaws are wired together, or any other airway obstruction is anticipated. Two types of maxillomandibular fixation (MMF) are available: Rigid MMF with jaw wiring, i.e. patients would be extubated with no ability to open their mouths and

**Table 7.7** Guidelines for extubation

| | |
|---|---|
| Decision based on | Individual case |
| | AIDAA guidelines Flow Chart 2 |
| | Cuff leak test |
| | Jaws wired - awake extubation |
| | Jaws not immobilized > Guedel airway/ nasopharyngeal airway |
| Stop | Induced hypotension |
| Keep ready | Difficult airway cart |
| | Appropriate anaesthetic drug drawn up |
| | Surgical team for tracheostomy |
| | Post op ICU bed |
| Avoid | Tight face mask ventilation |

MMF with elastics often applied, albeit later (from hours to 1 or 2 days) into the recovery phase where mouth opening will not be a problem.

- Guedel's airway or nasopharyngeal tube should be used to maintain the airway if jaws are not immobilized. A nasopharyngeal tube provides an extra dimension of safety in recovery.
- Nasal Endotracheal tubes removal should be gentle. To avoid passing of fresh tube through the vulnerable nasal mucosa, the ETT can be withdrawn into and left in oropharynx to serve as a nasopharyngeal airway. Submental ETT should be removed back from the oral cavity and closure of the submental incision done before the extubation.
- Consider extubation over a tube changer in case of difficult intubation or surgery.
- Avoid applying tight facemask to protect surgical correction after extubation.
- For reintubation, airway equipment / difficult airway chart should be available on standby and in case of failed extubation appropriate anaesthetic drugs drawn up in the required doses.
- In case of MMF, wire cutters or scissors should be available immediately for release of elastics band fixation.
- Until successful extubation and stabilization of patient, the surgical team should remain in the operating theatre.
- Before transfer to recovery, a short period of observation in the theatre should be followed.
- Handover and transfer to recovery should be done by the anaesthetist.
- Careful documentation of surgery details, vital signs, status at transfer, blood loss and replacement, drugs given, analgesia planned and expected problems should be done.

### 7.8.1 Handover from OT to Recovery Room/ICU

**Clinical Criteria for Shifting:**

- Patient should be awake and moving all 4 limbs
- Respiration should be regular with adequate depth
- Stable vital parameters
  - $SpO_2 > 95\%$ on room air
  - Pulse rate optimum for age
  - Respiratory rate < 30/min
  - Normothermic
- No active bleeding from surgical site

Anaesthesiologist should accompany patient to recovery

- Give handover to responsible personnel
- Handover should include
  - Name and age of patient
  - Surgery done
  - Any positive history and examination
  - Type of anaesthesia and drugs (time and dose) given, including analgesics.
  - Any intraoperative event
  - Clear postoperative orders
- Complete anaesthesia form and sign and name
- Nursing in the postoperative period should be in the reverse Trendelenburg position to decrease oedema and bleeding.
- In cases of Le Fort II and III fractures, one should be aware that the degree of oedema could worsen in the first 48 h.
- For close observation, some patients need to be admitted to a high dependency unit. Patients sent to ICU are those who remain intubated or ventilated.

In case of inadequate postoperative care facilities like an ICU, the patient may be required to be sent to another hospital (see appendix III and 1V).

## 7.9 Post-Operative Complications and Management

- Immediate
  - Airway Problems
  - Postoperative bleeding and haematoma
- Delayed
  - Nausea and Vomiting
  - Post-operative pain

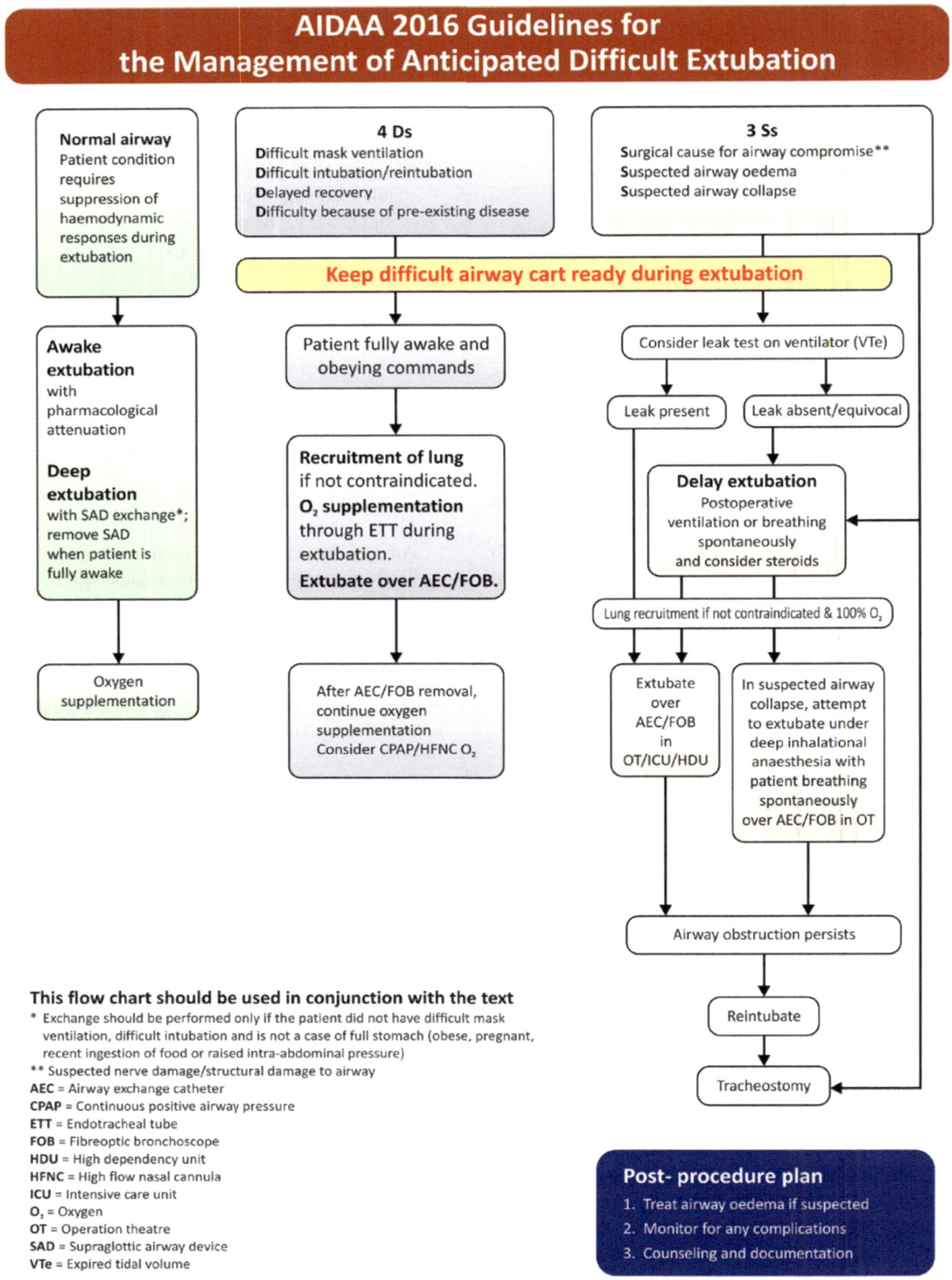


**Flow Chart 2** AIDAA Guidelines for the management of anticipated difficult extubation [22]

### 7.9.1 Airway Problems

In the post-anaesthesia care unit (PACU) the close monitoring of complications should be done, which can lead to airway obstruction such as soft-tissue swelling and formation of haematoma. Capnography may provide an earlier warning of serious problems than pulse oximetry when supplemental oxygen is being administered. Even in uncomplicated cases, the effects of residual anaesthetic agents on airway physiology are more pronounced in patients with MMF who may experience increased resistance to breathing.

### 7.9.2 Post-Operative Haematoma

Haematoma formation in the early postoperative period is an uncommon but potentially airway-threatening complication of some maxillofacial operations, notably neck surgery, thyroid resections and floor of mouth surgery. The rate at which airway compromise occurs is variable. Emergency decompression of the haematoma may be even done at the bedside. It involves removing the clips/sutures and manually evacuating the haematoma with a Yankaur sucker. However, this may not alleviate the airway obstruction adequately due to oedema that results from venous congestion. The airway needs to be secured urgently. The method of securing the airway should take into consideration information from the initial operation, but it is expected to be more challenging and may require expert airway management.

### 7.9.3 *Nausea and vomiting* [23]

Factors that predispose to PONV include the female gender, a history of motion sickness, a low threshold for nausea, preoperative anxiety, obesity and gastric distension. Volatile anaesthetic agents, nitrous oxide, opioid usage and intubation have also been implicated as has prolonged surgery, early oral intake and certain types of surgery, including maxillofacial surgery.

Vomiting in patients with MMF is dangerous as it may predispose to aspiration. If the jaws are wired together, there must be wire cutters immediately available, which accompany the patient from theatre, to the PACU, and also to the ward.

Elastics in MMF can be cut easily with ordinary scissors.

PONV prophylaxis is best given round the clock for the first 24 h and longer if opioids continue to be used. If treatment for PONV is required within 6 h of PONV prophylaxis, it should ideally be with a different class of anti-emetic drug to that used initially *(See Appendix I)*.

### 7.9.4 *Analgesia* [23–25]

After orthognathic surgery immediate postoperative pain is often not severe, and this is contributed to by the generous intra-operative use of local anaesthesia. A multi-modal analgesia approach should also be utilized perioperatively by combining opioids with paracetamol and non-steroidal anti-inflammatory drugs towards the end of the case.

Patient Control Analgesia (PCA): It allows the patient to self-administer intravenous analgesics by means of a computer-controlled pump. It administers the pre-programmed dose on demand by the individual.

## 7.10 Case Scenarios

Case 1: Problem-Based Learning Tool
Case 2: Multiple choice questions

### 7.10.1 Case 1: Cleft Palate

A 10-month-old child presents for surgery with a cleft palate

1. *What are the problems special for cleft babies*
- Regurgitation and repeated aspiration
- Repeated respiratory infections
- Airway obstruction
- Malnutrition/anaemia
- Associated syndromes

2. *What are the important features to look for during the pre- anaesthetic/presurgical evaluation?*
History–
- Feeding—Type of food, difficulty in swallowing, nasal regurgitation
- Repeated respiratory infections and/or hospitalization
- Airway obstruction especially during sleep (snoring or sleep apnoea)—position adopted when asleep
- Previous surgery as for repair of the cleft lip
- Episodes of cyanosis or referral to a cardiologist
- Birth history with details of ventilator requirements or neonatal ICU admission,
- Milestones and immunization

Examination

- Body weight, signs of malnutrition, dehydration or anaemia
- Pulse, BP and Room air saturation, temperature to be recorded
- Mouth opening, neck extension
- Respiratory system—signs of respiratory infection
- Rule out cardiovascular involvement
- Look for associated syndromes the most common of which are Pierre Robin Sequence, Treacher Collins syndrome and Down syndrome.

Investigations

- Hb,- nutritional anaemia is common
- Complete blood picture—white blood counts may be elevated due to repeated infections
- Bleeding parameters—to rule out coagulopathies
- Chest x-ray if repeated chest infections or respiratory signs present on clinical examination
- Cardiology consult: ECG and ECHO cardiogram if cardiac involvement suspected

In addition:

- Meet the parents, allay their anxiety and give full explanation of procedure.
- Explain fasting guidelines with details of timing of feeds
- Solids and milk feeds 6 h prior to surgery and clear fluids, especially with glucose/sugar, 2 h prior to surgery
- Document informed consent form.
- Discuss procedure and requirements with primary surgeon

3. *What preparations are necessary on day of surgery?*
Preparation: On day of surgery
- Ensure adequate help
- Ensure operating room temperature is not too cold
- Check Equipment and Drugs: Suction, Oxygen, Airway, Pharmacy (the pneumonic SOAP helps)
- Check anaesthesia machine
- Ensure that the difficult airway cart with rescue devices is available

*Monitors*: ECG, NIBP, Pulse Oximeter, $EtCO_2$, and airway pressure (once intubated)

4. *What are the problems that can present during anaesthesia?*
- Induction—intravenous or inhalational?
- Mask ventilation may be difficult especially in cases of facial cleft
- Laryngoscopy. The larynx is anterior, the tongue relatively large and laryngoscope tends to slip into the cleft
- Position of the patient in this case the trunk of the baby should be supported on a large pillow with the neck hyperextended and head stabilized within a head ring.
- Sharing the airway with the surgeon
  - kinking of tube when the gag is placed
  - accidental extubation during positioning of the baby or removal of the gag
  - tube may be pushed endobronchially resulting in one lung ventilation when gag is applied
  - throat pack/other packs may be left behind after surgery causing airway obstruction
- Intraoperative monitoring + access to the monitors difficult—so ensure they are fixed well and working well before patient is draped
- Access to the patient difficult, so make sure that intravenous access is good and fixed well before draping
- Analgesics like paracetamol and short-acting opioids like fentanyl may be used.
- Extubation is often more difficult than intubation. If there is any query regarding obstruction to the airway, place a nasopharyngeal airway and a tongue stitch prior to extubation.

5. *Could there be any problems post operatively? If so enumerate them.*
- Bleeding.
- Airway obstruction.
- Laryngospasm or post extubation stridor due to oedema of the upper airway: Treat with CPAP, humidified oxygen, aerosolized adrenaline, intravenous dexamethasone and nebulized steroids.
- Bronchospasm: Bronchodilators, oxygen and adrenaline, if severe.
- Aspiration: Suck out the mouth, nurse laterally, start antibiotics and chest.
- Physiotherapy along with nebulized bronchodilators.
- Electrolyte imbalance/hypoglycaemia: Send blood for investigations and correct
- Hypothermia/hyperthermia
- Seizures/Anticonvulsants: Rule out hyperthermia (tepid sponging and paracetamol) and hyponatraemia (intravenous normal saline).

### 7.10.2 Case–2: Polytrauma with Facial Injuries

A 27-year-old male presented with the history of polytrauma following a road traffic accident. He gives a history of brief period of loss of consciousness following injury. No history of seizures, or other comorbidities. On examination, his GCS was 15/15, and he was haemodynamically stable. Airway examination revealed restricted mouth opening of just one finger breadth, a short neck and a lacerated wound on the lower lip and chin with emphysema on the left side of the face extending into submandibular region. Cardiovascular, respiratory, abdominal and central nervous system examination was unremarkable. Blood investigations revealed increased CPK.

CT brain and spine showed a 3.5-mm extra-dural haemorrhage in the right temporal region, right frontal haemorrhagic contusion, an undisplaced fracture of the body of the mandible in bilateral parasymphyseal region with a displaced right zygomatic arch, a comminuted, mildly displaced fracture of right squamous temporal bone and undisplaced fracture of superior facet of C5 vertebra (Fig. 7.16).

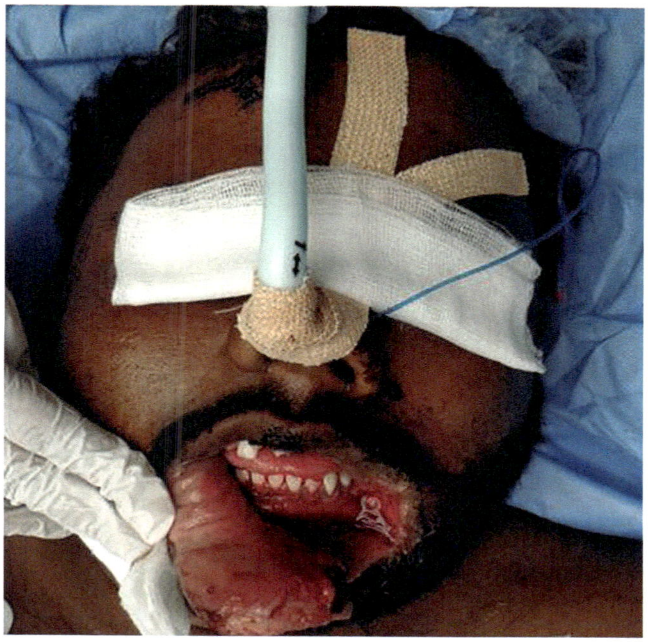



**Fig. 7.16** Photograph of a patient with polytrauma & facial injuries

*Questions*:

1. Following things are true about blunt trauma to face EXCEPT
   a. Cervical spine injury occurs in up to 10% of cases
   b. Drugs and alcohol could be a contributing factor
   c. Potential for injuries to other organs & massive blood loss
   d. Injuries in children are less severe than in adults

Answer: d) Injuries in children are usually more severe than in adults

2. In this patient, following could be cause of restricted mouth opening EXCEPT:
   a. Fracture Mandible
   b. Presence of trismus
   c. Cervical collar
   d # of superior facet of C5 vertebra

Answer: d) Fracture of Cervical vertebra usually does not restrict mouth opening

3. What is the reason for the presence of subcutaneous emphysema of the face in this patient?
   a. Pneumothorax
   b. Tracheal injury
   c. Soft-tissue injury
   d. # involving sinuses

Answer: d) Fractures involving air-filled sinuses around face can cause subcutaneous emphysema

4. What is the EXCEPTION to the bedside predictors of difficult intubation in a case like this?
   a. Receding mandible
   b. Facial injury
   c. Edentulous
   d. Cervical collar

Answer: c) Absence of teeth usually causes difficulty in ventilation rather than difficulty in intubation

5. Which of the following is most useful for detection of Extradural haematoma?
   a. CT scan of head
   b. MRI scan of head
   c. X-Ray Skull
   d. Careful clinical examination

Answer: a) A CT scan is more appropriate investigation in an emergency

6. What would be your preferred method for securing the airway?
   a. Conventional laryngoscopy with oral endotracheal intubation.
   b. Conventional laryngoscopy with nasal endotracheal intubation.
   c. Fibre optic bronchoscopy with nasal intubation.
   d. Conventional laryngoscopy with manual in line stabilization with nasal endotracheal intubation.

Answer: b) Conventional laryngoscopy with nasal endotracheal intubation

7. What would be your preferred airway device for securing the airway?
   a. Regular endotracheal tube
   b. Nasal RAE tube
   c. Oral RAE tube
   d. Reinforced cuffed endotracheal tube

Answer: b) Nasal RAE tube.

8. What do you anticipate with respect to airway in this case?
   a. Difficult mask ventilation
   b. Difficult laryngoscopy
   c. Both a) and b)
   d. Normal ventilation and laryngoscopy.

Answer: c) Both difficult mask ventilation and laryngoscopy.

9. The following monitoring would be useful during surgery in a case like this EXCEPT:
   a. Invasive arterial pressure
   b. Urine output
   c. Central venous pressure monitoring
   d. BIS monitoring

Answer: c) Central venous pressure monitoring would not add any additional value in a case like this

10. Where would you shift this patient after the surgery?
    a. General ward
    b. Special ward

c. ICU
d. HDU

Answer: d). HDU will be an appropriate place to monitor this patient post operatively

11. What is the most suitable method for pain relief in this patient?
    a. NSAIDs
    b. Nerve blocks
    c. Tramadol
    d. PCA Fentanyl

Answer: d) PCA fentanyl will be an appropriate choice as patient has multiple injuries and is being monitored in HDU.

12. Which intravenous fluid is appropriate during the surgery for this patient?
    a. Dextrose-containing solutions
    b. Balanced salt solutions
    c. Hypertonic saline
    d. Colloids

Answer: b) Balanced salt solutions

## Appendix I: Dosage of common Drugs

| Drug | Action/group | Dosage |
|---|---|---|
| Dexmedetomidine [11] | $\alpha_2$-adrenergic-agonists | Bolus: 1 mcg/kg over 10 mins followed by continuous infusion of 0.2-1mcgs/kg/h |
| Atropine | Anticholinergic | 0.5 mg I. V |
| Glycopyrrolate | Anticholinergic | Antisialagogue: 3-4 μ/kg I. M 30–60 min prior.<br>Bradycardia: 0.1 mg I.V repeated every 2 to 3 mins. |
| Topical Lignocaine | Local anaesthetic | Maximum safe dose: Adults: 9-10 mg/kg lean body weight.<br>Paediatrics: 4.5 mg/ kg |
| Dexamethasone | Adrenocortical steroid:<br>Anti-inflammatory dose<br>Antiemetic [14] | <br>0.1–0.2 mg/ kg<br>4–5 mg I.V |
| Ondansetron | Antiemetic—Serotonin antagonist | 0.1–0.2 mg/ kg |
| Prochlorperazine (Stemetil) | Antiemetic—Dopamine receptor antagonist | 0.25 mg/kg |
| Tranexamic acid [15] | Antifibrinolytic | 1. Bolus dose: 15 mg/kg can be repeated every 6–8 h (prior to incision) or<br>2. Continuous infusion during the surgery: 1 g over 10 mins followed by 1 gm over 8 h or 20–25 mg/kg followed by 1–2 mg/kg/h). |

## Appendix II: Commonly Used Drugs for Controlled Hypotension

| Drug | Administration and Dose | Advantages | Disadvantages |
|---|---|---|---|
| Vasodilators:<br>SNP | Infusion:<br>Up to 1.5mcgs/kg/min | Potent venous and arteriolar dilatation. | Reflex tachycardia.<br>Rebound hypertension.<br>Tachyphylaxis.<br>Cyanide toxicity. |
| NTG | Infusion: - 0.5–2 mcgs/kg/min | Venodilator | Reflex tachycardia.<br>Tachyphylaxis. |
| Adreno-receptor antagonists:<br>Selective:<br>∂ -selective:<br>Phentolamine | <br><br>Intermittent boluses: 2–5 mg. | <br><br>Vasodilatation. | |
| ß-selective:<br>Metoprolol<br>Esmolol | Intermittent boluses: 0.1 mg/kg.<br><br>Loading: 1 mg/kg over 1 min followed by Infusion: 0.5–1 mg/kg/h. | Heart rate control | Bronchospasm.<br>Negatively inotropic |
| Non-selective:<br>Labetolol | Boluses: 0.25 mg/kg followed by infusion: 0.5–2 mg/min | Vasodilatation + heart rate control | Bronchospasm |
| $\alpha_2$-adrenergic-agonists:<br>Clonidine | Infusion/boluses: 1mcgs/kg | Vasodilatation with heart rate control.<br>Analgesic properties | Post op sedation.<br>Rebound hypertension. |
| Dexmedetomidine | Bolus: 1mcgs/ kg over 10 mins followed by infusion of 0.3–1 mcg/kg/hr. | Vasodilatation with heart rate control.<br>Analgesic properties | Post op sedation. |
| Magnesium sulphate | Bolus: 20-60 mg/kg | Vasodilatation with heart rate control.<br>Analgesic properties | Prolonged neuromuscular block |

## Appendix III: Handover Form Used for Inter Hospital Transfer

***Patient details***

| Name: | Age: | Sex: M/F | MRN No: |
|---|---|---|---|
| Diagnosis: | | | |

| |
|---|
| Brief clinical history: |
| Clinical summary written by: |

| | |
|---|---|
| Reason for transfer: | |
| Transfer out hospital: | Referring doctor: |
| Transfer in hospital: | Accepting doctor: |
| Inter -hospital transfer consent taken: Y/N | |

***Vitals before transfer:***

| HR: /min | BP: mm Hg | RR: |
|---|---|---|
| SpO2: % | O2: l/min | AVPU score: |

Airway: Intubated and assisted / Intubated and spontaneous / Not intubated
Patent IV access:
Fluid on flow:
Medications on flow:
Monitors connected: ECG / Pulse oximetry / NIBP / Others

***Transfer details:***

| Departure time: | Arrival time : |
|---|---|

| |
|---|
| Duration of Transfer: |
| Accompanied by: |
| Critical events during transfer: |

***Vitals on arrival/admission:***

| HR: /min | BP: mm Hg | RR: |
|---|---|---|
| SpO2: % | O2: l/min | AVPU score: |

Airway: Intubated and assisted / Intubated and spontaneous / Not intubated
Patent IV access:
Fluid on flow:
Medications on flow:
Monitors connected: ECG / Pulse oximetry / NIBP / Others

***Handover details:***

Clinical summary: Y / N
Patient records: Y / N
Investigations: Y / N

| **Handing Over Doctor** | **Taking over doctor:** |
|---|---|
| Name: | Name: |
| Sign: | Sign: |
| Date & time: | Date & time: |

## Appendix IV: Inter-Hospital Transfer Guidelines

The transfer of the patient to a Centre where intensive care is available may sometimes be required if the facilities at the current hospital are inadequate. Most of these patients are critically ill and need the utmost care and planning to ensure safety during transfer. It is the responsibility of the referring team (surgeon as well as anaesthesiologist) to ensure a safe handover to the new treating team of doctors.

The following guidelines may be used to develop local protocols for inter-hospital transfer.

- The decision to transfer should be done by the treating team of doctors.
- Choose the appropriate hospital.
- The patient's family should be counselled by the treating doctor for the reason of transfer.
- Obtain consent from the patient's family after explaining the need as well as the risks involved in transfer.
- The administrative coordination between the two hospitals, e.g. checking the availability of beds, required doctors, equipment, etc. should be performed telephonically. The verbal consent to accept the patient by the destination hospital authorities should be done and documented.
- A short summary of the patient's clinical condition and handover document should be prepared.
- The transfer team should be identified. It should comprise at least 2 members who are adequately trained in handling sick patients, e.g. while transferring an intubated patient, the team should be trained in managing intubated patients. At least one doctor (preferably an anaesthetist) should accompany/supervise the patient during transfer especially sick patients.
- The departure checklist should include confirming the following:
  - Ambulance services.
  - Sufficient oxygen supply.
  - Shifting trolley.
  - Battery backup for equipment.
  - Mode of ventilation (for intubated patients).
  - Adequate monitoring (ECG, pulse oximetry, blood pressure).
  - Resuscitative medications (prefilled syringes).
  - Required paperwork—clinical summary, patient records and investigations.
  - Knowledge of destination hospital location and contact numbers.
  - Clinical stability of the patient should be confirmed before shifting.
- Patient should be stabilised before transfer. The following should be confirmed just before transfer—a patent IV line, a patent airway access, a functioning monitor with adequate battery backup. In case of an intubated patient –DO NOT EXTUBATE just prior to transfer.
- Note and record vital signs just before transfer.
- During transfer the vitals should be monitored continuously and documented frequently.
- Anticipation of problems during transfer and preparedness will help ensure safe transfer.
- Upon reaching the destination hospital, the transferring team should ensure that the patient is safely shifted to the desired critical care area and the hand-over formalities completed.

## References


1. Allman K, Wilson I. Oxford handbook of Anaesthesia. 3rd ed. Oxford, UK: Oxford University Press; 2011.
2. Shaw I, Kumar C, Dodds C, editors. Oxford textbook of Anaesthesia for Oral and maxillofacial surgery. Oxford, UK: Oxford University Press; 2010.
3. Sherwood MW, Douketis JD, Patel MR, Piccini JP, Hellkamp AS, Lokhnygina Y, et al. Outcomes of temporary interruption of rivaroxaban compared with warfarin in patients with nonvalvular atrial fibrillation: results from the rivaroxaban once daily, oral, direct factor Xa inhibition compared with vitamin K antagonism for prevention of stroke and embolism trial in atrial fibrillation (ROCKET AF). Circulation. 2014;129(18):1850–9.
4. Popat M. Difficult airway management. Oxford, UK: Oxford University Press; 2009.
5. American College of Surgeons Committee on Trauma. Advanced trauma life support for doctors. 6th ed. Chicago: American College of Surgeons; 1997.
6. Jacob R. Recognition and management of the difficult paediatric airway. In: Jacob R, editor. Understanding paediatric anaesthesia. 3rd ed. India: Wolters Kluwer (India); 2015. p. 184–94.
7. Kheterpal S, Martin L, Shanks AM, Tremper KK. Prediction and outcomes of impossible mask ventilation: a review of 50,000 anesthetics. Anesthesiology. 2009;110:891–7.
8. Reed MJ, et al. Can an airway assessment score predict difficulty at intubation in the emergency department? Emerg Med J. 2005 Feb;22:99–102.
9. Teasdale G, Jennett B. Assessment of coma and impaired consciousness. A practical scale. Lancet. 1974;2:81–4.
10. Mackay CA, Burke DP, Burke JA, Porter KM, Bowden D, Gorman D. Association between the assessment of conscious level using the AVPU system and the Glasgow coma scale. Pre-Hospital Immediate Care. 2000;4:17–9.
11. Chopra P, Dixit MB, Dang A, Gupta V. Dexmedetomidine provides optimum conditions during awake fiberoptic intubation in simulated cervical spine injury patients. J Anaesthesiol Clin Pharmacol. 2016;32:54–8.
12. Ramkumar V. Preparation of the patient and the airway for awake intubation. Indian J Anaesth. 2011;55(5):442–7.
13. Pavlakovic L, Lee G. Anaesthesia for maxillofacial surgery. Anaesthesia and intensive care medicine. 2014;15(8):379–84.
14. De Oliveira GS Jr, Castro-Alves LJ, Ahmas S, Kendall MA, RJ MC. Dexamethasone to prevent postoperative nausea and vomiting: an updated meta-analysis of randomized controlled trials. Anesth Analg. 2013 Jan;116(1):58–74.
15. WHO model list of essential drugs 17th list; March, 2011. http://www.who.int/medicines/publications/essentialmedicines/en/index.html

16. Rossaint R, Bouillon B, Cerny V, Coats TJ, Duranteau J, Fernández-Mondéjar E, et al. The European guideline on management of major bleeding and coagulopathy following trauma: fourth edition. 2016;20(1):100.
17. Rodrigo C. Induced hypotension during anesthesia with special reference to orthognathic surgery. Anesth Prog. 1995;42(2):41–58.
18. Bajwa S, Kaur J, Kulshrestha A, Haldar R, Sethi R, Singh A. Nitroglycerine, esmolol and dexmedetomidine for induced hypotension during functional endoscopic sinus surgery: A comparative evaluation. 2016;32(2):192–197.
19. Sajedi P, Rahimian A, Khalili G. Comparative evaluation between two methods of induced hypotension with infusion of Remifentanil and labetalol during sinus endoscopy. J Res Pharm Pract. 2016;5(4):264–71.
20. Morosan M, Parbhoo A, Curry N. Anaesthesia and common oral maxillo-facial emergencies. Continuing education in anaesthesia. Critical Care and Pain. 2012;12:5.
21. McDermott PJC. Reflex bradycardia in facial surgery. J Oral Maxillofac Surg. 1990;48(9):1015–6.
22. Kundra P, Garg R, Patwa A, Ahmed SM, Ramkumar V, Shah A, Divatia JV, Shetty SR, Raveendra US, Doctor JR, Pawar DK, Singaravelu R, Das S, Myatra SN. All India difficult airway association 2016 guidelines for the management of anticipated difficult extubation. Indian J Anaesth. 2016;60(12):915–21. https://doi.org/10.4103/0019-5049.195484.
23. Patel PK, Morris DE, Gassman A. Complications of orthognathic surgery. J Craniofac Surg. 2007;18(4):975–85.
24. Beck JI, Johnston KD. Anaesthesia for cosmetic and functional maxillofacial surgery. Continuing Education in Anaesthesia Critical Care & Pain. 2014;14(1):38–42.
25. Lupori JP, Van Sickels JE, Holmgreen WC. Outpatient orthognathic surgery: review of 205 cases. J Oral Maxillofac Surg. 1997;55:558–63.


## Additional Reading (Sub Mental Intubation)


Hernández AF. Sub-mental vs. retromolar intubation. Anaesthesia. 2006 Nov;61(11):1123–4.

Altemir FH, Montero SH, Peña MM. About submental intubation. Anaesthesia. 2003 May;58(5):496–7.

# Part IV

# Imaging in Oral and Maxillofacial Surgery

# Radiology for Maxillofacial Surgeons: The Essentials

8

Shyamsundar K. Joshi and Annie I. Kochuveettil

**Learning Objectives**

- To identify the strategies in building an effective working relationship with the imaging department and help plan appropriate imaging investigations.
- To understand the principles of various imaging techniques; the advantages and disadvantages of these techniques in varying clinical scenarios.
- To gain awareness about the benefits and risks of using ionizing radiation and understand the basic principles of radiation protection.
- To establish the role of imaging as a treatment guide following different maxillofacial surgeries.

## 8.1 Introduction

Accurate diagnosis is the mainstay of proper surgical management in a maxillofacial surgical patient. Definitive diagnosis may be possible in a few patients based on clinical evaluation in the outpatient department or emergency setup. Other cases may require the use of supplementary investigations, including radiological imaging.

Like other medical specialties, the scope of Radiology is vast, playing a significant role in disease management. Penning a chapter on Radiology for a clinical branch-like Maxillofacial surgery is an uphill task. As a clinician, the maxillofacial surgeon, after having made the diagnosis, has the desire to visualize and gain in-depth knowledge of the ongoing disease process within the patient. Radiology plays an important supporting role in helping the clinician visualize within the patient's body. It is hence necessary for clinicians to have basic knowledge of the key concepts of Radiology, helping them understand its applications in the diagnosis of a patient's clinical condition.

The scope of practice of a practicing MFS includes both surgical and nonsurgical problems that affect the orofacial region, and hence they need to be well versed with the imaging concepts of the head and neck region.

**Head and Neck Imaging**

Anatomy of the head and neck is complex and imaging in this region poses several challenges and an MFS needs to be cognizant of them.

Modern imaging has the unique advantage of being able to:

- Demonstrate intricate and critical anatomical structures packed in small compact space pockets.
- Define the anatomy pertinent to the region of clinical interest.
- Define the critical relation to vital structures like the brain and cerebral vessels.
- Define the related adjacent critical areas like the airway, orbital contents, and both intra- and extracranial neurovascular elements.
- Define the underlying pathological process.

Conventional Radiography is one of the modalities that have been available from early days, ever since X-rays were discovered by Wilhelm Conrad Roentgen in 1895. However, it is regarded as a poor choice for anatomical evaluation due to overlapping of anatomical structures especially in the head and neck region. Yet it still has a popular role in its own humble way. It is universally available, the least time-consuming imaging investigation, and gives a 'bird's eye view' of the region of interest. It provides instant practical

S. K. Joshi (✉) · A. I. Kochuveettil
Department of Radiology, SDM College of Medical Sciences and Hospital, Shri Dharmasthala Manjunatheshwara University, Dharwad, India



K. Bonanthaya et al. (eds.), *Oral and Maxillofacial Surgery for the Clinician*, https://doi.org/10.1007/978-981-15-1346-6_8

information on the status of the airway and osseous elements, helps inferring the underlying pathological process based on the presence of air pockets or bony destruction, and at times may even reflect systemic pathology. It guides the clinician as to the further steps to be taken for patient management or to the need for further imaging. Despite it being the era of advanced technology, conventional radiography should invariably be the first choice among imaging investigations. In cases of complex maxillofacial injuries and polytrauma, when the patient's clinical status demands the next level of investigation, CT may be performed first, bypassing conventional radiography.

Pioneers in the field of imaging had a yearning to develop modalities that could demonstrate finer anatomical details in the region of interest.

This, coupled with the technological evolution, has paved the way for the development of various radiological imaging technologies that include:

- Ultrasonography (USG)
- Color Doppler
- Computerized Tomographic (CT) scan
- Dentascan
- Cone beam CT
- PET scans
- Radioisotope scanning
- Magnetic Resonance Imaging (MRI)
- Functional imaging, etc.

These advances in imaging techniques have enabled the MFS to diagnose with greater confidence and refine their approach to surgical treatment. This has also led to a reduction in unexpected surprises springing up on the surgical table.

Considering that a range of imaging modalities are available, it is imperative that the MFS has basic knowledge about their functionality, being familiar with the advantages and disadvantages of each so that the appropriate imaging investigation that gives the most optimal information in a given clinical setup can be selected. The rationale behind choosing the right investigation is that it should be easily available, least time consuming, cause least possible discomfort to the patient and be economical. Appropriate use of the concerned imaging modality should provide the maximum possible anatomical and functional information. This is possible if a genuine effort is made by an MFS to understand the basic principles and other related components of specific diagnostic imaging relevant to his field of interest and establish a close rapport with the imaging department.

## 8.2 Requesting an Imaging Investigation

Prior to requesting a radiological investigation, the MFS needs to have a clear idea about the usefulness of an investigation, its limitations, and whether it will help to improve the patient outcome. A radiological imaging requisition must specify the choice of investigation and the surgeon's expectations from it, so that the information received strengthens his approach in treating the patient.

It must provide mandatory demographic and relevant clinical data, including the patient's symptoms, which primarily brought him to the MFS, their duration, clinical signs, and the clinician's differential diagnosis of the same. In addition to concentrating on the clinical data, entries made available through the Hospital Information system (HIS) and the Radiology Information system (RIS), accurate patient identification by the MFS is essential prior to referral to the imaging department.

## 8.3 Role of the Maxillofacial Surgeon (MFS) Vs. the Radiologist's expectation from the MFS

An MFS deals with patients suffering from maxillofacial disease processes, but being a clinician primarily he is expected to have basic knowledge of various systemic clinical problems as well. Systemic disease may manifest as disease in the maxillofacial region or vice versa. For instance, a cystic lesion in the jaw could be the primary radiographic finding in a patient suffering from hyperparathyroidism. Similarly, patients suffering from systemic diseases like osteopetrosis, fluorosis, fibrous dysplasia, and other marrow infiltrative disorders could also present with a disease in the maxillofacial region. Further, detection of congenital anomalies in the maxillofacial region is an indication for a more detailed survey to rule out associated anomalies elsewhere.

The surgeon should be able to identify radiological images, correlate the same with the report and the patient's clinical status, and focus on timely decision making and patient management, thus optimizing the patient's outcome. However, in a dire emergency when a radiologist's opinion is not available, or a delay is expected in obtaining the same, an MFS should be able to interpret radiographs that suggest life-threatening conditions like tension pneumothorax, aspiration bronchopneumonia, foreign body aspiration, or pulmonary edema among others. Imaging can help the MFS in narrowing down on the clinical diagnosis, in staging and evaluating the prognosis of a disease process, or in surgical planning by depicting the exact extent of a lesion after diagnosis is confirmed.

MFS' need to communicate with their radiology counterparts the expectations they have from imaging of a case so that the radiologist can provide the relevant anatomical and functional information from the region of interest. Each imaging modality has its own reporting language and the surgeon needs to be well versed with the language used and have a clear concept of principles of image formation, specific to the energy source used in the particular investigation.

## 8.4 Role of the Department of Imaging and the Radiologist

The responsibility of the imaging department is conducting the specified diagnostic imaging investigation, interpretation of the tests or procedures by the radiologist and providing the clinician with accurate reports of the performed investigation as early as possible. Clinical radiologists function as key members of multidisciplinary teams, being an integral part of patient care.

## 8.5 Energy Forms Used in Diagnostic Medical Imaging: Understanding the Basics

Different types of energies are used in diagnostic imaging. These energies are imperceptible to the human eye and when they are passed to the desired location in the body, they interact with the body tissues in different ways. The tissue interactions can reveal information about the tissue, but they need to be interpreted. Access to this information is possible only if it is converted into a visible form on a display system. In essence, the requirements for an imaging investigation are; a reliable and reproducible energy form, a subject (the patient) into whom the energy can be sent, and a format that can convert the invisible image into a visible display.

X-rays and gamma rays are photon energies and members of the electromagnetic spectrum having a wide range of wavelengths and frequencies. X-rays have very small wavelengths being lesser than 1 Å unit and greater than 0.1 Å units. This range of specific frequencies and wavelengths of X-rays give them special properties, gaining popularity in diagnostic imaging.

Gamma rays have shorter wavelengths and higher frequencies than X rays. They are used in nuclear medicine both for diagnostic and therapeutic purposes.

Conventional radiography, including mammography, fluoroscopy, computed tomography (CT), is a modality that generates images of the ionizing radiation. It works on the same basic principle, which essentially involves passing of an X-ray beam through the body followed by absorption and scattering of a portion of the X-ray energy by the body tissues and transmission of the resultant radiographic pattern formed by differential tissue absorption to a detector for recording or further computer processing.

The popularity of X-rays as an imaging modality is due to its optimum penetration power and photochemical and fluorescent properties. Its fluorescent property is useful in converting invisible images into visible light images, while the photochemical property is responsible for conversion of the visible light image into a permanent visible record called radiograph.

*Conventional radiography* includes plain radiographs of different body parts like chest, skull, PNS, etc., contrast studies of the gastrointestinal tract like Barium studies, contrast studies of the genitourinary tract like Intravenous urography (IVU), and contrast studies of the vascular system like Arteriography, Phlebography, etc.

*Fluoroscopy* involves a continuous display of real-time movements of moving structures as radiographic images on the monitor, e.g., act of swallowing, movement of the soft palate, movement of the temporomandibular joint, cardiac pulsations, diaphragmatic movements, etc.

*Computed Tomography* includes cross-sectional imaging with its modifications like 3D, Volume rendering, Multiplanar reconstruction images, C.T. angiography, etc.

*Ultrasound* imaging or sonography makes use of high-frequency sound waves that are transmitted from the transducer into the body. The reflection of these waves off the body structures forms the basis of ultrasound image formation. The information necessary for image production is provided by the amplitude of the reflected sound signal and the time taken for it to travel through the body. Commonly ultrasound is used in the imaging of the abdomen, fetus, breast, eye, heart, vessels, and the musculoskeletal system. In recent years, there has been much research into ultrasound of the maxillofacial region, and it has been found to have a range of unique applications, including the evaluation of cervical lymph nodes and the detection of space infections and cystic and solid lesions of the head and neck. In early cases of peripherally located carcinoma of the tongue, ultrasonography may be an initial mode of imaging for evaluation.

Ultrasound imaging is not associated with the same risks as ionizing radiation and is considered to be generally safe if used appropriately. Ultrasound energy does have the potential to produce biological effects on the body and can cause minimal heating of tissues and in certain cases produce tiny gas pockets in the tissues and body fluids known as cavitation.

*Magnetic resonance* imaging makes use of strong magnetic fields and radiofrequency energy to create images. The signals that produce an MR image originate from the protons present in water and fat molecules in the body. Application of a strong magnetic field by the MRI scanner causes the protons within the body to align themselves. Radiofrequency current is then passed into the patient's body creating a varying magnetic field that causes the protons to flip their spins. Turning off the radiofrequency pulse causes the protons to return to their normal spins, producing radio signals that are measured by receivers in the scanner and used to make digital images of the scanned area of the body.

Many forms of MRI exist, diffusion and functional MRI being the most common. Diffusion MRI helps in diagnosing disease processes like stroke that restricts diffusion of water molecules across body tissues, while functional MRI is used to visualize the functional activity of the brain. MRI does not use ionizing radiation but since it uses strong magnets, any form of metal implants like artificial joints and heart valves, pacemakers, cochlear implants, metal plates, screws, and rods do pose a hazard.

*Thermography* makes use of specialized cameras that can detect electromagnetic light energy in infrared wavelengths. Medical thermography produces a topographic heat map, displayed in the form of various color shades, based on the differential skin temperature at various dermatomes bearing resemblance to the visible image of the body. It is not a structural imaging technology providing information on structural changes like other modalities and does not provide a diagnosis, rather only aids in reaching a diagnosis. It is completely safe and painless, does not make use of any form of radiation, and is a unique form of imaging in that it can document pain, thus helping to differentiate malingering from an organic cause for the pain.

## 8.6 Basic Radiology for the Nonradiologist: What the MFS should know?

Plain radiographic film interpretation is an essential skill. The current implementation of electronic health records and digitization of the health care system has made radiographic images available throughout the hospital and an MFS may often have to interpret medical images. So, it is important that they know the basics of medical image interpretation, and this knowledge may prove to be crucial in an acute clinical setting. They should be aware of tissue appearances on radiographs and be capable of making a basic distinction between normal and abnormal.

Understanding the concept of density and contrast is fundamental to interpreting an X-ray image (radiographic image). Different body tissues, including bone, soft tissues, fat, and air, all attenuate the X-ray beam differently. Differential absorption of X-ray photons by the body tissues results in variable energy values of emerging photons producing an invisible image, which is converted into visible form as areas of different gray scales. The contrast on the image is the difference between adjacent densities. These densities range from white to black with varying gray shades in between them. If the densities of two tissues adjacent to each other are greatly different (say a white and a black density tissue), then they are said to have high contrast. If the densities of two tissues adjacent to each other are similar, then they are said to have low contrast. They appear similar in color, differing in their shades of gray. When two body structures of identical density are exactly side by side, the line of demarcation cannot be made out and whole of it appears as one structure.

Consider a chest radiograph. What do you think is the whitest component seen on the radiograph? Most commonly the answers given are heart, bones, below the diaphragm, and so on. Rarely does anyone mention that the "R" marker is the whitest. Similarly, if asked which the darkest component is, the popular answer given is, the lung surrounding the heart, very rarely does one mention that the air surrounding the chest is the darkest. Analyzing as to why the "R" marker is white and the air surrounding is dark, the reasoning is that the chest radiograph is nothing but a representation of the tissues in that region in various gray scales between extreme white and extreme dark, depending upon the variable absorption of X-ray photons in their path through the tissues.

The opacity produced on a radiograph by a specific body tissue is a representation of the actual penetrative ability of X-rays to pass through that tissue and then be incident on the film. Air and fat absorb less radiation, allowing more X-rays to pass through and be incident on the radiograph making their images appear black and pale gray, respectively. Bone and metal as is the "R" marker made of lead absorbs more radiation and so fewer X-rays are incident on the film making them appear white.

Continuing with the example of chest radiograph, what are branching structures that are seen in the lung fields? Are they arteries, veins, bronchi, lymphatics, or a combination of all these? The common answer given is bronchovascular. The correct answer is arteries and their branches, but not the bronchial tree. The explanation is simple. Air in the bronchi is surrounded by air in the alveoli and so no contrast exists between them and they are hence not seen. On the other hand, blood in the arteries is surrounded by air in the alveoli and hence they stand out. Veins do contain blood but are too less in number and do not significantly contribute to the branching structures. Lymphatics are too small to be detected.

If this basis of X-ray image formation is understood, you can easily interpret any radiographic image provided you have sound knowledge of the relevant anatomy, pathology, and pathophysiology.

## 8.7 Imaging Investigations

### 8.7.1 Imaging Investigations Using Ionizing Radiation (Photon Energies)

Electromagnetic radiation has a wide range of wavelengths ranging from being smaller than angstrom units to as large as many miles. Smaller wavelengths have greater energy and penetration power and are called photon energy meaning packets of energy and not particle energy. The two energies that are of concern in the present context are X-rays and Gamma rays. Passage of these energies through body tissues either for diagnostic or therapeutic purposes results in a series of events beginning with an incidence of the X-ray photon into tissue followed by sequential changes at molecular and atomic levels. The transformation of energy from the photon results in ionization, namely, in the discharge of an electron and a free radical. Hence, such energies are called ionizing radiation and the process involves breakage of enzyme bonds and formation of new molecules manifesting in the form of various repairable and irreparable biological effects.

The concept of photon energy and its effect on body tissues can be explained using the following example. Consider a hot iron ball being passed through a pile of corn (Fig. 8.1). The temperature of the ball after exiting the corn pile is grossly reduced. It is because the ball, during its transit through the pile, shares the energy with the corn in contact with it. The corn in very close contact to the ball is burnt to ashes, the corn a little farther away, is burnt to charcoal, corn still further away is converted to popcorn, while corn far away from the ball remains unaffected. The effect on the corn is directly proportional to the energy transferred from the hot iron ball to the corn. The same thing happens when photon energy passes through the body tissues with changes occurring at atomic level.

#### 8.7.1.1 X-Rays

X-rays are a form of electromagnetic radiation. Man-made X-rays are produced when fast-moving electrons undergo sudden deceleration on collision and interaction with the target anode in an X-ray tube. The electrons are emitted by the cathode, on being heated up by the electric current flowing through it.

Though conventional X-ray imaging has evolved over the past 100 years, the basic principle remains the same. On passage of an X-ray beam through the body, the beam is attenuated by the body's internal structures, being partly absorbed and partly scattered. The remnant of the X-ray energy is transmitted to a detector that records the image for later evaluation. The recording of the radiographic pattern may be on film or other electronic devices. The image created is due to weakening of the X-rays by tissues of varying density encountered along the beam's travel path. Bone being dense tissue, absorbs or attenuates a great deal of the X-rays, while soft tissue being much less dense attenuates or absorbs far less X-ray energy. These differences in absorption help in creating images that can clearly show normal tissue appearance as well as different forms of pathology.

Conventional radiography, fluoroscopy, and CT all work on the same basic principle differing only in their purpose. In radiography, a single image is recorded for later evaluation, in fluoroscopy X-ray images are displayed on a monitor in a continuous flow, thus allowing monitoring of a procedure or contrast passage in real time and in CT imaging a multitude of images are recorded as the detector rotates around the patient's body followed by reconstruction of the individual images as cross-sectional images of internal organs and tissues.

#### 8.7.1.2 Computerized Tomography (CT/Spiral CT)

Computerized axial tomography is a computer-controlled radiological study that produces a reconstructed image of a cross-sectional slice of the desired section of the body. Its features include the absence of superimposition, less scatter and better tissue differentiation of the anatomical slice, thinner slices producing a better reconstructed image. The major drawback of conventional radiography is the overlapping of anatomical structures resulting in difficulty in evaluation of desired structures in a particular plane. The imaging method 'Tomography' was introduced to overcome this drawback and involves imaging of anatomical structures at the desired plane with the blurring of overlapping structures. Classical conventional tomography had its own inherent drawbacks, which included poor-quality blurred images, high radiation dosage, and use of complicated techniques which led to it being replaced by tomography assisted by computer technol-

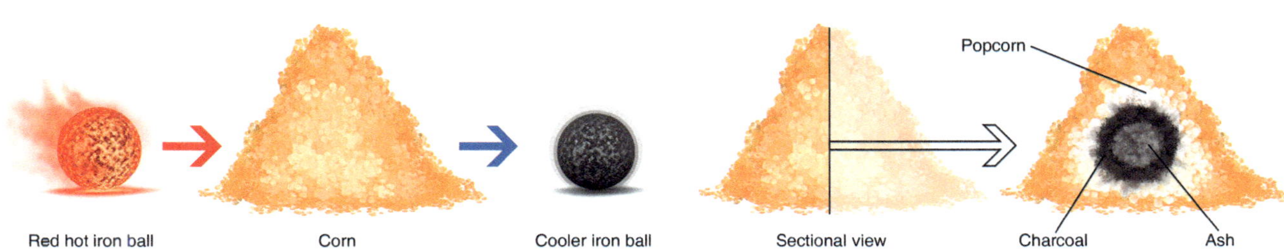


Fig. 8.1 Illustration of passing a hot iron ball through a pile of corn and its effect on the corn

ogy called 'Computer assisted Tomography' (CAT). With a rise in popularity, CAT has been replaced by the word C.T. and technological advances have resulted in the development of better equipment capable of scanning the entire body within a few seconds. This provides fine anatomical details of submillimetric structures, allows tracing of blood flow in all its phases, and also permits clear depiction of information related to moving structures like the heart in real time as well as their external and internal morphology. Two types of CT have been described based on the shape of the X-ray beam, the traditional fan beam CT and cone beam CT.

**CT Unit Components** (Fig. 8.2a, b)

The essential components of a CT unit include:

- **The X-ray tube**—a specialized tube of high heat loading and dissipating capacity with a very small focal spot, as a source of X-ray energy
- **Detectors** that receive and quantify the attenuated X-ray photons
- **A computer** of high capacity that evaluates attenuated photon energy from detectors, stores the values, and converts these values to sectional images
- **A console** that manipulates all data stored in the computer, helping in reconstructing the image at desired planes with volumetric imaging or multiplanar reconstruction, 3D and volume rendering, followed by projection of the desired structures based on their density values, etc.
- **A gantry** that houses X-ray tubes, detectors, and related cables with a central aperture for the patient's body to enter for sectional imaging
- **A moving table** or a couch that facilitates the movement of the body with extreme accuracy at even submillimetric increment

CT scans have many benefits that far outweigh their risk. It is quick and easy, widely available, and provides superior anatomic and bone details. It has Volume Rendering Technique (VRT), Maximum Intensity Projection (MIP), 3D and Shaded Surface Display (SSD) capabilities, provides multiplanar reconstruction images in desired planes, and is the modality of choice for follow-up studies. (Figs. 8.3a, b, 8.4a, b, 8.5a,b, 8.6a, b, 8.7a, b, 8.8a, b, 8.9a, b, 8.10, 8.11, and 8.12).

The possible risks of using CT imaging include exposure to ionizing radiation and the predicament of suffering an allergic reaction due to use of contrast media. One drawback of CT when compared to MRI is the lesser resolution of soft-tissue detail. Other disadvantages are the associated cost and the limitations of its use in the pediatric age group due to the need of sedation.

**CT Limitations**

Motion and beam-hardening artifacts used to be considered as major drawbacks, but they have been markedly minimized with advances in technology. A physical limitation is that the patient needs to weigh less than 300 to 400 lbs. For

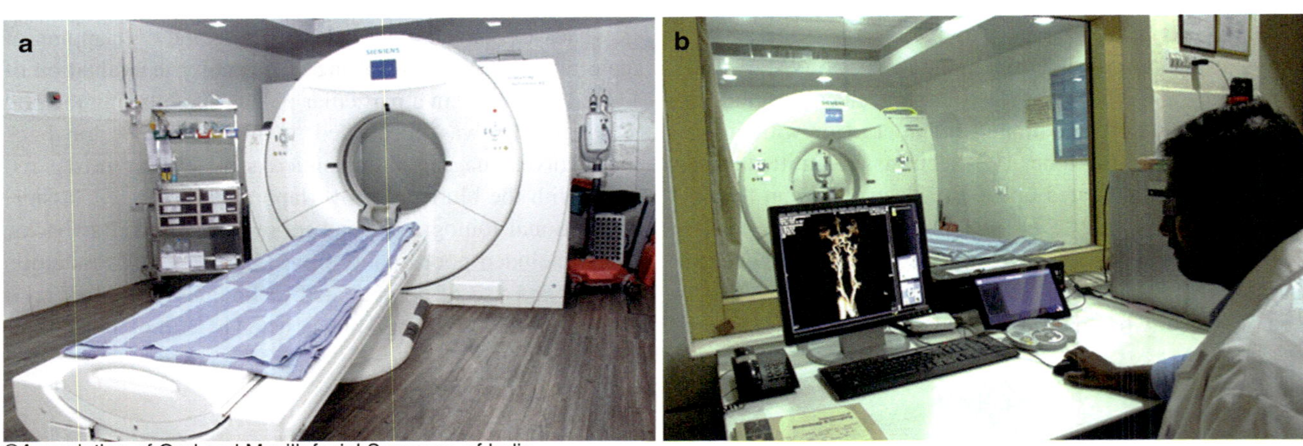




**Fig. 8.2** (**a**) CT room shows Gantry, Patient couch, Emergency crash trolley, Central suction, and Oxygen and Pressure Injector. (**b**) Control room showing a CT technician working with various controls and the image acquisition system

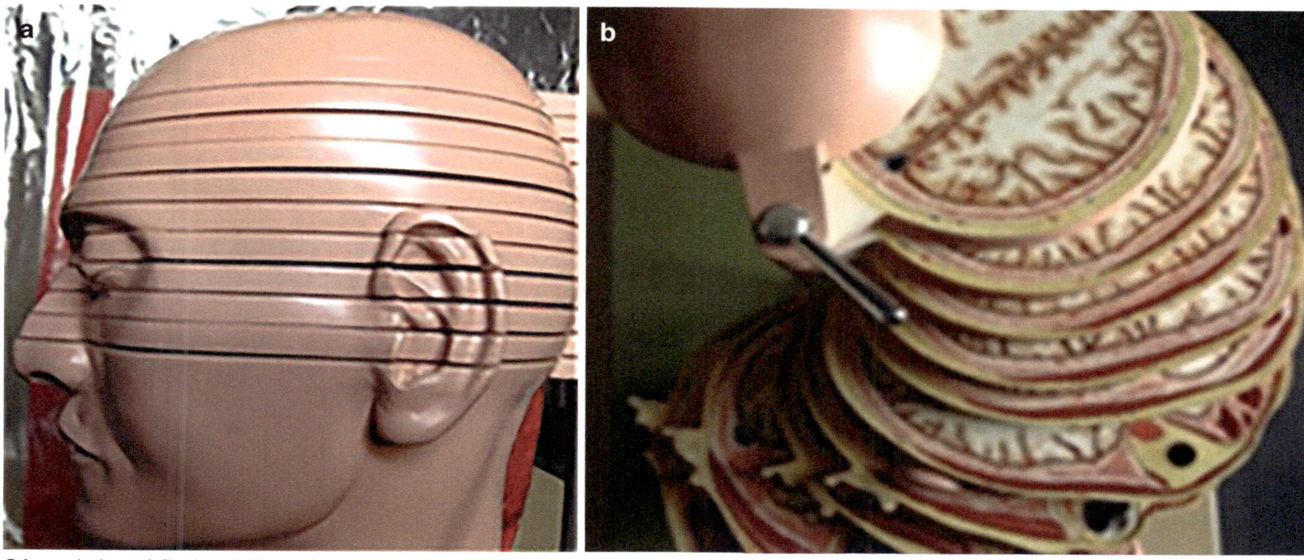




**Fig. 8.3** (**a**) Museum Model of head showing how axial slices are planned. The slice thickness varies from submillimeter to 10 mm, depending on the ROI (region of interest) and anatomical structure to be seen. (**b**) Stacked CT slices showing specific anatomy at a specific slice

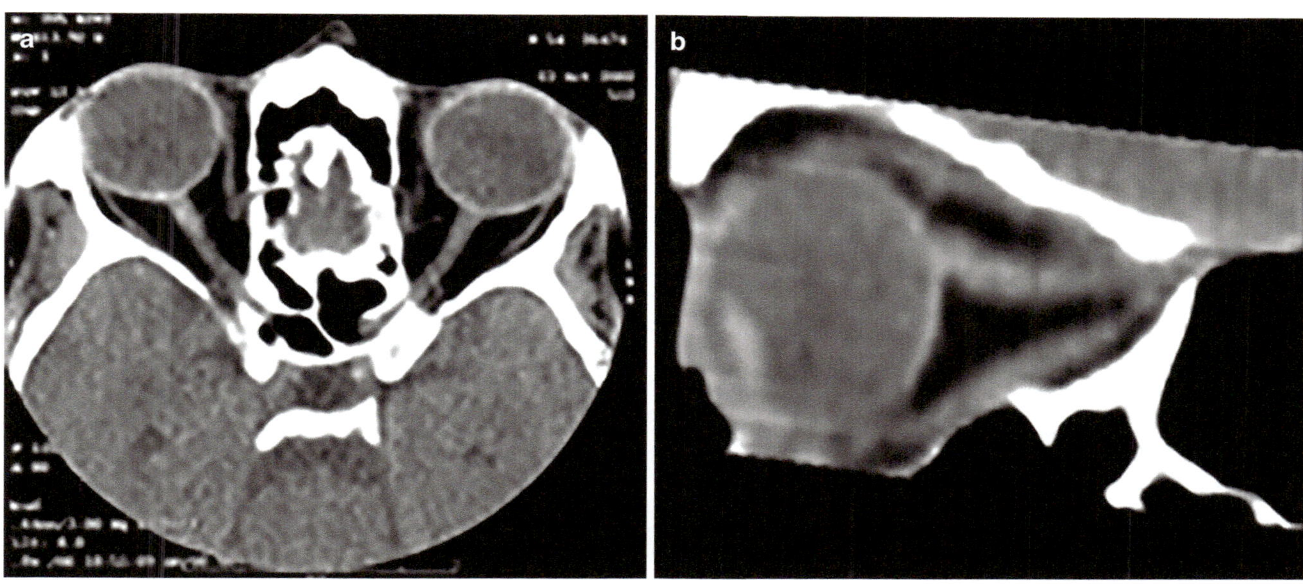




**Fig. 8.4** (**a**) CT axial primary slice soft-tissue window at the level of optic nerves showing mediolateral and anteroposterior relations and not superoinferior relations. (**b**) CT sagittal reconstructed image of the same patient at the level of optic nerve showing anterior, posterior, superior, and inferior relations

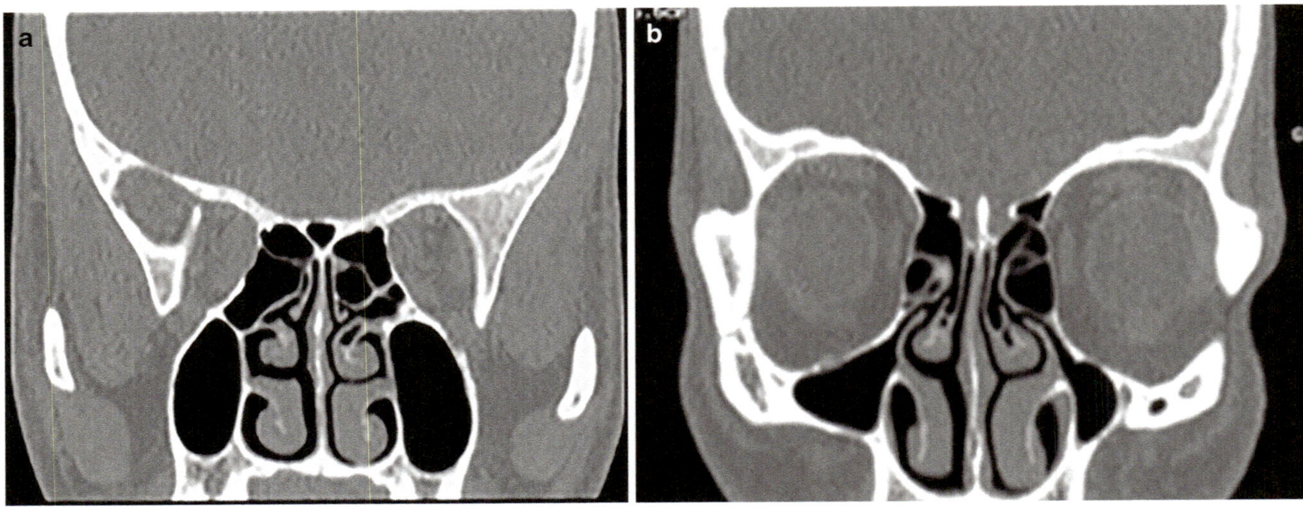




**Fig. 8.5** (**a**) and (**b**).CT coronal bone window primary images at different levels of paranasal sinuses

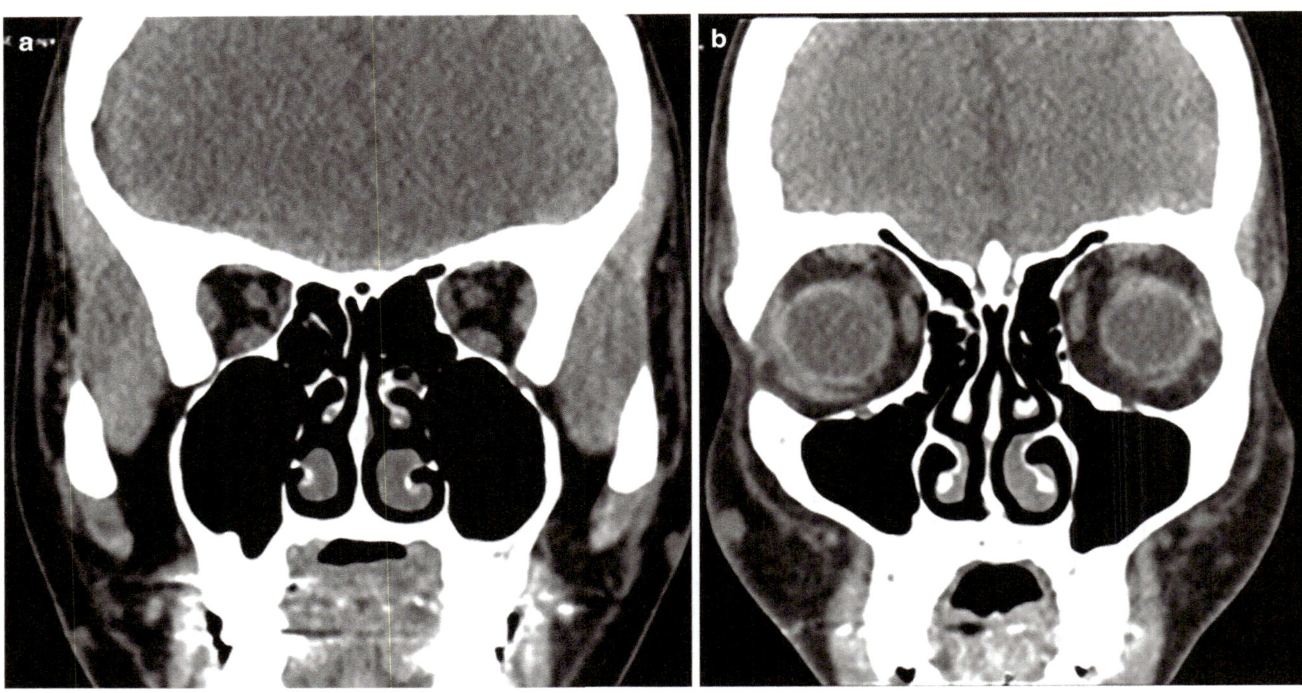




**Fig. 8.6** (**a**) and (**b**).CT coronal soft-tissue window primary images at different levels of Paranasal sinuses

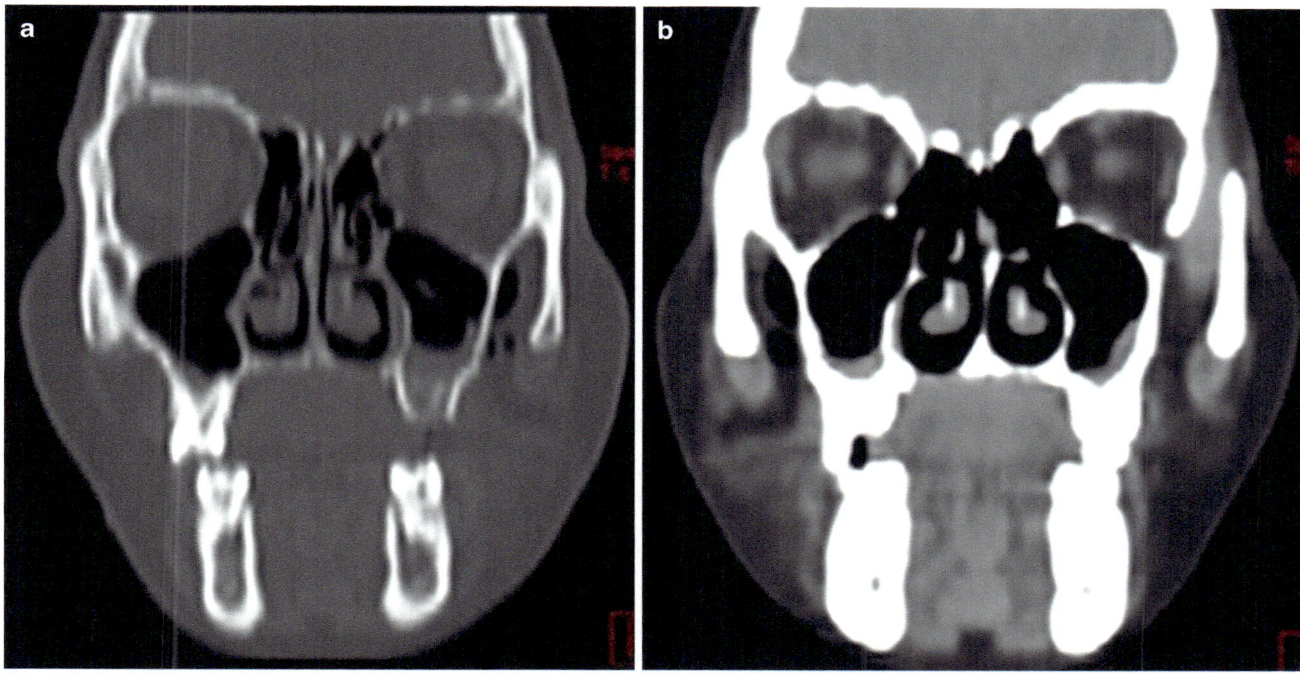




**Fig. 8.7** (**a**) and (**b**). CT reconstructed coronal images from thicker slices of paranasal sinuses at different levels. (**a**) bone window. (**b**) soft-tissue window. Note: coarse appearance

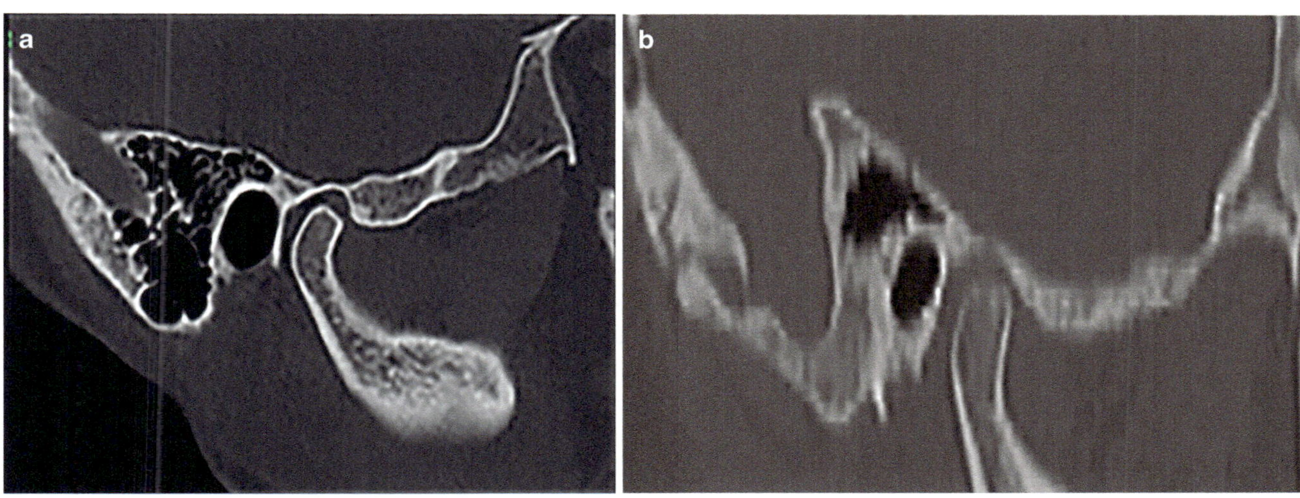




**Fig. 8.8** (**a**) CT direct slice of T.M. joint in its sagittal plane. Bone window. (**b**) CT reconstructed image from primary axial thick slices of T.M. joint in its sagittal plane. Note: coarse appearance

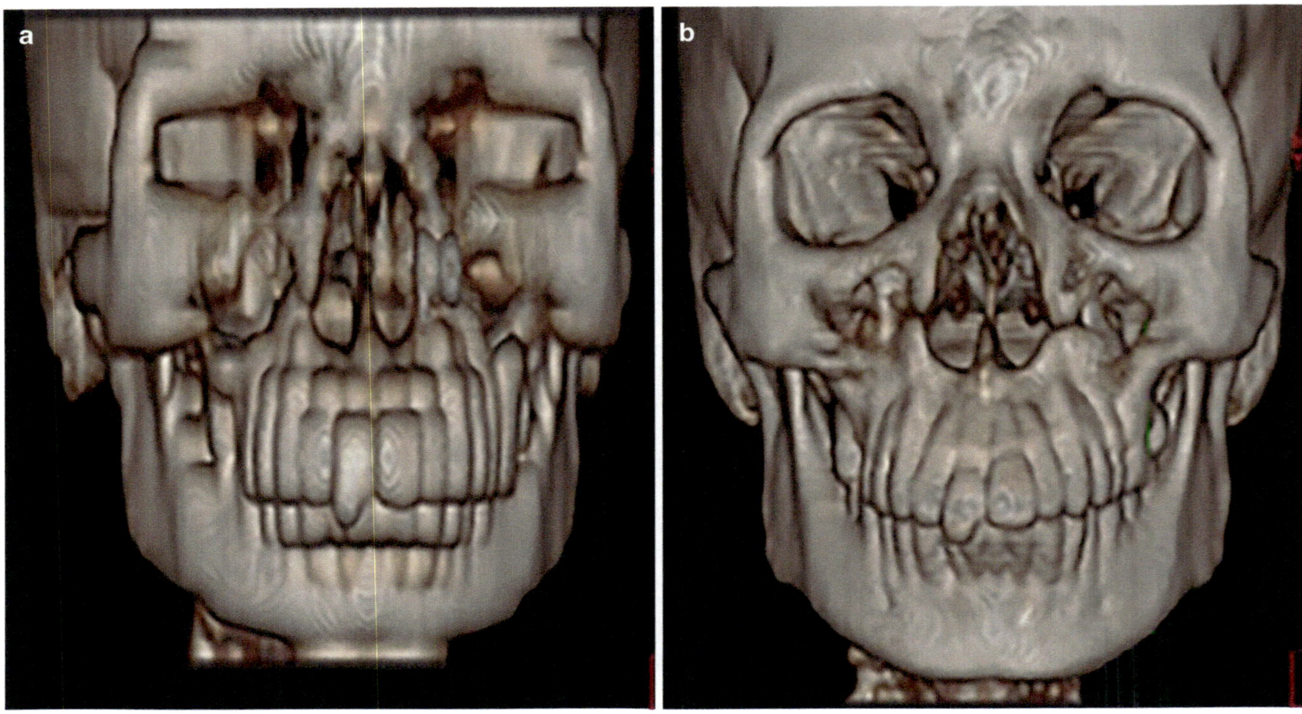




**Fig. 8.9** (**a**) CT 3D reconstructed image for surface bony details from thicker slices. Note: coarse appearance. (**b**) CT 3D reconstructed image from thin slices. Note: better and smoother image

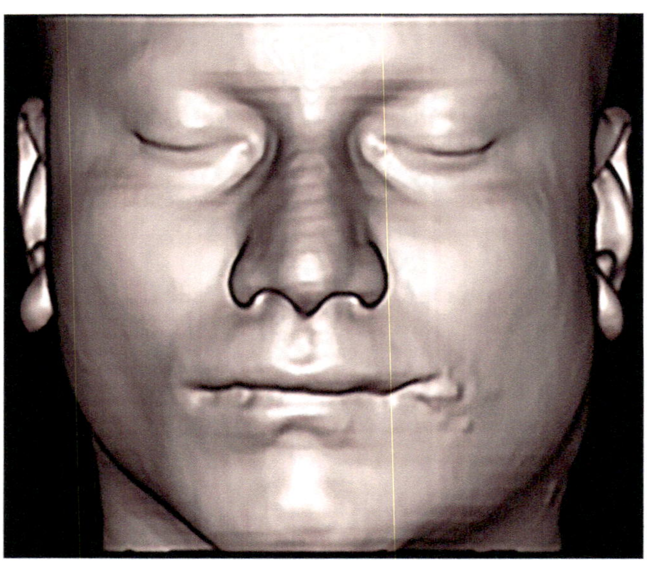



**Fig. 8.10** CT 3D surface rendering reconstructed image for surface soft-tissue details from thinner slices

CT imaging of the head region, axial and direct coronal slices are primarily possible, for the neck region, only axial slices are possible and in the temporomandibular joint region axial and direct sagittal slices are possible. It is through the raw data thus available that images are reconstructed in any desired plane.

**Dentascan**

*Basic principles of CT Orthopantomography (OPG) and Dentascan*

Conventional OPG is a first-level diagnostic exam that provides a gross panoramic view and just enough information about alignment of the teeth and any other related gross pathology. Unavoidable overlapping of some of the anatomical structures hinders accurate evaluation. To overcome these drawbacks, Dentascans and CT OPGs are used. They are extended applications of CT scan and involve the acquisition of thin axial submillimeter slices of the region covering the upper and lower jaws (Fig. 8.13). Reconstructed images obtained using these raw data image slices form the CT OPG or Dentascan image (Fig. 8.14a, b).

Coronal reconstructed images form the C.T. OPG (Fig. 8.15a, b, c). It is a second-level imaging technique wherein evaluation of the osseous elements of the maxilla and mandible is far better in comparison to conventional OPG. It provides the MFS with a better understanding of the morphology of the roots and the degree of contiguity between the roots and the mandibular canal. The information acquired is then used in planning and performing minimally invasive surgical procedures [1].

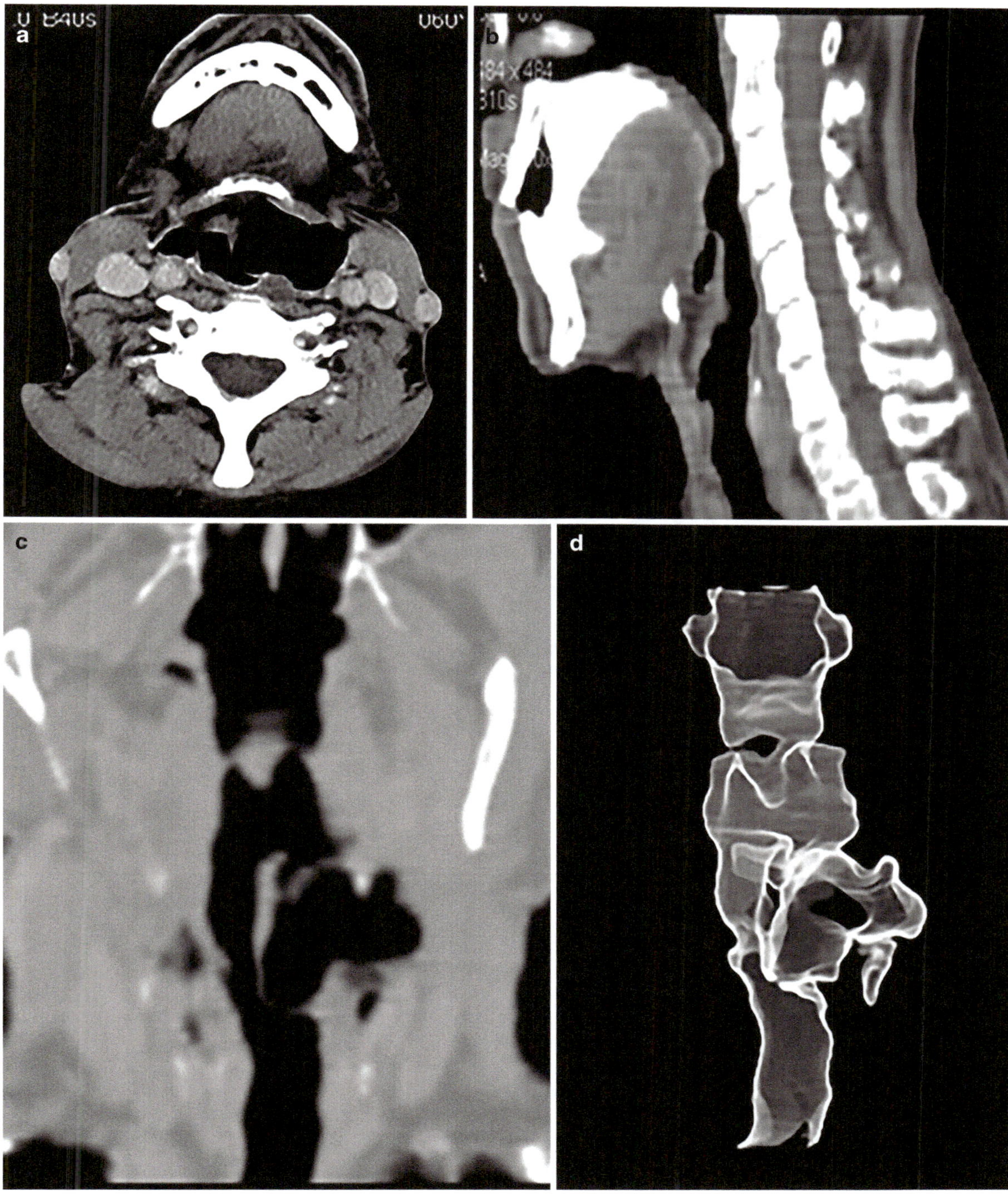




**Fig. 8.11** (**a**) CT Primary axial slice of neck at midlaryngeal level. (**b**) and (**c**) Sagittal and coronal reconstructed images from sequential CT primary axial slices. (**d**) CT Volume rendering technique (VRT) image of air column in the pharynx, larynx, and tracheal region as minimum density projection from primary axial slices (**a**). Note: Better visualization of laryngocele

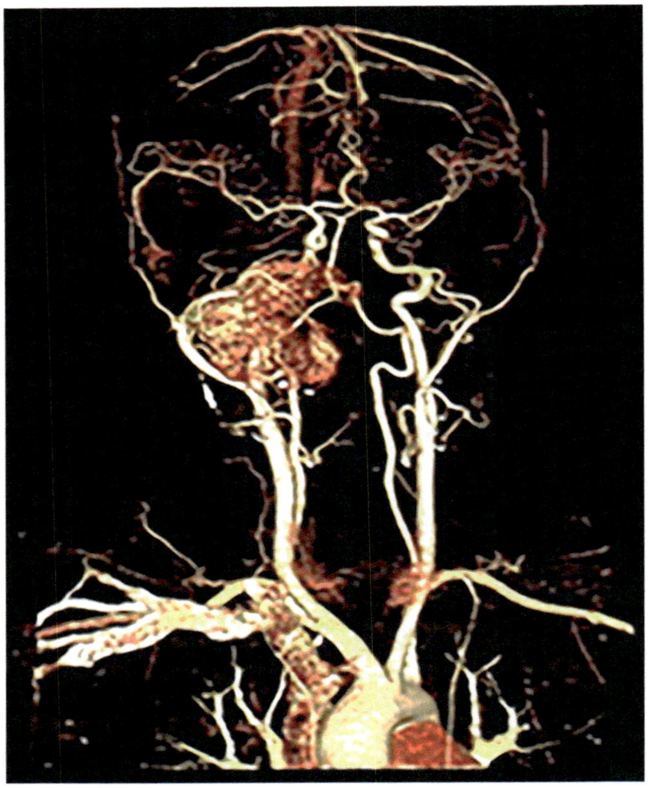



**Fig. 8.12** CT angiogram: 3D VRT (Volume Rendering Technique) displaying carotid arteries and its branches along with carotid body tumor. It is a reconstructed image from primary thin axial CT slices

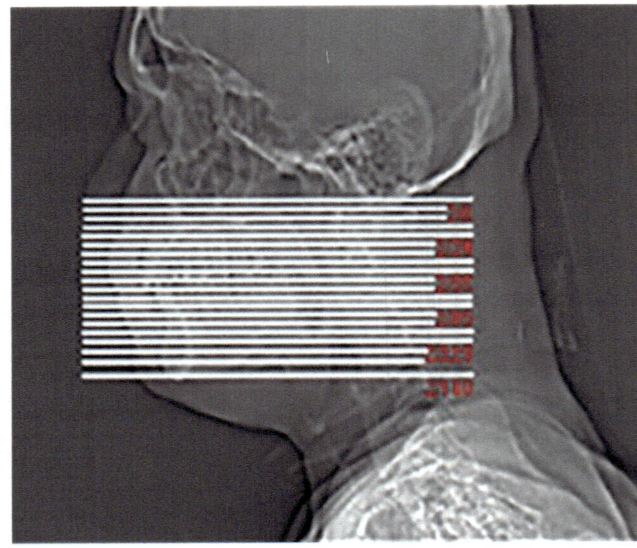



**Fig. 8.13** CT Scanogram for dentascan showing submillimeter axial slices planning in the region of maxilla and mandible

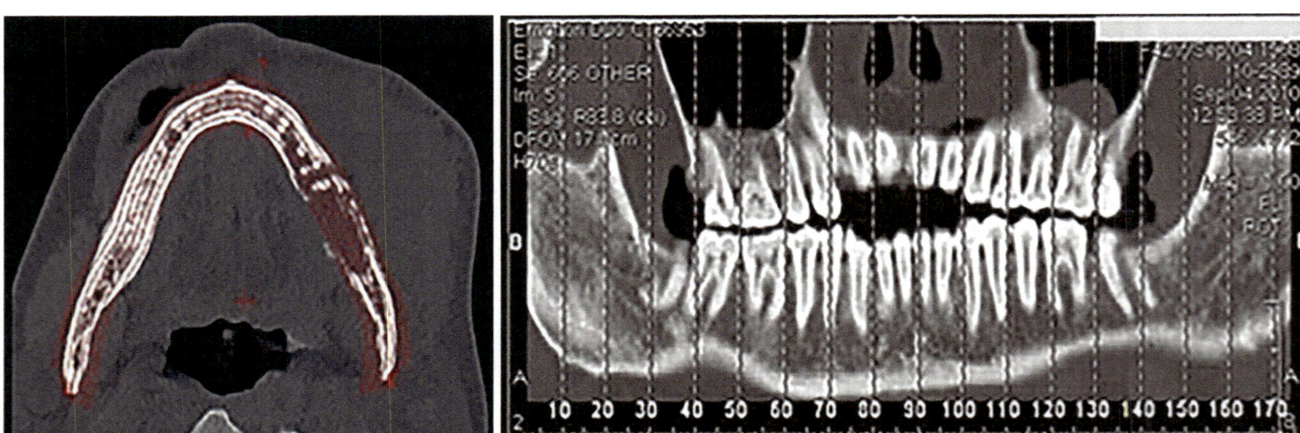




**Fig. 8.14** (**a**) and (**b**) .Reformatted panoramic CT images (**b**) are procured at desired plane of the jaw by curvilinear graphic lines drawn on the primary axial slice (**a**) selected

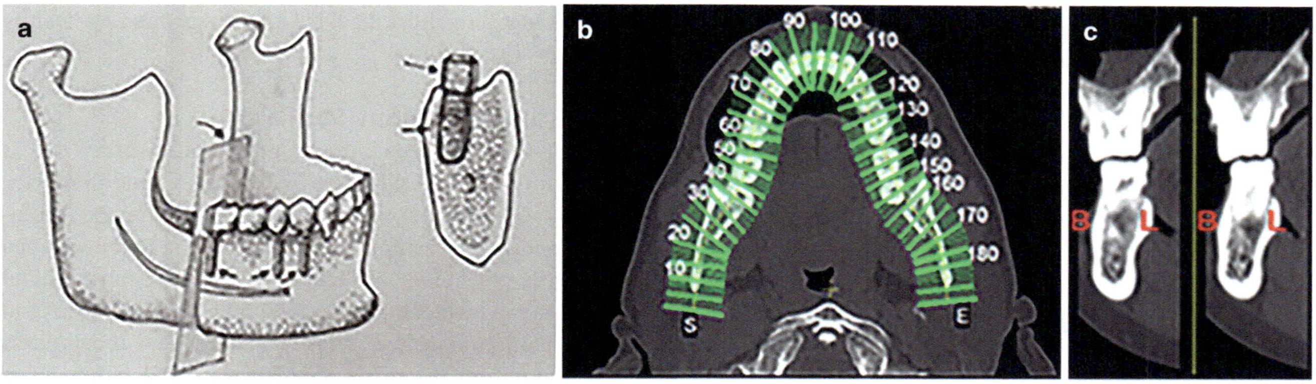




**Fig. 8.15** (**a**), (**b**), and (**c**). a and b show coronal plain image planning of individual tooth. c shows the coronal reformatted image of tooth

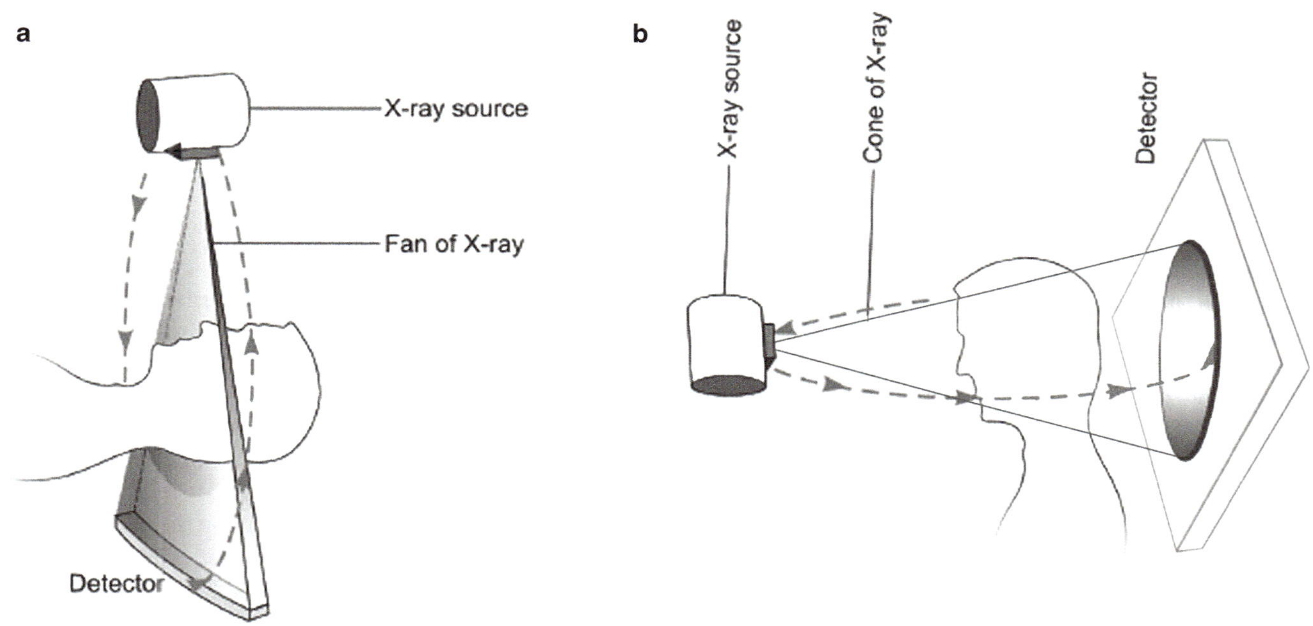




**Fig. 8.16** (**a**) and (**b**). Schematic diagram. (**a**) shows fan beam of X-rays from X-ray tube with curvilinear row of detectors. (**b**) shows cone beam of X-rays from X-ray tube with flat detector

## Cone Beam CT (CBCT)

*Indications for CBCT*

CBCT applications have proved helpful in a multitude of dental disciplines and the MFS needs to be aware of it. Its indications include periodontal and endodontic assessment, placement and evaluation of implants, evaluation of jaw bones, temporomandibular joints, bony and soft-tissue lesions, and alveolar ridge resorption and orthodontic evaluation.

### Working Principle and System Composition of CBCT System

As the name suggests, it is a form of computed tomography (CT). The basic process involved in CBCT is the scanning of the region of interest using a cone-shaped X-ray beam, making a single rotation around the vertical axis of the patient's head. The information obtained, from various angles about the structures in the region of interest, is in a digitized format relating to shape and density, which is then processed using

**Table 8.1** Comparison between CBCT and Fan Beam CT

| Fan Beam CT | CBCT |
|---|---|
| Conventional CT scanners make use of a fan beam and provide a set of consecutive slices of image. | CBCT makes use of a cone beam, which radiates from the x-ray source in a cone shape, encompassing a large volume with a single rotation. |
| Makes use of a lie-down machine with a large gantry | Makes use of a sitting up machine of smaller dimensions |
| Greater contrast and resolution | Ease of operation |
| Better differentiation between tissue types (bone, teeth, and soft tissue) | Commonly used for hard tissues Especially dental tissues |
| Higher radiation dose | Lesser radiation dose |
| Detector type X-axis only | Detector type X- and Y-axes |
| Volume acquisition requirements are sequential multiple gantry rotations | Volume acquisition requirements are single gantry rotations |
| Speed of examination is fast | Speed of examination is faster |

special software and a three-dimensional (3D) image is reconstructed [2].

CBCT occupies a special place in imaging of the Head and Neck region. It offers a number of advantages over traditional CT technology. It has a multitude of uses in the dental discipline, including dentoalveolar disease and anomalies, jaw tumors, vertical root and dentin fractures, among others. It has also had a positive impact on teaching students about oral and maxillofacial imaging making them adept at operating equipment and related instruments, resulting in greater accuracy in evaluation and analysis of the pathological characteristics of the disease process leading to a proper final clinical diagnosis. Both the traditional fan beam CT and CBCT are third-generation CT scanners but are different in some ways (Fig. 8.16a, b) (Table 8.1).

#### 8.7.1.3 Gamma Rays

Gamma rays are a form of Electromagnetic radiation (EMR). They are similar to X-rays but can be differentiated by the fact that they originate from the nucleus. Gamma-ray photons have the highest energy with their waves having the shortest wavelength in the EMR spectrum. The difference between the two is that X-rays are produced by accelerating electrons when they strike a target, while gamma rays originate from the nucleus of a radionuclide after radioactive decay. Gamma rays damage the DNA of cells and it is this action that is used in the treatment of cancerous tumors, care being taken not to affect the DNA of the surrounding healthy tissue cells [3].

#### 8.7.1.4 Nuclear Isotope Studies

Scintigraphy or radionuclide imaging is a modality that is readily available and relatively inexpensive. One drawback is that though it can provide specific information, the resolution is poor. It is a functional imaging modality and can assess early physiological changes even before bone mineral changes are evident. Bone scintigraphy is highly sensitive in detection of skeletal osteoblastic activity and the process involves uptake of the radiopharmaceutical Technetium-99 m (Tc-99 m), by the mineral component of the bone due to its affinity for bone. It has proven to be greatly useful in the study of malignant lesions and also in the evaluation of vascularized bone grafts used in reconstruction surgeries of the maxillofacial region [4]. Another use of radionuclide imaging is in evaluating patients with condylar hyperplasia. In these patients, radionuclide imaging of the temporomandibular joint is performed to exclude active condylar growth and in planning the extent of orthognathic surgery. A progressive condition necessitates the removal of the entire condyle and neck while trimming of the enlarged condyle suffices otherwise [5].

#### 8.7.1.5 Positron Emission Tomography (PET)

PET also is a functional imaging technique. It is unique in that it produces images reflecting in vivo changes in tissue metabolism, linking the changes to malignancy. Body images are produced when radiation is emitted from radioactive tracer substances like Carbon-11, Fluorine-18, Oxygen-15, or Nitrogen-13. When a positron emitted from the radioactive substance collides with an electron in the tissue, gamma rays are given off at the site, which are detected by a gamma detector. FDG-PET/CT fusion scans of the head and neck are not primarily for infection identification but for categorizing a clinically questionable lesion as malignant or not.

CT scans detect changes in body structure and only confirms the presence of a mass. PET scan is different from CT in that it can reveal the presence of disease earlier allowing for quicker diagnosis, can detect the extent of disease and whether a detected mass is benign or malignant, helps monitoring treatment and its effectiveness, and can detect abnormalities even before there is any anatomical change. This is based on the fact that glucose consumption by malignant cells and hence tissue is far higher than that of normal tissue.

The scan involves intravenous injection of a radiolabeled compound like 2-deoxy-2-(18F) fluoro-D-glucose (FDG). After uptake of the compound, it undergoes further break down in the cells. Since tumor cells have a high metabolic rate, it is also metabolized by the tumor cells. FDG is metabolized to FDG-6-phosphate, but the tumor cells are incapable of metabolizing it further and in consequence the FDG-6-phosphate accumulates and concentrates within the tumor cells. It is this accumulation that is detected and quantified. As compared to normal tissue, the uptake of FDG by malignant tissue is very high, making it a sensitive method to pick up early malignant tissue [6].

## 8.8 Radiation: Hazard Awareness and Principles of Protection

**Hazardous Nature of X-Rays**

When an X-ray photon is incident on tissue, it results in a series of changes at the molecular and atomic level. The transformed photon energy results in the discharge of an electron and a free radical, or ionization in other words. Ionization results in the production of a new molecule due to breakage of enzyme bonds manifesting in the form of different biological effects. These effects may be repairable when there is no appreciable damage, or irreparable when there is definite occurrence of damage, the adverse effect being cumulative in nature.

**Myths and Facts about radiation in the field of Diagnosis:** Many myths exist regarding radiation hazards associated with medical diagnostic imaging. Possible reasons for this are the available historical data, exaggerated social media reports, results of experimental studies and the complex nature of radiation biology making it difficult to evaluate its mechanism of action. Historical data relates to the reports of visible radiation hazards from studies on victims of the Hiroshima/Nagasaki bomb explosion in 1945 who were followed up for 15-18years. Exaggerated reporting by social media about nuclear reactor accidents like that at Chernobyl add to the existing myths. The extremely short time for which radiation interacts with matter ($10^{-5}$Sec) after absorption, makes it difficult to study the complex nature of radiation biology. The biological process of cell death can take days to months, carcinogenesis can take years to occur while generations may pass before a mutational change is seen.

In reality, the dose of received radiation from man-made X-rays that exist today is minute, in comparison with the massive radiation exposure that occurred in the aforementioned examples. It is true that in the infant stage following discovery of X-rays and its use in diagnosis, visible radiation hazards did occur, which was due to ignorance in the understanding of its potential hazards and the use of crude equipment resulting in high amounts of radiation leak. With passage of time, we have learnt to put the benefits of X-rays to full use, concurrently taking proper precautions to protect ourselves from its hazardous effects. Over the years, improvements in diagnostic equipment using ionizing radiation have led to the production of newer equipment providing the best possible image quality with minimal radiation exposure and improved devices that are protective against radiation. Yet, the fact remains that the best method to reduce the effects of radiation is using it only when it is an utmost necessity [7].

## 8.9 Imaging Investigations Not Involving Ionizing Radiation

### 8.9.1 MRI (Magnetic Energy Coupled with Radiofrequency Energy)

This imaging modality does not involve the use of ionizing radiation but makes use of magnetic and radiofrequency energy to obtain information of the internal organs. Components of an MRI unit include the magnet, the console, and the computer.

**Image Procurement by MRI**

Exploiting the body's magnetic property forms the basis of imaging using magnetic resonance. The human body is abundant in atoms with odd number of protons, or in other words ionized particles or charged atoms. A charged particle spinning around its own axis creates a magnetic field around itself behaving like a tiny bar magnet. Hydrogen represents one such atom that is present in water molecules and therefore in all body tissues.

The random orientation of the hydrogen atoms cancels out their magnetic fields and so there is no net magnetization at rest. When these protons are placed in a strong magnetic field, a net magnetization is produced that aligns parallel with the main magnetic field. To influence the human body, the external magnetic strength needs to be about 6000 to 80,000 times the earth's magnetic strength. The resultant net magnetization acts as the source of the MR signal and is used to produce MR images. Application of a radiofrequency (RF) pulse results in absorption of energy from the RF pulse causing the net magnetization to rotate away from the direction of the main magnetic field, the amount of rotation or flip angle depending on the strength and duration of the RF pulse. The strength and duration of the RF pulse can be controlled such that the net magnetization can be rotated to any angle [8]. Withdrawal of the RF pulse results in the liberation of energy, with the emission of signals based on the density of protons or hydrogen atoms. These signals are captured by the external antennae, fed into the computer, and processed to produce the image.

### Types of Magnets: Their Advantages and Limitations

- External magnets are of two types, the permanent magnet and the electromagnet.
- Permanent magnets are cheaper with no significant recurring cost. However, its limitations include limited strength of less than 0.5 tesla, heavy nature making transportation difficult, production of weak signals, and slower performance with limited range resolution.
- Electromagnets work by the passage of high current around ferromagnetic substances creating the required magnetic field. They are faster, have better resolution, produce better reconstructions, and are lighter than permanent magnets. The drawback is the production of large amount of heat that needs cooling using Liquid Helium. Other disadvantages include the high cost of infrastructure, high consumption of electricity, and recurring expenses.

### Preparing a Patient for an MRI

- Detailed history and clinical examination are mandatory.
- Specific history relating to previous surgery with the use of aneurysmal clips or metallic prosthesis needs to be ascertained.
- Patient compatibility for the procedure needs to be evaluated in view of the requirement of lying motionless for a minimum of 30 to 40 min, e.g., Orthopneic patients, COAD patients. Anesthesia might be required for agitated patients and infants.
- A double check for any metallic objects on the patient's body using a metal detector device is necessary.
- Claustrophobic patients need to be reassured and put at ease before the examination begins.
- The procedure needs to be explained in detail prior to the patient entering the MRI magnet room.

CT & MRI are complementary to each other. As far as the MFS is concerned, thin-slice CT with reconstruction is required while evaluating bony lesions, especially in cases of trauma. MRI on the other hand is good for evaluation of soft-tissue tumors and is contraindicated in penetrating injuries of the eye (Table 8.2).

**Table 8.2** CT and MRI: A comparison

| | CT | MRI |
|---|---|---|
| Multiplanar Imaging | Only axial slices are possible. Images need to be reconstructed in multiple planes following acquisition of primary axial sections. Direct sagittal and coronal slices are possible except for TM joint. | Direct multiplanar images can be primarily acquired in any desired plane. Excellent sectional images are possible. |
| Soft-tissue characterization | | Best with MRI than CT |
| Compact bone/ calcified lesions | Best analyzed by CT than MRI | |
| Bone marrow | | Assessment best with MRI than CT |
| Radiation | Ionizing radiation involved | No ionizing radiation involved |
| Motion artifacts | Relatively well managed with CT | Very sensitive to any kind of motion. May require anesthesia. Noisy breathing too may affect images |
| Time required | Faster, with whole body scan from vertex to toe taking 8–10 seconds | Takes longer. Minimum time required for scan of any part is 40–60 min |
| Contrast media | Invariably required and so contrast-related problems are unavoidable. | Contrast is less frequently used and is relatively safer. |
| Trauma | Best modality | |
| Ferromagnetic artifacts | | MRI is contraindicated in patients with pacemakers or recently placed implants. MRI compatible supportive gadgets: Pulse Oxymeter, anesthesia equipment, I.V. stands, etc. |

## How Does CT/MRI Differ from Conventional Radiography?

CT and MRI are sectional imaging methods, in which the whole body or the region of interest is sectioned into serial slices and further into cubes (Fig. 8.3a, b). Each slice surface represents the corresponding sectional anatomy with each slice being made up of small units or cubes with each cube representing the basic nature of the tissue in the digital form (Figs. 8.17 and 8.18a, b). Different modalities produce varied imaging appearances of the same structure. For instance, if a coconut is imaged using different modalities, the fine structural details of the interior of the tender coconut, and its contents are better seen on CT and MRI (Fig. 8.19a-c). Similarly, imaging of a pineapple in axial (Fig. 8.20a-d) and coronal planes (Fig. 8.21a-c) and using the volume-rendering technique (Fig. 8.22) reveals varied appearances on CT and different MRI sequences.

To summarize, in sectional imaging, the region of interest or the whole body is divided into slices and cubes with each cube representing the basic tissue of that region with thinner slices and smaller-sized cubes offering better resolution.

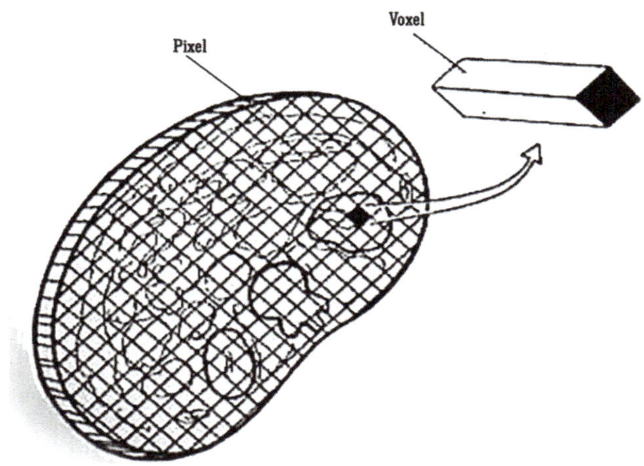




**Fig. 8.17** Each axial slice is divided into small cubes loaded with digitalized values representing corresponding tissue volume called voxel. Its surface represents a fraction of the grayscale image specific for that region called pixel. Thinner the slice and smaller the pixel, better is the resolution

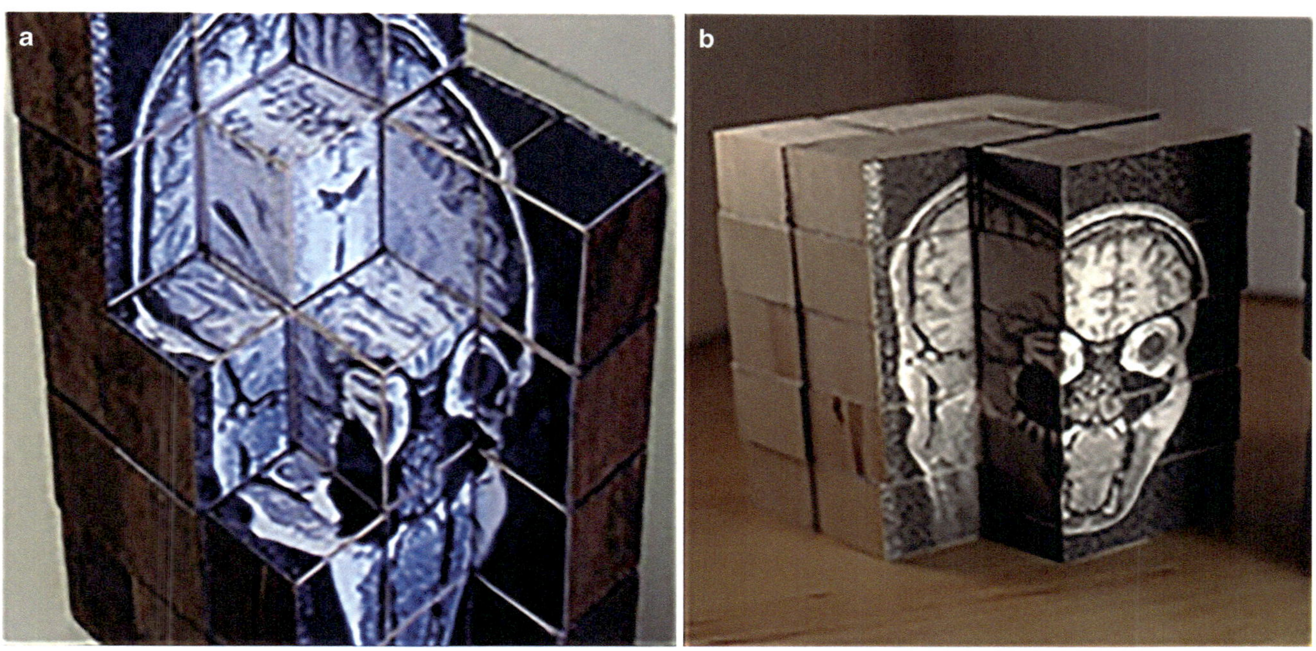




**Fig. 8.18** (**a**) and (**b**). Figures showing unit wise volumetric digitalized information of anatomical structures for retrieval and displayed as sectional anatomical slices

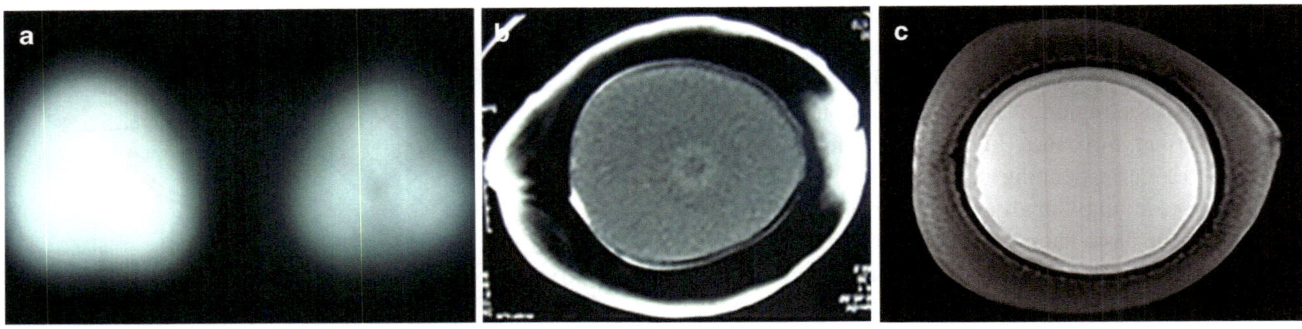



**Fig. 8.19** (**a**), (**b**), and (**c**). Imaging of tender coconut. (**a**) Conventional plain Radiograph. (**b**) CT Axial sectional imaging. (**c**) MRI sectional imaging. Note: added information with each of these modalities

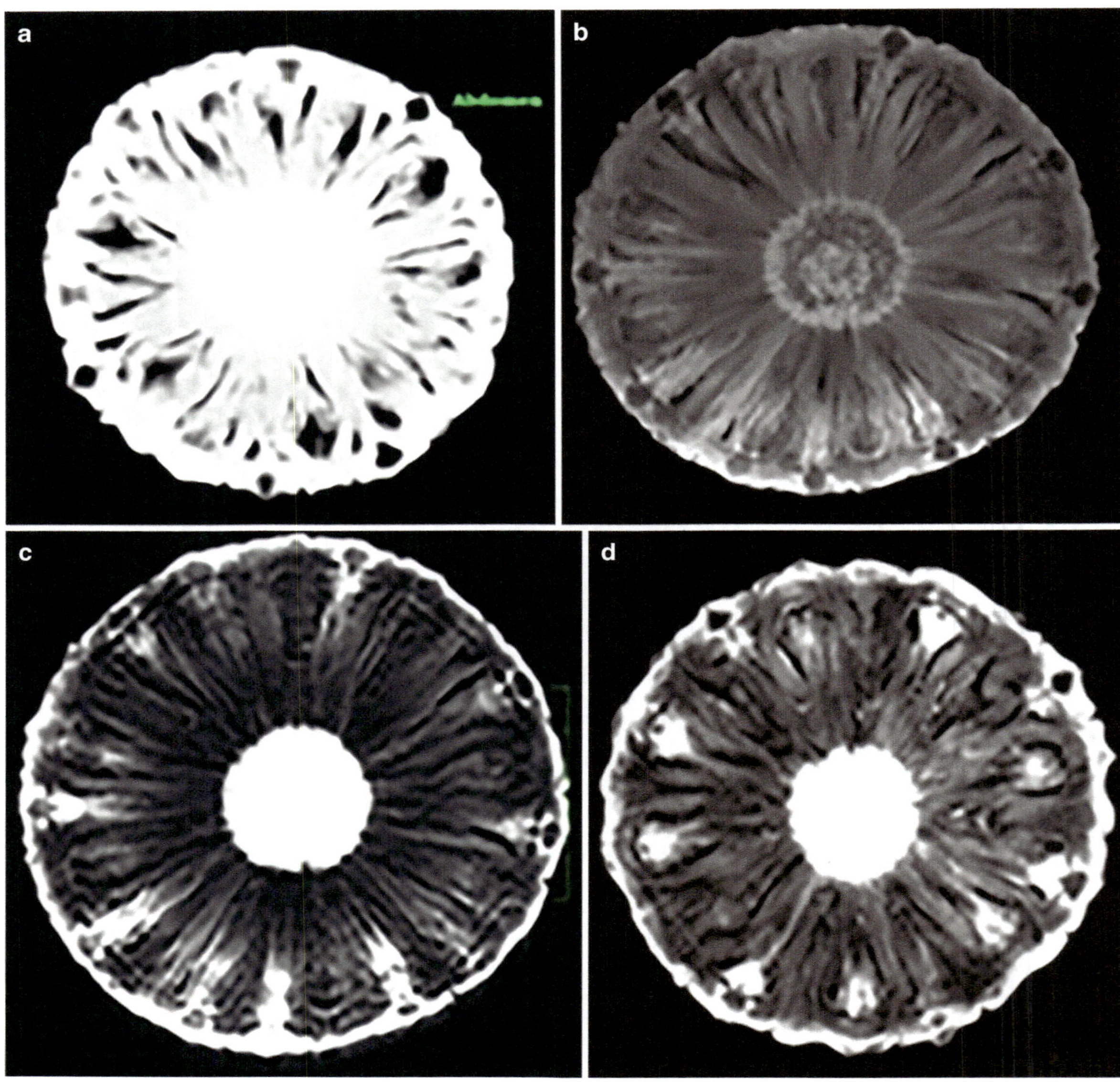



**Fig. 8.20** (**a**), (**b**), (**c**), and (**d**). Axial sectional images of pineapple taken at the same level (**a**) CT. (**b**, **c**, **d**) MRI various sequences. Note: superior soft-tissue resolution in MRI, highlighting various components of soft tissue in various sequences

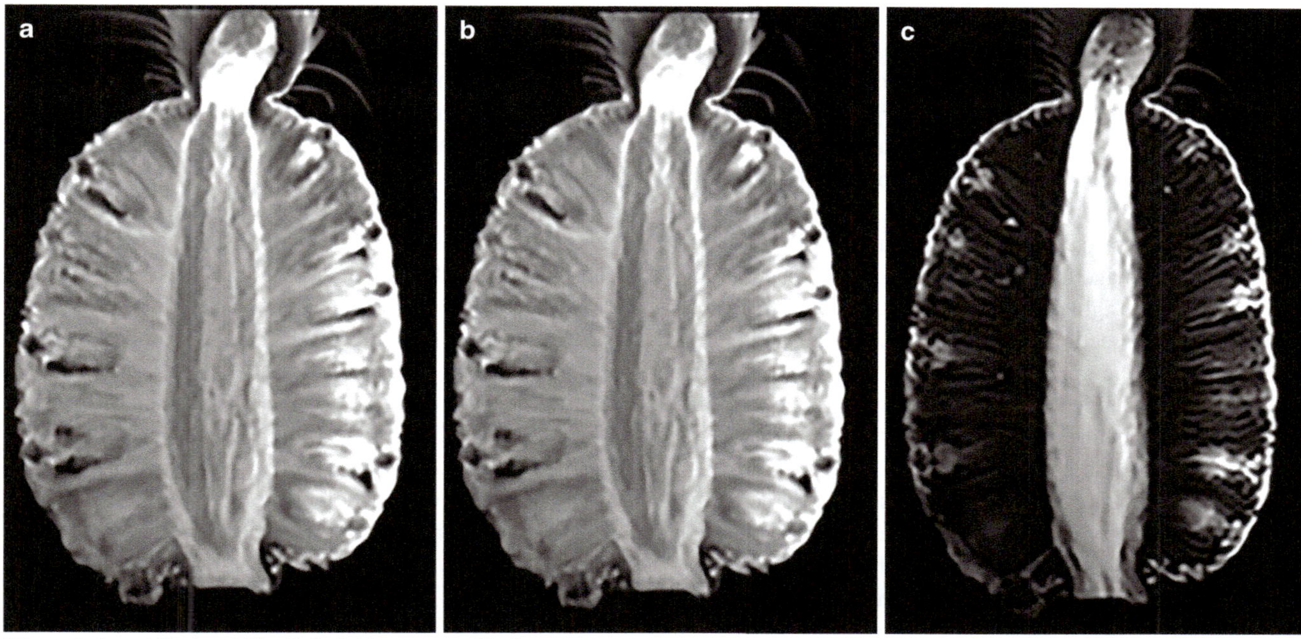




**Fig. 8.21** (**a**, **b** and **c**). Various sequences of MRI of a pineapple showing multiplanar capability to procure sections in any desired plane without reconstruction unlike CT

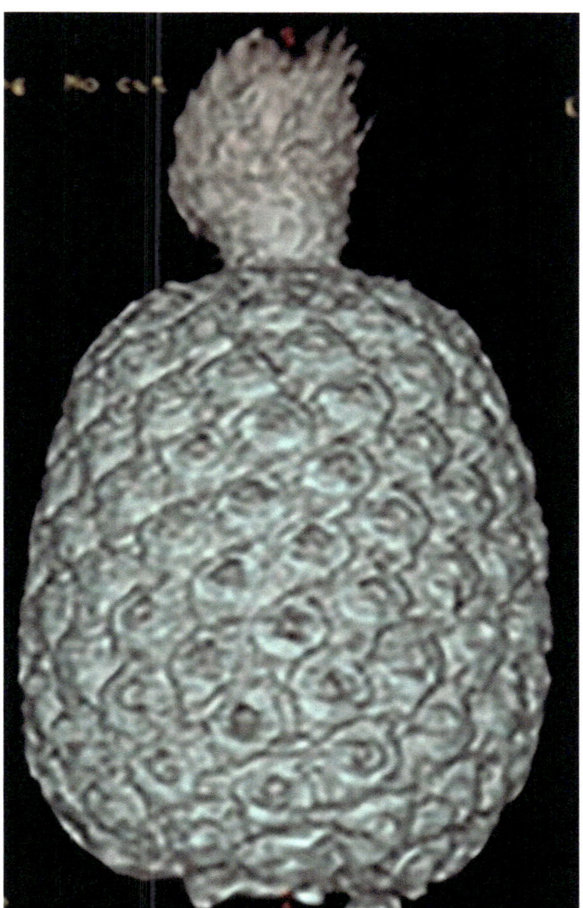



**Fig. 8.22** CT 3D surface rendering image of Pineapple

### 8.9.2 Ultrasound

It seems implausible that sound waves can produce informative images of internal organs of a human body. Yet it is true that technology has evolved so much over the years that it is now possible to obtain information of body structures using sound waves by making use of the echo and Doppler properties of sound waves.

Sound waves can be classified, based on their wavelength and frequency as audible sounds (20 to 2000 cycles/sec), infrasound (less than 20 cycles/sec), and ultrasound (>20,000 cycles/sec). Ultrasound in the range of 2 to 20 MHz is used in medical imaging [8]. The source of these ultrasound waves is piezoelectric crystals. These crystals have the special property of generating electrical pulses on being subjected to pressure. In addition, the passage of electricity through the crystals causes them to get compressed or deformed. Essentially, these crystals are unique in that they have the dual property of converting electrical energy into mechanical energy and mechanical energy into electrical energy. Intermittent passage of electrical current through the crystals makes them alternate between compression and relaxation, resulting in vibration of the crystal, in consequence producing sound energy of small wavelength in the ultrasound range.

Devices, equipped with piezoelectric crystals, having the capability to convert electrical energy to mechanical energy and finally to sound energy as well as having the reverse capabilities of converting sound energy to electrical energy, are termed as Transducers.

Sound waves are useful in imaging due to their property of echo/reflection and due to the Doppler effect. Echo property refers to the property of sound waves to get reflected at the interface of two media, the strength of the reflected sound echo depending on the density difference of the media through which they traverse. Reflected sound energy gets converted to mechanical energy and finally to electrical energy on striking the crystal, and this electrical energy is represented on a monitor as bright dots of variable gray scales.

Varying density interfaces throughout body tissues, produces variable image brightness with gray scales ranging between extreme bright dots to black dots, representing different organ or tissue sections. The Doppler effect of sound refers to the change in the apparent frequency of a wave when the observer and the source move toward or away from each other. Motion causes a change in pitch with a higher frequency being heard when the sound source approaches the observer, and a lower frequency being heard when the sound source moves away. This Doppler property is used in evaluating the direction and velocity of flow of blood in vessels. The transducer is considered as the fixed source of sound and the blood component, mainly the RBCs act as moving reflecting bodies. At a given point in the vessel by calculating the sudden change in the frequency of reflected sound, we can calculate the velocity of blood and also the direction of blood flow. This helps in the evaluation of percentage of stenosis in a vessel.

**B Mode**

A grayscale sectional image has specific echo texture based on tissue content with the display mode being called as the 'B' mode (Brightness mode) or grayscale mode. Higher sound frequency provides better image resolution with delineation of finer tissue components, however, at the expense of depth of penetration. Higher-frequency transducers (7 MHz to 20 MHz) are hence used for imaging superficial structures like cheek, the maxillofacial region, neck spaces, breast, thyroid, testis, eye, musculoskeletal system and skin, regions where finer analysis of tissue structure is expected. Deeper structures are evaluated by using transducers with frequency in the range of 2 to 5 MHz.

The relation between frequency, resolution, and depth can be understood well, using the hypothetical example of two friends—an ant and an elephant (Fig. 8.23a, b). Both of them are commanded to perform the same tasks, the first being to pick up and bring back a crystal of sugar dropped at a distance of 100 cm from the start line and the second to pick up and bring back a log of wood placed 100 meters from the start line. Both of them proceed to perform the first task. The ant being small is able to easily identify the sugar crystal and get it back; however, the elephant keeps moving around unable to identify the crystal. As to the second task, the ant is able to travel only a short distance after which it dies of exhaustion, unable to reach the log of wood while the elephant travels the distance with ease and brings back the log of wood.

The ant is comparable to the high-frequency short-wavelength sound wave that is able to travel a short distance and bring back finer information about superficial tissues. If, on the other hand, it travels a long distance all its energy is absorbed by interaction with tissues. The elephant is comparable to the low-frequency sound wave with long wavelength that can travel deeper into the tissues and get information of deep structures, but limited tissue details. In a clinical setup, both the ant (high-frequency sound) and the elephant (low-frequency sound) are essential for evaluation, depending on the clinical situation and region of interest.

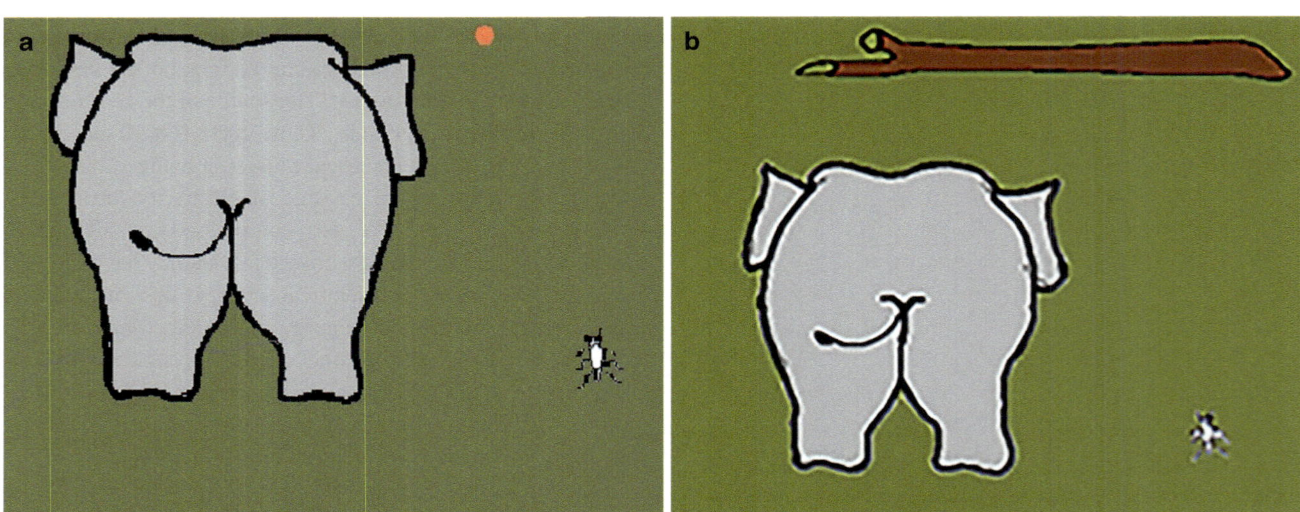




Fig. 8.23 (**a**) and (**b**). Example of an elephant and an ant demonstrating their varying capability in picking up large and small objects from varying distances—a pictorial representation for understanding the difference in the penetration capacity of high- and low-frequency sound waves. (Explained in the text)

**Color Doppler**
The display of flow of blood in a vessel is color coded. The flow toward the probe is depicted as red and flow away from the probe is blue. Arterial and venous flow, in a given anatomical region, is in opposite directions. Red generally represents flow in arteries, while blue represents venous flow. Turbulent flow is depicted using a mixture of colors.

**Power Doppler**
This display mode of Doppler conveys information about the overall flow in a given tissue, for instance, assessment of blood flow in a tumor. It helps to determine whether the tumor is hyper- or hypovascular.

**Strengths of Ultrasound**
- Ultrasound imaging is inexpensive and is free from the risk of radiation.
- Excellent soft-tissue resolution is possible and dynamic studies too can be performed under ultrasound guidance.
- It is the first line of investigation for hepatic, biliary, and renal disease and is an excellent modality for cyst imaging,
- Gynecological and prostate disorders are imaged using endocavitary ultrasound, Doppler studies allow assessment of blood flow, and real-time ultrasound imaging helps in guiding interventional biopsies and drainages.

**Weaknesses of Ultrasound**
- A long learning curve exists for some areas of expertise and image resolution is dependent on the machine that is available. Ultrasound does not give information of structure behind a bone and also gas filled structures.

**Specific Role of High-Resolution Ultrasonography (HRUSG) in the Maxillofacial Region**
HRUSG is a grossly underutilized modality in evaluating lesions of the maxillofacial region. This is due to the lack of awareness of its application. The tissues in the maxillofacial region are ideal for sonographic evaluation and hence is widely applied to help diagnose a number of clinical conditions. It can serve as the best possible initial parallel imaging investigation for all the superficial soft-tissue structures of head and neck region.

It is noninvasive and does not involve use of radiation. There are no contraindications to the use of ultrasound, and it can even be performed as a bed side examination. No prior specific preparation is required except for shaving of the beard, which might hamper the study. The study results are immediately available, and it is an excellent modality for evaluating various soft-tissue planes of the cheek. Evaluation of various anatomical spaces such as superficial masticator space, parotid space, carotid space, superficial neck spaces, visceral space, floor of the mouth, and all the infrahyoid neck spaces like the submandibular and sublingual spaces are possible using HRUSG, as are also pathologies like pre- and paravertebral abscesses, cellulitis, Ludwig's angina, and ranula [9].

High-resolution ultrasound is also capable of evaluating the nature of lymph nodes, assessing fluid and solid components and also assessing tissue vitality. Procedures like drainage of abscesses and biopsies can be conveniently performed under ultrasound guidance. Being a highly economical imaging modality, it is excellent for follow-up studies, excellent as a screening method, and at most times proves to be the conclusive examination [9].

**Drawbacks of Ultrasound Examination of the Maxillofacial Region**
Drawbacks include difficulty in assessing structures behind bony elements and structures containing gas. In case of huge masses, only partial information may be obtained, while short-necked individuals and obese patients are difficult to evaluate. Structures at the base of the skull cannot be evaluated as are structures medial to ramus. Another limitation is that ultrasound cannot provide information about structures behind bone or any gas-filled structure. Scanning using a hockey stick probe might help overcoming this limitation. Scans need to be performed by individuals having vast experience and expertise.

There needs to be an increase in awareness regarding the developments in the application of HRUSG in the maxillofacial region and a close interaction between the surgeon and the sonologist for creating an atmosphere of better understanding among them.

### 8.9.3 Thermography

Medical thermography is used for early preclinical diagnosis and treatment of homeostatic imbalances. It is noninvasive and safe since it does not use any radiation. It makes use of body heat to diagnose a wide range of health conditions. By using high-speed computers and thermal imaging cameras, body heat is processed and recorded in the computer as an image map that can be analyzed. The analysis is based on determining the presence of abnormal hot and cold areas that can relate to different conditions.

**Applications in the Maxillofacial Region**
A variety of conditions related to blood flow in the head and neck vessels can be assessed by thermal imaging. Easy visualization of facial blood vessels by thermography is possible because of its superficial location. Common venues of thermographic use in the head and neck region include evaluation of pain related to differentiation of different types of headache, facial nerve injury following a blow to the face or an accident, and visualization of disorders of the temporomandibular joint.

## 8.10 Role of Chest Radiograph in the Practice of Maxillo Facial Surgery

One of the most frequently requested investigations by an MFS is the Chest radiograph. Hence, interpretation of chest radiographic findings is of prime importance in determining the patient's clinical status.

### 8.10.1 Chest Radiographic Evaluation for Optimum Diagnostic Quality

An ideal chest radiograph, in terms of quality, is one that fulfills the following criteria (Fig. 8.24)

(a) Well-positioned patient without rotation.
  - *Purpose*—Avoiding problems related to improper positioning that can obscure certain lung regions like the hila and mediastinal lines, can prevent clarity of borders, or can result in distorted position of structures like the trachea, which can be misinterpreted as a paratracheal mass.
  - *Ideal radiograph*—The vertebral spinous processes are equidistant from the medial ends of the clavicle

(b) Proper lateral location of both scapulae on the radiograph.
  - *Purpose*—avoids superimposition of scapulae over the lung fields
  - *Ideal radiograph*—Medial border of the scapulae should be out of the lung field

(c) Inclusion of anatomical structures.
  - *Purpose*—inclusion of entire lung fields from apex to diaphragmatic domes
  - *Ideal radiograph*—must include the lower neck, both shoulders, lateral chest walls, and both diaphragms, including upper abdomen

(d) Proper identification references
  - *Purpose*—Proper patient and radiographic verification.
  - *Ideal radiograph*—must include the patient name, medical record number, date of acquisition, and the side marker (the most important of all)

(e) Optimum technical factors.
  - *Purpose*—Clear visualization of the normal anatomy or presence of any pathology
  - *Ideal radiograph*—
    - Posterior third of ribs faintly visible through heart shadow
    - Intervertebral spaces faintly visible through the heart shadow
    - Obtained in deep inspiratory effort as revealed by position of diaphragms

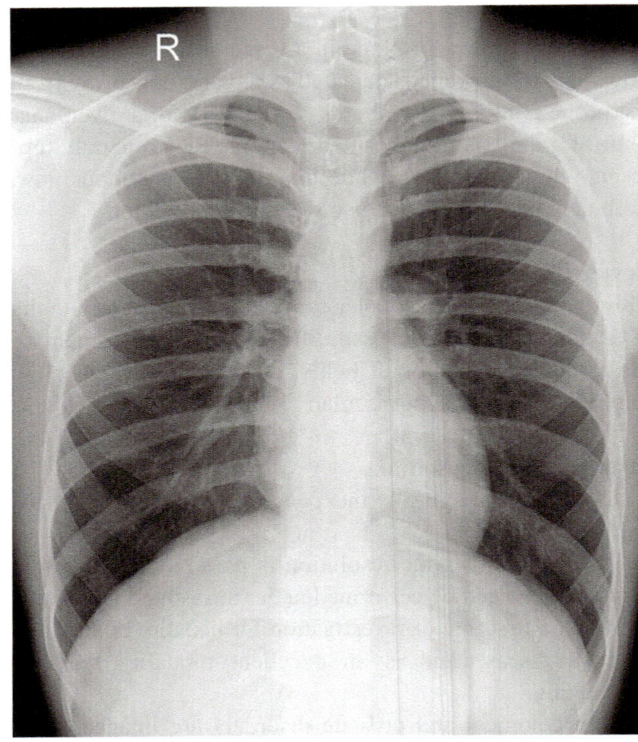




**Fig. 8.24** A Normal Chest Radiograph

### 8.10.2 Reading a Chest Radiograph: Interpretation Basics

The aim of reading a chest radiograph is to scan the whole image in a methodical way such that no anatomical part included in the radiograph is missed. While interpreting the radiograph, it is necessary for the interpreter to actually feel the structural component of the anatomical part being evaluated.

If, for example, a rib is being evaluated it needs to be traced, consciously keeping in mind, its component parts, the two cortical margins seen as white lines representing compact bone and the less dense central component representing marrow with fine normal trabeculae. This is in addition to evaluation of its number and shape. This meticulous evaluation will prevent missing of rib lesions and interpretation of the lesion is easier with prior knowledge of possible pathologies that affect ribs.

Many ways of methodical scanning have been documented in literature. The WHO-recommended method involves chest radiographic evaluation by beginning at one corner of the film, continuing to horizontally scan till the other corner, followed by sliding down and again continuing to scan toward the other edge, continuing till the whole of the radiograph has been scanned. As part of the examination, both sides of the chest must be compared.

It can be likened to the painting of a wall by a professional painter with a perfect finishing touch. Once the initial primary scan is complete, specific areas called the lawyer's zone or hidden areas of the lung need to be looked over a second time. These areas include both the hilar regions, both cardiophrenic regions, both apical and clavicular regions, and finally also through the heart and diaphragms.

### 8.10.3 Requesting a Chest Radiograph: Clinical indications

#### 8.10.3.1 Preoperative evaluation

i. Cleft lip and palate/any other congenital maxillofacial anomaly
ii. Infections of the maxillofacial region
iii. Known malignancy in maxillofacial region
iv. Trauma.

#### 8.10.3.2 Intra- / Postoperative recovery room

i. Sudden choking and breathlessness
ii. Sudden cyanosis
iii. Sudden cough
iv. Chest pain.
v. Fever
vi. Evaluation of chest tubes and catheters (suggested reference for further reading).

### 8.10.4 "The Chest Radiograph. A Mysterious Treasure"...the More you Search, the More you Find!!

#### 8.10.4.1 Consolidation

It is one of the most common terminologies used in Radiology. Clinicians and pathology textbooks, however, commonly use the term pneumonia. Any infection of the lung parenchyma is broadly referred to as pneumonia. Involvement of the alveolar components of the lung parenchyma by the infection is called parenchymal consolidation [10]. It is a disease process in which the air normally present within the small lung air sacs (alveoli) is replaced by liquids like pus, blood, or other fluids, or solids like tumor cells.

Radiologically, consolidation appears opaque [11]. Normally, the alveoli are filled with air and so the normal opaque pulmonary vasculature can be visualized against the dark background of air. However, as discussed earlier, the replacement of the air spaces by any form of fluid or solid material makes the normally visualized pulmonary vessels inapparent with the air containing bronchi being visualized against the opaque background, which is called the air bronchogram (Fig. 8.25a–c).

The consolidation process involving a single lobe and limited by a fissure is called as lobar pneumonia, while the involvement of the entire lung is known as whole-lung consolidation. At times, the process is not as uniform and is distributed in the form of patchy opacities with intervening nonopacified alveoli, an appearance referred to as the air alveologram, which is seen in Bronchopneumonia.

**Pulmonary Edema**

Maxillofacial surgeons are often faced with the problem of patients going into a state of sudden breathlessness in the postoperative recovery room for which the MFS asks for a portable chest radiograph. One of the most common causes of sudden breathlessness in the postoperative recovery room is pulmonary edema. The common confusion for which MFS postgraduates seek the radiologist's opinion is whether the cause of breathlessness is bronchopneumonia or aspiration bronchopneumonia.

In case of acute cardiogenic pulmonary edema caused either due to left ventricular failure or fluid overload, the characteristic radiographic abnormality would reveal bilateral symmetrical areas of consolidation predominantly in the

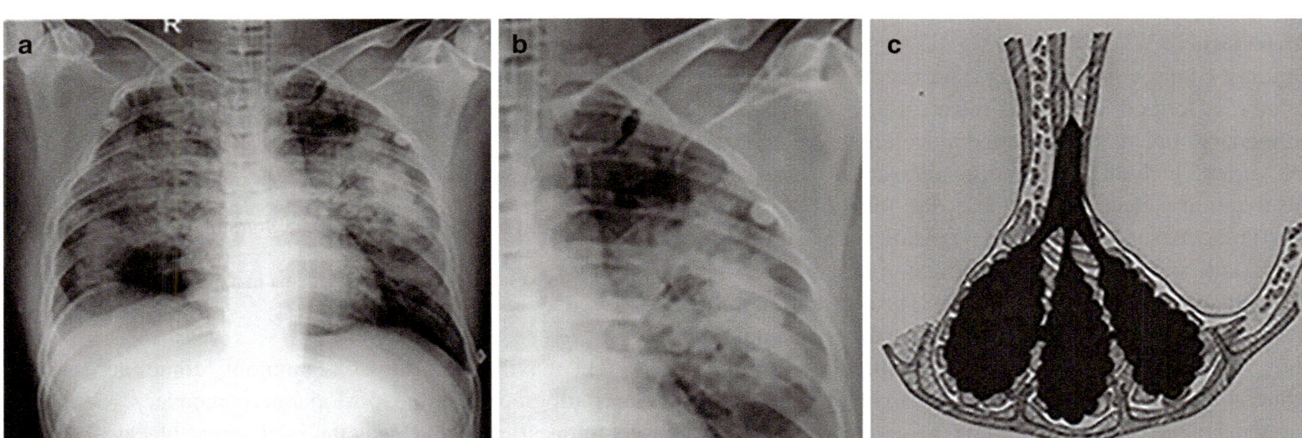




**Fig. 8.25** (**a**) and (**b**) Consolidation: Homogeneous opacities with "Air-bronchogram" sign. (**c**) Schematic diagram showing group of alveoli filled with fluid replacing normal air

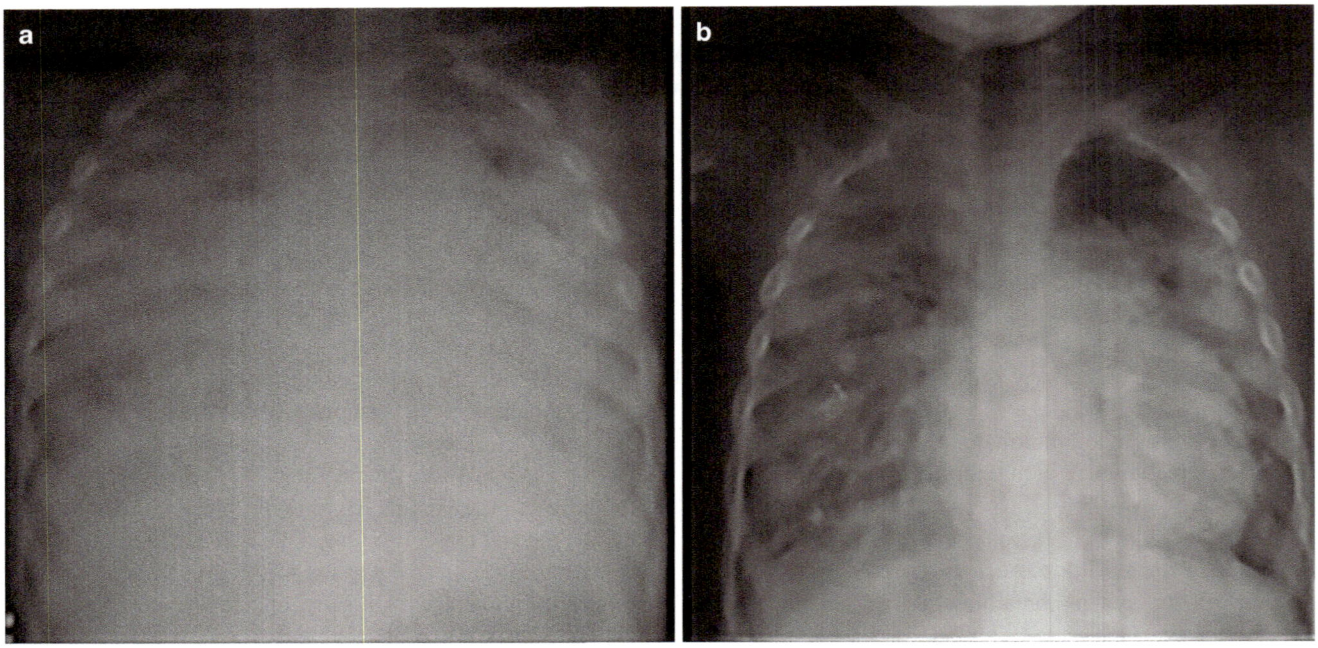




**Fig. 8.26** (**a**) Congestive cardiac failure with cardiomegaly and pulmonary edema. (**b**) Resolution of pulmonary edema after treatment

perihilar and lower lung zones [10] (Fig. 8.26a, b). Noncardiogenic pulmonary edema caused by different pathologies, including fluid overload, acute glomerulonephritis and adult respiratory distress syndrome among others, affects the permeability of the pulmonary capillary membrane (Fig. 8.27). The distribution can vary depending on the position of the patient. The opacities seen on the portable radiograph should not be confused with the appearance of pneumonia (Fig. 8.28).

Rare causes of unilateral pulmonary edema, including raised intracranial pressure and the administration of fluid through the central venous catheter inadvertently placed in the pulmonary artery, need to be kept in mind as well.

### Atelectasis

Diminished air within the lung associated with reduced lung volume is termed atelectasis manifesting radiologically as pulmonary opacity accompanied by volume loss. The causes are varied, including resorption, relaxation, adhesive and cicatrization atelectasis. Of these, the form of atelectasis a maxillofacial surgeon commonly deals with is resorption atelectasis, where there is an obstruction in the communication between the alveoli and trachea. The obstruction may be at any level from the common air way to the segmental bronchus; however, common air way obstruction resulting in bilateral atelectasis is a rare occurrence [11]. Radiologically, the appearance is that of a homogeneous opacity without an air bronchogram sign, with loss of lung volume and displacement of structures toward the opacity.

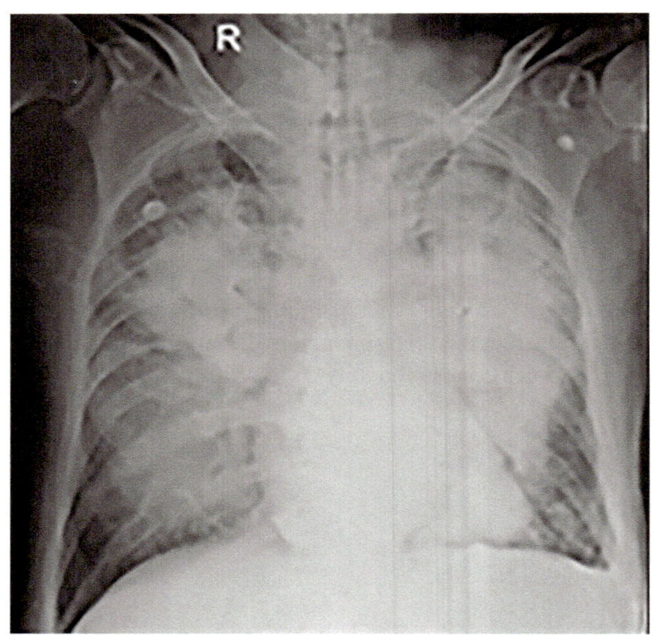




**Fig. 8.27** Noncardiac pulmonary edema in a patient with renal failure

The maxillofacial surgeon commonly comes across similar radiographs in the postoperative recovery room. The commonest cause of this is the inadvertent placement of the endotracheal tube into one bronchus, causing occlusion of the other bronchus, and resulting in atelectasis as a

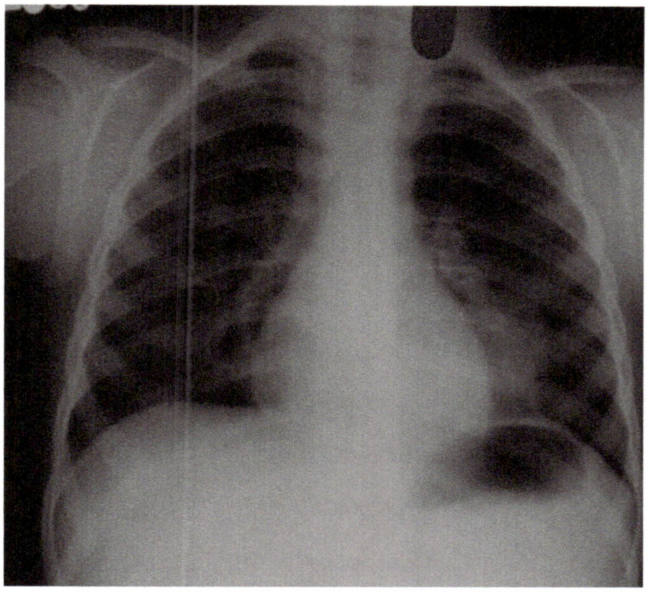



**Fig. 8.28** Aspiration Bronchopneumonia

consequence. Early detection and diagnosis with readjustment of the endotracheal tube is bound to be life saving, helping prevent long-term complications (Fig. 8.29a–c). Thick mucus plugs are other common occluding elements, seen in postoperative recovery rooms resulting in lobar or segmental opacities with loss of volume. Again, early detection and good respiratory physiotherapy are keys to improved lung compliance with a radiograph taken at a later date as follow-up.

**Relaxation Atelectasis**

Normally negative intrapleural pressure is caused by competing thoracic pressures. Lung elasticity and surface tension of the alveolar fluid create an inward tension, pulling the lung inward, which is countered by opposing forces from the pleural fluid and thoracic wall, the pleural cavity surface tension, and the parietal pleural attachment to the thoracic wall causing outward pull of the lungs. The outward pull is slightly higher than the inward pull with a negative intrapleural pressure of about -4 mm of Hg. When this intrapleural negative pressure is lost as occurs commonly in cases of pneumothorax or pleural effusion, the lung has a natural tendency to recoil, with the loss of lung volume being proportional to the amount of air or fluid collected in the pleural space [11].

**Pneumothorax**

The presence of air in the pleural space is called pneumothorax, the most common cause of which is trauma either accidental or iatrogenic. In the absence of such causes, it is called spontaneous pneumothorax. Radiological findings of pneumothorax include increased peripheral translucency, absence of lung markings within this area of translucency, and the identifiable visceral pleural margin of the collapsed lung (Figs. 8.30 and 8.31). The detection of a pneumothorax should prompt the search for an underlying cause like a fractured rib or a ruptured bulla or iatrogenic causes like a central venous catheter procedure. Associated lesions like pneumomediastinum and surgical emphysema should also be looked for.

A maxillofacial surgeon might have to read supine portable radiographs of patients presenting with clinical signs suggesting respiratory distress and the presence of pneumothorax might be missed. In such a scenario, the MFS should look for radiographic evidence of pneumothorax at sites adjacent to the diaphragmatic silhouettes on either side and the cardiophrenic and costophrenic angles and he should also be able to appreciate the appearance of an exceptionally sharp cardiac border [11]. The MFS needs to be aware that air trapped within the skin folds can mimic pneumothorax (Fig. 8.32).

Identification of an air fluid level would prompt the diagnosis of a hydropneumothorax. It is difficult to characterize the nature of the fluid as being transudate, exudate, blood, or chylous. An MFS may be unable to diagnose a hydropneumothorax, on an AP supine portable radiograph as the fluid level will not be identified. Here, the collapsed lung tends to float on the fluid, which is dependent posteriorly giving a veil effect (Fig. 8.33).

**Pneumomediastinum**

It is the collection of air within the pleural boundaries of the mediastinum and can arise secondary to barotrauma from mechanical trauma, intrathoracic, or iatrogenic trauma and infection or can occur spontaneously. A radiographic diagnosis of pneumomediastinum requires depiction of normal anatomic structures being outlined by air as they leave the mediastinum. The mediastinal air can cause elevation of the thymus, collect anterior or posterior to the pericardium, surround the pulmonary artery or its branches, or can collect adjacent to the major aortic branches or major bronchi (Fig. 8.34).

Most cases of pneumomediastinum described in maxillofacial surgery literature are as a result of dissection of air down the fascial planes of the neck. Chest radiographic findings need to be carefully examined to make the diagnosis of pneumomediastinum, which is crucial to the MFS in planning appropriate treatment of affected patients. On rare occasions, a significant amount of air in the mediastinum can cause vessel or tracheal obstruction and induce symptoms and signs of tamponade and decreased venous return.

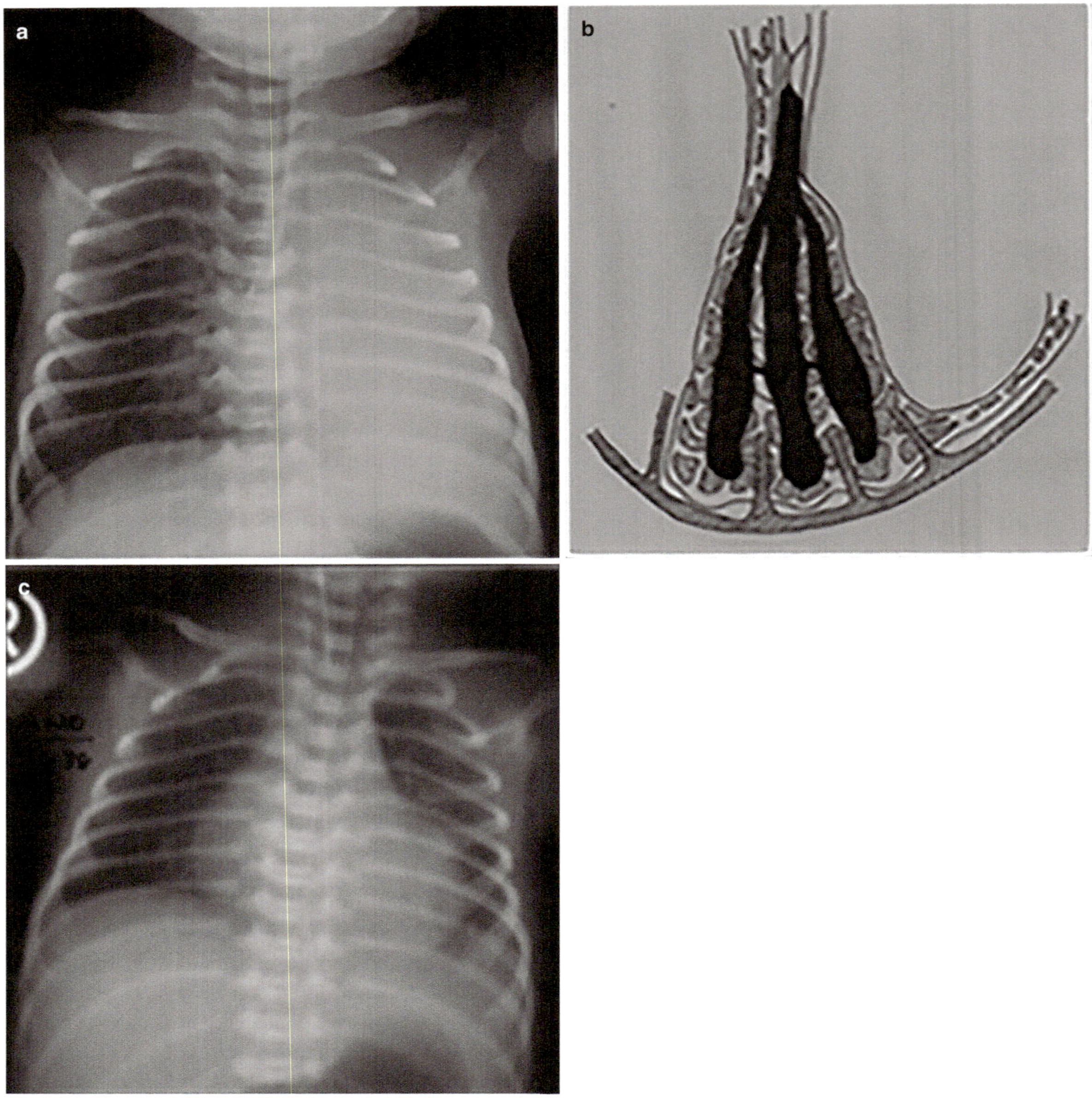




**Fig. 8.29** (**a**) Whole lung collapse: Left hemithorax is homogenously opaque with loss of volume of left lung with displacement of mediastinum to left. Note: Abnormal placement of endotracheal tube blocking the (Lt.) Bronchus. (**b**) Schematic diagram showing loss of volume of alveoli as seen in collapse with absence of air. (**c**) Reversion of normal left lung aeration after repositioning of endotracheal tube

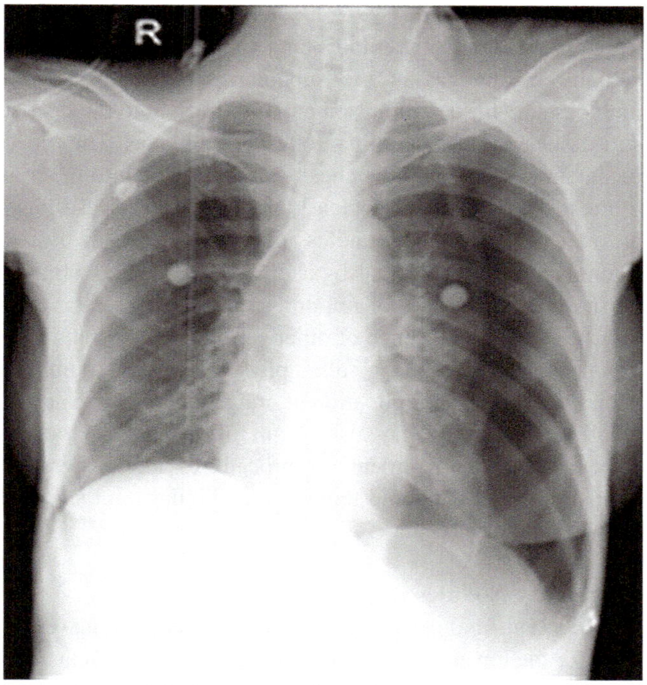




**Fig. 8.30** Left-sided pneumothorax

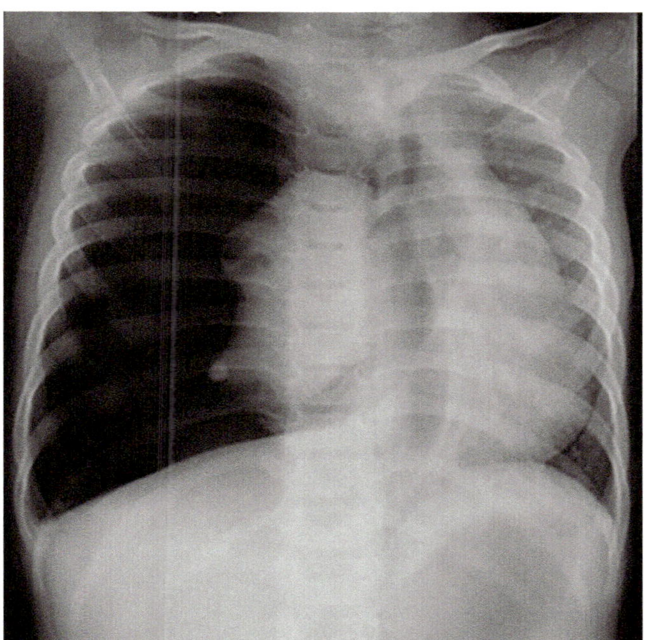



**Fig. 8.31** Right-sided tension pneumothorax

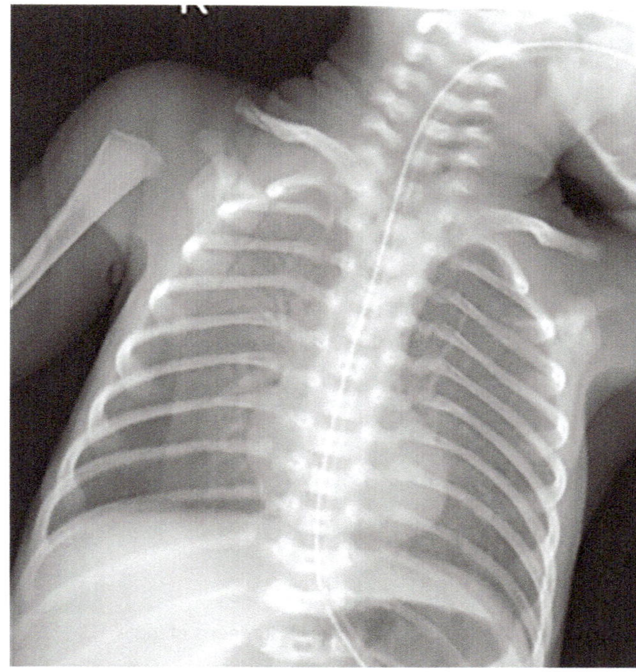



**Fig. 8.32** Right-sided pseudopneumothorax due to air trapped in skin fold

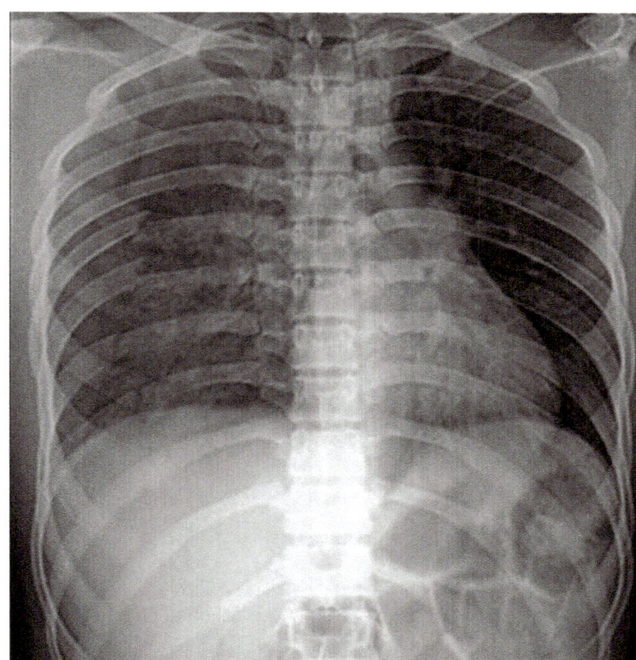



**Fig. 8.33** Right-sided hemopneumothorax with multiple rib fractures as seen in supine radiograph

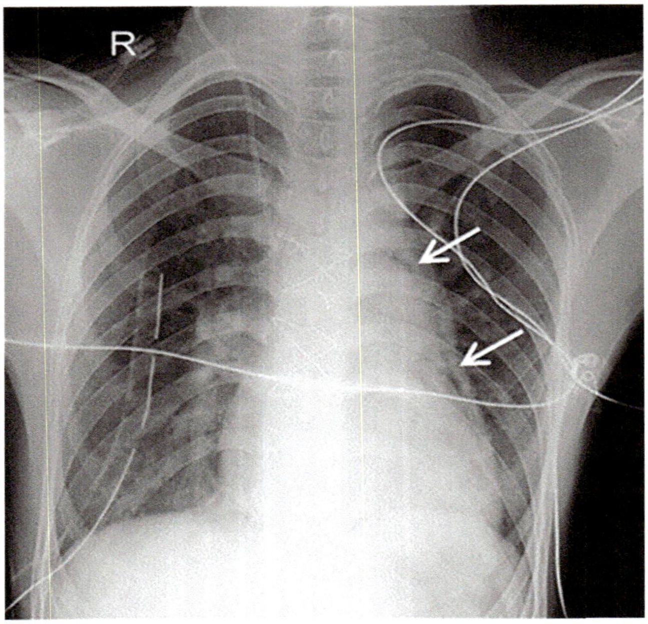




**Fig. 8.34** Pneumomediastinum. Air around the pulmonary artery and heart.

## Surgical Emphysema

Though subcutaneous emphysema or surgical emphysema actually means gas in the subcutaneous tissues, it also includes soft-tissue emphysema that dissects into the deeper soft tissues and musculature along fascial planes. The translucent air spreads over the chest wall and axilla into the root of the neck. Fascial planes clearly outline the pectoralis muscle and neurovascular bundles in neck (Fig. 8.35a, b). If trauma is the cause, the gas by itself may not need treatment, but its identification is of importance as it may be the only indication of the presence of other serious injuries requiring urgent management. Surgical emphysema can uncommonly occur as a serious complication of oral and maxillofacial surgical procedures. It may also occur following teeth extraction, endodontic treatment, or procedures like restorative dentistry, periodontal and temporomandibular joint surgery, or facial fracture repair.

## Pulmonary Nodules

For all intents and purposes, a nodule seen in the lung (especially in the lower zones) should be considered as metastasis unless proven otherwise, by a maxillofacial surgeon.

**Fig. 8.35** (**a**) and (**b**). Surgical emphysema with pneumothorax

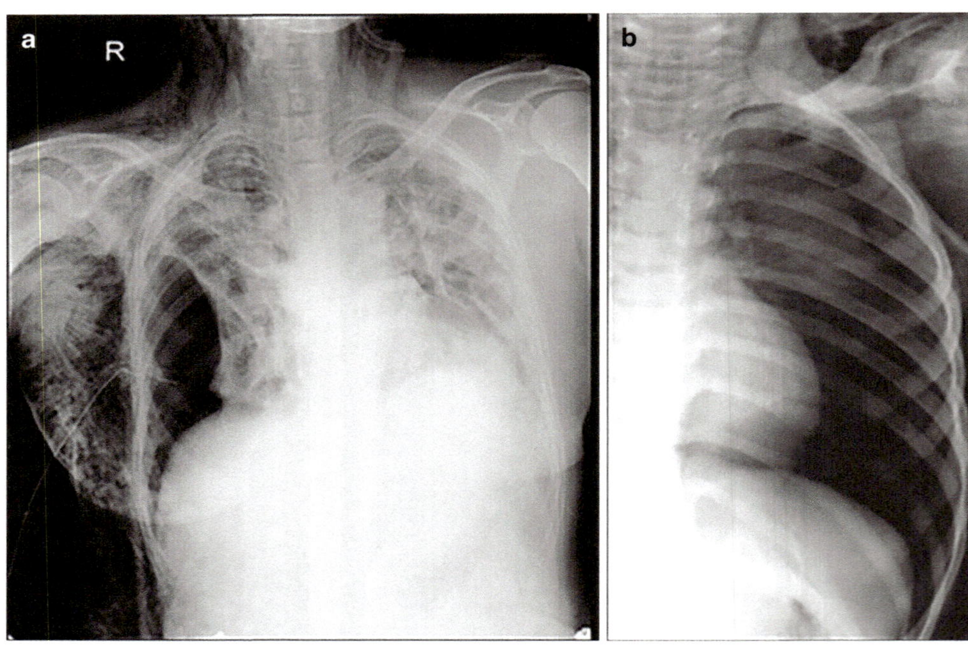

*Pulmonary nodules* can be characterized, based on some signature findings. In the absence of these findings, the nodule remains nonspecific. Common causes of pulmonary nodules are granulomas, bronchogenic cysts, hydatid cysts, hamartomas, pulmonary hematoma following laceration, rheumatoid nodules, fungal granulomas, and pulmonary metastasis.

*Tuberculomas* usually range in size from 1 to 3 cm in diameter, have central calcific lesions, and are surrounded by satellite scarred lesions. They are commonly seen in the upper zones, but they can occur anywhere in the lung (Fig. 8.36).

*Bronchogenic cysts* are well-defined nodules, around 3 to 4 cm in size, usually seen in the parahilar region, and are sometimes purely in the mediastinum (Fig. 8.37a–e).

*Hamartomas* are nodules that can occur anywhere in the lung having well-defined margins with central popcorn-like calcification (Fig. 8.38a, b).

*Hydatid cysts*, too, can occur anywhere in the lung. They have a stenciled outline and vary in size from 1 to 10 cms. The radiographic air crescentic sign is pathognomonic of a hydatid cyst, appearing like the arc of the moon caused by the separation of the endocyst from the exocyst. Continued separation of the endocyst from the exocyst results in an air fluid level typically called the 'water lily' appearance. Pulmonary hydatid cysts do not calcify.

Presence of a solitary nodule in the lower lung without any characteristic findings makes pulmonary metastasis a strong possibility, which should be further evaluated with imaging and HPR. Multiple nodules of varying sizes in the lower zones are very much suggestive of pulmonary metastasis.(Fig. 8.39a, b).

**Role of Chest Radiograph in Cases Developing Sudden Onset of Breathlessness in Postoperative Period**

1. Aspiration Bronchopneumonia
2. Pneumothorax
3. Foreign body (Fig. 8.40a–c)
4. Abnormal placement of Endotracheal Tube (Fig. 8.41)
5. Pleural effusion
6. Pulmonary edema and pulmonary embolism

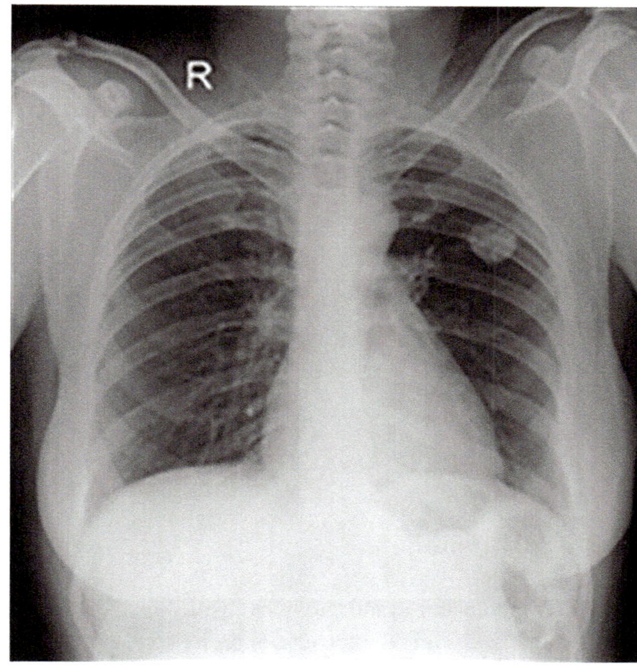




**Fig. 8.36** Pulmonary Nodule—Tuberculoma

A maxillofacial surgeon should be capable of identifying all of these causes of sudden onset of breathlessness in a postoperative patient in the event of the absence of availability of expert radiological opinion and act accordingly. They also need to be aware that patients on ventilators may develop ventilator-dependent complications.

**A glance into the future of imaging for Maxillofacial Surgeons**

1. Magnetization Transfer Imaging
   This is a modified MRI study that helps in
   - Prediction of whether the primary tumor is benign or malignant (possible in 80 to 90% cases).
   - Differentiation of reactive versus malignant adenopathy.
   
   This modality is still in the preliminary stage and needs further study.
2. MRI-guided biopsy procedures need MRI compatible equipment. The procedures are feasible and are usually done in cases that are not amenable to USG guidance.
3. Functional imaging of swallowing.

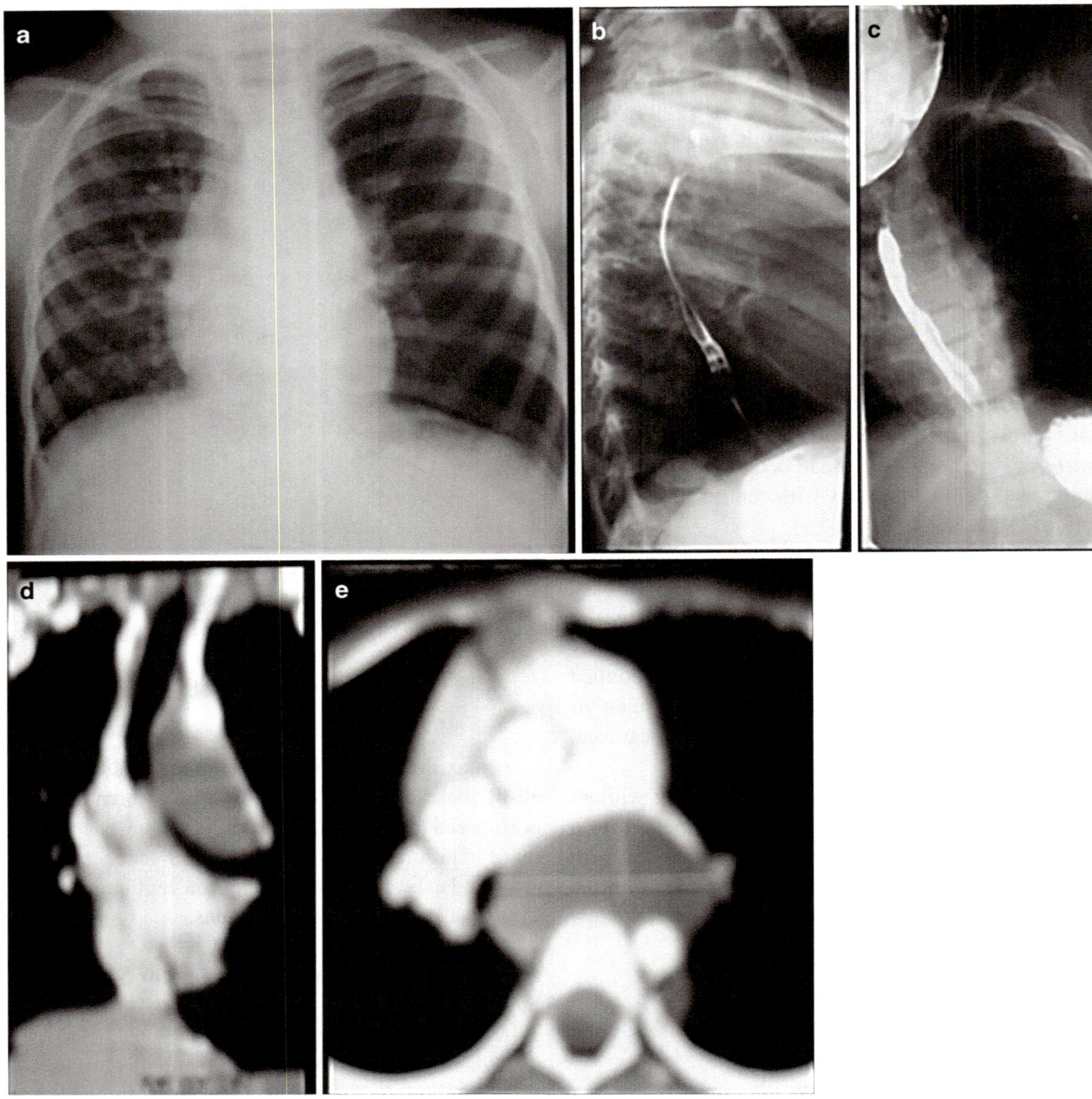




**Fig. 8.37** (**a**), (**b**), and (**c**). Preop chest radiographs of a patient with cleft lip presenting with dyspnea, more with changing position. (**d**) **and** (**e**) Mediastinal mass—Bronchogenic Cyst confirmed on CT

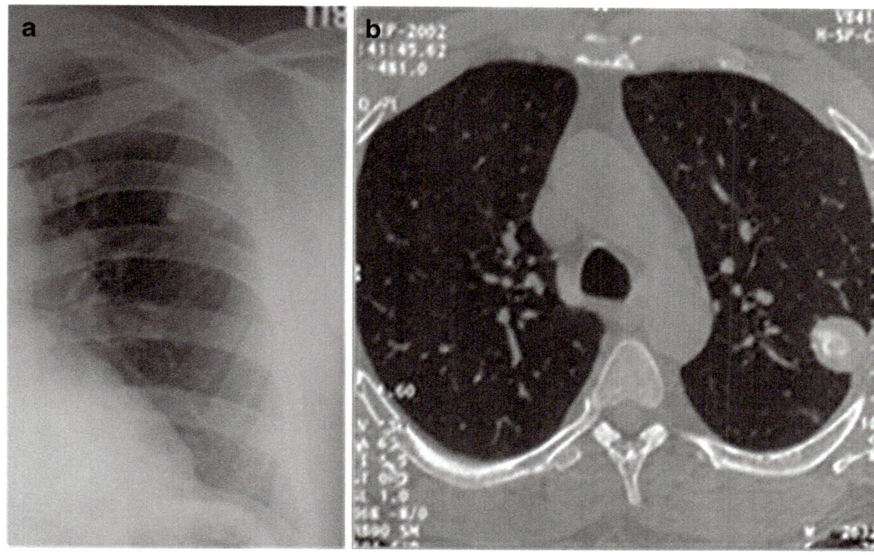




**Fig. 8.38** (**a**) Pulmonary Nodule-Hamartoma. (**b**) Confirmed on CT

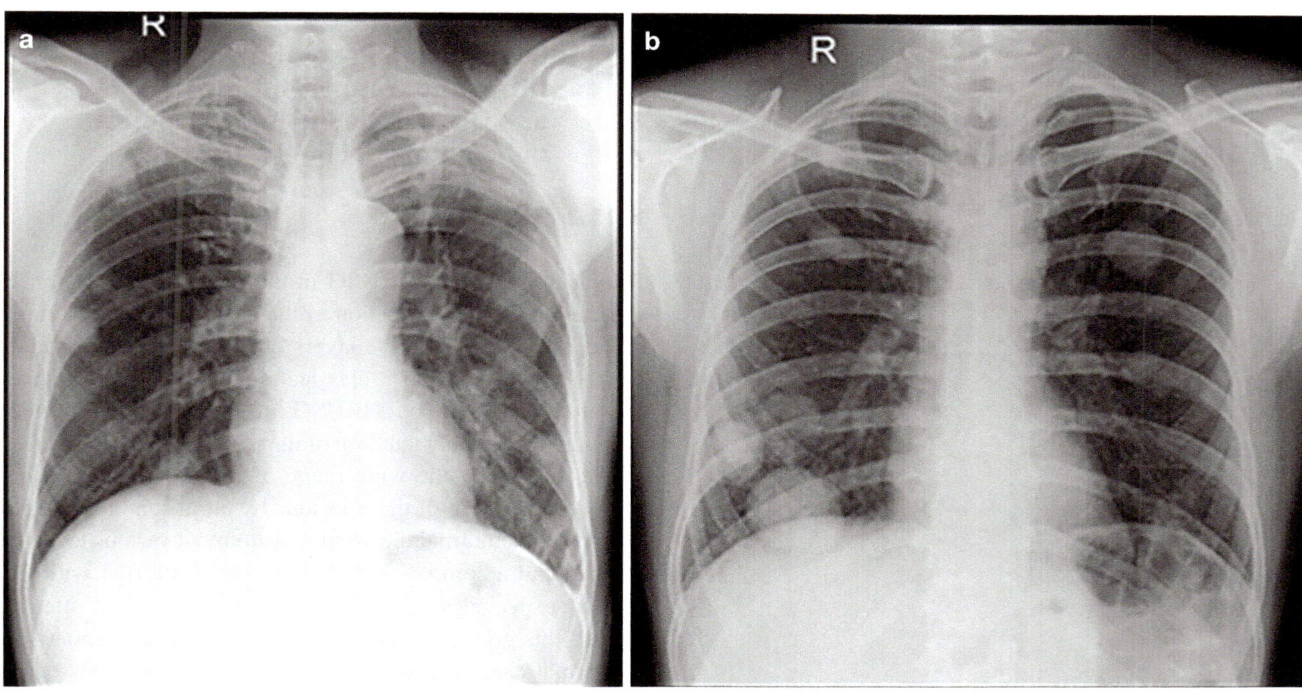




**Fig. 8.39** (**a**) and (**b**). Pulmonary metastasis

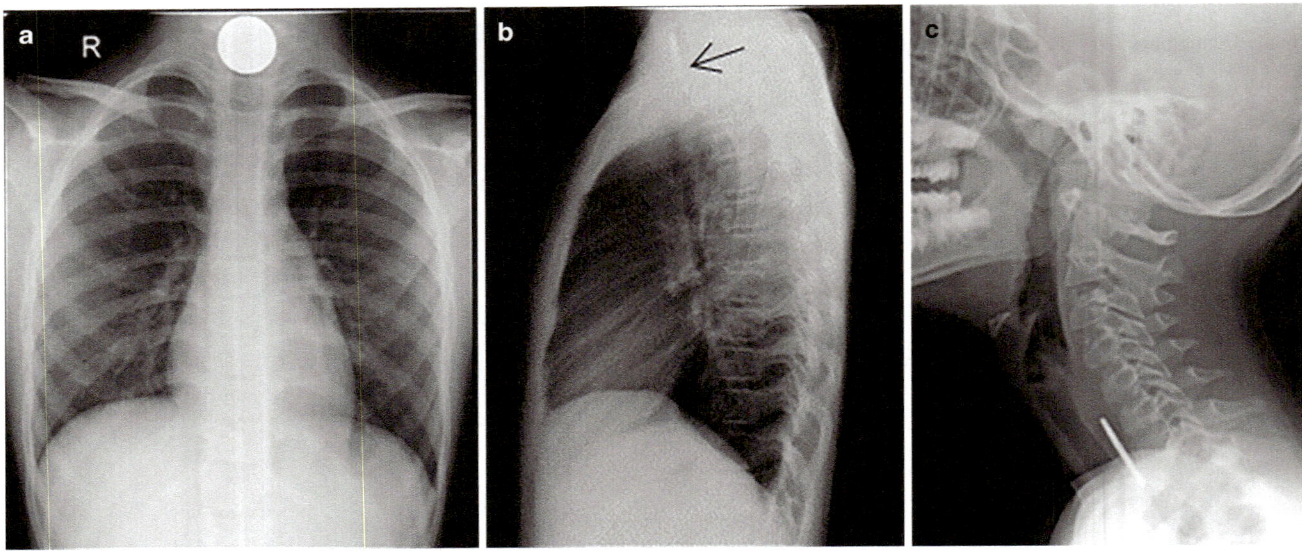




**Fig. 8.40** (**a**), (**b**), and (**c**). Foreign body, a coin in the cervical esophagus

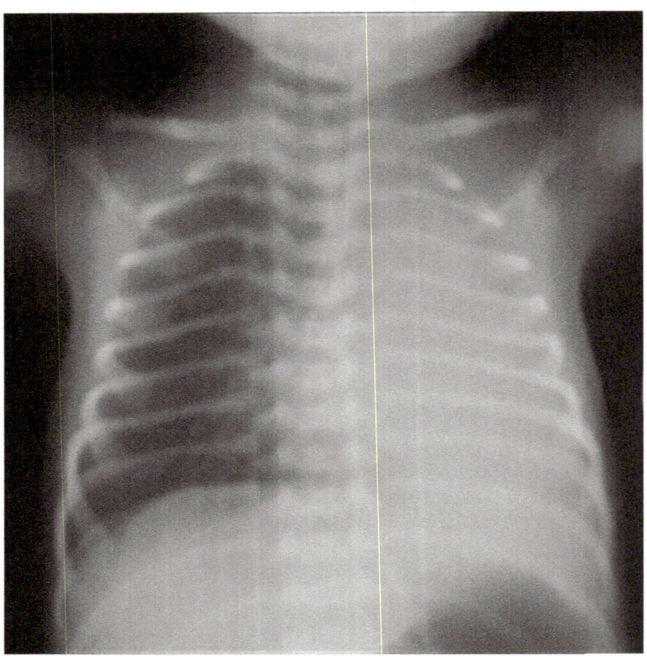



**Fig. 8.41** Abnormal placement of endotracheal tube with collapse of left lobe

## 8.11 Role of High Resolution Ultrasonography (HRUSG) as a Diagnostic Aid in the Practice of Maxillofacial Surgery

### 8.11.1 Preface

Primarily the use of HRUSG in the maxillofacial region is directed toward investigation of the cheek and the structures adjacent to it. Despite the layers of the cheek and the adjacent structures having a classical sonographic appearance, literature available on HRUSG of the cheek is limited. Having proper understanding of the relevant anatomy is critical in discerning the wide range of diseases affecting this region. Evaluation of these lesions by ultrasound is possible only once the normal ultrasound anatomy at various levels is defined and a comparison of the suspicious lesion with the normal expected appearance is made. An original attempt toward this goal was made at our institute with comparison of normal cadaveric sections at corresponding levels taken by HRUSG.

High-resolution ultrasonography has broad applications in the maxillofacial region especially in the cheek, which include evaluations of the unilateral or bilateral swollen cheek painful or pain less, restricted mouth opening, painful chewing without obvious clinical findings, and varied causes of facial swelling. Since early detection decisively influences patient prognosis in case of malignancy, it is one of the prime concerns in a presenting patient. Further, differentiation of lesions as being of benign, malignant, infective, or inflammatory etiology is important in deciding on a treatment plan. HRUSG should however be used to complement and not replace other imaging modalities as it does have its limitations.

Compared to other facial components, the cheek is predominantly composed of adipose tissue and is relatively small in size. Swelling of the cheek is easily visible and palpable in most patients presenting with cheek masses. Most lesions have nonspecific characteristics on computed tomography (CT) and magnetic resonance imaging (MRI). In contrast, HRUSG is ideal for evaluation of cheek lesions, because of its capability to differentiate between tissues like skin, fat, muscle, gland, ducts, and vessels especially since bony and gaseous interfaces are absent. Further, the superficial location of the cheek makes it easily accessible to ultrasound. Vestibule can be evaluated with fruit jelly technique obliterating the void space.

This short review attempts to aid the MFS in his understanding of HRUSG of the maxillofacial region, with special reference to the cheek.

## 8.11.2 Gross Cheek Anatomy

In simple terms, the cheek is the fleshy portion of the face, below the eye, extending from the angle of the mouth to the ear. Anatomically, it pertains to the buccomasseteric region comprising the buccal space and its contents, masseteric and buccinator muscles, the buccal fat pad, and Stenson's duct.

The region is continuous anteriorly with the lips. Its external anterior demarcation is formed by the nasolabial fold and groove extending from the side of the nose to the angle of the mouth. The mucosa lining the inner aspect of the cheek adheres to the buccinator muscle, while the gingival mucosa covers the mandibular and maxillary alveolar processes. The gingivobuccal sulcus is the junction formed between the gingival and buccal mucosae. The vestibule is the region of the mouth between the teeth, lips, and cheek, which is bound superiorly and inferiorly by buccal mucosal reflections onto the mandible and maxilla. Posteriorly the vestibule is continuous with the oral cavity proper (Fig. 8.42) [12, 13].

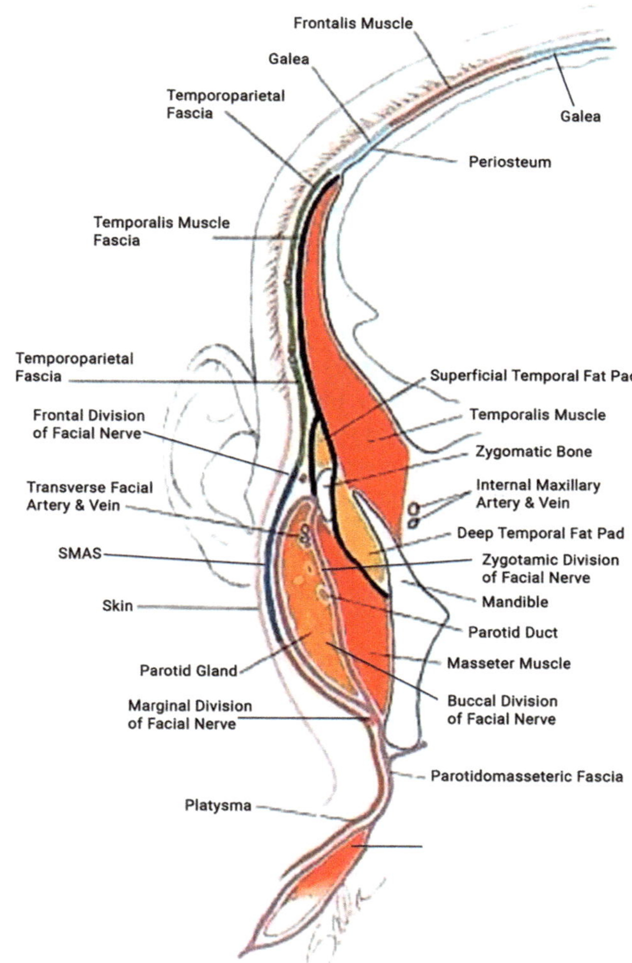




Fig. 8.42 Anatomical layers of the cheek

## 8.11.3 Floor of Mouth, Anatomy (Relevant to HRUSG)

The part of the oral cavity located underneath the tongue is called the floor of the mouth and it can be involved by a myriad of pathological processes. Superficial lesions involving the mucosal surface are easily visualized and may not need imaging. Disease involving the deeper structures of the floor needs to be evaluated by imaging, and HRUSG is many times the first line of investigation because of its superior soft-tissue differentiation capability, thus allowing for clear depiction of contents of the floor [14].

Inflammatory processes, malignancies, and vascular abnormalities can affect the floor contents, while certain conditions like ranula and obstruction of the submandibular gland are specific to this location [14].

### 8.11.4 Defining the HRUSG Anatomy of Maxillofacial Region (Predominantly Cheek)

**Normal Ultrasound Cheek**

Various cheek layers have varying sonographic echogenicity and echotexture, and hence ultrasound is an invaluable tool in the characterization and localization of cheek lesions.

Depending on tissue density, the sound wave transmission, absorption, or reflection capability of each tissue varies. Tissues, having high water content like blood, appear black and are called anechoic because they conduct sound waves well. In contrast, tissues that are poor conductors reflect most of the sound wave energy back to the transducer appearing bright and are termed hyperechoic, examples of which include bones, tendons, and fascial planes. Tissues like muscle reflect less of the sound wave energy and have a hypoechoic appearance. In the cheek, the mucosal and submucosal layers appear hyperechoic, the mucosa more so. Muscle tissue appears hypoechoic, while fatty tissue appears echogenic (Fig. 8.43).

Compared to other imaging modalities, ultrasound has proven to be superior as regards identification of small lesions, detection of lesion plane, and lesion characterization (Fig. 8.44).

The cheek layers and neighboring structures that can be identified by HRUSG are.

**Cheek**

- Skin
- Subcutaneous plane
- Buccal pad of fat
- Buccinator muscle
- Submucosal layer
- Mucosal layer
- Masseter muscle and its lateral relations.
- Temporalis muscle
- Temporomandibular joint (TMJ)

**Neighboring Structures**

- Vestibule
- Gingiva
- Buccogingival Sulcus
- Periodontal tissue, etc.
- Tongue, lips
- Floor of mouth, Sublingual space
- Submandibular space
- Parotid gland / duct
- Retromandibular space
- Interdental space
- Alveolar margin
- Mental foramina
- Infraorbital foramina
- External nose
- Various other facial planes and spaces
- Arteries

### 8.11.5 Techniques of HRUSG of Cheek

For ultrasound examination, the cheek is considered to be a rectangular area bordered as follows (Fig. 8.45).

- by an imaginary line beginning at the angle of mandible and extending along its lower border to the level of angle of mouth inferiorly,
- by an imaginary line beginning at the angle of mandible and running along the posterior border of the mandibular ramus to include the temporomandibular joint posteriorly,
- by an imaginary line along the zygomatic arch superiorly and,
- by an imaginary vertical line at the level of angle of mouth that joins the superior and inferior lines anteriorly [15].

Various techniques, including the resting (neutral) and Puffed (Blow out) cheek technique, the tongue touch technique, and fruit jelly technique, were experimented with, each having their own advantages and limitations [15].

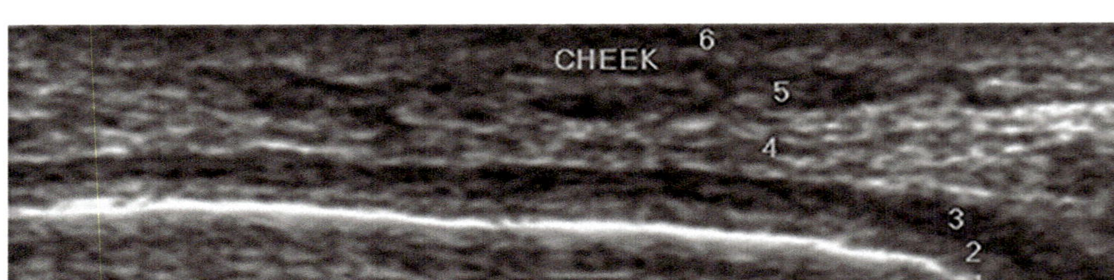


Fig. 8.43 Normal Cheek/ Buccal layers on ultrasound

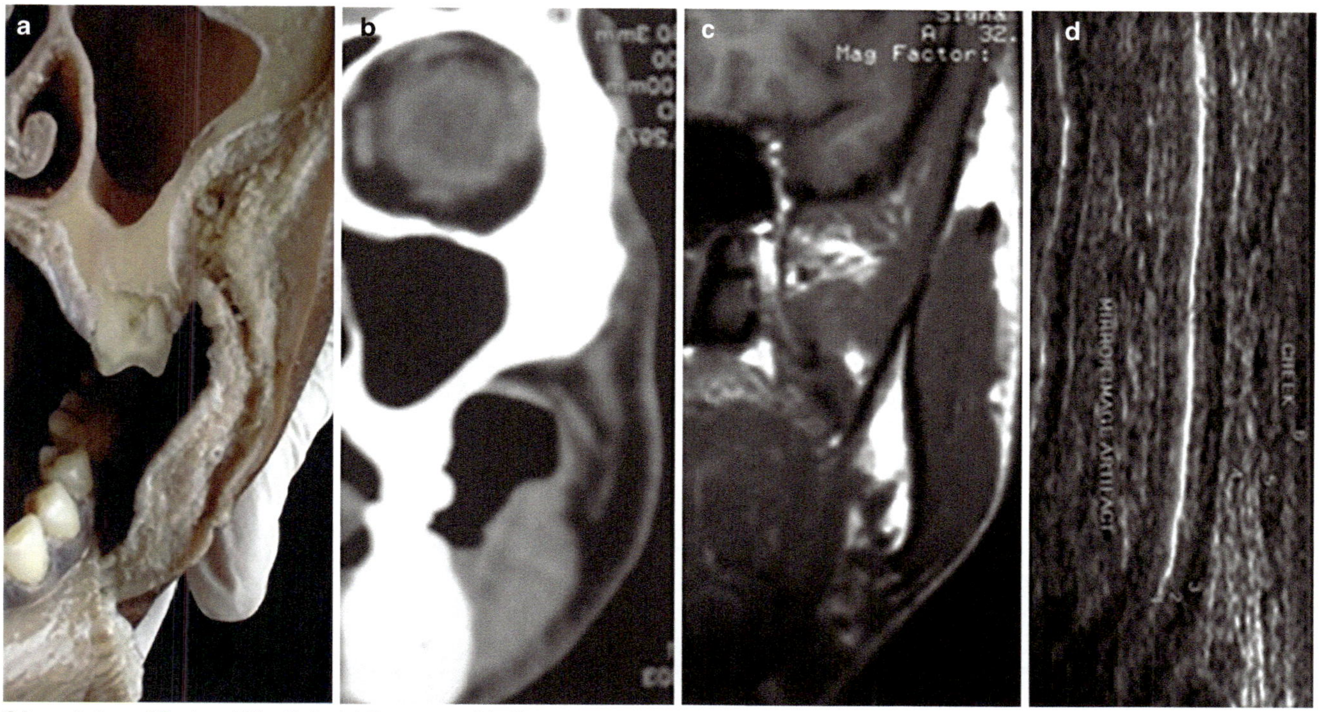




**Fig. 8.44** (**a-d**) Cheek anatomy—a comparison. Comparative cheek anatomy- (**a**) cadaveric specimen, (**b**) CT, (**c**) MRI, and (**d**) Ultrasound

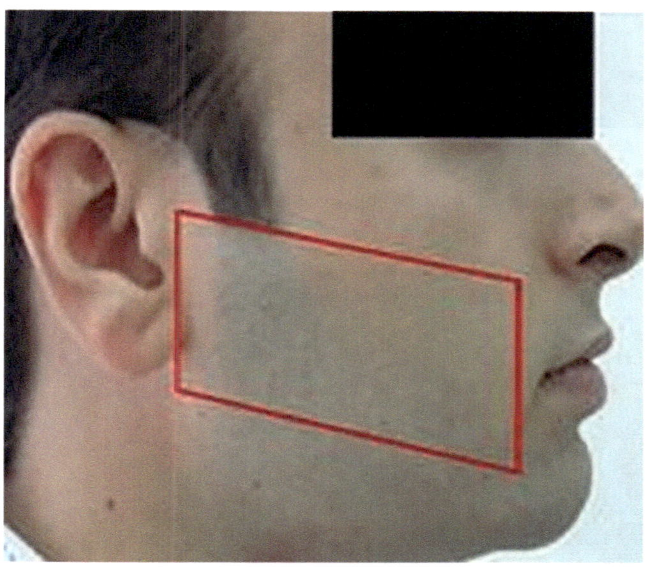



**Fig. 8.45** Area of Cheek ultrasound study

(a) *Resting (Neutral) and Puffed (Blow out) Cheek Technique* (Figs. 8.46 and 8.47).
   - Patient is instructed to blow, and ultrasound is performed in puffed cheek status.
   - Images obtained in axial and coronal planes.
     Advantage: Improved visibility of cheek layers and accurate definition of lesion size.
     Limitation: Occurrence of mirror image artifact.
     Less sensitivity in evaluation of lesions of the vestibule (gingivobuccal sulcus).

(b) *Tongue Touch Technique (*Fig. 8.48a–c).
   - Patient is instructed to feel the cheek lesion with the tongue.
   - Lesion is brought closer to the probe creating a better acoustic window.
   - Lesions of the superficial buccal mucosa and tongue lesions on its anterior half and corresponding lateral borders can be evaluated better.
     Advantage: Better visualization of lesion details.
     Limitation: Inaccessibility to tongue lesions along the posterior half and corresponding lateral borders.

(c) *Fruit Jelly Technique.*
   (Figs. 8.49a, b, and 8.50a–d)
   - Commercially available edible "Fruit jellies" are placed in the upper and lower gingivobuccal sulcus.
   - Patients are then instructed to close their mouth and ultrasound is performed.

   Advantages:
   - Useful in elderly and facial nerve palsy patients having difficulty holding puffed cheek for prolonged periods.
   - Absence of artifacts due to vestibular air.
   - Enhanced structural delineation and better evaluation of vestibular extension of lesion.

   Limitation: Inability to evaluate lesions involving far posterior aspect of Vestibule.

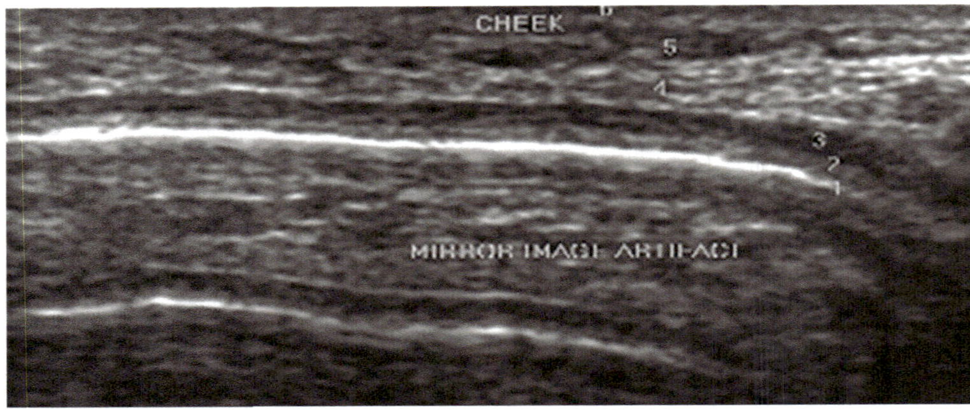




**Fig. 8.46** Cheek layers by "Puffed Cheek" Technique. (1) Mucosa. (2) Submucosa. (3) Buccinator. (4) Buccal fat. (5) Subcutaneous tissue. (6) Skin

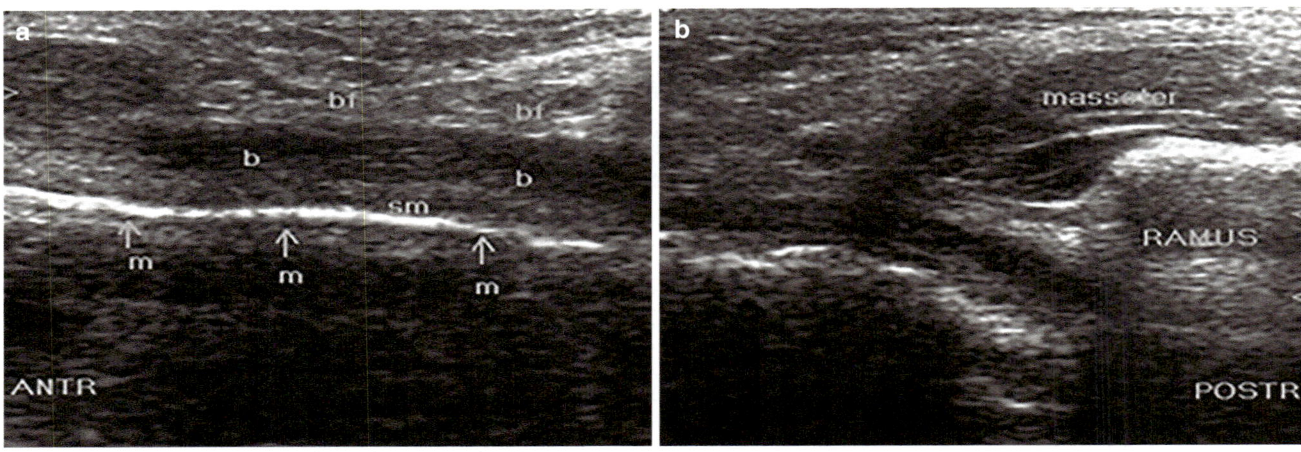




**Fig. 8.47** (**a**, **b**) Cheek layers by "Puffed Cheek" Technique. m-mucosa, sm-submucosa, b-buccinator, bf-buccal fat

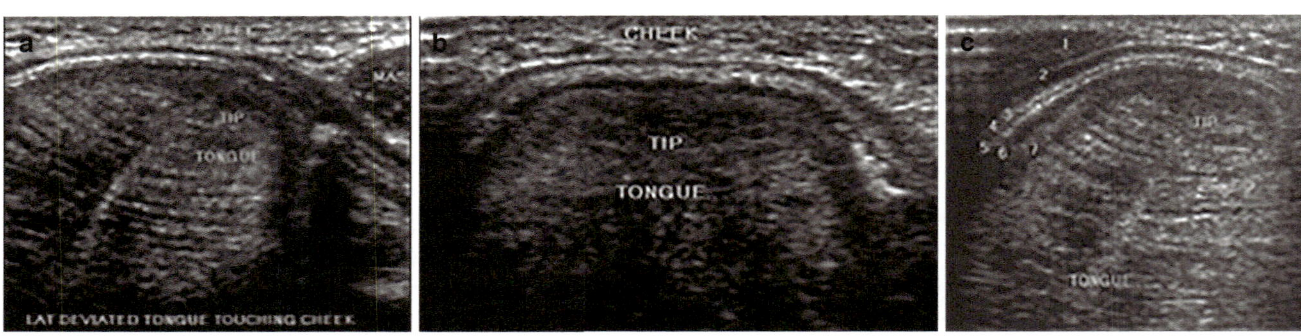




**Fig. 8.48** (**a**), (**b**), and (**c**). "Tongue Touch" Technique. Anterior tongue, its tip and lateral borders and cheek layers

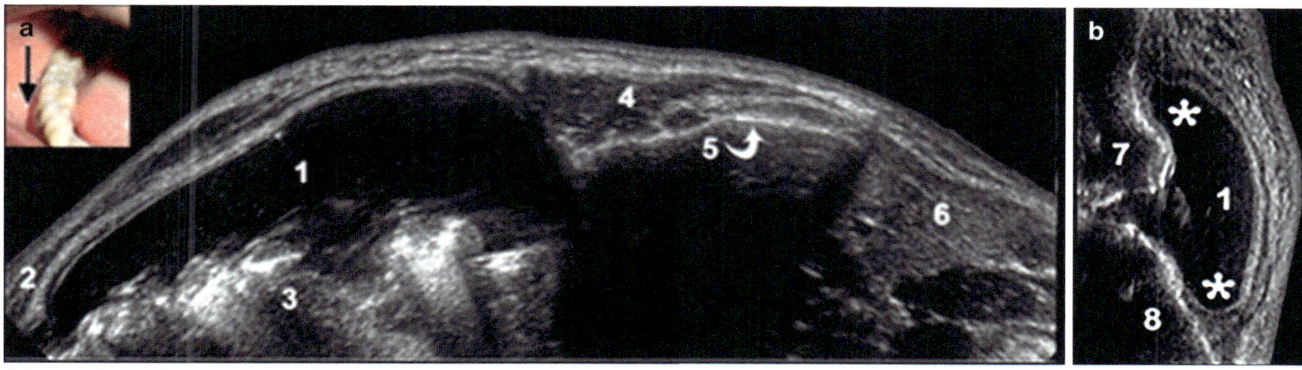




**Fig. 8.49** (**a**) Axial panoramic (**b**) Coronal Cheek layers by "Fruit Jelly" Technique. (1) Jelly (2) Angle of mouth (3) Alveolar process (4) Masseter (5) Mandible (6) Parotid (7) Maxilla (8) Mandible (Asterisk)- Upper and lower gingivobuccal sulcus

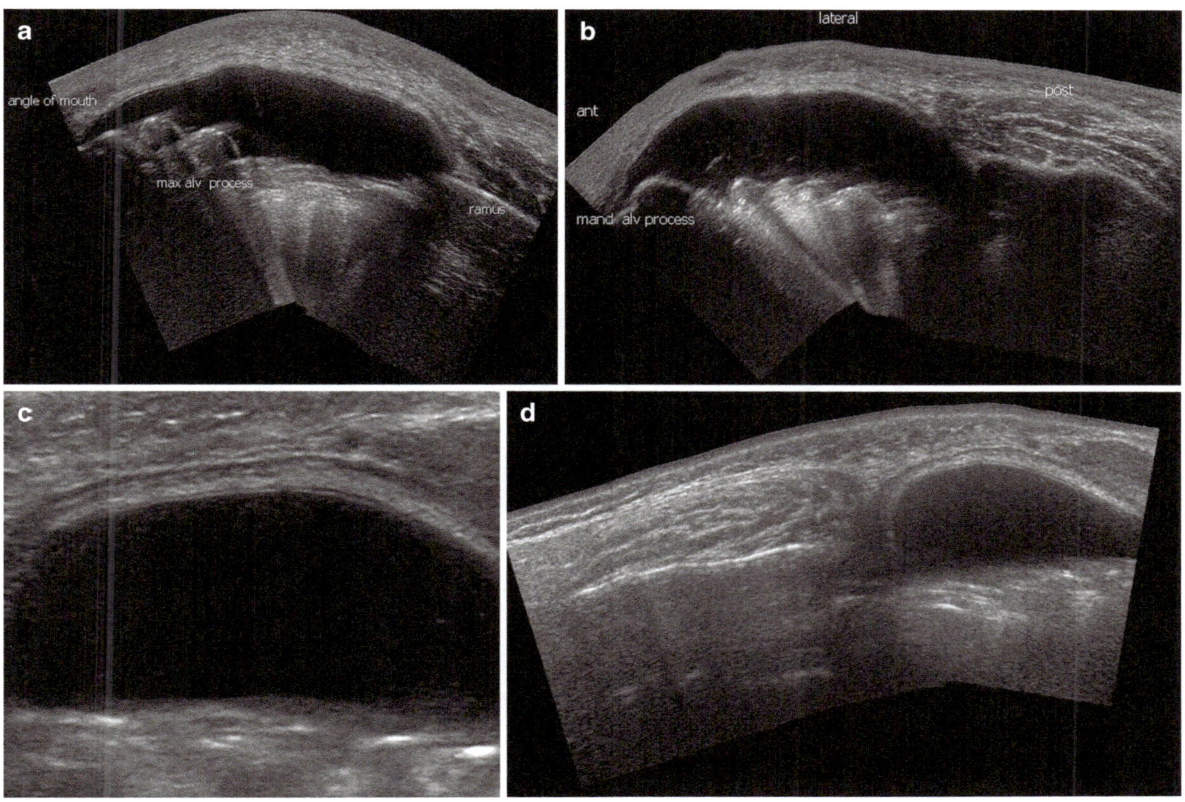




**Fig. 8.50** (**a, b, c**, and **d**).Cheek layers by "Fruit jelly" Technique. Panoramic axial slices. Coronal slices showing superior and inferior vestibules along with layers of cheek/alveolar surfaces

### 8.11.6 Case Presentation

**HRUSG Cheek: Scope of Use and Limitations**

Scope of practice of HRUSG cheek includes

- Cases where limitations are posed by the clinical presentation as in case of trismus or lesions that mimic others in their clinical presentation resulting in diagnostic difficulty
- Estimation of the extent of a lesion, thus helping in tumor staging
- Cases where the use of plain radiography is limited
- Inherent drawbacks of imaging modalities like CT and MRI and their high cost

**Limitations**

- Structures medial to the mandibular ramus
- Difficulty in obtaining information of intact bone
- Intra-articular structures of the temporomandibular joint
- Postoperative scar tissue or a large external wound
- Very thick patients, muscles, and nerves of the face

**Clinical Conditions that Can Be Evaluated**

- Swollen cheek: Painful, painless, unilateral, or bilateral.
- Limited mouth opening
- Painful chewing
- Swelling of the face involving the midline or parasagittal plane, floor of the mouth, TM joint region, submandibular region, nose, lip, gums, etc.
- Tongue lesions (Lateral margin).

**Notifiable Lesions**

- Cheek—Growth, hemangioma, lymphangioma, Oral submucous fibrosis, abscesses, discharging sinuses, etc.
- Masseter—evaluation of contraction, benign hypertrophy, trauma, Space infection, trauma, etc.
- Masticatory space.
- TMJ—swelling, click.
- Lytic lesions of jaws.
- Gum—evaluation. Lip lesions.
- Midline swellings.
- Tumor staging.
- Salivary gland.
- Space infections.
- Tongue.
- Lymph node evaluation.

1. **Inflammatory / Infective Pathology**
   (a) *Cheek cellulitis with evolving abscess (Fig. 8.51a–d).*

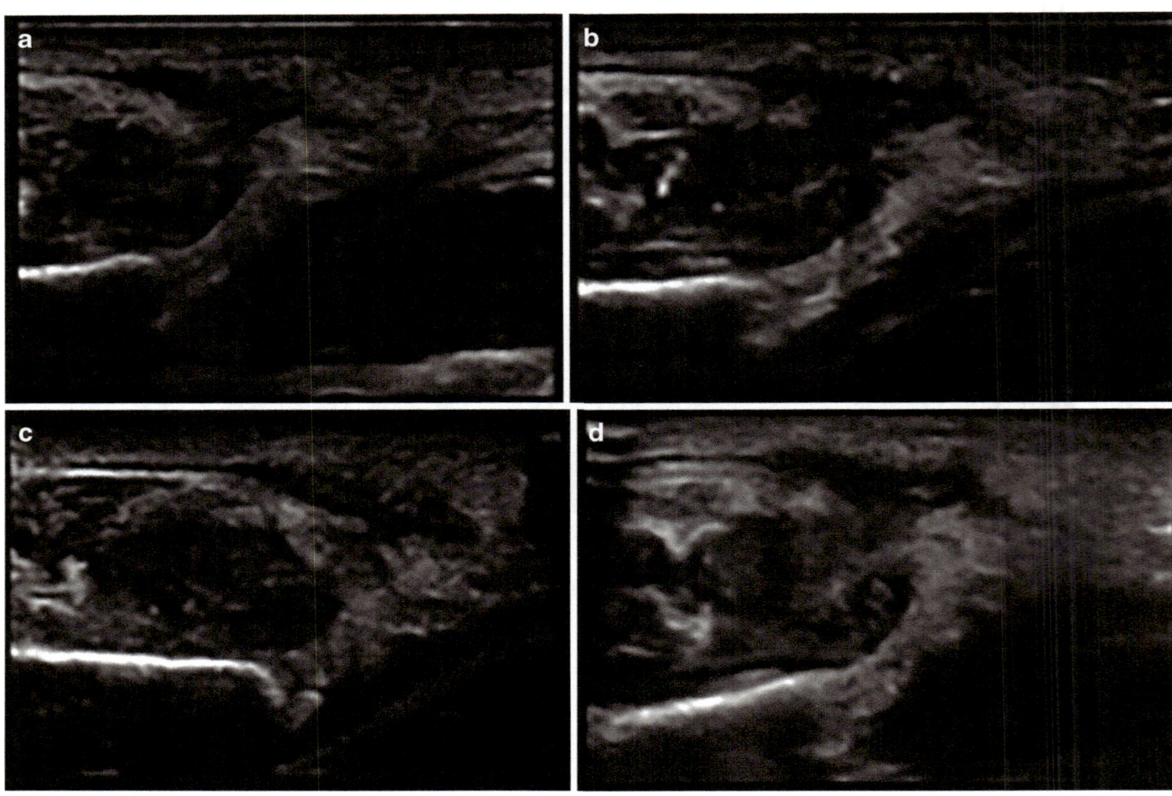




Fig. 8.51 (**a, b, c,** and **d**).Cheek cellulitis with evolving abscess. Diffuse soft-tissue thickening, edema of deep subcutaneous fat plane, edematous buccinators and submucosal plane with mild echogenic tracking collection within the fascial planes

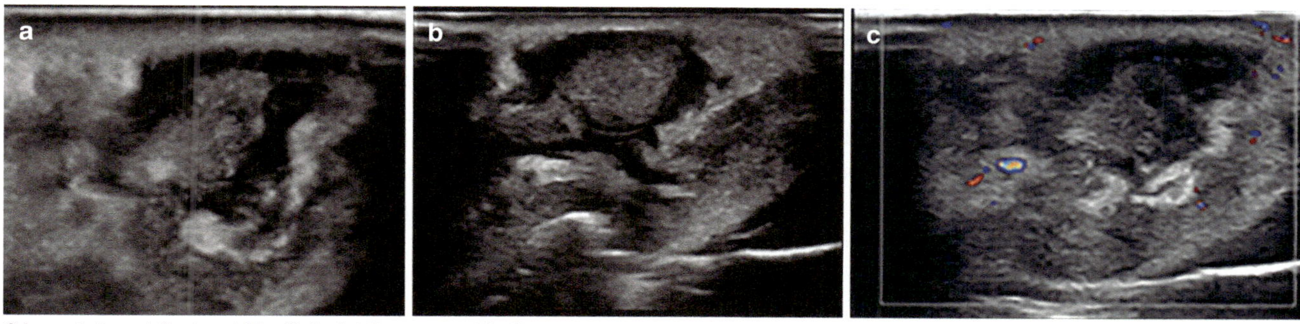


**Fig. 8.52** (**a, b** and **c**). Cheek abscess. Focal organized thick echogenic collection in the deep subcutaneous plane with minimal extension into buccinator muscle (45 year old male, with habit of chewing betel nut)

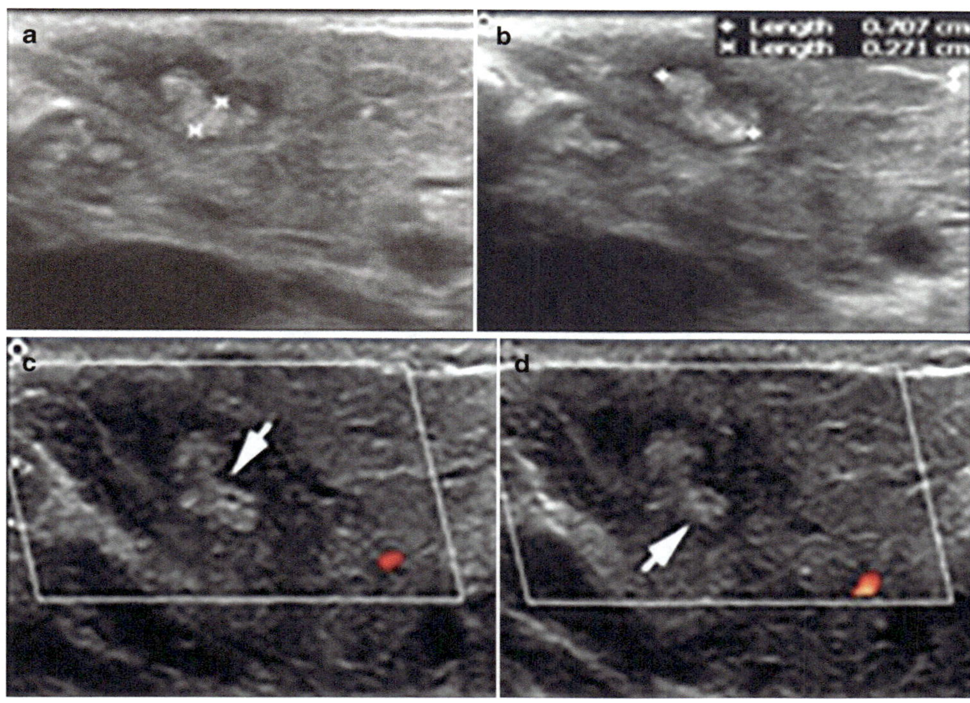



**Fig. 8.53** (**a–d**) Chronic osteomyelitis mandible. HRUSG showing hyperechoic lesion with hypoechoic halofungal granuloma

(b) *Cheek abscess (Fig. 8.52a–c).*
(c) *Chronic osteomyelitis mandible (Fig. 8.53a, b).*
(d) *Cysticercosis parotid (Fig. 8.54).*

2. **Benign Pathology.**
   (a) *Oral submucosal fibrosis (OSMF) (Fig. 8.55a–c).*
   (b) *Lesion at opening of Stenson's Duct (Fig. 8.56a, b).*
   (c) *Intraoral Mucocele (Fig. 8.57a, b).*
   (d) *Cheek lymphangioma (Fig. 8.58a–d).*
   (e) *Epidermoid cyst of cheek (Fig. 8.59a, b).*
   (f) *Painless unilateral swollen cheek (Intramasseteric lipoma) (Fig. 8.60).*
   (g) *Stenson's Duct calculus (Fig. 8.61a, b).*
   (h) *Polycystic disease of parotid (Fig. 8.62a, b).*

3. **Malignant Pathology.**
   (a) *Buccal mucosal malignancy with intact submucosa and buccinator (Fig. 8.63).*
   (b) *Buccal mucosal squamous cell carcinoma (Fig. 8.64 a-c).*

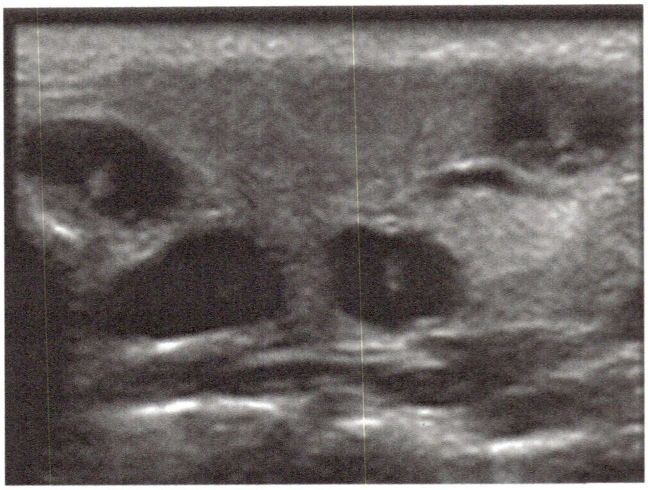



**Fig. 8.54** Cysticercosis parotid

(c) *Buccal mucosal carcinoma with mucosal and submucosal involvement, mandibular destruction and sparing of buccinator (Fig. 8.65).*
(d) *Buccal mucosal carcinoma comparative evaluation. (Fig. 8.66a, b).*
(e) *Superior vestibular malignant mass (Fig. 8.67a–c).*
(f) *Tongue malignancy-Tongue touch technique (Fig. 8.68a, b).*
(g) *Buccal malignancy with mandibular infiltration (Fig. 8.69a–d).*

4. **Vascular malformations**
   (a) *Arteriovenous malformation cheek (Fig. 8.70a–d).*
   (b) *Cheek hemangioma (Fig. 8.71).*

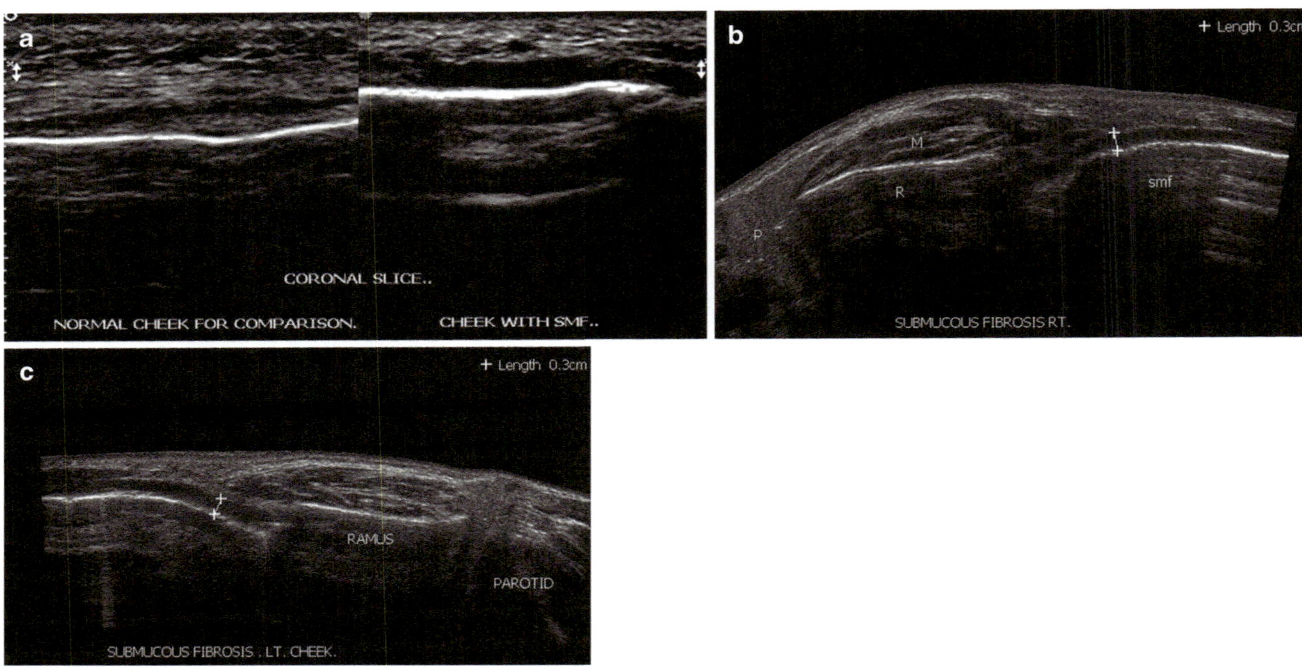




**Fig. 8.55** (**a, b** and **c**) Oral submucosal fibrosis. Axial slice showing thickening of the submucosal layer in OSMF in comparison to the normal thickness of the submucosal layer

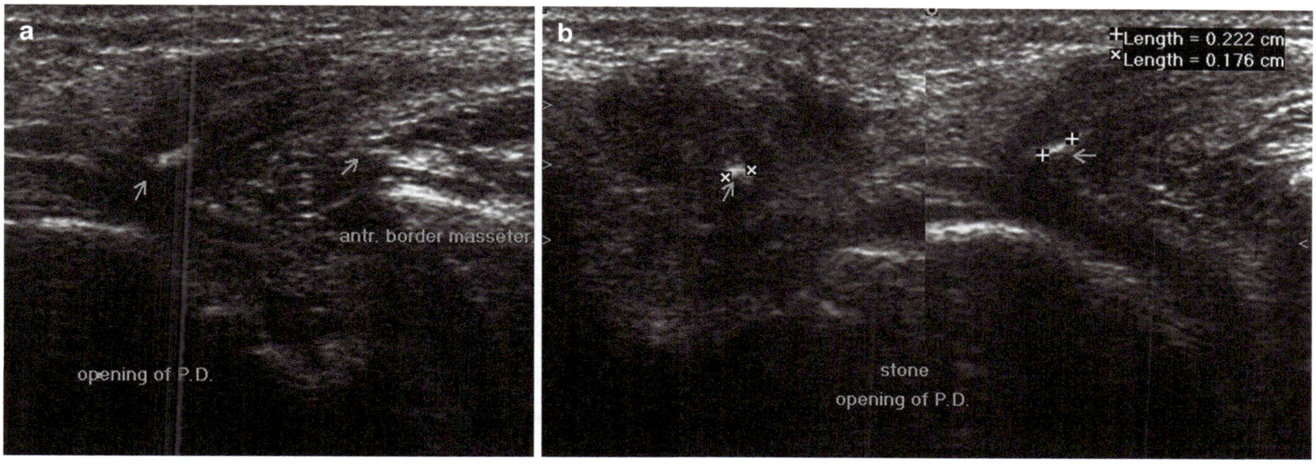




**Fig. 8.56** (**a**) and (**b**). Tiny calculus of about 1.2 mm revealed by HRUSG at Stenson's duct opening. (Pain while chewing food. No swelling)

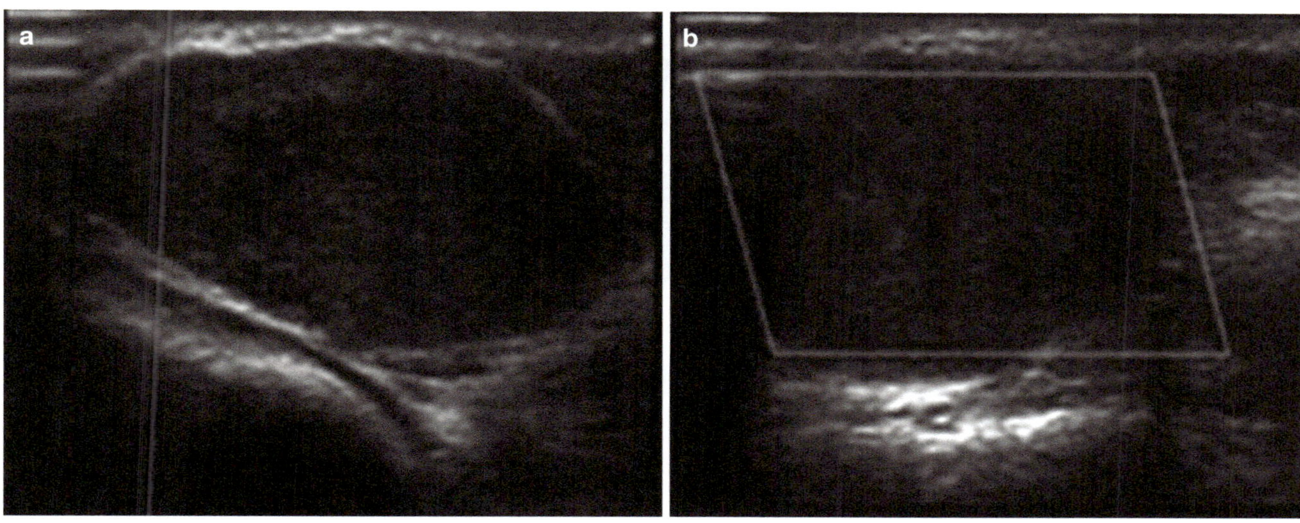




**Fig. 8.57** (**a**) and (**b**). Intraoral Mucocele. Well-defined cystic lesion in the submucosal layer with internal minimal echogenic contents. Possible diagnosis of mucocele given, later confirmed by HPR. (35 year old female, presenting with right-sided cheek swelling and mild pain)

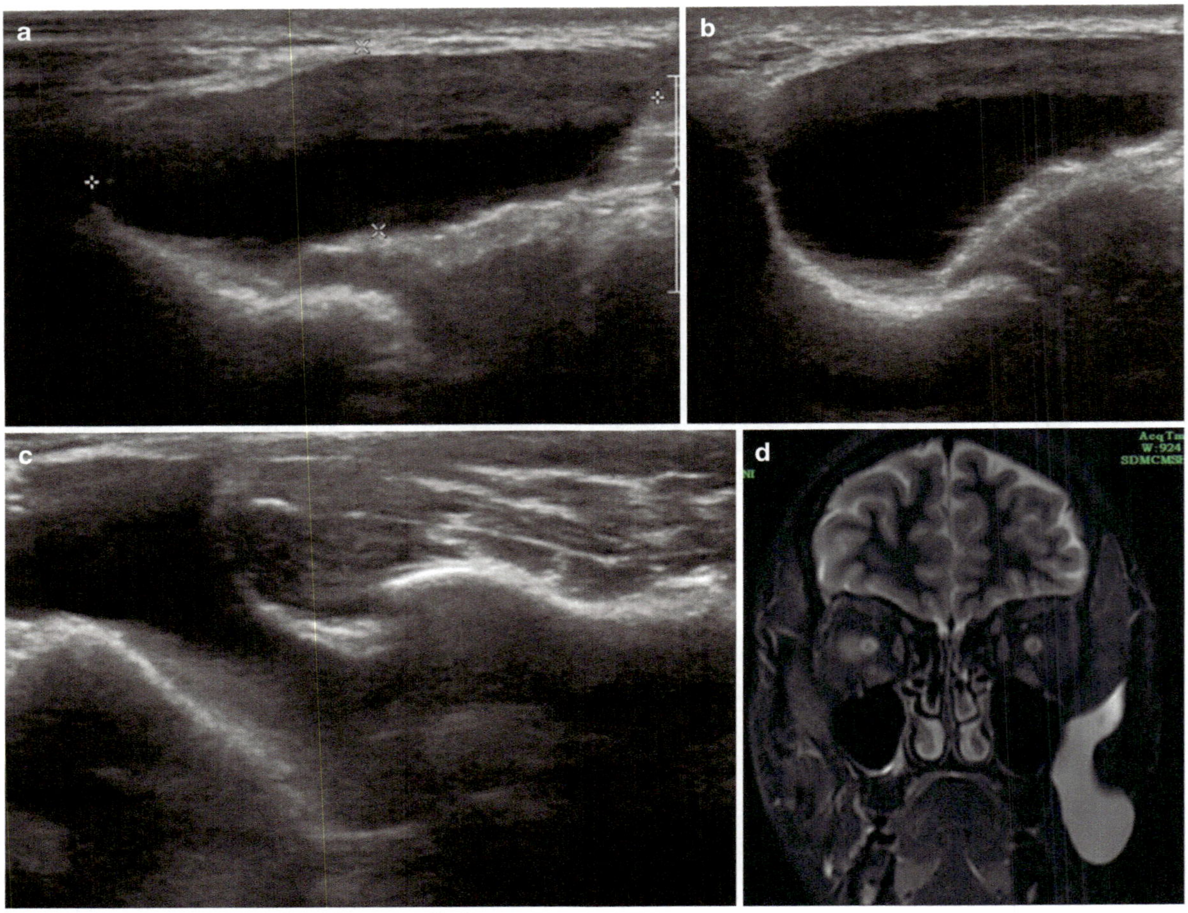




**Fig. 8.58** (**a, b, c,** and **d**). Cheek lymphangioma. Fluid-filled cystic lesion deep to submucosal layer with deep space extension adjacent to the masseter medial to mandibular ramus MRI coronal T2W imaging confirms hyperintense fluid along left side of cheek extending into infratemporal fossa (25 year old male, presenting with soft, painless swelling of left cheek)

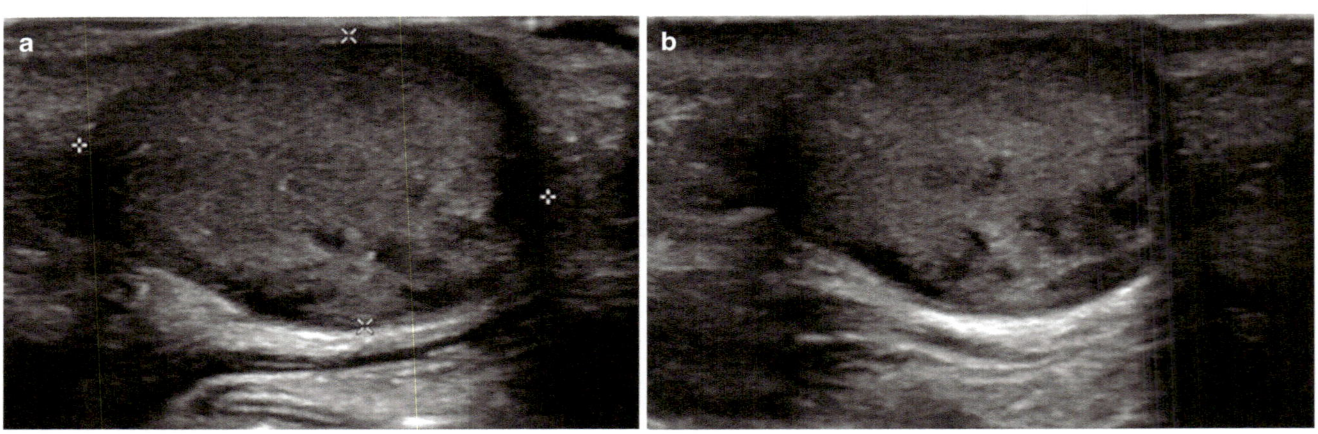




**Fig. 8.59** (**a**) and (**b**). Epidermoid cyst of cheek. Well-defined complex cystic lesion in the subcutaneous plane with internal echogenic contents causing displacement of underlying cheek layers (28 year old male presenting with painless left cheek swelling)

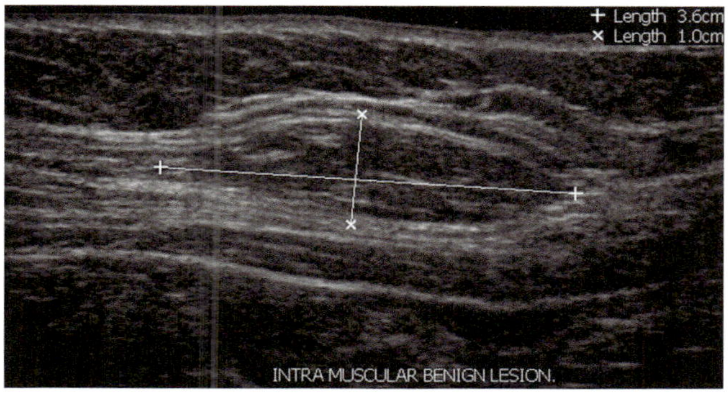




**Fig. 8.60** Intramasseteric Lipoma. Elongated intramuscular lesion isoechoic to the subcutaneous fat with internal echogenic strands representing intramasseteric lipoma. (30 year old female, presenting with painless swelling of cheek)

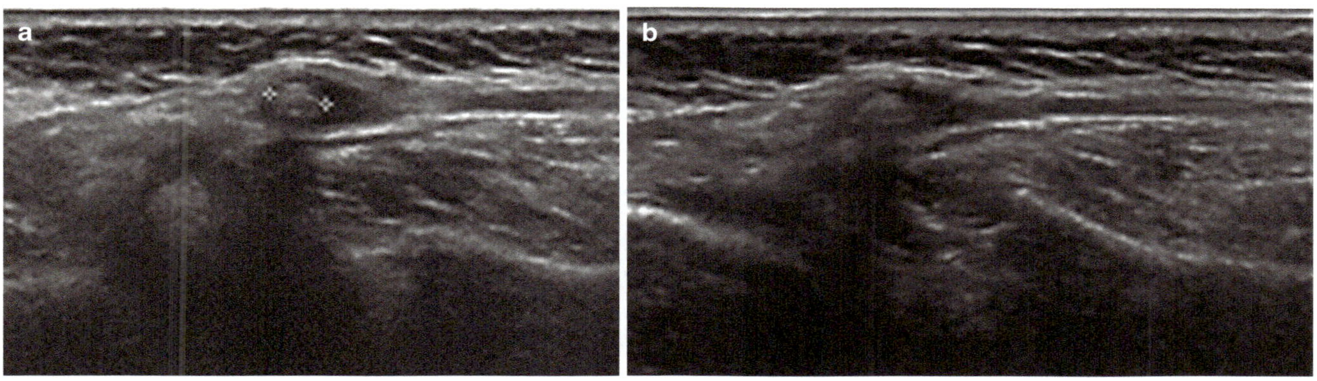




**Fig. 8.61** (**a**) and (**b**). Stenson's duct calculus. Hyperechoic calculus in the Stenson's duct with nondilated duct proximal to the calculus (23 year old male, with history of intermittent pain on right side of the cheek)

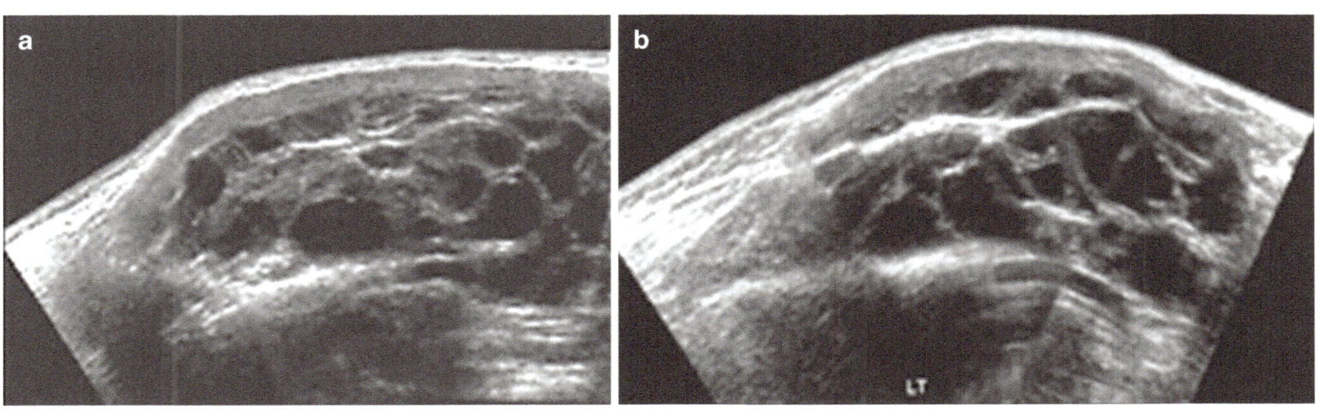




**Fig. 8.62** (**a**) and (**b**). Polycystic disease of parotid. (22 year old male Bilateral painless swollen cheek 7–8 yrs duration)

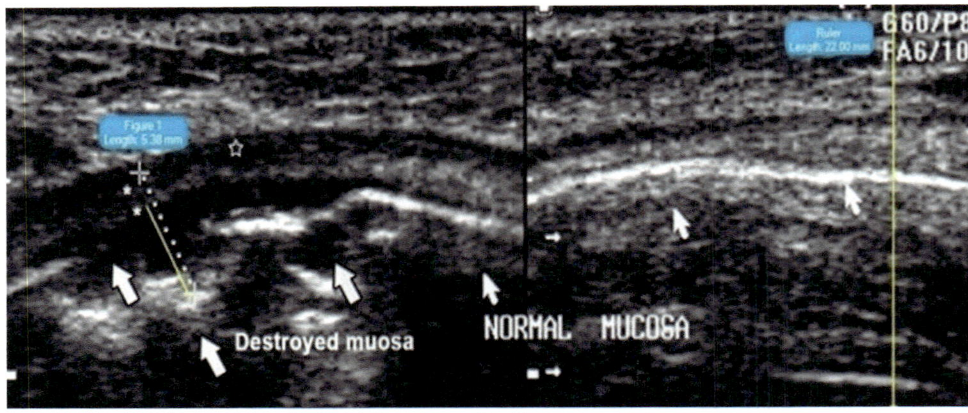




**Fig. 8.63** Buccal mucosal malignancy with intact submucosa and buccinator. Growth predominantly involving the mucosa, distinct from submucosa (between asterisk) buccinator (star) appears normal. (55 year old male with irritating nonhealing ulcer left cheek)

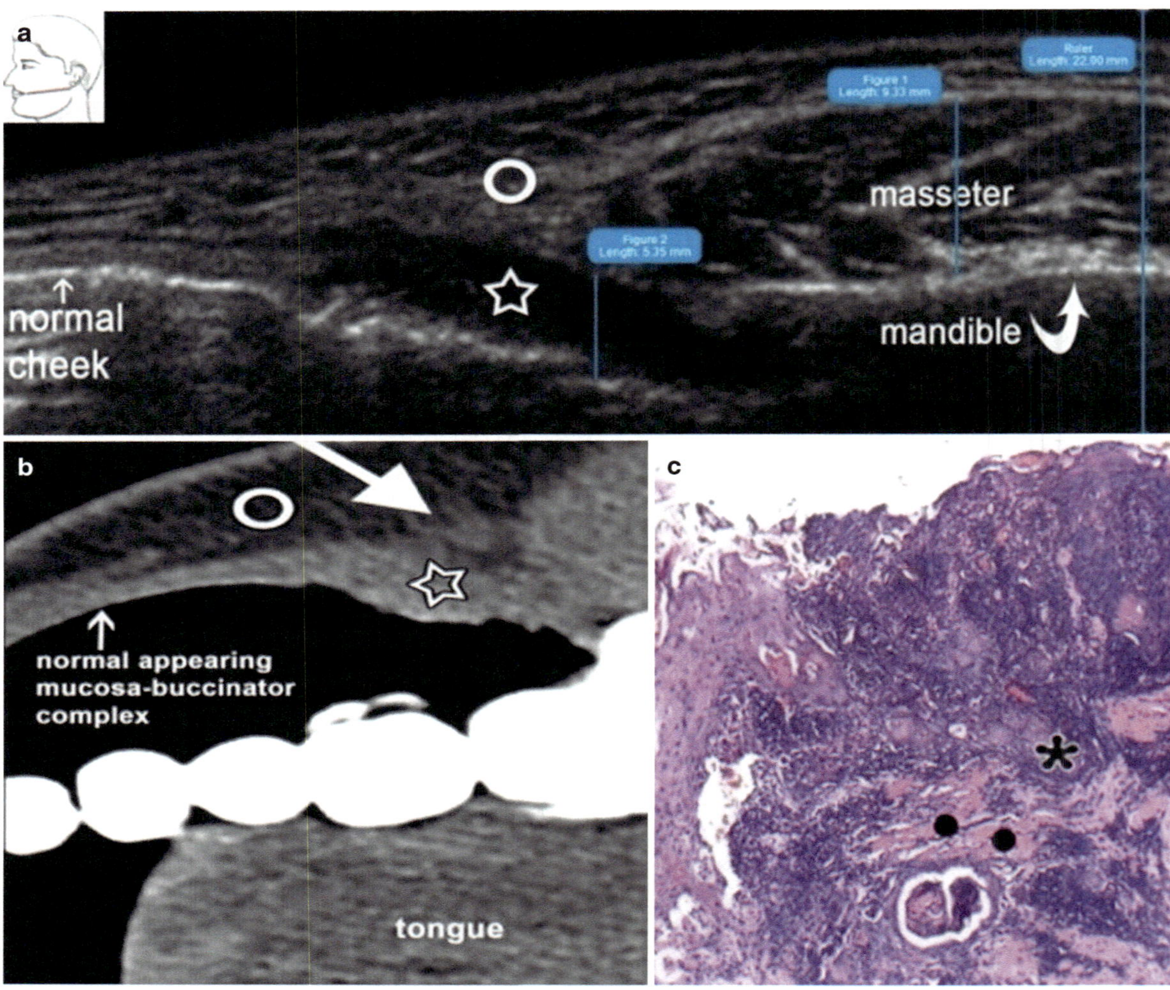




**Fig. 8.64** (**a**, **b**, and **c**). Early Carcinoma of the cheek better seen on HRUSG than by CT slice at the same level. Proved by Histopathology (52 year old male with squamous cell carcinoma of the buccal mucosa)

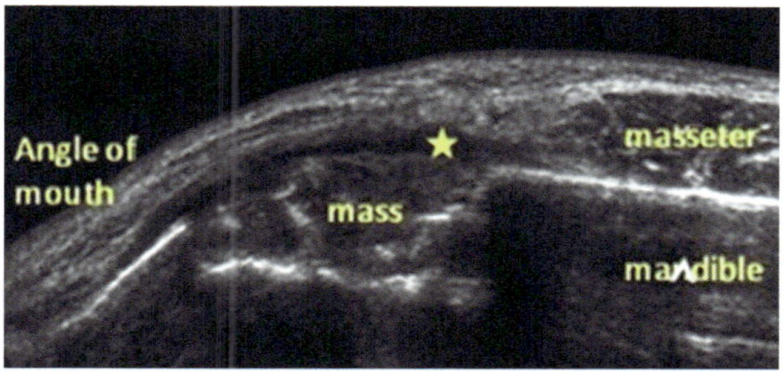




**Fig. 8.65** Buccal mucosal carcinoma

**Fig. 8.66** (**a**) Buccal mucosal carcinoma (Resting phase). (**b**) Buccal mucosal carcinoma (Fruit jelly technique). Patient was unable to perform the puffed cheek technique. Mass involving the mucosa, submucosa, buccinator, and fat

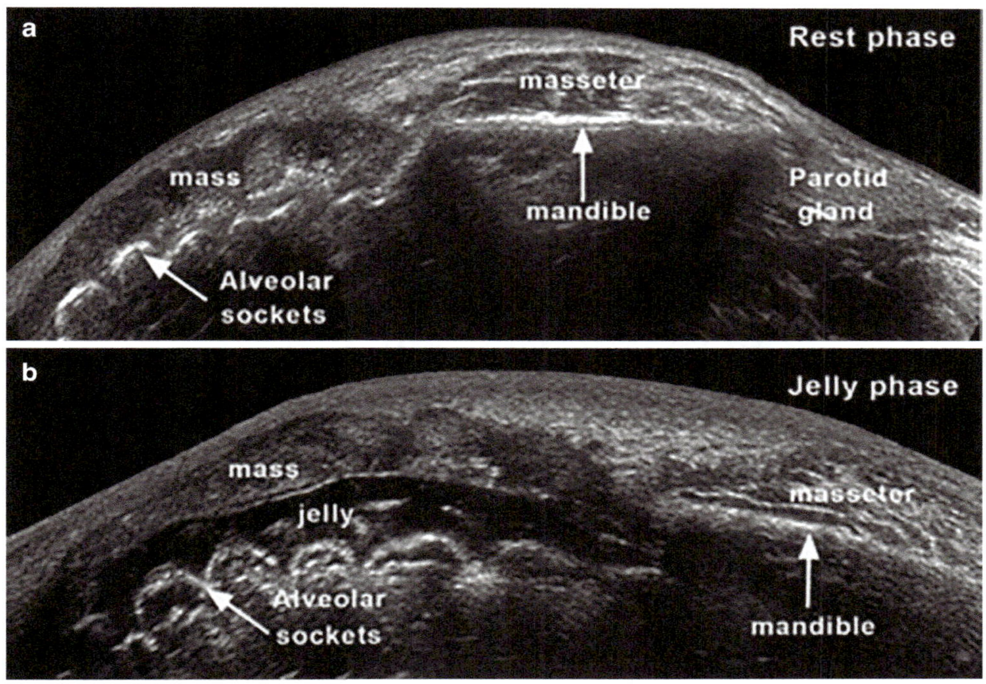

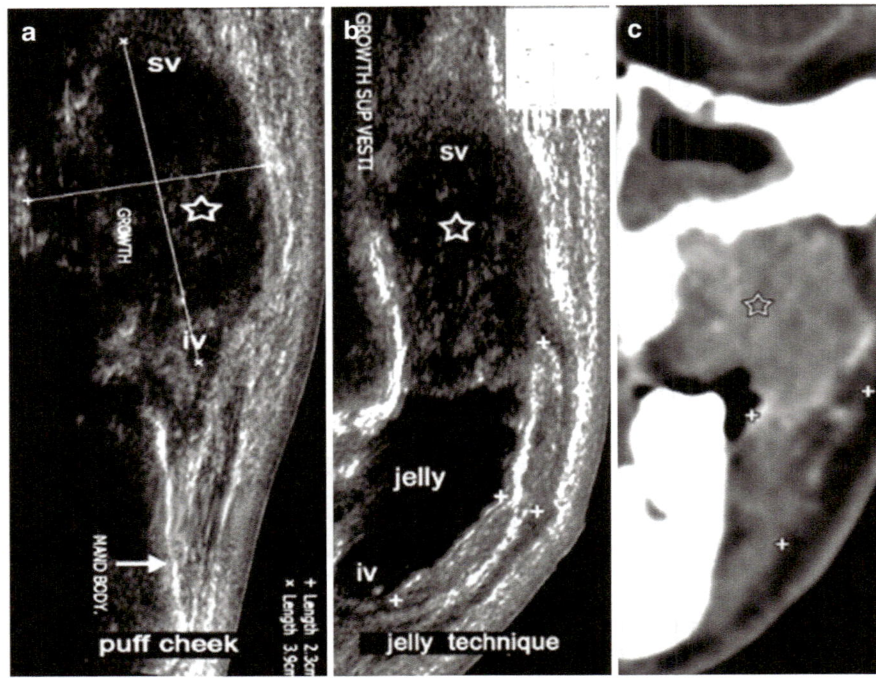




**Fig. 8.67** (**a, b** and **c**). Superior vestibular malignant mass. Coronal sections revealing predominantly hypoechoic, superior vestibular mass with irregular margins extending into cheek layers and causing underlying bony destruction. Comparison between (**a**) neutral cheek, (**b**) fruit jelly Technique and (**c**) CT

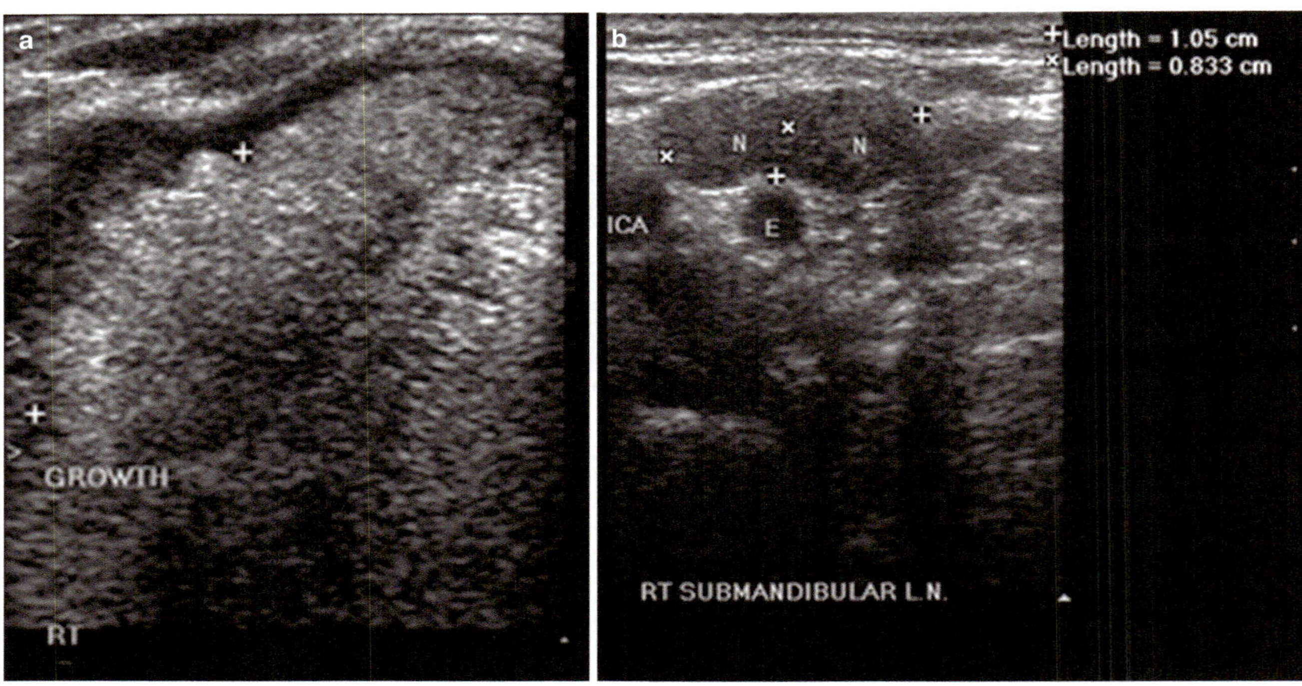




**Fig. 8.68** (**a**) and (**b**). Tongue malignancy against cheek wall. Irregular lesion along the Right anterolateral margin of the tongue by "Tongue touch" technique. Few enlarged lymph nodes are also noted with loss of hilar anatomy representing metastatic lymph nodes. (40 year old male, with complaint of swelling over the tongue)

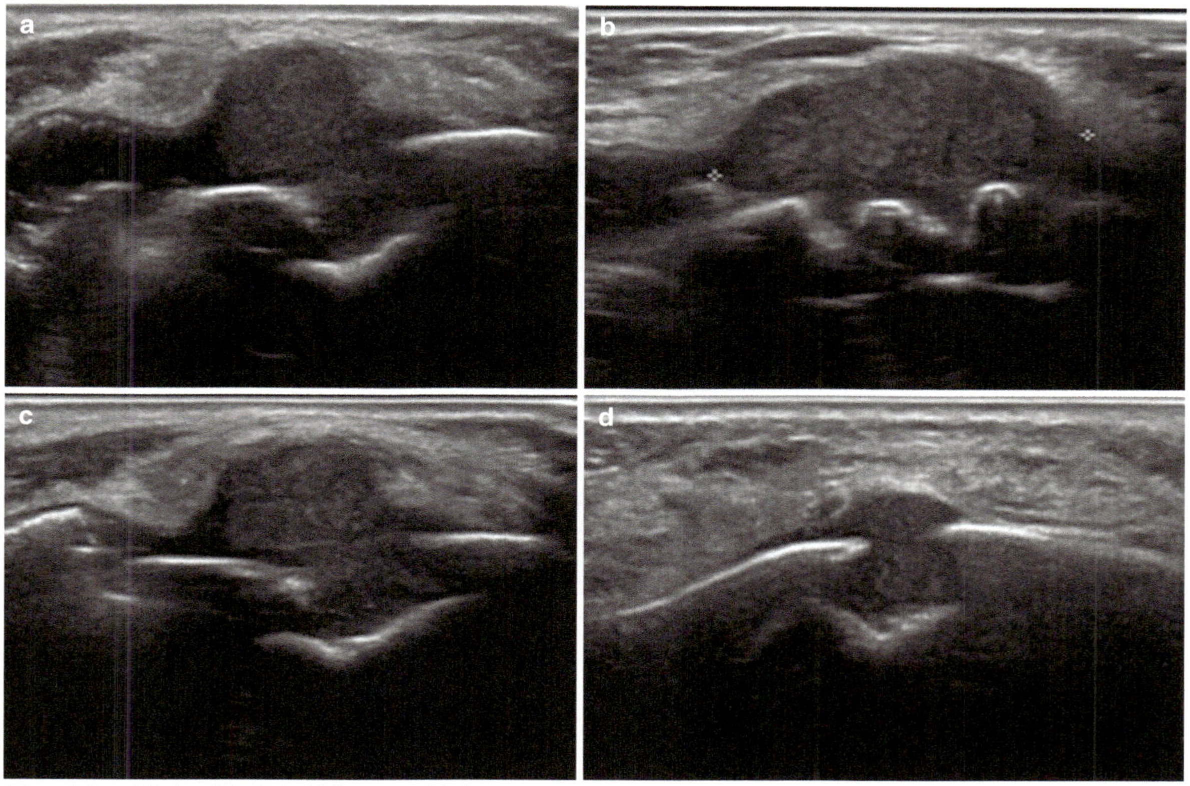




**Fig. 8.69** (**a, b, c,** and **d**) Buccal malignancy with mandibular infiltration. Heterogeneous mass lesion along the buccal mucosa extending into lower buccogingival sulcus with infiltration into submucosa and buccinator muscle. Focal cortical break is also noted in the mandibular bone with intraosseous infiltration. (48 year old male tobacco chewer presenting with right cheek swelling)

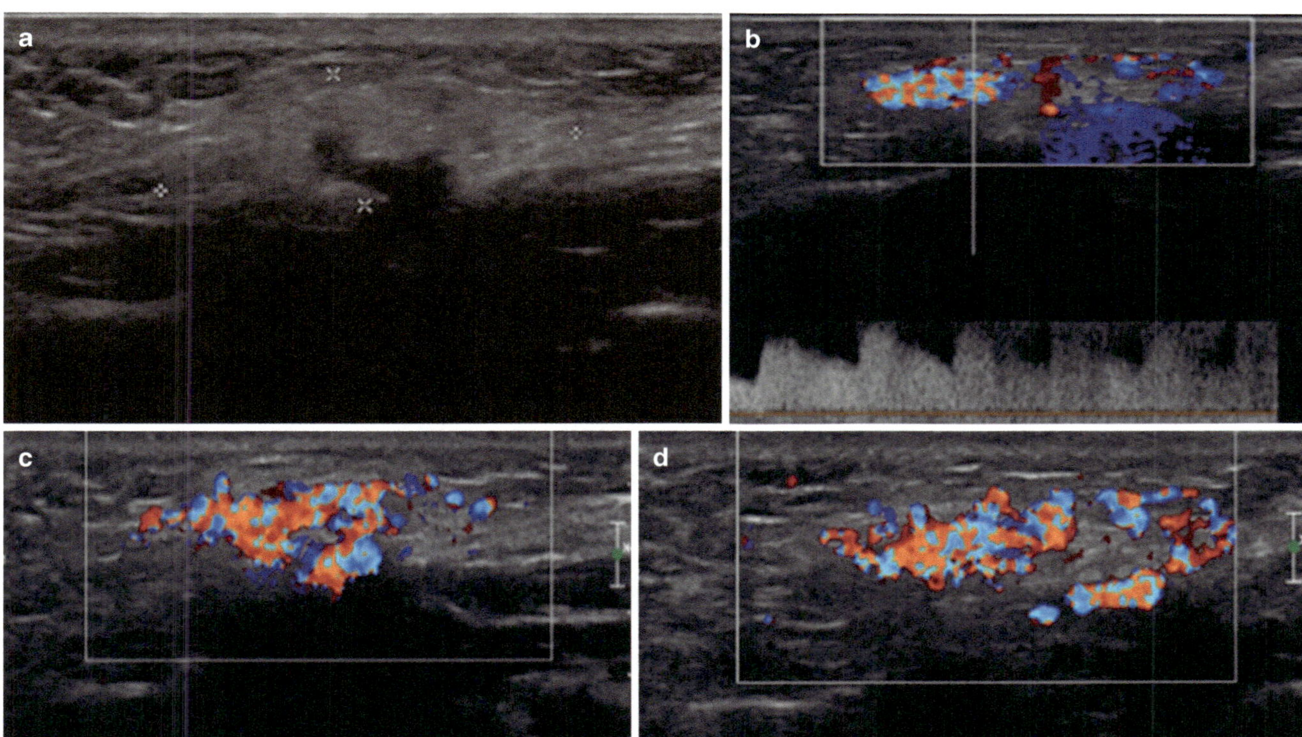




**Fig. 8.70** (**a, b, c,** and **d**) Arteriovenous malformation (AVM) cheek. Focal soft-tissue thickening with internal hypoechoic areas. Doppler study shows multiple vascular channels with high velocity, low resistance flow suggestive of AVM. (40 year old female presenting with history of swelling and intermittent pain)

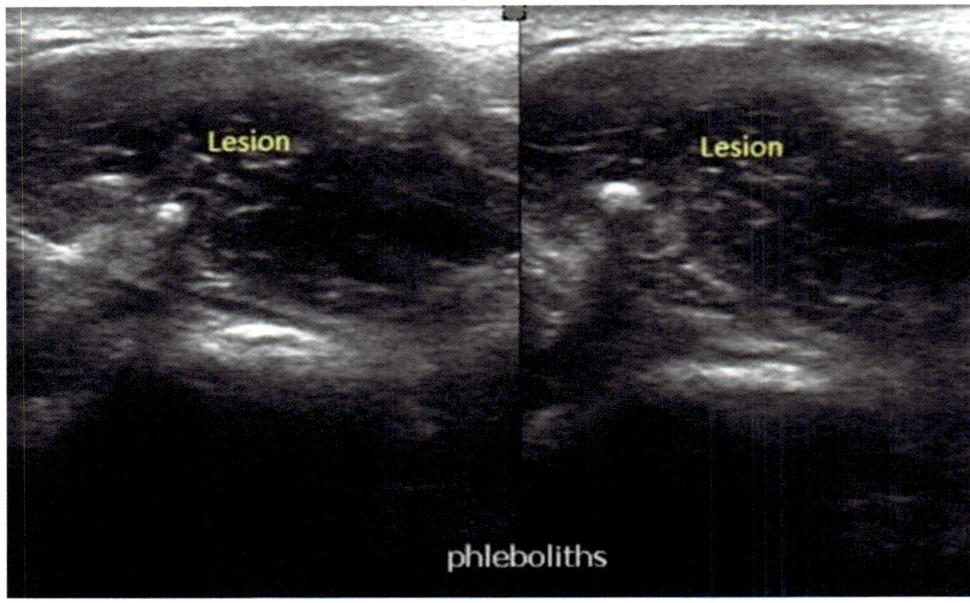




**Fig. 8.71** Cheek Hemangioma. Mixed echoic hemangioma with phlebolith. Absence of flow signals due to low-velocity flow

## 8.12 Conclusion

It is extremely difficult to limit radiology to a chapter and what has been written does not represent the whole of maxillofacial radiology. Only the relevant aspects and the bare minimum essentials of radiology for maxillofacial surgeons have been covered in this chapter. The entire range of radiology for maxillofacial surgeons, dealing with surgical problems pertinent to the maxillofacial region, would require more expansive and elaborate writing.

This chapter on radiology provides an outlook to the surgeon, who can proceed to applying radiology in his everyday surgical practice. In the event of encountering any lacunae in the book, the MFS must refer to the textbooks dedicated to maxillofacial radiology. Being a surgeon, the MFS should be aware of the use of the chest radiograph and its applications in his practice. The role of high-resolution ultrasonography has also been emphasized in this chapter. Dental radiology, both extra and intraoral, has not been included since all maxillofacial surgeons have extensive knowledge of the same in their surgical practice.

Since it is the MFS who is acquainted with the patient's clinical status, he must properly plan the imaging pathway for the patient. It is for this purpose that the MFS should be aware of the various imaging modalities as regards their nature, mode of image formation, their usefulness over other modalities, and their drawbacks. Radiation safety and cost effectiveness of a specific imaging modality also need to be kept in mind. The imaging method selected should be one that provides the required information within the shortest time possible, be the safest option for the patient, and be the most economical, while at the same time providing maximum information.

The MFS can commence with simple basic imaging methods like plain radiography or USG and later proceed to higher imaging methods in case the basic methods were not enough to satisfy the surgeon's needs for patient management. A recent costlier imaging method does not necessarily mean it is the best. Many times, it is the simpler basic imaging methods that provide more crucial findings that help in understanding complex disease processes.

**Acknowledgments** The authors would like to acknowledge & thank Dr Niranjan Kumar, M.Ch FRCS. ; Honorable Vice-Chancellor, Shri Dharmasthala Manjunatheshwara University for his valuable constructive suggestions and constant support towards this endeavour.

## References


1. Fusaro F, Constantinides F, Maglione M, Dalessadri D, Vettori E, Lenarda RDI. Comparison of orthopantomography (OPG) and computed tomography (CT) accuracy in predicting inferior alveolar nerve injury following lower third molar surgical extraction [Internet]. 2017 [cited 2019Jun3]. Available from: https://www.researchgate.net/publication/319548814_Comparison_of_orthopantomography_OPG_and_computed_tomography_CT_accuracy_in_predicting_inferior_alveolar_nerve_injury_following_lower_third_molar_surgical_extraction
2. Abramovitch K, Rice DD. Basic principles of cone beam computed tomography. Dent Clin N Am. 2014;58(3):463–84.
3. Lucas J.. What are gamma-rays? Available from: https://www.livescience.com/50215-gamma-rays.html
4. Ferreira RI, de Almeida SM, Boscolo FN, Santos AO, Camargo EE. Bone scintigraphy as an adjunct for the diagnosis of oral diseases. J Dent Educ. 2002;66(12):1381–7.
5. Appadurai R, Lingeshwar D, Venugopal S, Christina RD. Bone scintigraphy as a diagnostic tool in condylar hyperplasia [Internet]. 2017 [cited 2019Jun3]. Available from: http://www.joomr.org/article.asp?issn=2321-3841;year=2017;volume=5;issue=3;spage=84;epage=89;aulast=Appadurai
6. Griffeth LK. Use of PET/CT scanning in cancer patients: technical and practical considerations [Internet]. Proceedings (Baylor University. Medical Center). Baylor Health Care System; 2005 [cited 2019Jun4]. Available from: https://www.ncbi.nlm.nih.gov/pmc/articles/PMC1255942/
7. Williams N, O'Connell PR, McCaskie AW. Bailey and Love's short practice of surgery. 27th ed. New York: CRC Press; 2018.
8. Pooley RA. AAPM/RSNA Physics Tutorial for Residents Fundamental Physics of MR Imaging [Internet]. 2005 [cited 2019Jun3]. Available from: https://pubs.rsna.org/doi/pdf/10.1148/rg.254055027
9. Singh GP, Dogra S, Kumari E. Ultrasonography: maxillofacial applications. Annals of Dental Specialty. 2014;2(3):104–7.
10. Kumar V, Abbas AK, Aster JC. Robbins and Cotran pathologic basis of disease. 9th ed. Philadelphia: W.B. Saunders; 2015.
11. Fraser RS, Muller NL, Colman N, Pare PD. Fraser and Pare's diagnosis of diseases of the chest. 4th ed. Philadelphia: W.B. Saunders; 1999.
12. Christopoulos A. Mouth Anatomy [Internet]. Overview, Gross Anatomy: Oral Vestibule, Gross Anatomy: Oral Cavity Proper. 2015 [cited 2019Jun5].
13. Surgical fascial spaces [Internet]. online presentation [cited 2019 Jun 7];Available from: https://en.ppt-online.org/369373
14. La'Porte SJ, Juttla JK, Lingam RK. Imaging the Floor of the Mouth and the Sublingual Space [Internet]. RadioGraphics. 2011 [cited 2019Jun5]. Available from: https://pubs.rsna.org/doi/full/10.1148/rg.315105062
15. Joshi SK, Kamalapur MG, Joshi AS, Hallikeri K. Ultrasonographic evaluation of carcinoma of buccal mucosa: Ultrasound technique and evaluation of neoplastic conditions. J. Evid. Based Med. Healthc. 2016;3(34):1649–55.


## Further Reading


Mosier K. Functional imaging of swallowing. In: Mukherji SK, Casterlijins JA, editors. Head and neck imaging. Berlin: Springer; 2000. p. 79–86.

Yousem DM (2000) Magnetization transfer imaging of the Extracranial head and neck. In: Mukherji SK, Casterlijins JA (eds). Modern head and neck imaging. Springer, Berlin, pp1–16.

Sanjay N. Jain (2019) a Pictoral essay: radiology lines and tubes in the intensive care unit. Indian J Radiol Imaging. 2011;21:182–90.

# Part V

# Principles of Maxillofacial Surgery

# 9 Operating Room Protocols and Infection Control

Rishi Kumar Bali

## 9.1 Introduction

A study comprising data from 56 countries in 2004 stated that the annual major surgery volume was estimated to be 187–281 million operations, accounting for approximately one operation annually for every 25 human beings alive [1]. In subsequent studies, data were obtained from a total of 194 Member States of the World Health Organization for the years 2005–2012. According to these studies, 312.9 million operations took place in 2012, showing an increase from the 2004 estimate of 226.4 million operations. 6.3% and 23.1% of operations were carried out in *very-low* and *low*-expenditure countries representing only 36.8% (2573 million people) and 34.2% (2393 million people) of the global population of 7001 million people, respectively [2]. The incidence of postoperative infections reported among the developed countries like UK and USA was approximately 5% and 5–6%, whereas in developing countries like India it is much higher, accounting for approximately 10–25%. [3, 4].

The main problem encountered in the practice of surgical safety is that existing safety practices are not adequate in some countries. Lack of resources is the main reason behind this, particularly in developing countries. Good infection prevention and control is essential to ensure the safety of the patient undergoing any surgical procedure in the operating theater. The surgical site infections (SSIs) constitute 20% of the total hospital-acquired infections [4]. These infections cause substantial patient mortality and morbidity and burden healthcare systems with massive costs. Since these infections are primarily acquired during the operative procedure when the wound is still open, stringent protocols need to be followed at this point to minimize their onset.

R. K. Bali (✉)
Postgraduate Department of OMFS, DAV Dental college hospital, Yamunanagar, Haryana, India

## 9.2 Terminology

To establish surgical protocols, it is important to understand the basic concepts of sterilization, asepsis, and infection control. In this respect, the following terminologies are very commonly used:

**Antibiotics**
These agents are a by-product of certain microorganisms, which either have the capacity to destroy or inhibit the growth of other microorganisms at low concentrations.

**Anti-Infective**
A substance (or drug) capable of killing microorganisms or inhibiting their growth, in particular, pathogenic microorganisms. This is a general term used to encompass those drugs that specifically act on certain types of microorganisms, including antibacterial (antibiotics), antifungal, antiviral, and antiprotozoal agents.

**Antimicrobial Agent**
Any agent synthetically or naturally obtained that can destroy or attenuate the microorganisms.

**Antisepsis**
It is the process in which microbial agents on a living surface are either killed or their growth is arrested.

**Antiseptic**
These are the substances applied on the living tissues to reduce the possibility of infection, sepsis, and putrefaction by inhibiting the activity or growth of the microorganisms.

**Asepsis**
The state of being free from living pathogenic organisms.

**Aseptic**
Free of or using methods to keep free from microorganisms.



K. Bonanthaya et al. (eds.), *Oral and Maxillofacial Surgery for the Clinician*, https://doi.org/10.1007/978-981-15-1346-6_9

**Aseptic Processing**
It is defined as the processing and packaging of a sterile product into sterilized containers followed by proper sealing with a sterilized closure in a manner to control microbiological recontamination.

**Bactericide**
It is an antimicrobial agent that has the capacity to destroy both nonpathogenic and pathogenic organisms but may not destroy bacteria in spore form.

**Bacteriostatic**
It is an antimicrobial agent that inhibits the growth of microorganisms but is not capable of killing them.

**Bioburden**
The occurrence of viable microorganisms on a surface or object before the sterilization procedure.

**Biologic Indicator (BI)**
A standardized test preparation of bacterial spores used to demonstrate effective sterilizing conditions by providing a defined resistance to a specific sterilization process.

**Chemical Indicator**
These are agents or devices used to monitor or confirm the attainment of one or more of the parameters required for a satisfactory sterilization process or used in a specific test of the sterilization equipment.

**Chemisterilant**
It is an agent, chemical in nature with properties that kills all forms of microbial agents, including spores.

**Cleaning**
It is the process of removing all forms of foreign materials (from objects using detergents & water, soaps, and enzymes) by employing the mechanical action of washing or scrubbing the object.

**Contamination**
It is the process of entry of microbial agents into tissues or any aseptic environment.

**Crossinfection**
The spread of infection from one person, object or place to another.

**Decontamination**
The process by which a person or a surface is made free from all the agents that contaminate the surface and lead to the spread of infections. [5]

**Detergent**
It is a chemical agent with cleansing actions in dilute solutions, which, on combining with impurities and dirt, make them more soluble.

**Disease**
Disruption of the normal performance of the vital functions of a plant or animal by an infection.

**Disinfectant**
This is an agent, usually a chemical, applied on inanimate objects that destroys microorganism in the vegetative form but not the spores.

Chemical disinfectant agents are categorized into low level, intermediate, and high level (depending on the product claims and regulatory requirements in different parts of the world).

- High-level disinfection (HLD): It is a process in which a small number of spores or certain bacteria are killed by the use of certain antimicrobial agents at a specific temperature and appropriate concentration.
- Intermediate-level disinfection (ILD): It is a process in which vegetative forms of all microorganisms are destroyed but affect the activity of spores of certain bacteria.
- Low-level disinfection (LLD): It is a process in which vegetative forms of all microorganisms are destroyed having no activity on spores of bacteria at very low concentrations.

**Disinfection**
Antimicrobial process to remove, destroy, or deactivate microorganisms on surfaces or in liquids. Disinfection is often considered as a reduction of the numbers and types of viable microorganisms (or "bioburden") but may not be assumed to render the surface or liquid free from viable microbial contamination (in contrast to sterilization).

**Droplet Nuclei**
These are those particles of 1–10 μm that are implicated in the spread of airborne infections.

**Exogenous Infection**
The infecting microorganism comes from an external source.

**Fomites**
Any inanimate object that is capable of absorbing or transmitting infectious microorganisms from one person to the other.

**Fumigation**
The process of disinfecting or purifying an area or object with the fumes of certain chemical agents.

**Germicide**
Agents that are designed to kill and destroy pathogenic organisms on the surface of different things.

**Infection**
It is the process of invasion of the tissues by microorganisms and their multiplication in the body of the host to produce disease.

**Microorganisms or Microbe**
Microscopic organisms, which may exist in its single-celled form or in a colony of cells.

**Minimum Effective Concentration (MEC)**
The lowest concentration of a chemical or product, used in a specified process that achieves a claimed activity.

**Minimum Recommended Concentration (MRC)**
The lowest concentration of a chemical or product specified by the equipment manufacturer to be used in a process.

**Nosocomial**
This comes from two Greek words, i.e., "*nosus*" meaning "*disease*" and "*komeion*" meaning "*to take care of.*" Also known as "hospital-acquired infections." These are the infections originating or taking place in a hospital.

**Operating Room (OR)**
The operating room or operating theater is a facility within a hospital where surgical procedures are carried out in an aseptic environment.

**Pathogen**
A pathogen is a tiny living organism, such as a bacterium or virus that is capable of producing disease in an individual.

**Resistance**
It is the natural ability of the agent to oppose the effects of any harmful agents.

**Soil**
Natural or artificial contamination on a device or surface following its use or simulated use.

**Sterile Barrier System**
Packaging that prevents the ingress of microorganisms following a sterilization process, thereby preserving the sterile state.

**Sterilizer**
Equipment designed to achieve sterilization.

**Sterilizing Agent**
Physical or chemical agent (or combination of agents) that has sufficient microbicidal activity to achieve sterility under defined conditions.

**Septic**
Contaminated or infected.

**Spores**
These are the reproductive forms of some microorganisms that can survive harsh environmental factors and have the capability of developing into new viable microbes.

**Sterilization**
Sterilization is a process that destroys or removes all microbial life completely, including spores by means of certain chemical or physical processes.

**Sterile**
Free from living microorganisms.

**Sterilize**
Total destruction of all living forms.

**Vector**
It is an organism that does not cause disease itself but which spreads infection by conveying pathogens from one host to another.

**Virulence**
It is a pathogen's ability to infect, sustain, or spread infection in a living a host. Historical background of present day protocols is enumerated in Table 9.1.

## 9.3 Surgical Site Infections

Approximately 2–5% of all surgical patients tend to acquire surgical site infections (SSIs) [4]. In developed & high-income countries (HICs), SSIs are the second most common cause of healthcare-associated infections [6], whereas in Low- & Middle-Income Countries (LMICs) or underdeveloped & developing countries these infections are the most common ones. Thus, to reduce the risk of surgical site infections, a more systematic approach has to be adopted, based on proper knowledge regarding the status of the patient, type, & time of the operation, personnel involved and the health care facilities available during a surgical procedure. The main pathogenic source of surgical site infections is the endogenous flora (usually aerobic gram positive cocci) of the patient present in the skin, the mucous membranes, or the hollow viscera. The exogenous sources of infection include

**Table 9.1** Historical background leading to proper sterilization and disinfection protocols

| Year | Event |
|---|---|
| • First century BC. | *Varo and Columella* postulated that diseases were caused by invisible beings, "animals minutia," inhaled or ingested |
| • 500 AD | *Sushruta* instructed operating team members to clean and fumigate the operating theater with vapors of certain disinfectants prior to all surgical procedures |
| • 1493–1541 | *Paracelsus*, called the father of medicine, reformed pharmacopeia and introduced compositions of lead, copper, sulfur, iron, and mercury |
| • 1546 | *Fracastorious* proposed a "contagion vivum," as the possible cause of infectious diseases. |
| • 1827–1912 | *Joseph Lister*, "father of modern surgery," demonstrated that antisepsis could prevent infections; also known as "Listerian era" |
| • 1889 | *William Stewart Halsted* introduced rubber gloves for his scrub nurse |
| • 1882 | *Robert Koch* introduced the use of mercuric bichloride as antiseptic agents and isolated the bacilli of tuberculosis |
| • 1880s and 1890s. | Sterilization of instruments, hand washing, and the wearing of masks, caps, gloves, and gowns was introduced |

**Table 9.2** WHO: Ten essential objectives for safe surgery

(1) The operating team must ensure that the correct surgical procedure is to be carried out on the correct patient.
(2) The operating personnel should have adequate knowledge regarding the anesthesia, its methods of administration as well as its effects so that minimum pain is experienced by the patient.
(3) The operating personnel should be well prepared for any life-threatening conditions like loss of airway or respiratory function.
(4) The operating team should be prepared for risk of high loss of blood.
(5) The operating team should be well versed with the history of the patient in order to prevent or induce any allergic or adverse drug reactions that can cause a significant risk for the patient.
(6) Care must be taken to minimize the formation of surgical site infections by using proper measures.
(7) Proper care must be taken to not leave any instrument or any foreign material at the surgical site.
(8) All specimens should be carefully identified and secured for further investigations.
(9) Proper communication must be present among the operating team personnel for the safe conduct of the surgical procedure.
(10) A routine surveillance of the surgical volume, safety protocols, capacities, and the outcomes must be carried out by all the hospitals and the health care systems.

members of the surgical team, environment of the operating theater and tools, materials & instruments brought to the sterile zones during the surgical procedure. Various strategies employed to prevent or control the occurrence of surgical site infections include reducing the contamination by microorganisms on the sterile surgical instruments as well as the body of the patient, prophylactic preoperative antibiotic coverage, carrying out the surgical procedure carefully, proper handling of the operating room.

## 9.4 Surgical Safety

Surgical safety is of utmost importance in order to prevent major and life-threatening complications leading to undue loss of life and patient morbidity. Thus, a list of ten essential objectives with a surgical safety checklist have been elucidated by the WHO to be followed by all the personnel present in the operating room to reduce the risk of such complications [7] (Tables 9.2 and 9.3).

## 9.5 Environmental Control and Design

**Operating Room (OR)**

The operating room or operating theater is a facility within a hospital where surgical procedures are carried out in an aseptic environment. Since the operating theater is a highly sterile, aseptic, and restricted area in a hospital setting, it is mandatory for all the personnel concerned to have a proper understanding of the working of the operation theater abiding by certain laws, regulations, and professional guidelines. Integrated infection control in the operation theater is the key to decreasing morbidity and mortality among the patients undergoing surgery.

Following essentials must be present in an operating room:

- Adequate lighting
- Proper ventilation with 20 (ACH) air changes/hour
- Correct and sufficient instruments needed in the surgery
- Proper machines and equipment for monitoring the condition of the patients during the surgeries
- Emergency drugs and other items
- Separate rooms should be present to carry different procedures

- Location of the Operating Theater: The location of the operation theater should be such that adequate natural light and proper ventilation is present. For this, a two- or three-story building away from the general hustle and bustle of the hospital is preferred.
- Operation rooms: The standard recommended size of the operation theater is 6.5 m × 6.5 m × 3.5 m and can be modified as per requirement
- Doors and Windows: There should be separate entry and exit doors. The width of the door should be approximately

**Table 9.3** WHO's Surgical Safety Checklist

| Before induction of anesthesia | Before skin incision | Before patient leaves operating room |
|---|---|---|
| Sign in | Time out | Sign out |
| Patient has confirmed<br>• Identity<br>• Site<br>• Procedure<br>• Consent | Confirm all team members have introduced themselves by name and role | Nurse verbally confirms with the team<br>• The name of the procedure recorded<br>• The instrument, sponge, and needle counts are correct (or not applicable)<br>• How the specimen is labeled (including patient name)<br>• Whether there are any equipment problems to be addressed |
| Site marked/not applicable | Surgeon, anesthesia professional and nurse verbally confirm<br>• Patient<br>• Site<br>• Procedure | |
| Anesthesia safety check completed | Anticipated critical events<br>• Surgeon reviews: What are the critical or unexpected steps, operative duration, anticipated blood loss<br>• Anesthesia team reviews: Are there any patient -specific concerns<br>• Nursing team reviews: Has sterility (including indicator results) been confirmed? Are there equipment issues or any concerns? | Surgeon, anesthesia professional and nurse review the key concerns for recovery and management of this patient |
| Pulse oximeter on patient and functioning | Has antibiotic prophylaxis been given in the last 60 min?<br>• Yes / not applicable<br>Is essential imaging displayed<br>• Yes/not applicable | |
| Does patient have a known allergy<br>• No/yes<br>Difficult airway /aspiration risk<br>• No<br>• Yes, and equipment /assistance available<br>Risk of >500 ml blood loss (7 ml/kg in children)<br>• No<br>• Yes and adequate intravenous access and fluids planned | | |

1.2 to 1.5 m. Sliding doors are preferred than spring-loaded doors in order to minimize the generation of the air currents during the opening and closing of the doors. Windows made from glass are preferred, which are to be planned on one side only.

- The surface/flooring: The flooring must be such that it is nonslippery, strong, & with minimum joints to decrease the accumulation of dust and other tiny particulate matter within it.
- Walls: Washable light and soothing painted walls should be present
- Ceiling: Hard, impervious surface, plaster painted ceiling should be present.

**Different Zones of Operation Theater Complex**

There are four different zones observed in any operating room complex described on the basis of type of cleanliness present, presence or absence of microorganisms, and the different procedures to be carried out in each zone (Fig. 9.1).

1. *Protective zone*: It includes
   - Changing room for all the concerned persons
   - Transferring passage for the materials, equipment, and the patient
   - Rooms for administrative staff
   - Storage & record maintenance
   - Pre- and postoperative
   - Intensive and Coronary Care Units
   - Storage rooms to keep the sterilized objects
2. *Clean zone*: Links the protective zone to the aseptic zone
   - Clean rooms
   - Storage room for equipment
   - Rooms designed for surveillance, maintenance, and firefighting
   - Exit areas in case of emergencies exists

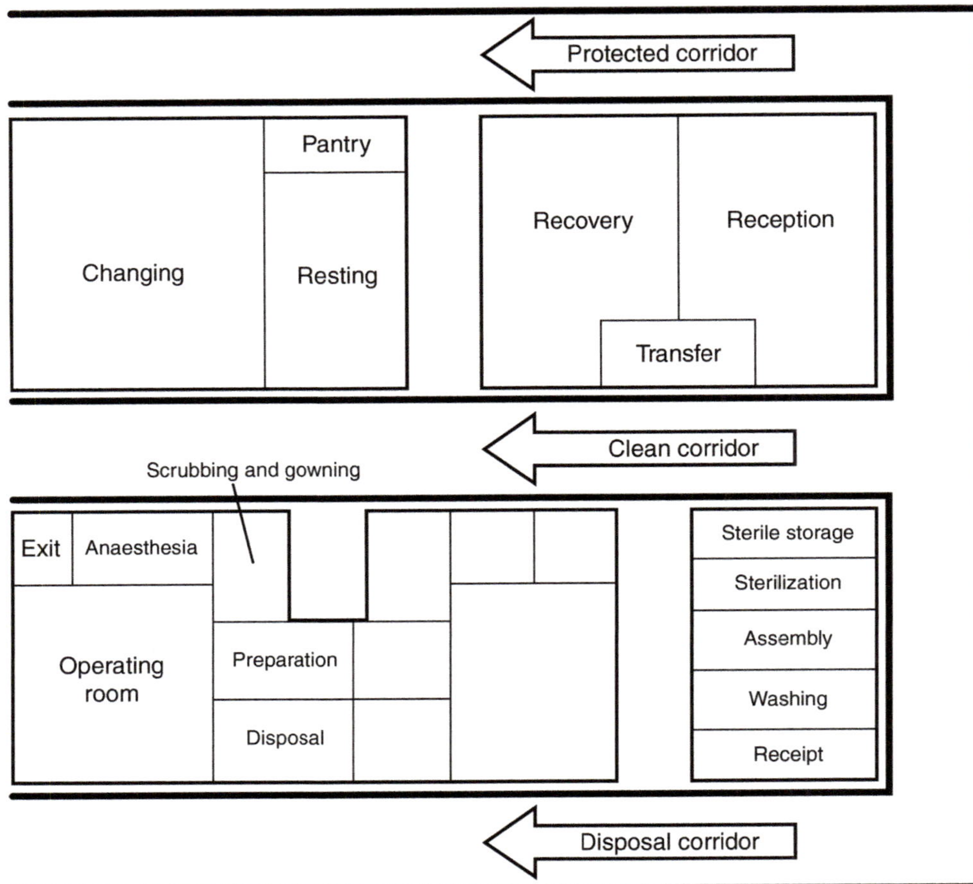


**Fig. 9.1** Different zones of operation theater complex

3. *Aseptic zone:* houses the operating rooms
4. *Disposal zone:* separate exit for disposing contaminated linen /used materials and instruments

**Important Points**

- The sterilized materials are transported from a sterile area to the operation theater on a covered cart, thus preventing any accumulation of the dust particles on their surfaces.
- Before entering the operation theater, all supplies/materials must be removed from their shipping or transported containers.
- All the blood-coated or soiled instruments/equipment must be transported in a covered wrap or container from the operating room to the decontamination or reprocessing area.
- Care must be taken that the soiled instruments/equipment must not to be stored with the sterilized goods.

**Maintenance in the Operation Theater**

- The machinery must be surveyed at least every week.
- Proper ventilation should be checked regularly and the filters should be changed as required.
- At the time of maintenance or inspection or observation of any fault in the working of the operation theater, the members of The Infection Control team should be informed. The theater should be thoroughly examined by the members of the team and appropriate measures must be taken to maintain the infection control protocols. The operation theater must only be functional after being carefully evaluated and cleared by the infection control team.
- Back-up facility for operation theater in all aspects should be present in any setup to provide any uninterrupted sessions at the time of maintenance or any fault observed.

## 9.6 Disinfection and Sterilization

Sterilization is the ultimate procedure in controlling the undesired activities of microorganisms that are outside of the human body. Its purpose in the operating field is to prevent the spread of infectious disease, and in surgery, it primarily relates to processing reusable instruments. Surgical instruments are an integral part of surgical field and, being reusable, have greater chances of spreading the microorganisms if any of the reprocessing steps fails. Steps of reprocessing include cleaning, repackaging, disinfection or sterilization, and reusing. Cleaning, being the first step in the cycle of reprocessing, is the major step in the removal of any organic matter present on the surface of the instruments. Any failure in the removal of the visible soil at the initial stage can create a discrepancy in the efficacy of the subsequent disinfection and sterilization procedures. Sterilization is more effective a process than disinfection. The process of disinfection is carried out with the use of various chemical agents. Chemical disinfecting agent necessarily does not kill all microorganisms or spores present on an inanimate object but instead reduces the number of microorganisms to a level that is not harmful to health. Depending on their potency against microbes, they are classified as *High-*, *Intermediate-,* or *Low-level* disinfectants.

The type of the sterilization procedures to be carried out for an object depends upon the classification of the instruments based according to the Spaulding Classification of the medical devices, the type of material of which the object is made of, the microorganisms to be present on the object, and availability of the sterilization methods and equipment (Table 9.4).

**Table 9.4** Spaulding Classification of Medical Devices And Level of Disinfection

- Critical: An instrument that has a direct contact with sterile tissues or vascular system [8]; such items are to be sterilized and made free from all microorganisms. Examples are extraction forceps, scalpel blades, bone chisels, periodontal scalers, surgical burs, needles
- Semicritical: An instrument that does not usually penetrate the sterile tissues but does come in contact with intact mucous membrane. These items are made free from microorganisms by high-level disinfection. Examples include endoscopes, amalgam condensers, air/water syringe, impression trays, dental hand piece, dental mirrors
- Noncritical: An instrument that does not touch the patient directly or come in contact with the intact skin only. These items may be cleaned or disinfected by low-level disinfection. Examples include light arm/handles, dental chair, dental X-ray equipment, chair side computers, chair switches.

**The Instrument Processing (Decontamination Steps)** (Fig. 9.2)

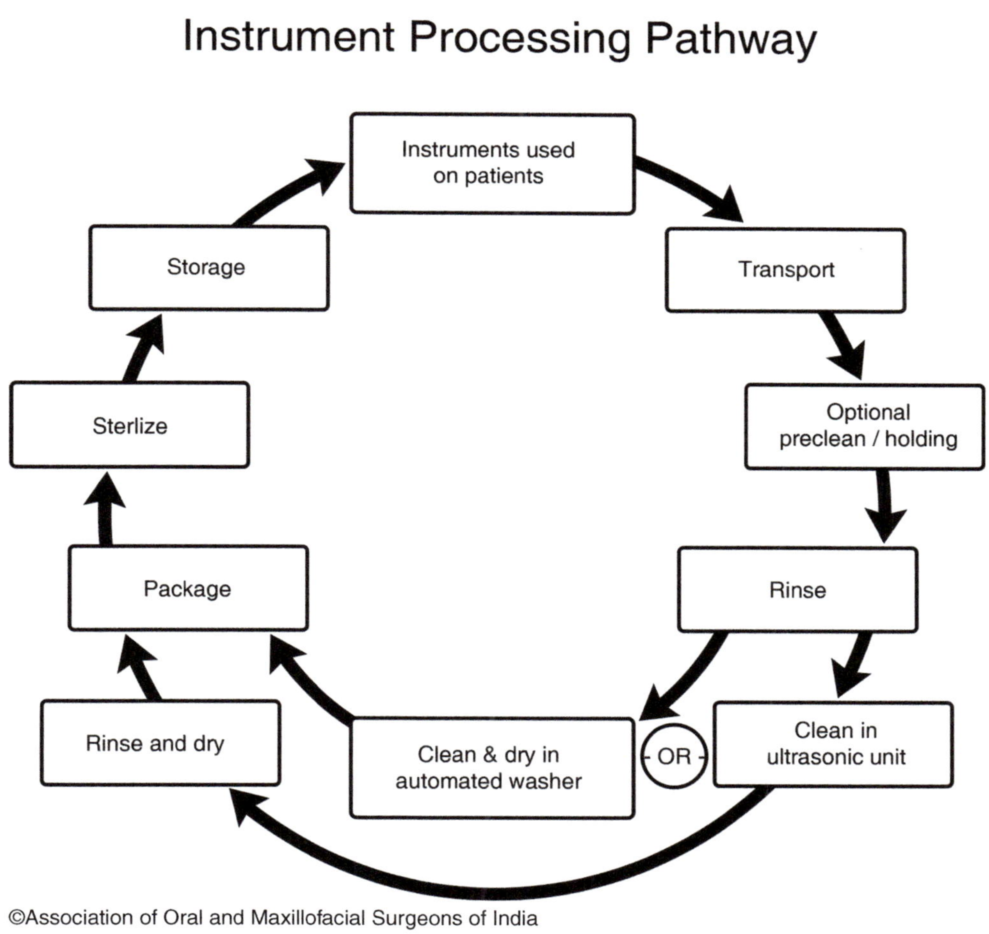


**Fig. 9.2** Instrument processing steps

Various methods of decontamination include.

- Physical cleaning.
- Water purification
- Ultrasonic cleaning
- Disinfection
- Antisepsis
- Sterilization

Processing of the clinical or surgical items is a two step procedure.

A. **Cleaning**, being the first step, is the most essential one, which is succeeded either by Disinfection or Sterlization
   - Cleaning is the process of removing all the foreign particles present on the surface of the object, which is accomplished by means of two main steps, i.e., cleaning by friction to remove foreign particles and rinsing away by fluids to remove the debris so cleaned.
   - If the objects to be sterilized, remain soiled with foreign materials, the microorganisms will be trapped in the organic matter and may interfere with the proper sterilization or disinfection procedure. Therefore, thorough cleaning should always precede the sterilization process.
   - Cleaning may be manual or mechanical and is normally accomplished by the use of water, detergents, and mechanical agents. Detergent is essential to dissolve proteins and oil that can reside on instruments and equipment after use.

1. *Mechanical cleaning*

   With the advancement in the sterilization equipment, most units are automated and there is very less handling of dirty equipment by the concerned staff. The equipment to be processed is placed in trays and is ready for washing.
   - *Washing machine*: It gives a cold rinse followed by a hot wash at 71 °C for 2 min. This is followed by a 10-second hot rinse at 80–90 °C and then by dry heat at 50–75 °C.
   - *Ultrasonicator*: The ultrasonicator is a device, which is extremely efficient in removing the debris. 0.44 W/cm$^3$ of power is used to remove the debris by the process of sonic waves produced. The solution used most often to clean is an enzymatic presoak (protease formula that dissolves protein).

2. *Manual cleaning*

   It is an active method that is carried out by thoroughly brushing the item with the help of a toothbrush under water to prevent the release of aerosols. The brush should be thoroughly cleaned after use and should be dried. The cleaned items are then dried and made ready for the proper sterilization procedure to be carried out depending upon the material of which they are made and the use they perform.

   Manual cleaning is necessary when:
   - Cleaning of instruments by mechanical means is not possible
   - Instruments to be cleaned are delicate in nature
   - Objects to be cleaned have a narrow lumen (Fig. 9.3)

3. *Soaking of instruments prior to cleaning:*

   There are times when cleaning alone cannot remove the debris present on the surface of the objects as the items become highly soiled with foreign materials. For this, it is sometimes necessary to soak instruments/objects prior to cleaning. A container having a deeper base is filled with detergent & water and all the instruments are kept in it for 3–5 min. The solution prepared is agitated by shaking it vigorously. The cleaned instruments are now removed from the container and placed over a tray for air drying.

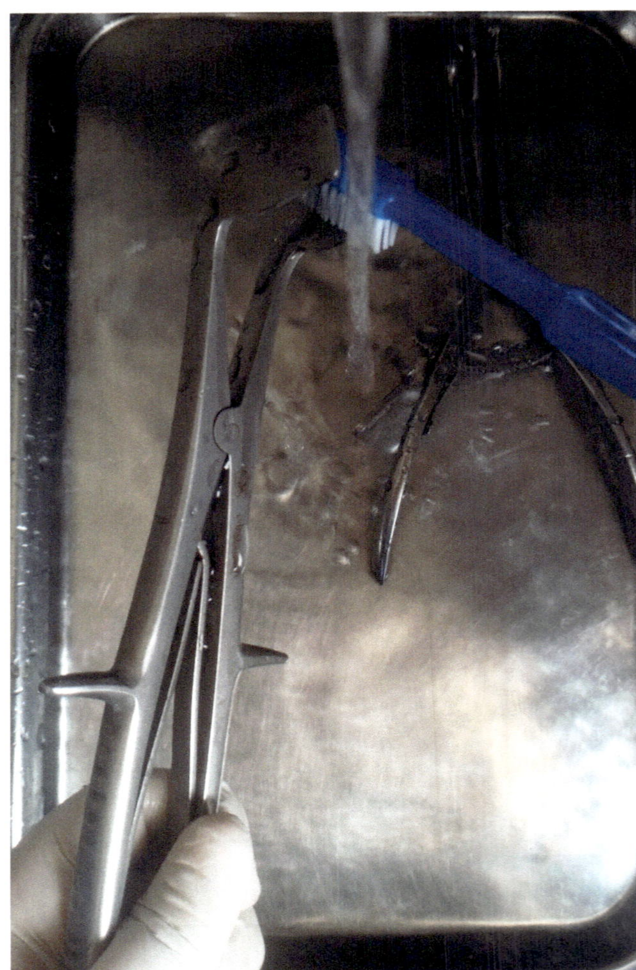



**Fig. 9.3** Manual Cleaning

B. **Disinfection and Sterlization**

- *Disinfection* can be achieved by either thermal or chemical processes. The thermal disinfection procedure is more easily controlled, more reliable, nontoxic and leaves no residue on the surface and is preferred more than chemical disinfection procedures. The main indication of chemical disinfectant use is the heat-sensitive objects. Chemical High-level disinfection (HLD):
  (a) Most commonly used for heat-labile instruments/objects (e.g., endoscopes) where single use is not cost effective.
  (b) Disinfectants used for this purpose are
    - Glutaraldehyde: 2% for 20 min.
    - Hydrogen peroxide: 6%–7.5% for 20–30 min.
    - Per acetic acid: 0.2–0.35% for 5 min.
    - Ortho-phthalaldehyde (OPA) for 5–12 min.
  (c) Steps:
    - All items to be disinfected are cleaned and dried.
    - Fresh disinfectant solution should be made each day in a sterile container. If a previously prepared solution is to be used, an indicator strip is dipped in the solution to check for the effectiveness of the solution.
    - Open all hinged instruments and disassemble whichever possible.
    - Place all items in the solution completely submerged in the container.
    - The container is covered and the instruments are allowed to soak in for 20 min.
    - Remove the items using dry, high-level disinfected pickups.
    - Rinse thoroughly with boiled water.
    - Air-dry by placing on disinfected tray.
    - Items disinfected are covered in a disinfected container and used within a week.

*Sterilization*

Sterilization is a method by which an article, medium, or surface is made free from all microbial invasions, including spores. The main aim of sterilization of instruments is proper delivery of sterilized instruments at the operating field, thereby maintaining a sterile environment and reducing the spread of infections from one person to another. Proper handling of the sterilized instruments is done by appropriate wrapping and storage of the instruments, thereby increasing the shelf life of the sterilized instruments. The instruments should be bagged or wrapped in a muslin cloth or clear pouches or paper before and after the procedure and the wrapping should be sealed with tape. No pin, staple, or any paper clips are to be applied on the wrapping as these may create small openings, which may allow entry of microorganisms, thereby hampering the process of sterilization. Sterilization is accomplished by:

1. *Steam sterilization (autoclaving):-*
   - This is the most simple and efficient means of sterilizing instruments. It is also commonly called steam sterilizing or autoclaving.
   - The steam autoclaves best suited for outpatient practice are usually made to operate in the following range.
     – Temperature 121 °C (250 °F) at a pressure of 15 pounds per square inch (psi) for 15 min.
     – Temperature 134 °C (270 °F) at a pressure of 30 psi for 3 min. This process termed "flash sterilization" has practical use in the operating room where fast sterilization of instruments may be necessary.
   - This combination of moisture and heat provides the bacteria-destroying power currently most effective against all forms of microorganisms.
   - Mainly used for items that are wrapped or porous.
   - Autoclaves are either classified as horizontal or vertical (based on design) and gravity displacement or vacuum type (based on functioning).
   - Autoclaves can also be classified as Type "N" and Type "B."
   - Type "N" autoclaves are the ones that do not remove air from the sterilization chamber with the help of a vacuum pump. These are used for solid loads.
   - Type "B" autoclaves remove air from the sterilization chamber with the help of a vacuum pump. Wrapped and hollow instruments, which can be sterilized and used later, are to be sterilized by this type of autoclave.
   - Importance of bagging the instruments for sterilization.
     – The main aim of bagging or wrapping the instruments prior to sterilization procedure decreases the chances of contamination of the items after the sterilization procedure is complete.
     – Two-layer wrapping of objects should be preferred and the materials used for this can be cotton fabric or muslin, paper, newspaper (Fig. 9.4).
   - Monitoring of sterilization.
   - Sterilization monitoring is a process by which adequate sterile environment and the effectiveness of the procedure is determined by assessing the biological, mechanical, and chemical parameters.
   - The most widely used and accepted parameter of assessing the sterilization procedures is the use of biological indicators (BIs) that directly inhibit the growth of highly resistant microorganisms, rather than merely testing the physical and chemical conditions necessary for sterilization. Since the spores present in a biological indicator are in a much higher number and are highly resistant by nature compared to the other and common microorgan-

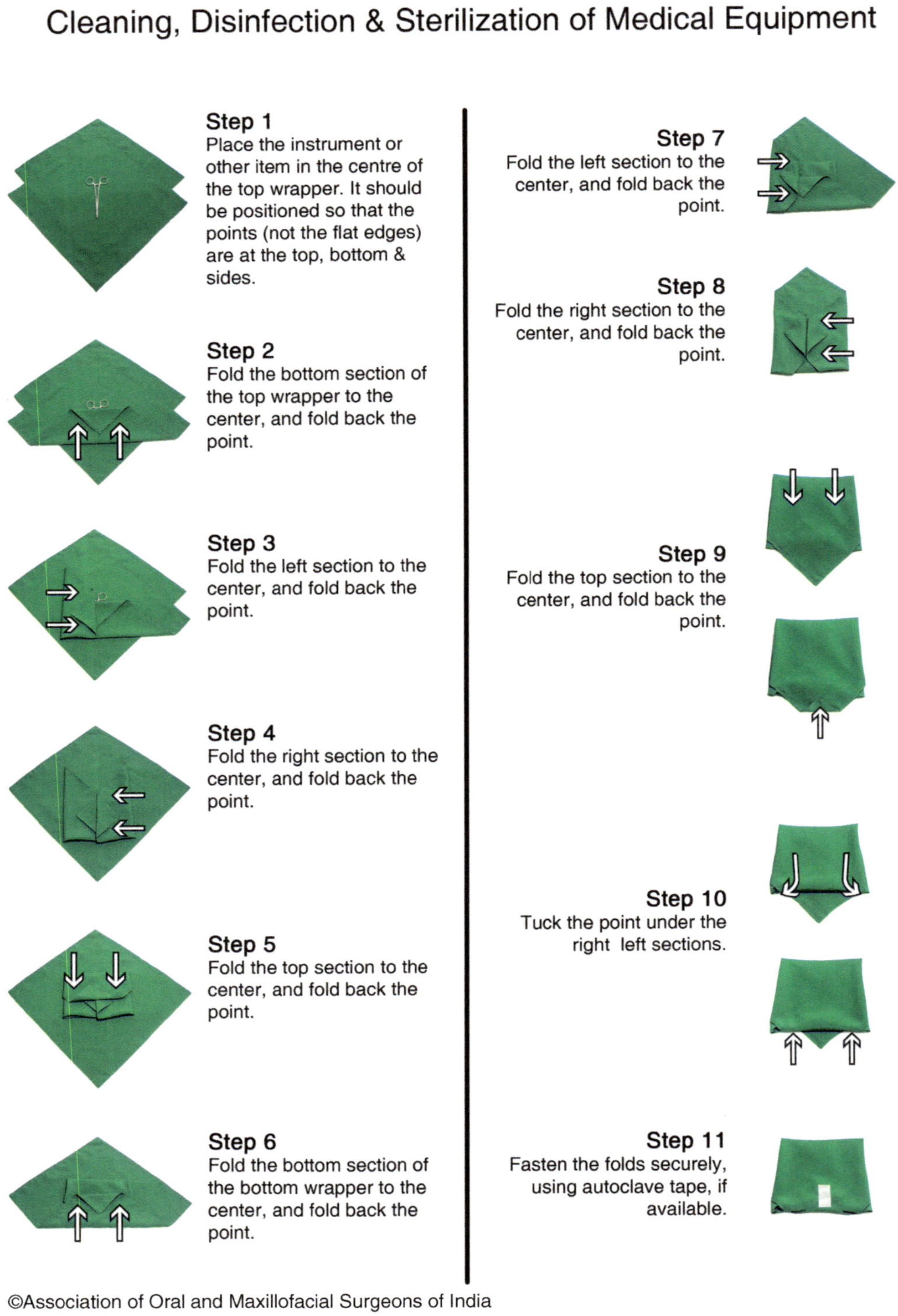


**Fig. 9.4** Diagram depicting the way the instruments are wrapped for sterilization

isms found on items used for the patient, an inactivated biological indicator indicates that the other microorganisms are killed depicting an effective sterilization procedure. A control BI, from the same lot as the test indicator and not processed through the sterilizer, should be incubated with the test BI; the control BI should yield positive results for bacterial growth.

- Assuring the temperature & the cycle time, and observing the gauges or display for the pressure on the sterilization equipment for each set of items to be sterilized come under the mechanical monitoring of sterilization.
- Certain chemical agents are used to check the efficacy of the sterilization procedure being carried out by undergoing chemical changes in their properties on

being exposed to the sterilizing conditions. These chemical agents are called the chemical indicators and these include TST (Time-Steam-Temperature) Strip. This TST strip is to be placed in a big surgical wire basket and when exposed to a critical time, steam, and temperature it undergoes a change in color from yellow to dark blue indicating complete sterilization procedure. Another strip is to be used when double-layered packing of instruments in crepe paper is done to assess the parameters inside the sterilizer.
- Another form of sterilizing monitor is the use of the external indicators. These are usually in the form of Tapes. The main indication of the complete sterilization procedure is the change in color of the strips of the tape from yellow to dark brown or black.
- *How to store the sterilized instruments/objects*
  - There must be a separate area for storing of the sterile instruments and single-use (disposable) products.
  - The storing of the bagged sterilizer objects can be depicted either by the date on which they are sterilized or the procedure for which it is to be used or an event causing it to become contaminated.
  - All the packed items must be carefully inspected before using to verify the integrity of the outer covering and the condition of the packing (dry/wet).
  - Once the packing is assessed and if any breach is seen in the packing, the wrapping should be replaced and the instruments again sent for the sterilization procedure.
  - All the sterilized instruments must be kept in covered drawers.
- Care must be taken that all instruments should be placed away from the place where chances of getting wet are higher.
- *Expiry of the sterilized instruments*
- The expiry of the materials and objects undergoing the sterilization procedure depends on the type and time of the sterilization process, the efficacy of the process, and the handling of the sterilized instruments.
- Once all the sterile conditions are met, 4 weeks is the maximum time for which the items are considered sterilized and safe for use. However, the contaminated instruments are preferred processing and sterilization prior to every procedure.

2. *Ethylene oxide:*
   - It is used for sterilization of heat-labile and moisture-sensitive items, supplies, and equipment.
   - The operating cycle ranges from 2–24 h and it is a relatively expensive process.
   - It can be used for glass, paper surfaces, clothing, plastics and metals, food stuffs, and dental equipment.
   - It is unsuitable for fumigating rooms because of its explosive property.
3. *Dry heat:*
   - It may be used for sterilization of instruments with cutting surfaces.
   - No corrosion occurs with this method of sterilization.
   - Dry heat sterilization, which usually occurs consists of hot air oven has typical cycles of 1 h at 171 °C or 2 h at 160 °C.
   - Air is a poor conductor of heat and requires a long time for getting the instruments effectively sterilized.
4. *Chemical sterilization and disinfection:*
   - This is also a choice for some limited circumstances.
   - Some instruments cannot be subjected to high temperatures and in a field environment chemical sterilization may have to be used.
   - The disinfectant must remain in contact with the surface for appropriate time.
   - Disinfectants include Chlorine solutions, 2–3.2% glutaraldehyde, iodophors, and phenols.

## 9.7 Operating Room Decorum

1. *Hand hygiene:*

Hand hygiene by operation theater persons is the most efficient way to reduce the risk of spread of infections.

2. *Surgical hand wash:*
   - Surgical hand wash or surgical hand rub should be carried out prior to the procedure in order to decrease the residing flora of the hand.
   - Steps:
     - All jewellery from wrists and hands must be removed.
     - The temperature of water is to be adjusted so that it is slightly warm. Hands and forearms are to be washed 5 cm above the level of the elbows to remove any particles of dirt.
     - Before performing the first scrub of the day, a nail cleaner is used to clean the fingernails and the nail beds.
     - The nails should be cut short and no nail polish should be used.
     - Antimicrobial agent is to be applied on the hands and in circular motion; lathering should begin at the finger tips of one hand and between the fingers, continuing from the fingertip to 5 cm above the elbow. The same process is to be repeated for other arm and hand.
     - The rubbing should be done for a period of 3–5 min.
     - Each arm is to be washed separtely at the level of elbow, starting at the fingertips.
     - One side of the sterile towel is used to dry the fingertips up to the elbow of one hand and the other side is used to dry the same on the other hand.

3. *Barrier techniques:*
   Barrier techniques are useful where the chances of spread of infection are higher.
   (a) Head Cover
   Prior or during the procedure, all facial and head hair should be tied properly and covered by means of head covers. Ideally head covers should be disposable and made of soft, nonporous cloth like material. If one has long hair, the hair should be tied in a bun. In situations where tying a bun is not possible, use of helmets or hoods or headgears is of utmost significance.
   (b) Masks
   - Tuberculosis is one of the most common infectious diseases that can spread through airborne route,
   - The main aim of using a mask is the prevention of transmission of infectious agents from the member of the operating team to the patient's wounds and also protecting the operating team members from the splashes and sprays from the patient.
   - The masks, which are disposable in nature, are always preferred.
   - The mask should be made of synthetic fibers, must be flat with two or three pleats that expand to cover the area up to chin, and should have filters of polypropylene or polyester (Fig. 9.5).

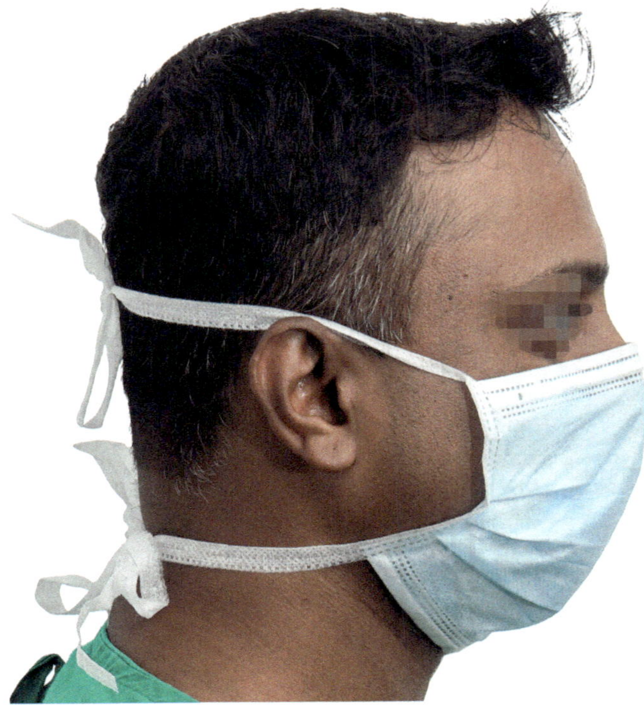



**Fig. 9.5** Surgical Mask

   (c) Scrub suits and cover gowns
   These are the pair of garments to be worn over, or instead of regular clothing of the persons involved in the surgical procedures to protect the transmission of any infectious agent present on the regular clothing from the operating personnel to the patient or any other personnel. These should have a simple design, should be comfortable, should be easy to clean and wash, should be economical, easily replicable if damaged and should have minimal place for the contaminants to hide.
   (d) Surgical gowns
   These are a loose pair of clothing to be worn over the scrub suits or cover gowns at the time of the surgery to protect both the patient and the operating personnel from transfer of microorganisms, blood or body fluids, and another particulate matter.
   Steps of wearing gown:
   - Dry the hands completely and hold the gown in such a manner that it is at the least risk of contamination.
   - Slip arms into the sleeves through the armholes, keeping at the shoulder level and away from the body.
   - Hold arms out and slightly up.
   - The circulating person must pull the gown over the shoulders touching only inside of the gown.
   All the belts and loops are to be tied securely (Fig. 9.6).
   (e) Gloves
   They help to protect the operator from infection by bacteria and viruses from patient's blood. Gloving is essential to protect both the surgeon and the patient from blood-borne viruses and to prevent wound from becoming contaminated with the surgeon's skin flora. The "open gloving" and "closed gloving" technique of donning the gloves should be employed for wearing gloves.
   - Steps in wearing gloves by Open Gloving Technique
     - Handwashing must be performed under aseptic conditions.
     - Inspect the outer covering for the integrity. Open the first nonsterile packaging by peeling it completely off the heat seal exposing the inner sterile wrapper, but without touching it.
     - The inner sterile packing is kept on a dry area, without touching the outer surface. Open the package and fold it toward the bottom so as to unfold the paper and keep it open.
     - By using index finger and thumb of one hand, the folded edge of the glove is grasped.
     - In a single movement the other hand is slipped into the glove.
     - The second glove is picked by using the cuff of the other glove and sliding the fingers of the gloved hand into it.

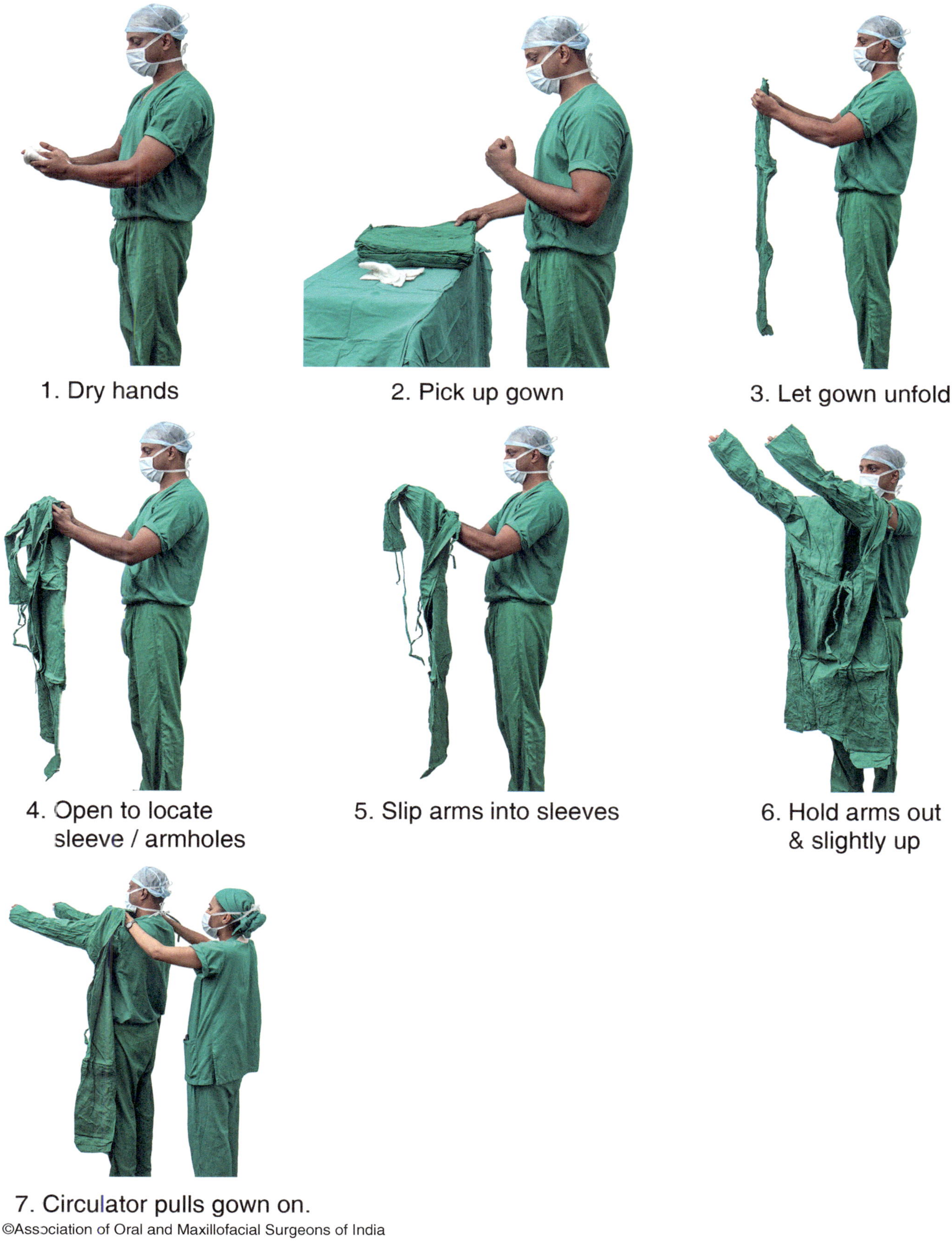


Fig. 9.6 Putting on the sterile gown

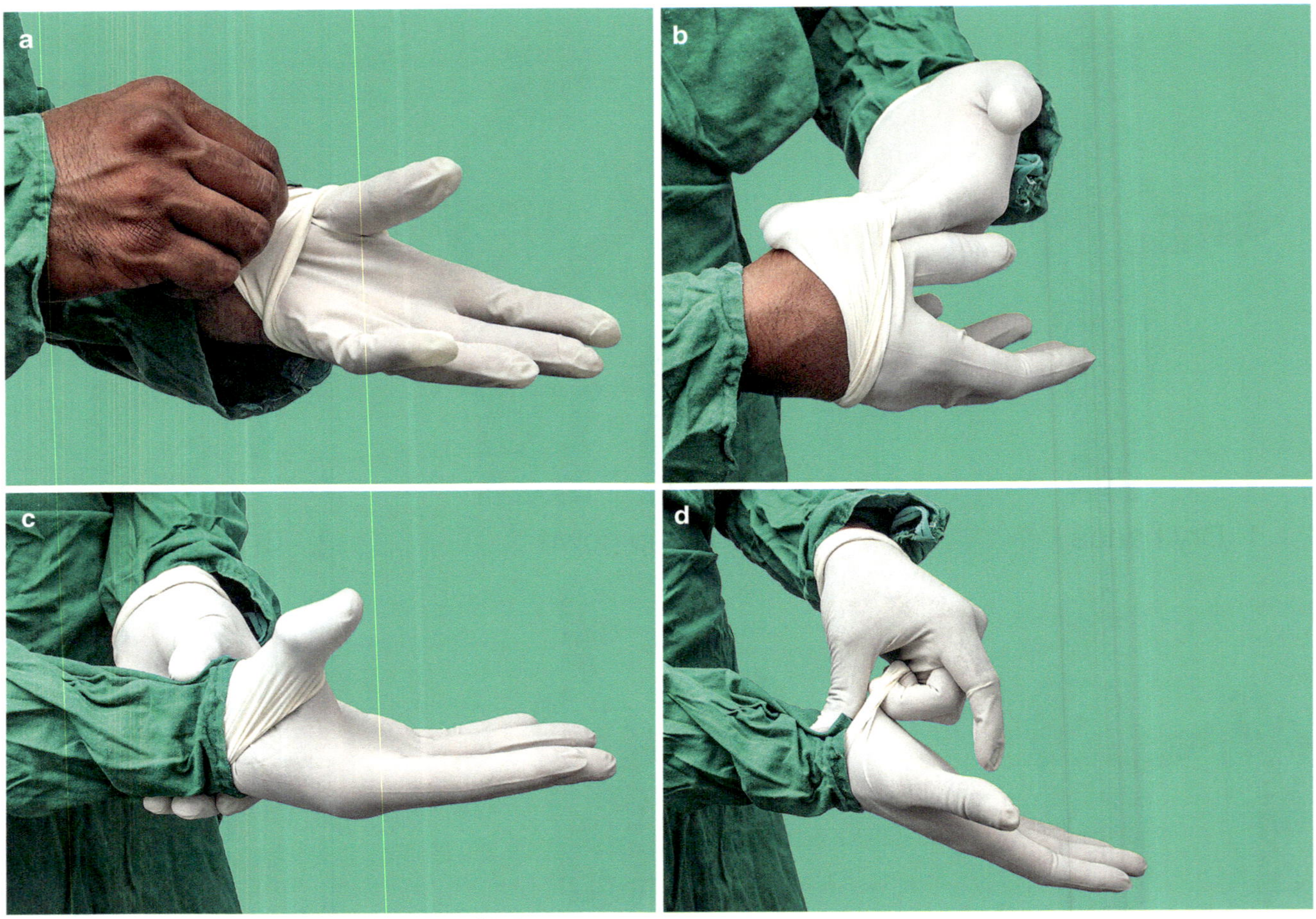



**Fig. 9.7** Putting on sterile gloves by open gloving technique

- In a single movement, slip the second glove on to the ungloved hand while avoiding any contact/resting of the gloved hand on surfaces other than the glove to be donned (Fig. 9.7).

- Steps of wearing gloves by closed gloving technique
  - If the cuffs are not fitting, a tuck is taken in each gown.
  - The circulating person should open the outer covering of the glove and should flip them onto the sterile field.
  - The inner packing containing the gloves is opened carefully and the glove is picked up by the folded cuff edge with the hand covered by the sleeve.
  - The glove is placed on the sleeve of the opposite gown, the palm facing downwards, with the fingers of the glove pointing toward the shoulder.
  - The gloves should be placed in such a manner that the rolled cuff edge of the gloves connects the sleeve to the gown cuff. Bottom cuffed and rolled edge of the glove is grasped at the bottom with the index finger and thumb.
  - With the opposite hand, the outermost edge of the cuff of the gloves is held taking care that the uncovered fingers are not exposed by it.
  - Stretch the glove over the hand
  - By using the opposite hand covered with sleeve, both the cuffs of the sleeve and the glove are seamed and the glove is pulled over the hand.
  - The same procedure is to be followed for the other hand. The fingers are adjusted to properly fit in the glove (Fig. 9.8).

4. The role of drapes:

   Drapes are used during surgical procedure to protect the contacting of the unprepared surfaces/areas and maintaining the sterility of environmental, equipment, and the surrounding of the patients.

   The different drapes available are:-

   - Towel drapes, which are used for squaring off the operative site, wrapping syringes & small instruments, and

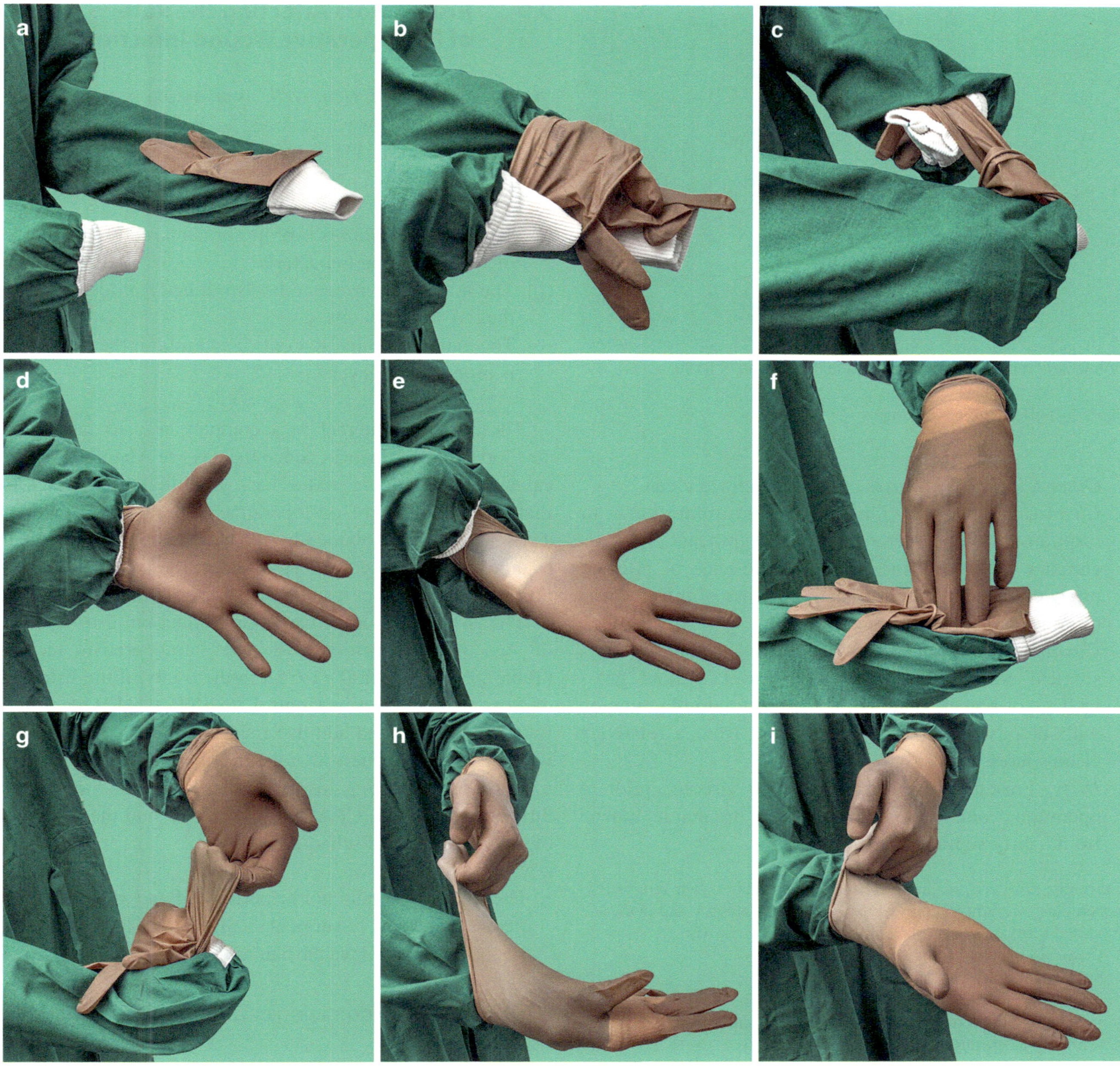




**Fig. 9.8** Putting on sterile gloves by closed gloving technique

drying of the hands. These must be more resistant to water and must be made of cotton compared to linen.

- Lap sheets are used for covering the patient. They are large and long, usually made of lightweight cotton, and provide limited protection and coverage to the patients or staff or the surface areas.
- Site drapes are made of cotton and have a circular opening in the center that is placed over the prepared operative site. These drapes are primarily intended for use with minor surgical procedures (Fig. 9.9).

## 9.8 Classification of Surgical Wounds

A widely used classification of surgical wounds is based on an estimate of likelihood of bacterial contamination of the operative site. In 1964 [9], National Academy of Sciences/ National Research Council defined five general classes of operations:

1. *Refined-Clean:* Elective operations not drained and primarily closed.

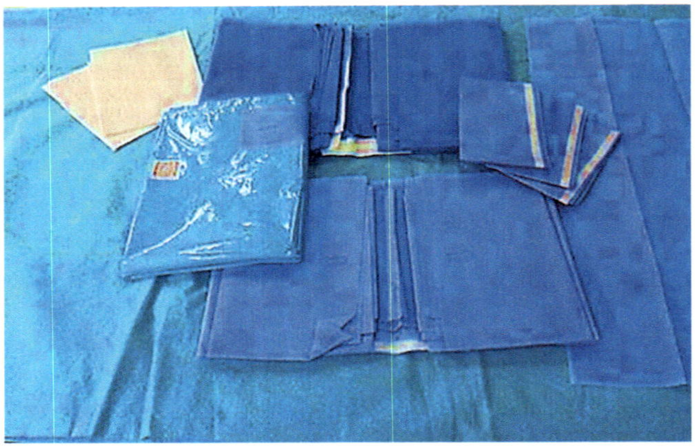

©Association of Oral and Maxillofacial Surgeons of India

**Fig. 9.9** Different types of drapes

2. *Other-Clean:* Clean cases other than refined clean.
3. *Clean-Contaminated:* Oral cavity, gastrointestinal, or respiratory tract entered without significant spillage, entrance of genitourinary tract in presence of infected urine, entrance of biliary tract in presence of infected bile or minor break in technique.
4. *Contaminated:* Major break in operative techniques (e.g., surgical entrance of unprepared bowel without gross spillage of bowel contents); acute bacterial inflammation without pus; fresh, traumatic wound from a relatively clean source.
5. *Dirty:* Presence of pus or perforated viscous (prior to operation), old traumatic wound, or traumatic wound from a dirty source.

Currently, this classification has been condensed into four groups for general use, without a subdivision of the clean category and in the modified form it is categorized into four categories [10]

1. *Clean sites (wounds):*
   - Elective (not urgent or emergency).
   - Primary closed.
   - No acute inflammation or transection of tracheobronchial, biliary, gastrointestinal, oropharyngeal tracts.
   - No technique breaks.
2. *Clean-contaminated sites (wounds):*
   - Emergency or urgent cases that are otherwise "clean."
   - Elective procedures.
   - Reoperation via "clean incision" within 7 days.
   - Blunt trauma, intact skin, and negative exploration.
3. *Contaminated sites (wounds):*
   - Acute nonpurulent inflammation.
   - Major technique break or major spill from hollow organs.
   - Entrance of genitourinary or biliary tracts in presence of infected urine or bile, respectively.
   - Penetrating trauma less than 4 h old.
   - Chronic open wounds to be grafted or covered.
4. *Dirty sites (wounds):*
   - Purulence or abscess.
   - Preoperative perforation of tracheobronchial, biliary, gastrointestinal, oropharyngeal tracts.
   - Penetrating trauma more than 4 h old.

## 9.9 Risk Factors Affecting the Rate of Postoperative Wound Infections

*"Cut Well, Sew Well, Heal Well"* is an axiom favored by surgeons but is not always destined to be true. Altemeir and Culbertson (1965) [11] depicted that the risk of infection varies:

(a) The risk of infections is proportional directly to the dose of contamination to bacteria.
(b) The microbial virulence is also directly proportional to the risk of infections.
(c) The patient's ability to control and inhibit the resistance is proportional inversely. [12]

These factors interact in a complex way to fasten the development of infection. Since the days of Altemeier, clinical and epidemiologic studies have identified the risk factors that affect the rate of postoperative surgical site infection. This can be best explained by the classical epidemiological triangular model, i.e., model of interaction between agent host and environment resulting in disease (Fig. 9.10).

The risk of postoperative wound infection also depends on the patient factors, pre and intraoperative factors (Table 9.5). Haley et al. (1985), in the Study of the Efficacy of Nosocomial Infection Control "(SENIC)," [13] identified four independent and additive risk factors for postoperative wound infection. These factors are operation on the abdomen, operation lasting for more than 2 h, contaminated or dirty wounds (NRC CLASSIFICATION), and the presence of more than three discharge diagnoses.

- Hair removal should not be performed on routine basis to decrease the risk of surgical site infection. Razors should not be used to remove the hair as they increase the chances

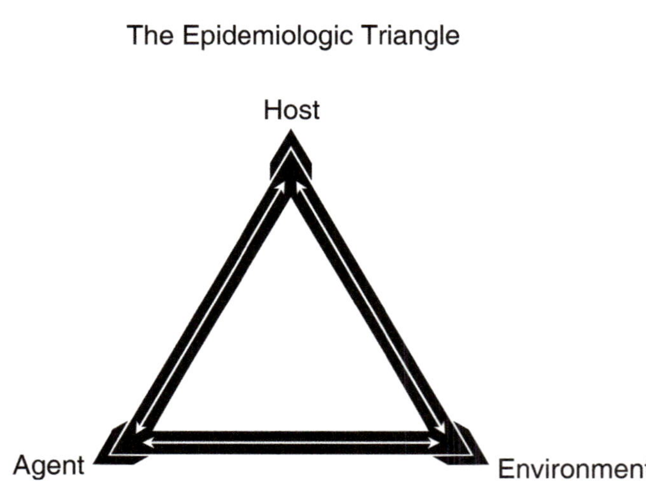


©Association of Oral and Maxillofacial Surgeons of India

**Fig. 9.10** Classical Epidemiological triangle

**Table 9.5** Factors that predispose a patient to infection

| *Patients factors* | Preoperative factors | Intraoperative factors |
|---|---|---|
| *Age*<br>• Malnutrition<br>• Obese persons<br>• Underlying diseases<br>• Hidden infections<br>• Immunosuppressive therapy<br>• Any recent surgery<br>• Longstanding illness | • Longer duration of hospital admission<br>• Improper scrubbing prior to procedure<br>• Removal of hair<br>• Preoperative prophylactic coverage | • Contamination at the time of procedure<br>• Longer duration of the procedure<br>• Any foreign object<br>• Transfusion reactions occurring at the time of the procedure |

of infections [14]. Electric clippers with disposable heads must be used only for removing hair few hours prior to the surgical procedure.

- The treatment protocols and the condition of the patient during the hospital stay make them more prone to the spread of infections.
- Wound dressings: Cover surgical incisions with an appropriate interactive dressing at the end of the operation.

## 9.9.1 Factors Influencing the Development of Nosocomial Infections

### 9.9.1.1 The Microbial Agent

Hospital infections occur as a result of a variety of microorganisms. The microorganisms causing the disease may be divided into the following categories:

1. Conventional pathogens are the ones that are capable of causing a disease in normal and healthy person.
2. Conditional pathogens are the ones that initiate the onset of a disease in persons who have decreased immunological response to infection or when implanted directly into sterile area or tissues.
3. Opportunistic pathogens are the ones that normally do not harm its host but can cause disease when the host's resistance to the microorganisms is low.

During the stay in a hospital, the patient comes in contact with various kinds of microbial agents (such as viruses, fungi, parasites, and bacteria), which are the main cause of the occurrence of infections in a patient. This exposure is not the only reason for the development of hospital-acquired infections. The other possible reasons are the host's natural defense mechanisms (healthy/compromised/immunosuppressed), conditions present in a hospital environment, microbiology of the microbial agents (characteristic features), infective material present on the microbial agent, resistance to the antimicrobial agents, and other factors. The hospital-based infections may be a result of the spread of infection from one person to the other or by the residential flora of the patient or from any contaminated sources or from sources of the external origin (e.g., airborne diseases).

Following are the factors that are the main sources of spread of hospital-based infections:

### 9.9.1.2 Susceptibility of the Patient

Patient factors that lead to the occurrence of infection are age, host's immune response, presence of any disease, and interventions, which either help in diagnosing or treating any condition. Patients, either infant or older individuals, are at a higher risk of acquiring infections. Patients having a compromised immune system, undernourished, having some underlying chronic disease (AIDS, leukemia, malignant tumors, renal failure, diabetes mellitus, etc.), undergoing irradiation therapy, all at the highest risk of being infected by the hospital-based infections. Certain processes like catheterization, biopsy, intubations, etc. make the patient more vulnerable to these infections.

### 9.9.1.3 Resistance of the Bacteria

Resistance of bacteria to antimicrobial agents is seen with the prolonged or prophylactic use of these agents. The microbial agents present normally in the human flora have both sensitive and resistant strains. Some antimicrobial agents have their action on sensitive strains by suppressing their activity, whereas the resistant strains are still active. These active resistant strains are the major cause of the development of resistance against the antimicrobial agents. Examples of resistant microbial agents are Multiresistant Klebsiella, strains of pneumococci, staphylococci, etc. In low-income or middle-income countries, this is the major problem faced due to unavailability and unaffordability of the better drugs.

### 9.9.1.4 Month of Operation

The possible explanation for increased infection rates in summer is the relatively high environmental temperature leading to humid climate, resulting in excessive sweating. In addition, excessive sweating results in the displacement of bacteria lodged in skin appendages to the surface.

### 9.9.1.5 Use of Electric Cautery

The use of electric cautery for cutting and coagulation during surgery causes more inflammation; more necrosis and abscess than the conventional use of scalpel and thus it increases the susceptibility of tissue for infection. Soballe et al [15], in their experimental study, found that electric cautery lowers the contamination threshold for infection of laparotomies and concluded that electric coagulation current should be used only when the need for meticulous hemostasis outweighs the considerably increases risk of infection.

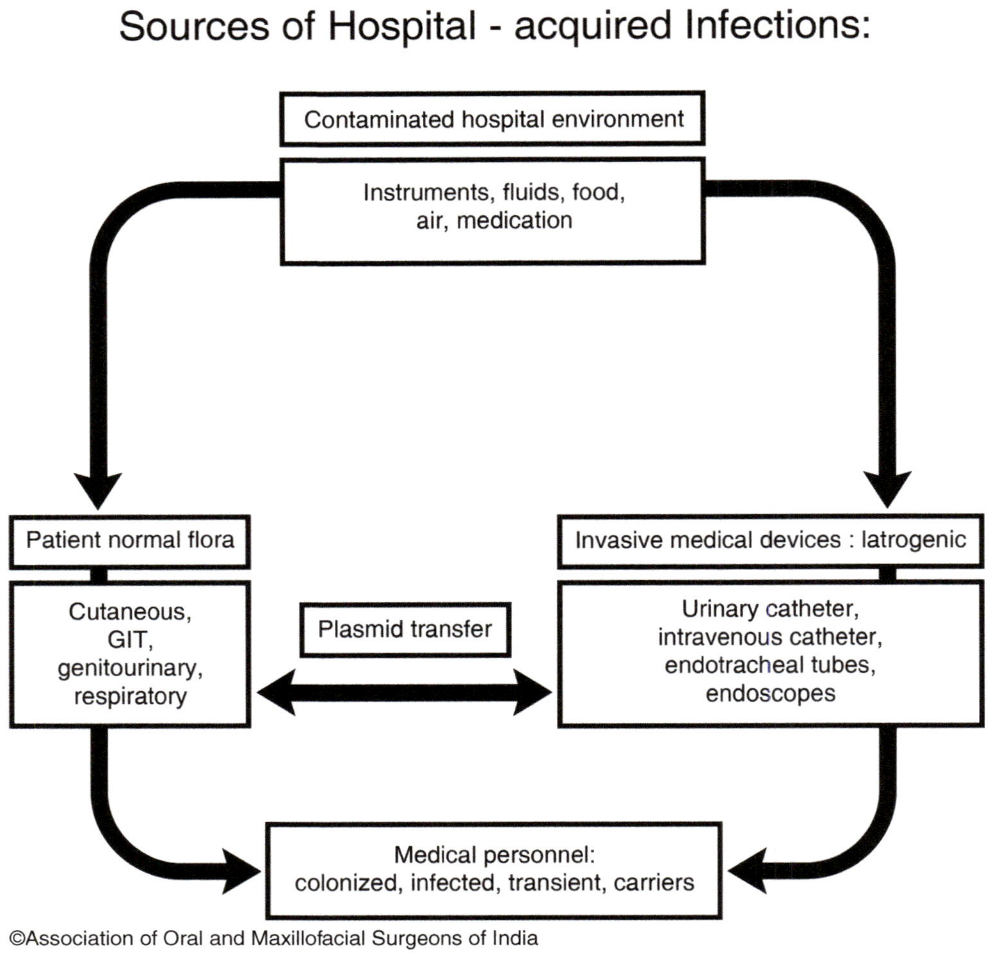


**Fig. 9.11** Sources of hospital-acquired infections

#### 9.9.1.6 Duration of Operation

There is a direct correlation between the infection rate and time taken for the procedure. This may be the result of the more complicated operations being of longer duration, increased wound contamination from airborne bacteria, increased damage to the tissues due to large exposure of the wound, and increased manipulation; moreover, local resistance of tissue is reduced due to drying.

#### 9.9.1.7 Spread of Infection

The microbial agents are spread by different ways in a health care setup. The different ways with which the agents can spread are contacting, droplets, airborne route, via vehicle, and vector-borne (Fig. 9.11).

Sources of the infectious agents are either external, i.e., from one person to the other, or from the hospital's environment; or internal, i.e., within the patient himself.

- *Contacting* is the most frequent and important route of spread of infections. It is further of two types, i.e.
  – *Direct* contacting is the spread of infection directly from the person infected from the infection to other normal who has increased chances of being infected. It also occurs among two patients where one acts the source of microbial agents and the other becomes the one to receive the infection.
- *Indirect* contacting is the spread of infection indirectly from one person/object to the other. It involves contact of a susceptible host with a contaminated intermediate object. Droplets spread results due to generation of droplets from the source person mainly during coughing, sneezing, and talking, and during the performance of certain procedures such as bronchoscopy, which can travel a shorter distance via air and get deposited on the body of the other susceptible person.
- *Airborne transmission* results from spreading of small particulate matter (approximately 5 pm or smaller in size) through the air, which remain suspended in the air for a longer period of time. These particles are passed from one individual to the other by the process of inhalation of

these particles. The main diseases to be spread via the airborne route are Tuberculosis, Influenza, Common cold, etc.
- *Vehicle spread* is the spread of infectious microbial agents to the individuals by means of contaminated items such as food, water, medications, devices, and equipment.

*Vector*-borne transmission occurs when vectors such as mosquitoes, flies, rats, and other vermin transmit microorganisms.

## 9.10 COVID 19 and Maxillofacial Surgery

The occupational risk of acquiring viral diseases has been well known in Maxillofacial Surgery [16]. The WHO announced the Corona virus pandemic also known as COVID-19 as a public health emergency of international concern on January 30, 2020.

Coronaviruses are RNA viruses infecting many species of animals including humans, name coronavirus was derived from corona meaning crown like because of the morphology observed for these viruses in the electron microscope. This family of viruses includes Middle East Respiratory Syndrome (MERS-CoV), Severe Acute Respiratory Syndrome (SARS-CoV), and novel Coronavirus (n CoV).

Coronavirus is enveloped having round, spherical, or sometimes pleomorphic structure, with size ranging from 80 to 120 nm in diameter, containing a positive-strand RNA. The virus is made up of lipid bilayer envelop, membrane protein, and nucleocapsid, these structures also protect the virus when the virus is outside the host cell. The lipid bilayer forms the viral envelop which anchors the membrane protein, envelop protein, and the spike protein. The spike protein (S-protein) is responsible for the crown-like structure of the coronavirus as it forms the protrusions from the surface which bind to the host cells.

### 9.10.1 Mode of Transmission of SARs-CoV 2

Human to human transmission is due to respiratory droplet transmission and contact transmission. Spread occurs through coughing, sneezing, spitting, contacting the body fluids of the infected patient. The COVID-19 can remain infectious on inanimate surfaces from 2 h to 9 days, depending on the humidity, temperature, surface type, and viral load [17]. It has become an occupational threat to health care providers worldwide.

Some of the known routes of spread of infection to health care providers are:

- Manual ventilation with a bag and mask
- Intubation
- Open endotracheal suctioning
- Bronchoscopy
- Cardiopulmonary resuscitation
- Sputum induction
- Surgery on the lungs
- Nebulizer therapy
- Noninvasive positive pressure ventilation (BIPAP, CPAP)
- An autopsy on the lungs
- High-speed devices such as those used for surgery, post-mortem
- Dental procedures

Aerosols generating procedures (AGP) create widespread environmental contamination and therefore pose a greater risk of transmission of infection to healthcare workers. Oral and maxillofacial surgeons are particularly vulnerable to this transmissible disease by way of the droplet or aerosol transmission due to the area of work and the type of instrumentation [18].

The incubation period is long and unpredictable ranging from 0 to 27 days with a mean of 6.4 days. Recent studies have shown that asymptomatic patients and those within the incubation period are also potential spreaders of the disease [19].

### 9.10.2 Symptoms

Symptoms may range from mild symptoms to severe respiratory distress and some patients may be asymptomatic.

- Common symptoms may include fever, cough, fatigue, shortness of breath, loss of taste, and smell.
- Less common symptoms may include myalgia, headache sore throat, and chills.
- Rare symptoms may include nausea, vomiting, nasal congestion, diarrhea, palpitation, and chest congestion.

### 9.10.3 Radiographic Findings

- **Chest X-ray** may show findings that of atypical pneumonia showing bilateral consolidations in lateral lower lobes, bronchovascular thickening.
- **Chest CT** ground-glass opacity and areas of consolidation laterally.

### 9.10.4 Testing and Laboratory Findings

The real time polymerase chain reaction (RT-PCR) of respiratory secretions from bronchoalveolar lavage, endotracheal aspirate, and nasopharyngeal or oropharyngeal swab is the definitive test.

Other laboratory findings include lymphopenia, increased prothrombin time, and mildly raised CRP and ESR.

### 9.10.5 General Preventive Measures

COVID 19 has shifted the focus on teleconsulting which includes tele screening, telemedicine, and triage. Telemedicine should be practiced whenever possible to decrease the footfall.

Thorough history should be obtained from the patient regarding COVID 19 illness and elective procedures should be postponed and only emergent conditions should be taken up for surgery.

Patient should be called on the basis of appointments, time between two appointments should be sufficient enough to perform all necessary sanitization measures and ensure minimal patient to patient overlap. In the waiting area, posters should be displayed to encourage hand hygiene and the wearing of masks and the area should be well ventilated. A minimum of 2 m distance should be maintained between the individuals.

Extraoral radiographs should be preferred as an alternative to intraoral periapical radiographs.

In the operatory there should be minimum personnel present, Air Conditioners should be avoided, doors and windows are advised to be kept open. The operating room should be spacious with adjoining two rooms for donning and doffing of the PPE's. No touch sensor-based sanitizer dispenser should be installed at the entry and exit of OR [20].

All the surfaces of equipment like OR table, motor drills etc., should be covered with plastic sheets and sheets to be changed after every patient.

OT's should be equipped with HEPA filter (0.1 micron efficiency) and high frequency of air changes (ideally 25 per hour) should be ensured to reduce the viral load [20].

High-volume suctions should be used with one-third of suction jars prefilled with povidone-iodine solution.

The Povidone Iodine solution has been shown to have significant viricidal activity up to 3 h and it has been advised to coat the oral cavity and nasal passages of both the patient and the operating team before the surgery [21, 22].

Fogger machines with 0.5% sodium hypochlorite can be used for sterilization of dental chairs, tables, doors, doorknob, etc. [20]. One-minute contact of the chemical ensures viral kill.

### 9.10.6 Personal Protective Equipment

- Masks including three-ply surgical masks, N95, N99 (FFP3), and the Powered air-purifying respirators (PAPR's) provide viral filtration in the increasing order. It is important to mention that N95 masks were not found to be adequate to prevent transmission in Chinese surgeons and PAPR's had to be used to prevent transmission from COVID patients [23].
- Surgical gloves.
- Goggles and cover all gowns.
- Triple protection gowns and face shield protect the surgeon from exposure to any kind of infected aerosols, body fluids of the patient. Disposable gowns are made of nonwoven material and protect from liquid penetration. Personal protective equipment like basic kit 45 GSM, medium kit 70 GSM for surgery, and advance kit for ICU 180 GSM are recommended to be worn [20].

### 9.10.7 Specific Precautions to Be Taken During Surgery

- Surgery on COVID patient should be performed in a negative pressure theater or in airborne infection isolation room [20].
- Focus should be on minimally invasive techniques whenever possible which could reduce the time of surgery and/or reduce aerosol generation.
- Local anesthesia with appropriate sedation should be preferred over GA.
- The surgeon should enter the theater after 20 min following intubation with complete PPE to minimize the exposure to aerosols [23].
- Scalpels should be preferred over cautery.
- Use of high-power drills, oscillating saw, and forceful irrigation should be avoided.
- Absorbable sutures should be used to avoid unnecessary trips of the patient [18].

As the COVID-19 situation is a dynamic evolving one and there is no definitive treatment available proper planning and implementation of infection control protocols are key to preventing transmission of the disease in the Maxillofacial settings.

## 9.11 Control of Nosocomial Infections

CDC elucidated certain guidelines to check the nosocomial infections in the Study on efficacy of nosocomial infection control (SENIC). These guidelines have decreased the emergence of hospital-acquired infections by a greater number. However, any breach in the infection control procedures can lead to spread of such infections.

Certain conditions leading to improper infection control and spread of such infections are:

1. Improper sterilization and disinfection procedures.
2. Presence of contaminants in the food or water

3. Environment of the health care setup.
4. Untrained and inadequate personnel
5. Insufficient knowledge of Infection control principles and practices among the staff.
6. Antibiotic abuse both in the community and in the hospital.

### 9.11.1 Prevention from Nosocomial Infections

Following are the steps that can be taken by the staff in a hospital setup to prevent the spread of such infections:

- Isolation rooms for persons suffering from contagious diseases such as COVID 19 and tuberculosis.
- Hand-scrubbing practices prior to performing any procedure.
- Disinfecting all the areas in a health care setup.
- Adequate sterilization and disinfection protocols to be followed everywhere.
- The wound dressings should be changed at an appropriate time with the use of proper agents.
- The antimicrobial agents should be carefully used. Prolonged use should be avoided whenever possible to avoid the emergence of the resistance.
- Proper management of the biomedical waste.

## 9.12 Conclusion

Preventing and controlling infections is the key factor in improving care and ensuring safety of both the patient and the health care worker. Infection control addresses factors related to the spread of infections within the operation theater complex (whether patient-to-patient, from patients to staff and from staff to patient, or among staff), including prevention (via hand hygiene/hand washing, cleaning/disinfection/sterilization, vaccination, monitoring).

Integrated infection control in the operation theater has various aspects, ranging from its designing ,environmental cleaning , management of biomedical waste and adherence to theatre attire. Use of Personal Protective Equipment (PPE) including gloves, gowns, face masks ,respirators and full face visors are essential to minimize risks of occupational infections. Whether in developed or developing country, where resources are limited, thorough knowledge about the principles of infection control and a little ingenuity will suffice to solve the problem of hospital-acquired infections.

Surgical site infections are a result of microbial invasion in a sterile atmosphere. The main sources of microbial invasion in the operating theater include the atmosphere of the operating theater, the medical and the paramedical staff present at the time of the procedure, surgical instruments, and the patient at times also. Proper designing of operation theater, appropriate microbiological monitoring, proper sterilization, and strict adherence to barrier techniques form the basis to prevent infections in an operating environment.

## References


1. Weiser TG, Regenbogen SE, Thompson KD, Haynes AB, Lipsitz SR, Berry WR, Gawande AA. An estimation of the global volume of surgery: a modelling strategy based on available data. Lancet. 2008 Jul 12;372(9633):139–44.
2. Weiser TG, Haynes AB, Molina G, Lipsitz SR, Esquivel MM, Uribe-Leitz T, Fu R, Azad T, Chao TE, Berry WR, Gawande AA. Size and distribution of the global volume of surgery in 2012. Bull World Health Organ. 2016 Mar 1;94(3):201.
3. Bali R, Sharma P, Nagrath S, Gupta P. Microbial isolations from maxillofacial operation theatre and its correlation to fumigation in a teaching hospital in India. Journal of maxillofacial and oral surgery. 2014 Jun 1;13(2):128–32.
4. de Lissovoy G, Fraeman K, Hutchins V, Murphy D, Song D, Vaughn BB. Surgical site infection: incidence and impact on hospital utilization and treatment costs. Am J Infect Control. 2009 Jun 1;37(5):387–97.
5. Block SS. Definition of terms. Disinfection, sterilization, and preservation. Philadelphia: Lippincott Williams & Wilkins. 2001:19–28.
6. Bratzler DW, Houck PM, Workgroup SI. Antimicrobial prophylaxis for surgery: an advisory statement from the National Surgical Infection Prevention Project. Am J Surg. 2005 Apr 1;189(4):395–404.
7. Safety WP, World Health Organization. WHO guidelines for safe surgery: 2009: safe surgery saves lives. Geneva: World Health Organization; 2009.
8. Petersen BT, Chennat J, Cohen J, Cotton PB, Greenwald DA, Kowalski TE, Krinsky ML, Park WG, Pike IM, Romagnuolo J, Rutala WA. Multisociety guideline on reprocessing flexible gastrointestinal endoscopes: 2011. Gastrointest Endosc. 2011;73(6):1075–84.
9. B'erard F. Postoperative wound infections: the influence of ultraviolet irradiation of the operating room and of various other factors. Ann Surg. 1964;160(1):1–92.
10. Knight R, Charbonneau P, Ratzer E, Zeren F, Haun W, Clark J. Prophylactic antibiotics are not indicated in clean general surgery cases. Am J Surg. 2001 Dec 1;182(6):682–6.
11. Altemeier WA, Culbertson WR, Hummel RP. Surgical considerations of endogenous infections—sources, types, and methods of control. Surg Clin N Am. 1968 Feb 1;48(1):227–40.
12. Cheng H, Chen BP, Soleas IM, Ferko NC, Cameron CG, Hinoul P. Prolonged operative duration increases risk of surgical site infections: a systematic review. Surg Infect. 2017 Aug 1;18(6):722–35.
13. Haley RW, Culver DH, Morgan WM, White JW, Emori TG, Hooton TM. Identifying patients at high risk of surgical wound infection: a simple multivariate index of patient susceptibility and wound contamination. Am J Epidemiol. 1985;121(2):206–15.
14. Edmiston CE, Lee CJ, Krepel CJ, Spencer M, Leaper D, Brown KR, Lewis BD, Rossi PJ, Malinowski MJ, Seabrook GR. Evidence for a standardized preadmission showering regimen to achieve maximal antiseptic skin surface concentrations of chlorhexi-

dine gluconate, 4%, in surgical patients. JAMA Surg. 2015 Nov 1;150(11):1027–33.
15. Soballe PW, Nimbkar NV, Hayward I, Nielsen TB, Drucker WR. Electric cautery lowers the contamination threshold for infection of laparotomies. Am J Surg. 1998 Apr;175(4):263–6.
16. Bali R, Sharma P, Garg A. Incidence and patterns of needlestick injuries during Intermaxillary fixation. Br J Oral Maxillofac Surg. 2011;49:221–4.
17. Kampf G, Todt D, Pfaender S, Steinmann E. Persistence of coronaviruses on inanimate surfaces and their inactivation with biocidal agents. J Hosp Infect. 2020;104(3):246–51.
18. Bali RK, Chaudhry K. Maxillofacial surgery and COVID-19, The pandemic!! J Maxillofac Oral Surg. 2020;19(2):159–61.
19. Meng L, Hua F, Bian Z. Coronavirus disease 2019 (COVID-19): Emerging and future challenges for dental and oral medicine. J Dent Res. 2020;99(5):481–7.
20. Datarkar A, Purohit S, Tayal S, Bhawalkar . Operating room protocols in OMFS during Corona virus (Covid-19) pandemic. J Maxillofac Oral Surg. 2020;19(3):327–31.
21. Eggers M, Koburger-Janssen T, Eickmann M, Zorn J. In vitro bactericidal and virucidal efficacy of povidone-iodine gargle/mouthwash against respiratory and oral tract pathogens. Infect Dis Ther. 2018;7:249–59.
22. Kirk-Bayley J, Challacombe S, Sunkaraneni V, Combes J. The use of povidone iodine nasal spray and mouthwash during the current COVID-19 pandemic may protect healthcare workers and reduce cross infection. Br Dent J. 2020;228(12):902.
23. https://aocmf3.aofoundation.org/#o=News%20Date%20Facet,Descending. Accessed 30 Mar 2020

## Additional Reading

Surgical site infections: prevention and treatment. https://www.nice.org.uk/guidance/cg74

# Pharmacotherapy in Oral and Maxillofacial Surgery

# 10

Latha P. Rao

The human fascination—and sometimes infatuation—with chemicals that alter biological function is ancient and results from long experience with, and dependence on, plants. Many plants produce harmful compounds for defense that animals have learned to avoid and humans to exploit [1]

## 10.1 Introduction

With phenomenal increase in the knowledge about mechanism of action of chemical compounds and rapid introduction of new drugs, pharmacology—the science of drugs—has become increasingly important to all health professionals. Practice of maxillofacial surgery utilizes drugs either as primary treatment modality or as a facilitator of surgical procedures. A detailed description of the pharmacodynamics & pharmacokinetics of these drugs is beyond the scope of this chapter. The readers are encouraged to refer to the standard textbooks of pharmacology for the same.

## 10.2 Antimicrobial Agents

Infections caused by microorganisms have threatened human life since time immemorial. Some of the organisms had the potential to spread from one infected person to another at an alarming rate causing worldwide pandemics and epidemics. With the discovery of the first antibiotic, "the magic bullet"—Penicillin, patients could effectively be cured of many life- threatening infections [2].

Antimicrobial agents are of the few classes of drugs that effectively treat the etiology of conditions and not simply alleviate the symptoms of the diseases.

### 10.2.1 Definition

The term antibiotic was first used by Selman Waksman et al. to describe any substance produced by a microorganism that is antagonistic to the growth of other microorganisms in high dilution [3]. This definition excluded substances like gastric juices and hydrogen peroxide that kill bacteria but are not produced by microorganisms. It also excluded synthetic antibacterial compounds like the sulfonamides. In current usage, however, the term "antibiotic" is applied to any medication that kills bacteria or inhibits their growth, regardless of whether that medication is produced by a microorganism or not.

### 10.2.2 Classification

The antibiotics have been classified in many ways, based on their chemical nature, mechanism of action, type of organisms against which primarily active spectrum of activity, etc. (Table 10.1). The antibiotics exert their remarkably specific action on the microorganisms, sparing the host, due to their selectivity for target components, which are either absent or not very important in humans. Among these targets are bacterial and fungal cell wall synthesizing enzymes, the bacterial ribosome, the enzymes required for nucleotide synthesis and DNA replication, etc.

### 10.2.3 Oral Microflora

The infectious diseases associated with the oral and maxillofacial region have unique microbiological features because of the abundance and variety of microorganisms in this region. The normal flora of the oral cavity consists of up to $10^{11}$ bacteria per gram of tissue, with anaerobic bacteria predominating [4]. Although the subtypes and proportions of organisms differ, the general pattern of the indigenous

L. P. Rao (✉)
Department of craniomaxillofacial surgery, Aster Medcity, Kochi, Kerala, India



K. Bonanthaya et al. (eds.), *Oral and Maxillofacial Surgery for the Clinician*, https://doi.org/10.1007/978-981-15-1346-6_10

**Table 10.1** Different classes of antibiotics—based on their chemical structure and mechanism of actions

| Class of antibiotics | Common examples | Mechanism of action | Bacteriostatic / Bactericidal |
|---|---|---|---|
| *Beta lactams*—most widely used | (a) Penicillins<br>(b) Cephalosporins | Inhibit bacterial cell wall synthesis | Bactericidal |
| *Sulfonamides*—first commercial antibiotics | (a) Sulfanilamide<br>(b) Sulfadiazine<br>(c) Sulfizoxazole | Prevent bacterial growth and multiplication | Bacteriostatic |
| *Aminoglycosides* | (a) Streptomycin<br>(b) Neomycin<br>(c) Kanamycin<br>(d) Paramomycin | Inhibit bacterial protein synthesis | Bactericidal |
| *Tetracyclines*—more chances of resistance formation | (a) Tetracyclines<br>(b) Doxycycline<br>(c) Oxytretracycline | Inhibit bacterial protein synthesis | Bacteriostatic |
| *Chloramphenicol*—first line of drug only in conjunctivitis | | Inhibit bacterial protein synthesis | Bacteriostatic |
| *Macrolides*—second most prescribed | (a) Erythromycin<br>(b) Clarithromycin<br>(c) Azithromycin | Inhibit bacterial protein synthesis | Bacteriostatic |
| *Glycopeptides*—last-resort drugs | (a) Vancomycin<br>(b) Teicoplanin | Inhibit bacterial cell wall synthesis | Bactericidal |
| *Ansamycins*—have antiviral activity also | (a) Geldanamycin<br>(b) Rifamycin<br>(c) Naphthomycin | Inhibit bacterial RNA synthesis | Bactericidal |
| *Quinolones*—rapid development of resistance | (a) Ciprofloxacin<br>(b) Levofloxacin<br>(c) Trovafloxacin | Inhibit bacterial cell wall synthesis | Bactericidal |
| *Streptogramins* - two groups of antibiotics that act synergistically | (a) Pristinamycin I A<br>(b) Pristinamycin II A | Inhibit bacterial protein synthesis | Bactericidal |
| *Oxazolidinones*—potent last-resort drugs | (a) Linezolid<br>(b) Posizolid<br>(c) Tedizolid<br>(d) Cycloserine | Inhibit bacterial protein synthesis | Bacteriostatic |
| *Leptopeptides*—instances of resistance rare | (a) Daptomycin<br>(b) Surfactin | Disrupt multiple cell-membrane functions | Bactericidal |

microflora is similar in healthy individuals. However, systemic diseases and concurrent use of medications result in the presence of unusual organisms as part of the normal flora and an increase in diseases caused by normal organisms that usually are considered to have low pathogenicity. Usually, the microorganisms are held in check by the body's defense mechanisms. When these mechanisms are impaired, infection may result from an otherwise minor bacterial exposure.

The pathobiology of mixed odontogenic infection is relatively clear. The early cellulitis is the result of streptococci, the moderate-to-severe infection is caused by a combination of aerobic and anaerobic bacteria, and the well- circumscribed chronic abscess is caused primarily by anaerobic bacilli alone [5]. A complex mix of strict anaerobes and facultative anaerobes account for most of the odontogenic infections. Empirical antibiotic choices can be made in this situation where the microbiological pattern is well established (Table 10.2).

### 10.2.4 Guidelines to the Therapeutic Use of Antibiotics

Understanding that infections are ultimately dealt by the host's immune systems, and antibiotics play only an adjunctive role, is critical. Antibiotic therapy should be reserved for those with clearly established infection. Surgical treatment of the infection also should be initiated as early as possible.

Antibiotics help in preventing infections after a contamination has happened or they can abort a developing infection, if administered early. Antibiotics should not be used as a substitute for the needed surgical treatment.

In most clinical situations, it is easy to determine whether a patient has an infection—local and systemic findings would point to the diagnosis. Diagnostic difficulty arises when a patient who has had a maxillofacial procedure performed, during the second or third day after surgery, develops swelling and pain. Similarly, elevated temperature and white blood cell count also may be found. Surgical insult and

**Table 10.2** Efficacy of commonly used antibiotics against head and neck pathogens and dosage

| Antibiotics | Aerobes | Staphylococcus | Anaerobes | Dose |
|---|---|---|---|---|
| Penicillin | Excellent | No action | Guarded against prevotella, porphyromonas, fusobacterium, bacteroides | Penicillin G- 6,00,000 – 1,200,000 u q4h im/iv<br>Penicillin V – 250-500 mg q6h orally |
| Amoxycillin / clavulanate | Excellent | Active | Guarded against prevotella, porphyromonas, fusobacterium, bacteroides | 375-625 mg q8h orally<br>1.2 g q8h im/iv |
| Cefuroxime | Excellent with all except guarded action against capnocytophaga and no action against eikenella | Active | No action against prevotella, porphyromonas, fusobacterium, bacteroides | 1.5 g q8h im/iv |
| Erythromycin | Good, guarded against capnocytophaga & eikenella | Active | Guarded action against fusobacterium, no action against prevotella, porphyromonas, bacteroides | 250-500 mg q6h orally<br>1-4 g /day in divided doses q6h iv for severe infections |
| Clindamycin | Excellent | Active | Active | 150–300 mg q8h orally<br>1200–2400 mg /day in divided doses q8h for severe infections |
| Ciprofloxacin | Good | Guarded action | Guarded action | 500 mg q12h orally<br>400 mg q12h iv |
| Metronidazole | No action | No action | Active | 400 mg q8h orally<br>500 mg q8h iv |

prolonged general anesthesia often result in these symptoms. Clinical judgment is important in making the diagnosis, and the clinician should weigh all information available before making the diagnosis of infection.

There are a few basic guidelines to be followed in the administration of antibiotics (Table 10.3).

### 10.2.5 Consistency in Route of Administration

In severe infection, parenteral antibiotics are needed to get adequate blood levels. But with an initial response within couple of days, one is always tempted to switch to oral administration. When this is done, the infection may recur because blood levels achieved with oral dose are suboptimal. Maintenance of peak blood levels of antibiotic, until eradication of bacteria, is important, which may take 5–6 days. After the fifth day of parenteral administration, the blood levels achievable with oral administration are usually sufficient.

### 10.2.6 Cross-allerginicity between Penicillins & Cephalosporins

A frequently asked question about penicillin allergic patients is whether the cephalosporins can be used safely. Overall the frequency of crossallergenicity between the two groups of drugs is low (7–18%) [10, 11]. Cross-allergenicity appears to be most common among penicillin, aminopenicillins, and early-generation cephalosporins, which share similar R-1 side chains; this is thought to increase the risk of cross-reactivity. Patients with a history of anaphylaxis to penicillins should not receive first- or second-generation cephalosporins, while third- and fourth-generation cephalosporins should be administered with caution, preferably in a monitored setting.

### 10.2.7 Patient Monitoring

The patient should be monitored for the response to treatment and any deterrent should be identified and rectified. A second empirical choice should be avoided, if at all possible because the likelihood of success is substantially less. Repeat cultures may also be attempted.

In some cases, the patient may respond well to the empirical antibiotics, but the culture and sensitivity report would reveal that the organisms isolated are resistant to the antibiotics being used. The combined surgical and antibiotic treatment, along with natural host defenses, would have resulted in resolution of infection. The antibiotic may or may not have played an important role. The antibiotic that was clinically effective for the patient should be continued despite the contradictory data.

## 10.3 General Considerations in the Prophylactic Use of Antibiotics

The original guidelines for timing and use of antibiotics to prevent infection postoperatively were established by Burke and Miles et al.'s experimental observations [12, 13]. They

**Table 10.3** Guidelines for the use of antibiotics

1. *Empirical therapy*
2. *Identification* of the organisms—obtain culture & sensitivity in
   (a) Compromised host defenses
   (b) Persistence of infection in spite of appropriate antibiotics & surgical therapy.
   (c) Postoperative infection
   (d) Suspected cases of actinomycosis, osteomyelitis
3. Use of *specific narrow-spectrum antibiotic*—to prevent/minimize bacterial resistance [6] & superinfections [7].
4. Reserve *combination therapy* for:
   (a) Patient with life-threatening sepsis of unknown cause
   (b) Increased bactericidal effect against a specific organism is required
   (c) Prevention of rapid emergence of resistant bacteria—e.g., tuberculosis
   (d) Empiric treatment for certain odontogenic infections—that are rapidly progressing posteriorly around the neck space
5. Use of antibiotics with proven history of success
6. Use of the least toxic antibiotic
7. Use of a *bactericidal* rather than a bacteriostatic drug
8. *Proper administration*: Dose, time interval, route of administration, & consistency in the route of administration
9. Cost of the antibiotics
10. *Patient compliance*—decreases with increasing number of pills [8]
11. *Patient monitoring*—initially a subjective sense of feeling better, then look for reduction in swelling, pain, & temperature [9]
12. *Causes of failure of antibiotic therapy*:
    (a) Inadequate surgical intervention –
        (i) Failure to drain pus,
        (ii) Increasing pressure inside tissue spaces,
        (iii) Retained nonvital tissue or foreign body.
    (b) Other sources of infection—IV catheter, Foley's catheter
    (c) Reduced or compromised host defenses—immunocompromised, malnourished, dehydrated patients
    (d) Mistakes in antibiotic administration
        (i) Improper route of administration,
        (ii) Inadequate dosage,
        (iii) Patient noncompliance,
        (iv) Incorrect carrying out of physician's orders.
    (e) Wrong culture report or misinterpretation of the culture report

noted that antibiotics must be given within 4 h after injection of bacteria into a surgical site to prevent the aggressive level of infection that occurs when no antibiotics are administered.

Antibiotic prophylaxis entails administering the antibiotic appropriate for the potential microbial contamination before the surgical insult, at a high enough dosage to establish an appropriate bacteriologic titer [14].

1. *Indications for antibiotic prophylaxis* [15, 16] are given in Table 10.4.
2. *Condition & bacterial contamination of the surgical area*: Surgical wounds are generally classified into clean, clean–contaminated, contaminated, and dirty/infected [16–18] (Table 10.5).

   With judicious use of antibiotics, the infection rates are known to be lesser [16, 18].

**Table 10.4** Indications for antibiotic prophylaxis

1. Compromised host defenses
   (a) Physiological—old age, obesity, malnutrition
   (b) Disturbances in circulation—massive transfusion, recent surgery
   (c) Disease related—poorly controlled diabetes, cancer, leukemia, alcoholic cirrhosis, end-stage renal diseases
   (d) Compromised immunity—multiple myeloma, total body irradiation, splenectomy
   (e) Immunosuppressants—cytotoxic drugs, glucocorticoids, azathioprine, cyclosporine
2. Potential for bacterial contamination of a sterile field
3. Procedures with high infection rate
4. Surgical procedures in which there is a high mortality / morbidity rate following infection
5. When a foreign body is inserted into the tissues

**Table 10.5** Classification of surgical wounds

| Type | Incidence of infection (values given for general surgical cases) | Examples for the types of surgical wounds in maxillofacial surgery |
|---|---|---|
| Clean | 1-5% | Temporomandibular joint surgery, facial cosmetic surgery |
| Clean–contaminated | 3-11% | Orthognathic procedures, extractions |
| Contaminated | 10-17% | Maxillary fracture with active maxillary sinusitis |
| Dirty wound | >27% | Mandibular fracture through an infected third molar socket |

**Table 10.6** Need for postoperative antibiotics

| | |
|---|---|
| 1 | Compromised immunity |
| 2 | Inflammation at the surgical site |
| 3 | Evidence of wound dehiscence |
| 4 | Active periodontal disease |
| 5 | Poor oral hygiene |
| 6 | Inadequate surgical skill |
| 7 | Prolonged surgery |
| 8 | Wound contamination during surgery |

3. The *selected antibiotic should be bactericidal* against the most common microorganisms that cause infection in the oral cavity. The bactericidal antibiotics rely less on the host defense mechanisms providing faster results [18].
4. The *concentration of antibiotics* in the tissue should be sufficient to fight the bacteria that may enter the surgical wound at incision or during the course of surgery. To achieve a blood concentration of *three-four fold that of minimum inhibitory concentration*, the antibiotic is typically given at twice the treatment dose *1 h prior to surgery* [14, 16].
5. Usually antibiotics can be administered as a single preoperative dose. In cases where the surgeon feels that postoperative infection is a high possibility, the drug can be *extended postoperatively as deemed necessary* [19] (Table 10.6).

One must be vigilant in identifying cases where antibiotics are required for the success of surgery, as antibiotic usage and overusage have considerable risks [6, 7, 20, 21]—gastrointestinal disturbances, toxicity reactions, antibiotic resistance and superinfections, anaphylaxis, pseudomembraneous colitis, etc.

### 10.3.1 Prophylactic Uses of Antibiotics in Maxillofacial Surgery

Infection, one of the most common postoperative complications, can be prevented by the timely use of appropriate antibiotic. In spite of many studies in literature, a definitive conclusion cannot be made regarding the need for antibiotic prophylaxis in maxillofacial surgery and, if needed, the dose required. The antibiotic prescription pattern is still hugely based on personal preferences and shows wide regional variation, which many a time is inappropriate. The drugs would be initiated either at an incorrect time, or would be continued beyond the time required, and this has greatly contributed to the emergence of resistant bacteria [6].

Prophylactic use of antibiotics should be evidence based taking into consideration the effectiveness and the possible adverse outcomes of antibiotic therapy. Moreover, a thorough knowledge of the likely organisms involved in the infection is needed to prevent the prescription of unsuitable antibiotics. Antibiotics, if needed, should have a spectrum of activity that involves streptococci, anaerobic Gram-positive cocci, and anaerobic Gram-negative rods, which are considered the most pathogenic for oral infections and should be bactericidal and the least toxic agents available - amoxicillin being the most common choice of the clinicians [12, 18].

The need for antibiotic prophylaxis and the preferable drugs for wisdom teeth removal, orthognathic surgery, dental implants, maxillofacial trauma, and in special circumstances like patients with diabetes mellitus, patients—pre- and post-organ transplant, rheumatic heart disease—valve replacements, oncological surgery & reconstruction, cleft surgeries, etc. are mentioned in the following sessions.

### 10.3.2 Antibiotic Prophylaxis in the Surgical Removal of Wisdom Teeth

Though one of the most commonly performed minor oral surgical procedures, the reported infection rate with the removal of mandibular third molars is ≤10% [22]. However, the rate can be as high as 25% when the patient's immunity is compromised [20]. The infection rate associated with the corresponding procedure in maxilla is quite low, <1% [20, 22]. The higher rate of postoperative infection in relation to mandibular third molar has been attributed to the reduced vascularization and the gravity-induced pooling of bacterial-rich saliva.

The prophylactic use of antibiotics in wisdom teeth removal had been an issue of many debates. There are studies for [20, 23] and against [24, 25] the practice of antibiotic prophylaxis in third molar removal. Considering the potentially contaminating oral environment in which the third molar removal is carried out, it is reasonable to favor antibiotic prophylaxis. Moreover, since the postoperative infection and alveolar osteitis, an inflammatory response whose etiology could be traced to bacterial contamination and fibrinolysis of the socket blood clot, cause debilitating pain and severe functional impairment, it is only prudent to consider the use of prophylactic antibiotics.

Studies have shown that preoperative administration of antibiotics reduces the postoperative infection when administered 1-2 h prior to the procedure [26, 27]. Amoxicillin/amoxicillin—clavulanic acid is the widely used antibiotic in the prophylaxis for the surgical removal of impacted teeth [28] and when given as a single dose preoperatively is found to reduce postoperative infection and alveolar osteitis [21]. But certain other studies have failed to show a considerable difference between amoxicillin, clindamycin, metronidazole, and placebo in terms of postoperative infection rates [25]. Studies have found topical tetracycline [29], chlorhexidine irrigation [30],& metronidazole dressings [31]into the mandibular third molar sockets, effective in reducing the postoperative infection & the incidence of dry socket. Review of literature does not give definite indication to use of antibiotics as prophylaxis in healthy patients or asymptomatic impacted teeth and in case of the removal of maxillary wisdom teeth [22].

Studies have advocated the use of antibiotic prophylaxis in immunocompromised patients to prevent infection after surgical removal of impacted teeth [22].

Two recent meta-analyses [28, 32] summarize the antibiotic prophylaxis in wisdom teeth removal (Table 10.7).

### 10.3.3 Antibiotic Prophylaxis in the Placement of Dental Implants

Dental implants play a crucial role in the successful restoration of missing dentition. The success rate of dental implants is high, with only 0-10% of reported failure rates [33]. However, risk of failure is high during the first year after implant placement [34]. The implant surfaces can become colonized by oral and perioral microorganisms during surgery (perioperative contamination) [35]. This can lead to pain, swelling, bone loss, and eventually failure of implants. The failure of the dental implants is multifactorial (Table 10.8).

**Table 10.7** Antibiotic prophylaxis in wisdom teeth removal—Key points

| | |
|---|---|
| 1 | Factors influencing the rate of postoperative infection [20, 32] *may need to consider postoperative antibiotics*<br>History of pericoronitis<br>Smoking<br>Old age<br>Poor oral hygiene<br>Duration of surgery<br>Amount of bone removal<br>Presence of foreign bodies—hemostats or devitalized bone fragments<br>Operator skill |
| 2 | Amoxicillin & Amoxicillin—clavulanic acid equally effective [28] |
| 3 | Systemic administration more effective [32] |
| 4 | Single preoperative dose: 30–90 min prior to procedure [18, 32] |
| 5 | Usually double the usual strength is given preoperatively [18, 26] |
| 6 | Antibiotics reduce incidence of alveolar osteitis [21]. |
| 7 | Topical tetracycline [29], chlorhexidine [30], & metronidazole [31] effective in reducing the infection rate |
| 8 | Preoperative and extended postoperative doses may be required in immunocompromised patients [22] |
| 9 | No antibiotic prophylaxis required in removal of asymptomatic mandibular third molars and maxillary third molars in healthy individuals [22] |

**Table 10.8** Factors affecting the survival of implants [33, 34]

| | |
|---|---|
| Local factors | 1. Pre-existing infections<br>2. Quality & quantity of bone<br>3. Bone grafts—autogenous vs allogenic<br>4. Ill-fitting prostheses<br>5. Bad oral hygiene<br>6. Irradiated bone |
| Systemic factors | 1. Immunocompromised diseases<br>2. Diabetes<br>3. Long-term steroids<br>4. Malnutrition<br>5. Elderly patients<br>6. Smoking |
| Surgical factors | 1. Incorrect instruments<br>2. Overheating during placement<br>3. Lack of attention to sterility.<br>4. Increased duration of the procedure [20]<br>5. Operator skill [20] |

Hence all these local, systemic, surgical, and procedural factors contributing to implant failure should be eliminated before considering infection as the reason for failure [33].

Because of the morbidity associated with infection of the implants, antimicrobial therapy is routinely used with the aim of prevention of surgical site infection. Though by definition, dental implant placement is a clean-contaminated surgery with 3–11% chances of infection, the infection rate can be brought down to about 1% by proper patient selection, attention to surgical details, and by judicious use of antibiotics [18].

There are studies supporting antibiotic use to reduce implant failures [33, 34] and studies that fail to show any added benefits of antibiotics against implant failurte [36]. Few other studies have observed similar failure rates for the implants with a single preoperative dose and routine use of antibiotic for 7 days [37].

The currently advocated dose of antibiotic prophylaxis for implant surgery is 2–3 g of amoxicillin 2 h prior to multiple implant placement, especially along with bone graft [33]. If the patient is allergic to penicillin group, 600 mg clindamycin should be given 1 h before surgery. For sinus augmentation, 1.2 g of amoxicillin/clavulanic acid starting day before the surgery is the prophylaxis of choice [33]. Chlorhexidine gluconate mouth rinses have been known to reduce the number of pathogenic microorganisms, by lysing the bacterial cell membranes, and by virtue of its substantivity, can get retained in the oral soft tissues and get released slowly for up to 12 h [30, 33]. The key points in the antibiotic prophylaxis for dental implants are given in Table 10.9.

### 10.3.4 Antibiotic Prophylaxis in Orthognathic Surgery

Orthognathic surgical procedures aim to correct the facial deformities and malocclusion, thereby improving the functional disorders of the stomatognathic system. It is an elective procedure, usually carried out in young healthy adults. It is considered as a clean-contaminated procedure with a reported infection rate of 3–11% [18, 39]. But certain studies have reported the rate of infection after orthognathic surgery to be as high as 6–33.4% [39]. The postoperative infection was found to be related to poor oral hygiene and the habit of smoking.

The surgical site infections (SSIs) that develop can be incisional SSIs and organ and space SSIs [40]. Both types of SSIs can occur after orthognathic surgery and may develop within the first few weeks after surgery. The development of SSIs increased the total length of hospital stay and expenditure. Though the potential for postoperative infections after orthognathic surgery is known for a very long time, a consensus has not yet been achieved with regard to the drug that is useful, the dose, and the duration of administration.

The specific orthognathic procedure that has been associated with higher infection rate was mandibular sagittal split osteotomy, especially where a transbuccal approach had been adopted for fixation [38]. Increased rate of infection associated with mandibular procedures has been attributed to the diminished vascularity of mandible in comparison with maxilla and pooling of food and saliva along the vestibular incision line in the mandible. Till the incision seals off, oral microflora can freely enter the deeper tissues from the pooled saliva. Though concomitant extractions, especially of partially erupted mandibular third molars had been implicated as a risk factor for the development of postoperative infec-

**Table 10.9** Antibiotic prophylaxis in dental implants—Key points

| |
|---|
| *Care to be taken* [35]:<br>Through oral prophylaxis & measures to improve oral hygiene<br>Stabilize oral focus of infection<br>Procedure in a well-monitored asceptic environment—disinfection, draping, hand scrubbing, sterile gowns & gloves, sterile instruments<br>Prevent contamination of implants with contact with skin, infected oral mucosa, & sinus lining<br>Bactericidal antibiotic with coverage against pathogenic oral microflora [12, 18, 33]<br>Preoperative administration of antibiotics—1 h before the procedure, twice the therapeutic dose [18, 33]—Amoxicillin 2gm, / clindamycin 600 mg 1 h prior to surgery<br>Chlorhexidine gluconate rinses—hugely effective in controlling the immediate local infection [30, 33]. |
| 1 *Only Chlorhexidine 0.12% rinse twice daily in healthy individuals* [33]<br>(a) Simple implant,<br>(b) Short duration,<br>(c) No bone graft,<br>(d) Sterile environment is ensured.. |
| 2 *Single preoperative dose + Chlorhexidine 0.12% rinse twice daily in healthy individuals* [33]<br>(a) Multiple implants with minimal tissue reflection,<br>(b) Immediate extraction & implant placement,<br>(c) Socket bone grafting. |
| 3 *Single preoperative dose + 3 doses / day X 3 postoperative days + Chlorhexidine 0.12% rinse twice daily in healthy individuals* [33]<br>(a) Multiple implants with extensive tissue reflection,<br>(b) Multiple extractions & implant placement,<br>(c) Bone grafting—allografts,<br>(d) Long duration. |
| 4 *Single preoperative dose + 3 doses / day X 5 postoperative days + Chlorhexidine 0.12% rinse twice daily* [33]<br>(a) In medically compromised patients,<br>(b) Extensive tissue reflection,<br>(c) Full arch implants,<br>(d) Block bone grafting—autografts,<br>(e) Indirect sinus floor lift procedures,<br>(f) Active periodontal disease. |
| 5 *Loading dose on the previous day + 3 doses / day X 5 postoperative days + Chlorhexidine 0.12% rinse twice daily* [33]<br>In sinus lift procedure |

tion, studies were not able to support or refute this [38, 41] Longer surgeries involving multiple/segmental procedures also show a higher rate of infections [12, 18, 38].

Use of various antibiotics has been proposed—penicillin [42], ampicillin [43], amoxicillin with or without clavulanate [43], clindamycin [42], or a member of the cephalosporin group [19, 41]. Literature fails to report a significant difference in the infection rate when using a penicillin or nonpenicillin group of antibiotics or among the various types of penicillins [18, 19, 44]. Based on the bacteriological studies, penicillin, amoxicillin, or amoxicillin—clavulanic acid or cephalosporins is commonly recommended in the preoperative antibiotic prophylaxis for orthognathic surgery [19, 38, 41–44].

The preoperative single dose of antibiotic increases the level of the drug in circulation prior to incision. Whether short-term antibiotics (single dose or dose × 24 h) [ 42] or extended-term antibiotics (for more than 24 h) [ 41, 43] is beneficial in the prevention of postoperative infection after orthognathic surgery is still a debatable question [19, 38, 41, 44].

### 10.3.5 Is Antibiotics Needed when Bone Plates and Screws Are Being Inserted?

One question that keeps on surfacing is whether prophylactic antibiotics are needed in cases where bone plates and screws are used to hold the bony segments together. Any foreign body inserted into the body, be it a medical device or implant, may elicit a foreign body reaction. Moreover, the microorganisms can colonize on the implant surface in a biofilm, while they are being inserted, and as the physical presence of the implants may compromise the blood supply to the region, thereby reducing the delivery of body's immune cells to the region and resulting in infections at the host –implant interface by normal flora with low virulence [45, 46]. The oral biofilm and its toxins, adhered to the surface of titanium plates and screws used for stabilization of osteotomy segments, could be a source of local or regional infectious complications [19]. Hence, the use of antibiotic prophylaxis is justified.

*Take-home points regarding antibiotic prophylaxis in orthognathic surgery are mentioned in* Table 10.10.

### 10.3.6 Antibiotic Prophylaxis in Maxillofacial Trauma

In today's world of fast-moving vehicles and expressways, hundreds of thousands of people get involved in road traffic accidents. Head and face are among commonly injured body parts. Both the soft and hard tissues of the face may be involved in the trauma. Firearms, contact sports, and interpersonal violence are other reasons for facial injuries. The management of these injuries should follow protocols and be done in a systematic manner. With advances in anesthetic and surgical techniques and availability of better implant materials with favorable metallurgy, open reduction and internal fixation (ORIF) has become the norm. The reestablishment of form, function, & cosmesis is of paramount importance. To arrive at this goal, the probable complications of ORIF need to be prevented or managed correctly. Of the various complications reported, none has generated more interest and controversy than the occurrence of postoperative infection. By adhering to the standard surgical protocols and strict aseptic techniques, the occurrence of postoperative

**Table 10.10** Antibiotic prophylaxis in orthognathic surgery—Key points

| | |
|---|---|
| 1. | Risk factors for SSIs [47, 48]<br>(a) Longer surgery;<br>(b) Short-term antibiotic prophylaxis;<br>(c) Extraction of a third molar during surgery;<br>(d) Greater number of osteotomies performed;<br>(e) Older age;<br>(f) Smoking;<br>(g) Poor oral hygiene;<br>(h) Compromised immune system. |
| 2 | Orthognathic surgery - clean–contaminated wound—with the osteotomized maxilla / mandible exposed to oral / nasal / antral cavities [48].—Antibiotics needed |
| 3 | Need for antibiotics in presence of bone plates & screws [45, 46]. |
| 4 | Loading dose of double strength 1 h prior to incision [18]. |
| 5 | Confusion between—single loading dose + short-term doses × 24 h vs long-term antibiotics for more than 24 h [19, 44].<br>Commonly isolated organisms—aerobic bacteria—streptococci (43%) & anaerobic bacteroides (50%) [18, 39] |
| 6 | Amoxicillin / amoxicillin—clavulanic acid—best suited [19, 42–44]. |
| 7 | Higher infection rate—mandibular osteotomies with transbuccal approach for fixation [38]. |
| 8 | Longer procedures & segmental osteotomies—more prone for infection [38]. |
| 9 | Concomitant removal of mandibular third molars does not increase the risk for postoperative infection [39], though may cause issues with fixation. |

infection can be brought down considerably. But the presence of the microorganisms in the oral cavity and facial skin and possible contamination from environment necessitate the consideration of antibiotics in the maxillofacial trauma management.

Though prophylactic antibiotics were considered essential in the management of maxillofacial trauma for many years [18], the evidence for this preventive intervention was weak and confusing. Among facial fractures, mandibular fractures are most commonly studied, because of the compound nature of the fractures, except in the ramus—condyle unit, where the fractures usually do not communicate with the external environment. Fractures of the mandibular condyles or Lefort fractures of maxilla are rarely infected when compared with the fractures involving mandibular angle, body, or symphysis [49, 50].

The decision to use antibiotic prophylaxis depends on whether the fracture is an open or closed type and whether it is going to be managed with open or closed reduction. Open procedures were four times more commonly prone to postoperative infections according to a few studies [41, 51, 53, 54], whereas certain other studies reported no difference between the patients treated with closed reduction and maxillomandibular fixation and those who underwent open reduction and internal fixation [54]. The microbiology of the infected fractures was mixed and responded to beta-lactam antibiotics well.

**Table 10.11** Antibiotic prophylaxis in maxillofacial trauma—Key points

| | |
|---|---|
| 1. | Risk factors for SSIs [22, 32, 51, 56]<br>(a) Longer surgery;<br>(b) Older age;<br>(c) Smoking;<br>(d) Poor oral hygiene;<br>(e) Compromised immune system. |
| 2 | Mandibular fractures/ fractures of the teeth-bearing area—open / compound fractures.—Antibiotics needed [49, 50, 53, 54]. |
| 3 | Need for antibiotics in presence of bone plates & screws [45, 46] |
| 4 | Loading dose of double strength 1 h prior to incision [18, 56]. |
| 5 | Beta-lactam antibiotics—preferred [56]. |
| 6 | Higher infection rate—in fractures involving mandibular teeth–bearing areas [49] |
| 7 | Longer duration of antibiotics in immunocompromised patients [49, 52]. |
| 8 | Chances of infection more with open reduction than in those treated with closed reduction with no antibiotic prophylaxis [16, 50, 51]. But with single dose of perioperative antibiotics, no significant difference between closed & open reduction [51, 54] |
| 10 | Delayed healing and increased infection rate with tobacco smoking [51]. |

Studies have shown that single dose of preoperative antibiotic prophylaxis is sufficient to prevent wound infection [51, 54]. If the surgery extends beyond the half-life of the antibiotic, the antibiotic can be redosed [51]. The need for postoperative antibiotics in the maxillofacial trauma too has been extensively studied [16, 49, 53, 55, 56]. These studies reported no statistically significant difference in the development of SSIs between the patients who had received perioperative antibiotics and those who had received extended antibiotics in the postoperative period.

Longer antibiotic usage has been advocated in the immunocompromised patients [32, 52, 56]. The habit of tobacco smoking was found to have a deleterious effect on the healing of mandibular fractures by inducing hypovascularity and prolonged inflammation [54]. The other major factors, which contribute to the occurrence of SSIs, are poor oral hygiene, extremes of age and malnutrition [22, 32].

*Important points mentioning the need for antibiotics in the management of maxillofacial trauma are given in* Table 10.11.

### 10.3.7 Diabetes Mellitus & Antibiotic Prophylaxis in Maxillofacial Surgery

Diabetes mellitus is a metabolic disorder resulting in elevated glucose levels, due to inadequate insulin secretion (type I) or reduced insulin secretion with an accompanying insulin resistance (type II). Diabetic patients pose a special challenge to the surgeon as the balance between the insulin they can secrete and the hyperglycemia induced by surgical stress-adaptive hormones catecholamines, cortisol, growth hormone, and glucagon is lost. Patients, who are nondiabetic, usually are able to handle this glucose overload effectively, whereas diabetic patients may have issues resulting in cardiovascular complications, infection, and reduced rates of wound healing. Moreover, the defective polymorphonuclear leukocytes function and macro- and microvascular dysfunction resulting in compromised local circulation increases the susceptibility to infections [57]. With the vast microbiological colonization of the oral cavity, it has always been assumed that maxillofacial surgical procedures carry a high risk of infection and prolonged or delayed wound healing. The guidelines as to the prophylactic use of antibiotics in diabetic patients had been vague as "….are more prone to infection necessitating routine antibiotic prophylaxis for all maxillofacial procedures" [58].

In many of the literature surveys, authors have noted that well-controlled diabetic patients are at no increased risk of postoperative infection than normal healthy patients and delayed wound healing is not a pressing concern due to the rich vascularity of the region [59, 60]. Antibiotic prophylaxis is warranted only in conditions where a normal patient also would benefit from it. Poorly controlled diabetic patients would require normalization of their hyperglycemic state prior to elective procedures. In emergency situations, antibiotic prophylaxis prior to the surgical incision is desirable and attempts should be made to control the glycemic level during the peri- and postoperative period [58–60].

### 10.3.8 Antibiotic Prophylaxis in Head and Neck Oncology

Head and neck oncology patients usually require a major surgical procedure +/– with radiation therapy. The surgical site tends to be large, the surgical time and postoperative immobilization period longer. The surgical management attempts at removal of the tumor, clearance of the neck nodes, and involves an additional surgical site from where flap is harvested for reconstruction—either microvascular flaps or pedicled ones [61]. The large wound area exposed to local flora of the oral cavity and the skin is at risk of wound contamination and infection. Nosocomial infections are known to run a protracted course and pre-existing general comorbidities further increase the morbidity and, thus, the hospital expenses associated with these surgeries.

The reasons for increased infection rate are mainly the number of procedures carried out in the same operation (excision, neck dissection, tracheostomy, and distant flap harvest), the pooling of saliva due to difficulty in swallowing, leading to aspiration, and the inability in obtaining a watertight closure when the flap is inset in the recipient bed leading to salivary leak and contamination of neck wounds with saliva [62, 63].

**Table 10.12** Key points in oral oncology & antibiotic prophylaxis

| |
|---|
| Increased risk of SSIs [62]<br>Multiple procedures done at a single operation,<br>Large wound area,<br>Long procedure,<br>Tobacco & alcohol abuse<br>Immunocompromised patients |
| Probable pathogens [62] - Escherichia spp. & staphylococcal spp |
| Preferred antibiotic [62] - ampicillin & sulbactum |
| Bartella et al. (2017) [62] - Statistically significant reduction in infectious complications with postoperative antibiotics |

The need for antibiotic prophylaxis is well established in the oncologic surgery, but the need for a long postoperative course of antibiotics is still debated upon. There are studies, which have shown benefits of prolonged antibiotics in preventing postoperative infections like pneumonia, urinary tract infections, sepsis, and SSIs in patients who had oral squamous cell carcinoma [64], and there are studies, which have shown no extra benefits of prolonged postoperative antibiotics [63, 64].

Escherichia spp. and Staphylococcus spp. are predominantly responsible for the infections and in 72% were sensitive to ampicillin & sulbactum [62].

*A few key points, which would be beneficial in making a decision, are given in* Table 10.12.

### 10.3.9 Antibiotic Prophylaxis in Cleft Surgeries

Orofacial clefting is one of the more common congenital anomalies and cleft lip & palate deformity is the most common among them. Management of cleft lip & palate deformity involves staged procedures and spans over 12–16 years. The management aims at correction of the deformity so that function and cosmesis are restored as much as possible and the psyche of the individual is minimally scarred. Postoperative infections can result in wound breakdown, poor speech & esthetics, and nasal regurgitation of food in cleft lip and palate patients.

Various authors had reported on obtaining swabs from nose and oral cavity to identify the possible pathogens and using antibiotics according to the culture reports before cleft lip and palate repair [65–67]. The pathogenic bacteria isolated from the swabs were Staphylococcus aureus and beta hemolytic streptococci [67]. But later studies demonstrated that there were not many differences between the group that underwent swab acquisition and corresponding antibiotics therapy and the group that didn't receive any antibiotics in terms of postoperative complications [68]. The rate of complications was found to be independent of the potential pathogens in the mouth [65].

*Factors, which have been implied as contributing factors to wound dehiscence, are given in* [66, 67] Table 10.13.

**Table 10.13** Factors contributing to wound dehiscence in cleft surgeries

| |
|---|
| Wide clefts |
| Closure under tension |
| Bilateral clefts |
| Long duration of surgery |
| Poor technique—traumatized nasal mucosa |
| Independent of potential oral pathogens |

In a recent prospective study, Azner et al. (2015) noted a statistically significant reduction in the incidence of palatal fistulas with 5 days of postoperative antibiotics [69]. But 80% of their control group, who had received no postoperative antibiotics, too healed without any complications. Both study and control groups had received a single dose of cefuroxime 30 mg / kg body weight, before incision. The use of one dose of antibiotics before incision has been advocated by other authors also and may be more effective in preventing complications related to wound infection than a prolonged course of postoperative antibiotics [68].

### 10.3.10 Organ Transplant and Antibiotic Prophylaxis

The concept of organ donation had always excited mankind. Twentieth century saw developments that made the dream of replacing a diseased organ with a healthy one a reality. Understanding the human immunology and the development of powerful immunosuppressant drugs laid the foundation for modern transplant medicine, making transplantation of kidney, liver, lungs, and heart a successful treatment option. As the transplant science advanced, so did the numbers and life span of transplant patients and their need for dental/maxillofacial surgical procedures. As these patients are on immunosuppressants, they are more prone to opportunistic infections and their sequel. Hence, care must be given to treat or remove the existing/potential sources of infection before the transplant procedures.

In a pretransplant patient, the need for maintaining oral hygiene should be stressed upon. The treating physician should be consulted with regard to the fitness to undergo the planned procedures and the safety of using any drugs if required. Drugs, which have a hepatic metabolism or renal clearance, should be used with caution in patients with compromised liver or kidney function. The selection of antibiotics is made after careful evaluation of the existing pathology and the chances of spread of infection with the planned dental treatment.

In the immediate post-transplant period—the first 3 months post-surgery, the graft, and the patient are very vulnerable to any insult—graft anastomoses are susceptible to endarteriris due to bacterial colonization as they are not yet fully epithelialized. Hence, only emergency procedures should be done. Any acute orofacial infection developing should be managed aggressively, surgical drainage, culture and sensitivity of the organism, and appropriate antibiotics would be required [70]. After 3 months, elective, noninvasive procedures can be carried out. Since the patients who have undergone organ transplantation are immunosuppressed and are at high risk of infection, prophylactic antibiotics need to considered for any invasive dental procedures, even after 6 months. Beta-lactam antibiotics are relatively safer to be used in renal and hepatic transplant patients [71]. But for those with meticulous oral hygiene, there is no consensus regarding the need for antibiotic prophylaxis for minimally invasive procedures [71]. The decision to use antibiotics should be done on a case-to-case basis.

*Important points to be kept in mind while contemplating antibiotic prophylaxis in organ transplant patients are given in* Table 10.14.

**Table 10.14** Key points—organ transplant and antibiotic prophylaxis

| |
|---|
| Pretransplant patients—stress on<br>1. Elimination of potential focus of infection,<br>2. Oral hygiene,<br>3. Liver / kidney friendly drugs. |
| Post-transplant patients: |
| Immediate postop:<br>1. Only emergency procedures,<br>2. Aggressive management of infections. |
| 3 months postop—noninvasive elective procedures |
| 6 months postop—invasive elective procedures under antibiotics |
| Beta-lactam antibiotics - relatively safer to be used in renal and hepatic transplant patients [72] |
| No consensus on minimally invasive procedures in patients with meticulous oral hygiene [71] |

## 10.4 Infective Endocarditis

Bacterial endocarditis, a rare but life-threatening condition, was initially described by Lewis & Grant in 1923 [72]. They suggested that bacteria released into the blood stream after a dental procedure colonize on the heart valves or the endocardium. The bacteremia associated with infections of skin and soft tissues, genitourinary tract, and gastrointestinal tract are also known to result in infective endocarditis (IE). Bacteria can gain direct access to the bloodstream through the indwelling catheters. The American Heart Association (AHA) came up with the first guidelines to reduce the risk of IE following invasive procedures in 1955 [73]. The AHA guidelines have been updated regularly since then and the latest one was released in 2007 [74]. The 2007 guidelines categorized cardiac conditions into having a low risk, moderate risk, and high risk of developing IE and advocated the use of antibiotic prophylaxis only in

**Table 10.15** High-risk cardiac conditions, which require antibiotic prophylaxis [75]

| |
|---|
| Prosthetic cardiac valves |
| Congenital heart diseases—unrepaired, with palliative shunts or conduits or repaired with prosthetic material or those repaired, but with residual defects |
| Previous IE |
| Cardiac transplants who have developed valvulopathy |

high-risk-category patients (Table 10.15) who were to undergo dental procedures that involved the manipulation of gingival tissues or the periapical region of teeth or incision of the oral mucosa.

The guidelines prescribed a single dose of antibiotic 30-60 minutes prior to the procedure—Amoxicillin 2 g PO, Cephazolin/Cephtriaxone 1gm IV/IM, or Clindamycin 600 mg PO/IM/IV, depending on whether the patient is unable to take oral preparations or is allergic to penicillin or not [74]. The reason for the revision of the antibiotic policy was predominantly the observation that IE is more likely to result from transient bacteremias caused by routine daily activities, like chewing food, and by regular oral hygiene care. The authors concluded that maintaining optimal oral hygiene is more important in reducing the risk of IE and the adverse effects of antibiotics exceeded the benefits of antibiotic prophylaxis. The British Society for Antimicrobial Chemotherapy (BSAC) also recommend antibiotic prophylaxis only in those who have a history of healed IE, prosthetic heart valves, and surgically constructed conduits [75]. The advice to the patient is to concentrate on achieving and maintaining meticulous oral hygiene as this has been found to reduce the risk of IE. Similar observations were made by the National Institute for Health and Care Excellence (NICE) [76] and the European Society of Cardiology (ESC) [77].

There has been a rising concern over the potential for an increased incidence of IE and a worse prognosis for the diseased since the guideline changes by the AHA, NICE, ESC, BSAC. Several studies have been carried out to assess the impact of these changes on the disease incidence in adults and pediatric population. Whereas earlier studies showed not much difference pre- and post-guideline changes in incidence [78], recent studies have noted a definite increase in the incidence of IE post-guideline changes [79]. Sakai et al. in 2017, though noting no change in the incidence and severity of IE in pediatric patients, pre- and post- guideline changes, reported an increase in the viridans group streptococci (VGS)–induced IE in older age group [79]. The data from these studies point to the need for further investigation into the effectiveness of 2007 guidelines, though it has been argued that the increase in IE incidence may be related to the increasing life span of the patients with congenital heart diseases and prosthetic devices and increase in the number of invasive procedures being performed on them.

## 10.5 Postoperative Pain Management in Maxillofacial Surgery

The International Association for the Study of Pain (IASP) defines pain [80] as: "an unpleasant sensory and emotional experience associated with actual or potential tissue damage or described in terms of such damage."

Pain is the most debilitating postoperative symptom and its control or elimination is usually the primary goal in postoperative management of a patient. Inadequate pain control resulting in patient distress is the most common cause of an increased length of hospital stay. The postoperative pain, inflammatory in character, is a temporary one persisting only until healing. But severe, acute, repetitive, postoperative pain increases the risk of the pain becoming chronic and may lead to allodynia and hyperalgesia [81]. Orthognathic surgery patients may continue to feel the pain even after 1 year of surgery [82]. Hence, appropriate pain management is critical to achieving a successful surgical outcome. Prevention of pain is more efficient than the treatment of pain. For this, an understanding of basic pathophysiology behind pain mechanism is important.

## 10.6 Pathophysiology of Postoperative Pain

Pain is initiated by the excitation of nociceptors, receptors that respond to noxious - mechanical, thermal, and chemical stimuli. Sensory nociception is disproportionately greater in the head and oral cavity when compared with other parts of the body. Often a patient's overanxiety about undergoing an elective surgery would result in an increased intensity of the perceived pain [83].

Surgical insult results in tissue trauma and initiates a chain of inflammatory events, causing a release of chemical substances responsible for nociceptor excitation. Trauma releases tissue phospholipids, which are converted into arachidonic acid due to the action of phospholipase A2 and the consequent conversion of this substance into prostaglandins, prostacyclins, and leukotrienes due to the action of cyclooxygenase (Cox) and lipoxygenase enzymes. These locally released chemical mediators sensitize the nociceptors and cause vasodilatation, with a consequent increase in cell permeability and edema. Trismus after a maxillofacial surgery is a sequela to the postoperative edema around the masticator muscles and is aggravated by pain [84]. The physiological responses to tissue trauma, pain & edema, can be managed successfully by inhibiting the pathways that produce the chemical mediators, before the occurrence of surgical trauma (Fig. 10.1).

Similarly, mechanisms, which enhance the endogenous pain inhibition and anxiolysis and patient education, can

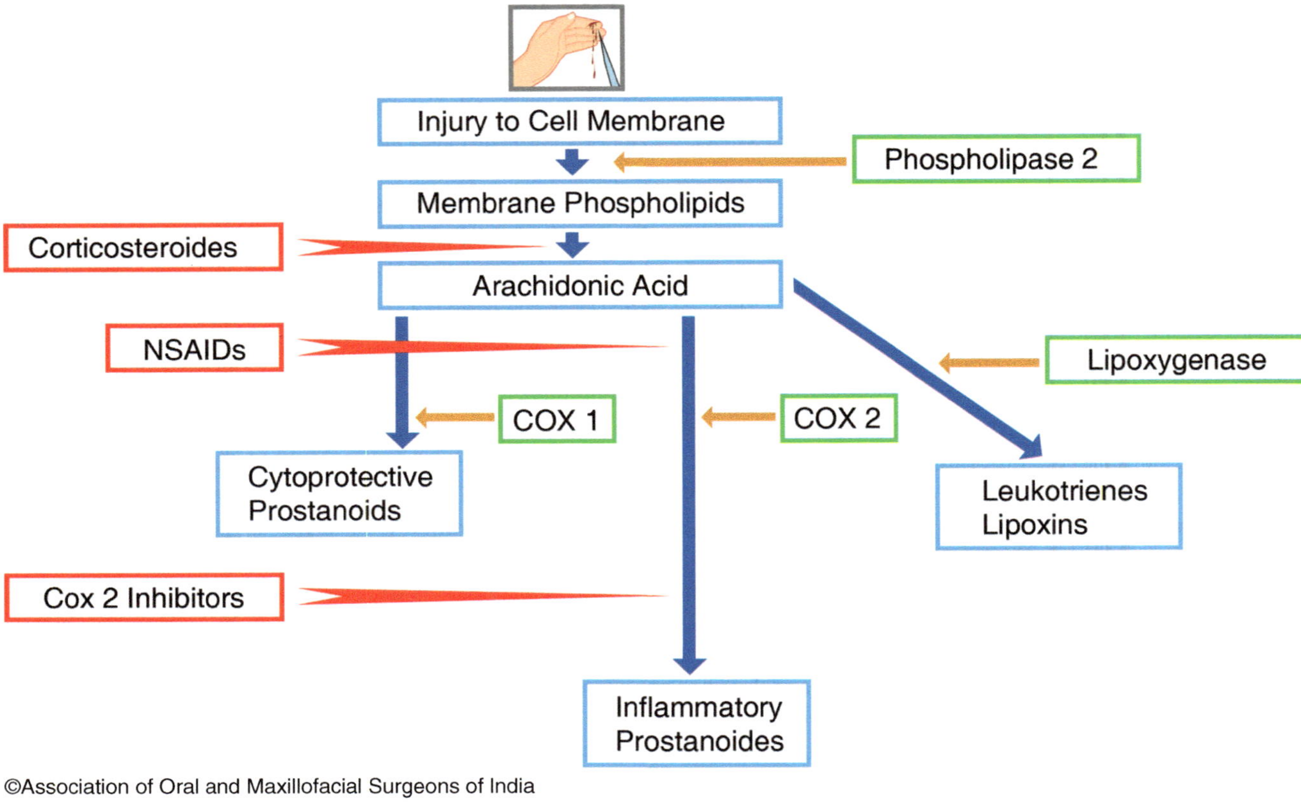


**Fig. 10.1** Pharmacologic interventions in arachidonic acid metabolism

modify cortical processing of pain perception [85]. All these measures collectively lead to an efficient postoperative pain management.

### 10.6.1 Pre-Emptive Analgesia

Postoperative pain has a protective function as it allows for undisturbed healing of the operated tissue by restricting movements. The aim of postoperative pain management is to reduce pain significantly, but not to eliminate it completely [86]. Overall postoperative pain experience could be reduced by paying attention to lessening of the pain during the surgical procedure itself. Pre-emptive analgesia is defined as an antinociceptive treatment that is started preoperatively and is active during surgery, reducing the physiological consequences of nociceptive transmission [87]. Since the introduction of the concept of pre-emptive analgesia by Woolf in 1983, many attempts to reduce the pain by using analgesics and adjunctive measures, such as the administration of long-acting local anesthesia, corticosteroids, and intraoperative nitrous oxide analgesia, have been reported [88]. These should be given before the surgical incision and should be timed so that the maximum plasma concentration of the drug is reached at the time of surgical incision. This will prevent the release of the inflammatory mediators, giving immediate analgesic effects. The use of IV analgesia has an added benefit over oral administration, as following oral administration analgesics reach maximum concentration after 1.5 h, whereas intravenous administration results in maximum concentration in a short period.

Numerous studies have shown beneficial effects of the preoperative administration of ibuprofen with paracetamol [89] piroxicam [90], ketorolac [91], meloxicam [92], parecoxib [93], and dexamethasone with rofecoxib [94]. There had been contradictory reports also in which the authors fail to find a clear-cut benefit for pre-emptive NSAIDS [95, 97]. The authors state that the pre-emptive intake of analgesics should not be used in all patients as a general rule. They base their recommendations on the lack of enhanced analgesic effects and on the potential adverse effects such as increased intraoperative bleeding [95].

Despite the confusion regarding the effectiveness of the pre-emptive analgesia, it has been strongly advised to start systemic analgesics before the local anesthesia effect wears off and/or give a nerve block with long-acting agent like bupivacaine [86].

**Table 10.16** Predictors of postoperative pain

| Patient-related factors | Surgical indicators |
|---|---|
| Age [98, 99] | Major surgeries—long duration |
| Female sex [98] | Bony surgery > soft tissue surgery [100] |
| Anxiety & apprehension, fear of the procedure | Bi-jaw surgery vs single jaw surgery |
| Pre-existing or chronic pain | Mandibular surgery > maxillary surgery |
| Preoperative use of opioids / neuropathic analgesics [98] | Oncological surgery |
| | Emergency procedures [101] |

### 10.6.2 Postoperative Pain Management

Postoperative analgesia has traditionally been achieved by prescribing analgesics with instructions to take as and when necessary. Experience with this approach was that many patients would not take the medication until the onset of significant pain. This practice earned the maxillofacial surgery the reputation of being an extremely painful one. The truth is that the postoperative pain management can be successfully achieved by carefully planning the delivery of the pain control measures at the appropriate time in the peri- and postoperative periods.

Pain perception is a subjective feeling, which is amplified by many factors and identification of the patients who are "at risk" for the development of severe postoperative pain would help in charting out an individualized management plan [97] (Table 10.16).

Identifying predictors of postoperative pain in patients before surgery, educating patients at the preoperative visit regarding the expected pain, and presenting the postoperative pain management plan will prepare patients better and relieve some of their anxiety regarding the procedure. An increased awareness of the importance of the psychological factors will allow more effective pain management.

### 10.6.3 Pharmacological Management of Postoperative Pain

The postoperative pain management is usually done with opioids and nonsteroidal class of anti-inflammatory drugs.

#### 10.6.3.1 Opioids

Opioids have been in use for moderate-to-severe pain relief for a long period. References to opium poppy can be found in Sumerian and Egyptian culture, as back as 300 BC. The opium poppy, Papaver somniferum, gives rise to more than 20 different alkaloids [100]—morphine and codeine being the main ones (Table 10.17).

**Table 10.17** Opioid analgesics

| Drug name | Dose |
|---|---|
| Codeine | 15–60 mg orally q4-6h |
| Hydrocodone | 5–10 mg orally q3h |
| Oxycodone | 5–7.5 mg orally q6h |
| Meperidine | 50–150 mg orally q3–4h |
| Pentazocine | 50 mg orally q3–4h |
| Tramadol | 50-100 mg q4–6h, max 400 mg /day |

**Table 10.18** Side effects of opioid analgesics

| |
|---|
| Respiratory depression |
| Sleepiness |
| Constipation |
| Nausea & vomiting |
| Addictive potential [102] |
| Drug overdose death [103] |
| Pharmacological tolerance ➔ opioid-induced hyperalgesia [102, 104] |

Opiate alkaloids exert their action by acting on the opioid receptors- μ, κ, δ (mu, kappa, and delta), which otherwise provide sites for activation of endogenously released opioid substances - beta-endorphins, enkephalins, and dynorphin compounds, which produce endogenous central analgesia. Opiate agonists produce analgesia by inhibiting excitatory neurotransmission of substance P, acetylcholine, noradrenaline, and dopamine.

Unfortunately, opioid use, even when prescribed for short periods, comes with certain risks (Table 10.18).

For these reasons, most opioid agents used in outpatient postsurgical pain management are formulated in combination with non-narcotic analgesics [104]. This formulation potentiates the analgesic effects of the individual agents within the formulation while minimizing the side effects of pure opioid administration [105].

#### 10.6.3.2 Tramadol

Tramadol, a synthetic substance with both opioid and non-opioid properties, is structurally related to codeine. It exhibits antidepressant and anxiolytic-like effects, in addition to analgesic action. It is considered safe for long-term use unlike NSAIDs with their potential for impairment of renal function and gastrointestinal complications, and with respect to other opioid medications for its low addiction rate and favorable safety profile. The most common adverse effect of tramadol is nausea and vomiting, especially with oral administration. Tramadol is contraindicated in patients with poorly controlled epilepsy because of its excitatory serotonergic effects. It is available either as a single drug or in combination with acetaminophen. Submucosal injection of tramadol at the extracted site of third molars has been proven effective in reducing the postoperative pain [106]. It suffers no side effects of systemic administration.

#### 10.6.3.3 Nonsteroidal Anti-Inflammatory Drugs (NSAIDs)

NSAIDs have been in use for the treatment of pain, fever, and inflammation since late 1800 [107]. The anti-inflammatory and analgesic properties of these drugs without the side effects and the addictive potential of opioids have made this class of drugs the first choice in ambulatory dentoalveolar procedures (Table 10.19).

They are a group of chemically heterogeneous compounds with several similar pharmacologic actions like anti-inflammatory, antipyretic, analgesic, and antiplatelet actions. They primarily act at the site of tissue injury by inhibiting the synthesis of prostaglandins within the endoperoxide pathway (Fig. 10.1).

**Table 10.19** Nonsteroidal anti-inflammatory drugs

| Drug name | Action | Analgesic Dose |
|---|---|---|
| Salicylic acid derivative—Acetyl salicylic acid | Analgesic, anti-inflammatory, antiplatelet, antipyretic—Nonselective cox inhibitor | 325-650 mg orally q4h / 1000 mg orally q6h. |
| Propionic acid derivative—Ibuprofen | Analgesic, anti-inflammatory, antipyretic—Nonselective cox inhibitor | 400–600 mg orally q4–6h |
| Propionic acid derivative—Naproxen | Analgesic, antipyretic—Nonselective cox inhibitor | 550 mg orally initially, then 275 mg orally q6–8h |
| Acetic acid derivative—Keterolac | Analgesic, antipyretic—Nonselective cox inhibitor | 30 mg IV or 60 mg IM q6h / 20 mg orally initially, then 10 mg orally q4–6h |
| Acetic acid derivative—Diclofenac | Analgesic, anti-inflammatory—Nonselective cox inhibitor | 50–75 mg orally/IV q12h |
| Oxicams—Piroxicam | Analgesic, anti-inflammatory—Nonselective cox inhibitor | 10-20 mg orally q 12 h |
| N- phenyl—anthranilates—Mefenamic acid | Analgesic, anti-inflammatory—Nonselective cox inhibitor | 500 mg load, then 250 mg q6h orally |
| Celecoxib | Cox 2 inhibitor | 200 mg orally q24h / 100 mg orally q12h |

Historically, majority of the NSAIDs were nonselective COX inhibitors with side effects related to the blockade of cytoprotective prostanoids - gastric irritation, increased bleeding time, and renal impairment. Over the past few years, selective COX2 inhibitors have been developed, which block the COX-2–mediated prostaglandins while maintaining the physiologically beneficial effects of the COX-1 isoenzyme [108].

Overall, NSAIDs are safe drugs to be used in the management of acute/postoperative pain. Parenteral use of NSAIDs has shown to be more effective in pain control [109]. About 60% of the patients would respond to the first NSAID, and the rest would show benefit with another NSAID. Ibuprofen is a widely used NSAID, with proven efficacy [110]. About 5% people experience "aspirin-sensitive asthma," probably due to the inhibition of Cox enzyme. Because of the probable mechanism of inducing asthma, it is felt that selective Cox 2 inhibitors may not cause asthmatic attacks [111].

#### 10.6.3.4 Paracetamol

Paracetamol or acetaminophen is a widely available analgesic with an antipyretic action. It acts by inhibition of the COX-3 isoenzyme, reducing the production of prostanoids in the central nervous system. This central inhibition explains the antipyretic action of paracetamol. Paracetamol shows an excellent result in relieving mild-to-moderate pain relief and fever [112]. When used in combination with other analgesics, it shows superior analgesic power, thereby reducing the dose of opioids required [96].

### 10.6.4 Guidelines to the Use of Analgesics

Since there is no definitive evidence or clear algorithms, the selection of NSAIDs, to a large extent, depends on clinical experience and side effects. Patient convenience and cost also play a minor role in the selection of analgesics.

Laskarides (2016), in his review on control of dental pain, puts forward his observations (Table 10.20) [113].

#### 10.6.4.1 Analgesic Ladder

WHO initially described the concept of "pain ladder" in their guidelines for the use of drugs for the management of cancer pain [114]. The concept has been now accepted in the management of all types of pain [104]. The concept is based on the use of first line of drugs for the mild-to-moderate pain and then climb the ladder to more potent drugs if pain still persists. Please see chapter on postoperative care, to view the analgesic ladder.

**Table 10.20** Key points in using analgesics

| | |
|---|---|
| 1 | Care to administer correct dose of opioids [100–103] |
| 2 | Opioids + NSAIDs—centrally acting - + peripherally acting analgesia ➜ moderate-to-severe pain relief |
| 3 | Tramadol—opioid & nonopioid properties—safe for long-term use [106]. |
| 4 | Ibuprofen—excellent analgesia, transition drug to wean off form opioids [110, 113]. |
| 5 | Use NSAIDs with caution—cardiovascular conditions & gastric irritation. |
| 6 | Paracetamol, tramadol, & short-acting opioids—drugs of choice [113]. |
| 7 | NSAIDs drug interactions –<br>Sulfonyl urea & other hypoglycemic agents<br>Oral anticoagulants<br>Phenytoin<br>Sulfonamides |
| 8 | Paracetamol + NSAIDs—superior analgesic power [89, 112]. |
| 9 | Maximum daily dose of paracetamol 4 g decides the dose of combination therapy [113]. |

#### 10.6.4.2 Preventive /Protective/Multimodal Analgesia

Pain is multifactorial in origin and multiple techniques and drugs may be required to achieve control over it. The simultaneous use of different classes of analgesics and techniques has been called preventive, protective, or multimodal analgesia [115] This approach uses a combination of drugs that act at different sites of action on the nervous system by different mechanisms to prevent peripheral and central sensitization of pain. It results in additive analgesia, but with lowered side effects than the single agents when used alone. Intraoperative local anesthesia followed by a range of analgesic drugs have been found to be effective in controlling the pain in day cases and reduces the need for opioid analgesics [116].

The complex surgeries involving multiple surgical sites as in head and neck oncological cases and craniofacial surgeries would gain hugely from the administration of multimodal analgesia. Multimodal analgesia can be successfully achieved by combining the currently available analgesic modalities (Table 10.21).

**Table 10.21** The analgesics and adjuncts that can be used in multimodal analgesia [117]

| Drugs | Examples | Mechanism of action |
|---|---|---|
| A. Opioids [102]. | Codeine, Hydrocodone Tramadol | Inhibits excitatory neurotransmission of substance P, acetylcholine, noradrenaline, & dopamine. |
| B. Local anesthesia [86, 118] techniques. | Bupivacaine, levobupivacaine & ropivacaine—nerve blocks & infiltration | Blocks the pain transmission |
| C. Acetaminophen [112]. | Weak analgesic | IV administration raises the plasma & CSF concentration rapidly to achieve adequate analgesia |
| D. Nonsteroidal anti-inflammatory drugs (NSAIDs) [108, 110]. | Ibuprofen, Diclofenac, Mefenamic acid, nasal spray of ketorolac | Blocks arachidonic acid metabolism |
| E. Cyclooxygenase (COX)-2-specific inhibitors [108]. | Celecoxib | Cox 2 inhibitor |
| F. Adjuncts. | | |
| 1. *Steroids* [80]. | Dexamethasone, hydrocortisone | Blocks lipoxygenase & cox pathways |
| 2. N-methyl-d-aspartate *(NMDA). Antagonists* [97, 115, 117] | Ketamine | Effects on central sensitization & neural modulation |
| 3. *Alpha – 2 agonists* [97, 115, 117]. | Clonidine, Dexmedetomidine | Sedative and analgesia-sparing effects via central actions in the locus ceruleus and in the dorsal horn of the spinal cord, respectively |
| 4. *Anticonvulsants* [97, 115, 117]. | Gabapentin, pregabalin | Inhibits central sensitization through presynaptic or postsynaptic inhibition of calcium influx, which inhibits the release of neurotransmitters |

#### 10.6.4.3 Patient-Controlled Analgesia (PCA)

Patient-controlled analgesics are intravenous agents, delivered through a microprocessor-controlled infusion pump, in which a predetermined dose can be delivered by the press of a button, and a lockout time can be set, so that patient cannot overdose himself [119]. PCA is usually used in patients who are distressed at the thought of postoperative pain. Fentanyl, morphine, & combinations are the usually used medications. Though PCA was initially thought to reduce the patient pain perception, thereby reducing the length of stay (LOS), studies have failed to show any statistically significant difference in the pain score and the LOS between the PCA group & non-PCA group of patients after orthognathic surgery [119, 120]. This could be attributed to the fact that the subjects in the PCA group were predominantly bijaw surgery patients for whom the surgical time was longer and the surgical procedure resulted in more tissue injury. But from patient's perspective, PCA is the preferred method, as they feel in charge of their own pain control [121].

## 10.7 Corticosteroids in Maxillofacial Surgery

When tissue damage occurs as a result of injury, body's natural defense mechanism is inflammation and body tries to heal. But overt inflammation results in pain, edema, and limitation of movement, trismus. These symptoms may not be evident immediately, but peak after the second day, returning to normal by seventh postoperative day [122]. Corticosteroids suppress the inflammation (Fig. 10.1) by interfering with the capillary dialatation, fluid transduation, fibrin deposition, leukocyte migration, and phagocytosis. Under normal nonstressful conditions, the body produces approximately 15 to 30 mg of hydrocortisone/cortisol per day. During stressful situations, 300 mg of hydrocortisone per day can be produced. Generally speaking, to suppress inflammation, the dose of exogenous corticosteroids must exceed the normal physiological amounts of hydrocortisone released [123].

The first reported clinical use of the anti-inflammatory properties of corticosteroids was in the treatment of rheumatoid artritis [124], following which its efficacy was tried in maxillofacial surgical procedures. The use of steroids and their effectiveness have been extensively studied in the third molar surgeries—the most commonly performed maxillofacial surgical procedure [125]. Markiewicz et al. noted that postoperative findings of swelling, trismus, and pain were significantly lower in the group who received corticosteroids, than in the control group in the immediate postoperative period (1–3 days) [126].

The use of dexamethasone and methyl prednisolone, in controlling the postoperative sequel of third molar surgery when these drugs are administered via parenteral [127], oral [128] submucosal [129, 130] and topical [131] routes, has been reported.

*Studies have evaluated different formulations, dosages, and routes and sites of administration of corticosteroids, without any consensus*. (Table 10.22).

Dexamethasone has a longer duration of action than methylprednisolone and is considered more potent. Intralesional/intramasseteric injection of dexamethasone is found to be better than the intravenous or parenteral administration in controlling postoperative edema & trismus and has an additional benefit of being given through an already-anesthetized area [130, 132].

Almeida et al. (2019) [133] failed to note any benefit of submucosal injection of steroid at the local site. Authors gave the reason for this as the displacement of the medicine from the local site when mucoperiosteal flap is reflected to expose the tooth. Similarly, the merits of intravenous administration of steroids perioperatively in major surgeries have been questioned by a group of authors [134]. Kainulainen et al. [134] reported infectious complications—pneumonia, gastrostomy site infections, & surgical site infections in oncological cases.

Though the reduction of edema brings about some reduction in discomfort, steroids alone do not have a clinically significant analgesic effect [130, 135] This has been attributed to the inability of the steroids to block the production of neurotransmitters by the injured tissues and central sensitization to pain. The combination of dexamethasone with tramadol or diclofenac sodium has been proven more effective in controlling postoperative pain and trismus, as opposed to corticosteroids alone [136]. Alexander & Throndson [127] summarized few salient points with regard to usage of steroids, based on their review (Table 10.23).

**Table 10.22** Commonly used steroids with their anti-inflammatory potency& equivalent dose and commonly used doses [1]

| Drug | Duration of action | Anti-inflammatory potency | Equivalent dose | Dose |
|---|---|---|---|---|
| Dexamethasone | Long acting | 25 | 0.75 mg | 0.5–5 mg /day PO, 4–20 mg /day IV |
| Betamethasone | Long acting | 25 | 0.75 mg | 0.5–5 mg /day PO, 4–20 mg /day IV |
| Prednisolone | Intermediate acting | 4 | 5 mg | 5–60 mg /day PO<br>10–40 mg / day IM or IV |
| Methyl prednisolone | Intermediate acting | 5 | 4 mg | 4–32 mg /day PO |
| Triamcinolone | Intermediate acting | 5 | 4 mg | 4–32 mg /day PO<br>5–40 mg intra-articular |
| Hydrocortisone | Short acting | 1 | 20 mg | 100 mg IV/IM bolus |

**Table 10.23** Summary of corticosteroid use in maxillofacial surgery

| | |
|---|---|
| 1 | Preoperative intralesional / parenteral administration of steroids to reduce the inflammation associated with surgery [125, 132]. |
| 2 | No adrenal suppression with small doses [125] |
| 3 | Long-term use—adrenal suppression interference with immune system & infection [126] |
| 4 | Usually tapering of dose is not required for short-term uses [137] |
| 5 | Contraindications [138]:<br>Active tuberculosis<br>Active viral / fungal infections<br>Active acne vulgaris<br>Primary glaucoma<br>Patients with psychoses |
| 6 | Use with care [138]:<br>Diverticulitis<br>Peptic ulcers<br>Cushing's syndrome<br>Renal insufficiency<br>Uncontrolled hypertension<br>Uncontrolled diabetes mellitus<br>Pregnancy & lactation<br>Chronic infections<br>Myasthenia gravis |
| 8 | Exogenous steroid dose > endogenous cortisol level [123, 138] |

## 10.8 Conclusion

Maxillofacial surgical practice involves use of many therapeutics to facilitate the treatment or promote healing. A careful evaluation of these drugs or reported literature, a detailed knowledge about their side effects, interactions with other chemicals, and how any alterations in the patient's physiology enhance or suppress the mechanism of action of these drugs is needed before their use or prescription. It is always prudent to remember that no medicine is without side effects and the benefits of using them should be weighed against the risks involved.

## References


1. Dandon RH, Brual LL. Goodman & Gilman's manual of pharmacology and therapeutics. 2nd ed. New York: McGraw Hill Education; 2014.
2. Gaynes R. The discovery of penicillin—new insights after more than 75 years of clinical use. Emerg Infect Dis. 2017;23(5):849–53.
3. Waksman SA. What is an antibiotic or antibiotic substance? Mycologia. 1947;39(5):565–9.
4. Salit IE. Diagnostic approaches to head and neck infections. Infect Dis Clin N Am. 1988;2:35–55.
5. Kuriyama T, Karasawa T, Nakagawa K, Saiki Y, Yamamoto E, Nakamura S. Bacteriologic features and antimicrobial susceptibility in isolates from orofacial odontogenic infections. Oral Surg Oral Med Oral Pathol Oral Radiol Endod. 2000;90:600–8.
6. Paterson SA, Curzon MEJ. The effect of amoxicillin versus penicillin V in the treatment of acutely abscessed primary teeth. Br Dent J. 1993;174:443–9.
7. Chang C, et al. Overview of penicillin allergy. Clinic Rev Allerg Immunol. 2012;43:84–97.
8. Raz R, Elchanan G, Colodner R, et al. Penicillin V twice daily vs four times daily in the treatment of streptococcal pharyngitis. Infect Dis Clin Pract. 1995;4:50–4.
9. Martin MP, Longman LP, Hill JB, et al. Acute dento alveolar infections: an investigation of the duration of antibiotic therapy. Br Dent J. 1997;183:135–7.
10. DePestel DD, et al. Cephalosporin use in treatment of patients with penicillin allergies. J Am Pharm Assoc. 2008;48:530–40.
11. Kelkar PS, Li JT. Cephalosporin allergy. N Engl J Med. 2001;345:804–9.
12. Burke JF. The effective period of preventative antibiotic action in experimental incisions and dermal lesions. Surgery. 1961;50:161–8.
13. Miles AA, Miles EM, Burke J. The value and duration of defense reaction of the skin to the primary lodgment of bacteria. Br J Exp Pathol. 1957;38:79–96.
14. Classen DC, Evans RS, Pestotnik SL, et al. The timing of prophylactic administration of antibiotics and risk of surgical-wound infection. N Engl J Med. 1992;326:281–6.
15. Pallasch TJ. Antibiotic prophylaxis: the clinical significance of its recent evolution. J Calif Dent Assoc. 1997;25(619–24):26–32.
16. Kamolratanakul P, Jansisyanont P. A review of antibiotic prophylaxis protocols in oral and maxillofacial surgery. J Oral Maxillofac Surg Med Pathol. 2018;30:395–404.
17. Garner JS. CDC guideline for prevention of surgical wound infections, 1985. Supersedes guideline for prevention of surgical wound infections published in 1982. (originally published in November 1985). Revised. Infect Control. 1986;7:193–200.
18. Peterson LJ. Antibiotic prophylaxis against wound infections in oral and maxillofacial surgery. J Oral Maxillofac Surg. 1990;48:617–620.
19. Tan SK, Lo J, Zwahlen RA. Perioperative antibiotic prophylaxis in orthognathic surgery: a systematic review and meta-analysis of clinical trials. Oral Surg Oral Med Oral Pathol Oral Radiol Endod. 2011;112:19–27.
20. Sancho-Puchades M, Herraez-Vilas JM, Berini-Aytes L, Gay-Escoda C. Antibiotic prophylaxis to prevent local infection in Oral surgery: use or abuse? Oral Med Oral Patol Oral Cir Bucal. 2009;14:E28–33.
21. Lewis MAO, McGowan DA, Macfarlane TW. Short – course, high-dosage amoxicillin in the treatment of acute dento-alveolar abscess. Br Dent J. 1986;161:299–302.
22. Lodi G, Figini L, Sardella A, Carrassi A, Del Fabbro M, Furness S. Antibiotics to prevent complications following tooth extractions. Cochrane Database Syst Rev. 2012;11:CD003811.
23. Figueiredo R, Valmaseda-Castellon E, Formoso-Senande MF, Berini-Aytes L, GayEscoda C. Delayed-onset infections after impacted lower third molar extraction: involved bacteria and sensitivity profiles to commonly used antibiotics. Oral Surg Oral Med Oral Pathol Oral Radiol Endod. 2012;144:43–8.
24. Sekhar CH, Narayanan V, Baig MF. Role of antimicrobials in third molar surgery: prospective, double blind, randomized, placebo-controlled clinical study. Br J Oral Maxillofac Surg. 2001;39:134–7.

25. Adde CA, Soares MS, Romano MM, et al. Clinical and surgical evaluation of the indication of postoperative antibiotic prescription in third molar surgery. Oral Surg Oral Med Oral Pathol Oral Radiol. 2012;114(5 Suppl):S26–31.
26. Lacasa JM, Jimenez JA, Ferras V, Bossom M, Sola-Morales O, Garcia-Rey C, et al. Prophylaxis versus pre-emptive treatment for infective and inflammatory complications of surgical third molar removal: a randomized, double-blind, placebo-controlled, clinical trial with sustained release amoxicillin/clavulanic acid (1000/62.5 mg). Int J Oral Maxillofac Surg. 2007;36:321–7.
27. Pasupathy S, Alexander M. Antibiotic prophylaxis in third molar surgery. J Craniofac Surg. 2011;22:551–3.
28. Menon RK, Gopinath D, Li KY, et al. Does the use of amoxicillin/amoxicillin–clavulanic acid in third molar surgery reduce the risk of postoperative infection? A systematic review with meta-analysis. Int J Oral Maxillofac Surg. 2018;48(2): 263–73.
29. Poeschl PW, Eckel D, Poeschl E. Postoperative prophylactic antibiotic treatment in third molar surgery–a necessity? J Oral Maxillofac Surg. 2004;62:3–8. Discussion 9
30. Larsen PE. The effect of chlorhexidine rinse on the incidence of alveolar osteitis following the surgical removal of impacted mandibular third molars. J Oral Maxillofac Surg. 1991;49:932–7.
31. Lyall JB. Third molar surgery: the effect of primary closure, wound dressing and metroniadazole on postoperative recovery. J R Army Med Corps. 1991;137:100–3.
32. Ren Y-F, Malmstrom HS. Effectiveness of antibiotic prophylaxis in third molar surgery: a meta-analysis of randomized controlled clinical trials. J Oral Maxillofac Surg. 2007;65(10):1909–21.
33. Resnik RR, Misch C. Prophylactic antibiotic regimens in oral implantology: rationale and protocol. Implant Dent. 2008;17:142–50.
34. Rasmusson L, Roos J, Bystedt H. A 10-year follow-up study of titanium dioxide-blasted implants. Clin Implant Dent Relat Res. 2005;7(1):36–42.
35. Friberg B. Sterile operating conditions for the placement of intraoral implants. J Oral Maxillofac Surg. 1996;54:1334–6.
36. Esposito M, Coulthard P, Oliver R, Thomsen P, Worthington HV. Antibiotics to prevent complications following dental implant treatment. Cochrane Database Syst Rev. 2003:CD004152.
37. Hossein K, Dahlin C, Bengt A. Influence of different prophylactic antibiotic regimens on implant survival rate: a retrospective clinical study. Clin Impl Dent Rel Res. 2005;7(1):32–5.
38. Davis CM, Gregoire CE, Steeves TW, et al. Prevalence of surgical site infections following orthognathic surgery: a retrospective cohort analysis. J Oral Maxillofac Surg. 2016;74:1199–206.
39. Chow LK, Singh B, Chiu WK, Samman N. Prevalence of postoperative complications after orthognathic surgery: a 15-year review. J Oral Maxillofac Surg. 2007;65:984–92.
40. Horan TC, Gaynes RP, Martone WJ, Jarvis WR, Emori G. CDC definitions of nosocomial surgical site infections, 1992: a modification of CDC definitions of surgical wound infections. Infect Control Hosp Epidemiol. 1992;13(10):606–8.
41. Danda AK, Ravi PE. Ectiveness of postoperative antibiotics in orthognathic surgery: a meta-analysis. J Oral Maxillofac Surg. 2011;69:2650–6.
42. Posnick JC, Choi E, Chavda A. Surgical site infections following bimaxillary orthognathic, osseous genioplasty, and intranasal surgery: a retrospective cohort study. J Oral Maxillofac Surg. 2017;75:584–95.
43. Danda AK, Wahab A, Narayanan V, Siddareddi A. Single-dose versus single-day antibiotic prophylaxis for orthognathic surgery: a prospective, randomized, double-blind clinical study. J Oral Maxillofac Surg. 2010;68:344–6.
44. Brignardello-Petersen R, Carrasco-Labra A, Araya I, Yanine N, Cordova Jara L, Villanueva J. Antibiotic prophylaxis for preventing infectious complications in orthognathic surgery. Cochrane Database Syst Rev. 2015;1:CD010266.
45. Mangram AJ, Horan TC, Pearson ML, et al. Guideline for prevention of surgical site infection, 1999. Centers for Disease Control and Prevention (CDC) hospital infection control practices advisory committee. Am J Infect Control. 1999;27:97–132.
46. Peel TN, Buising KL, Choong PF. Prosthetic joint infection: challenges of diagnosis and treatment. ANZ J Surg. 2011;81:32–9.
47. Fridrich KL, Partnoy BE, Zeitler DL. Prospective analysis of antibiotic prophylaxis for orthognathic surgery. Int J Adult Orthodontics Ortho Surg. 1994;9(2):129–31.
48. Laskin DM. The use of prophylactic antibiotics for the prevention of postoperative infections. Oral Maxillofac Surg Clin North Am. 2003;15:155–60.
49. Abubaker O, Rollert MK. Postoperative antibiotic prophylaxis in mandibular fractures: a preliminary randomized, double-blind, and placebo-controlled clinical study. J Oral Maxillofac Surg. 2001;59:1415–9.
50. Haug RH, Assael LA. Infection in the maxillofacial trauma patient. In: Topazian RG, Goldberg MH, Hupp JR, editors. *Oral and Maxillofacial Infections*. Ed 4. Philadelphia: PA, Saunders; 2002. p. 359–80.
51. Andreasen JO, Jensen SS, Schwartz O, Hillerup Y. A systematic review of prophylactic antibiotics in the surgical treatment of maxillofacial fractures. J Oral Maxillofac Surg. 2006;64:1664–8.
52. Dillon JK, Christensen B, McDonald T, et al. The financial burden of mandibular trauma. J Oral Maxillofac Surg. 2012;70:2124–34.
53. Shridharani SM, Berli J, Manson PN, et al. The role of postoperative antibiotics in mandible fractures: a systematic review of the literature. Ann Plast Surg. 2015;75:353–7.
54. Gaal A, Patel Y, Smiley N, et al. Limiting antibiotics when managing mandible fractures may not increase infection risk. J Oral Maxillofac Surg. 2016;74:2008–18.
55. Baliga SD, Bose A, Jain S. The evaluation of efficacy of post-operative antibiotics in the open reduction of the zygomatic and mandibular fracture: a prospective trial. J Maxillofac Oral Surg. 2014;13:165–75.
56. Miles BA, Potter JK, Ellis E. The efficacy of postoperative antibiotic regimens in the open treatment of mandibular fractures: a prospective randomized trial. J Oral Maxillofac Surg. 2006;64:576–82.
57. Goodson WH III, Hunt TK. Wound healing and the diabetic patient. Surg Gynecol Obstet. 1979;149:600–8.
58. Zoeller GN, Kadis B. The diabetic dental patient. Gen Dent. 1981;29:58–61.
59. Rahimi-Nedjat RK, Sagheb K, Pabst A, et al. Diabetes and hyperglycemia as risk factors for postoperative outcome in maxillofacial surgery. J Surg Res. 2017;217:170–6.
60. Ramaraj PN, Cariappa KM. Is there a need for antibiotic prophylaxis after routine dental extraction in diabetic patients? Br J Oral Maxillofac Surg. 2006;44:421.
61. Lee DH, Kim SY, Nam SY, Choi SH, Choi JW, Roh JL. Risk factors of surgical site infection in patients undergoing major oncological surgery for head and neck cancer. Oral Oncol. 2011;47:528–31.
62. Bartella A, Kamal M, Teichmann J, et al. Prospective comparison of perioperative antibiotic management protocols in oncological head and neck surgery. J Cran-Max-Fac Surg. 2017;45:1078–82.
63. Zhang Y, Dong J, Qiao Y, He J, Wang T, Ma S. Efficacy and safety profile of antibiotic prophylaxis usage in clean and clean-contaminated plastic and reconstructive surgery: a meta-analysis of randomized controlled trials. Ann Plast Surg. 2014;72:121–30.
64. Ariyan S, Martin J, Lal A, Cheng D, Borah GL, Chung KC, et al. Antibiotic prophylaxis for preventing surgical-site infection in plastic surgery: an evidence-based consensus conference statement from the American Association of Plastic Surgeons. Plast Reconstr Surg. 2015;135:1723–39.

65. Mercer NSG. The use of preoperative swabs in cleft lip and palate repair. Br J Plast Snrg. 2002;55:176–7.
66. Moss ALH. The use of preoperative swabs in cleft lip and palate repair. Br J Plast Surg. 2002;55:533–4.
67. Chuo CB, Timmons MJ. The bacteriology of children before primary cleft lip and palate surgery. The Cleft Palat-Craniofac J. 2005;42(3):272–6.
68. Rennie AL, Treharne LJ, Richard B. Throat swabs taken on the operating table prior to cleft palate repair and their relevance to outcome: a prospective study. Cleft Palate Craniofac J. 2009 May;46(3):275–9.
69. Aznar ML, Schönmeyr B, Echaniz G, et al. Role of postoperative antimicrobials in cleft palate surgery. Plast Recon Surg. 2015;136(1):59e–66e.
70. Douglas LR, Douglass JB, Sieck JO, Smith PJ. Oral management of the patient with end-stage liver disease and the liver transplant patient. Oral Surg Oral Med Oral Pathol Oral Radiol Endod. 1998;36:55–64.
71. Guggenheimer J, Mayher D, Eghtesad B. A survey of dental care protocols among US organ transplant centers. Clin Transpl. 2005;19:15–8.
72. Lewis T, Grant RT. Observations relating to subacute infective endocarditis. BrHeart J. 1923;10:21–77.
73. Jones TD, Baumgartner L, Bellows MT, et al. Prevention of rheumatic fever and bacterial endocarditis through control of streptococcal infections. Circulation. 1955;11:317–20.
74. Wilson W, Taubert KA, Gewitz M, et al. American Heart Association. Prevention of infective endocarditis: guidelines from the American Heart Association: a guideline from the American Heart Association rheumatic fever, endocarditis and Kawasaki disease committee, council on cardiovascular disease in the young, and the council on clinical cardiology, council on cardiovascular surgery and anesthesia, and the quality of care and outcomes research interdisciplinary working group. JADA. 2008;139(suppl):3S–24S.
75. Gould FK, Elliott TSJ, Foweraker J, et al. Guidelines for the prevention of endocarditis: report of the working party of the British society for antimicrobial chemotherapy. J Antimicrob Chemother. 2006 57:1035–42.
76. Prophylaxis against infective endocarditis. National institute for health and care excellence. 2008.
77. Habib G, Hoen B, Tornos P, et al. Guidelines on the prevention, diagnosis, and treatment of infective endocarditis (new version 2009): the task force on the prevention, diagnosis, and treatment of infective endocarditis of the European society of cardiology (ESC). Endorsed by the European society of clinical microbiology and infectious diseases (ESCMID) and the international society of chemotherapy (ISC) for infection and cancer. Eur Heart J. 2009;30:2369–413.
78. Pasquali SK, He X, Mohamad Z, et al. Trends in endocarditis hospitalizations at US children's hospitals: impact of the 2007 American Heart Association antibiotic prophylaxis guidelines. Am Heart J. 2012;163:894–9.
79. Sakai Bizmark R, Chang R-KR, Tsugawa Y, et al. Impact of AHA's 2007 guideline change on incidence of infective endocarditis in infants and children. Am Heart J. 2017;189:110–9.
80. Pain terms: a list with definitions and notes on usage. Recommended by the IASP Subcommittee on taxonomy. Pain. 1979;6:249–52.
81. Feizerfan A, Sheh G. Transition from acute to chronic pain. Contin Educ Anaesth Crit Care Pain. 2015;15:98–102.
82. Luo Y, Svensson P, Jensen JD, et al. Quantitative sensory testing in patients with or without ongoing pain one year after orthognathic surgery. J Oral Facial Pain Headache. 2014;28:306–16.
83. Desjardins P. Patient pain and anxiety: the medical and psychologic challenges facing oral and maxillofacial surgery. J Oral Maxillofac Surg. 2000;58(2):1–3.
84. Pedersen A. Interrelation of complaints after removal of impacted mandibular third molars. Int J Oral Surg. 1985;14:241–4.
85. Crane M, Green P, Gordon N. Pharmacology of opioid and non-opioid analgesics. Oral Maxillofacial Surg Clin N Am. 2001;13:1–13.
86. Coulthard P, Bailey E, Patel N, Coulthard MB. Pain pathways and pre-emptive and protective analgesia for oral surgery. Oral Surg. 2013;7(2):74–80.
87. Woolf CJ, Chong MS. Preemptive analgesia treating postoperative pain by preventing the establishment of central sensitization. Anesth Analg. 1993;77:362–79.
88. Woolf CJ. Evidence for a central component of postinjury pain hypersensitivity. Nature. 1983;306:686–8.
89. Viswanath A, Oreadi D, Finkelman M, Klein G, Papageorge M. Does pre-Emptive Administration of Intravenous Ibuprofen (Caldolor) or intravenous acetaminophen(Ofirmev) reduce postoperative pain and subsequent narcotic consumption after third molar surgery? J Oral Maxillofac Surg. 2019;77(2):262–70.
90. Hutchison GL, Crofts SL, Gray IG. Preoperative piroxicam for postoperative analgesia in dental surgery. Br J Anaesth. 1990;65:500–3.
91. Ong KS, Seymour RA, Chen FG, Ho VC. Preoperative ketorolac has a preemptive effect for postoperative third molar surgical pain. Int J Oral Maxillofac Surg. 2004;33:771–6.
92. Aoki T, Yamaguchi H, Naito H, Shiiki K, Izawa K, Ota Y, Sakamoto H, Kaneko A. Premedication with cyclooxygenase-2 inhibitor meloxicam reduced postoperative pain in patients after oral surgery. Int J Oral Maxillofac Surg. 2006;35:613–7.
93. Desjardins PJ, Grossman EH, Kuss ME, Talwalker S, Dhadda S, Baum D, Hubbard RC. The injectable cyclooxygenase-2-specific inhibitor parecoxib sodium has analgesic efficacy when administered preoperatively. Anesth Analg. 2001;93:721–7.
94. Moore PA, Brar P, Smiga ER, Costello BJ. Preemptive rofecoxib and dexamethasone for prevention of pain and trismus following third molar surgery. Oral Surg Oral Med Oral Pathol Oral Radiol Endod. 2005;99:e1–7.
95. Møiniche S, Kehlet H, Dah JB. A qualitative and quantitative systematic review of preemptive analgesia for postoperative pain relief: the role of timing of analgesia. Anesthesiology. 2002;96:725–34.
96. Aznar Arasa L, Harutunian K, Figuereido R, et al. Effect of preoperative ibuprofen on pain and swelling after lower third molar removal: a randomized controlled trial. Int J Oral Maxillofac Surg. 2012;41:1005–9.
97. Evans SW, McCahon RA. Management of postoperative pain in maxillofacial surgery. Br J Oral Maxillofac Surg. 2019;57(1):4–11.
98. De Cosmo G, Congedo E, Lai C, et al. Preoperative psychologic and demographic predictors of pain perception and tramadol consumption using intravenous patient-controlled analgesia. Clin J Pain. 2008;24:399–405.
99. Coulthard P, Haywood D, Tai MA, Jackson-Leech D, Pleuvry BJ, Macfarlane TV. Treatment of postoperative pain in oral and maxillofacial surgery. Br J Oral Maxillofac Surg. 2000;38(6):588–92.
100. Mobini A, Mehra P, Chigurupathy R. Postoperative pain and opioid analgesic requirements after orthognathic surgery. J Oral Maxillofac Surg. 2018;76:2285–95.
101. Moore PA, Hersch EV. Analgesic therapy in dentistry - from a letter to the editor to an evidence-base review. Dent Clin N Am. 2019;63:35–44.
102. Fletcher MC, Spera JF. Management of acute postoperative pain after oral surgery. Dent Clin N Am. 2012;56:95–111.
103. Rudd RA, Seth P, David F, Scholl L. Increases in drug and opioid involved overdose deaths—United States, 2010-2015. Morb Mortal Wkly Rep. 2016;65:1445–52.

104. Patel N, Bailey E, Coulthard P. Opioids for pain after oral surgery. Oral Surg. 2013;7(4):196–202.
105. Moore RA, Derry S, McQuay HJ, Wiffen PJ. Single dose oral analgesics for acute postoperative pain in adults. Cochrane Database Syst Rev. 2011;9:CD008659.
106. Ceccheti MM, Negrato GV, de Melo Peres MP, et al. Analgesic and adjuvant anesthetic effect of submucosal tramadol after mandibular third molar surgery. Oral Surg Oral Med Oral Path Oral Radiol. 2014;117(3):e249–54.
107. Power I, Barratt S. Analgesic agents for the postoperative period: nonopioids. Surg Clin North Am. 1999;79:275–95.
108. Moore P, Hersh E. Celecoxib and rofecoxib, the role of COX-2 inhibitors in dental practice. J Am Dent Assoc. 2001;132: 451–6.
109. Seymour RA, Moore U, Hawkesford J, Coulthard P, Jackson-Leech D, Thomas D, Hill M, Combs ML, Renton T, McGurk M. An investigation into the efficacy of intravenous diclofenac in post-operative dental pain. Eur J Clin Pharmacol. 2000 Sep;56(6-7):447–52.
110. Derry CJ, Derry S, Moore RA, McQuay HJ. Single dose oral ibuprofen for acute postoperative pain in adults. Cochrane Database Syst Rev. 2009;3:CD010210.
111. Gyllfors P, Bochenek G, Overholt J, et al. Biochemical and clinical evidence that aspirin intolerant asthmatic subjects tolerate the cyclooxygenase 2-selective analgesic drug celecoxib. J Allergy Clin Immunol. 2003;111:1116–21.
112. Weil K, Hooper L, Afzal Z, et al. Paracetamol for pain relief after surgical removal of wisdom teeth. Cochrane Database Syst Rev. 2007;3:CD004487.
113. Laskarides C. Update on analgesic medication for adult and pediatric dental patients. Dent Clin N Am. 2016;60:347–66.
114. World Health Organization. WHO Pain Ladder. 2013. Available from URL: http://www.who.int/cancer/palliative/painladder/en/.
115. Buvanendran A, Kroin JS. Multimodal analgesia for controlling acute postoperative pain. Curr Opin Anaesthesiol. 2009;22:588–93.
116. Yong SL, Walsh T, Coulthard P. Protective analgesia for postoperative pain following third molar surgery [protocol]. Cochrane Database Syst Rev. 2010;9:CD008692.
117. Rosero EB, Joshi GP. Preemptive, preventive. Multimodal Analgesia Plast Recon Surg. 2014;134:85S–93S.
118. Rood JP, Coulthard P, Snowdon AT, Gennery BA. Safety and efficacy of levobupivacaine for postoperative pain relief after the surgical removal of impacted third molars: a comparison with lignocaine and adrenaline. Br J Oral Maxillofac Surg. 2002 Dec;40(6):491–6.
119. Chang FSC, Burrows A, Gebauer DP. Patient-controlled analgesia and length of hospital stay in orthognathic surgery: a randomized controlled trial. J Oral Maxillofac Surg. 2019;77:818–27.
120. Geha H, Nimeskern N, Beziat J. Patient-controlled analgesia in orthognathic surgery: evaluation of the relationship to anxiety and anxiolytics. Oral Surg Oral Med Oral Pathol Oral Radiol Endod. 2009;108:e33–6.
121. Hudcova J, McNicol ED, Quah CS, Lau J, Carr DB. Patient controlled opioid analgesia versus conventional opioid analgesia for postoperative pain. Cochrane Database Syst Rev. 2006;4:CD003348.
122. Peterson LJ. Postoperative patient management. In: Peterson LJ, Ellis E, Hupp JR, Tucker MR, editors. Contemporary oral and maxillofacial surgery. 3rd ed. St Louis: Mosby; 1998. p. 251.
123. Gilman AG, Rall TW, Nies AS, et al. The pharmacological basis of therapeutics (ed 8). New York, NY: Macmillan; 1990. p. 1436–52.
124. Axelrod L. Adrenal corticosteroids. In: Miller RR, Greenblatt, editors. Handbook of drug Therauv. New York. NY: Elsevier; 1979. p. 809–40.
125. Beirne OR, Hollander B. The effect of methylprednisolone on pain, trismus, and swelling after removal of third molar. Oral Surg Oral Med Oral Path. 1986;61:134–8.
126. Markiewicz MR, Brady MF, Ding EL, Dodson TB. Corticosteroids reduce postoperative morbidity after third molar surgery: a systematic review and meta-analysis. J Oral Maxillofac Surg. 2008;66(9):1881–94.
127. Alexander RE, Throndson RT. A review of perioperative corticosteroid use in dentoalveolar surgery. Oral Surg Oral Med Oral Pathol. 2000;90:406–15.
128. Montgomery MT, Hogg JP, Roberts DL, et al. The use of glucocorticosteroids to lessen the inflammatory sequelae following third molar surgery. J Oral Maxillofac Surg. 1990;48:179–87.
129. Pedersen A. Decadronphosphate in the relief of complaints after third molar surgery. Int J Oral Maxillofac Surg. 1985;14:235–40.
130. Grossi GB, Maiorana C, Garramone RA. Effect of submucosal injection of dexamethasone on postoperative discomfort after third molar surgery: a prospective study. J Oral Maxillofac Surg. 2007;65:2218–26.
131. Messer EJ, Keller JJ. The use of intraoral dexamethasone after extraction of mandibular third molar. Oral Surg Oral Med Oral Pathol. 1975;40:594–8.
132. Brucoli M, De Andreis M, Boffano BP, et al. Comparative assessment of dexamethasone administration routes for the management of postoperative symptoms following third molar surgery. J Stomatol Oral Maxillofac Surg. 2019.
133. de Almeida AC, Lemos CAA, de Moraes SLD, et al. Efficacy of corticosteroids versus placebo in impacted third molar surgery: systematic review and meta-analysis of randomized controlled trials. Int J Oral Maxillofac Surg. 2019;48:118–31.
134. Kainulainen S, Lassus P, Suominen AL, et al. More harm than benefit of perioperative dexamethasone on recovery following reconstructive head and neck cancer surgery: a prospective double-blind randomized trial. J Oral Maxillofac Surg. 2018;76:2425–32.
135. Dionne RA, Gordon SM, Rowan J, et al. Dexamethasone suppresses peripheral prostanoid levels without analgesia in a clinical model of acute inflammation. J Oral Maxillofac Surg. 2003;61:997–1003.
136. de Sousa Santos JAS, DaSilva LCF, de Santana Santos T, et al. Comparative study of tramadol combined with dexamethasone and diclofenac sodium in third-molar surgery. J Cranio-Maxillo-Facial Surg. 2012;40:694–700.
137. Matheny JL. Adrenocorticosteroids: systemic and topical therapy. In: Holroyd SV, Wynn RL, Requa-Clark B, editors. Clinical pharmacology in dental practice. 4th ed. St Louis: Mosby; 1988. p. 238–45.
138. Butler RCD, Vorono AA, Finstuen K. Dosage effects of pulsed steroid therapy on serum cortisol levels in oral and maxillofacial surgery patients. J Oral Maxillofac Surg. 1993;51:750–3.


## Additional Reading


*Odontogenic microbiological spectrum.*

Lewis MAO, Macfarlane TW, McGown DA. A microbiological and clinical review of acute dentoalveolar abscesses. Br J Oral Maxillofac Surg. 1990;28:359–66.

Poeschl PW, Spusta L, Russmueller G, Seemann R, Hirschl A, Poeschl E, et al. Antibiotic susceptibility and resistance of the odontogenic microbiological spectrum and its clinical impact on severe deep space head and neck infections. Oral Surg Oral Med Oral Pathol Oral Radiol Endod. 2010;110:151–6.

*Antibiotic prophylaxis.*

Moreno-Drada JA, Garcia-Perdomo HA. Effectiveness of antimicrobial prophylaxis in preventing the spread of infection as a result of oral procedures: a systematic review and meta-analysis. J Oral Maxillofac Surg. 2016;74:1313–21.

*Antibiotics in third molar surgery.*

Bezerra TP, Studart-Soares EC, Scaparo HC, Pita-Neto IC, Batista SH, Fonteles CS. Prophylaxis versus placebo treatment for infective and inflammatory complications of surgical third molar removal: a split-mouth, double-blind, controlled, clinical trial with amoxicillin (500 mg). J Oral Maxillofac Surg. 2011;69:e333–9.

Monaco G, Tavernese L, Agostini R, Marchetti C. Evaluation of antibiotic prophylaxis in reducing postoperative infection after mandibular third molar extraction in young patients. J Oral Maxillofac Surg. 2009;67:1467–72.

Lopez-Cedrun JL, Pijoan JI, Fernandez S, Santamaria J, Hernandez G. Efficacy of amoxicillin treatment in preventing postoperative complications in patients undergoing third molar surgery: a prospective, randomized, double-blind controlled study. J Oral Maxillofac Surg. 2011;69:e5–14.

*Antibiotics in implants.*

Chrcanovic BR, Albrektsson T, Wennerberg A. Prophylactic antibiotic regimen and dental implant failure: a meta-analysis. J Oral Rehabil. 2014;41:941–56.

*Antibiotics in orthognathic surgery.*

Bentley KC, Head TW, Aiello GA. Antibiotic prophylaxis in orthognathic surgery: a 1-day versus 5-day regimen. J Oral Maxillofac Surg. 1999;57(3):226–30. Discussion 230-2

Tan SK, Lo J, Zwahlen RA. Are postoperative intravenous antibiotics necessary after bimaxillary orthognathic surgery? A prospective, randomized, double-blind, placebo-controlled clinical trial. Int J Oral Maxillofac Surg. 2011;40:1363–8.

Brignardello-Petersen R, Carrasco-Labra A, Araya I, et al. Antibiotic prophylaxis for preventing infectious complications in orthognathic surgery. Cochrane Database of Systematic Reviews. 2015.

Lindeboom JA, Baas EM, Kroon FH. Prophylactic singledose administration of 600 mg clindamycin versus 4-time administration of 600 mg clindamycin in orthognathic surgery: a prospective randomized study in bilateral mandibular sagittal ramus osteotomies. Oral Surgery, Oral Medicine, Oral Pathology and Radiology and Endodontics. 2003;95(2):145–9.

*Steroids in third molar surgery.*

Graziani F, D'Aiuto F, Arduino PG, et al. Perioperative dexamethasone reduces post-surgical sequelae of wisdom tooth removal. A split-mouth randomized double-masked clinical trial. Int J Oral Maxillofac Surg. 2006;35:241–6.

Lim D, Ngeow WC. A comparative study on the efficacy of submucosal injection of dexamethasone versus methylprednisolone in reducing postoperative sequelae after third molar surgery. J Oral Maxillofac Surg. 2017;75:2278–86.

*Steroids in orthognathic surgery.*

Dan AEB, Thygesen TH, Pinbolt EM. Corticosteroid administration in oral and orthognathic surgery: a systematic review of the literature and meta-analysis. J Oral Maxillofac Surg. 2010;68:2207–20.

# 11 Wound Closure and Care in Oral and Maxillofacial Surgery

Ravi Veeraraghavan

## 11.1 Wound Management

Management of soft tissue wounds needs a careful assessment of the wound, a good understanding of wound types and healing as well as adequate knowledge and skill for wound care. The various steps in wound care include cleansing and debridement, hemostasis, tetanus immunization and antibiotic medication and wound closure.

Wound closure can be accomplished in diverse ways, but suturing remains the mainstay. A wide variety of materials are available for wound suturing. One has to choose the right material and technique depending on the wound type and closure needs. Alternate techniques such as staples, tapes and adhesives are fast gaining popularity.

Wounds are treated by

1. Cleansing and debridement,
2. Haemostasis,
3. Tetanus immunisation,
4. Wound dressings,
5. Wound closure,
6. Antibiotic medication.

## 11.2 Wound Closure

Artificial closure of the wounds is required if significant connective tissue is exposed. Wound closure leads to faster wound healing with reduced complications. Even though suturing is the mainstay of wound closure, other alternatives are fast gaining popularity.

**Electronic Supplementary Material** The online version of this chapter (https://doi.org/10.1007/978-981-15-1346-6_11) contains supplementary material, which is available to authorized users.

R. Veeraraghavan (✉)
Department of Oral and Maxillofacial Surgery, Amrita School of Dentistry, Ernakulam, India

### 11.2.1 Purposes of Wound Closure

Before going into the intricacies of material selection and techniques of wound closure, one needs to be clear about the actual need for artificially closing a wound. The main indication for wound closure is significant exposure of connective tissue. In general, there are five reasons behind the concept of wound closure.

1. *Healing by Primary Intention*
   This is the most important purpose of wound closure. The open wounds, which are likely to heal by secondary intention, are made to heal in a 'more' primary manner by the intervention of wound closure. This hastens the healing process and also reduces scar formation, with resultant advantages in aesthetic and functional facets.
2. *Coverage of Deep Tissues*
   When the epithelium is breached and connective tissue is bared, it exposes the inner tissues to mechanical and biological threats. This threat becomes even more serious when deeper structures such as the viscera or bone is exposed.
3. *Prevent Contamination*
   An open wound is under constant attack by the pathogenic microorganisms, more so in the oral cavity. Such relentless contamination is likely to lead to a full-blown infection and/or delayed healing. Sooner the wound is closed, the lesser the risk of major contamination.
4. *Haemostasis*
   This is not one of the primary purposes of wound closure. But sutures may help in impeding blood loss by preventing mechanical disturbance to the clot.
5. *Prevention of Dead Space*
   If only the superficial cutaneous sutures are placed over a deep wound, a dead space can result beneath the surface. This condition usually leads to wound breakdown and/or wound infection. Dead space is prevented by closing the deep tissues in multiple layers.


K. Bonanthaya et al. (eds.), *Oral and Maxillofacial Surgery for the Clinician*, https://doi.org/10.1007/978-981-15-1346-6_11

## 11.3 Wound Suturing

Suturing is the process of wound closure by holding the edges of the wound together using a thread. This thread, called a 'suture', is used to approximate the wound edges together and to hold them in position till the tissue healing is sufficiently advanced to maintain themselves in the corrected anatomic position and alignment to each other. The surgeon uses a 'suture needle' to pass the thread through the tissues on either side of the wound so as to hold the separated edges in the proper position.

### 11.3.1 Suturing Instruments

Apart from the suture thread and needle, some instruments are used to perform the suturing process. Commonly used instruments include a needle holder, a tissue holding forceps and a pair of scissors.

#### 11.3.1.1 Needle Holder

The needle holder (needle driver) is the primary instrument used for suturing. Similar to a haemostat, it is used to grasp and manipulate the suture needle to which the thread is attached. A needle holder has three parts—a pair of beaks, a joint ('pivot') and a pair of handles with rings. Many designs are available, examples being Webster, Halsey and Mayo-Hegar. Most designs have a serrated or cross-hatching pattern of teeth for the beaks. This helps to grip the needle securely without damaging it. A locking mechanism similar to haemostats is present to lock the needle grasp.

The classical way to hold the instrument is to engage the handle-rings with the thumb and the fourth finger. The middle finger is used for support and the index finger is used to direct or orient the instrument in the required direction. Alternatively, while suturing on tough tissues, one may be 'palmed', i.e. may be held against the palm with fingers around. While palming the needle holder, some surgeons still rest the fourth finger lightly in the handle-ring.

#### 11.3.1.2 Tissue Holding Forceps

The pickup forceps are used to delicately handle and manipulate the wound edge which is being sutured. The fine-toothed Adson forceps is the workhorse for most interior and cutaneous wound closures. The forceps is held in the non-dominant hand and is used to grasp, lift and evert the wound edge so that the surface is made more amenable to a perpendicular needle entry. Fine skin hooks may also be used for the same purpose.

#### 11.3.1.3 Suture Cutting Scissors

The suture cutting scissors is used to cut the suture thread tags after the knot is tied. It is also used to cut the thread during suture removal.

These scissors should be differentiated from scissors used for cutting tissue. Many of them have specifically designed blades and tips, which are uniquely shaped to lift and grasp up the handing tags or the tied suture thread away from the tissue and to cut it safely without injuring the tissues. Short and long versions are available. The tip may be straight or curved and may have a sharp slot for the thread to be cut. Some manufacturers have incorporated a cutting component in the needle holder itself, using which the surgeon can cut the suture tag without switching instruments.

### 11.3.2 Suture Needles

The suture needles help to pass the suture threads through tissues. In ancient days, needles were made of natural materials such as bones, ivory, horns, wood or thorns. In fact, eyed needles from as early as 30,000 AD have been unearthed. Later, metals such as silver, copper and aluminium bronze were used. The modern needles are diligently shaped and contoured as per use and are smooth and strong so that they withstand the stresses of suturing and least traumatic to tissues at the same time.

The suture needle has three parts: the tip, the body and the suture attachment. Made of stainless steel or carbon steel, they are thin, smooth and sharp, designed to pass through tissues with ease (Fig. 11.1).

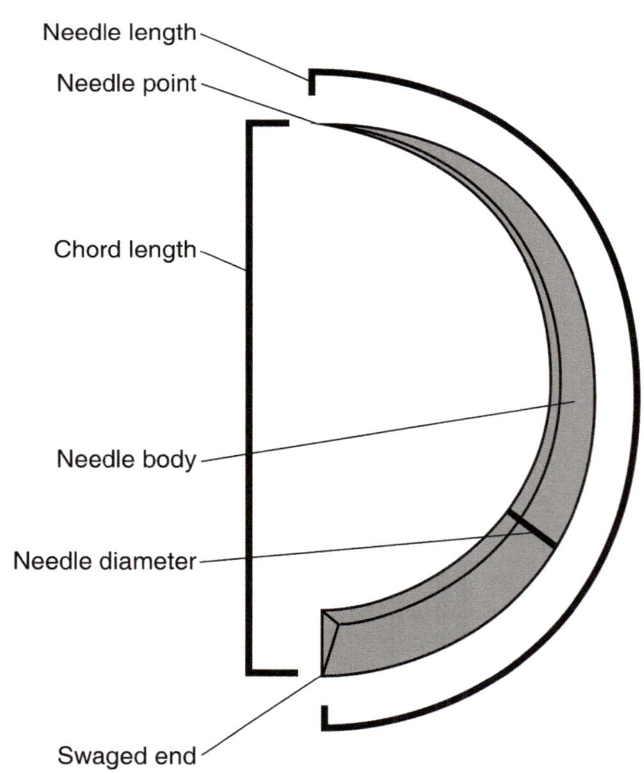




**Fig. 11.1** Parts of suture needle

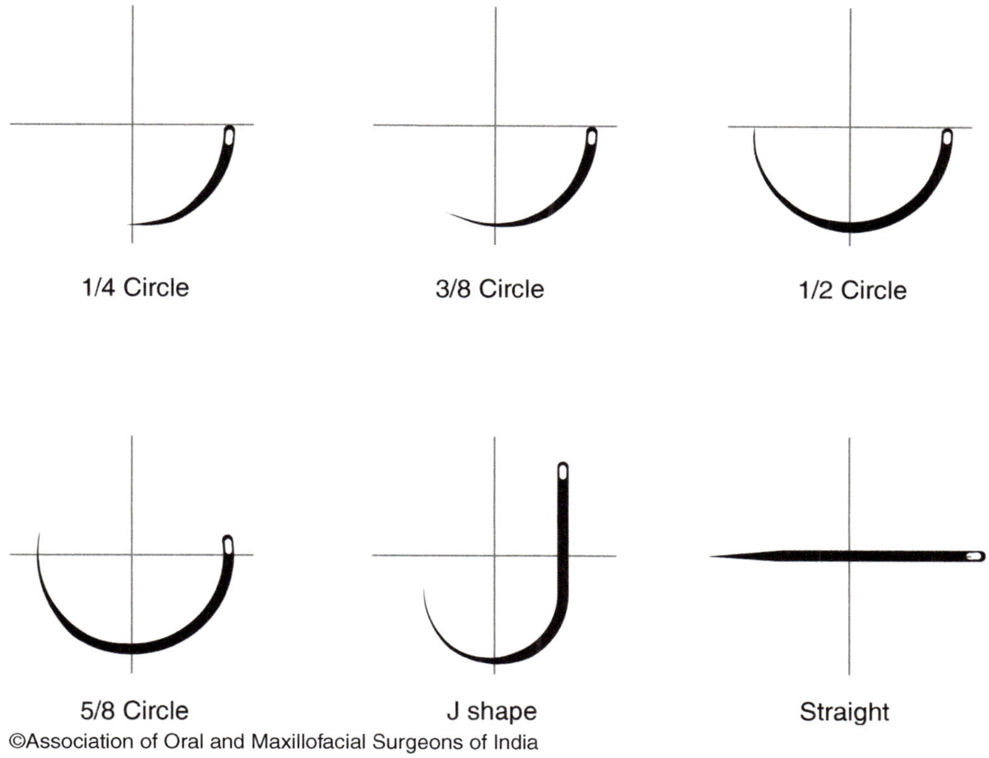


Fig. 11.2 Needle shapes/curvature

#### 11.3.2.1 Needle Shape

The suture needles are usually curved as an arc of a circle. Straight needles, though available, have very limited practical applications. The curvature is described as the span of the arc, in terms of ¼, $^{3}/_{8}$, ½ and $^{5}/_{8}$ of a circle. Most of the regular suturing in oral and maxillofacial surgery is done with half circle needles. A smaller arc such as $^{3}/_{8}$ can be used for suturing flat skin surfaces. Longer arc, i.e. $^{5}/_{8}$ circle, needles are used in narrow tunnelled surgical fields such as in cleft palate or inside the nose (Fig. 11.2).

The cross section and the tip of the needles can be widely varied. Depending on these aspects, the suture needles can be.

1. Round bodied,
2. Conventional cutting (Fig. 11.3) or
3. Reverse cutting.

Round bodied needles are generally used to suture viscera and other internal structures such as muscle and fascia. It can also be effective on non-keratinised mucosa. The tip of the round-bodied needle can be blunt or sharp. The blunt tip needle is specifically used in the inner abdominal wall and in friable tissues. The sharp tip is used for most other purposes. But even the sharp tip is hard to pass across the skin and keratinised mucosa. The shape of the 'cutting' needle overcomes this problem. In the cutting needles, the needle cross section is a triangle, with the inner curve side being pointed and the outer convex side flat. This shape enables the needle to 'cut' through the dense tissues to make the needle passage easier. But the cutting design presented a new problem. Even under minimum tension, the needle behaved like a knife, and the sharp edge often tended to lacerate the tissue resulting in a 'cut-through' of the wound edge. This was solved by the reverse-cutting design, wherein the inner curve is flat and the outer curve is pointed. This helps to retain the cutting nature while avoiding the risk of wound edge laceration. In oral and maxillofacial surgery, the tissues encountered may be keratinised (skin, gingiva and palate) or non-keratinised (buccal mucosa, floor of mouth and lips). Mostly, reverse-cutting needles are now being used since they are well-suited to pass through all oral tissues without causing inadvertent tears.

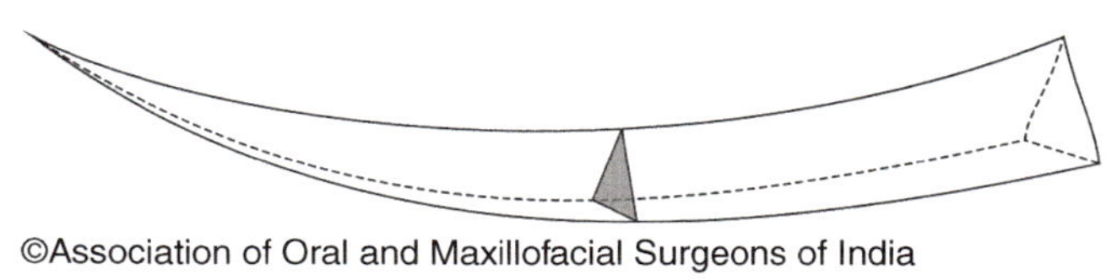


Fig. 11.3 Needle cross section of a conventional cutting needle

#### 11.3.2.2 Needle Size

The suture needle size generally depends on the size of the suture. In general, smaller the suture size, smaller the needle. It is important to recognise the various dimensions of a needle.

The 'needle length' refers to the end-to-end measurement along the curve of the needle. The straight line distance from the tip to the other end is called 'chord length'. The chord length determines the bite-width of the needle in the tissues. The bite-depth into the tissue is defined by the 'chord diameter' which is perpendicular from the chord length to the centre of the needle body. Needle diameter and needle radius are dimensions which refer to the cross-sectional thickness and not to the needle curve.

#### 11.3.2.3 Eyed vs Swaged Needles

The eye of the needle is a small hole at one end for attaching the suture thread. This necessitates an increase in the needle thickness at the attachment end, increasing the risk of potential tissue trauma. The suture is passed through the eye, and may then be tucked or tied for better retention. Both tucking and tying further increases the tissue drag and causes additional trauma. The attached suture now follows the needle through the tissues. The eyed needles are cheaper and can be reused after resterilisation.

Modern suture needles do not have an eye. Instead, the suture thread is sealed inside the needle for a permanent attachment. This mechanism, called 'swaging', reduces the tissue trauma significantly as the needle diameter is not increased for thread attachment. Further, only a single thread strand passes through the tissue at all times. So these needles are often called 'atraumatic needles'. The swaged needle with thread is available as a sterile pack, and cannot be reused.

## 11.4 Suture Thread

Many different types of suture threads are available for use. Each type has its specific benefits and indications for application (Table 11.1).

A basic classification divides them into 'natural' and 'synthetic'. Suture materials sourced from natural sources include catgut, steel and silk. Synthetic plastic materials such as nylon, polypropylene and polymers of glycolic acid, lactic acid, etc., have become popular in recent decades.

Suture materials can also be classified as absorbable and non-absorbable. Absorbable sutures hold the tissues together till they have healed sufficiently to withstand normal stress, and are then absorbed by the tissues where they are embedded. Non-absorbable sutures, on the other hand, are not absorbed, and they should be removed after the initial stabilisation of the wound edges has occurred. In reality, most or all natural materials will get absorbed by the body in due course of time. Thus, for clinical practice, a suture is considered non-absorbable if it retains its tensile strength in tissues for more than 60 days.

**Table 11.1** Suture material classification

| Basis of classification | Types |
|---|---|
| Source | Natural, synthetic |
| Absorbability | Absorbable, non-absorbable |
| Thread size | 3, 2, 1, 0, 1–0, 2–0, 3–0..........................11–0 |
| Filament type | Monofilament, multifilament (braided) |

According to the filament type, the sutures may be monofilament or multifilament. A monofilament suture is essentially a single strand of fibre. This simple structure enables these sutures to pass through tissues with least resistance. Though this makes it the material of choice in delicate tissues such as the vascular tissues, there are some notable drawbacks. The handling and knot-tying are generally more taxing, and the knot has less friction to keep its position. In addition, the cut edges tend to be stiff leading to probable irritation of movable and delicate regions like the tongue and buccal mucosa.

The multifilament sutures are made of multiple fibre strands, which are either coated or braided together to make one fine thread. The process of braiding bestows a higher tensile strength as well as better pliability and flexibility. This improves the handling characteristics and the ease of knot-tying. They also better resist the tendency of the knot to untie itself. The cut edges are usually smooth and soft, and are not irritating to oral tissues. The disadvantages of multifilament sutures include the higher risk of harbouring pathogens in its structure and the tendency to 'wick' the oral fluids into deeper tissues through the suture track. This, in turn, can lead to occurrence to unaesthetic suture tracks visible on the skin.

### 11.4.1 Suture Thread Size

The suture thread is available in different thicknesses. The thickness is usually mentioned as 'number of zeroes'. This system follows the U.S. Pharmacopeia, and has gained wide acceptance. The most commonly used thread size for intraoral use is mentioned as 3–0 or 000 size. Sutures are available from size 6 to 11–0 (Table 11.2).

**Attributes of an Ideal Suture Material**

1. Sterile or sterilisable,
2. Good handling characteristics,
3. Ensure a secure knot,
4. Adequate tensile strength,
5. Retention of strength during the healing phase,
6. Rapid absorption after healing.
7. Stay inert in tissues without causing antigenicity or other adverse tissue reaction.

**Table 11.2** Suture sizes—U.S. Pharmacopeia designation and equivalent metric measurements

| USP designation | 11–0 | 10–0 | 9–0 | 8–0 | 7–0 | 6–0 | 5–0 | 4–0 | 3–0 | 2–0 | 0 | 1 | 2 | 3 |
|---|---|---|---|---|---|---|---|---|---|---|---|---|---|---|
| Diameter (mm) | 0.01 | 0.02 | 0.03 | 0.04 | 0.05 | 0.07 | 0.1 | 0.15 | 0.2 | 0.3 | 0.35 | 0.4 | 0.5 | 0.6 |

It is beyond the purview of this chapter to go into the details of all the types of suture materials available in the market, chemical structure, method of resorption, qualities, indications, advantages, etc. Details of few suture materials widely used in oral and maxillofacial surgery are given below.

### 11.4.2 Natural Absorbable Sutures (Absorbed by Proteolysis)

The absorbability characteristics of many natural materials had been recognised for millennia. All absorbable natural suture materials contain predominantly collagen. Over the years, they have progressively fallen out of favour due to the risk of antigenicity and adverse tissue reaction [1].

#### 11.4.2.1 Catgut

Catgut has been the most popular material in this group. Its use has been prevalent at least from the time of Galen of Pergamon (200 AD). This material is made of tissue taken from the submucosal layer of sheep intestine or from the serosal (adventitial) layer of the cattle small intestine intima. The collagen strands are twisted together and the resultant thread is precision-ground to form a monofilament. Catgut has long been a popular fibre to make string instruments and tennis racquets. For many centuries, catgut (surgical gut) had been the only absorbable suture material available. The absorption is by proteolytic biodegradation brought about by proteolytic enzymes.

Performance-wise, catgut has good flexibility but relatively poor tensile strength, poor knot stability and high tissue reactivity. Full tensile strength remains only for 7 days.

#### 11.4.2.2 Chromic Catgut

It has been found that many poor characteristics of catgut can be overcome by impregnating the suture material with chromic salts. This modified product, called chromic catgut, has higher tensile strength and delayed absorption time. Chromic catgut retains its maximum tensile strength for about 2 weeks. It also has reduced tissue reaction as compared to plain gut.

Manufacturers package catgut sutures soaked in the disinfectant isopropyl alcohol solution to retain the flexibility and to increase shelf life. This necessitates rinsing of the suture in sterile saline to remove the irritant alcohol before use. Some manufacturers use a glycerine coating on chromic catgut to do away with the alcohol in packaging. Glycerine-coated chromic gut is smoother and thicker and has better handling characteristics.

### 11.4.3 Natural Non-absorbable Sutures

These are the oldest suture materials known to mankind. People tended to use any threaded material known to them for holding the wound edges together. Non-absorbable natural materials include cotton, linen, steel and silk.

#### 11.4.3.1 Cotton and Linen

Cotton and linen sutures primarily contain cellulose polymer. Both the materials get absorbed in due course, but are considered non-absorbable because of delayed absorption time. Cotton is sourced from the hair of the cotton seed while linen is made from flax. The fibres are twisted to form a suture. It has good tensile strength, but there is moderate tissue reaction. Handling is average but knot-holding is good. Linen has the advantage that it gains tensile strength when wet.

Cotton and linen have largely fallen out of favour because of adverse tissue reactions and the high 'wicking' effect which causes seepage of fluids into the suture track.

#### 11.4.3.2 Silk

Silk has been a well-known textile material from fourth millennium BC. It is produced by the silkworm larvae to form the cocoon. Natural silk is a protein fibre, the main components being fibroin and sericin. Fibroin forms the basic structure and contributes to the tensile strength. Sericin is a gum layer which holds the strands together. The silkworm larvae are cultivated and once they start pupating, the cocoons are dissolved in boiling water to extract the individual fibres which are fed into the spinning reel. To make it suitable as a medical product, the sericin protein component is later removed by a degumming process.

Silk is the most widely used natural non-absorbable suture material. Surgical silk is made from the larvae of the silkworm *Bombyx Mori*. The silk suture consists of a group of strands braided around a core and has a wax or silicon coating. It is usually dyed black in colour for better visibility.

The most impressive property of the silk suture is the ease of handling. It is extremely pliable and smooth and has good knot-holding capability. But the tensile strength is pretty low. The other drawbacks include high levels of tissue friction, capillary action and tissue inflammatory response. The wax coating helps to counteract all these negative attributes.

Silk is now not considered an appropriate material for cutaneous suturing, except on specific sites such as eyelids and lips. It is very often used for ligating blood vessels and for hitching drains. It is the most popular material used in dentistry. Its soft and pliable nature makes it suitable for use in oral mucosa which is mobile and wet.

### 11.4.4 Synthetic Non-absorbable Sutures

#### 11.4.4.1 Polyamide/Nylon (Ethilon, Dermalon)

Nylon belongs to the first generation of commercially successful synthetic thermoplastic polymers, having started production in 1927. It is made of repeated units linked by aliphatic or aromatic amide links (polyamide). It has been a very versatile material and has been used as fabric, fibres, films, coatings and moulded shapes for wide applications in diverse fields.

Nylon surgical sutures were introduced in 1940. Monofilament nylon sutures are very popular for cutaneous suturing. The main advantages are their high tensile strength, exceptional elasticity and low tissue reaction. The elasticity helps the material to accommodate tissue swelling and maintain wound edge apposition. The nylon sutures are dyed black in colour.

The biggest shortcoming of this material is its shape memory, which negatively affects its knot-tying and knot-holding properties. Often, one needs 3–4 knots to hold a stitch in place. Also, the monofilament may be stiff. Multifilament nylon sutures are available with increased pliability and handling features. Addition of fluid (alcohol) in the package reduces the shape memory and improves pliability.

#### 11.4.4.2 Polypropylene (Prolene, Surgipro)

Polypropylene is another thermoplastic polymer used as a non-absorbable suture material. It is produced by chain-growth polymerisation of the monomer propylene. It is pigmented blue to enhance visibility, hence the name polypropylene blue.

Similar to nylon, polypropylene has a very high tensile strength, excellent elasticity and minimal tissue reaction. It can extend up to 30% without breakage, making it highly suitable for suturing cutaneous wounds. The shape memory is also similar to nylon and can contribute to knot slippage. This feature, though, is advantageous in subcuticular suturing since it slides out smoothly during suture removal.

The excellent mechanical properties and inert nature have made polypropylene the material of choice in stressful sites. It is widely used in the management of hernia and vaginal prolapse, often in the form of a mesh in addition to sutures.

#### 11.4.4.3 Polyester (Ethibond, Surgidac, Dacron)

Polyester is a general term used for any organic polymer which has an ester functional group in the main chain. More specifically, the term is used for the material polyethylene terephthalate. It is a type of petroleum-based plastic, made by mixing ethylene glycol and terephthalic acid. Because of its durability, cleanability, anti-wrinkle and quick-drying characteristics, it swiftly made a name in the textile industry as a reliable material.

Polyester is a non-absorbable, braided, surgical suture with high tensile strength and low tissue reactivity. The braided nature adds to enhanced handling, knot-tying and retentivity. Thus, it combines the positive features generally attributed to monofilaments and multifilaments. It is thus the suture of choice in cardiovascular surgery, prosthetic implants and facelifts.

Polyester braided sutures are usually dyed green in colour. They may be coated or uncoated. The uncoated variant has a rough surface which produces drag in the tissues. The coating is made of PTFE or polybutylate.

#### 11.4.4.4 Polybutester (Novafil, Vascufil)

Polybutester is a relatively new thermoplastic material with unique stress-strain properties. It is a copolymer comprised of polybutylene terephthalate and poly teramethylene ether glycol, and is coated with polytribolate. The polybutester monofilament sutures are designed to have high strength, elasticity and pliability. The flexibility and lack of memory allow it to be handled with ease resulting in a high knot security. The unique features have made this a popular material for abdominal wound closure.

The elasticity of polybutester is phenomenal. It can stretch 50% of its length at initial loads. It has a biphasic expansion curve wherein it expands well in response to initial stress and maintains pressure without cutting the tissue, and at the same time withstanding creep by not undergoing permanent deformation even under constant pressure.

#### 11.4.4.5 Polytetrafluroethylene (Gore-Tex, Cytoplast, Coreflon, Teflon)

Polytetrafluroethylene (PTFE) is a synthetic material which has found extensive application globally. It is a fluoropolymer of tetrafluoroethylene (-$CF_2$-$CF_2$-), made by free-radical polymerisation of monomer units. PTFE is a strong, tough, waxy, non-flammable material popular for its non-stick properties.

PTFE suture is considered as the ideal material for oral surgeries, especially for dental implant surgeries. It is inert, non-absorbable and monofilament in nature. The strong fluoro-carbon bond is thought to be the reason for its inertness. Unlike other synthetic monofilament sutures, PTFE is smooth, supple and soft. The cut ends cause no irritation to delicate oral tissues. It has no shape memory. It is well tolerated in the oral cavity and has excellent handling, knot-tying and knot-holding abilities. Thus, it has most of the positive attributes of braided sutures, at the same time avoiding the risk of bacterial contamination by wicking effect.

#### 11.4.4.6 Stainless Steel

Surgical stainless steel non-absorbable surgical suture is composed of 316 L austenitic stainless steel. It can be monofilamentous or multifilamentous. The obvious advantages of stainless steel sutures are strength and low tissue reaction. Its drawbacks include very poor flexibility that makes it highly demanding in suturing skills. Incorrect technique can cause an excessive pull or tear on the tissues resulting in necrosis of wound edges. Barbs at the end can cause glove punctures and trauma to adjacent tissues.

Stainless steel suture is used in sternal closure and in orthopaedic procedures involving cartilage and tendon repair. It is also sparingly used for abdominal wound closure and hernia repair.

### 11.4.5 Synthetic Absorbable Sutures (Absorbed by Hydrolysis)

Till polyglycolic acid sutures were introduced in the 1970s, all absorbable sutures were natural. The synthetic absorbable sutures are all polymers based on glycolic acid, l-lactic acid, paradioxanone, trimethylene carbonate and e-caprolactone [2]. They are sterilised either by ethylene oxide gas or by gamma radiation. These polymers have definite advantages over chromic catgut in clinical use. They are much stronger, evoke minimal tissue reaction, stay longer before absorption and leave no reactive changes after they are resorbed. They are absorbed typically by hydrolysis reaction which breaks the polymer chains. The hydrolysis end products are $CO_2$, $H_2O$ and the monomer.

#### 11.4.5.1 Polyglycolic Acid (Dexon, PolySyn, PGA)

Polyglycolic acid suture, introduced in the early 1970s, was the first absorbable synthetic suture material. It is braided homopolymer of glycolic acid. The uncoated version is beige in colour while the polycaprolate-coated product may be undyed or dyed green, violet or bicoloured. When compared to catgut, the tensile strength and knot security are excellent. It retains 65% of its tensile strength after 2 weeks, by which time catgut would have lost all its strength.

The polylycolic acid soon became very popular but fell out of favour later as better products were developed in due course of time.

#### 11.4.5.2 Polyglactin 910 (Vicryl, Polysorb)

Polyglactin 910 is a synthetic heteropolymer consisting of 90% glycolic acid and 10% lactic acid. Introduced in 1974, this is a multifilamentous, braided suture with a lubricant coating of polyglactin 370 (30:70 ratio) and calcium stearate. The final product is usually dyed violet in colour, but an undyed beige version is also available. Polyglactin 910 is among the most popular absorbable sutures used for surgical wound closure today.

The main advantages of polyglactin over polyglycolic acid include consistently higher residual tensile strength and faster absorption. The absorption happens between 40 and 70 days. The coating ensures smooth passage. Since the coating is made of similar material, the risk of flaking is very low. Calcium stearate used in the coating is an absorbable organic lubricant. The shelf life of polyglactin is as high as 5 years.

As the material became very popular and widely used, manufacturers began to bring out modified products providing specific benefits. One of them is a monofilament version which does not require a coating. Another one is an 'antibacterial suture' with embedded triclosan, which is said to be very effective in preventing surgical site infections. Yet another useful modification is 'rapidly absorbing polyglactin' (Vicryl Rapide/Velosorb Fast). By treating the coating with γ-radiation, it is made to lose strength by second week and is fully absorbed by sixth week. This variant is widely used in oral surgery, where faster resorption is desired.

#### 11.4.5.3 Polydioxanone (PDS, PDO)

Polydioxanone was the first monofilament suture available of large size (larger than 3–0). It is a polyester product and is synthesised through the ring opening of the monomer paradioxanone (1, 4-dioxan 2-one). As a monofilament suture, it has much less drag through the tissues than polyglactin or polyglycolic acid. Since it retains its tensile strength over a long span of time (80% strength at 2 weeks and 60% after 6 weeks), it is considered a better alternative to polyglactin for suturing of fascia.

A modification called PDS II is chemically similar but is annealed above melting temperature to soften the external surface, imparting improved flexibility to the final product.

#### 11.4.5.4 Poliglecaprone 25 (Monocryl/Biosyn/Petcryl Mono/Monoglyde)

Often seen as the monofilament alternative to polyglactin, poliglecaprone is a segmented block polymer consisting of 75% glycolide and 25% ε-caprolactone. It is available as an undyed or a violet dyed version. The key feature that differentiates poliglecaprone from other monofilament sutures is the high level of pliability and handling properties. This is achieved through the formation of an interim soft polymer chain 'pre-polymer' which is high in caprolactone. In the ensuing stages of manufacturing, more glycolide is added to supplement hard segments to the pre-polymer. In this way, we get a final product with high tensile strength without compromising on the pliability.

The tensile strength of the undyed poliglecaprone suture degrades to 50% in 1 week and 30% in the second week. The dyed version retains 70% strength after 1 week. Complete absorption by hydrolysis happens in about 100 days.

##### 11.4.5.5 Polyglyconate (Maxon)

This copolymer has a molar ratio of 64% glycolic acid and 36% trimethylene carbonate. It is an uncoated monofilament which may be undyed or dyed dark green. Polyglyconate has good handling properties. But its main advantage is the retention of tensile strength over a long time span. It retains at least 50% of its strength 4 weeks after implantation, making this an excellent choice in situations where long-term retention is needed. The slow absorption makes it relatively unsuitable for subcuticular sutures, since the dyed suture may be visible under the surface.

##### 11.4.5.6 Glycomer 631 (Biosyn)

It is a synthetic absorbable coated monofilament polyester suture. It is a tri-block copolymer and contains glycolide (60%), trimethylene carbonate (26%) and p-dioxanone (14%). It may be undyed or dyed violet. It has high flexibility, low memory and minimal tissue reactivity.

It passes through the tissues easily but has poor knot-holding capability. Degradation and absorption are similar to polyglactin. Full absorption is complete in around 100 days.

##### 11.4.5.7 Polyglytone 6211 (Caprosyn)

Polyglytone 6211 is the only suture available with four different monomers in its core structure. It is a polyester copolymer of glycolide, caprolactone, trimethylene carbonate and lactide in the ratio 6:2:1:1. It is a monofilament, uncoated, absorbable suture which is undyed or dyed violet.

Polyglytone 6211 is a suture for the short-term approximation of tissues. Because of its quick disintegration, it offers an inert alternative to catgut that can evoke inflammatory response. Its strength decreases to 50–60% at 5 days and to 20–30% at 10 days post-implantation.

## 11.5 Knot-Tying

The suture knot-tying can be accomplished by using an instrument (usually the needle holder) or using hands. Three main techniques are described.

### 11.5.1 Two-Handed Tie

The two-handed tie is cumbersome and is not routinely used. The suture is tied together by holding one tag in each hand and intertwining them.

### 11.5.2 One-Handed Tie

The one-handed tie is the most popular hand-tie method. It is quicker and can be accomplished in a smaller space. One end of the suture thread tag ('the long end') is held with thumb and forefinger of the dominant hand. The other side tag ('the short end') is placed a bit distal to the first tag, running in the same direction. The middle finger is folded and is used to guide the short end around the long end, and then the two tags are pulled away.

### 11.5.3 Instrument Tie

Instrument tie is the most popular technique for tying a suture knot. The long end is wrapped around the needle holder. Then the needle holder beaks are opened to grasp the short end, which is then pulled to form a tie. One such tie is called a 'throw'.

## 11.6 Suture Knots

The suture thread tags are intertwined to form a knot. The knot should be firm and tight, and should not lie on the wound/incision line. It is important that the knot stays tight and maintains strength during the healing phase. Knot slippage or breakage before healing can be detrimental to the wound. In general, knot security is higher for braided and uncoated sutures because of higher friction coefficient.

The knots placed for the surgical suturing are of simple design. Those employed commonly are the square knot, surgeon's knot and granny's knot. These three variants are very similar to each other and differ from each other only in minor aspects.

### 11.6.1 Square Knot/Reef Knot

A square knot is among the simplest of the knot designs. It involves a simple intertwining of the two threads. This 'half-hitch' knot (one 'throw' around the instrument) need to be complemented with an additional similar throw to make it secure. Preferably the second hitch should be in the opposite direction, i.e. if the first throw is in clockwise direction, the second one should be in anticlockwise orientation.

The classical square knot formed by a clockwise and a counterclockwise hitch can be further complimented by more similar hitches in alternatively changing directions.

### 11.6.2 Surgeon's Knot

A surgeon's knot is a minor modification of the square knot in which the initial intertwining is doubled. This is accomplished by doubling the first throw, by doing two turns of the thread around the instrument. This is followed by a regular second throw in the opposite direction.

### 11.6.3 Granny's Knot

In the granny's knot, two initial throws are placed in the same direction, followed by a third throw in the opposite direction.

**Principles of Wound Suturing**

Regardless of the specific technique, some basic principles are to be followed while performing a suturing procedure. It is to be remembered that these are only general principles, and can be modified or rejected in specific situations depending on the clinical context.

1. The suture needle is to be held with the needle holder about ¾$^{th}$ of the distance from the needle tip.
2. The selected suture size should be the smallest possible which will hold the wound edges securely.
3. The needle tip should enter the tissue perpendicular to the tissue surface.
4. The needle penetrations should be at equal distances from the wound edge on both sides of the wound. The actual distance depends on the suture/needle size but is generally agreed to be 2–3 mm.
5. The passage of the needle through the tissues should follow the curvature of the needle.
6. When one side of the wound is fixed to the underlying tissues, one should first engage the mobile wound edge.
7. When one side of the wound is thicker than the other, the thinner wound edge should be engaged first.
8. When one side is deeper and the other more superficial, the deeper side should be engaged first.
9. The depth of needle penetration should be more than the distance from wound edge to needle penetration point. This will ensure eversion of wound edges.
10. The sutures should ensure proper tissue approximation of wound edges at the same time avoiding excessive tension on the tissues. Excessive tissue tension can lead to blanching, tear and necrosis. In case the edges are not approximating passively, the flaps may be undermined to achieve better mobilisation so that a tension-free closure can be achieved.
11. The knot should lie on one side of the wound, and not over the wound edges.
12. The spacing between the individual sutures depends on the type of tissue and the size of sutures. Generally placed 3–4 mm apart, they should be closer together at areas of underlying muscular activity and when the sutures are smaller in size.

## 11.7 Specific Suturing techniques [3] (Video 11.1)

There are quite a large number of techniques available to stitch a wound. Only the commonly used methods are mentioned.

**Factors to Be Considered on Specific Material and Technique**

1. Type of tissue,
2. Type of wound,
3. Time available,
4. Aesthetic requirements,
5. Functional needs,
6. Likely tension on the wounds.
7. Expected time for tissue healing.

### 11.7.1 Simple Interrupted Suture

A simple interrupted suture ('simple loop') is the most common method to suture a wound. This is the simplest design of wound closure. The suture passes once through each side of the wound in a simple loop and is then tied in a knot above the surface. Multiple such ties are made over the length of the wound, resulting in several independent sutures collectively securing the tissue edges together. The same technique is frequently employed for internal suturing of tissue layers also [4].

The needle penetrates the surface 2–3 mms away from the wound edge on one side and proceeds into the subcutaneous tissue. The curve of the needle is then used to pass it through to the subcutaneous tissue on the opposite side. The needle then exits through the surface. The initial and final tags, now outside of the tissues, are then tied in a knot. The configuration inside the tissue is thus in the form of a loop. If the wound sides are of unequal depth, then the needle should travel deeper in the lower side while staying superficial on the higher side. This will help to correct the depth disparity and ensure proper surface levelling.

This technique is easy to learn and employ. This suture provides good tensile strength and carries minimal risk of wound oedema or impaired circulation. Several adjustments to the design are possible with this method depending on the wound characteristics. Since there is a series of multiple sutures, even if one suture fails, the others may provide sufficient strength to keep the wound edges together (Fig. 11.4).

The major drawback of this method of suturing is the high possibility of 'rail-road track' shaped scars caused due to the ingrowth of epithelium into the suture tracks. There is also a tendency to cause 'wound inversion' (depression of the surface at the wound site) due to tissue contracture during healing. The inversion can be prevented by making the suture configuration 'flask-shaped' inside the tissues, by making the needle travel farther laterally away from the wound within the tissues. When compared to continuous suturing techniques, the interrupted method is more time-consuming as it requires many more knots need to be tied.

### 11.7.2 Simple Buried Suture

The buried suture is a modification of the simple interrupted suture and is reserved for stitching the inner (deeper) tissue layers. The only difference is that the knot ends up in the tissues deeper to the suture loop, i.e. away from the surface. In essence, this is a simple interrupted suture in the reverse orientation.

The wound edge is first reflected using fine forceps or hooks. The needle is then inserted into the underside of the dermis on one side. The needle then proceeds along its curvature to exit in the wound edge more superficial to the initial bite. The needle then pierces the dermis wound edge (near the surface) on the opposite side, proceeds in a path mirroring its motion in the first side and comes out at a deeper point which corresponds to the first bite. Though the tie is done outside, the knot gets buried deep inside the tissues as it is tightened (Fig. 11.5).

This technique is extremely useful in suturing the inner tissue layers before the surface closure. As the knot is buried deep, it does not interfere with the closure of superficial layers. This aspect is extremely useful while closing cutaneous facial wounds.

Two major drawbacks have been observed with this suture. One is a skin dimpling which typically happens if the suture arc inadvertently involves the epidermis. Another problem is the tendency for wound inversion to occur. Small modifications such a set-back dermal buried suture or a vertical mattress buried suture can be employed to overcome this

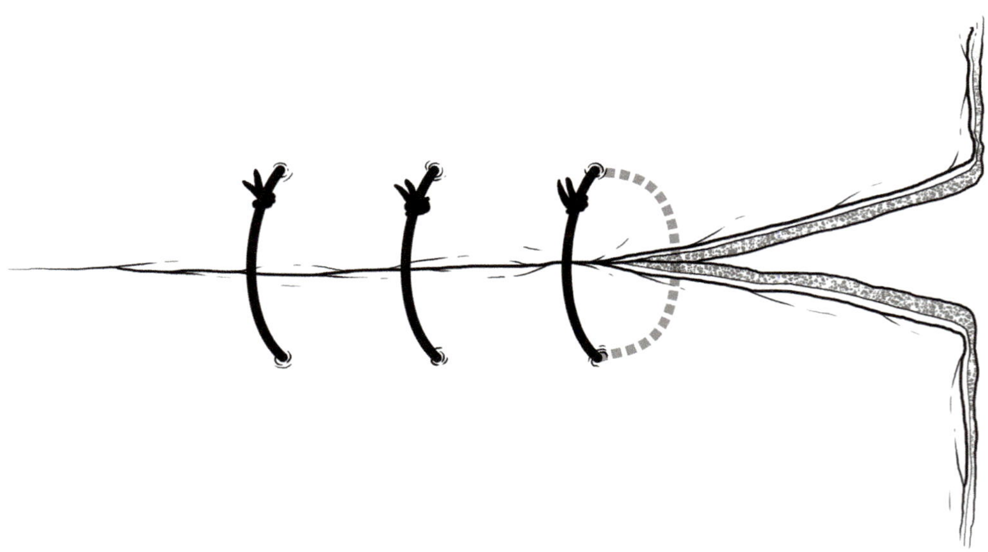

Fig. 11.4 Simple interrupted suture technique

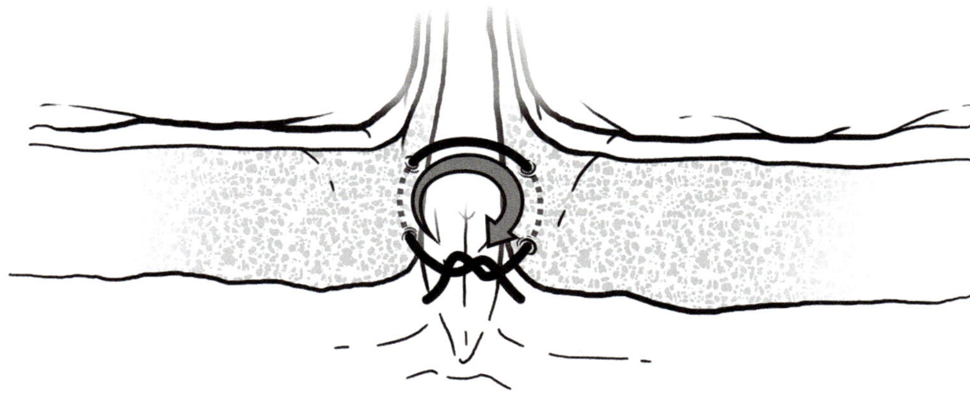


**Fig. 11.5** Buried suture

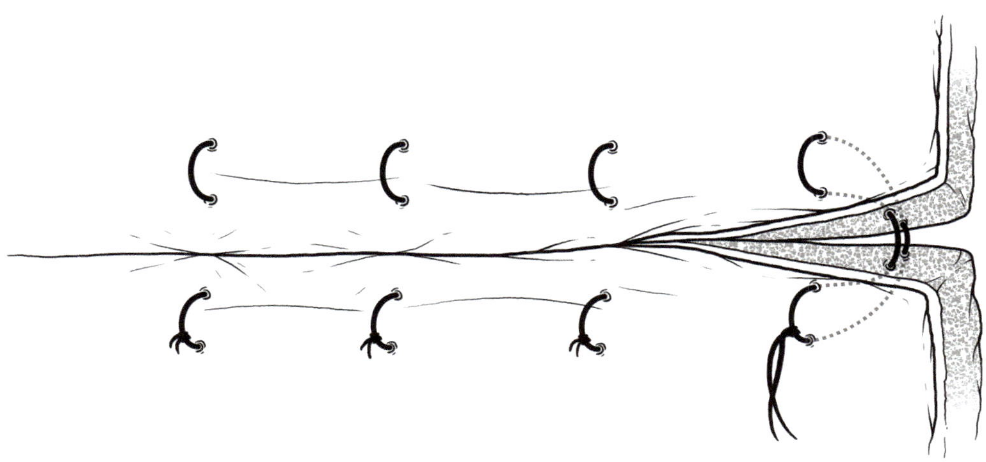


**Fig. 11.6** Vertical mattress suture

problem. These modifications attempt to pass the bridging suture segments to be deeper, thus resulting in wound eversion.

### 11.7.3 Vertical Mattress Suture

The vertical mattress suture is in part similar to simple interrupted sutures but includes an additional suture bridge close to the wound edge. Also known as Donati Suture, or 'far-far, near-near' suture, this is the most frequently used suturing technique to obtain wound eversion [5]. This suture design is very popular in abdominal and limb surgeries.

The needle is first penetrated far from the wound edge (about 6 mm), and then proceeds through the deeper tissue to the opposite side and emerges out at an equal distance from the edge. The needle is then reinserted at a point closer (2–3 mm) to the wound edge on the second side itself. It is then rotated superficially through the tissues and is exited on the other side at a corresponding near point. This results in a double bridging of the wound, one deep in the tissues and another superficial and nearer to the wound edge. Thus, both tags of the thread are now on one side of the wound. They are tied together gently (Fig. 11.6).

The primary advantage of this suture is the resultant wound eversion. This eversion is expected to compensate for the anticipated contracture occurring along the wound margin. As the suture is bridging the wound twice, the binding strength is more. Elimination of dead space is another obvious advantage. The suture thread does not pass the wound edge on the surface, minimising the chance of track marks.

On the flip side, fine wound edge approximation is almost never achieved with this suture. Excessive tightening could lead to over-constriction and sometimes exposure of the raw area. This may necessitate placement of additional interrupted sutures for better results.

The vertical mattress concept can be used in a buried suture situation also by ensuring that the more superficial suture thread passed back to the first side in a path parallel to the first, deeper suture bridge. This will result in a better wound eversion.

### 11.7.4 Simple Continuous Suture

Simple continuous suture ('running loop', 'standard running suture') is a good method for rapid closure of small wounds. It gives an even distribution of tension all along the wound span. It combines many benefits of the simple interrupted sutures with the additional advantage of a quicker finish.

The technique is very simple. The first part follows the same process as a simple interrupted suture. The first knot becomes the anchoring knot for the ensuing running line. The tags are not cut and the longer tag (with the needle) is used for making the remaining loops. The needle is inserted back into the tissues a few millimetres away from the first piercing. Then the needle (followed by the thread) passes through the tissues in a path parallel to the first loop. Once it comes out of the second loop, it is not tied. Instead, the loop is tightened and the thread crosses over obliquely across the wound and enters the tissue surface again, a few millimetres away from the second piercing. This process continues over and over until one reaches the other end of the wound. As the last loop goes through the tissues, the thread is only partially pulled through, leaving some loose thread on the opposite side. The suture is then tied to this loose thread for the final knot. Thus, the suture material runs across the wound in repetitive loops, and there are only two knots—one at either end (Fig. 11.7).

The obvious advantages of this technique are the quickness of suture placement and the ease of avoiding many knots. Also, if the tissue wells up in one site, the remaining part of the suture can provide some compensatory slack.

The principal drawback is that the integrity of the entire suture line is vested in just two knots. Any breakage to the suture at any point leads to the entire line getting untied. Since the loops are in continuous succession, fine-tuning of design for each loop is not possible. Also, since the tension is the same across all loops, the areas of the wound with greater tension, usually the central part, may tend to gape.

### 11.7.5 Locking Continuous Suture

This is a variation of the simple continuous suture technique used for surface wounds. Each loop of the continuous suture is 'locked' on itself before making the next loop. This is the most popular continuous suturing technique especially for closing wounds over long spans. As with other superficial continuous sutures, this method is frequently used as a surface layer after the internal tissue layers have been closed.

Similar to the simple continuous technique, the first loop is passed and the knot tied. After the second loop has gone through the tissues and exited, the suture is not immediately tightened. The needle and the leading thread it is made to pass through the earlier loop. After making this 'lock', the suture is tightened and is then passed into the tissues for the third loop. The assistant should maintain this tension until the next loop is passed. This process is repeated for the entire line of succeeding loops (Fig. 11.8).

The locking helps to align the tissues in a proper anatomic orientation perpendicular to the wound. There is an added haemostatic effect due to the tension on tissues. Uniform degree of tension is maintained across all the loops. At the same time, the running locks partially detach the tension on the individual loops from one another. Thus, to an extent, individual control of tension depending on the site can be obtained.

This technique inherits the main disadvantage of the simple continuous sutures of being dependent on only two knots, and the risk of complete loss of suture integrity in case of breakage at any point. The locks, if they are too tight, may cause vascular compromise of underlying tissues.

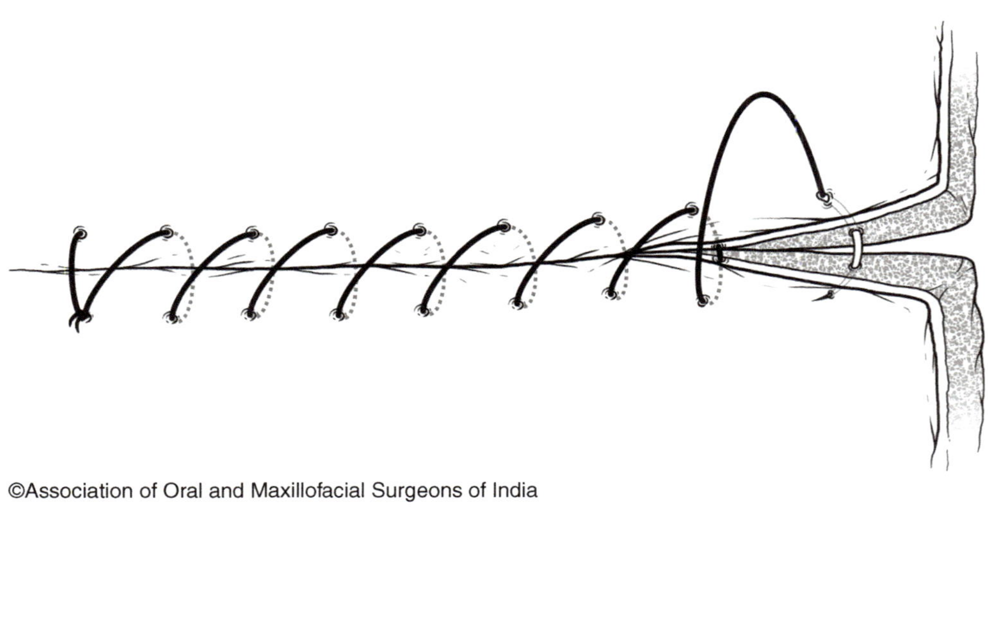

Fig. 11.7 Simple continuous suture

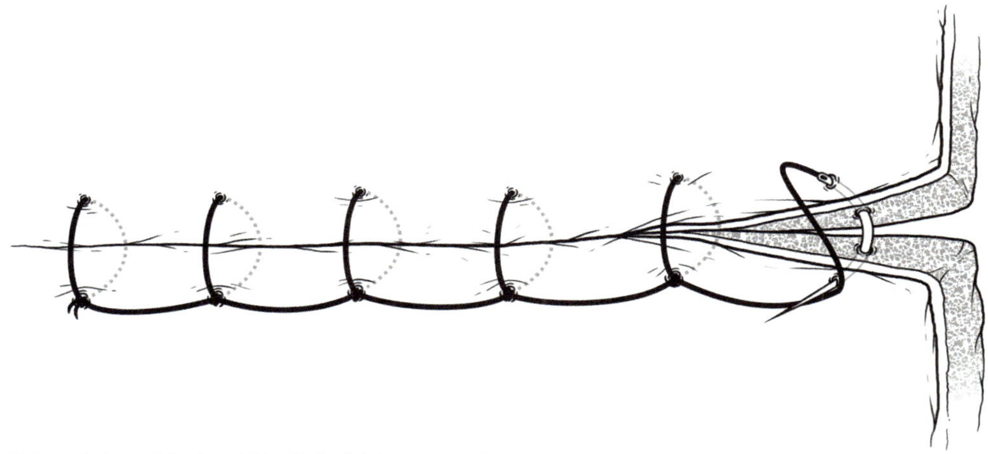



**Fig. 11.8** Locking continuous suture

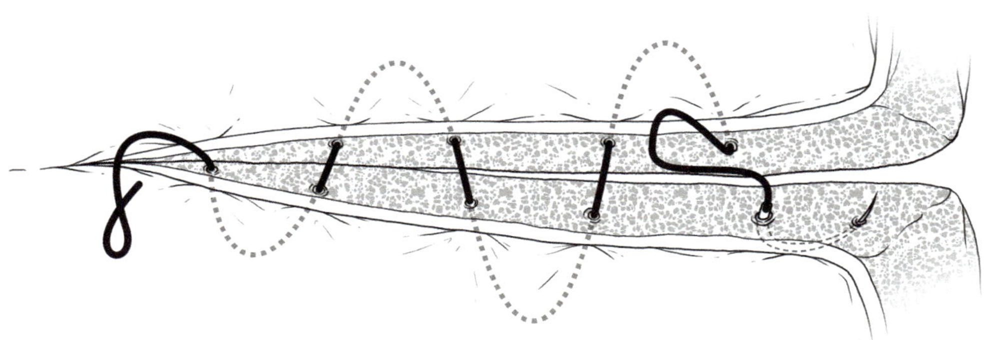



**Fig. 11.9** Subcuticular suture

### 11.7.6 Subcuticular Suture

This is a mostly buried, continuous, epidermal wound closure which is used for surface closure. The suture ends exit a few mms away from the wound corner. The subcuticular suture is employed only after the deeper structures and dermis have been secured well with absorbable sutures. It is popular as an aesthetic suture for face [6].

The suture may be absorbable or non-absorbable, and is usually thin (size 5–0 or 6–0). The needle insertion is at one end of the wound, 2–5 mm away from the apex. It is passed along the curve into the wound, where it exits in the interior, close to the apex. Then the needle is inserted again into the dermis on any one side of the wound edge walls. Thereafter, it passes horizontally parallel to the surface, and following the needle curve to come out into the wound interior a small distance away. The same step is then repeated on the other side of the wound. This process is repeated till one reaches the other end of the wound, wherein the needle is made to pierce the far end apex and to come out in the surface. This last step is a mirror image of the initial steps. Then each of the suture tags on both sides is tied separately on to itself. Alternatively, the tags may be secured with adhesive strips, surgical tape or tissue glue (Figs. 11.9 and 11.10).

The biggest advantage of this technique is the much decreased risk of scars. The close approximation achieved in the dermis region makes the need for a further surface suturing unnecessary. The tension is aligned centrally across the wound and is evenly distributed all along the length of the suture. Also, this technique is highly suitable in cases where the suture material is required to stay in place for a long period of time.

On the negative side, the subcuticular suture takes longer time to perform. Leaving a large quantity of foreign material in situ can increase the risk of foreign body reaction and infection. If non-absorbable material is used, there is a minor risk of long and thin suture track following removal. If absorbable material is used, an undyed suture should be chosen to prevent cutaneous visibility. Incorrect technique can leave small segments of exposed raw area, which need to be addressed with additional surface sutures.

### 11.7.7 Purse-String Suture

This is essentially a modification of the simple continuous suture, and is designed to reduce the size of a two-dimensional surface defect. It is not a cosmetically superior technique and is rarely used in the face. The purse-string effect causes a puckering in the surrounding skin tissue. But this is an effective method to reduce wound area. It may also be used to achieve haemostasis.

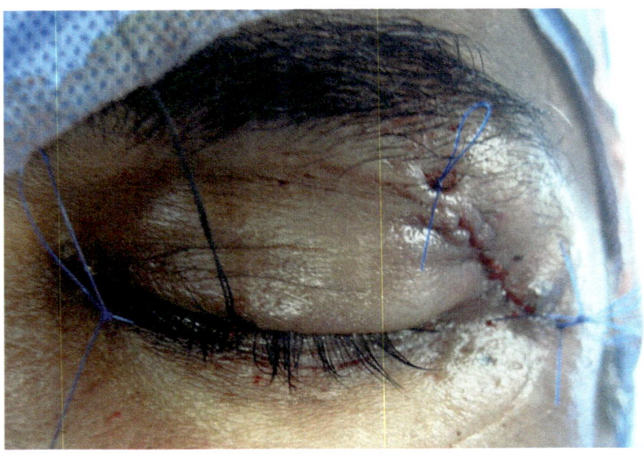



**Fig. 11.10** Subcuticular suture at the subciliary incision site and at the pre-existing lateral orbital laceration in a case of zygomatic complex fracture fixation

At first, the wound edges of the defect need to be freshened and underlined. The needle and thread is passed along the edge of the defect in a course running parallel to the wound edge. Thereafter, it continues in a series of loops running along the edge of the surface wound along its entire circumference. As the thread completes the full distance and reaches near the initial needle entry, it is pulled taut, leading to complete or partial closure of the wound. Then the tags are tied together.

### 11.7.8 Three-Point Suture

Also known as 'tip stitch' or 'half-buried horizontal mattress suture', this technique is used for managing a situation where three ends of the tissue have to be sutured together. In maxillofacial surgery, this situation is encountered while repairing V-shaped lacerations and while closing flaps with sharp corners (such as the triangular flap at the vermilion border for cleft lip repair)

This suture is placed only after the flaps are brought into position using buried dermal sutures. The surface suture thread is used, that is, 6–0 for face and 3–0 for scalp. The needle is first inserted into one side of the non-flap side of the wound. It follows the needle curve to exit in the inner aspect of the wound. The next tissue insertion is into the superficial dermis of the flap tip. Then the needle passes horizontally and comes out through the dermis on the other side of the flap tip. After releasing from the flap tip, it re-enters the dermis of the non-flap side on the other side and comes out through the skin at a point corresponding to the initial entry. The tags are then knotted together (Figs. 11.11 and 11.12).

**Fig. 11.11** Three-point suture technique

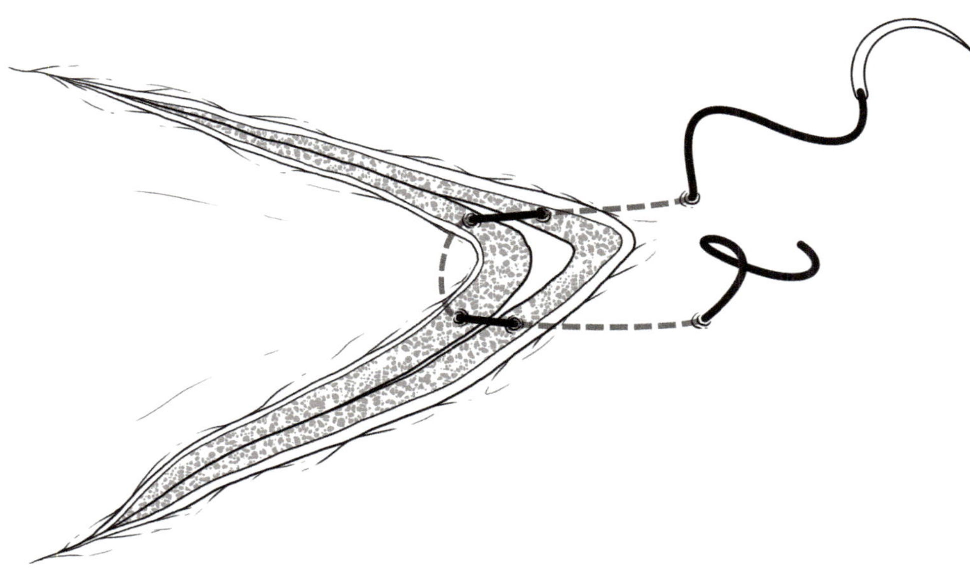

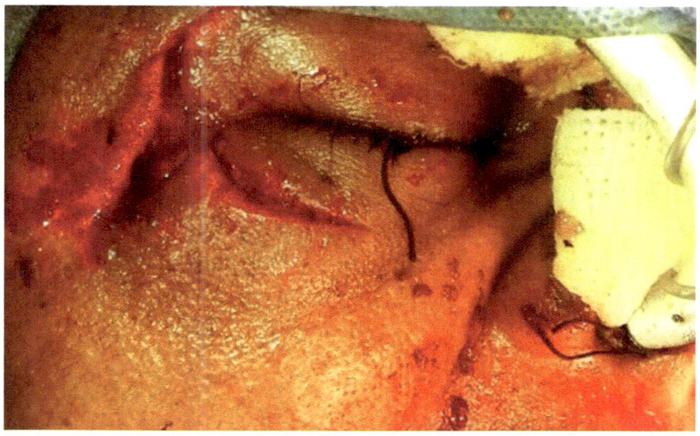



**Fig. 11.12** A laceration that needs three-point suturing

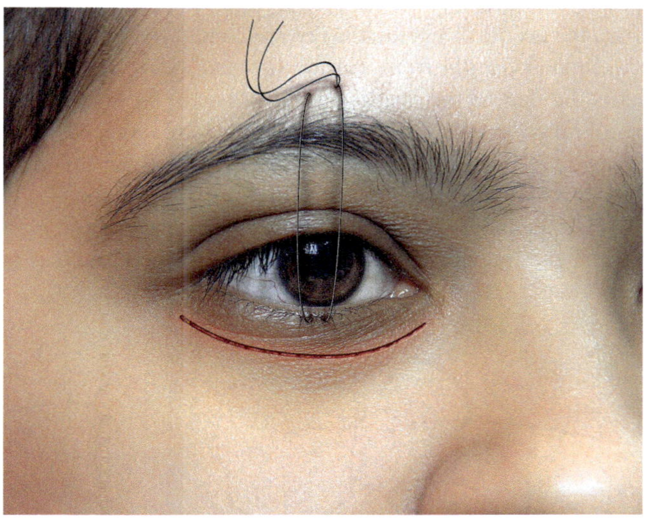



**Fig. 11.13** Frost suture

### 11.7.9 Frost Suture

The Frost suture is a temporary eyelid suspension suture, used to ensure proper lower eyelid placement during the post-operative period [7].

After the closure of the lower eyelid incision, a needle bite is taken on the tarsal plate or just inferior to it. Then a second bite is taken just above the eyebrow, ensuring the anatomic position and alignment of the lower lid. These tags are then tied or secured with tapes or tissue glue (Fig. 11.13).

These sutures may be removed on third post-operative day, but need to be kept longer if there has been significant trauma to the tissues.

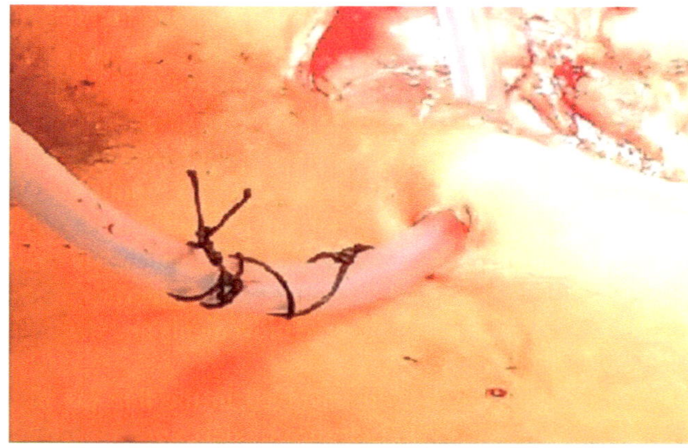



**Fig. 11.14** Drain anchoring suture

### 11.7.10 Drain Anchoring Suture

Different types of drains are used in surgery, such as corrugated rubber drain, the suction drain, intercostal drain, etc. After the drain has been inserted, it needs to be securely fixed to the body to prevent displacement.

The most common means to secure drains is the Roman Garter method, which uses silk sutures. A strong bite is first taken on the skin near the drain entry site. After making a knot, the two suture tags go around the drain tube in a series of windings. A knot may be tied after each 2 or 3 turns around the tube. The large number of windings around the tube increases the friction, holding the tube in position without dislodgement (Fig. 11.14).

Other techniques which have been described include the use of nylon suture, safety pin, drain clip, adhesives and Tie-lok.

## 11.8 Dentoalveolar Suturing

The tissues and the surgical environment in the dentoalveolar region are different from other parts of the body. Consequently, the wound closure requirements also differ. Wound closure in dentoalveolar surgery involves suturing in situations such as

1. Suturing of buccal and/or lingual flaps back to its place after dentoalveolar surgery around teeth or implant accessories.
2. Wound closure after tooth extraction.
3. Flap closure in edentulous ridge.

In most cases, the needle passage is through keratinised mucosa with little or no subcutaneous tissue, obviating the need for multilayered closure. The presence of teeth or artificial crown on one side of the flap forces the surgeon to innovate on the basic suture design. Another difference is when the extraction wound is closed—the wound is usually closed only at the edges and is largely left open in the middle. Also, the suture site will have to endure itself in a challenging environment with the presence of saliva, food materials and a very dynamic milieu where tongue movements and masticatory forces abound [8].

If marginal gingiva is not involved in the flap (as in a semilunar flap), the wound closure models are usually not different from the general cutaneous designs which were discussed in the previous section.

### 11.8.1 Simple Interrupted Suture (Interdental Suture)

As in any case of wound closure, the simple interrupted suture is the mainstay in closing dentoalveolar flaps [9]. In general, it involves suturing the detached interdental papillae together. The needle passes from the buccal aspect of the buccal flap, emerges on the inside of the flap and then passes between the tooth roots to enter the inner aspect of the lingual flap. As it pierces the lingual flap and emerges through the mucosa, the needle is turned back and is taken back via the interdental region to the buccal side. The two suture tags are then tied together. Thus, the knot remains on the buccal side and is accessible for removal.

If only one flap (usually buccal) has been raised, the needle can still pass through the attached lingual flap and the suture design stays the same. In post-extraction wounds also, the procedure is the same, and the tooth socket space is not totally closed.

### 11.8.2 Interrupted Reversing Suture

In this modified interrupted suture, the direction of the needle is reversed for engaging the lingual papilla. Once it passes through the buccal papilla and reaches the lingual side, the needle orientation is reversed and it is made to enter the lingual papilla from outside (lingual side). The needle exits the flap on the inside, passed across to the buccal side and is then tied. Thus, both the papillae are engaged in an 'outside-to-inside' orientation, ending in a figure-of-eight formation in the vertical plane (Fig. 11.15).

This technique is especially useful in cases where both buccal and lingual flaps are raised during surgery, such as in periodontal surgeries.

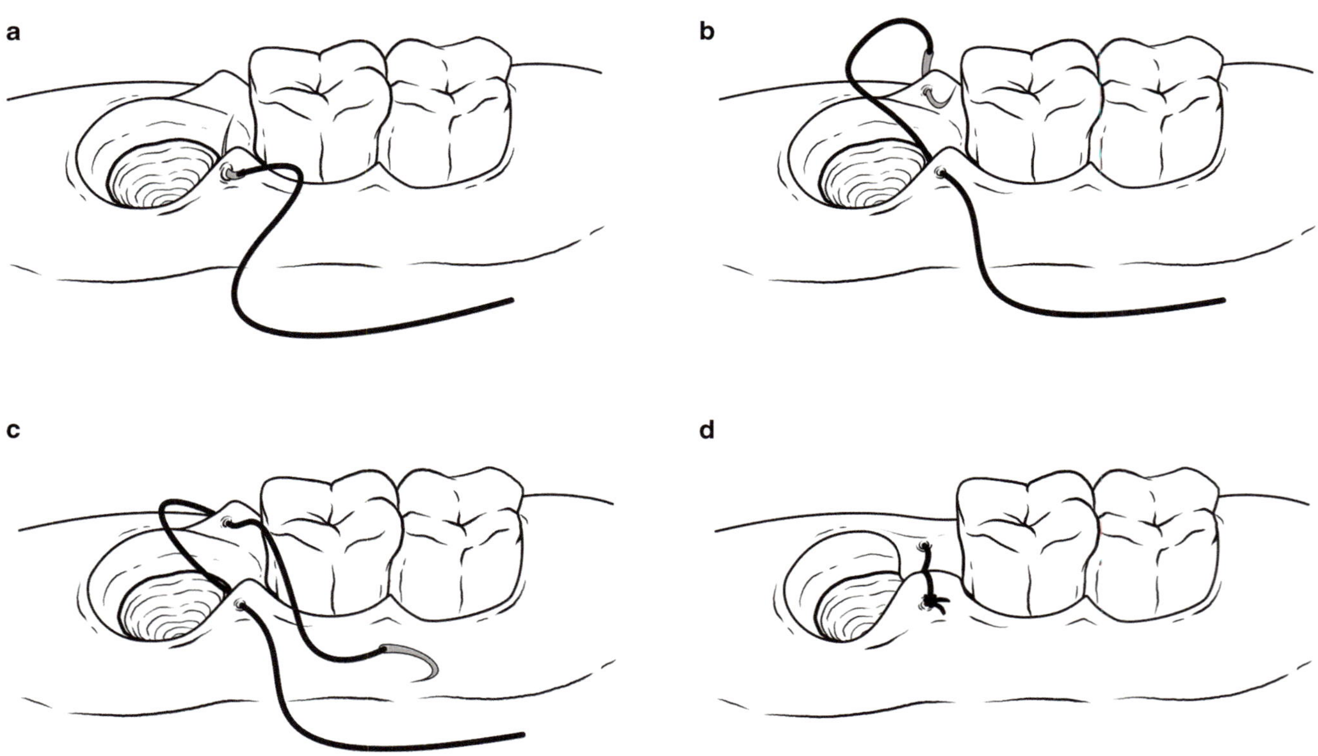




**Fig. 11.15** Interrupted reversing interdental suture

### 11.8.3 Vertical Mattress Suture

Vertical mattress technique in dentoalveolar surgery is a modification of the papilla-attaching simple interrupted technique. After the initial passage of the needle through the buccal and lingual papillae, the needle is turned back and picks a small bite at the tip of the lingual papilla before passing back to the buccal side. Then it again pierces the tip of buccal papilla before knot-tying.

While this technique helps in pressing the papilla into the interdental space, it is not a popular technique because of the difficulty in getting a solid bite at the papilla tip without 'cutting through'. Obviously, one needs to use an atraumatic needle with a small thread (4–0 or smaller) for this purpose.

### 11.8.4 Horizontal Mattress Suture

This is a two-dimensional suturing technique where the suture thread is spread in a horizontal fashion in the tissues. It is not very popular for general cutaneous suturing but is especially useful in dentoalveolar surgery.

When closing flaps in edentulous areas, the needle first passes through both flaps. Then it is reinserted into the flap on the same side, a little distance away from the earlier exit point. The reinserted needle now passes through both flaps and emerges out a similar distance away from the initial entry point. Both the thread tags, now on the same side, are tied together (Fig. 11.16).

In dentulous areas, this technique sutures two adjacent papillae together, eventually tying four papillae segments around a tooth in a horizontal square fashion. To close extraction wounds, only the papillae are approximated and the tooth socket space is not closed completely.

The advantage of this technique is that a single horizontal mattress suture serves like two separate interrupted sutures, thus helping to reduce the number of sutures. It compresses the wound from four corners and helps in haemostasis. It also results in some degree of wound eversion.

### 11.8.5 Horizontal Mattress Modification: Dental Anchor Suture

In this modification, the suture does not pass through the lingual soft tissues. After passing through the buccal papilla, the suture passes through the interdental region into the lingual side. Without engaging the lingual papilla, it goes around the tooth and comes back to the buccal side via the interdental space on the other side. Then it engages the buccal papilla before being tied. In this way, it secures the papilla to the bone using the tooth as its 'anchor'.

This technique can also be used in a reversing fashion, where only the papilla on the lingual side is engaged and the buccal side papillae are not pierced.

### 11.8.6 Horizontal Mattress Modification: Mattress Sling Suture

This technique attempts to combine the benefits of vertical mattress suture with those of horizontal mattress suture. The basic technique goes similar to the horizontal mattress but the final tag re-enters the buccal papilla at the tip and traverses a reverse path around the tooth to exit near the initial entry. In this way, it ensures the engagement of both buccal papillae in a vertical mattress fashion.

### 11.8.7 Horizontal Mattress Modification: Figure-of-Eight Suture (Cruciate Mattress Suture/Cross Suture)

The figure-of-eight suture is the most popular modification of the horizontal mattress technique. This is used mostly in closure of extraction wounds, and never in the presence of teeth at the wound site.

The needle first penetrates the buccal papilla on one side and then the lingual papilla. Then the thread crosses across the edentulous site, and the needle is reversed in orientation to pierce the buccal papilla of the other side from outside

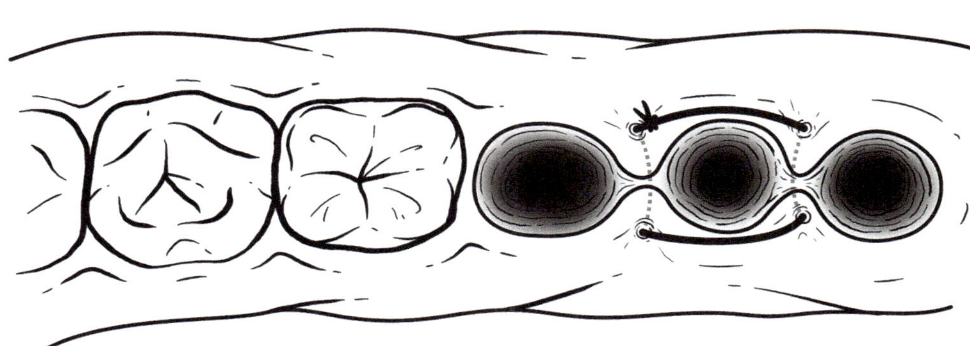

Fig. 11.16 Horizontal mattress suture (extraction wound)

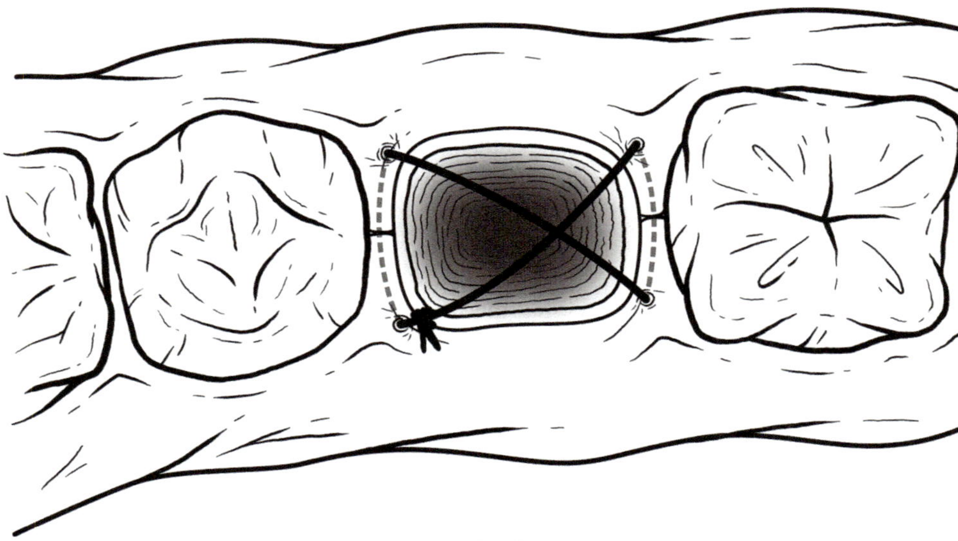
©Association of Oral and Maxillofacial Surgeons of India

**Fig. 11.17** Figure-of-eight suture

(buccal side) to pass through the lingual papilla and exit on lingual side. Then the thread passes across the site to be tied with the initial tag. The suture thus ends with the appearance of suture material crossing the wound site in a 'cross' shape (Fig. 11.17).

Many surgeons consider the figure-of-eight suture to be the most comprehensive way to suture a single tooth extraction site. This method ensures an even tension on the tissues from four corners, effectively constricting the wound. There is a positive effect on haemostasis also, due to the tension on the flap and due to its presence a mechanical barrier to clot loss.

### 11.8.8 Simple Continuous Suture

The continuous sutures are almost exclusively used for edentulous situations including post-extraction closure. After making a conventional interrupted suture knot, the longer tag is not cut and is instead used to make a series of 'running loops' approximating the succeeding pair of papillae one after the other. Gentle tension must be maintained on the thread to keep the loops tight while the needle passes through the next tissue. Knots are not tied for each loop but is done only at the other end of the long wound. Some surgeons prefer to tie a knot after 3 or 4 running loops. In the end, the part of the suture passing through the inner tissues are perpendicular to the wound, and the superficial, exposed parts lie across the wound in an oblique fashion.

The continuous sutures save time and effort while closing wounds of long span. It also ensures an even distribution of tension across the wound. The obvious disadvantage is the fact that if one loop or part of the suture is compromised (by untying, cutting through or loosening), the entire suture line gets loosened.

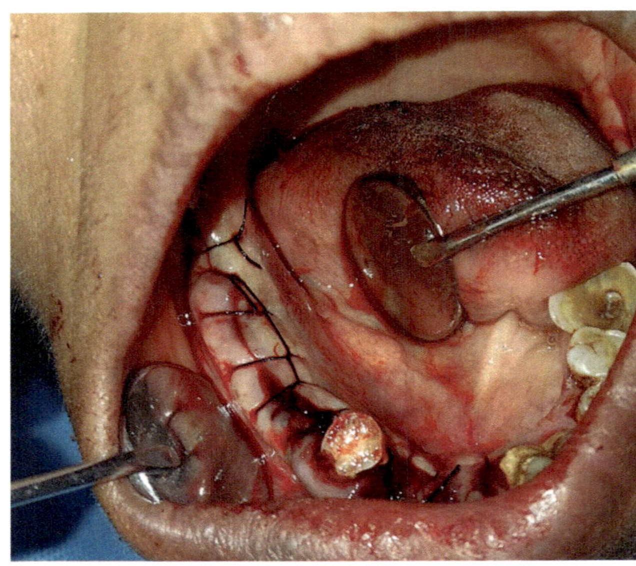
©Association of Oral and Maxillofacial Surgeons of India

**Fig. 11.18** Continuous locking suture (dentoalveolar)

### 11.8.9 Continuous Locking Suture

The continuous locking suture is a continuous suture in which a 'lock' is incorporated by passing the thread under the previous loop before it is pulled through the tissue. It is important to keep maintaining the tension on the previous loops as the needle makes the next pass through the tissue (Fig. 11.18).

This technique ensures a better orientation of the sutures with respect to the wound. The superficial, exposed parts of the suture are oriented perpendicular to the wound, leading to better anatomic wound approximation.

## 11.9 Suture Removal

Non-absorbable sutures on skin and mucosa should be removed after the wound surface has achieved initial stability. The timing of suture removal is very important. They should remain in tissue long enough to prevent dehiscence and scar spread. On the other hand, early removal reduces tissue reaction and suture marks.

Sutures on facial skin and in oral cavity are usually removed in 5–7 days. The recommended interval is 3–5 days for eyelids, 7 days for neck and 7–10 days for scalp. Those on trunk and limbs should remain in place for 10–14 days.

The suture line is cleansed with antiseptic. The knot is grasped and is pulled away mildly from the surface and to one side of the wound. An uncontaminated segment of the thread is exposed on the other side by this pull. The thread is cut at this segment near to the surface. Then the suture is pulled out, making sure that no contaminated (exposed) part is ragged through the tissues.

In the case of a continuous suture, every single loop should be cut and pulled out separately. A subcuticular suture is removed by cutting the knot off at any one end, and then pulling the suture out gently from the other end. It is important to make sure that the suture does not break within the tissues.

## 11.10 Other Wound Closure Methods

### 11.10.1 Staples

The use of specialised staples for wound closure was popularized in 1900s by the Hungarian surgeon Hümér Hültl, known as the 'father of surgical stapling'. Compared to suturing, surgical stapling is a quicker method to close the skin in large wounds, and the inflammatory response is relatively less. Staples provide good wound edge eversion without strangulation of the tissue. It is an excellent method to employ in cases which require quick wound closure and where aesthesis is not a major concern [10] (Fig. 11.19).

Though titanium staples were initially used, almost all of the contemporary hardware is stainless steel. However, titanium retains the advantages of being biocompatible and MRI-compatible. Bioresorbable staples, based on polyglycolic acid, are also available. The stapler devise itself may be of stainless steel (reusable) or plastic (disposable), into which the disposable staple cartridges can be loaded.

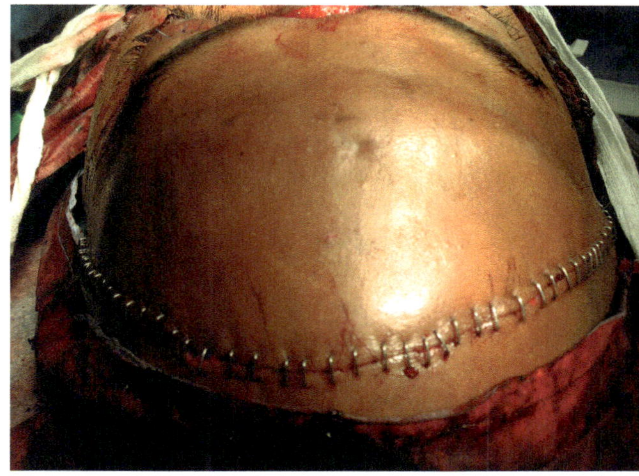



**Fig. 11.19** Stapled scalp incision in a coronal approach

In maxillofacial surgery, staples are frequently used to close scalp wounds and neck incisions, following the closure of internal layers with conventional sutures. Staples are also popular in reconstructive surgery to secure skin grafts and to close the flap donor sites. They are not generally used to close facial wounds, since there is a tendency to produce 'rail-road track' scars. Skin staples are removed after 7-10 days with a specialized staple remover device.

### 11.10.2 Tapes

Different types of surgical adhesive tapes are used to effect wound closure, to reduce tension on sutured wounds and to reinforce wound site after suture removal.

The indications of this method for wound closure per se are limited. Tapes can be used to close superficial lacerations where tissue tension is minimal. They are also employed in the closure of superficial layer after buried dermal sutures have been employed for wound edge approximation and tension reduction. A major indication is its use an additional reinforcement and protection over sutured wounds. The advantages of using tapes for wound closure are.

(a) They are rapid and easy to perform.
(b) The tape application is painless (patient anxiety and discomfort are minimal).
(c) Residual suture track scars are avoided.
(d) There is no need for a review visit to remove the tape.
(e) Tapes, being non-invasive, are less prone to infection than other methods.
(f) They are suitable for thin, fragile skin of the elderly and infants.

On the other hand, there are significant limitations to the use of tapes to close wounds. The most obvious contraindication is an area under significant tension. Tapes are difficult to apply on to highly convex surfaces, irregular wounds and in areas of tissue laxity. They do not attach well to wet surfaces (e.g. oral mucosa). They may get detached easily in hairy areas and those which tend to sweat.

These tapes are typically made of synthetic reinforced material with a hypoallergenic adhesive and are made porous to make them 'breathable' for skin. Some products are made elastic to account for oedema tension while some have incorporated antibiotic to reduce the incidence of surgical site infection. Modifications of tape-based wound closure include incorporation of a zip-lock mechanism and a clip attachment, both techniques designed to pull the wound edges together for better approximation.

### 11.10.3 Adhesives

The use of tissue adhesives is an efficient way to close wounds in select cases. Just like surgical tapes, tissue adhesives can be used to approximate wounds that do not require deep-layer closure and do not have significant tension on the edges [11].

All currently available tissue adhesives are chemically cyanoacrylates (esters of cyanoacrylic acid). These compounds were discovered by Ardis in 1949 and were first used in surgery by Coover in 1959. These are chemically similar to methacrylates, the only difference being the methyl ($CH_3$) group substituted with cyano/nitrile (CN) group. The water present on the skin or mucosal surface activates the acryl groups in the resin to rapidly polymerise and form long, strong chains. Three types of tissue adhesives are currently available for clinical use—2-octyl cyanoacrylate, N-butyl-2-cyanoacrylate and isoamyl 2-cyanoacrylate. The adhesion involves two mechanisms—mechanical interlocking into the surface irregularities and chemical covalent bonding with the nucleophilic amine groups on skin surfaces.

Tissue adhesives are mainly used to treat superficial skin tears (that do not extend past the dermis) and for surface closure after the deeper layers are secured with sutures. Other indications include stabilisation of bone fragments during plating, sealing of CSF leaks and sinus perforations, attaching grafts, achieving peripheral nerve reanastomosis and closure of dentoalveolar flaps [12]. They are also widely used to achieve haemostasis at surgical sites and as a biologic cover on ulcers. The relative contraindications include wounds over or near joints and wounds under significant static or dynamic skin tension. Also animal bite wounds, crushed wounds and wounds in high friction areas and those with cross mucocutaneous borders are not considered suitable for a closure using adhesives.

The procedure for using the tissue adhesives for surface closure involves thorough cleaning and haemostasis. Though moisture is a prerequisite for adhesion, the presence of excessive water or blood at the site is detrimental to a good result. The surface is dried before applying the adhesive in at least three to four thin layers along the length of the wound's surface. It is advisable to extend it approximately 5–10 mm from each side of the wound. The edges of the wound are held together for at least 1 minute as the adhesive dries.

The main advantages of tissue adhesives over other wound closure methods are the rapidity and painless application [13]. In addition, the suture track scars are avoided, leading to a much better cosmetic result. The risk of suture site infection is also found to be less. The material sloughs off in 5–10 days, as the skin sheds.

The obvious disadvantage is that it cannot be used in areas of tension. Additionally, there is a minor risk of toxicity and foreign body reactions. If the clinician's gloved fingers, gauze or plastic instruments contact the tissue adhesive during application, these materials may adhere to the patient's skin.

## 11.11 Conclusion

Wound care primarily involves measures to ensure that the wound heals quickly without going through adverse situations such as infections. Along with mechanical debridement, antibiotic medication and dressings, the various wound closure methods form the foundation of wound care practices. Depending on the patient needs and the wound types, one should choose from a wide variety of materials and techniques to implement effective wound closure.

## References


1. Buckley MJ, Keller JC. Emerging biomaterials and tissue engineering. Oral Maxillofac Surg Clin North Am. 2002 Feb;14(1):ix.
2. Herford AS, Haug RH. Emerging biomaterials and techniques in tissue regeneration. Oral Maxillofac Surg Clin N Am. 2017;29(1):1–120.
3. Kandor J. Atlas of suturing techniques. Approaches to surgical wound, laceration, and cosmetic repair. New York: McGraw-Hill; 2016.
4. Hupp JR. Guide to suturing. Section 2. J Oral Maxfac Surg. Aug 2015;73(Suppl 1):9–35.
5. Kudur MH, Pai SB, Sripathi H, Prabhu S. *Sutures* and *suturing* techniques in skin closure. Indian J Dermatol Venereol Leprol. 2009;75(4):425–34.
6. Gusman DN. Suture materials and techniques. In: Lower extremity soft tissue and cutaneous plastic surgery, vol. 1. Nottingham: Saunders; 2012. p. 77–100.

7. Connolly KL, Albertini JG, Miller CJ, Ozog DM. The suspension (frost) suture: experience and applications. Dermatol Surg. 2015 Mar;41(3):406–10.
8. Koshak HH. Dental suturing materials and techniques. Glob J Otolaryngol. 2017;12(2):1–11. GJO.MS.ID.555833
9. Griffin TJ, Hur Y, Bu J. Basic suture techniques for oral mucosa. Clin Adv Periodontics. 2011, Nov;1(3):221–32.
10. Iavazzo C, Gkegkes ID, Vouloumanou EK, Mamais I, Peppas G, Fallagas ME. Sutures versus staples for the management of surgical wounds: a meta-analysis of randomized controlled trials. Am Surg. Sept 2011;77(9):1206–21.
11. Tuptis A, Salma I. Fibrin sealant in maxillofacial surgery (literature review). https://www.rsu.lv/en/scientific-papers/fibrin-sealant-maxillofacial-surgery-literature-review. 2015.
12. Kaderi MA, Menaka KB, Metgud RM, Gharat MR, Naik PS, Ajmani JM, et al. In-vitro evaluation of antibacterial potential of cyanoacrylate tissue for intra-oral wound closure. J Dent Mater Tech. Sep 2017;6(4):163–9.
13. Oladega AA, James O, Adeyemo WL. Cyanoacrylate tissue adhesive or silk suture for closure of surgical wound following removal of an impacted mandibular third molar: a randomized controlled study. J Craniomaxillofac Surg. 2019 Jan;47(1):93–98.

# Postoperative Care of the Maxillofacial Surgery Patient

# 12

J. Naveen Kumar and Poornima Ravi

Postoperative care of the patient encompasses the time from the completion of the surgical procedure to the complete return of the patient to the normal physiological state. This is divided into three phases. Phase I is early recovery and takes place in the postanesthesia care unit (PACU). Phase II is intermediate recovery, and takes place in the ward. Phase III is late recovery that occurs after discharge.

## 12.1 Assessment of the Patient After Surgery

### 12.1.1 Assessment of the Patient Immediately After Surgery

Postoperative care of the patient begins immediately after the surgical procedure has been completed, even before the anesthesia is reversed. The first step is clearing the airway of blood and debris. Maxillomandibular fixation and occlusal splints, if placed earlier need to removed [1]. The next step is the removal of the throat pack.

#### 12.1.1.1 Care of the Airway

The decision to extubate or not must be made in conjunction with the anesthetist. Cases in which there is a high risk of airway edema will require the ET tube to be retained [1]. These include:

- Space infections compressing on the airway, e.g. Ludwig's angina.
- Severe facial trauma where there is likelihood of blood ooze, edema, or tongue fall back.
- Prolonged surgery, e.g. Free flap reconstructions.

In other cases, the patient may be extubated on the table. Awake extubation is usually preferred for head and neck surgery. The patient may be extubated when the following criteria are met [1]:

- No bleed from surgical site or secretion in the oropharynx.
- Patient is able to follow verbal commands.
- Patient is able to sustain head lift for at least 5 seconds.
- Patient is breathing on his own, with respiratory rate less than 24/min, tidal volume greater than 5 ml/kg, and Spo2 > 90%.

Once the extubation is done, an oropharyngeal airway can be inserted to prevent clenching of teeth and the tongue from falling back, which can cause obstruction. Alternatively, a nasopharyngeal airway can be used in case the surgeon deems oral cavity unfit for manipulation using the former. This must remain in place until the patient is conscious and obeys commands.

Some patients, such as those who have undergone extensive face and neck resection, may have required a tracheostomy prior to surgery. The tube must be secured after surgery by taping the stay sutures to the neck or chest. Tracheostomy care in the postoperative period is critical; a blocked or dislodged tube can have disastrous consequences [2].

1. The tube must be checked at frequent intervals.
2. The tube stoma must be covered with a humidifying bib, or a moist gauze.

J. N. Kumar (✉)
Oral and Maxillofacial Surgery, Sri Ramachandra Institute of Higher Education and Research, Chennai, India
e-mail: naveenkumarj@sriramachandra.edu.in

P. Ravi
Department of Oral and Maxillofacial Surgery, SRM Dental College, Ramapuram, Chennai, Tamil Nadu, India



K. Bonanthaya et al. (eds.), *Oral and Maxillofacial Surgery for the Clinician*, https://doi.org/10.1007/978-981-15-1346-6_12

3. The tube must be suctioned regularly to prevent clogging due to secretions. The suction catheter must be inserted to half of its length, which will correspond to the carina (Patients usually cough when this point is reached). Suction is then applied while simultaneously withdrawing the catheter.
4. To break up secretions, small quantities of sterile water can be syringed in and suctioned immediately.

#### 12.1.1.2 Need for Ventilation in the PACU

In some instances, ventilation may be required even after anesthetic recovery. Some examples include:

1. Patients who have history of COPD.
2. Severe trauma or infection.

While monitoring the patient who is on a ventilator, it is important to be aware of the various modes that the ventilator operates on [3]. These have been summarized in Table 12.1. Patients who have been on the ventilator for long periods of time need to be weaned off slowly. OMF surgeons frequently come across such patients in neurosurgical ward having concomitant traumatic brain injuries and craniomaxillofacial fractures. This may be done by setting the ventilator in CPAP mode (Continuous Positive Airway Pressure). This allows the patient to breathe, with the ventilator taking over if the patient is unable to do so.

#### 12.1.1.3 Monitoring in the PACU

Once the patient has been shifted to the recovery room, the cardiac monitor and pulse oximeter must be attached for proper monitoring. The following parameters must be monitored continuously:

- *Oxygen Saturation:* Hypoxia can occur in the postoperative period and the patient must be kept on oxygen for 1–2 h (2–6 L/min) to prevent this. Oxygen may be delivered using a face mask or through nasal prongs.
- *Pulse, blood pressure:* Increase in these parameters may indicate pain. Serious complications (Infarction, Malignant hyperthermia) may produce a drastic change in these parameters and must be recognized.
- *ECG waveform:* To monitor cardiac status.
- *Postanesthesia tremors/shivering:* This can occur on the table during recovery from anesthesia. It can occur if the patient is hypothermic, and is commonly associated with the use of halogenated anesthetics. Management consists of rewarming the patient. Tramadol and meperidine may be used to stop uncontrollable shivering [4].

The suction apparatus must be kept handy to evacuate blood ooze or secretions that may hamper the airway. It is advisable to avoid Maxillomandibular fixation (MMF) in the immediate postoperative period; if required, this may be done after 24 h.

Detailed surgical notes must also be recorded, along with the number and type of implants that were used. Postoperative instructions must also be documented in detail. A list of notes to be completed by the surgeon before leaving the operation theater complex is summarized in Table 12.2.

#### 12.1.1.4 Briefing the Patient and Family

Immediately after the surgery, the surgeon must interact with the patient's immediate caregivers, giving them the details of the procedure, and any anticipated complications.

#### 12.1.1.5 Discharge from PACU to Ward

This is done when the patient has regained consciousness, with adequate respiratory function and stable vitals. Decisions can be made based on a standard scoring system, such as the Aldrete scoring system [5]. The scoring system which was originally proposed in 1970, underwent modifications in 1995 and 1999. The various factors considered

**Table 12.1** Ventilator modes and settings

| Ventilator mode | Type of setting | Description/indications |
|---|---|---|
| Volume control | Continuous mandatory ventilation (CMV) | Patients with respiratory muscle weakness or LV dysfunction<br>If patient breathes rapidly, may cause hyperinflation and respiratory alkalosis |
| | Synchronous intermittent mandatory ventilation (SIMV) | Patient breathes partially on their own; meant for patients who breathe rapidly on CMV<br>Mandatory breaths are synchronized with spontaneous breathing |
| Pressure control | Pressure controlled ventilation (PCV) | Patients with neuromuscular disease but normal lungs who can control volume. |
| | Pressure support ventilation | Used during weaning, patient determines respiratory volume and frequency, but the ventilator provided continuous positive airway pressure (CPAP) |

**Table 12.2** Checklist for completion before leaving the theater complex

| Checklist to complete before leaving the OT |
|---|
| Surgical notes |
| Details of implants and hardware used |
| Postoperative instructions to be followed by nursing staff |
| Postoperative fluid management instructions |
| Postoperative medication dose and schedule |
| Biopsy requisition form |
| Requisition form for aspirates/swabs and others |
| Investigation requisition form |

**Table 12.3** Subjective assessment of the patient

| Subjective parameters evaluated | Assessment made |
|---|---|
| Pain (use visual analog scale- VAS/ faces scale) | Whether the pain medication is adequate or whether it needs to be increased or discontinued (see Sect. 12.2.2.1) |
| Nausea/vomiting | If the patient has experienced this, assess the need for antiemetics, and insertion of nasogastric tube to decompress the stomach. (Sect. 12.2.5.5) |
| Mobility | The patient must be encouraged to sit up and walk by the first postoperative day. (Section IID) |
| Function- e.g. swallowing, speech, nerve function | It is important to evaluate branches of the facial nerve and trigeminal nerve that may have been at risk of damage during surgery |
| Passing urine/stools/ flatulence | Inability to pass urine may indicate inadequate fluid therapy, and may lead to acute renal failure. (see Sect. 12.2.5.6)<br>Inability to pass stools may be a sign of paralytic ileus; may occur after iliac crest harvest |

are patient activity, respiration, circulation, consciousness, $O_2$ saturation, pain, surgical site bleeding, and nausea/vomiting. Patients scoring greater than 9 on this scale can be moved to the ward for the next phase of care. Readers are advised to refer the article for getting a detailed idea of the scoring table.

**Table 12.4** Objective assessment of patient

| Objective parameters evaluated | Assessment made |
|---|---|
| *Vital signs* | |
| Temperature<br>Pulse<br>Blood pressure<br>Respiratory rate | Is postoperative fever present? If so, it must be worked up (Sect. 12.2.5.2)<br>Changes in pulse and blood pressure have several causes (Sect. 12.2.5.3)<br>If abnormal, evaluate whether the patient has respiratory distress (Sect. 12.2.5.4) |
| *Fluid input/output* | |
| | Is the input adequate? (Sect. 12.2.1)<br>Is urinary output adequate? This helps assess renal function(Sect. 12.2.5.6) |
| *Surgical site evaluation* | |
| | The wound must be inspected, and assessed for healing. (Sect. 12.3) |

**Table 12.5** Postoperative investigations

| Investigation | Indications |
|---|---|
| Hemoglobin | If there has been extensive blood loss during surgery, to determine the need for blood transfusion. |
| Serum electrolytes | Suspicion of electrolyte imbalances (seizures, palpitations, muscle cramps) |
| WBC TC/DC | Suspicion of spreading infection |
| Chest x-ray | Suspicion of atelectasis/aspiration pneumonia |
| OPG/other facial radiographs | To check the accuracy of reduction and status of plating. |

### 12.1.2 Comprehensive Assessment of the Patient in the Ward

This is done according to the SOAP format [6]. SOAP is an acronym for Subjective, Objective, Assessment, and Plan. In Subjective evaluation, the patient must be asked if they have any complaints. Specific complaints are recorded. In Objective evaluation, a thorough evaluation of the patient is done by the physician. This includes evaluation of the vital signs, fluid intake and output, as well as an assessment of the surgical site. Helpful information may be obtained from the TPR chart, input/output chart, and nurses' notes. Based on the subjective and objective evaluation, the patient's current status is assessed (Tables 12.3 and 12.4). This is used to formulate a plan.

#### 12.1.2.1 Postoperative Investigations

Sometimes investigations may be required in the postoperative period, either to check the health status of the patient or to confirm the diagnosis of certain complications. A list of investigations that may be ordered and the indications for the same are summarized in Table 12.5.

## 12.2 Formulating a Plan of Care Based on Assessment

### 12.2.1 Fluid Therapy in the Postoperative Period

The patient is usually 'nil per mouth' for a few hours prior to surgery and after surgery. Apart from this, there is a loss of blood and body fluids in any surgery, which requires replacement. It is therefore essential to infuse intravenous fluids during this period [7, 8]. This is done for two purposes.

**Replacement** Any fluid deficit that has occurred must be replaced by infusion. This could have occurred during either of the following periods:

- Preoperative period: This could be due to
  - NPO status.
  - Blood or fluid losses that may have occurred due to trauma, burns, etc.
- Intraoperative period: Surgical blood loss of greater than 500 ml or 7 ml/kg requires replacement.

**Maintenance** This is to maintain the ongoing fluid requirements, till the patient resumes oral intake of fluids. Maintenance fluids are essential to maintain proper pH and electrolyte balance and for adequate organ perfusion.

#### 12.2.1.1 Types of Fluids Used

There are three types of fluids than can be used—crystalloids, colloids, blood and blood products. The preference of one type of fluid over another has several controversies, and there are no clear-cut guidelines available [9]. A few indications for each fluid type are given below.

**Crystalloids**

Crystalloids are balanced salt solutions with or without the addition of a buffering agent. When infused into the bloodstream, crystalloids tend to leave the capillaries and enter the extravascular fluid compartment. Crystalloid infusion will increase fluid in the extravascular tissues and does little to expand the circulating blood volume. In maxillofacial surgery, crystalloids are favored as maintenance fluids during the postoperative period.

**Colloids**

Colloids are protein-containing solutions. Since these proteins have a large molecular size, under ordinary circumstances, these are prevented from crossing the capillary endothelial cells and going into the extravascular space. Therefore, they tend to expand vascular volume alone. Colloids are mostly used in the intraoperative period if there has been significant blood loss and the plasma volume needs to be expanded. It is not common to use colloids in the postoperative setting.

Commonly used iv fluids are listed in Table 12.6.

**Table 12.6** Commonly used postoperative IV fluids

| IV Fluid | Composition (in meq/l) | Indications | Risks |
|---|---|---|---|
| *Crystalloids* | | | |
| Lactated Ringers (RL) | Na –130; Cl –109; K –4; Ca –3; Lactate –28 | Fluid of choice in postoperative maintenance | Lactic acidosis if liver function is poor |
| Dextrose Normal Saline (DNS) | Na –154; Cl –154; Dextrose –50 g | Alternative to RL | Hyperchloremic acidosis |
| Normal Saline (NS) | Na –154; Cl –154 | Alternative to DNS in diabetics | Hyperchloremic acidosis |
| 5% Dextrose (D5W) | Dextrose 50 g | Replacing free water deficit | Hyperglycemia in diabetics |
| *Colloids* | | | |
| Hetastarch | 6% hydroxyethyl starch | Plasma volume expansion | Nephrotoxicity, coagulopathy |

#### 12.2.1.2 Strategy for Estimating Fluid Requirement

1. The input-output chart must be verified before determining the fluid requirement. This will help to estimate fluid excess (positive balance), or deficits (negative balance) and plan requirements.
2. Calculate the Estimated Fluid Requirement (EFR) for each hour:
   This is done using Holliday and Segar's formula (The 4-2-1 rule) [10].
   - First 10 kg: 4 cc/kg.
   - Next 10 kg: 2 cc/kg.
   - Above 20 kg: 1 cc/kg.

   E.g. a 60 kg adult will require $(4 \times 10) + (2 \times 10) + (1 \times 40) = 40 + 20 + 40 = 100$ ml/h.
3. Calculate the total Estimated Fluid Deficit: This depends on the number of hours from the last oral intake to the next oral intake. For example, if the patient has not had oral intake for 12 h:
   EFD = EFR × no. of NPO hours = $100 \times 12 = 1200$ ml.
4. Estimate the surgical blood loss. If crystalloids are used to replace this blood loss, for a particular volume of blood, three times the volume of crystalloids are used for replacement. If colloids are used, the same volume is sufficient.
5. Estimate the amount of fluids that have already been infused during anesthesia.
6. Total postsurgical fluid requirement:
   EFD+(blood loss × 3)−fluids replaced during surgery.
   In the above scenario, if 300 ml of blood was lost, and one liter of fluid was infused during surgery, then:

   Total postsurgical fluid requirement:
   $1200 + (300 \times 3) - 1000 = 1200 + 900 - 1000 = 1100$ ml.

#### 12.2.1.3 Liberal Versus Restrictive Fluid Therapy

In recent years, the above method of estimating fluid requirements has been criticized, as it tends to overestimate the amount of fluids needed by a patient [11]. Excessive fluid infusion may cause fluid shift into the extravascular compartment, which in turn can result in overload complications such as renal injury, acute respiratory distress syndrome, etc. On the other hand, liberal fluid infusion can reduce postoperative complications such as nausea, vomiting, and drowsiness.

For major systemic surgeries, the current trend is either to follow a 'restrictive' approach or a goal-directed therapy. Goal-directed therapy measures hemodynamic parameters such as stroke volume, and fluids are given accordingly. While this has been found useful in major surgeries, particularly abdominal surgeries, there is no evidence on its effectiveness in postoperative recovery for maxillofacial surgery. A liberal approach may be preferred for most kinds of

**Table 12.7** Risks vs. benefits of blood transfusion

| Risks of blood transfusion | Benefits of blood transfusion |
|---|---|
| Transmission of infections that cannot be identified by screening (cytomegalovirus, Epstein-Barr virus, B-19 parovirus, dengue, chikungunya, HHV-8, malarial parasite) | Better functional status |
| Transfusion reactions | Lower morbidity and mortality (for levels below 7.0 mg/dl) |

**Table 12.8** Indications for postoperative blood transfusion

| Postoperative hemoglobin level | Risk factors/compensatory mechanisms present | Transfusion requirement |
|---|---|---|
| <6 g/dl | | Required |
| 6–8 g/dl | No risk factors | Not required |
| | Presence of risk factors (coronary artery disease, heart failure, cerebrovascular disease/limited mechanisms of compensation) | Required |
| | Presence of symptoms indicative of hypoxia (physiological transfusion triggers: Tachycardia, hypotension, electrocardiographic signs of ischemia, lactic acidosis, etc.) | Required |
| 8–10 g/dl | Presence of symptoms indicative of hypoxia (physiological transfusion triggers: Tachycardia, hypotension, electrocardiographic signs of ischemia, lactic acidosis, etc.) | Required |
| | Absence of above symptoms | Not required |
| >10 g/dl | | Not required |

maxillofacial surgery, which generally fall under low or intermediate risk procedures. Nevertheless, as long as postoperative fluids are being administered, the patient must be monitored for signs of overhydration such as peripheral edema, dyspnea, high blood pressure, and a bounding pulse. If any of these are present, the current fluid regimen must be reassessed [12].

#### 12.2.1.4 Transfusion of Blood and Blood Products

Postoperative blood transfusion is rarely required in routine maxillofacial surgery. It has been stated that the risks of blood transfusion outweigh the benefits [13] (See Table 12.7), and currently a restrictive approach to blood transfusion is favored.

If there has been extensive blood loss during surgery, or preexisting anemia, the postoperative hemoglobin must be assessed, and the decision to transfuse is based on this level [14]. This is described in Table 12.8.

### 12.2.2 Postoperative Medication

The maxillofacial surgeon must be aware of the type and dosage of medication that is required in the immediate postoperative period. Pain control and prophylaxis against infection are the most important factors to be kept in mind while prescribing medication.

#### 12.2.2.1 Pain Control

Pain control is an important goal after every surgical procedure as it can not only affect the patients' attitude, but it can also impair oxygenation and thereby delay wound healing. The pain must be assessed subjectively, by asking the patient to rate their pain on a standard scale (e.g. Visual Analogue scale or Faces pain scale). If the patient is in pain, pain medication must be increased or changed.

Preemptive analgesia is an evolving, controversial technique that involves the administration of analgesics prior to the onset of noxious stimuli. This is believed to limit the sensitization of the nervous system, thereby reducing the need for postoperative analgesia [15]. One effective preemptive technique is the infiltration of a long-acting local anesthetic, such as bupivacaine, into the incision site before closure. This provides effective pain relief throughout the postoperative period.

In the postoperative period, various classes of analgesics may be used [16]. Some of the commonly used analgesics are summarized in Table 12.9.

The best method of choosing the appropriate analgesic is using the WHO analgesic ladder (Fig. 12.1). If the pain is not well controlled, the patient can move to the next step of the ladder. Once the pain is controlled, patients must be weaned by moving down the ladder [17]. This step ladder approach is just a broad lattice and has its own share of controversies and modifications. Readers are encouraged to read appropriate references for getting a broader picture of the analgesic ladder and a detailed discussion is beyond the scope of this chapter.

**Patient-controlled Analgesia** Postoperative patients often require immediate pain relief at varied intervals. PCA allows the use of iv pumps which, when the patient presses a button, allows a bolus dose of analgesic to be delivered for immediate relief [18]. This allows analgesics to be tailored to the patients' requirements and also records the amount of opioid being administered per day.

#### 12.2.2.2 Anti-inflammatory Drugs

The role of corticosteroids in postoperative care is controversial. Corticosteroids are potent anti-inflammatory agents and are often used after surgery. It has been established that corticosteroids reduce pain and inflammation [19]. There is also evidence that single doses of steroids can reduce postoperative nausea and vomiting, and improve fatigue after surgery. However, the benefit of extended doses of steroids seems controversial and comes with the risk of impaired wound healing, infectious complications, and hyperglycemia. It is

**Table 12.9** Analgesics commonly used for postoperative pain control

| Drug | Classification | Dosage and frequency | Precautions and adverse effects |
|---|---|---|---|
| Diclofenac | NSAIDS (aryl acetic acid derivatives) | 75 mg bd adults<br>1.5 mg/kg bd children | Has been linked to adverse cardiovascular events—Avoid in patients with heart disease<br>Gastric ulceration and bleeding may worsen<br>Nephrotoxic; avoid in patients prone to kidney disease |
| Aceclofenac | | 100 mg bd adults<br>Safety not established in children | Less than diclofenac, mild GI symptoms have been reported |
| Ketorolac | NSAIDS | 20–30 mg q6hr<br>0.5 mg/kg q6hr | GI symptoms, hypertension reported in few patients |
| Acetaminophen (paracetamol) | NSAIDS (Para-amino phenol derivative) | 0.5–1 g tds adults<br>10–15 mg/kg children | Hepatotoxicity |
| Tramadol | Synthetic opioid | 50 mg bd or sos<br>Safety not established in children. | May worsen nausea and vomiting. Like all opioids, respiratory depression is higher. |
| Morphine | Natural opioid | 0.2–0.8 mg/kg bd | Respiratory depression, nausea, vomiting, constipation. Not suitable in immediate postop as consciousness cannot be evaluated |

therefore recommended that steroids be used only till the first postoperative day. Dexamethasone 8 mg is generally used twice a day. For single day dosing, taper is not generally required.

Enzymatic anti-inflammatory medication is also used to reduce postoperative edema [20]. These include serratiopeptidase (10 mg tds) or trypsin:chymotrypsin (chymoral, 100,000 IU). However, its efficacy is based mostly on anecdotal reports and there is hardly any scientific evidence to back its use.

#### 12.2.2.3 Antibiotic Prophylaxis

The use of antibiotic prophylaxis (for wound infections) in maxillofacial surgery is a controversial area. Literature evidence is insufficient to ascertain whether prophylaxis is required or not, and the duration of prophylaxis has no definite guidelines. Based on recent systematic reviews, Table 12.10 sums up current recommendations [21, 22].

Preferred antibiotics for prophylaxis include:

Amoxicillin-Clavulanate 1.2 mg IV bd.
Amoxicillin 500 mg per oral tds (OR) Cefotaxime 1 g IV bd with Metronidazole 500 mg IV tds.
Prophylaxis must be started 30–90 min before the surgical procedure. The postoperative regimen has no clear guidelines, but must continue for at least 24 h after the procedure. After this, the wound must be monitored for infection, and therapeutic antibiotics may be instituted only if required. This section is covered in more detail in Chap. 10, of this book

#### 12.2.2.4 Medication to Prevent Postoperative Gastritis and Vomiting

Preoperative and intraoperative fasting, as well as drugs used in the postoperative period, can induce gastric irritation in the surgical patient. To counter this, drugs that reduce the acidity of gastric secretions may be used. Ranitidine, a H2 blocker, may be used in a dose of 50 mg bd. An alternative drug is Pantoprazole, which may be used in a dose of 40 mg once a day.

Prevention of postoperative nausea and vomiting is an important factor in postoperative care. One of the important drugs used for the management of PONV is Ondansetron, which is given in a dose of 4 mg [23]. This is usually a rescue medication and is not given on a routine basis.

#### 12.2.2.5 Drugs for Thromboprophylaxis

Patients undergoing prolonged surgery or hospitalization may be at increased risk of developing thromboembolic events, namely deep vein thrombosis and pulmonary embolism. Additional risk factors include smoking, pregnancy, oral contraceptives, and malignancy. These patients must be placed on thromboprophylactic drugs. In indicated cases, TED (thromboembolic deterrent) stockings have to be used in the postoperative patients. The guidelines are summarized in Table 12.11 [24].

#### 12.2.2.6 Other Drugs That May be Required Based on the Patients' Medical History

If the patient has other medical comorbidities, medication that was being taken prior to the procedure may need to be continued or modified. It is best to confer with the patients' physician to determine the dosage and kind of drugs needed. These have been summarized in Table 12.12.

### 12.2.3 Nutritional Status in the Postoperative Period

Maxillofacial surgical procedures provide a unique challenge to the nutritional status in the postoperative period. Pain and edema in the oral region often prevent the patient

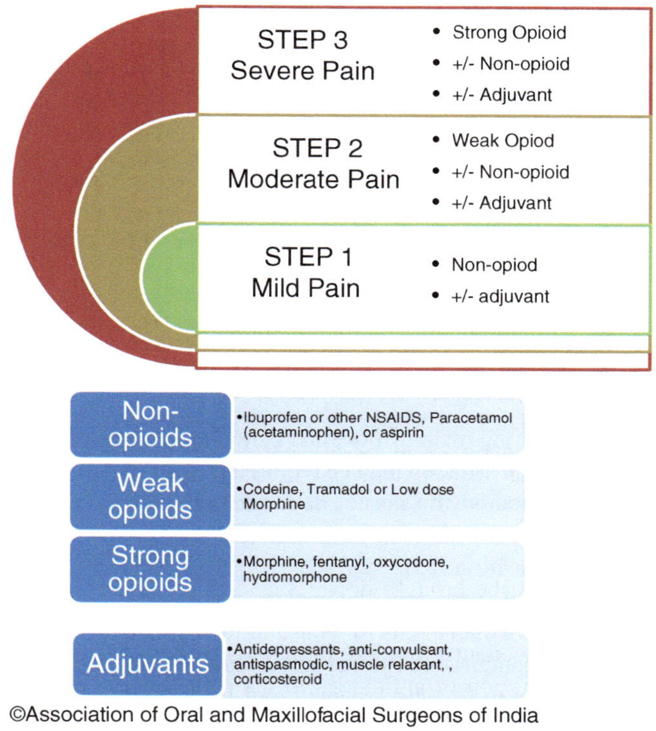


**Fig. 12.1** WHO analgesic ladder

**Table 12.10** Recommendations for antibiotic prophylaxis

| Type of surgery | Recommendation for antibiotic prophylaxis |
|---|---|
| Orthognathic surgery | Strongly recommended |
| Trauma—compound fractures | Recommended |
| Resections involving oral and cervical region | Recommended |
| Reconstruction | Weak evidence; physician judgment |
| Cleft surgery | Weak evidence; physician judgment |
| Minor oral surgery | Weak evidence; physician judgment |

**Table 12.11** Thromboprophylaxis guidelines

| Risk level | Criteria | Thromboprophylaxis required |
|---|---|---|
| Low | Minor surgery, age < 40 yrs., no additional risk factors | Early and persistent mobilization |
| Moderate | Minor surgery in age 40–60 yrs., with risk factors<br>Major surgery <40 yrs., no risk factors<br>Patients with medical illnesses or burns, with one risk factor<br>Neurosurgical patient with one risk factor | Low molecular weight heparin, <3400 units per day<br>OR intermittent pneumatic compression devices |
| High | Minor surgery >60 years<br>Major surgery >40 years with risk factors<br>Patients with malignancy<br>Patients with medical illness or burns with two or more risk factors<br>Neurosurgical patient with two or more risk factors<br>Trauma patients with one or more risk factors | Low molecular weight heparin, >3400 units per day<br>OR intermittent pneumatic compression devices |
| Highest | Patients with multiple risk factors, pelvic and lower extremity trauma or surgery, head injuries | Low molecular weight heparin, >3400 units per day AND intermittent pneumatic compression devices |

from taking food comfortably, and there is a tendency to eat less or not at all. In patients with intermaxillary fixation, there is an inability to open the mouth and chew food. In certain kinds of surgery, such as reconstructive flaps involving the oral region, the patient is asked to avoid taking food by mouth at all to prevent the possibility of infection and flap failure in the postoperative period.

It is important, however, that the nutritional status is maintained. Inadequate nutrition has been shown to increase morbidity and mortality and can delay wound healing. It also increases the patient's susceptibility to infection. In the young, healthy adult patient, nutritional support may not be required, as the body compensates for decreased intake by increased glycogenolysis, gluconeogenesis, lipolysis, and amino acid oxidation. However, in young children, patients

**Table 12.12** Additional drugs that may be required in the postoperative period

| Medical comorbidity | Drugs to be administered |
|---|---|
| Diabetes mellitus | Insulin based on insulin sliding scale |
| Patient with chronic hypertension | Patient's regular antihypertensive regimen to be restarted within 24 h |
| Patient on anticoagulants | Low molecular weight heparin for 24 h, after which warfarin should be resumed |
| Patient on long-term steroids | Hydrocortisone 50 mg three times a day, (equivalent to dexamethasone 2 mg) in addition to patient's normal dose, for up to 72 h |

with preexisting malnutrition, and patients with wasting diseases, supplementation may be required for even routine procedures. Patients who do not have adequate oral intake for 7–14 days (3–10 days in children) will require support to avoid malnutrition [25].

Nutritional status must be evaluated in the postoperative patient. This usually calls for consultation by a dietician. For long-term patients, nutritional status can also be measured using certain tools. The accepted tool for assessment is the subjective global assessment scale [26].

In patients on intermaxillary fixation, the classic use of the nasogastric tube must be discouraged. Patients may be educated on taking food through the retromolar region, using a feeding tube. NG tubes may be reserved for cases in whom oral feeds are contraindicated to avoid infection. Nutritionally complete formulas (e.g. Ensure) are available for enteral feeds. The patient may be started on 50 ml formula every 4 h, and this may be gradually increased in 50 ml increments until the desired target is achieved. After each feed, the tube must be flushed with 30 ml water to prevent blockage.

In cases of extensive neck surgery, where swallowing may be impaired, percutaneous gastrostomy (PEG) or jejunostomy tubes may be placed. For these tubes, infusion feeds (at the rate of 20 ml/h, increased in 20 ml increments every 4 h) may be given.

Total parenteral nutrition is usually not preferred because it has been linked to higher rates of infectious complications as compared to enteral nutrition. Patients who have complete block of the gastrointestinal system or those who cannot tolerate or retain enteral feeds are candidates for TPN. Dextrose solutions are preferred, with a dose of 10–20 g/kg/day of glucose. This is used in conjunction with amino acid solutions (0.5–3.5 g/kg/day) and lipid emulsions (50 ml/hr) [25].

### 12.2.4 Postoperative Mobilization of the Maxillofacial Surgery Patient

After the surgical procedure, early mobilization is recommended for all patients. Early mobilization is believed to enhance recovery by reducing the incidence of postoperative complications. It reduces secretions in the lungs, accelerates peristalsis, and improves venous blood flow to the extremities, thereby preventing thrombophlebitis and deep vein thrombosis [27]. Immobilization increases the risk of complications such as DVT and pressure sores. It can also lead to urinary retention.

For most maxillofacial procedures, the patient may be allowed to sit up with legs dangling 6 h after surgery. The patient may be mobilized within 24 h, and it is recommended that they ambulate every 4–6 h (during waking hours) till discharge. Caution must be employed in patients who have had grafts or flaps taken from the fibula. While the early mobilization protocol must be followed, protected weight bearing may be employed.

For patients who require prolonged bed rest, the use of alternating pressure mattresses or gel mattress overlays must be considered to prevent pressure sores.

Chest physiotherapy forms an important component of postoperative care. The in-hospital patient is prone to increased lung secretions and infections, which may be cleared using chest physiotherapy.

### 12.2.5 Management of Complications in the Postoperative Period

#### 12.2.5.1 Sudden Airway Obstruction

Maxillofacial surgery and surgery to the neck carry a risk of edema and hematoma developing in the postoperative period that can compress on the airway. The airway must be monitored closely, both in the immediate postoperative period and during the stay in the ward.

If the patient presents with hypoxia and airway obstruction, the head tilt-chin lift-jaw thrust maneuver must be employed. The airway must be checked manually and cleared of obstruction such as vomitus or blood. If the airway obstruction is at or above the oropharynx, insert an airway (such as Guedel's) to keep the passage patent. If there is a hematoma compressing the airway, surgical sutures must be removed to allow a release of pressure. In extreme cases, emergency airway procedures such as cricothyroidotomy may need to be performed.

#### 12.2.5.2 Fever in the Postoperative Period

Fever is defined as a rise in body temperature above 38 °C (100.4 °F). Postoperative fever represents a diagnostic challenge for most surgeons. Although most cases of fever are self-limiting, some can be serious and need urgent intervention. The timing of postoperative fever often gives a clue as to its diagnosis and management [28, 29].

**Immediate Fever (During Surgery or Within the First 24 h).**

Fever in the immediate postoperative period is most likely to be an inflammatory response to surgery. The surgical procedure causes *release of pyrogenic cytokines*, which stimulate the anterior hypothalamus to release prostaglandins, causing a rise in body temperature. The extent of fever depends on the amount of tissue trauma, but usually resolves in 24 h. Laboratory and diagnostic workup is not warranted for this kind of fever.

Occasionally, immediate fever can occur due to more serious reasons, and it is important to identify these. *Malignant hyperthermia* is a rare, life-threatening disorder that can manifest in susceptible individuals when they are exposed to inhalational anesthetics, or succinylcholine. There is an immediate rise in body temperature during or up to 1 h after surgery. It may be recognized by an immediate rise in $ETCO_2$, tachypnea, tachycardia, and muscle rigidity. Prompt intervention is required to avoid muscle lysis and organ system failure. Treatment involves immediate intravenous Dantrolene sodium (2.5 mg/kg), repeated every 5 min till reversal occurs, or till the maximum dose is reached (10 mg/kg).

If the fever occurs during or immediately *after a blood transfusion*, it is a sign of transfusion reaction. Transfusion of incompatible (mismatched) blood can cause a severe hemolytic reaction, which, in addition to fever, can present with dyspnea, fever, and myoglobinuria. In such cases, the transfusion must be discontinued immediately. Sometimes, febrile reactions can also occur with compatible blood, due to reaction of recipient antibodies with antigens in the transfused blood. This fever will be accompanied by headache, nausea, and vomiting. Slowing the transfusion may suffice, but it must be stopped if the reactions become severe.

*Adverse drug reactions* can rarely cause fever. This is usually a diagnosis of exclusion, and if suspected, all drugs must be discontinued one at a time to identify the offender. If replacement is necessary, a chemically unrelated drug must be used.

### Early Postoperative Fever (24–48 h After Surgery)

A serious cause of postoperative fever in this time period is *deep vein thromboembolism*. This must be suspected if the patient has known risk factors, such as a history of smoking, malignant disease, prolonged surgery, advanced age, or prolonged immobility after surgery. Diagnosis is made by ultrasound or impedence plethysmography. If present, prompt systemic anticoagulation must be started to avoid fatal pulmonary embolism. The use of Homan's sign (Pain in the calf on forced dorsiflexion of the foot) is no longer recommended because of the risk of dislodging the thrombus into circulation. A suspected PE may be confirmed with a ventilation-perfusion (V/Q) scan of the lungs.

*Thrombophlebitis* can also cause a rise in body temperature. Any iv line in place for more than 24 h can cause phlebitis. This presents with pain, erythema, and edema at the affected site. The iv line must be removed and replaced, and anti-inflammatory drugs may be given. A topical ointment containing heparin and benzyl nicotinate (thrombophob) may be applied locally.

*Atelectasis* was once thought to be a cause of fever, but it is now believed that fever and atelectasis are unrelated, though they can coexist. *Aspiration pneumonia* is more likely to be a respiratory cause of fever, but it presents 3–5 days after surgery.

### Delayed Postoperative Fever (After 48 h)

*Surgical site wound infections* can result in fever 3–5 days after surgery. The surgical site must be examined for pain, swelling, and pus discharge if fever occurs during this period. If an infection is present, it must be managed as detailed in the following sections.

*Aspiration pneumonia* can occur if the gastric fluid is aspirated into the lungs, owing to a depressed cough reflex after surgery. The risk increases in patients on maxillomandibular fixation.

### Fever Beyond Fifth Postoperative Day

Fever beyond the fifth postoperative day is usually a sign of systemic infection and needs a diagnostic workup. The most common infections that can occur are *urinary tract infection* and *upper respiratory tract infection*.

Indwelling urinary catheters are the main source of UTIs. Women are at greater risk because they have a shorter urethra; however, both genders can develop UTI if the catheter is in place for more than 72 h. Concomitant signs such as burning sensation on passing urine may be present. Urine will appear cloudy. Diagnosis is best confirmed by urine culture; empirical antibiotics may be started in the meantime.

Respiratory tract infections can range from sinusitis to hospital-acquired pneumonia. In Hospital Acquired Pneumonia (HAP), chest auscultation may reveal crackles or rales, and diagnosis is made by chest x-rays. Treatment is by empirical antibiotics.

A rare infection that can occur beyond the fifth day is *necrotizing soft tissue infection*. Although this is more common after colorectal surgery, cervical necrotizing infection has been reported after maxillofacial surgery as well [30]. Diagnosis may be made by detecting subcutaneous 'gas' on x-rays or CT imaging. Treatment involves the use of broad spectrum antibiotics and fluid resuscitation.

With all systemic infections, blood culture must be done to rule out sepsis. It is also important to monitor the patient's vitals closely to ensure that the patient does not go into septic shock.

> It may be of interest to know that in the literature there is a mnemonic of 6 W's, with regard to causes of postoperative fever. The W's being *Waves* (ECG changes, MI), *Wind* (atelectasis, pneumonia), *Water* (UTI), *Wound* (surgical site infection), *Walking* (Venous thromboembolism), *Wonder* drugs(drug-related fever).

The workup for postoperative fever is shown in Fig. 12.2.

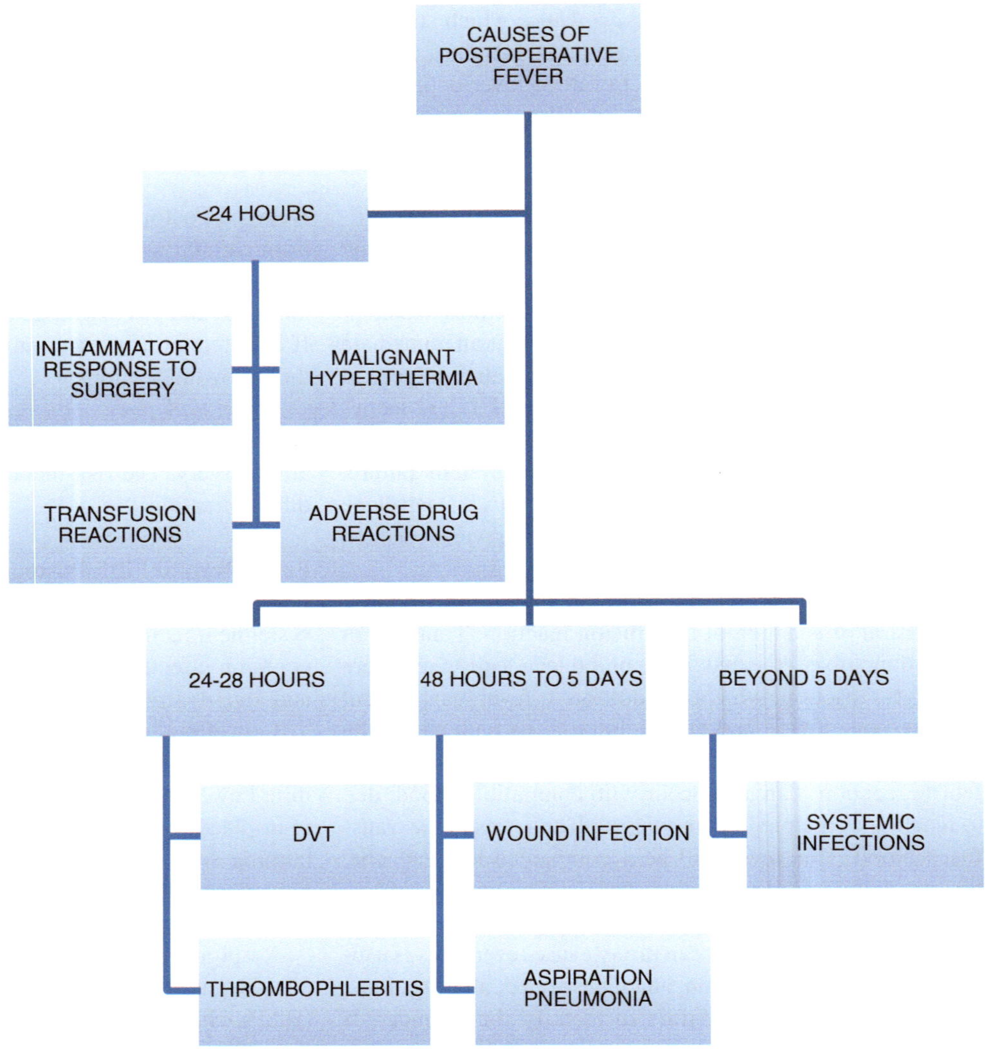


**Fig. 12.2** Postoperative fever workup

### 12.2.5.3 Changes in Pulse and Blood Pressure

Any gross deviation from the normal vital signs must be looked into. Changes in pulse (tachycardia or bradycardia) are usually associated with changes in the other vital signs as well, and these must therefore be evaluated first.

Hypotension in the postoperative period can occur due to several causes [6] (Fig. 12.3). Hypotension is usually the result of reduced plasma volume; this may be due to inadequate fluid resuscitation, or ongoing blood loss. Excessive usage of opioid analgesics may also cause a fall in blood pressure. A myocardial infarction and blood sepsis may also present with hypotension. Hypotension with tachycardia can be a sign of developing shock; which must be treated immediately with a fluid challenge (rapid bolus of fluid). Regardless of the cause, hypotension must be managed by increasing fluid input and supplemented by high-flow oxygen to improve the perfusion.

Raised blood pressure usually occurs in patients who have had preexisting hypertension. If the patient has a history of ischemic heart disease or cerebrovascular disease, it must be managed with appropriate medication, to reduce the risk of developing myocardial infarction or stroke postoperatively. Sometimes, hypertension may occur in healthy adults with no history. In these cases, it could reflect pain and anxiety, or distension of the bowel and/or bladder. Excessive fluid resuscitation may also result in hypertension [6].

### 12.2.5.4 Changes in Respiration

Increase in respiratory rate (tachypnea) is usually a sign of respiratory distress, and may be accompanied by decreased

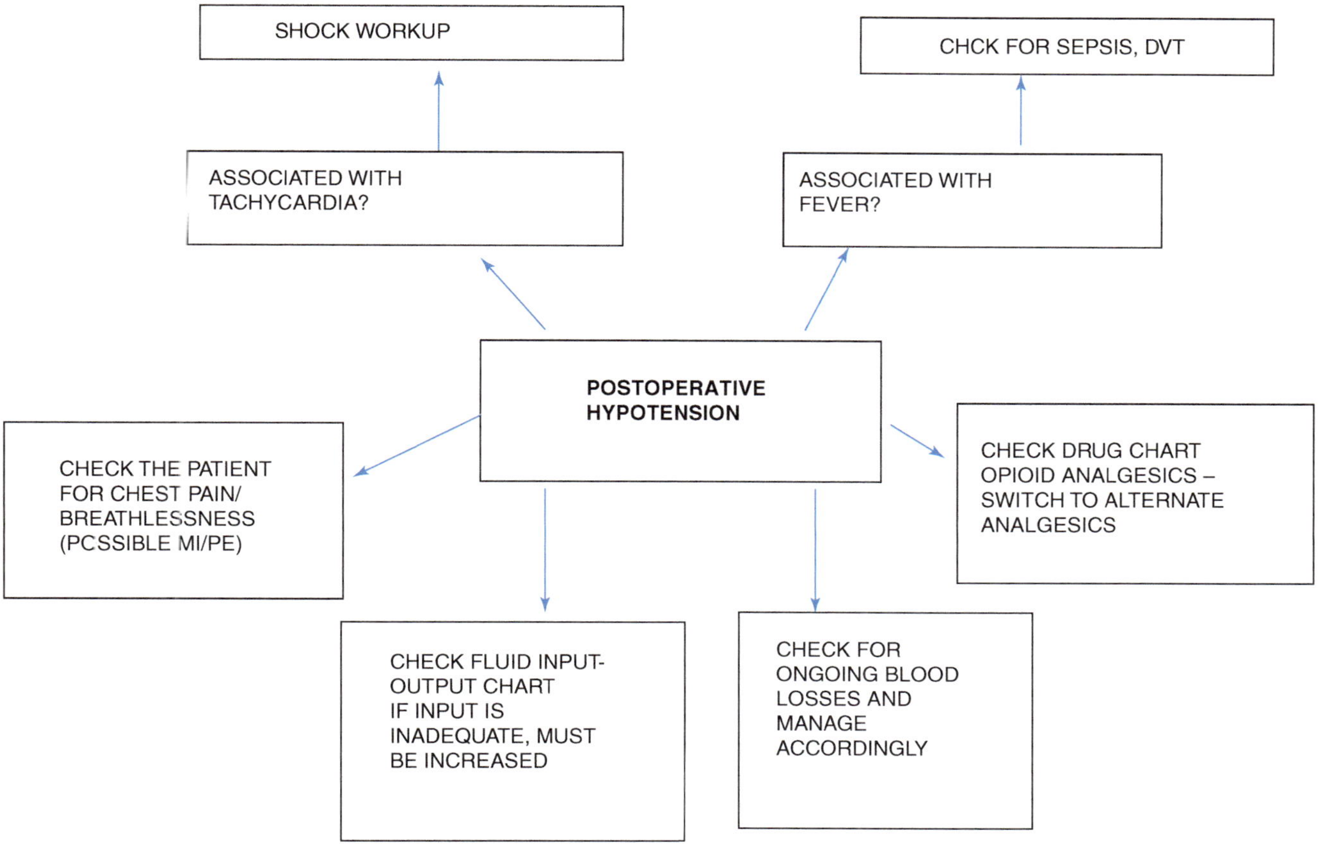




**Fig. 12.3** Postoperative hypotension workup

oxygen saturation, and use of accessory muscles of respiration [6]. Sudden acute shortness of breath may be a sign of pulmonary embolism. Gradual onset that occurs within 2–5 days of surgery is commonly due to atelectasis. Atelectasis is the collapse of a small segment of the lung and commonly occurs after general anesthesia. Atelectasis after maxillofacial surgery may be obstructive in nature, occurring secondary to epistaxis or mucus secretion. Another reason for the slow onset of respiratory distress is Acute Respiratory Distress Syndrome (ARDS), which can occur secondary to hypovolemia, sepsis, or trauma. Respiratory infection and cardiac causes such as myocardial infarction or cardiac failure can also alter respiratory rate. The various causes are illustrated in Fig. 12.4.

If a person experiences shortness of breath, high-flow oxygen must be started, and a chest x-ray and EKG must be taken. Laboratory tests including cardiac enzymes and arterial blood gases must be performed to ascertain the cause. If sputum is present, it must be sent for culture and gram staining.

#### 12.2.5.5 Postoperative Nausea and Vomiting

This is a common complication that occurs due to activation of the nucleus tractus solitarius and vomiting center by inhalational anesthetics. Patients who undergo maxillofacial surgery, particularly orthognathic surgical procedures, are at increased risk of developing postoperative nausea and vomiting, due to accumulation of blood in the throat. It can affect 20–80% of all patients, the risk being higher in young patients, females in the first 8 days of their menstrual cycle, and obese patients [23]. This complication is best managed symptomatically using antiemetics such as ondansetron and metoclopramide.

#### 12.2.5.6 Oliguria and Acute Renal Failure

The normal urine output is 1 ml/kg/h in infants, 0.5 ml/kg/h in children, and at least 400 ml/day in adults. Any drop below this level is referred to as oliguria and this must be addressed to prevent acute kidney injury (AKI). AKI is diagnosed as oliguria, along with serum creatinine levels 1.5 times above baseline [6]. The various causes of postoperative oliguria and management are outlined in Table 12.13.

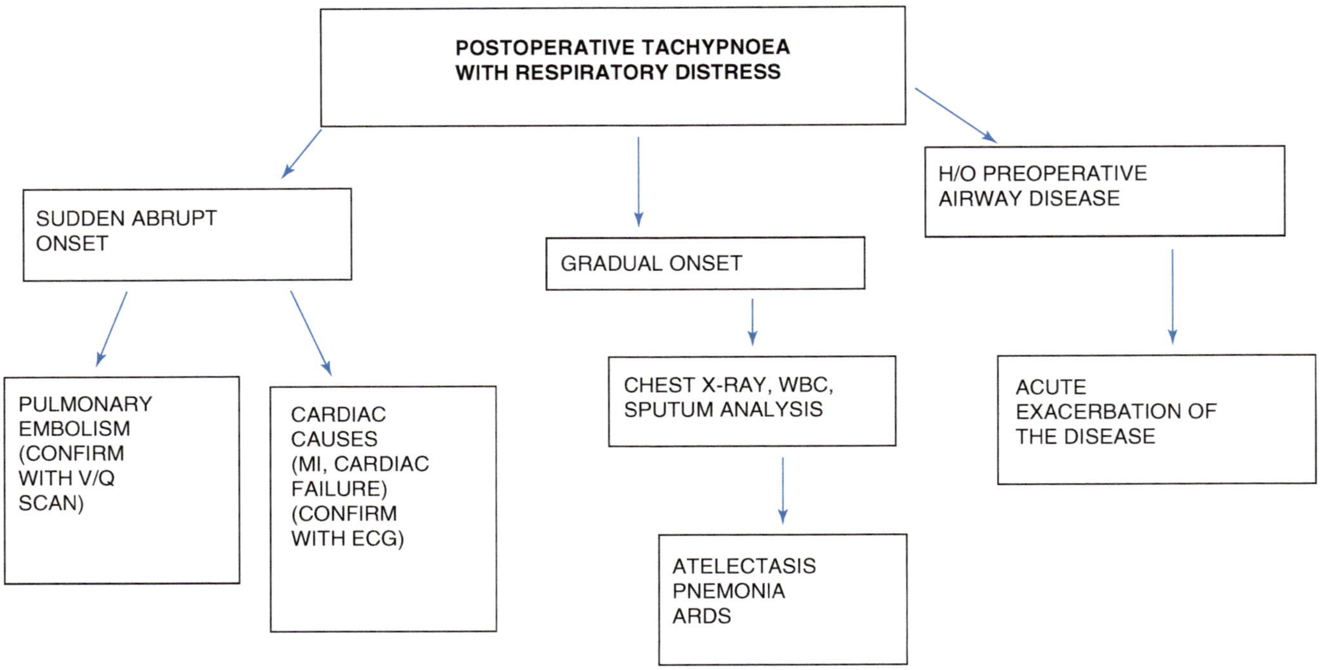




**Fig. 12.4** Postoperative respiratory distress workup

**Table 12.13** Types of postoperative oliguria and management

| Type of oliguria/ AKI | Cause | Management |
|---|---|---|
| Prerenal | Hypovolemia | Fluid challenge of 250 ml iv fluid over 1 h |
| | Hypotension | Address the cause of hypotension |
| Renal | Nephrotoxic drugs: NSAIDS, aminoglycosides, steroids | Discontinue the offending drug |
| | Sepsis | Aggressive treatment with broad spectrum antibiotics and fluid resuscitation |
| Post-renal | Blocked Foley's catheter<br>Blocked ureter | Relieve obstruction |

## 12.3 Care of the Surgical Wound Site

### 12.3.1 Immediate Care in the Operating Room

Care of the surgical wound site begins even before closure of the wound has been completed. It may be necessary to place drains or catheters within the wound.

**Surgical Drains**

A drain is a device that is intended to evacuate fluids and air from the surgical wound site. By evacuating accumulated pus, blood, and serous fluid, they help prevent infection of the surgical site. By evacuating air, they help eliminate dead spaces, which results in faster wound healing.

The various kinds of drains are summarized in Table 12.14. Drains may be classified as:

- Active drains: These work under negative pressure and actively remove fluids and air from the surgical site.
- Passive drains: They drain fluids passively, and are dependent on gravity. Passive drains may be open or closed.

Technique of inserting a surgical drain:

- The drain must be inserted before the last layer of sutures is placed.
- The drain tube has a needle at one end and perforations at the other end.
- The needle is inserted from the deeper edge of the surgical wound, and pulled out through the skin surface, about 2 cm away from the wound margin. The end with the perforations must remain within the surgical site.
- The exit of the needle must be in a dependent area, lower than the incision line.
- The needle is cut off from the tube and discarded safely.
- The drain tube is secured with sutures to the skin surface.
- The bulb or container is deflated completely, to ensure negative pressure, and is then attached to the exit end of the tube.
- Dressing with betadine gauze is done around and over the drain tube.

**Table 12.14** Types of drains

| Type of drain | | Example | Indications for use | Image |
|---|---|---|---|---|
| Active | | Jackson-Pratt drain | Inserted into the surgical site to drain blood and serous fluid; to eliminate dead spaces | 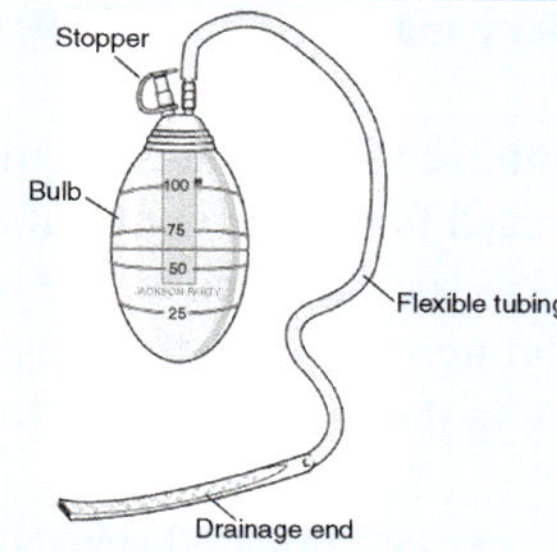  |
| | | Hemovac | | 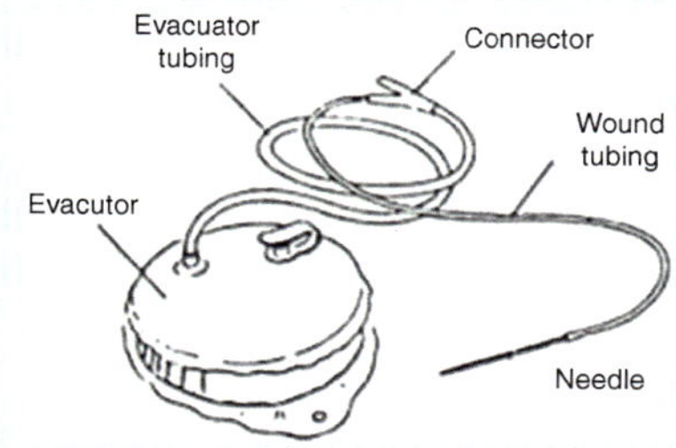  |
| Passive | Open | Corrugated rubber drain | To drain pus from infected abscesses and anatomical spaces | 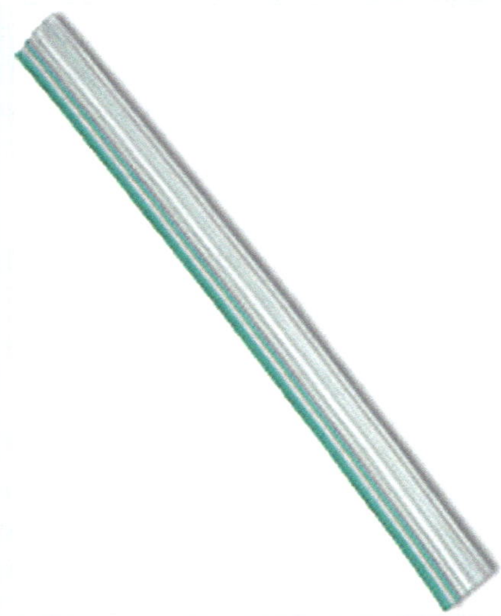 |
| | | Penrose drain | | 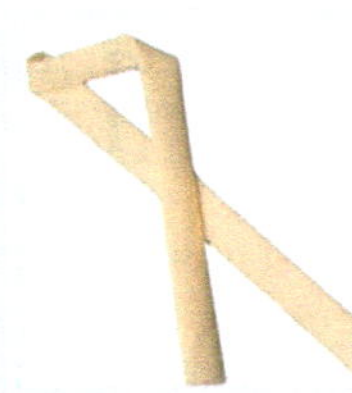 |
| | Closed | Nasogastric tube, Foley's catheter | To drain body secretions (gastric fluid, urine) | 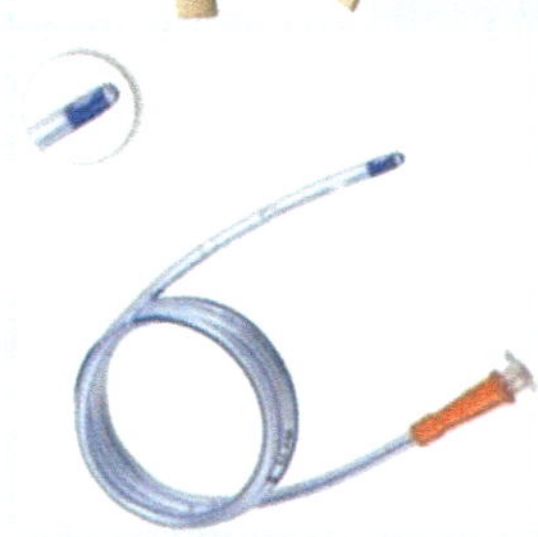 |

**Surgical Site Catheters**

Catheters may be inserted directly into the surgical site beneath the skin sutures. These may serve the following purposes:

- Analgesia: An intravenous cannula inserted into the surgical site may be used for delivering local analgesia. Long-acting anesthetics, such as ropivacaine and bupivacaine, are delivered through this into the surgical site. This is especially useful in the iliac crest after harvest of autogenous bone.
- Local antibiotic therapy: Infected spaces or osteomyelitic bone may benefit from local antibiotics that are delivered via catheters.
- Marsupialization: Decompression of a cystic lesion may be followed by catheter insertion into the cystic cavity. This allows continued drainage of fluid from the cyst.

**Wound Dressing**

Once complete suturing of the wound has been completed, appropriate dressing of the wound site must be carried out. Various types of dressing material are available [31]. These are detailed in the Chap. 11 on soft tissue injuries and management.

### 12.3.2 General Guidelines for Postoperative Wound Care [32]

- Aim to leave the wound undisturbed for at least 48 h after surgery.
- Premature removal of the wound dressing may, however, be required in certain situations. These include:
- Excess exudate or blood soaking through the dressing.
- Suspicion that the wound site is infected (e.g. Postoperative fever with no other attributable cause).
- The dressing is no longer serving its purpose (e.g. Falling off).
- If the wound dressing is being changed, check if there is excess exudate or devitalized tissue that may delay wound healing. If these are present, the wound must be cleansed. This is done by gentle irrigation of saline (for the first 48 h) or clean tap water (after 48 h) using a syringe. The wound must never be swabbed with gauze, as this can delay healing.

**Postoperative Care of Drains and Catheters**

- The drain must be monitored every 4 h and more frequently if the discharge from the wound is excessive.
- The drain container must be evacuated at least once every day.
- Once the drain fluid collection goes below 25–50 ml/day, the drain may be removed.

Surgical site catheters must be removed by the third postoperative day.

### 12.3.3 Surgical Site Complications

**Postoperative Bleeding, Hematoma, and Seroma**

Bleeding after surgery is classified as primary (occurs during or immediately after the surgical procedure), reactionary (occurs after few hours, possibly due to slipped ligatures), and secondary (occurs after few days, commonly due to infection). Active, ongoing bleeding is referred to as hemorrhage.

Hematoma refers to a clotted collection of blood below the tissues, which occurs due to damage to vessel walls. Most hematomas are self-limiting. Larger hematomas can be treated with ice packs or compression dressings. Analgesics may be given if the swelling is painful. Hematomas in the submandibular and neck region, or other regions which can potentially compress the airway, must be drained surgically.

Seromas are collections of serous fluid that generally develop 5–7 days after surgery. They are more common in extensive surgeries, particularly in neck dissection, where lymph nodes have been removed. Small seromas resolve over time. If the seroma is large and painful, the fluid may be aspirated and a pressure dressing can be applied.

**Infected Wound**

As maxillofacial procedures are clean-contaminated surgeries, they carry a higher risk of developing infection as compared to clean surgeries. Signs and symptoms of an infected wound include:

- Unexplained fever 3–5 days after surgery.
- Localized pain at the wound site.
- Erythema around the wound.
- Wound dehiscence, with pus discharge from the wound.

If the wound appears infected, a few sutures must be removed and pus must be drained out. A swab must be sent for culture and sensitivity testing, and the patient must be started on empirical antibiotics. The patient must be monitored closely for signs of systemic infection. The infected wound can be treated by local debridement and antibiotic irrigation.

**Wound Dehiscence**

This generally occurs as a result of one of the above complications, most commonly subacute infection. Sometimes, however, it may simply be the result of excessive wound tension due to inadequate tissue undermining. If the wound is uninfected less than 24 h postoperatively, re-suturing may be attempted. Otherwise, the wound is best left to heal by secondary intention. Resistant wound dehiscence may lead to orocutaneous communications and may become difficult to handle. The decision to either allow these to granulate or surgically provide a cover depends on individual scenarios.

## 12.4 Postoperative Care for Specific Types of Surgeries

While the general rules apply to all kinds of surgeries, there may be extra measures which are required in each specific surgery type. These are outlined below [2].

**Postoperative Care for the Trauma Patient**

- In the immediate postoperative period, the airway must be monitored. This may get compromised due to bleeding or edema.
- For fractures of the zygoma and orbit, monitoring for retrobulbar hemorrhage is important. This can be diagnosed by the three Ps—pain (in the orbit), proptosis, and pupillary defects [33]. The postoperative care team is generally required to check papillary reflexes on an hourly basis for the first 6 h which can be relaxed to once in 2 h for the next 6 h. Any impending sign of diminishing vision or pupillary inactivity is brought to the notice of the consultant and steps initiated accordingly.
- Assess and document paresthesia along any nerves involved in the fractured segment. This includes the inferior alveolar nerve for mandibular fractures and infraorbital nerve for zygomaticomaxillary complex fractures.
- The accuracy of reduced fractures must be checked on the first postoperative day using radiographs. For fractures involving the dentoalveolar segments, occlusion may be used as a guide.

**Postoperative Care for Orthognathic Surgery Patients**

- As with trauma patients, airway compromise due to bleeding and edema must be monitored.
- Considerable facial swelling is common. Ice packs and systemic steroids can help reduce swelling.
- Occlusion must be checked on the first postoperative day, and elastics must be placed if required. Class II elastics are placed from the upper anterior teeth to lower posterior teeth. Class III elastics are placed from lower anteriors to upper posterior teeth.

**Postoperative Care for Oncology and Reconstruction Patients**

- These patients usually undergo extensive surgery that lasts for hours, and will therefore need intensive monitoring in the postoperative period. Tracheostomy care may be required (See Sect. 12.1.1).
- Most of these patients will be unable to feed properly till wound healing is complete. Ryle's tube or PEG insertion must be done on the day of surgery or the first postoperative day.
- Patients must be on DVT prophylaxis. The malignancy, prolonged surgery, and in-hospital stay increase the risk of the patient developing DVT.

**Flap Monitoring**

- Reconstructed flaps must be monitored for vitality. If the blood supply to the flap is lost due to thrombi, it may be salvageable within the first 48 h. Periodic monitoring ensures prompt surgical intervention if the need arises.
- Flaps may be monitored using a handheld Doppler. Capillary refill may be assessed for flaps which are not buried. The needle prick test is simple, but must be done only to confirm congestion or loss of vitality.
- Flaps must be monitored hourly for the first 24 h, and 4 hourly for the next 48 h.

## 12.5 Postoperative Complications Specific to each Type of Surgery

Table 12.15 lists the complications that may be encountered with each specific surgery.

## 12.6 Criteria for Discharging the Patient

Prolonged hospital stay increases the patient's risk of developing nosocomial infections. Therefore, the patients must be discharged as soon as feasible. Criteria for discharge are as follows:

- Patient is hemodynamically stable, and all vitals are stable.
- Patient can take nutrition independently or with the aid of a caregiver.
- Wounds are healing well with no signs of infection.

Discharge summary: This is a record given to the patient, detailing the diagnosis, procedure performed, and any implants that were used. Instructions and medications to be taken must also be noted.

Follow-up appointments must be made for review. In case facial and neck incisions were placed, an appointment for suture removal must be given.

**Table 12.15** Specific postoperative complications

| Type of surgery | Complication | Management |
|---|---|---|
| Trauma | Malunion/nonunion | Reopen, remove cause of malunion, induce bleeding, use of graft |
| | Ptosis, diplopia, enophthalmos (orbital and ZMC repair) | Secondary surgical correction |
| | Persistent paresthesia | Palliative |
| TMJ surgery/ condylar fractures | Frey's syndrome (gustatory sweating) | Botox injection, surgical intervention |
| | Sialocele, salivary fistula | Debride the fistula lining and keep the area clean till healing occurs. |
| | Facial nerve palsy | Temporary—Palliative care<br>Permanent—Facial nerve reanimation |
| Orthognathic surgery | Condylar malpositioning leading to anterior open bite (BSSO) | Re-surgery, removal of plates, repositioning the condyle and re-fixation |
| | Inferior alveolar nerve paresthesia | Palliative management |
| | Alar base widening (maxillary surgery) | Alar cinching |
| | Nasal septal deviation | Septoplasty |
| | Aseptic necrosis of segment | Removal and reconstruction |
| | Malocclusion | Orthodontic treatment |
| Neck dissections | Chyle leak | Chyle duct repair |
| | Shoulder syndrome (spinal accessory nerve damage) | Physiotherapy |
| | Paresthesia of sensory nerves, e.g. greater auricular, lingual nerves | Palliative |
| | Carotid blowout | Surgical emergency, immediate repair needed. |

## 12.7 Conclusion

Postoperative care requires a thorough understanding of the patient, the procedure they have undergone, and the expected outcome. Surgeons must realize that more often it may be the first experience for a patient in going under the knife and lying at the ICU or ward. Hence, a perfect coherence of scientific and psychological views is required of the surgical team at all levels. The chapter emphasizes the need for comprehensive management of the maxillofacial patient at the ward after their procedure. The reader is expected to understand that outcome depends, but not ends at operating room or ward/ICU.

## References


1. Ogle O. Postoperative care of oral and maxillofacial surgery patients. Oral Maxillofac Surg Clin North Am. 2006;18(1):49–58.
2. Cascarini L, Schilling C, Gurney B, Brennan P. Oxford handbook of oral and maxillofacial surgery. Oxford: Oxford University Press; 2018 August 2.
3. Chatburn RL, Primiano JF. A new system for understanding modes of mechanical ventilation. Respir Care. 2001 Jun;46(6):604–21.
4. Buggy DJ, Crossley AW. Thermoregulation, mild perioperative hypothermia and post-anaesthetic shivering. Br J Anaesth. 2000 May 1;84(5):615–28.
5. Aldrete JA. The post anaesthesia recovery score revisited [letter]. J Clin Anesth. 1995;7:89–91.
6. Williams N, O'Connell PR, editors. Bailey & love's short practice of surgery. 26th ed. Boca Raton, FL: CRC Press; 2013 Feb 18.
7. Alfonsi P. Postanaesthetic shivering. Epidemiology, pathophysiology and approaches to prevention and management. Minerva Anestesiol. 2003;69:438–41.
8. Giannakopoulos H, Albakoff J. Fluid and electrolyte management and blood product usage. Oral Maxillofac Surg Clin North Am. 2006;18:7–17.
9. Kayilioglu SI, Dinc T, Sozen I, Bostanoglu A, Cete M, Coskun F. Postoperative fluid management. World J Crit Care Med. 2015;4(3):192–201.
10. Chesney RW. The maintenance need for water in parenteral fluid therapy, by Malcolm A. Holliday, MD, and William E. Segar, MD, Pediatrics, 1957; 19: 823–832. Pediatrics. 1998 Jul 1;102(Supplement 1):229–30.
11. Doherty M, Buggy D. Intraoperative fluids: how much is too much? Br J Anaesth. 2012;109(1):69–79.
12. Della Rocca G, Vetrugno L, Tripi G, Deana C, Barbariol F, Pompei L. Liberal or restricted fluid administration: are we ready for a proposal of a restricted intraoperative approach? BMC Anesthesiol. 2014;14(1):62.
13. Chao J. Transfuse or not to transfuse: for postop anemia. Am J Clin Med. 2011;8(1):11–4.
14. Liumbruno GL, Bennardello F, Lattanzio A, Piccoli P, Rosetti G. Recommendations for the transfusion management of patients in the peri-operative period. III. The post-operative period. Blood Transfus. 2011;9:320–35.
15. Ong CK, Lirk P, Seymour RA, Jenkins BJ. The efficacy of preemptive analgesia for acute postoperative pain management: a meta-analysis. Anesth Analg. 2005 Mar 1;100(3):757–73.
16. Coulthard P, Haywood D, Tai M, Jackson-Leech D, Pleuvry B, Macfarlane T. Treatment of postoperative pain in oral and maxillofacial surgery. Br J Oral Maxillofac Surg. 2000;38(6):588–92.
17. Vargas-Schaffer G. Is the WHO analgesic ladder still valid? Twenty-four years of experience. Can Fam Physician. 2010 Jun 1;56(6):514–7.
18. Grass JA. Patient-controlled analgesia. Anesth Analg. 2005 Nov 1;101(5S):S44–61.
19. Fleischli J, Adams W. Use of postoperative steroids to reduce pain and inflammation. J Foot Ankle Surg. 1999;38(3):232–7.
20. Bhagat S, Agarwal M, Roy V. Serratiopeptidase: a systematic review of the existing evidence. Int J Surg. 2013;11(3):209–17.
21. Escobar JIS, de Velasco AAF. Antibiotic prophylaxis in Oral and maxillofacial surgery. Med Oral Patol Oral Cir Bucal. 2006;11:E292–6.

22. Kreutzer K, Storck K, Weitz J. Current evidence regarding prophylactic antibiotics in head and neck and maxillofacial surgery. Biomed Res Int. 2014;2014:1–7.
23. Dobbeleir M, De Coster J, Coucke W, Politis C. Postoperative nausea and vomiting after oral and maxillofacial surgery: a prospective study. Int J Oral Maxillofac Surg. 2018;47(6):721–5.
24. Lachiewicz PF. Comparison of ACCP and AAOS guidelines for VTE prophylaxis after total hip and total knee arthroplasty. Orthopedics (Online). 2009 Dec 1;32(12):74.
25. Fang J, Chirag D, Dym H. Nutritional aspects of care. Oral Maxillofac Surg Clin North Am. 2006;18(1):115–30.
26. da Silva FJ, Daniel de Mello P, Daniel de Mello E. Subjective global assessment of nutritional status – a systematic review of the literature. Clin Nutr. 2015;34(5):785–92.
27. Dolgun E, Giersbergen M, Aslan A, Altınbaş Y. The investigation of mobilization times of patients after surgery. Asian Pac J Health Sci. 2017;4(1):71–5.
28. Ansari R. Fever work-up and management in postsurgical oral and maxillofacial surgery patients. Oral Maxillofac Surg Clin North Am. 2006;18(1):73–9.
29. Jadwani S, Bansod S, Chug A, Misra B. Management of postoperative fever in oral and maxillofacial surgery patients. Asian J Oral Maxillofac Surg. 2010;22(1):2–6.
30. Tung-Yiu W, Jehn-Shyun H, Ching-Hung C, Hung-An C. Cervical necrotizing fasciitis of odontogenic origin: a report of 11 cases. J Oral Maxillofac Surg. 2000;58(12):1347–52.
31. Ovington LG. Advances in wound dressings. Clin Dermatol. 2007 Jan 1;25(1):33–8.
32. Yao K, Bae L, Yew WP. Postoperative wound management. Aust Fam Physician. 2013;42(12):867–70.
33. Bater MC, Ramchandani PL, Brennan PA. Post-traumatic eye observations. Br J Oral Maxillofac Surg. 2005 Oct 1;43(5):410–6.

# Part VI

# Dentoalveolar and Oral Surgery

# Principles and Techniques of Exodontia

# 13

Anuj Jain

## 13.1 Introduction

Exodontia is the removal of tooth from its socket in the alveolar bone with the help of anesthesia. It is a challenging procedure in itself as the dental surgeon has to work in an oral cavity, access to which is restricted by patient's lips and cheeks. Also, the movement of the tongue and the jaw makes the procedure troublesome. Another factor which complicates the procedure is saliva. The oral cavity communicates with the pharynx which further communicates into larynx and esophagus, due to which there is always a potential risk of aspiration or deglutition of the extracted tooth. Hence, it is of paramount importance that the exodontia must be performed judiciously and be based on sound surgical principles.

Apart from the competence and practical skills of the dental surgeon, patient's cooperation also holds the key to an uneventful extraction of a tooth. Patient's cooperation is dependent on various factors like misinformation, myths, anxiety, pain phobia, patient's previous exodontia experiences, and trust over the operator. A dental surgeon must have a calm, patient, and reassuring approach towards the patient to gain his/her confidence. This empathetic nature of the doctor must be superadded with good principles of patient management and pharmacokinetics. This combination helps in controlling patient's anxiety and fear toward the procedure.

## 13.2 Definition

Exodontia or tooth extraction is defined as the painless removal of a whole tooth or tooth root, with minimal trauma to the investing tissues, so that the bone heals uneventfully and no postoperative prosthetic problem is created [1].

A. Jain (✉)
Oral and Maxillofacial Surgeon, Department of Trauma and Emergency Medicine, All India Institute of Medical Sciences, Bhopal, Madhya Pradesh, India

## 13.3 History

The thought of how extractions were performed in eleventh century is disturbing. The operator used to hold the patient's head between his knees, the soft tissue was cut with a sharp scalpel, and the tooth was pulled out in single direction. Often the wound was cauterized with a red hot iron and a repellent mouthwash was prescribed [2].

Historically, dental extractions were carried out as a prophylactic as well as therapeutic treatment for a variety of illnesses. Before the discovery of antibiotics, exodontia was a preferred treatment. Dentistry was not a separate profession at that time and mainly the barbers were extracting the tooth popularly known as 'barber surgeons'. They used to hang rows of rotten teeth outside their shops to advertise their services as tooth pullers [3].

Various kinds of instruments were used in different geographical areas of the globe and can be grouped as forceps, pelicans, keys, screws, and elevators. The modern-day forceps have been evolved over time and are highlighted in Table 13.1.

Regarding Indian history, Sushruta is to be credited for his description of surgical instruments. He highlighted two types of instruments viz. 'Yantra or blunt' and 'Shastra or sharp'. And among the category yantra, 'dantasanka' – a special forceps for extraction of teeth is described [6]. Vagbhata, around 650 AD, described forceps for extraction of tooth [7].

## 13.4 Applied Surgical Anatomy

*Knowledge of Anatomy is the foundation for an uneventful surgery.*

The jaw bones namely maxilla and mandible harbor the teeth in their respective alveolar process within the shape-appropriate sockets designed by nature. Sharpey's fibers of periodontal ligament attach the teeth to their alveolar sockets with the joint called gomphosis.



K. Bonanthaya et al. (eds.), *Oral and Maxillofacial Surgery for the Clinician*, https://doi.org/10.1007/978-981-15-1346-6_13

**Table 13.1** Evolution of dental forceps

| | | |
|---|---|---|
| 1 | Seventeenth Century BC | It can be assumed that extractions were carried out considering the prominent carvings of forceps on the walls of Egyptian caves in the work of Edwin Smith Papyrus [4]. |
| 2 | Fifth century BC | Hippocrates referred that the dental forceps have been discovered in Greece. These forceps were made up of Iron and called 'Odontagra' [4]. |
| 3 | Fourteenth century | Guy de Chauliac invented pelicans for dental extraction. They were named after the bird from their resemblance to the shape of the beak. The early drawing of the pelican showed a straight shaft, a wheel-shaped bolster, and a single claw attached to the shaft by a rivet [2]. |
| 4 | Sixteenth century | Pierre Fauchard, 'father of modern dentistry', modified the pelican with proper dimensions and advised regarding patient and operator position. His pelican was double hooked and held the tooth firmly, following which 'shaking' of tooth was done to achieve extraction [5]. |
| 5 | Eighteenth century | Dental key (also known as clef de Garengeot, fothergill key), an instrument modeled after a door was popular. It was first inserted horizontally into the mouth, then its claw would be tightened over the tooth to be extracted. Once secured, rotation movements were carried out to loosen the tooth. It was continuously modified for better results; however, its use was often associated with complications [2]. |
| 6 | By the end of the nineteenth century | The introduction of modern-day forceps was made popular notably by sir John tomes making the dental key obsolete [2]. |

### 13.4.1 **Maxilla** (Fig. 13.1)

It is a paired bone forming the midface of a person, bearing upper teeth separating the oral cavity from the nasal cavity and maxillary sinuses. Compared to the mandible, it is composed of spongier bone with thinner cortical plates. Palatal processes extend from both the maxillary bone and meet in the midline to form the roof of the oral cavity. The branches of *Maxillary Nerve* innervate the maxillary teeth and their periodontium (Table 13.2).

Exodontia becomes easier in maxilla due to following reasons:

1. The maxilla is characterized by thin cortical plates with spongier bone due to which the alveolar sockets expand easily on the application of pressure, facilitating extraction.
2. Due to thin cortical plates, mere para periosteal infiltrations of local anesthetic solutions produce adequate anesthesia to perform a dental extraction. However, in cases where adequate anesthesia is not achieved, a nerve block is desirable.
3. Maxilla has better vascularity as compared to mandible due to which the healing is faster with minimum complications.

Following factors complicate exodontia of maxillary teeth:

1. Use of heavy elevators is associated with the risk of fracture of the alveolar bone. Hence, their use must be judicious.
2. The root apices of maxillary molars are in close proximity to the floor of maxillary sinus with a thin bone separating them. Due to which there are chances of.
   (a) Oroantral communication during the extraction of maxillary molars.
   (b) Spread of periapical infection into the sinus leading to odontogenic maxillary sinusitis.
   (c) Displacement of the root into maxillary sinus if injudicious retrieval is attempted in the event of a root fracture.
3. The maxillary third molar is present in the maxillary tuberosity as it is the last tooth to erupt. There are high chances of maxillary tuberosity fracture in patients with unfavorable and bizarre root patterns especially in the elderly as the tuberosity is made up of spongy bone.

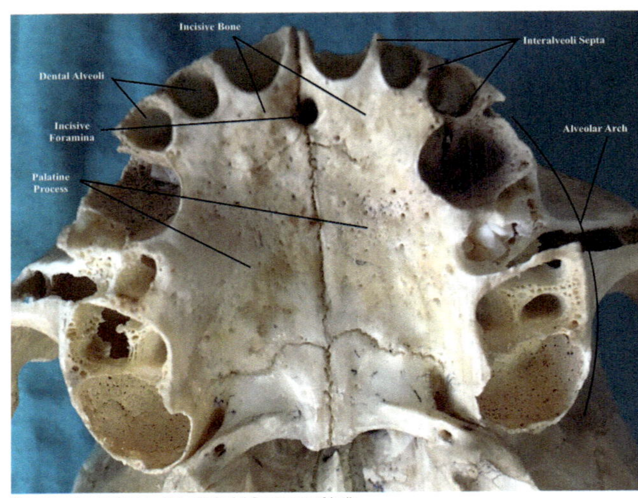



**Fig. 13.1** Alveolar process of maxilla

### 13.4.2 **Mandible** (Fig. 13.2)

It is horseshoe shaped, mobile and the heaviest bone of the craniofacial skeleton. Compared to maxilla, it has less spongy bone as well as vascularity and has thick cortices. The branches of *Mandibular Nerve* innervate the mandibular teeth and their periodontium (Table 13.3).

**Table 13.2** Nerve supply of maxillary teeth with periodontal tissue

| Teeth | Nerve supply | Nerve blocks |
|---|---|---|
| Central incisor | ASAN: Tooth and its buccal soft tissue<br>Anastomosis with opposite side<br>NPN: Palatal soft tissue | Infraorbital nerve block<br>Local infiltration on buccal aspect<br>Nasopalatine nerve block |
| Lateral incisor and canine | ASAN: Tooth and its buccal soft tissue<br>NPN: Palatal soft tissue | Infraorbital nerve block<br>Nasopalatine nerve block |
| Premolars | MSAN: Tooth and its buccal soft tissue<br>GPN: Palatal soft tissue | Infraorbital nerve block<br>Greater palatine nerve block |
| First molar | MSAN: Mesiobuccal root<br>PSAN: Tooth and its buccal soft tissue<br>GPN: Palatal soft tissue | Local infiltration on buccal aspect<br>Posterior superior alveolar nerve block<br>Greater palatine nerve block |
| Second and third molar | PSAN: Tooth and its buccal soft tissue<br>GPN: Palatal soft tissue | Posterior superior alveolar nerve block<br>Greater palatine nerve block |

Abbreviations: *ASAN* Anterior Superior Alveolar Nerve, *NPN* Nasopalatine Nerve, *MSAN* Middle Superior Alveolar Nerve, *GPN* Greater Palatine Nerve, *PSAN* Posterior Superior Alveolar Nerve

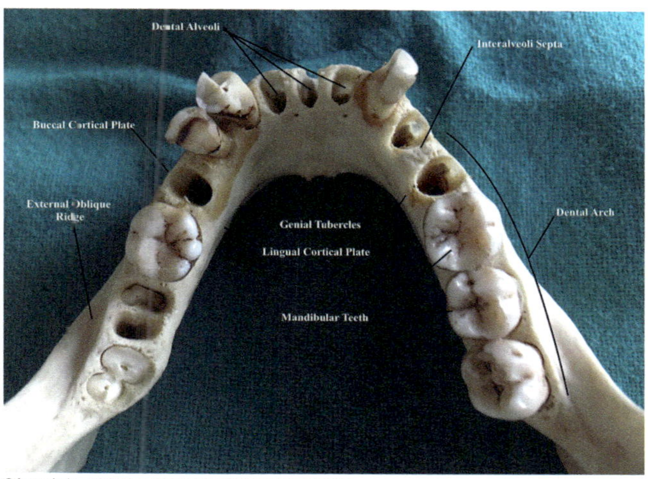




**Fig. 13.2** Alveolar process of mandible

**Table 13.3** Nerve supply of mandibular teeth with periodontal tissue

| Teeth | Nerve supply | Nerve blocks |
|---|---|---|
| Incisors and canine | Inferior alveolar nerve: Teeth<br>Mental nerve: Buccal soft tissue<br>Lingual nerve: Lingual soft tissue | Inferior alveolar nerve block<br>Mental nerve block<br>Lingual nerve block |
| Premolars and molars | Inferior alveolar nerve: Teeth<br>Long Buccal nerve: Buccal soft tissue<br>Lingual nerve: Lingual soft tissue | Inferior alveolar nerve block<br>Long Buccal nerve block<br>Lingual nerve block |

Following factors complicate exodontia of mandibular teeth:

1. Presence of thick cortical plates makes it a requirement to apply more pressure for luxation and extraction of teeth as the sockets do not expand readily.
2. Due to less vascularity, healing is slower as compared to maxilla.
3. Mandible is depressed when the mouth is open. Hence, there are high chances of temporomandibular joint injury or dislocations if the mandible is unsupported with the application of forces in a long-standing procedure.

### 13.4.3 Teeth

Apart from the bone, the anatomy of teeth also plays a pivotal role in an uneventful extraction. The shape of crown and roots must be assessed carefully, preoperatively. A narrow tapering crown requires the use of a lighter beaked forceps whereas a bulbous crown needs to be extracted using heavy beaked forceps. If the tooth is multirooted, it offers more resistance than a single-rooted tooth and cannot be extracted using a rotational force, as such a motion will lead to root fracture. In cases where the roots are divergent, the application of heavy forces will lead to root fracture. Dilacerated roots are also prone to fracture on the application of injudicious forces. Also, a more careful approach is required while extracting non-vital and endodontically treated teeth, as they fracture readily due to their fragile and brittle nature secondary carious undermining and loss of pulpal tissue.

## 13.5 Indications for Exodontia

Extraction of the teeth can be either prophylactic or therapeutic. Following are the indications for exodontia (Box 13.1).

1. *Dental Caries*: Extensively damaged teeth due to caries which cannot be preserved/restored by any conservative or endodontic procedure. (Fig. 13.3a).
2. *Pulp Pathology*: Pulpal necrosis or any pulpal pathology which cannot be treated by endodontic therapy (Fig. 13.3b).
3. *Severe Periodontal Disease*: Periodontally compromised teeth with mobility and irreparable loss of periodontal tissue (Fig. 13.3c).
4. *Periapical Pathology*: To prevent the spread of infection, in cases where all the reparative measures for periapical pathology have failed (Fig. 13.3d).
5. *Orthodontic Reasons*: There are a few conditions when a tooth is indicated for extraction during the course of orthodontic treatment.
   (a) Malposed teeth: The teeth which are misaligned and cannot be reoriented within the proper arch form with orthodontic treatment.
   (b) Creation of Space: To gain space to align malposed teeth. In such cases, premolars are commonly extracted.
   (c) Serial Extractions: During the mixed dentition stage, a few deciduous teeth are extracted in a sequential manner to avoid malocclusion in permanent dentition as the child grows.
6. *Preprosthetic Extractions*: Total extraction for the fabrication of a complete denture or extraction of a few undesirable teeth to provide better design and stability to a removable partial denture.
7. *Fractured Teeth*: The teeth which are fractured and cannot be conserved (Fig. 13.3e).
8. *Root Fragments*: Root fragments which may cause various problems like recurrent ulcerations under a denture, initiation of bony pathologies, and numbness if in close proximity to nerve. However, considerably small asymptomatic root fragments may be left alone but the patient needs to be kept under regular follow-up (Fig. 13.3f).
9. *Supernumerary Teeth*: These teeth may be malposed or impacted. They predispose to malocclusion, pain, periodontal disturbance, pathologies, or sometimes esthetics. If there is no advantage in retaining a supernumerary tooth, it must be subjected to extraction (Fig. 13.3g).
10. *Retained Decidous Teeth*: Deciduous teeth which are retained beyond the age of exfoliation.
11. *Impacted Teeth*: Teeth impacted in the jaw and creating discomfort to the patient or identified incidentally and found to be initiating some pathological changes within the bone (Fig. 13.3h).
12. *Tooth in fracture line* (Fig. 13.3i): The extraction of tooth in fracture line has always been controversial. In earlier times, all the teeth in fracture line were extracted but in recent times a more conservative approach is advocated. The teeth in fracture line are indicated for extraction if the tooth is a source of infection at the site of the fracture, the tooth itself is fractured, or the retention of the tooth in fracture line may interfere with the fracture reduction or healing.
13. *Teeth associated with pathologies* (Fig. 13.3j): Teeth involved in cyst formation and associated with other pathologies like tumors, osteomyelitis, or neoplasms.
14. *Teeth in firing line of radiations*: In the past, prophylactic extractions were carried out before the patient was subjected to radiation therapy. This practice was done as the effects of radiation, such as loss of vascularity of bone and radiation caries of the tooth, leading to a risk of osteoradionecrosis. However, with betterment in technology, it is not commonly practiced anymore.

Indications of Exodontia

1. Dental Caries
2. Pulp Pathology
3. Severe Periodontal Disease
4. Periapical Pathology
5. Orthodontic Reasons
6. Preprosthetic Extractions
7. Fractured Teeth
8. Root Fragments
9. Supernumerary Teeth
10. Retained Decidous Teeth
11. Impacted Teeth
12. Tooth in Fracture Line
13. Teeth associated with pathologies
14. Teeth in firing line of radiations



**Box 13.1** Indications of exodontia

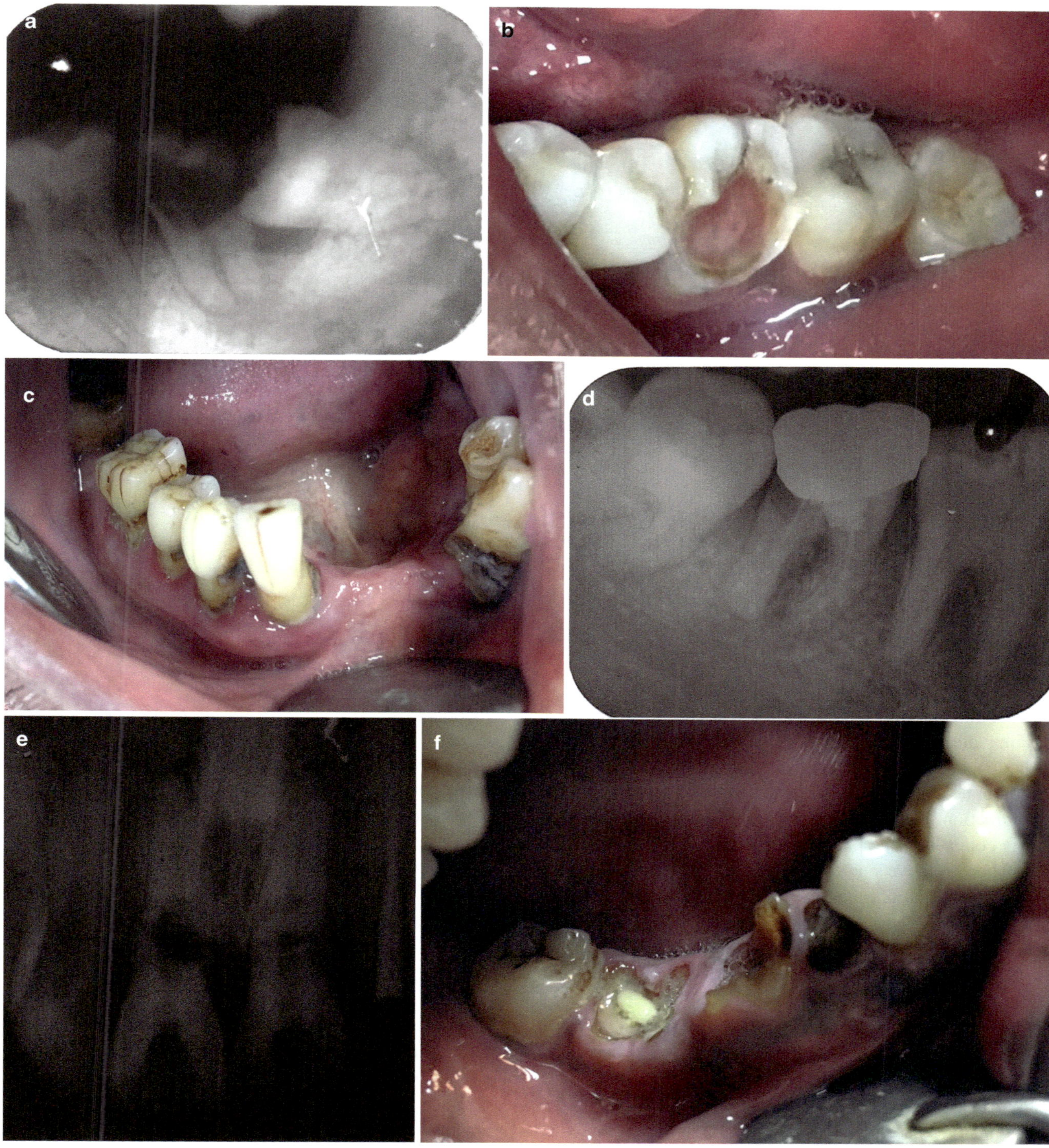


**Fig. 13.3** (**a**) Intraoral periapical radiograph showing grossly carious second molar indicated for extraction. (**b**) Clinical Photograph showing pulpal pathology. (**c**) Clinical Photograph showing generalized periodontitis. (**d**) Radiograph showing developing root caries following endodontic treatment. (**e**) Radiograph showing fractured central incisors. (**f**) Clinical Photograph showing root pieces. (**g**) Clinical Photograph showing supernumerary teeth. (**h**) OPG showing impacted mandibular canine. (**i**) OPG showing left mandibular third molar in fracture line. (**j**) OPG showing cyst associated with impacted maxillary canine

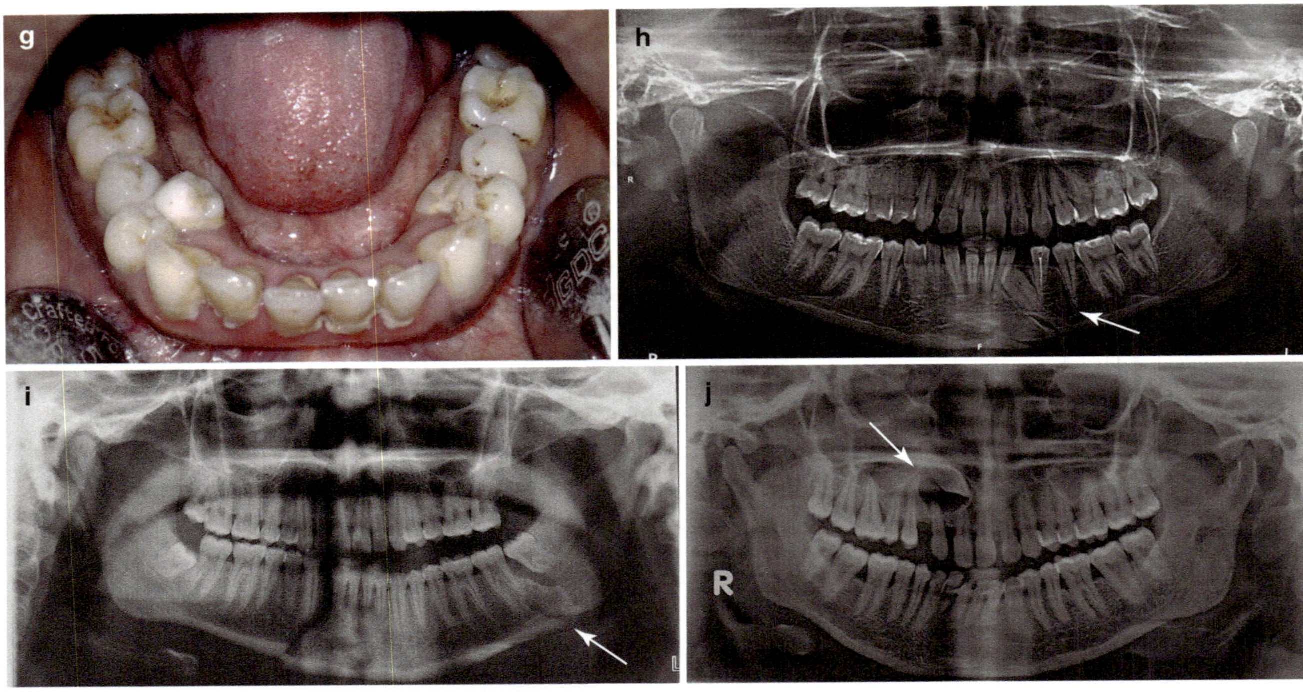




**Fig. 13.3** (continued)

## 13.6 Contraindications for Exodontia

A tooth may be indicated for extraction, but the presence of certain factors makes it contraindicated for extraction at that particular time. Any medical disorder in an uncontrolled, severe, or acute state may become a relative contraindication for extraction. However, once the underlying medical condition is controlled, the patient may be fit to undergo extraction. These relative contraindications may be classified as systemic or local contraindications.

### 13.6.1 Systemic Contraindications

Any uncontrolled systemic disease becomes a relative contraindication.

1. *Neurological disorders* like stroke and epilepsy.
2. *Pulmonary disorders* like bronchial asthma, tuberculosis, chronic obstructive pulmonary disease, and pulmonary effusion.
3. *Cardiovascular disorders* like hypertension, cardiomyopathy, valvular disorders, ischemic heart disease, and chronic cardiac failure.
4. *Hepatic disorders* like acute liver infections and liver cirrhosis.
5. *Renal disorders* like glomerulonephritis, uremia, and chronic renal failure.
6. *Metabolic disorders* like diabetes mellitus, thyrotoxicosis, Addison's disease, myxedema, and long-term steroid therapy.
7. *Hematologic disorders* like severe anemia, leukopenia, thrombocytopenia, pancytopenia, leukemia, agranulocytosis, patients on anticoagulant drugs, and bleeding and clotting disorders.
8. *Immunocompromised patients*.

### 13.6.2 Local Contraindications

1. *Tooth in a malignant growth*: Cases where a tooth is associated with a malignant tumor is generally mobile due to the destruction of periodontal tissues because of the underlying disease process and patients often insist for extraction. Extraction of such tooth must be considered as a relative contraindication because extraction may cause seeding of malignant cells into the capillaries subsequently leading to distant metastasis of the tumor [6].
2. *Tooth associated with vascular lesions*: There is a high risk of catastrophic bleeding while extracting the tooth associated with vascular lesions like hemangiomas, aneurysms, arteriovenous malformations, etc. Hence, such extractions should be carried out while treating the pathology in a controlled environment.
3. *Tooth in close proximity to vital structures*: The extraction should be avoided to prevent injury to vital structures.

However, if it is unavoidable, may be performed, but meticulously.

4. *Tooth in an irradiated jaw*: An irradiated jaw is highly avascular; carrying out the extraction of a tooth in such condition is associated with a high risk of osteoradionecrosis. However, such a tooth can be extracted after a considerable period of time following radiation therapy [8].
5. *Tooth with an acute infection*: If a tooth associated with acute infective pathology is extracted, there is a risk of extension of infection into deeper tissue planes due to loss of natural barriers during surgery. Also, there are chances of ingress of microorganisms into blood stream resulting in bacteremia. This may cause pyrexia and bacterial endocarditis in susceptible patients. Hence, in such a situation, the tooth must be extracted under proper antibiotic coverage. Apart from antibiotics, local measures for the drainage or decompression of the infective pathology should be carried out if possible. This relieves the pain and discomfort of the patient [9].

## 13.7 Armamentarium for Exodontia [10, 11]

### 13.7.1 Forceps

Forceps are the basic instruments used to perform exodontia. They are based on principles of simple machines. Forceps are designed to provide adequate access to the targeted tooth without injuring the neighboring tissues. Forceps basically have three components: (Fig. 13.4).

- The handle: Handle is the area of forceps from where the operator holds the instrument in a palm grip. It has serrations to facilitate firm grip. It is longer as compared to the beaks, corresponding to the longer arm of the lever, providing maximum mechanical advantage.
- The Hinge: It the area where the beaks and handle unite with each other and this part corresponds to the fulcrum of the lever.
- The beaks: Beaks are shorter as compared to the handle and correspond to the short arm of the lever, providing maximum mechanical advantage. The beaks of maxillary forceps are parallel to the handle, whereas the beaks of mandibular forceps are at a right angle. This helps in the application of beaks parallel to the long axis of the tooth. The beaks are curved and designed specifically for different teeth for proper two-point contact. The outer surface of beaks are smooth and tapering, facilitating wedging between the tooth and alveolar process. However, the inner surface of beaks are serrated to provide a firm grip over the tooth.

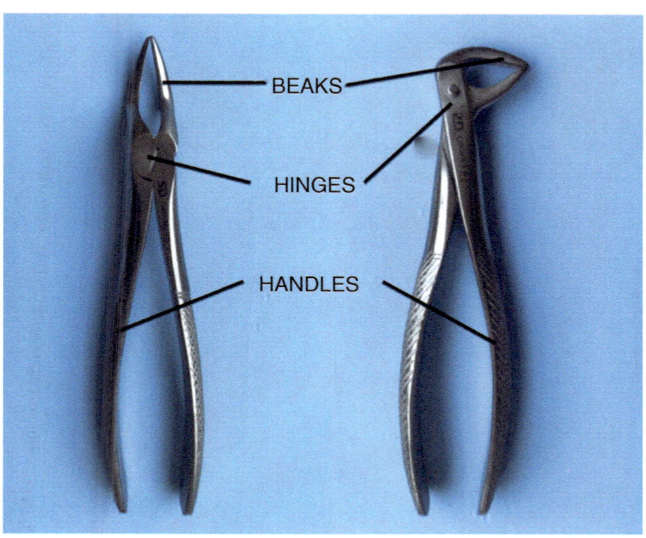




Fig. 13.4 Components of forceps

The forceps are of two types:

1. English Pattern: These forceps have a hinge that is directed vertically to the handles of the forceps.
2. American Pattern: These forceps have a hinge that is directed in a horizontal direction with the handles of the forceps.

Tables 13.4 and 13.5 describe various maxillary and mandibular forceps with their salient features, respectively.

Maxillary forceps must be held in a 'palm up' position (Fig. 13.7a) and mandibular forceps must be held in a 'palm down' position (Fig. 13.7b). These forceps majorly apply five different motions: (Fig. 13.8).

1. Apical pressure: With the force in this direction, the tooth movement is minimal in apical direction; however, the socket expands due to insertion of beaks in the periodontal ligament space. Also, the center of rotation of tooth displaces apically, resulting in less amount of force at the apical portion of root preventing it from getting fractured. (Fig. 13.9).
2. Buccal/Labial pressure: This results in expansion of buccal cortical plate, specifically at the crest of the ridge. However, at the same time, it results in lingual apical pressure. However, excessive pressure must be avoided to prevent fracture of buccal bone and the apical portion of the root.
3. Palatal/Lingual pressure: Similar to the buccal/labial pressure, but in opposite direction aiming in the expansion of lingual cortical plate.
4. Rotational pressure: Here the tooth is rotated resulting in internal socket expansion and tearing of periodontal ligaments. This force must only be applied to the teeth with single and conical roots. Teeth with multiple or dilacerated roots are prone to fracture on the application of this force.

**Table 13.4** Maxillary forceps with their salient features

| Sr. No. | Forceps | Description | Use |
|---|---|---|---|
| 1 | Maxillary anterior forceps (Fig. 13.5a) | Beaks are approximated with each other and handle is straight | Extraction of maxillary incisors and canines. |
| 2 | Maxillary premolar forceps (Fig. 13.5b) | Beaks do not approximate. Handle has concavity on one side to provide better grip and access. | Extraction of maxillary premolars. |
| 3 | Maxillary molar forceps (Fig. 13.5c) | These are paired forceps having asymmetrical and broader beaks. Beak is pointed on one side which engages the buccal bifurcation of roots and blunt on the other side engaging palatal root. Handle is similar to that of premolar forceps. | Extraction of maxillary molars. |
| 4 | Maxillary cow horn forceps (Fig. 13.5d) | These are also paired forceps having beaks that resemble the horns of the cow, pointed on one side engaging buccal bifurcation and notched on the other engaging palatal root. | Extraction of maxillary molars with extensive loss of coronal structure. |
| 5 | Maxillary third molar forceps (Fig. 13.5e) | Beaks are curved and angulated to engage the crown of third molars. Handle is long for accessing the posterior region. | Extraction of maxillary third molars |
| 6 | Maxillary bayonet forceps (Fig. 13.5f) | Beaks of the forceps are narrow, symmetrical, and approximating. Handle is angulated to provide access to posterior areas as well. | Extraction of maxillary roots. |

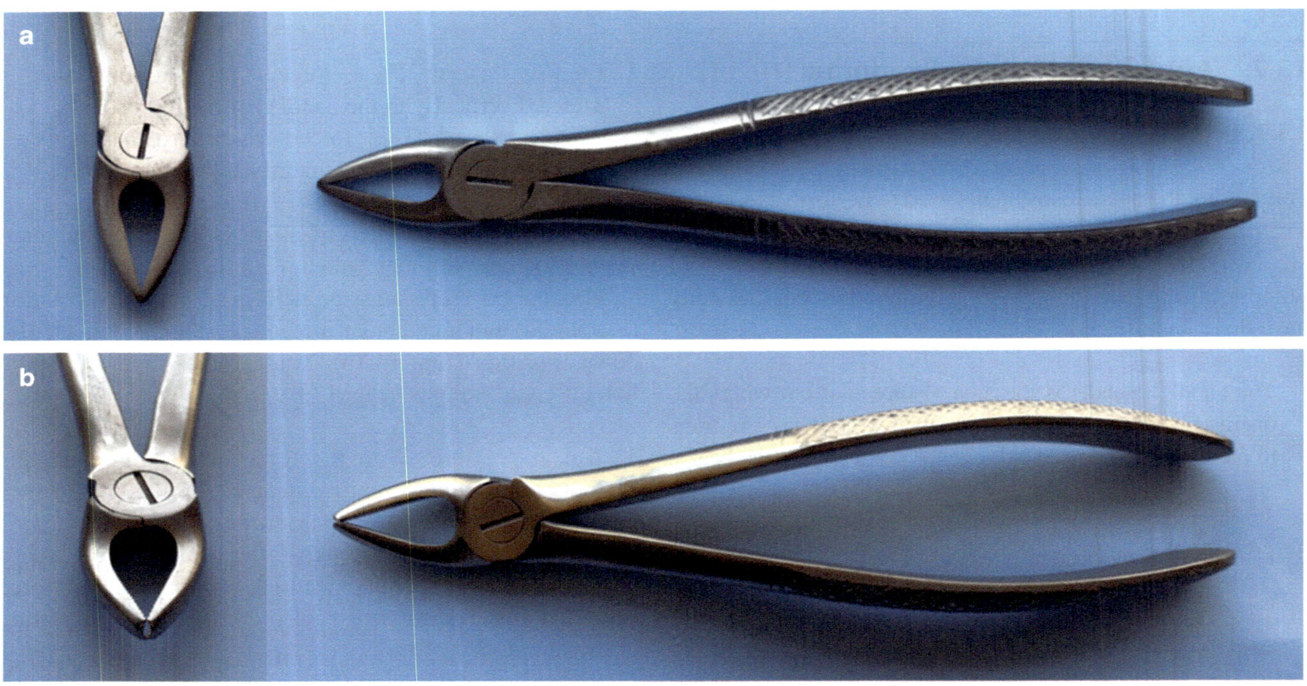


**Fig. 13.5** (**a**) Maxillary anterior forceps, (**b**) Maxillary premolar forceps, (**c**) Maxillary molar forceps, (**d**) Maxillary cow horn forceps, (**e**) Maxillary third molar forceps, (**f**) Maxillary bayonet forceps

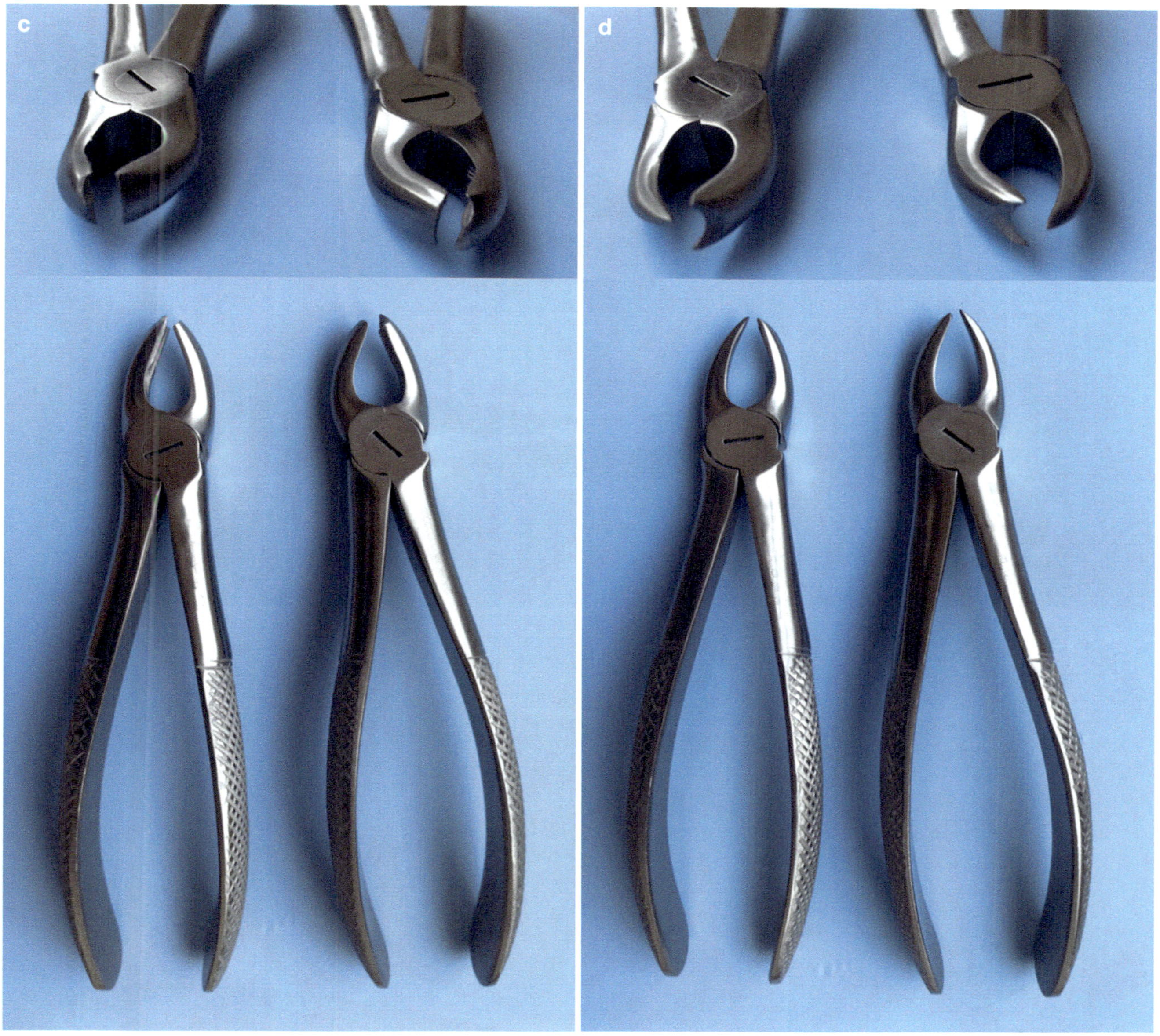


Fig. 13.5 (continued)

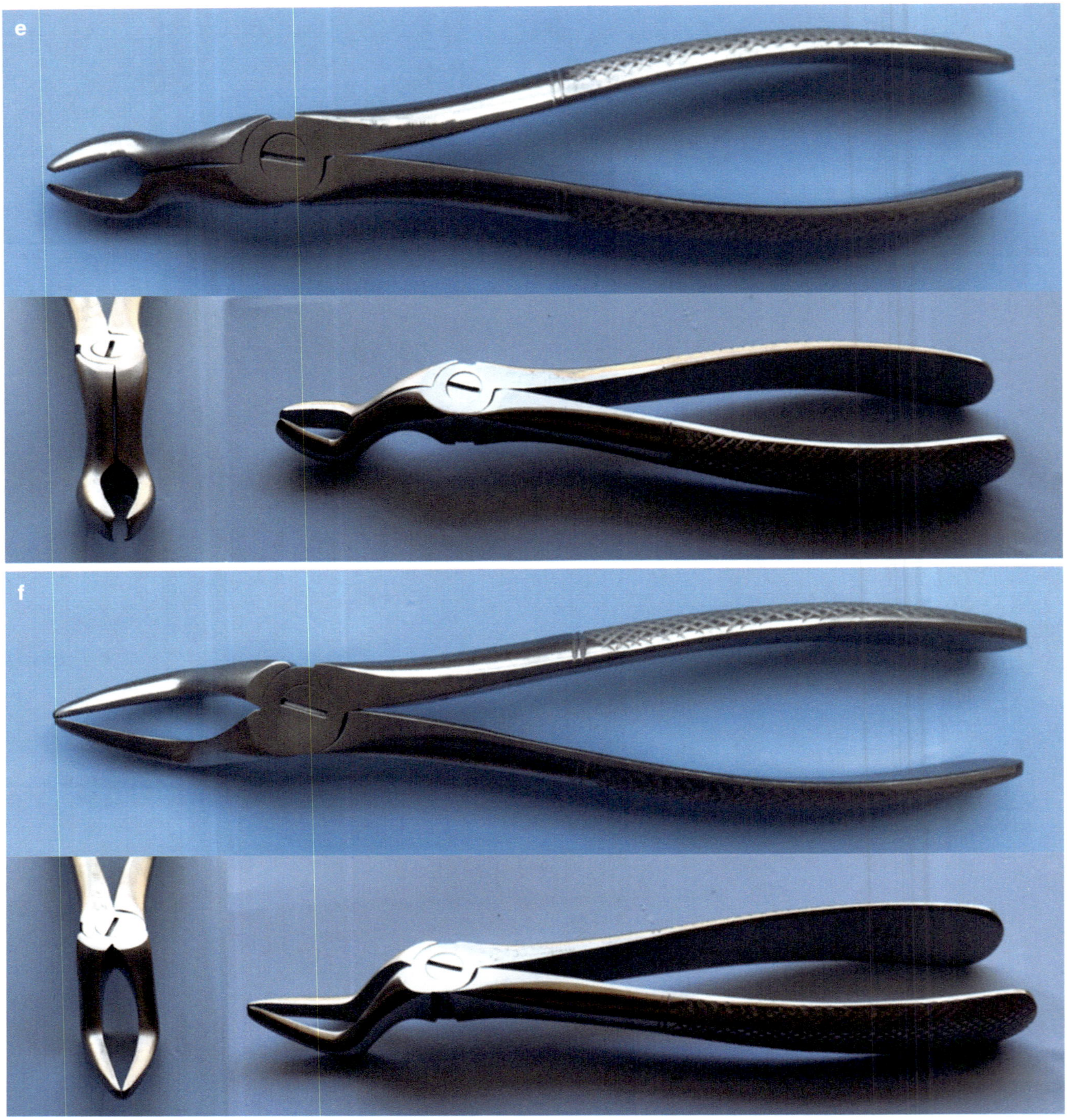




**Fig. 13.5** (continued)

Table 13.5 Mandibular forceps with their salient features

| Sr. No. | Forceps | Description | Use |
|---|---|---|---|
| 1 | Mandibular anterior forceps (Fig. 13.6a) | Beaks are perpendicular to handle, approximating each other, and handle is straight with no curvature | Extraction of mandibular incisors and canines |
| 2 | Mandibular premolar forceps (Fig. 13.6b) | Beaks do not approximate. Handle is similar to the anterior forceps | Extraction of mandibular premolars |
| 3 | Mandibular molar forceps (Fig. 13.6c) | Beaks are broader with triangular projections to engage the buccal and lingual furcations | Extraction of mandibular molars |
| 4 | Mandibular cow horn forceps (Fig. 13.6d) | Beaks are pointed and conical resembling the horns of cow. Beaks engage the furcations | Extraction of mandibular molars with extensive loss of coronal structure |
| 5 | Mandibular third molars (Fig. 13.6e) | These are paired forceps having an angulated beak to reach up to the mandibular third molars. Both beaks have triangular projections to engage the buccal and lingual furcation | Extraction of mandibular third molars |
| 6 | American pattern mandibular molar forceps (Fig. 13.6f) | Beaks are similar to that of mandibular molar forceps except that they are facing forward toward each other at right angles | Extraction of mandibular molars |

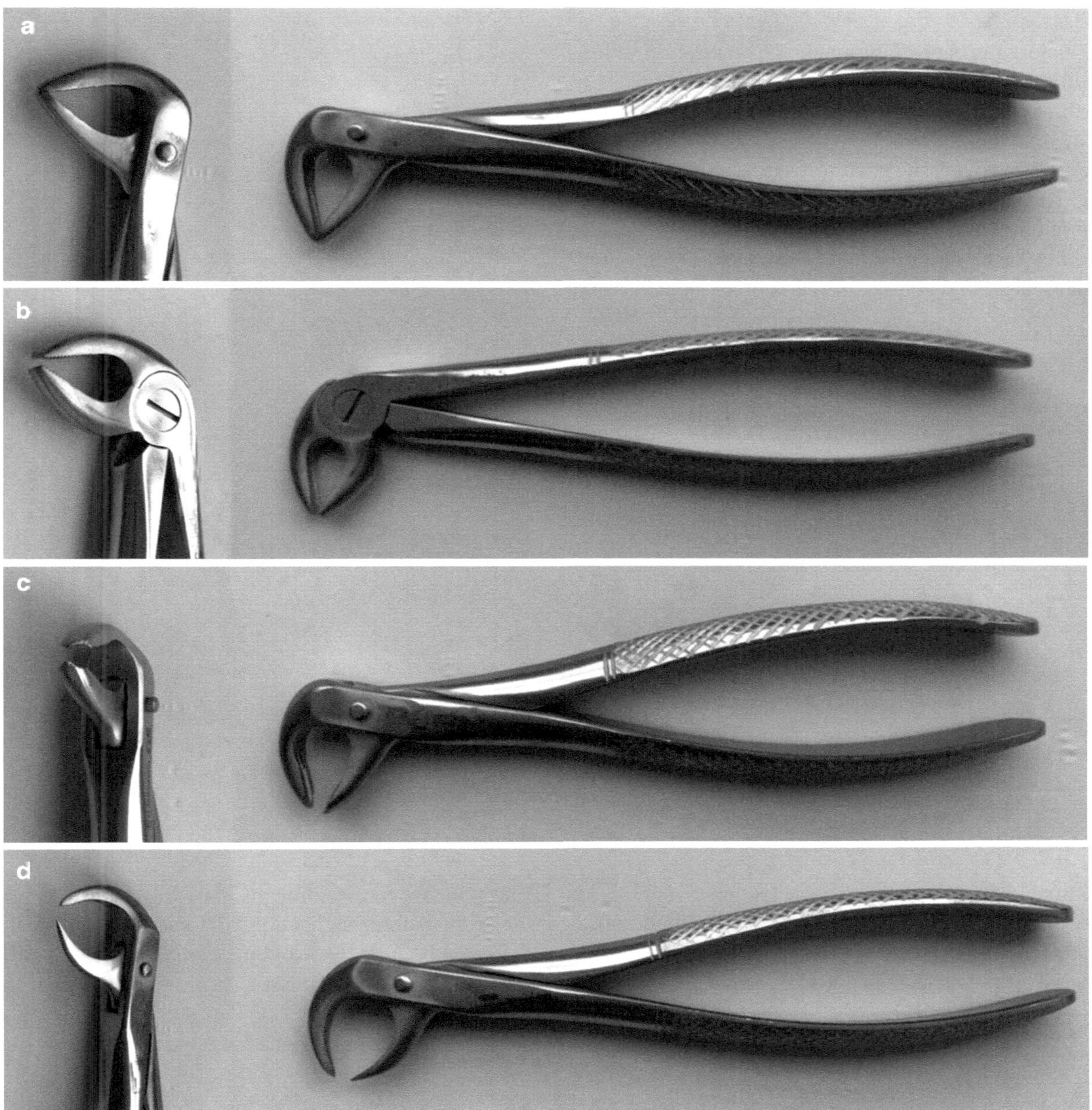

Fig. 13.6 (**a**) Mandibular anterior forceps, (**b**) Mandibular premolar forceps, (**c**) Mandibular molar forceps, (**d**) Mandibular cow horn forceps, (**e**) Mandibular third molar forceps, (**f**) Mandibular molar forceps (American pattern)

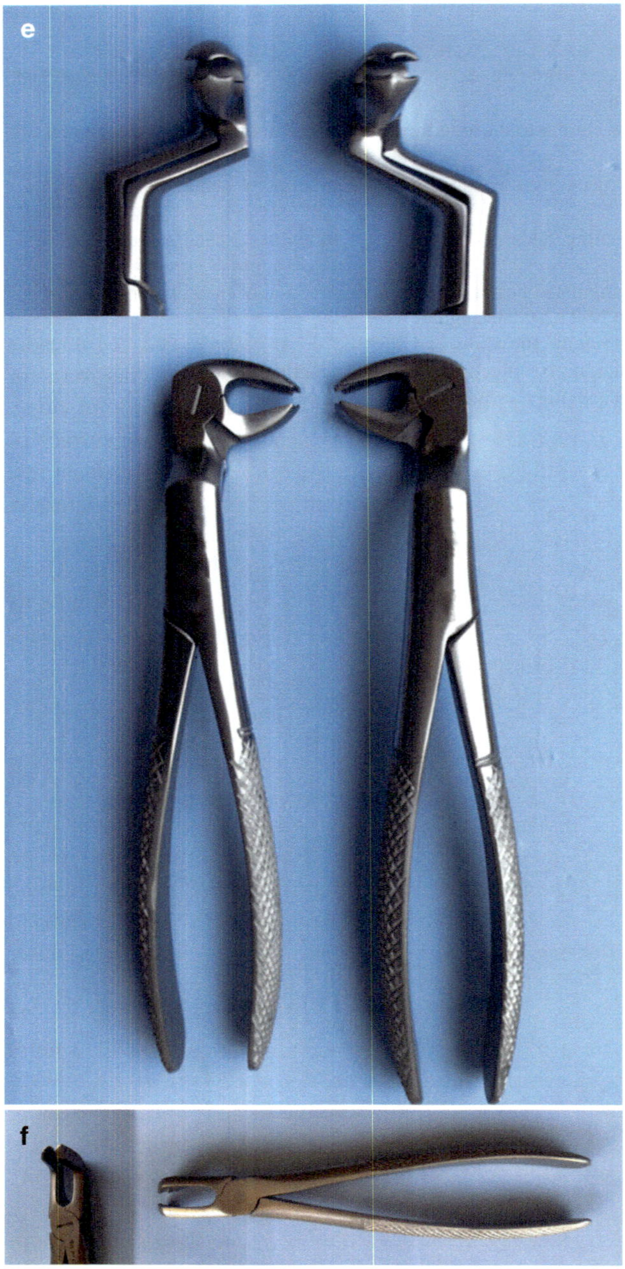


©Association of Oral and Maxillofacial Surgeons of India

**Fig. 13.6** (continued)

5. Tractional forces: This delivers the tooth out of the socket. This force should be gentle and the tooth should not be pulled out of the socket. However, if excessive force is required, other maneuvers must be carried out to improve luxation.

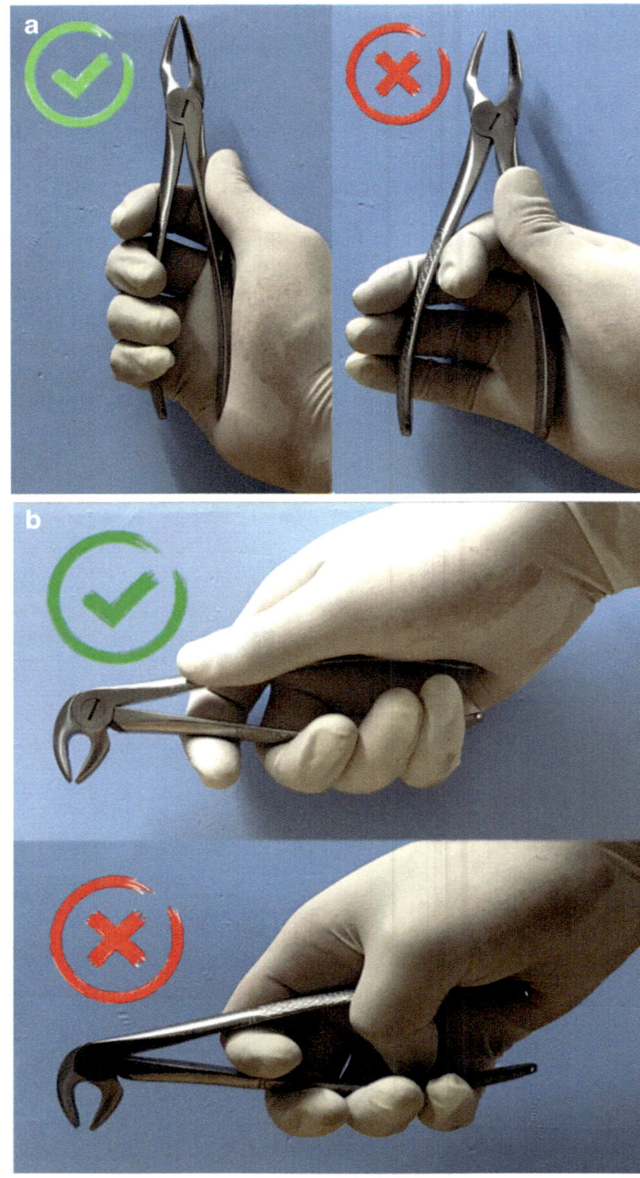


©Association of Oral and Maxillofacial Surgeons of India

**Fig. 13.7** (**a**) Correct way of holding maxillary forceps, (**b**) Correct way of holding mandibular forceps

### 13.7.2 Elevators

Elevators are the instruments used for luxating (loosening) the teeth before application of forceps making extraction easier, subsequently avoiding complications like fracture of crowns, roots, and bone. They are also used to remove fractured or surgically sectioned roots. Elevators are single-bladed instruments designed for specific purposes deliver-

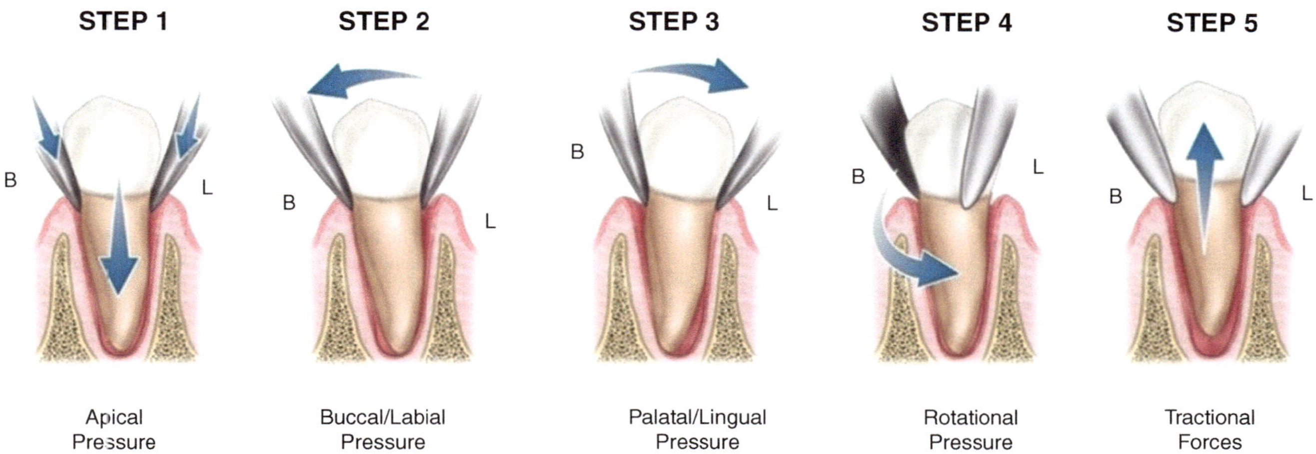




**Fig. 13.8** Sequential motions performed using forceps

**Fig. 13.9** Center of rotation of tooth gets displaced apically when the forceps is inserted beyond cementoenamel junction

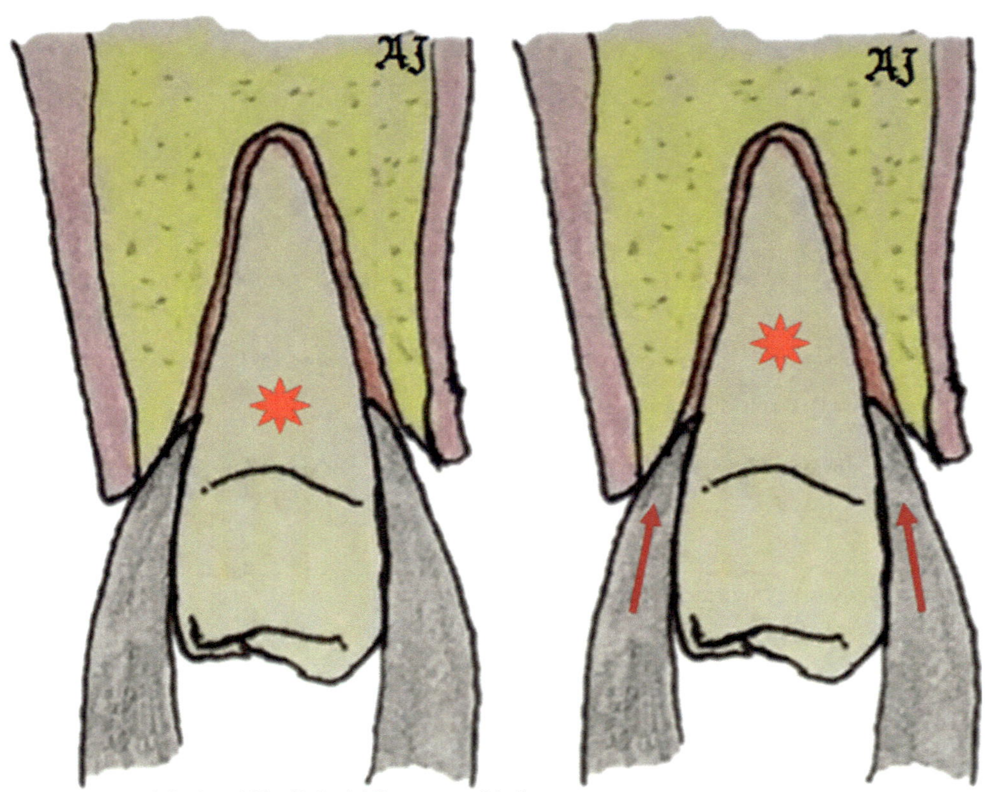




ing maximum mechanical advantage with minimum efforts. Elevators have three components (Fig. 13.10):

- Handle: It is of generous size for proper grip and delivering adequate but controlled force. Handle can be a continuation of the shank or at a right angle to the shank.
- Shank: It connects the handle with the working end or blade of the elevator. It is strong enough to transmit the force from the handle to the blade.
- Blade: It is the working end of the instrument and transmits the force to the tooth, bone, or both to achieve the desired action.

Table 13.6 highlights various types of elevators used for exodontia and Fig. 13.12 shows the proper way to hold an elevator.

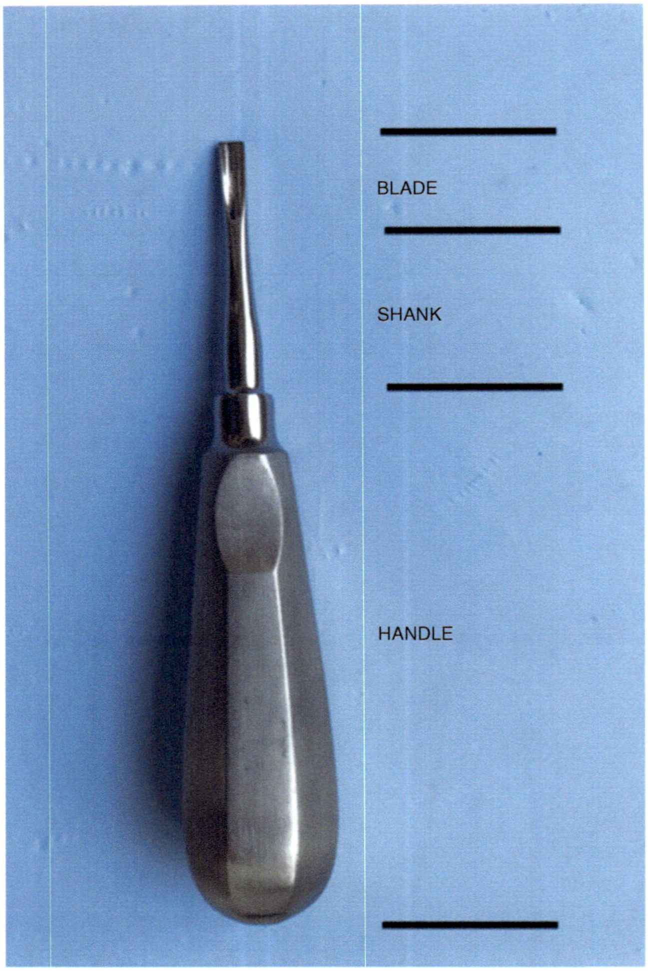




**Fig. 13.10** Components of elevator

Elevators works on principles of

1. Wedge
2. Lever
3. Wheel and Axle
4. Combination of the above

**Table 13.6** Elevators with their salient features

| Sr. No | Elevator | Description | Use |
|---|---|---|---|
| 1 | Straight elevator (Fig. 13.11a) | The blade, shank, and handle are in one line. Blade is pointed with one surface serrated and other convex. | Luxation of maxillary and mandibular teeth |
| 2 | Coupland elevator (Fig. 13.11b) | The blade, shank, and handle are in one line. Blade is sharp and straight cut having one surface concave and other convex. | Acts as a wedge to create purchase. Splitting of tooth |
| 3 | Apexo elevator (Fig. 13.11c) | These are paired elevators with blade at an angulation of 45° to shank. This facilitates its reach up to roots' apical region. | Extraction of root pieces |
| 4 | Cross Bar elevator (Fig. 13.11d) | These are paired elevators with blade at a right angle to shank and shank at a right angle to handle. The blade is triangular with slight curve and pointed tip. | Extraction of mandibular roots |
| 5 | Cryer elevator (Fig. 13.11e) | There are paired elevators similar to cross bar elevator. The only difference is that the handle is parallel to the shank. | Extraction of roots Elevation of upper third molars |
| 6 | Warwick James elevator (Fig. 13.11f) | The blade is short with a rounded end and the handle is flattened. There are three elevators, two angled (mesial and distal) and one straight. | Extraction of retained roots, deciduous teeth, maxillary third molars, and teeth with less resistance |
| 7 | Root tip elevator or root fragment ejector (Fig. 13.11g) | It can be a single or double ended instrument similar to Apexo elevators. The only difference is that they are smaller with more pointed blades | Removal of apical root tips/fragments of roots |

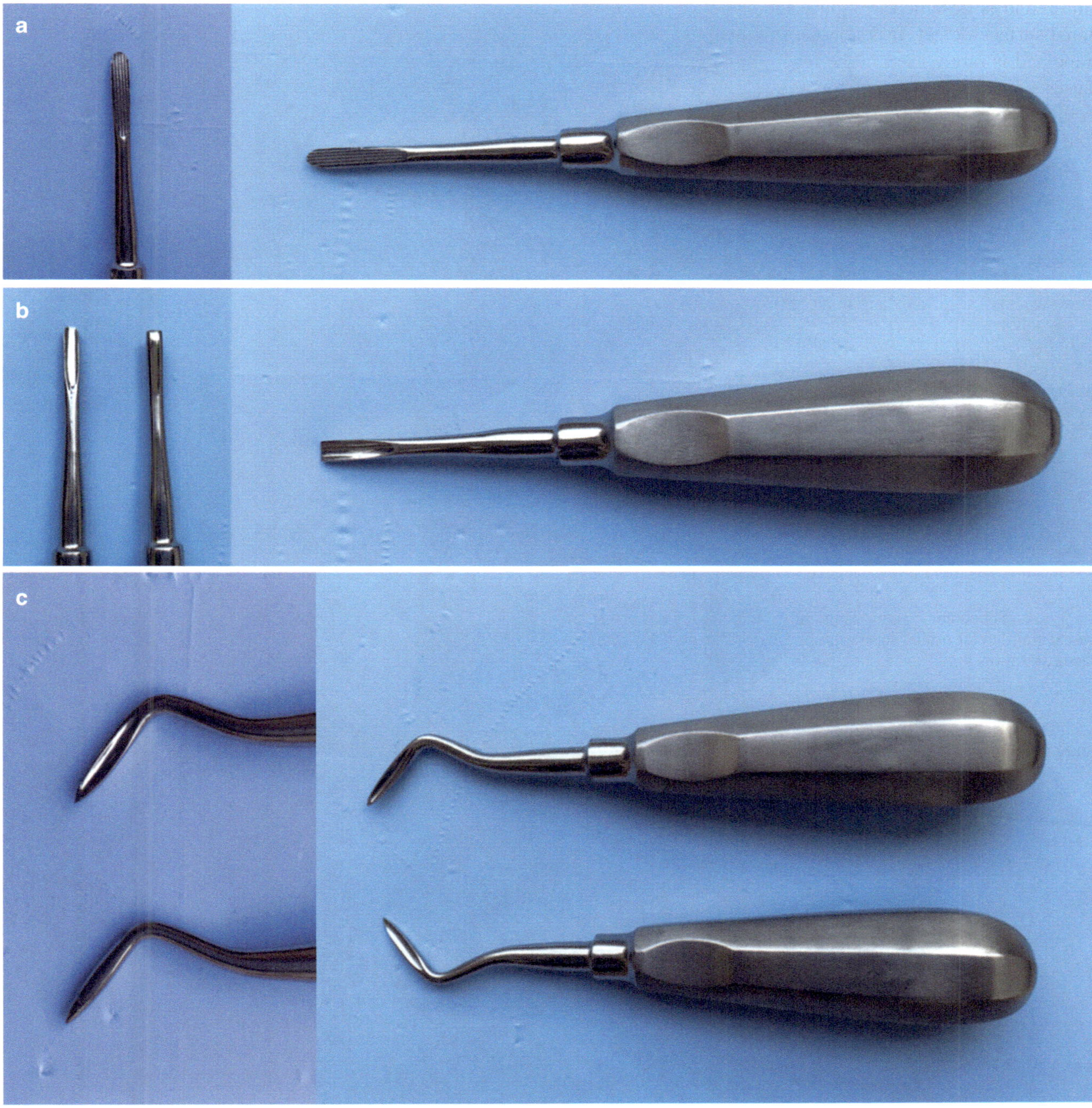


Fig. 13.11 (**a**) Straight elevator, (**b**) Coupland elevator, (**c**) Apexo elevator, (**d**) Cross bar elevator, (**e**) Cryer elevator, (**f**) Warwick James elevator, (**g**) Root tip elevator

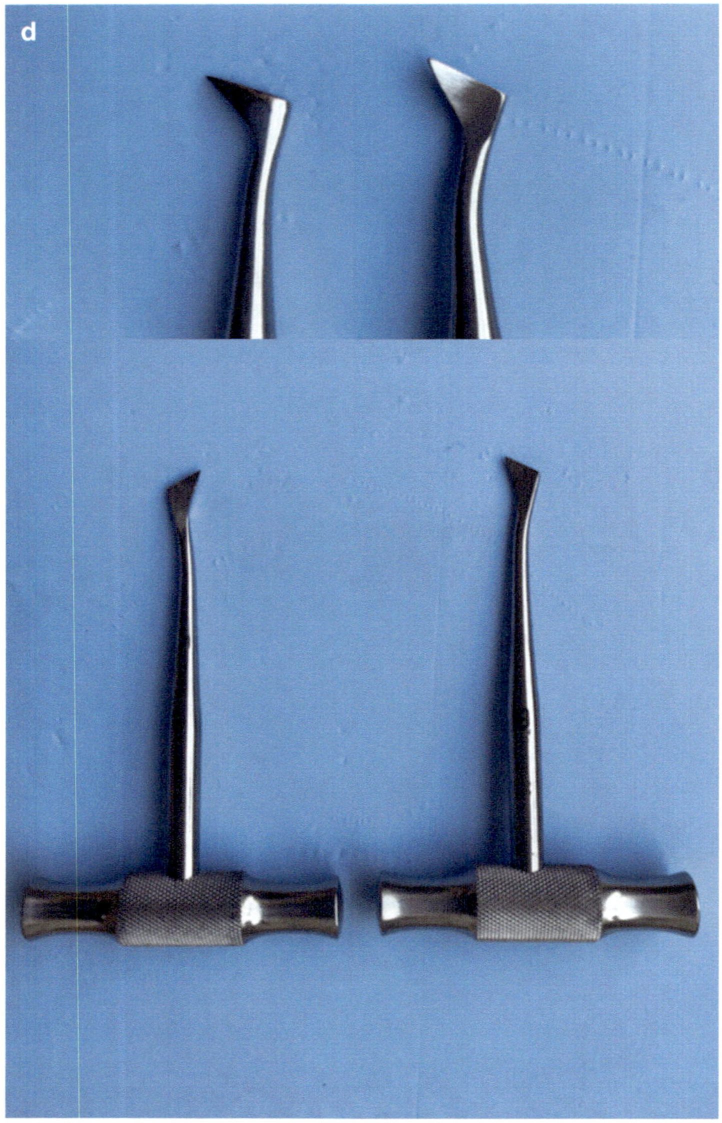

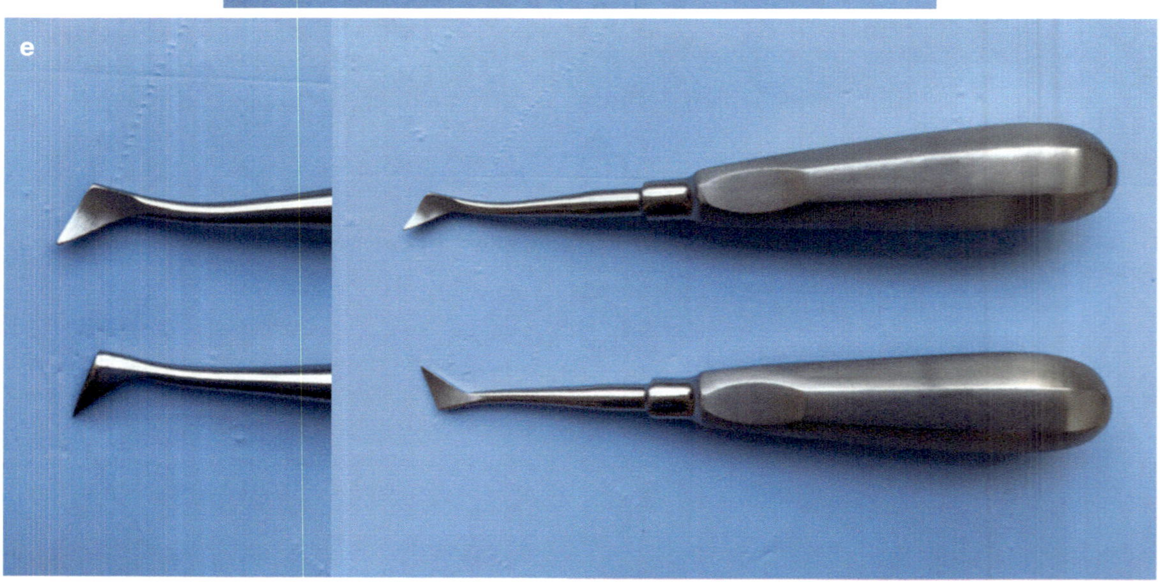

Fig. 13.11 (continued)

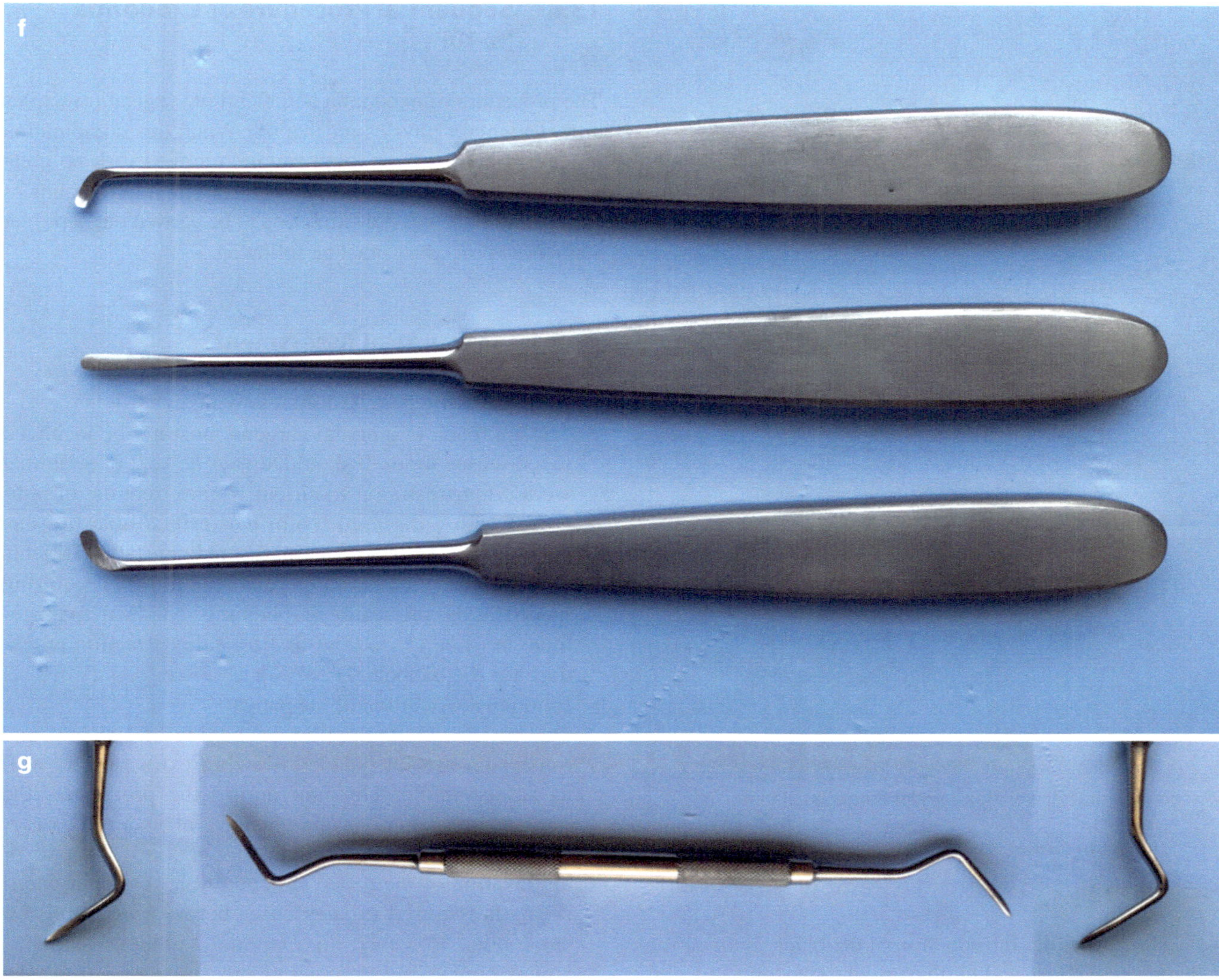



**Fig. 13.11** (continued)

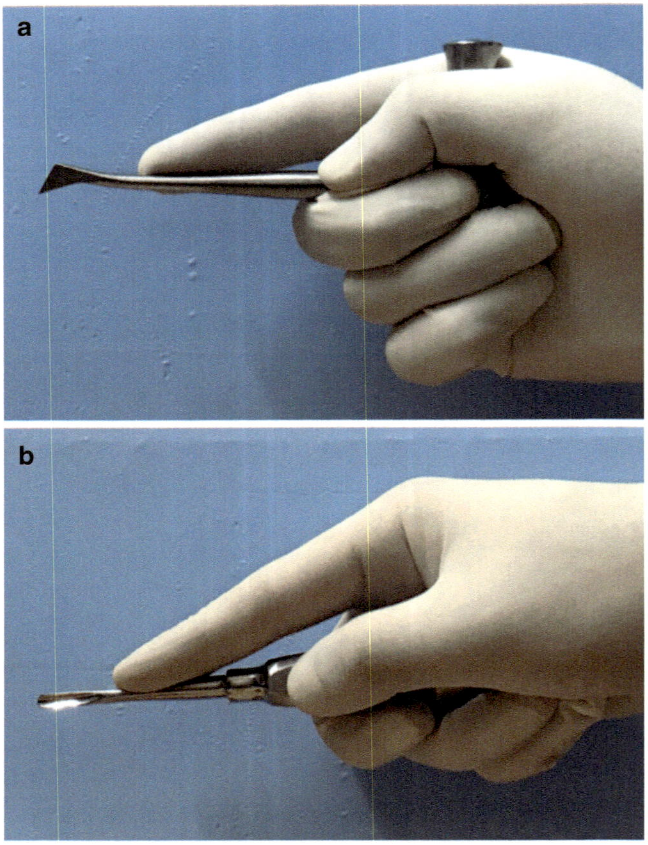




Fig. 13.12 (**a**, **b**) Correct way of holding an elevator

1. Wedge Principle: Introduction of the blade of an elevator between the bone and tooth parallel to the long axis of the tooth is wedging. A wedge is basically a movable inclined plane which overcomes a larger resistance at right angle to the applied effort. The resistance has its effect on the slant side when the effort is applied at the base of the plane (Fig. 13.13a and b).
2. Lever Principle: The elevator is the lever of first class. To gain mechanical advantage in first-class lever, the effort arm must be longer (3/4th of the total length) than the resistance arm divided by the fulcrum which lies on the bone (Fig. 13.14a and b).
3. Wheel and Axle Principle: In this principle, the effort is applied to the circumference of a wheel, which turns the axle generating the force to raise a weight (Fig. 13.15).

## 13.8 Sequential Procedure of Exodontia [6, 10]

The procedure of exodontia is a blend of surgical principles and elementary physics mechanics. When this combination is applied efficiently, a tooth can be removed with no great difficulty and finesse without requiring a large amount of force. For an uneventful extraction to be carried out, a proper sequential procedure must be followed.

### 13.8.1 Presurgical Assessment

- Presurgical Medical Risk Assessment:
  The approach of a dental surgeon must not be localized to a diseased tooth. It should always be kept in mind that we are not treating a tooth but we are treating an individual with a diseased tooth. It is critical that the surgeon must examine the patients' medical status. Patients may suffer from a variety of medical ailments requiring modification in treatment planning. Medical management must be carried out first for safe extraction procedure for the patient.
- Emotional Condition of the patient:
  Due to various myths like weakening of eyesight and impact on mental health following extraction as well as severe intolerable pain during the procedure, the patients are generally apprehensive to undergo extraction. Such patients are liable to go into syncope or aggravation of their medical condition. A proper counseling is required in such cases before proceeding for exodontia. However, in extremely anxious patients, where counseling is not enough, premedication like Diazepam/Alprazolam (Anxiolytics) for reduction of anxiety may be considered.
- Extraoral Examination:
  The patient must be examined for the presence of any extraoral swelling, cellulitis, abscess, or lymphadenopathy. Presence of any swelling is suggestive of extension of infection into surrounding soft tissue space which may require another surgical procedure. Presence of trismus must also be examined as it affects the access to the tooth to be extracted.
- Intraoral Examination:
  It includes an examination of the size of the tongue, bulky buccal fat pad, and hyperactive gag reflex as these fac-

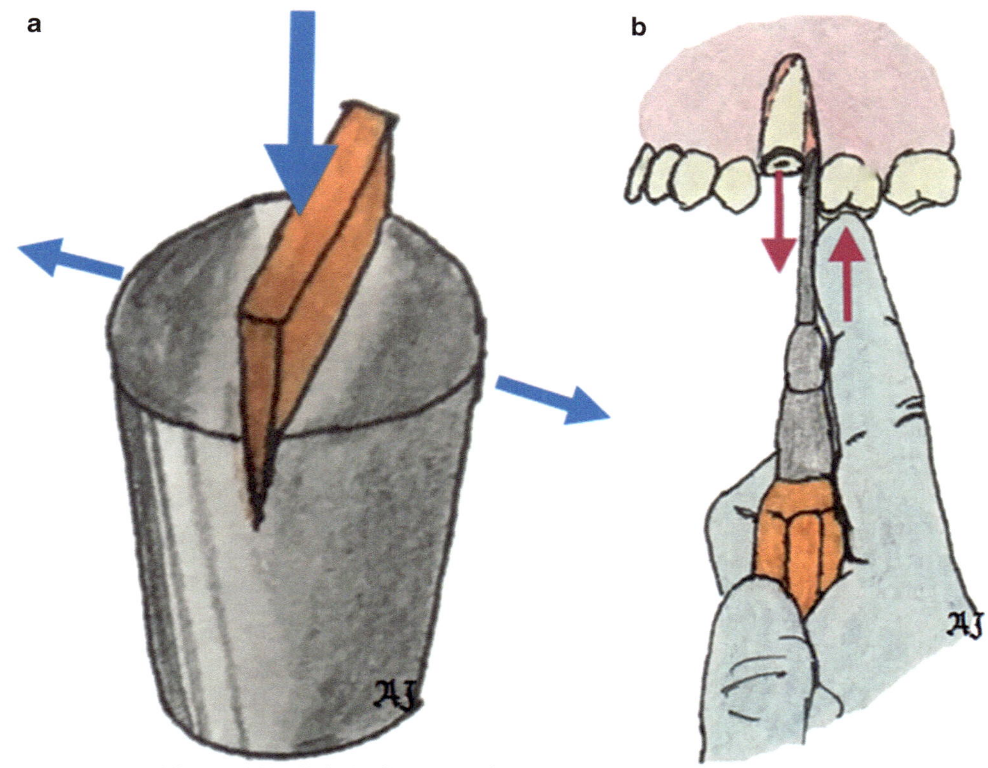


©Association of Oral and Maxillofacial Surgeons of India

**Fig. 13.13** (**a**) Wedge principle where a wedge is used to expand, split, and displace portions of the substance that receives it, (**b**) The blade of the elevator is used as a wedge to displace the tooth root out of the socket

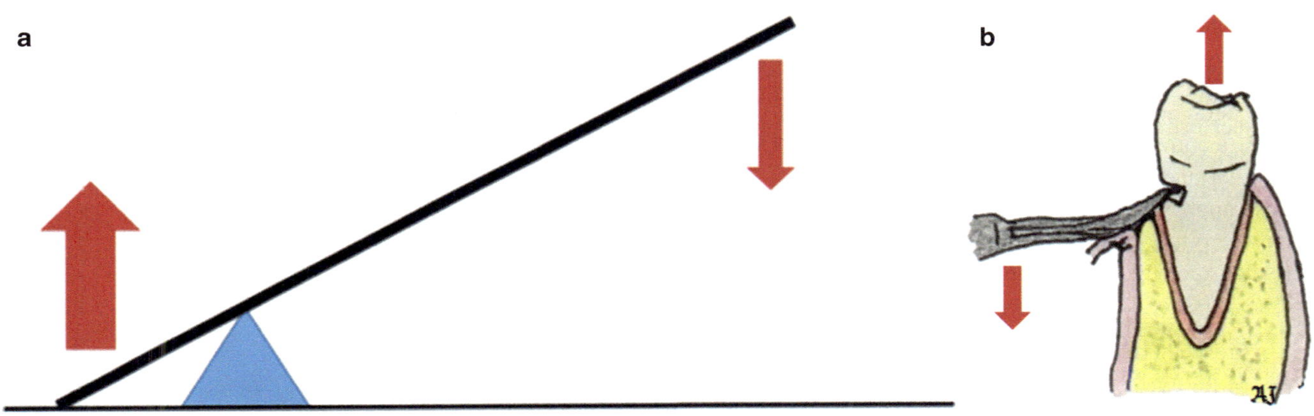


©Association of Oral and Maxillofacial Surgeons of India

**Fig. 13.14** (**a**) The small force and large movement transformed to small movement and large force by the first-class lever, (**b**) The tooth is elevated out of the socket where the bone acts as a fulcrum

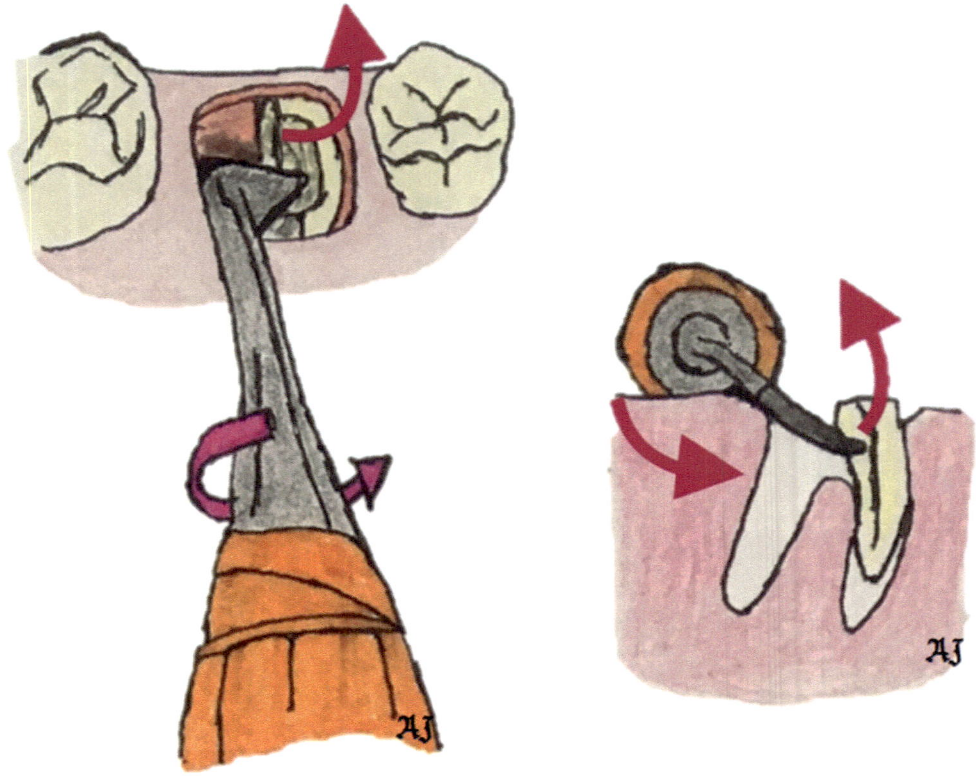

**Fig. 13.15** The elevator acting on the principle of Wheel and Axle aids in retrieval of root from the socket



tors may hamper the access to the surgical site. Acute signs of infection like inflammation, edema, and pus discharge must also be assessed and the procedure must be performed under local antiseptic care and antibiotic coverage.

- Examination of the tooth in question.

  This step includes a thorough examination of

  - Crown size
  - Form
  - Shape
  - Presence of caries
  - Mobility
  - Previous endodontic therapy
  - Tooth Angulation
  - Malposition

  These factors play a significant role in the extraction procedure. The status of the adjacent tooth should also be examined as in its absence the interdental bone cannot be used as a fulcrum. Moreover, if it is carious, there are chances of fracture of the adjacent tooth while application of elevator in the interdental space.

- Radiographic Examination.

  It is advisable to take a proper radiograph for any tooth which is to be extracted. Generally, an intraoral periapical radiograph provides accurate and sufficient details of the tooth, its root/s, and the surrounding tissue.

  Examination of the following factors must be done:

  - Configuration of roots
  - Size of roots
  - Shape of roots
  - Number of roots
  - Root form
  - Presence of dilacerations
  - Resorption
  - Hypercementosis

  A proper radiograph also gives an idea regarding the proximity of the root to the vital structures such as inferior alveolar neurovascular bundle and maxillary sinus. Moreover, the condition of surrounding bone can also be identified for the presence of sclerotic bone or periapical pathologies like cyst, abscess, or granuloma.

### 13.8.2 Treatment Planning

As the proverb says '*Failing to plan is planning to fail*', it is of paramount importance to device a proper treatment plan before carrying out an extraction procedure. The degree of difficulty must be anticipated during the pre-extraction period. On assessment, if it is believed that the degree of extraction is high or the initial attempts of extraction confirm it, a deliberate surgical approach must be planned. A large amount of force during simple exodontia must be avoided as it may injure local soft tissue and damage surrounding bone and teeth. There are also chances of crown fracture which makes the procedure more difficult. Also, the application of excessive force aggravates the intraoperative and postoperative discomfort of the patient.

### 13.8.3 Administration of Local Anesthesia

Extraction of the tooth can be effectively carried out under local anesthesia. Hence, administration of local anesthesia must be carried out with proper technique and appropriate agent. For different teeth, different nerve blocks are to be given (Tables 13.2 and 13.3). Once the local anesthesia, nerve block and/or local infiltration is administered, surgeon must wait for it to act and confirm the same by subjective and objective tests.

### 13.8.4 Surgeon and Patient Preparation

The principle of universal precaution states that all the patients must be viewed as having blood-borne diseases that can be transmitted to the surgical team and other patients. Hence, to avoid transmission of diseases, a surgeon and the assistant must wear surgical gloves, surgical mask, eye-wear with shields, surgical cap, and a long-sleeved surgical gown. Before the patient is subjected to the extraction procedure, a sterile drape should be put over the patient's chest to decrease the risk of contamination. It is advisable to reduce the bacterial contamination in the patient's mouth by making him/her rinse the mouth vigorously using an antiseptic rinse like chlorhexidine prior to the procedure. Some surgeons prefer to keep a partially unfolded 4 × 4 inches' gauze loosely into the back of the mouth to prevent the tooth or its fragment from potential aspiration or swallowing. However, it should not be kept posterior enough to trigger gag reflex.

### 13.8.5 Position of Operator, Patient, and Chair

The positions of the operator, the patient, and the chair are very important for comfortable and successful extraction. The best position is one that is comfortable for both the patient and surgeon and which allows the surgeon to have maximum control during the procedure.

**Table 13.7** Chair and patient positions for extraction

| | Maxillary extraction | Mandibular extraction |
|---|---|---|
| Operator standing | • Chair tipped backward<br>• Maxillary Occlusal plane at 45° to the floor<br>• Patient's mouth should be at the level between the operator's shoulder and elbow | • Upright position<br>• Mandibular occlusal plane parallel to floor<br>• Patient's mouth should be at the level slightly below the operator's elbow |
| Operator sitting | • Supine position (10° to ground)<br>• Patient's mouth should be at the level of operator's elbow | • Supine position (20°–30° to ground)<br>• Patient's mouth should be at the level slightly above the operator's elbow |

**Table 13.8** Operator's standing position for extraction

| Teeth | Position for right handed operator | Position for left handed operator |
|---|---|---|
| All maxillary teeth and mandibular anterior teeth | 7 O′ clock – 8 O′ clock | 4 O′ clock – 5 O′ clock |
| Mandibular left posterior teeth | 7 O′ clock – 8 O′ clock | 1 O′ clock |
| Mandibular right posterior teeth | 11 O′ clock | 4 O′ clock – 5 O′ clock |

- Chair and Patient's Position (Table 13.7).
- Operator's Position (Table 13.8) (Figs. 13.16 and 13.17).

### 13.8.6 Exodontia Procedure

Choosing the correct technique and following fundamental principles, leading to an atraumatic extraction. The three fundamental requirements for a good extraction are:

(a) Adequate access and visualization of the surgical field.
(b) An unimpeded pathway for the removal of the tooth, and
(c) Use of controlled force to luxate and remove the tooth.

Dental extractions are based on three mechanical properties, which are as follows:

1. *Expansion of alveolar socket*: The tooth itself is used as a dilating instrument to expand the alveolar socket in order to permit the removal of its harbored tooth. This is performed mainly in 'intra-alveolar exodontia' by holding the tooth firmly with a forceps and carrying out lateral movements in buccal and lingual directions (Fig. 13.18). This expansion depends on the elasticity of the bone which is maximal in young bone and decreases with age. Dilatation of socket results in microfractures in the bony

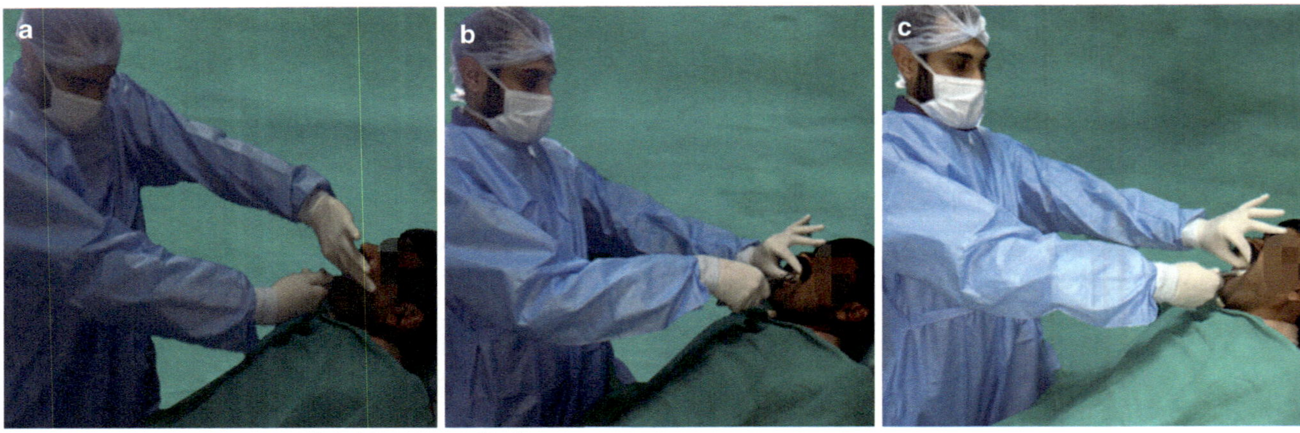



**Fig. 13.16** Operator's position for maxillary teeth extraction, (**a**) Right posterior, (**b**) Anterior, and (**c**) Left posterior

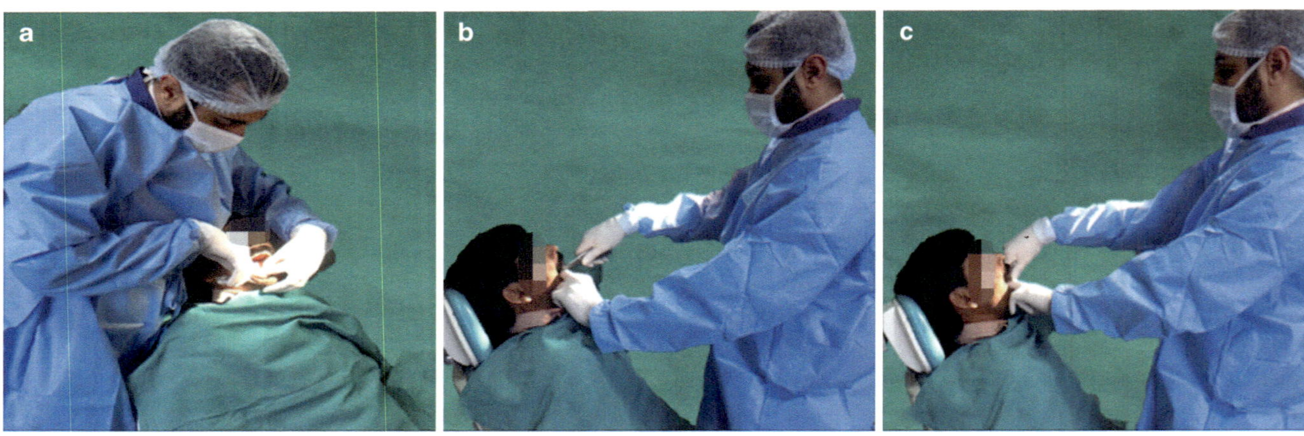



**Fig. 13.17** Operator's position for mandibular teeth extraction, (**a**) Right posterior, (**b**) Anterior, and (**c**) Left posterior

wall and interradicular septa. The bony fragments retain the periosteal attachment in almost all the cases and hence must be digitally compressed unless an implant placement is planned.

2. *Use of Lever and Fulcrum*: This principle is used to luxate the tooth or root and force it out of the socket along the path of least resistance. This principle is the basic factor which governs the use of elevators to extract tooth or tooth root (Fig. 13.14b).
3. *Insertion of a wedge of wedges*: Insertion of wedge between the tooth/root and bony socket wall leads to the rise of tooth in the socket (Fig. 13.19). Lesser the elasticity of bone, more are the effects of wedging. This is the reason that sometimes on application of blades of forceps, the conical rooted mandibular premolars shoot out of the sockets.

The two methods of exodontia are as follows:

1. *Intra-alveolar Exodontia*: This method of extraction is also referred to as closed method or routine exodontia, usually practiced for extraction of erupted and intact tooth with enough structure to grasp with a forceps and pull the tooth out of alveolar socket. Instruments used are forceps or elevators or both. This technique is the most frequently used technique for almost every extraction. However, if the operator believes that the extraction will require an excessive force or if a substantial amount of crown is missing or covered by tissue, an open technique may be opted.

5 sequential steps are to be followed for exodontia by closed technique (Fig. 13.20). Other than these 5 steps, the opposite hand also plays a vital role during the procedure which is highlighted in Table 13.9.

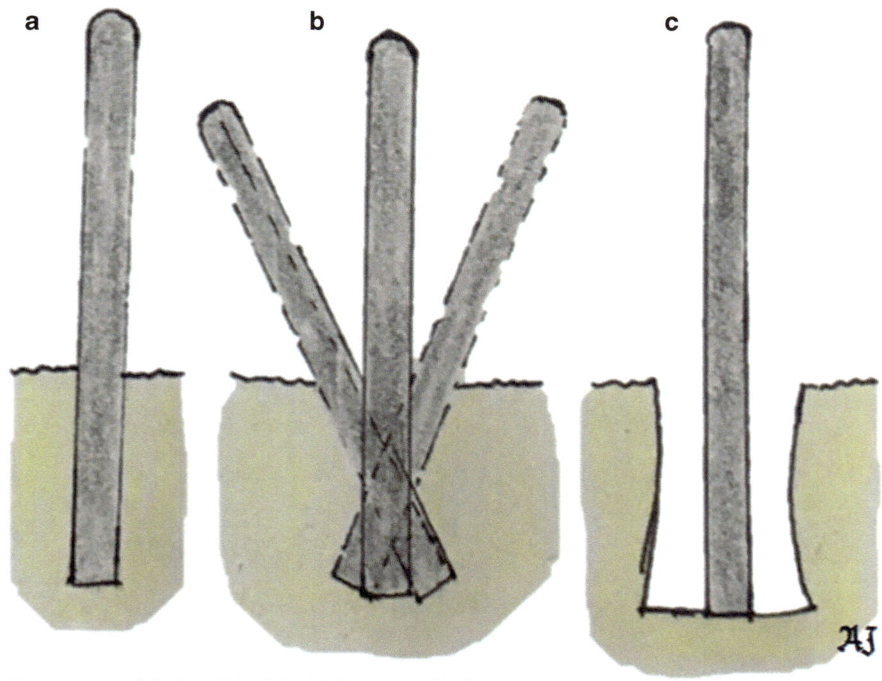




**Fig. 13.18** (**a**) Exodontia by expansion of bony socket is similar to the removal of a post embedded in the ground, (**b**) The post is moved laterally in a to and fro motion, (**c**) This results in displacement of soil surrounding the post and permitting the post to be removed out

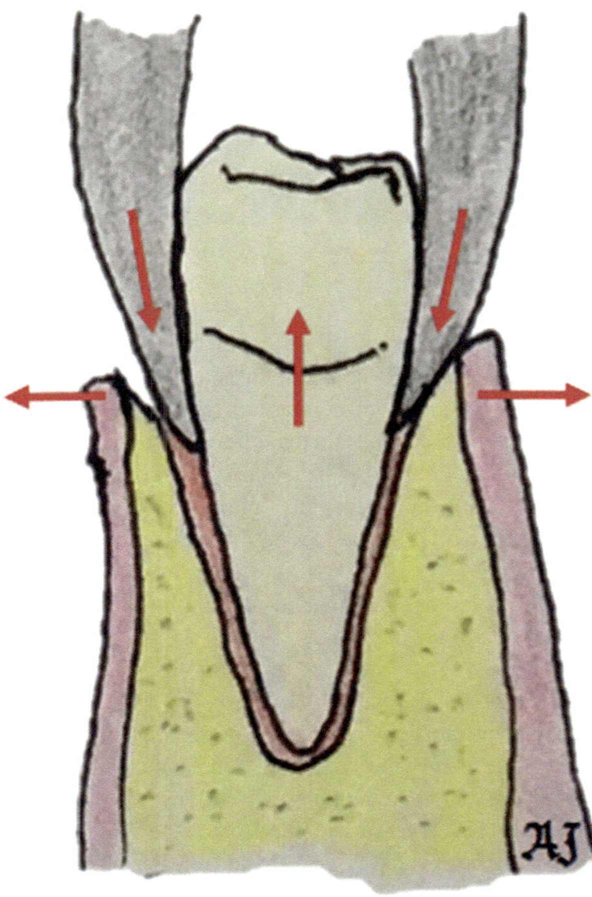




**Fig. 13.19** Insertion of wedge-shaped forceps blades resulting in rise of the tooth in the socket

2. *Transalveolar Exodontia:* This method includes removal of alveolar bone to access and extract the tooth. It is generally practiced for extraction of impacted teeth, root pieces, or teeth with unfavorable root form. It is often termed as surgical extraction or complicated exodontia. Indications for open technique are enlisted in Box 13.2. For an open technique exodontia, 5 steps are to be followed: (Fig. 13.23) (Clinical Case, Fig. 13.24a–f).

## 13.9 Various Mucoperiosteal Flap Designs for Transalveolar Extraction

Transalveolar exodontia necessitates incision making and subsequent mucoperiosteal flap reflection for adequate exposure of the underlying alveolar bone. The flap must be an adequate sized full-thickness mucoperiosteal flap with a broader base which is made on intact bone, avoiding injury to the local vital structures. The various types of flaps used in transalveolar exodontia are:

1. *Envelope Flap:* When a crevicular incision without any releasing incision is given, it produces an envelope flap. Usually, this flap provides adequate access to perform the surgery (Fig. 13.25a).
2. *Triangular Flap:* When a crevicular incision has one vertical releasing incision, it produces a triangular flap. It is also known as a two-sided or three-cornered flap. The three corners are posterior end of the crevicular incision, inferior

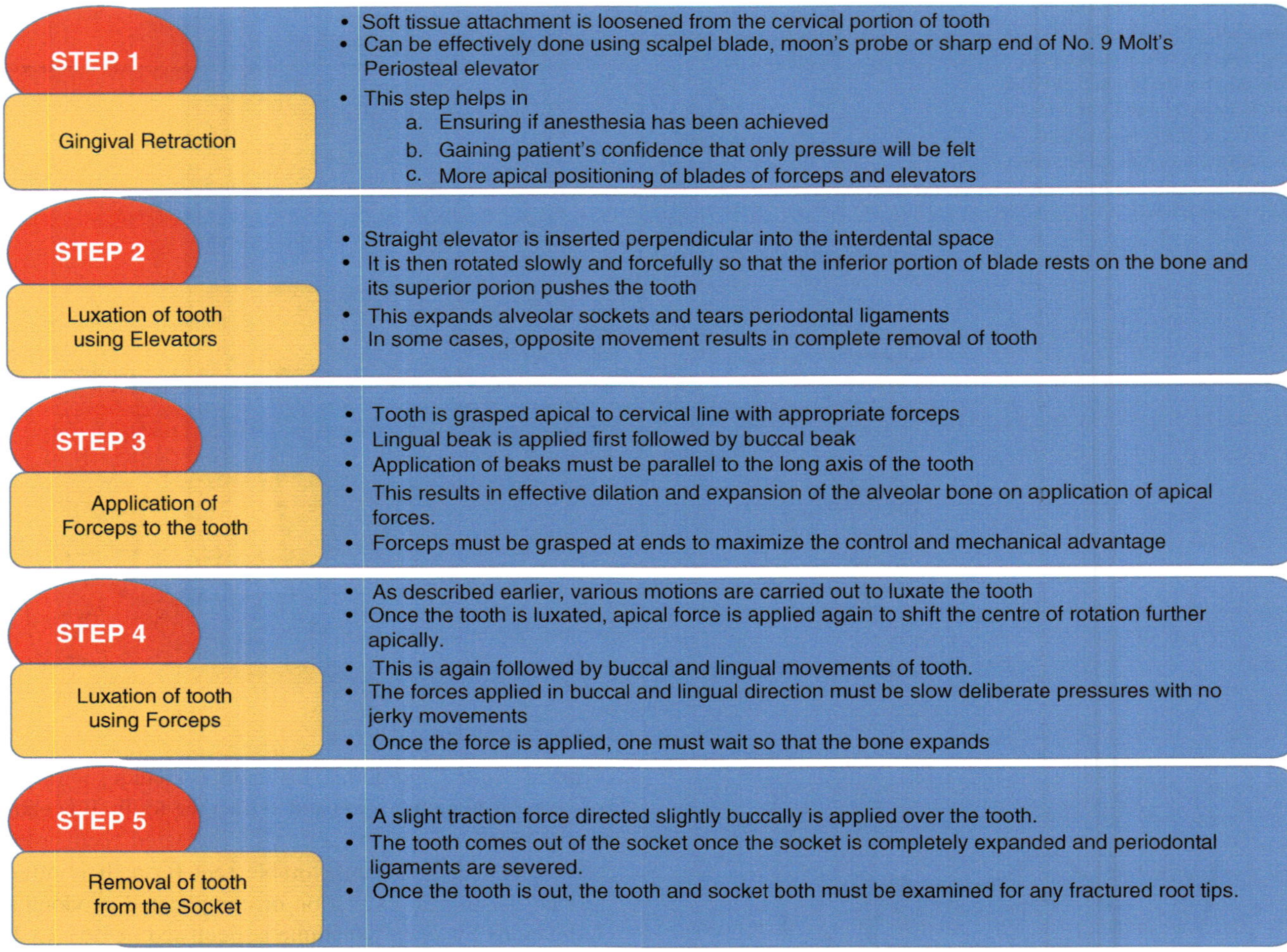




**Fig. 13.20** Steps for Intra-alveolar exodontia

**Table 13.9** Role of opposite hand during exodontia

| Functions of opposite hand | Grasp of opposite hand |
|---|---|
| • Reflection of soft tissues of the cheeks, lips, and tongue<br>• Protection of other teeth from the forceps<br>• Stabilization of patient's head (along with opposite arm)<br>• Supporting the jaw during mandibular extraction<br>• Supporting the alveolar process providing tactile information regarding expansion | • Pinch grasp: While extracting maxillary teeth, the operator grasps the alveolar bone around the tooth to be extracted by a pinch grasp (Fig. 13.21)<br>• Sling grasp: While extracting mandibular teeth, the operator grasps the alveolar bone around the tooth to be extracted by a sling grasp (Fig. 13.22) |

aspect of vertical releasing incision, and the superior aspect of the vertical releasing incision. When a greater exposure is required, this flap is preferred (Fig. 13.25b).

3. *Trapezoidal Flap:* When a crevicular incision has two vertical releasing incisions on either sides, it produces a trapezoidal flap. It is also known as a three-sided or four-cornered flap. Two corners are at the superior aspect of the releasing incisions and the other two corners are at the ends of the crevicular incision. The vertical releasing incisions are not vertically placed but are directed obliquely to allow a broader base (Fig. 13.25c).

Transalveolar or complicated exodontia can be further described in two types.

1. *Complicated Exodontia of Single rooted tooth.*
   It starts by incision making and reflecting a sufficiently large flap to provide adequate visualization and access. Mostly an envelope flap is preferred which is extended at least two teeth anterior and one tooth posterior to the tooth that has to be extracted. If required, a releasing incision can be placed. Once the flap is reflected adequately and the surgical site is exposed sufficiently, extraction of the tooth/root must be performed by using one of the various options.

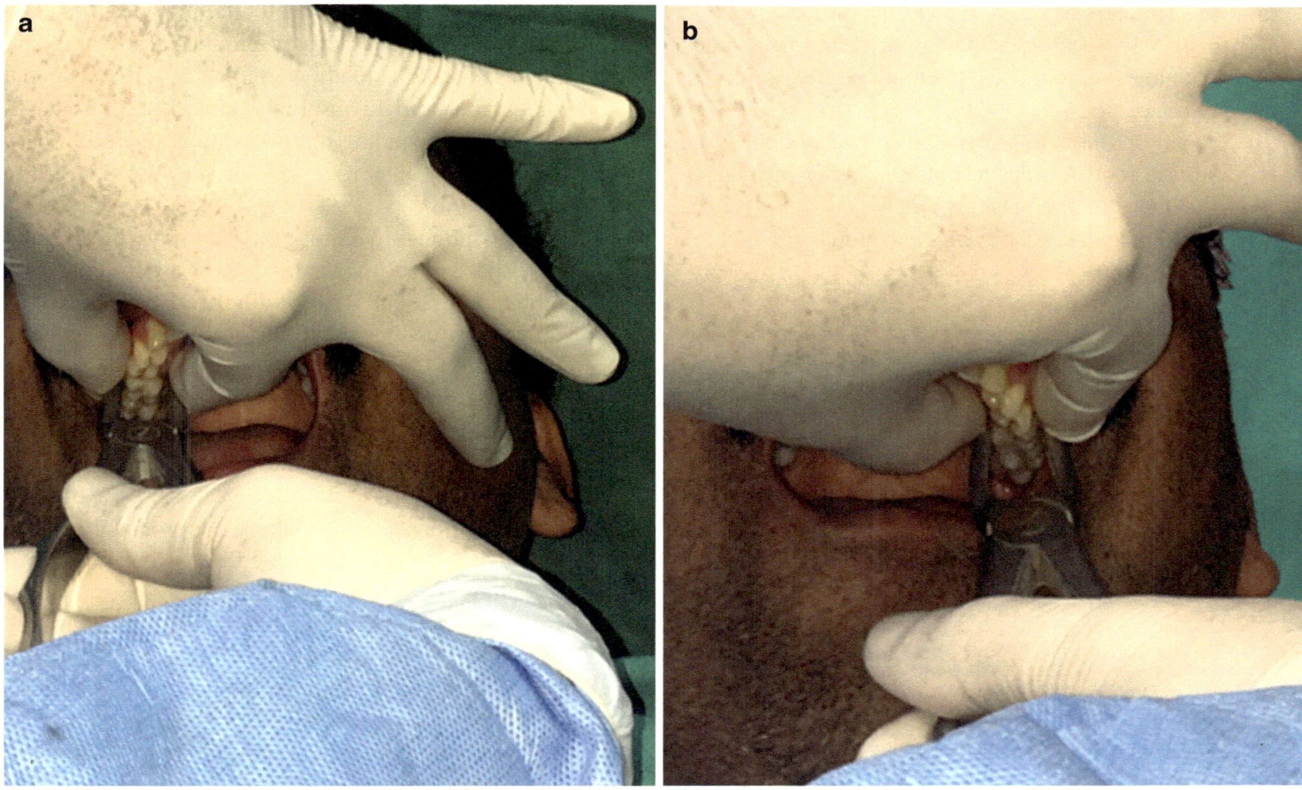




**Fig. 13.21** Pinch grasp for maxillary teeth (**a**) Right posterior, (**b**) Left posterior

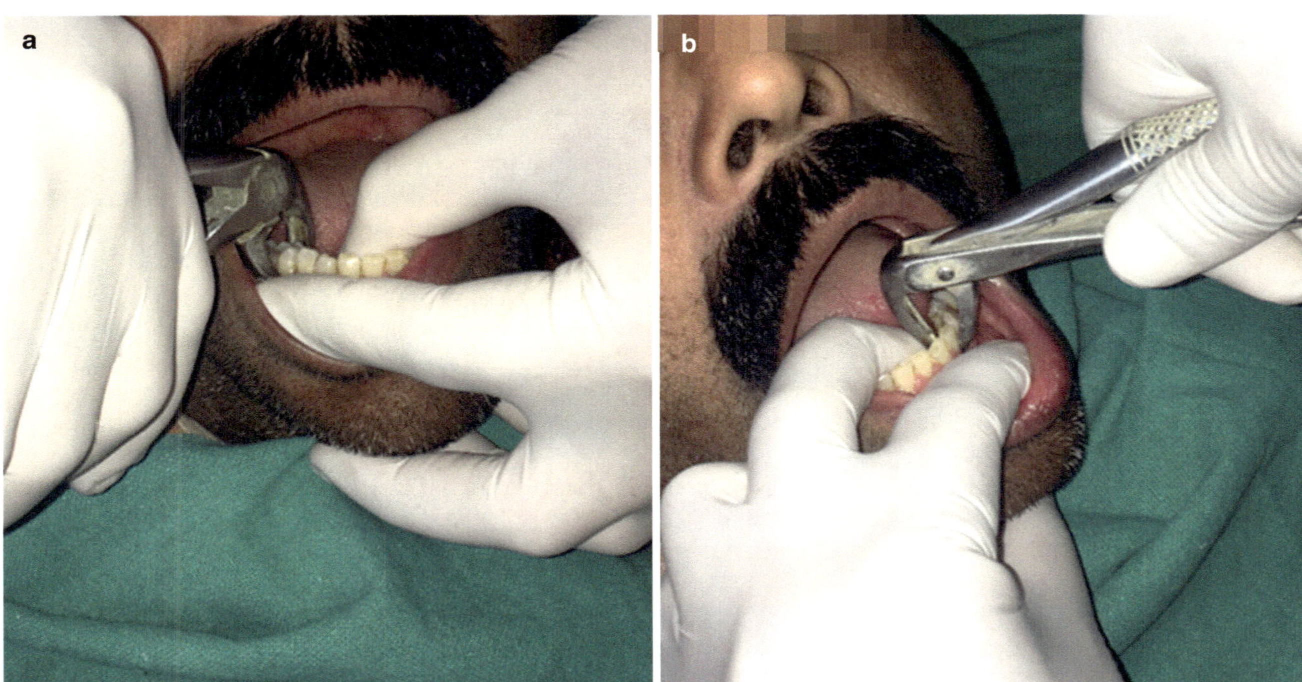




**Fig. 13.22** Sling grasp for mandibular teeth (**a**) Right posterior, (**b**) Anterior

(a) First option is to reseat the extraction forceps under direct visualization achieving a better mechanical advantage and removing the tooth without removing any bone.

(b) Second option is to grasp a bit of buccal bone along with the root in order to obtain a better mechanical advantage. In this case, a small amount of buccal bone is pinched off and removed along with the tooth (Fig. 13.26a).

Indications of Trans alveolar exodontia

- Teeth with Severely undermined crown
- Fractured teeth
- Endodontically treated teeth
- Root pieces
- Teeth with unfavourable root form like bulbous or dilacerated roots
- Multiple divergent roots
- Ankylosed teeth
- Hypercementosis
- Presence of dense bone
- Malposed tooth
- Impacted tooth
- Tooth in proximity to vital structures
- Long standing tooth with grossly carious crown



**Box 13.2** Indications of transalveolar exodontia

(c) Third option is to push the tooth out of the socket by inserting a straight elevator into the periodontal ligament space of the tooth. A small to and fro movement should be used to insert the straight elevator as a wedge by expanding the periodontal ligament space to displace the root in an occlusal direction (Fig. 13.26b).

(d) Fourth option is to remove the bone covering the buccal aspect of root with the help of a bur along with ample irrigation. The width of the bone to be removed must be essentially equal to the mesiodistal width of the root. Also, the amount of bone to be removed in the vertical dimension should be approximately one half or two thirds the length of the root (Fig. 13.26c). Removal of this much amount of bone minimizes the force necessary for the displacement of the root, making the procedure easier. The extraction can be carried out using forceps or elevator.

(e) In some cases, removal of the root is still difficult even after the removal of bone. In such cases, a purchase point can be made in the most apical position of the exposed root with the help of a round bur. This purchase point must be 3 mm in diameter and deep

**STEP 1** — Incision and Flap Reflection

- Based on basic principles of flap designing, an incision is placed and a full thickness mucoperiosteal flap is elevated.
- Adequate buccal cortical bone is exposed to access the tooth/root.

**STEP 2** — Removal of Bone

- The bone is removed from buccal aspect using chisel or burs.
- When an intact tooth is present, root is exposed below the cementoenamel junction.
- In case of root piece, enough root structure is exposed to create purchase point.

**STEP 3** — Odontectomy

- When an intact tooth is present, the crown can be sectioned and removed first.
- This is mainly done when the path of removal of crown and roots are different.
- Once the crown is removed, the roots are addressed.

**STEP 4** — Removal of Tooth

- A hole is drilled in the tooth to engage the tip of the elevator. This hole is called 'Purchase Point'
- It must be deep enough to engage the elevator tip and must be drilled in healthy root to avoid fragmentation.
- In case of multiple roots, they can be sectioned and removed separately.

**STEP 5** — Closure

- After the tooth is removed completely, wound debridement, curettage of granulation tissue, removal of loose and sharp bony fragments, rounding off socket margins, gentle irrigation with normal saline and finally closure using suture is done.



**Fig. 13.23** Steps for transalveolar exodontia

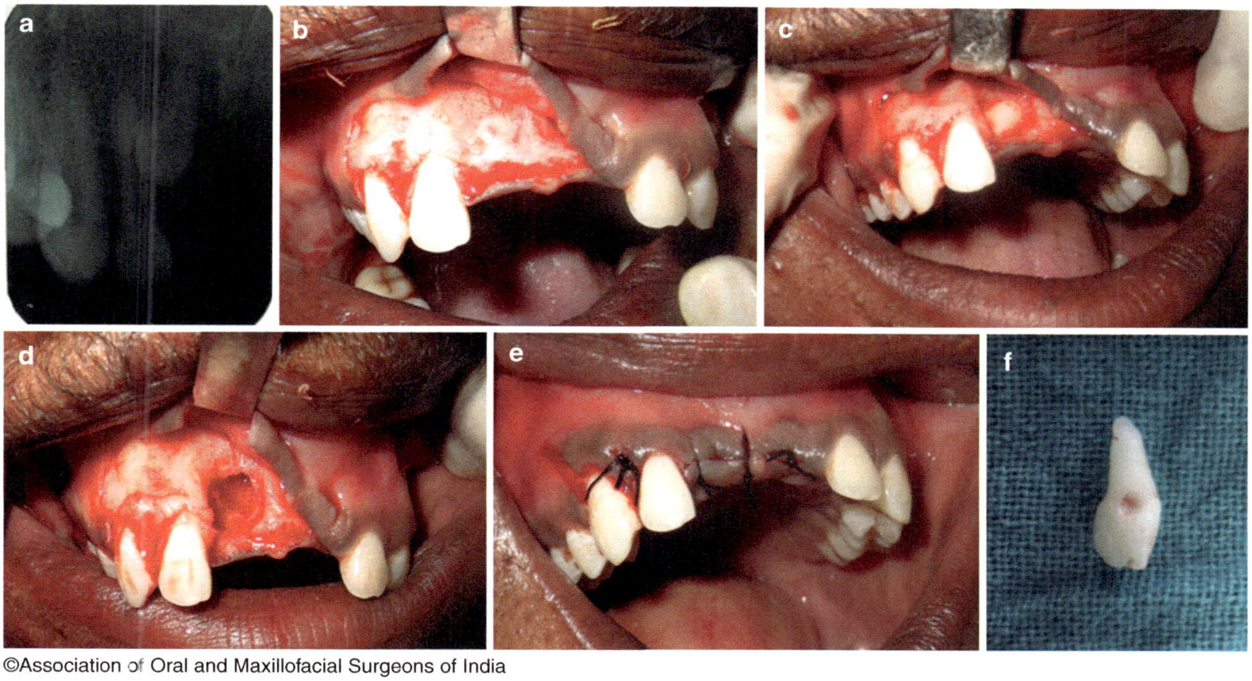


**Fig. 13.24** Transalveolar extraction of impacted tooth: (**a**) IOPA showing impacted tooth, (**b**) Incision and flap reflection (Triangular flap), (**c**) Bone removal, (**d**) Extraction socket (**e**) Closure, (**f**) Extracted tooth

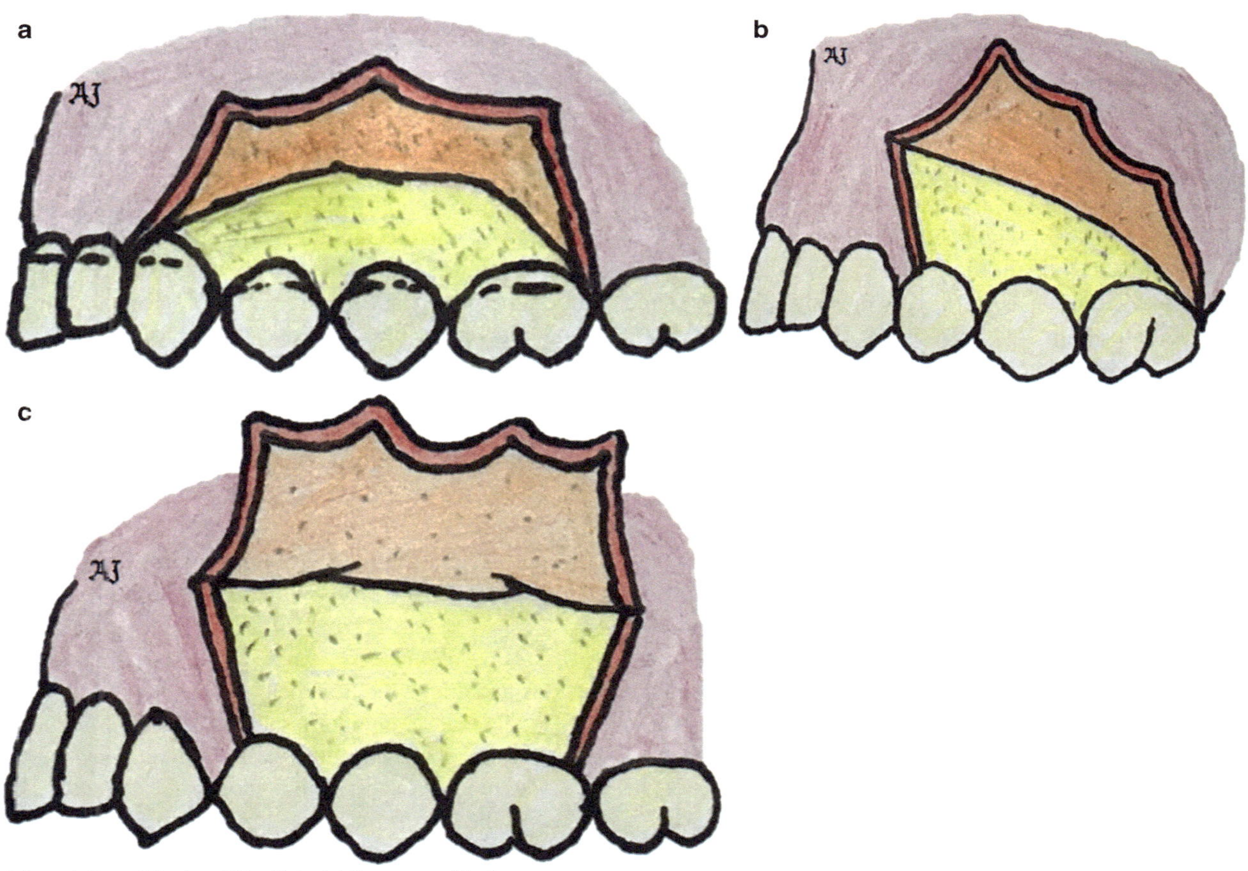


**Fig. 13.25** (**a**) Envelope flap, (**b**) Triangular flap, (**c**) Trapezoidal flap

enough to engage the tip of an instrument to be used for elevation of the tooth.

Once the tooth is delivered, the sharp bony edges must be smoothened using a bone file and the whole surgical site must be thoroughly irrigated using copious amount of sterile saline. The flap must be repositioned and sutured into place.

2. *Complicated exodontia of multirooted teeth.*

   If a treatment plan of complicated exodontia is devised for a multirooted tooth, it is extracted with the same technique as of single-rooted tooth. The only difference is that the tooth is divided using a bur to convert into two or three single-rooted fragments (odontectomy). Following incision and flap reflection, once the tooth is converted into multiple single-rooted fragments, the extraction procedure is carried out in a similar way as of single-rooted tooth. Also, the immediate postoperative procedures like smoothening of bony fragments, irrigation, and closure also remains the same. The following text describes different techniques of splitting a multirooted tooth in different scenarios.

   (a) Mandibular molar with intact crown: First step involves the exposure of bifurcation by removing a small amount of crestal bone. The tooth is usually sectioned buccolingually to split the tooth into mesial and distal halves (Fig. 13.27a). These halves are then mobilized using a straight elevator and are treated as two single-rooted teeth. These teeth are then extracted with the help of mandibular premolar forceps.

       Alternatively, mesial root is sectioned using a bur to convert the molar into single-rooted tooth (Fig. 13.27b). The tooth along with distal root is removed with the help of forceps followed by the removal of mesial root. This mesial root is extracted with the help of a Cryer elevator.

   (b) Mandibular molar with lost crown: The roots are separated in a buccolingual direction with the help of a bur in two separate mesial and distal roots (Fig. 13.27c). A small straight elevator is inserted in between the roots and rotated to mobilize the roots and elevate the mesial root. With the help of the Cryer elevator, the mesial root is delivered out of the socket by engaging the tip into the created purchase point and rotating in a wheel-and-axle manner. The distal root is then extracted by inserting the opposite member of the Cryer instrument into the empty socket and rotating again in a wheel-and-axle manner through the interradicular bone.

   (c) Maxillary molar with an intact crown: The roots of maxillary molar are three in number and are divergent. Sometimes, an open technique of extraction causes less morbidity than the closed technique as the extraction of maxillary molar requires excessive force during forceps' extraction. Once the flap is raised, a small amount of crestal bone is removed to expose the trifurcation. With the help of a straight bur, the mesiobuccal and distobuccal roots are sectioned horizontally at the level of trifurcation. This separates the two buccal roots converting the molar into single-rooted tooth (Fig. 13.27d). The molar with palatal root is then extracted using the maxillary molar forceps with gentle but firm bucco-occlusal forces. The two buccal roots are then mobilized with the help of a straight elevator. These roots are then delivered out with the help of a straight or Cryer elevator. The operator must take precaution to maintain controlled force in an apical direction during removal of these roots using the straight elevator as maxillary sinus might be in a close proximity to these roots. Uncontrolled and excessive force may result in an oroantral communication or displacement of the root into the sinus.

   (d) Maxillary molar with lost crown: A small amount of buccal bone is removed to expose the roots and is divided into two buccal and palatal roots (Fig. 13.27e). The roots are mobilized with the help of a straight elevator and are extracted with the help of bayonet forceps or Cryer elevators. Generally, buccal roots are approached first followed by palatal root.

During exodontia, once completed either by closed technique or by open technique, a few important things must be kept in mind which are listed in Box 13.3 and the patient should be instructed properly as listed in Box 13.4. During exodontia, either closed or open, an assistant may be really helpful and plays an important role during the procedure (Box 13.5).

## 13.10 Multiple Extractions

If multiple adjacent teeth are indicated for extraction, a few key points are to be taken into consideration.

1. Soft tissue must be reflected to expose the crestal bone around all the teeth in the quadrant.
2. If removal of any tooth requires excessive force, a small amount of buccal bone should be removed to prevent fracture and excessive bone loss.
3. All the teeth must be luxated well enough before extraction.

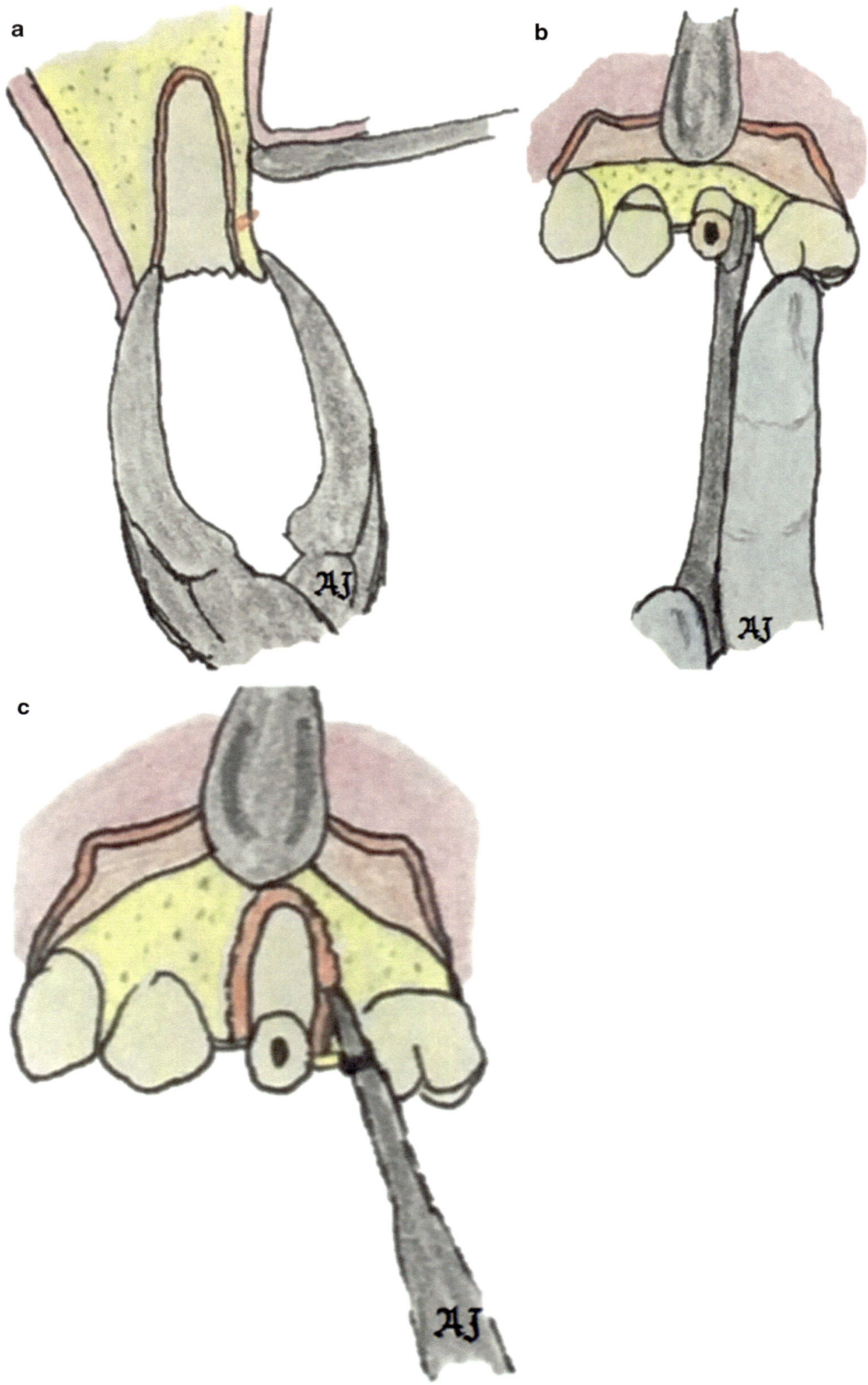




**Fig. 13.26** (**a**) A small portion of buccal bone is grasped along with the root in cases when the root is fractured at the level of alveolar bone (Alveolar Purchase Technique), (**b**) A small straight elevator is being used to luxate the broken root, (**c**) Bone is removed from the buccal aspect of the root using a bur

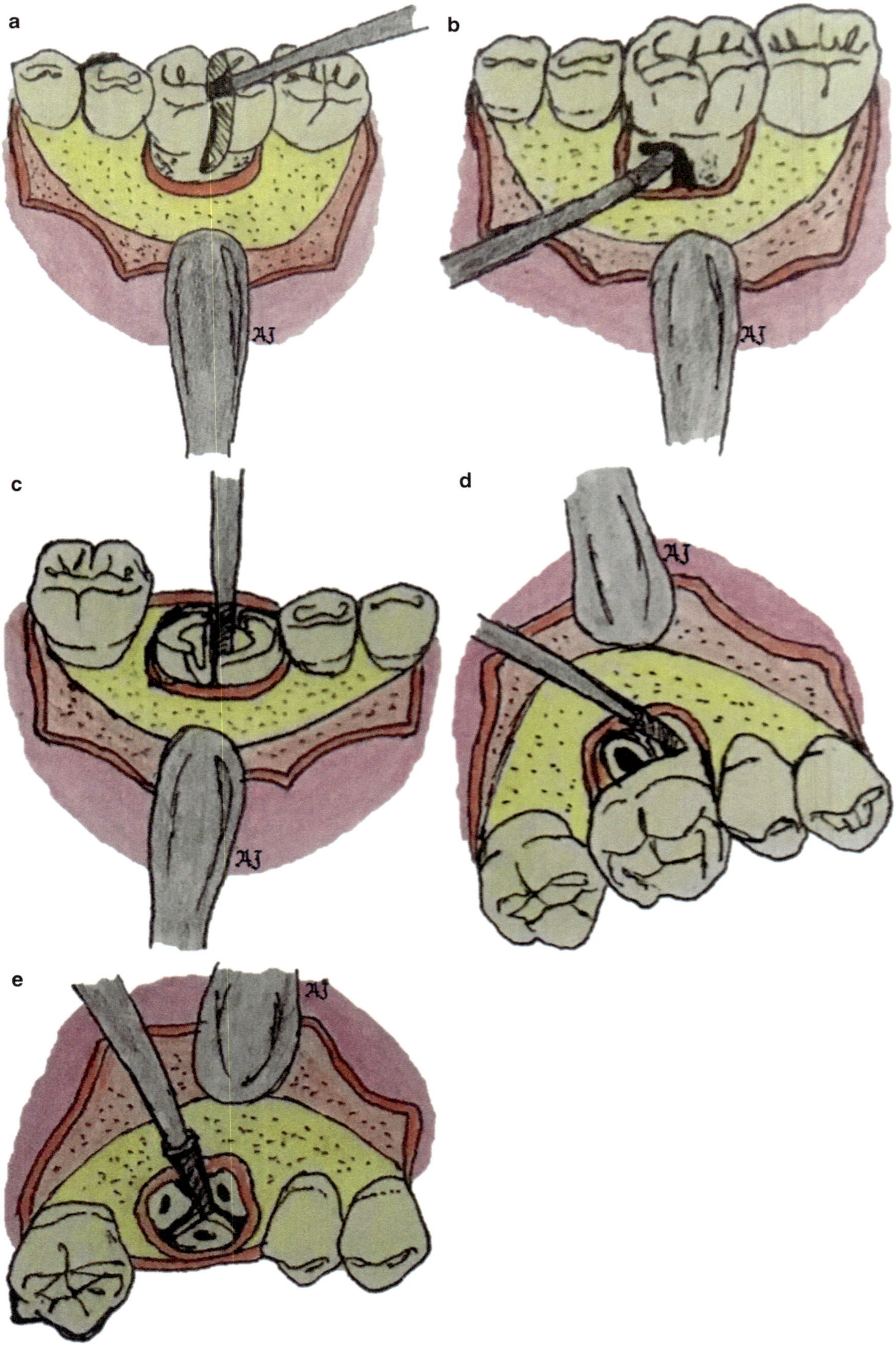




**Fig. 13.27** (**a**) Sectioning of tooth into mesial and distal halves, (**b**) Separation of mesial root from the tooth, (**c**) Separation of roots of mandibular molar, (**d**) Buccal roots are sectioned from the tooth, (**e**) Separation of roots of maxillary molar

**Box 13.3** Immediate post-extraction care

Immediate Post-extraction Care

- Inspect the tooth and root to ensure complete removal
- Visualize the socket by thoroughly drying the socket and the adjacent field
- Inspect the socket for excessive bleeding which could be due to injured vessel (forceful bleeding) or friable granulation tissue (steadily flowing blood) and curette the socket
- Inspect for foreign bodies like fragments of tooth, calculus tags, granulation tissue, sharp bony fragments and remove using a mosquito artery if present
- Palpate the edges of socket to rule out any sharp bony margins. If present smoothen them using a file
- Compress the expanded socket with digital pressure (simple alveoloplasty). Not recommended if implant is planned
- Application of pressure pack to arrest bleeding using a moistened sterile gauze rolled over cotton wool
- Loose approximating sutures are placed following extraction to stop bleeding and prevent food impaction if required.
- Analgesics can be prescribed to the patients



**Box 13.4** Postoperative instructions

Post-operative Instructions

- Maintenance of pressure pack for 30 – 60 minutes (Initial clot is soft and friable. Clot retraction takes 30-45 minutes)
- Swallow the saliva and not to spit or rinse till 24 hours post extraction
- Soft and cold diet for 24 hours so as not to disturb the clot and for vasoconstriction
- Warm saline rinses after 24 hours to enhance healing of socket
- Avoid smoking as it may dislodge the clot and lead to bleeding
- No hot fomentation, only cold compressions in the immediate post-operative phase



4. Maxillary teeth are extracted first because.
   (a) Infiltration anesthesia has a more rapid onset in maxilla leading to early start of the procedure.
   (b) Profound anesthesia is lost early in maxilla.
   (c) If mandibular teeth are extracted first, debris such as fractured crowns, bone chips, and portions of restorative material may fall in the empty mandibular sockets during extraction of maxillary teeth.
5. Hemostasis must be achieved with maxillary sockets before the extraction of mandibular teeth as the hemorrhage may interfere with mandibular surgery.
6. Extraction should be started with the most posterior teeth as it allows the effective use of dental elevators to luxate and mobilize the teeth.
7. While extracting multiple mandibular anterior teeth, an elevator is inserted between the two adjacent teeth and is rotated. This movement luxates both the teeth simultaneously aiding in the extraction of both the teeth. This technique is known as Stobies technique.
8. Canine is the most difficult tooth to extract, hence it should be extracted last.

Role of Assistant during Exodontia

- Helping surgeon to visualize or gain access to the surgical site
- Suction away blood, saliva and irrigating solutions
- Helps in protecting the teeth of opposite side
- Stabilize the head of the patient
- Support the jaw of the patient
- Psychological and Emotional support for the patient



**Box 13.5** Role of assistant

9. If maxillary and mandibular teeth of one side are to be extracted in one sitting, the sequence of extraction recommended is: Maxillary Posterior Teeth – Maxillary Anterior Teeth – Maxillary Canine – Mandibular Posterior Teeth – Mandibular Anterior Teeth – Mandibular Canine.
10. Post-extraction, the buccal and lingual plates are repositioned to the original position using digital pressure unless implants are planned.

11. If removable partial or complete dentures are planned, the undercuts and bony spicules must be identified and primary alveoloplasty must be carried out.
12. Soft tissue must be inspected for excessive granulation tissue; if present, it should be removed as it may prolong postoperative hemorrhage.
13. Papillae should be sutured in position. Primary closure must not be performed at the cost of vestibular depth, because if the vestibular depth decreases, it may interfere with denture construction.

## 13.11 Extraction of Root Fragments and Tips

Ideally, when the apical one-third of the root (3–4 mm) is fractured, it should be removed as it may act as a septic focus or may result in the formation of cyst or other pathologies. To extract these root tips, the two most important requirements are excellent light and excellent suction with a tip of small diameter.

Once the fracture of root tip has been diagnosed, the operator must reposition the patient to achieve proper visualization and suction. Initially, closed technique must be attempted; if unsuccessful, then the open technique must be carried out for retrieval of root tip.

- Initial attempt of root tip removal must be made by vigorous irrigation of the socket using normal saline. Following irrigation and suction, the socket must be inspected properly to check if the root has been removed or not.
- If unsuccessful, the root tip may be teased out of the socket with the help of a root tip elevator (Fig. 13.28a). The blade of the elevator is inserted in the periodontal ligament space and the root is teased out of the socket gently. Root tip elevator is a delicate instrument; hence excessive force must be avoided as it may result in bending or fracture of the blade. For larger fragments, a small straight elevator may also be used.
- If the closed technique is unsuccessful, the operator must shift to an open technique. A full-thickness mucoperiosteal flap is elevated and reflected to expose the buccal bone. The buccal bone is removed using a bur to expose the root fragment. The root is then delivered buccally with the help of an elevator (Fig. 13.28b). The socket is irrigated, flap is repositioned, and closure is performed.
- If the buccal bone has to be preserved, a modification of open technique can be performed. This technique is known as open window technique. In this technique, once the flap is reflected, the apical area of the root fragment is identified and a hole is drilled with the help of a bur. This exposes the root tip. An elevator is inserted through this hole and the root fragment is guided out of the socket (Fig. 13.28c and d).

However, if the risk during retrieval of root fragment is comparatively more than the benefit of its removal, it is advisable to leave the root in situ. If the surgeon decides to retain the root, it should be documented and informed to the patient. The criteria for retaining the root are highlighted in Box 13.6. The policy of dealing with fractured apical root tips of maxillary molars and the management of root tips displaced into the antrum is elaborated in Chap. 24 of this book.

## 13.12 Extraction During Menstruation

If permissible, extractions should be avoided during menstruation because during this period there is a high level of estrogen circulating in the blood streams which results in increased tissue bleeding. Menstrual cycle could be a determinant risk factor for alveolar osteitis. Also, both exodontia and menstruation are stressful conditions, it is better not to subject the patient to increased stresses [12].

## 13.13 Extraction During Pregnancy

*Pregnancy*: Second trimester is considered to be relatively safer for carrying out minor oral surgeries. However, in other trimesters, if the potential risk of retaining the tooth outweighs the complications of performing the surgery, one must plan to carry out extraction with the utmost care and avoiding use of drugs and radiographs as much as possible. Caution should be exercised to evaluate teratogenic potential of drugs when prescriptions are warranted.

During first trimester, the fetus is at risk of developmental defects if the extraction is carried out as it undergoes organogenesis. The best course of action is to prevent the patient from all kinds of infection. During the third trimester, there are chances of premature labor or even an abortion. However, if an exodontia is planned, the patient must be kept in a left lateral position. If the patient is maintained in a supine position, there are chances of obstruction of venous return resulting in supine hypotension syndrome [13, 14].

## 13.14 Healing of Extraction Socket [15]

Along with understanding the general principles of exodontia, it is pivotal for a dental surgeon to thoroughly know the phenomenon of healing of extraction wounds. An extraction socket heals in a similar fashion as any other wound in the body except for minor variations which occur due to the anatomic structures in and around the socket.

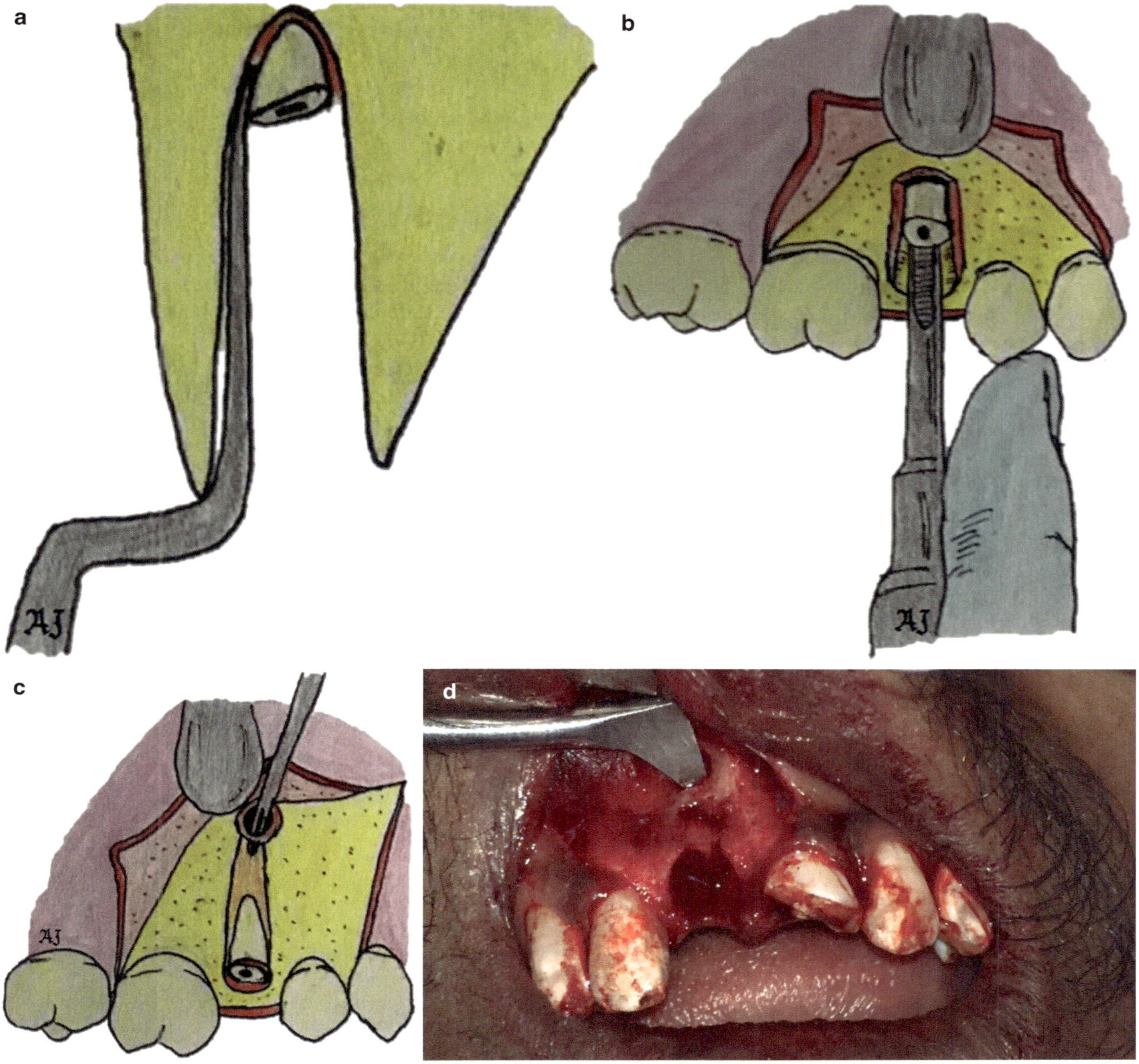




**Fig. 13.28** (**a**) The root tip elevator is inserted into the periodontal ligament space to elevate the root tip, (**b**) Open technique for removal of fractured root fragment, (**c**) Open Window technique for removal of fractured root fragment, (**d**) Clinical picture of open window technique

**Box 13.6** Criteria for retaining root piece

Criteria for leaving root piece in situ

- If it is small (<2 – 3mm in length)
- If it is deep seated
- If it requires excessive bone removal
- If it is not infected
- If there is no presence of periapical infection
- If it is in close proximity to vital structures which may be injured during retrieval
- If during exploration there are chances of its displacement to adjacent anatomical spaces.

Blood present in the socket immediately after extraction of tooth coagulates and red blood cells become entrapped in the fibrin meshwork. This initial time period postextraction is critical because if the clot dislodges, healing becomes delayed and painful. Alterations in the vascular bed such as vasodilatation along with engorgement of blood vessels of periodontal ligament and transport of leukocytes around the clot occur during first 24–48 hours. A thick layer of fibrin covers the clot which shows signs of contractions. This clot forms a scaffold over which cells associated with healing grow.

In the first week following extraction, fibroblasts from remnants of PDL begin to grow in the periphery of clot and a thick layer of leucocytes gather over the clot. Osteoclastic activity starts in the crest of alveolar ridge. Blood clot undergoes organization by fibroblast and endothelial cell proliferation, signaling the growth of small capillaries in the PDL area.

Epithelial proliferation over the surface of the clot increases during the second week of healing leading to a more organized blood clot with new capillaries in the center. Remnants of PDL undergoing degeneration are no longer visible. Margins of alveolar socket appear frayed due to osteoclastic activity. Surfaces of small wounds epithelize completely by this time.

By the third week, fibrin meshwork of the original clot is replaced by mature granulation tissue. Young trabeculae formed by osteoblasts derived from pluripotent cells of PDL form around the periphery of wound. Crest of alveolar bone appears rounded due to resorption. All kinds of wound epithelize by this stage of healing.

Wound enters the final stage of healing in the fourth week. There is deposition and resorption of bone of alveolar socket which continues for several weeks. Newly formed bone is poorly calcified; therefore, the bone after extraction becomes radiographically evident only after 6–8 weeks. Loss of crestal and buccal bone during transalveolar extractions leads to smaller alveolar ridges post healing.

## 13.15 Complications of Exodontia [10]

Surgical procedures are associated with complications and exodontia is no different. Various complications related to exodontia are highlighted in Table 13.10.

Modalities to manage hemorrhage are as follows:

- Pressure packing.
- Injecting local anesthetic solution containing vasoconstrictor.
- Curettage of granulation tissue.
- Suturing.
- Use of resorbable oxidized cellulose (Surgicel) or gelatin foam (Gelfoam).
- Mechanical obstruction using bone wax.
- Tying or coagulation of visible blood vessel.

*Displacement of tooth in Antrum*: Operator must be careful while extracting maxillary molars to avoid displacement of tooth/root into maxillary antrum. Excessive and uncontrolled force in the apical direction may lead to displacement of tooth/root in the maxillary sinus. If displaced, it can be retrieved by carrying out sinus exploration [16].

*Displacement into adjacent spaces*: Tooth/root might get displaced into adjacent anatomic spaces. If it happens, retrieval must be attempted. However, delayed retrieval can also be done as foreign body reaction aids in localization of the tooth/root [17].

*Loss of tooth in pharynx*: During exodontia, if the tooth is lost in pharynx, one must get a chest radiograph done to rule out aspiration. If the tooth is aspirated, bronchoscopy has to be done for retrieval of tooth [18].

*Injury to Temporomandibular Joint*: It is mainly due to the application of excessive forces while extracting mandibular teeth and failure to support mandible. It can be avoided by using mouth gags and supporting mandible properly. Unsupported mandible may lead to dislocation of temporomandibular joint. If occurred, it must be reduced immediately by mechanical reduction.

**Table 13.10** Complications of exodontia

| Complications |
|---|
| 1. General complications |
| (a) Postoperative pain |
| (b) Hemorrhage |
| 2. Problems with tooth being extracted |
| (a) Root fracture |
| (b) Root displacement in adjacent spaces or antrum |
| (c) Loss of tooth in pharynx |
| 3. Injury to adjacent teeth |
| (a) Fracture or dislodgement of adjacent tooth restoration |
| (b) Luxation of adjacent tooth |
| (c) Extraction of wrong tooth |
| 4. Injury to soft tissue |
| (a) Abrasion |
| (b) Puncture wound |
| (c) Tear of mucosal flap |
| 5. Injury to osseous structure |
| (a) Fracture of alveolar process (Fig. 13.29) |
| (b) Fracture of maxillary tuberosity (Fig. 13.30) |
| 6. Injury to adjacent structures |
| (a) Injury to regional nerves |
| (b) Injury to regional vessels |
| (c) Injury to Temporomandibular joint |
| 7. Oroantral communication and fistula |
| 8. Fracture of mandible |
| 9. Delayed healing and infection |
| (a) Infection |
| (b) Wound dehiscence |
| (c) Dry socket (Fig. 13.31) |
| (d) Osteomyelitis |

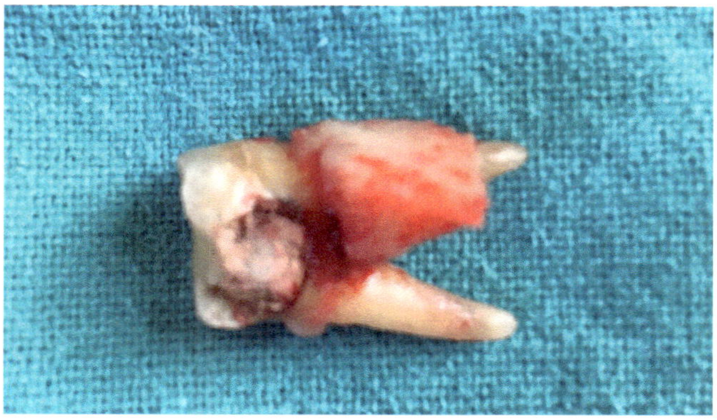

©Association of Oral and Maxillofacial Surgeons of India

**Fig. 13.29** Fractured alveolar process

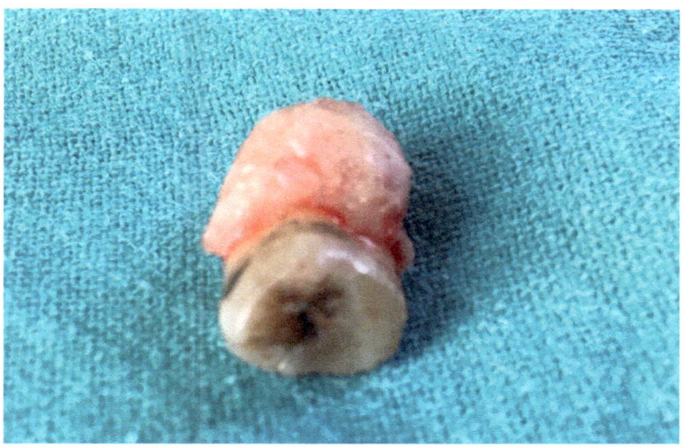

©Association of Oral and Maxillofacial Surgeons of India

**Fig. 13.30** Fractured maxillary tuberosity

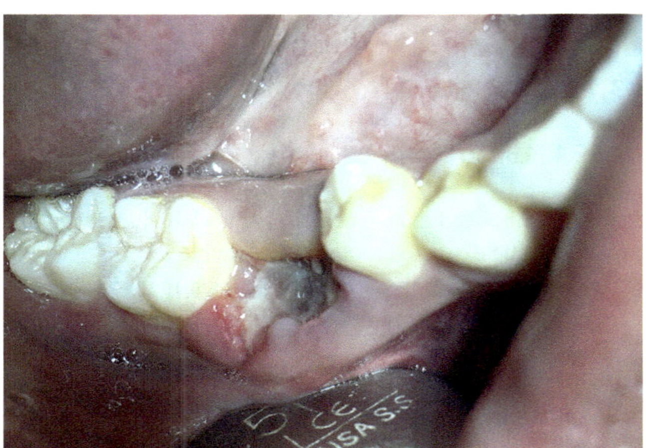

©Association of Oral and Maxillofacial Surgeons of India

**Fig. 13.31** Dry socket

*Hemorrhage*: It is classified as

1. Primary hemorrhage: bleeding at the time of surgery.
2. Reactionary hemorrhage: it is seen a few hours after surgery due to cessation of vasoconstriction of damaged blood vessels.
3. Secondary hemorrhage: evident up to 14 days post-operatively due to infection.

Mechanical reduction is done by an operator standing in front of the patient and holding the mandible with both hands. The thumbs should be placed over the external oblique ridge/molars and the fingers holding the lower border of mandible. Once held firmly, mandible should be moved in inferior, posterior, and superior directions in a sequential manner [6].

*Oroantral Communication and Fistula*: Oroantral communication (OAC) is a pathologic communication between oral cavity and maxillary antrum; however, once epithelized, it is termed as oroantral fistula (OAF). OAC must be closed immediately if it is larger than 5 mm. In cases of OAF, fistulectomy followed by closure is the treatment of choice [19].

Refer the Chap. 24 on oroantral communication and fistula for further reading.

*Dry Socket*: Dry socket or alveolar osteitis denotes delayed healing with moderate to severe pain. Birn's, hypothesis is the most accepted explanation of dry socket. It states that trauma and inflammation cause release of stable tissue activator from adjacent bony socket and soft tissue. Tissue activator converts plasminogen to plasmin which causes lysis of blood clot and pain. Management of dry socket involves relief of pain and ameliorating healing. A loose dressing composed of zinc oxide and oil of cloves on cotton wool is tucked into socket. Analgesic tablets and warm saline rinses are prescribed and patient is kept on regular follow-up [20, 21].

*Osteomyelitis*: It is 'an infection of the bone and the bone marrow which can be caused by an infection in the body spreading in the blood stream from point of origin to the bone'. Appropriate antibiotics for an extended period of time is the line of treatment. In chronic cases, surgical debridement becomes mandatory [22, 23].

## 13.16 Technological Advances in Exodontia Techniques [24]

Evolution never stops, this can be prominently justified by the fact that a variety of new techniques and instruments have been introduced to revolutionize the field of oral and maxillofacial surgery. Some of the technological advancements for dental extraction are highlighted here.

### 13.16.1 Powered Periotome

It is an electric unit which contains a controller box with adjustable power settings and a periotome mounted on a handpiece that is activated by a foot control. Use of standard periotome is cumbersome as the force delivered is uncontrolled; however, this powered periotome is characterized by complete control over the force delivery and the depth to which it travels into the periodontal ligament space.

This device functions by wedging and severing mechanisms. The thin metal blade of periotome is wedged into the periodontal ligament space in a circumferential manner severing the Sharpey's fibers. Once most of the Sharpey's fibers are severed, tooth can be extracted with minimal lateral movement. Hence, it allows flapless removal of tooth maintaining the periosteal blood supply with reduced risk of fracture of buccal or lingual cortical plate and decreased postoperative pain and discomfort.

### 13.16.2 Physics Forceps (Fig. 13.32)

Golden–Misch [25, 26] based on Class I lever mechanics designed the Physics Forceps to perform exodontia atraumatically. These forceps have a bumper which acts as a fulcrum, is placed at the mucogingival junction on the facial aspect applying steady, unrelenting pressure. Other than the bumper, there is a lingual beak, which is positioned on lingual or palatal root, making a single point contact with the tooth.

Due to the pressure applied by the bumper, periodontal ligament is traumatized resulting in the release of hyaluronidase. Once the enough chemical breakdown of periodontal ligament is achieved by the hyaluronidase, the tooth is released from its attachment to the alveolus aiding in easy removal. Physics forceps releases more hyaluronidase than conventional forceps in a shorter period of time, resulting in more efficient extraction of tooth with minimal trauma to the alveolar bone.

### 13.16.3 Use of Implant Drills for Extraction Prior to Implant Placement

Yalcin and colleagues [27] suggested a novel and minimally invasive technique to perform exodontia with minimal risk of damaging the thin buccal bone. The implant's drills were inserted into the root canals making the roots walls thin leading to extraction with application of much less force.

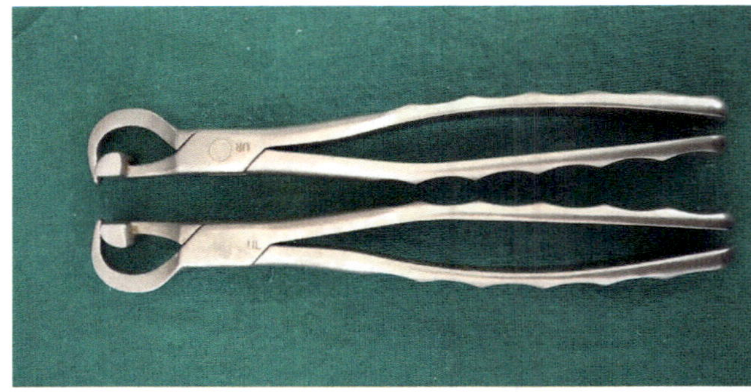



Fig. 13.32 Physics forceps

### 13.16.4 Use of LASER

Laser offers a noncontact and low vibration bone cutting without any visible, negative, and thermal side effects. Er:YAG laser can be used for surgical extractions to ablate the covering bone layer by layer exposing the portion of the root. Once the tooth/root is uncovered, they can be conventionally removed [28]. However, laser osteotomies are time consuming and require constant suctioning to achieve a dry field for effective cutting.

### 13.16.5 Piezo Surgery

Piezo surgery is very effective in bone cutting as it works selectively without injuring any soft tissue structure. Hence, it is very advantageous over the conventional burs which have potential to cause injury to soft tissue. Also, a clearer field is obtained while using piezo surgery. However, the time required while using piezo surgery is more [29].

## 13.17 CASE Scenario

### CASE 1 [18, 30]

Patient is subjected to an extraction of a tooth and during the procedure, the extracted tooth is lost leaving an empty alveolar socket. The tooth is nowhere to be seen in the oral cavity neither it could be found in the surrounding area.

Possibilities:

1. Aspiration of the tooth.
2. Ingestion of the tooth.

Clinical Features:

- *Aspiration.*

  Signs and symptom of aspiration depends on the site where the tooth is present. A laryngotracheal obstruction presents with dyspnea, cough, and stridor. It also results in difficulty in breathing with or without cyanosis. Chocking is also characterized by the sign of hands clutched to the throat, depending on whether the chocking is partial or complete. However, tooth in bronchus is associated with cough, diminished airway entry, dyspnea, and wheezing. Sometimes, the patient may remain asymptomatic for several months if the aspirated tooth is very small. However, long-term retention may result in late complications including postobstructive pneumonia, atelectasis, bronchiectasis, pneumothorax, hemorrhage, lung abscess, vocal cord paralysis, and death.

- *Ingestion.*

  Generally, the passage of ingested tooth through the gastrointestinal tract is uneventful. In cases of obstruction, the most frequently noticed symptoms are dysphagia and odynophagia. Esophageal obstruction presents with gagging, coughing, chest pain, drooling of saliva, nausea, hematemesis, regurgitation, muscular incoordination, and incessant twitching. Abdominal pain is one of the symptoms other than fever, nausea, vomiting, and abdominal distensions in cases of abdominal impactions.

Management:

- Patient must be kept in a Reverse Trendelenburg position.
- If the patient has visible Airway Obstruction, he must be asked to cough and Heimlich maneuver must be attempted to relieve obstruction.
- If the object is dislodged, it should be identified and confirmed. If not, then cricothyroidectomy must be done to secure airway. If not possible in the clinic, then the patient must be rushed to the emergency unit for securing airway.
- In cases with no airway obstruction, the entire oral cavity must be examined. If the object is found, it should be identified and confirmed.
- If the object is not found in the oral cavity, the patient must be subjected to Chest radiography and Ultrasonography Abdomen.
- For radiolucent objects, bronchoscopy and Computed Tomography of Chest and Abdomen are preferred.
- If the object is in respiratory tract, bronchoscopy must be planned for retrieval.
- If the object is in Esophagus, Endoscopic removal must be done.
- If the object is in Gastrointestinal tract (GIT), beyond esophagus, patient must be monitored for 2 weeks with serial radiographs. Stool examination must be done till the object is expelled.
- If the object is retrieved, identify and confirm.
- If the object is not retrieved, radiographic examination must be repeated.
- Radiographic examination reveals the absence of object in GIT, it should be assumed that the object has passed out. The patient must be reassured, however, must be kept on follow-up.
- If the radiographic examination reveals the presence of object in GIT, the patient must be referred to a gastroenterologist for removal either by surgery or by endoscopy.
- During the whole process, the patient must be reassured time and again.

## CASE 2 [31]

A 33 year-old male reported with a chief complaint of a firm, diffuse swelling of size approximately 2 × 1 cm in left mandibular body region with occasional pus discharge from the extraoral skin fistula (Fig. 13.33a). He also complained of associated intermittent pain and fever.

### History

On further questioning, he revealed that he had visited a private clinic 6 months back for the complaint of dental caries. Following clinical and radiographic examination, the dentist had planned to extract the tooth. To the patient's knowledge, the extraction was done uneventfully, but one root was lost during the procedure. Patient was prescribed with antibiotics and analgesics for a period of 5 days. The patient became apprehensive and uneasy in the following days. The fear of further complications kept him from visiting the dentist again and the condition went on worsening. Finally, after 6 months, he reported to an oral and maxillofacial surgeon.

### Investigations

An orthopantomogram was taken which revealed a displaced root fragment in left first molar region. (Fig. 13.33b).

### Diagnosis

Displacement of Mandibular molar root in buccal space.

### Management

After obtaining patient's consent, under antibiotic coverage and local anesthesia, surgical exploration was done through the existing skin fistula extraorally. With the digital pressure, the root piece was delivered out (Fig. 13.33c). Curettage and debridement was done carefully and patient was kept on follow-up. Closure was not performed. Antibiotics, analgesic, and nonsteroidal anti-inflammatory drugs were prescribed postoperatively. Patient recovered without further incident. In the late period of follow-up, no complication was observed except extraoral scarring.

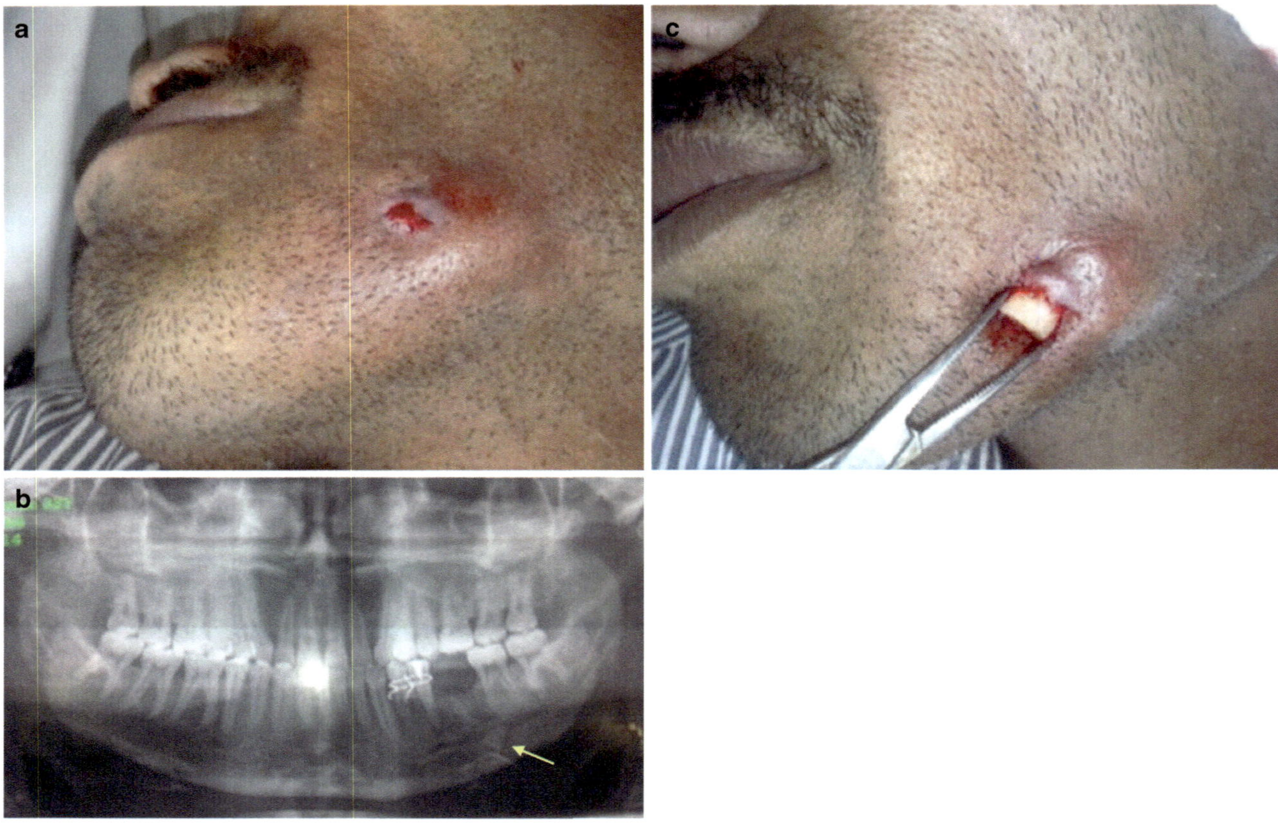

**Fig. 13.33** (**a**) Patient with extraoral swelling and skin fistula. (**b**) Orthopantomogram showing displacement of left first mandibular molar root into adjacent space. (**c**) Retrieval of root from buccal space

## References


1. Howe GL. The extraction of teeth. 2nd ed. Bristol: J Wright; 1974.
2. Bennion E. Antique dental instruments. London: Sotheby's Philip Wilson Publishers; 1986.
3. Kumar A. Dentistry in historical perspective. IJOCR. 2013;1(2): 51–4.
4. Ring ME. Dentistry: An illustrated history. New York/St Louis, Toronto: Harry N Abrams/The CV Mosby Company; 1992.
5. Atkinson HF. Some early dental extraction instruments including the pelican, bird or axe? Aust Dent J. 2002;47(2):90–3.
6. Borle RM. Textbook of oral and maxillofacial surgery. 1st ed. New Delhi: Jaypee Brothers Medical Publishers; 2014.
7. Teja MV, Teja TS, Shetty S, Kashyap R. The rise of Indian orthodontics: a historical perspective. J Ind Orthod Soc. 2013;47(3):113–20.
8. Koga DH, Salvajoli JV, Alves FA. Dental extractions and radiotherapy in head and neck oncology: review of the literature. Oral Dis. 2008 Jan;14(1):40–4.
9. Johri A, Piecuch JF. Should teeth be extracted immediately in the presence of acute infection? Oral Maxillofac Surg Clin North Am. 2011 Nov;23(4):507–11.
10. Hupp J, Ellis E III, Tucker M. Contemporary oral and maxillofacial surgery. 6th ed. London: Elsevier, RELX; 2017.
11. Moore UJ. Principles of oral and maxillofacial surgery. 6th ed. Hoboken: Blackwell Science; 2011.
12. Eshghpour M, Rezaei NM, Nejat A. Effect of menstrual cycle on frequency of alveolar osteitis in women undergoing surgical removal of mandibular third molar: a single-blind randomized clinical trial. J Oral Maxillofac Surg. 2013 Sep;71(9):1484–9.
13. Beard RW, Roberts GM. Supine hypotension syndrome. Br Med J. 1970 May 2;2(5704):297.
14. Steinberg BJ, Hilton IV, Iida H, Samelson R. Oral health and dental care during pregnancy. Dent Clin N Am. 2013 Apr;57(2):195–210.
15. Farina R, Trombelli L. Wound healing of extraction sockets. Endod Top. 2012;25:16–43.
16. Fickling BW. Oral surgery involving the maxillary sinus. Ann R Coll Surg Engl. 1957 Jan;20(1):13–35.
17. Huang IY, Wu CW, Worthington P. The displaced lower third molar: a literature review and suggestions for management. J Oral Maxillofac Surg. 2007 Jun;65(6):1186–90.
18. Elgazzar RF, Abdelhady AI, Sadakah AA. Aspiration of an impacted lower third molar during its surgical removal under local anaesthesia. Int J Oral Maxillofac Surg. 2007;36:362–4.
19. Dym H, Wolf JC. Oroantral communication. Oral Maxillofac Surg Clin North Am. 2012 May;24(2):239–47.
20. Tarakji B, Saleh LA, Umair A, Azzeghaiby SN, Hanouneh S. Systemic review of dry socket: aetiology, treatment, and prevention. J Clin Diagn Res. 2015 Apr;9(4):ZE10–3.
21. Houston JP, McCollum J, Pietz D, Schneck D. Alveolar osteitis: a review of its etiology, prevention, and treatment modalities. Gen Dent. 2002 Sep–Oct;50(5):457–463. quiz 464–5.
22. Lorè B, Gargari M, Ventucci E, Cagioli A, Nicolai G, Calabrese L. A complication following tooth extraction: chronic suppurative osteomyelitis. Oral Implantol (Rome). 2013 Oct 15;6(2):43–7.

23. González-Navarro B, Arranz-Obispo C, Albuquerque R, Jané-Salas E, López-López J. Osteomyelitis of the jaw (with pathological fracture) following extraction of an impacted wisdom tooth. A case report. J Stomatol Oral Maxillofac Surg. 2017 Oct;118(5):306–9.
24. Weiss A, Stern A, Dym H. Technological advances in extraction techniques and outpatient oral surgery. Dent Clin N Am. 2011 Jul;55(3):501–13.
25. Golden RM, inventor; GoldenMisch Inc, assignee. Dental plier design with offset- ting jaw and pad elements for assisting in removing upper and lower teeth utilizing the dental plier design. US patent 6,910,890. June 28, 2005.
26. Misch C, Perez H. Atraumatic extractions: a biomechanical route. Dent Today. 2008;27:8.
27. Yalcin S, Aktas I, Emes Y, et al. A technique for atraumatic extraction of teeth before immediate implant placement. Implant Dent. 2009;18:6.
28. Giovannacci I, Giunta G, Pedrazzi G, Meleti M, Manfredi M, Migliario M, Brucoli M, Greco Lucchina A, Mortellaro C, Vescovi P. Erbium yttrium-aluminum-garnet laser versus traditional bur in the extraction of impacted mandibular third molars: analysis of intra- and postoperative differences. J Craniofac Surg. 2018 Nov;29(8):2282–6.
29. Badenoch-Jones EK, David M, Lincoln T. Piezoelectric compared with conventional rotary osteotomy for the prevention of postoperative sequelae and complications after surgical extraction of mandibular third molars: a systematic review and meta-analysis. Br J Oral Maxillofac Surg. 2016 Dec;54(10):1066–79.
30. Yadav RK, Yadav HK, Chandra A, Yadav S, Verma P, Shakya VK. Accidental aspiration/ingestion of foreign bodies in dentistry: a clinical and legal perspective. Natl J Maxillofac Surg. 2015;6:144–5.
31. Jain A. Accidental displacement of mandibular first molar root into buccal space: a unique case. J Stomatol Oral Maxillofac Surg. 2018;119(5):429–31.

## Articles for Additional Reading

Dym H, Weiss A. Exodontia: tips and techniques for better outcomes. Dent Clin North Am. 2012;56(1):245–66.

Araújo MG, Silva CO, Misawa M, Sukekava F. Alveolar socket healing: what can we learn? Periodontol 2000. 2015;68(1):122–34.

Nayyar J, Clarke M, O'Sullivan M, Stassen LF. Fractured root tips during dental extractions and retained root fragments. A clinical dilemma? Br Dent J. 2015;218(5):285–90.

Lodi G, Figini L, Sardella A, Carrassi A, Del Fabbro M, Furness S. Antibiotics to prevent complications following tooth extractions. Cochrane Database Syst Rev. 2012;11:CD003811.

# 14 Management of Impacted Third Molars

George Varghese

## 14.1 Introduction

Even as the scope of practicing oral and maxillofacial surgery grows and continues to evolve, the mainstay of practice remains dentoalveolar surgery. In this area, the surgical removal of impacted teeth is one of the commonest procedures that is performed. Among the teeth that are commonly impacted, the mandibular molars rank first, followed by the maxillary third molars and the maxillary canines. Less commonly, impaction of other teeth such as the mandibular canines, maxillary and mandibular premolars, and the second molars are also seen.

### 14.1.1 Terminology

The term impaction comes from the term "impactus," which is of Latin origin. Its general usage refers to the failure of an organ or structure in achieving its normal position because of an abnormal mechanical condition.

Archer [1] defined impacted tooth as a tooth that is partially or completely unerupted and is positioned against another tooth or bone or soft tissue so that its further eruption is unlikely.

Lytle [2] proposed a definition that is intimately related to that of Archer. An impacted tooth is a tooth that has failed to erupt into its normal functional position beyond the time usually expected for such appearance. Eruption may have been prevented by adjacent hard or soft tissue including tooth, bone, or dense soft tissue.

Andreasen et al. [3] defined impaction as a cessation of the eruption of a tooth caused by a clinically or radiographically detectable physical impediment in the eruption path or by an ectopic position of the tooth.

- An *unerupted tooth* is the one lying within the jaws, entirely covered by soft tissue, and partially or completely covered by bone. This tooth is undergoing the eruption process and will probably erupt into occlusion based on clinical and radiographic findings.
- A *partially erupted tooth* is one that has failed to erupt fully into a normal position. The term implies that the tooth is partly visible or in communication with the oral cavity.
- An *impacted tooth* is a tooth which is prevented from completely erupting into a normal functional position. The reason may be due to lack of space, obstruction by another tooth, or an abnormal eruption path.

### 14.1.2 Incidence of Impaction

***Archer observed that the following types of teeth, in order of frequency, are most likely to be impacted:***
maxillary third molars,
mandibular third molars,
maxillary cuspids,
mandibular bicuspids,
mandibular cuspids,
maxillary bicuspids,
maxillary central incisors,
maxillary lateral incisors.

**Electronic Supplementary Material** The online version of this chapter (https://doi.org/10.1007/978-981-15-1346-6_14) contains supplementary material, which is available to authorized users.

G. Varghese (✉)
Principal, Professor and Head, Department of Oral and Maxillofacial Surgery, Pushpagiri College of Dental Sciences, Tiruvalla, Kerala, India


K. Bonanthaya et al. (eds.), *Oral and Maxillofacial Surgery for the Clinician*, https://doi.org/10.1007/978-981-15-1346-6_14

## 14.2 Management Techniques for the Impacted Tooth

Although the standard management strategy is usually considered to be surgical removal of the impacted tooth, the following methods listed below also should be considered depending upon the case:

1. Conservative method—Leaving the tooth alone with regular follow-up clinically and radiographically. For instance, a deeply asymptomatic third molar may be left as such especially in an older age group patient.
2. Operculectomy—This procedure can be considered in a mandibular third molar that has partially erupted, and has sufficient space to come into occlusion, but is prevented from doing so by thick overlying mucoperiosteum. If the tooth still fails to erupt fully, it has to be considered for removal.
3. Autogenous transplantation—Occasionally, the third molars can be considered for autogenous transplantation, usually to a first molar socket site. Because of the low success rate with such procedures, it is not widely used except in special circumstances.
4. Orthodontically guided eruption—This is usually suited to impacted maxillary and mandibular canine teeth. Orthodontic guidance enables the tooth to reach a functional position within the arch. This technique can also be applied to impacted premolars and, in some instances, even impacted mandibular molars.
5. Procedures that activate eruption—When indicated, these are usually applied to developing teeth.

### 14.2.1 Controversies on Prophylactic Removal of Third Molars

The benefits of prophylactic surgical removal of impacted third molars that are disease-free is quite controversial [4–6]. There are opinions that retaining the teeth may be more cost-effective than prophylactic removal, at least in the short to medium term. Nevertheless, there may still be clinical situations that demand prophylactic surgery. Each clinical scenario needs an individualized evaluation and the consequences of all management techniques must be discussed with the patient. Thomas Dodson in [4] brought out a classification based upon the presence/absence of symptoms and the presence/absence of disease. He proposed to use this method to decide on the removal vs retention of third molars.

## 14.3 Etiology of Impaction

Generally, the third molars or the wisdom teeth are the last teeth to erupt and they erupt between 18 and 25 years of age. Since they erupt at about the time when the youth goes off into the world to become "wise," the name "wisdom teeth" was used.

A number of theories have been put forth to explain the phenomenon of impaction. The following are the most commonly accepted ones:-

1. Discrepancy between the tooth size and the arch length.
2. Differential growth pattern of the mesial and distal roots.
3. Delayed maturation of the third molar—dental development of the tooth lags behind the skeletal growth and maturation.
4. Incidence of extraction of permanent molars is decreased in the mixed dentition period, providing less room for eruption of third molars. This is very pertinent in the present day due to better awareness of the population and dental treatments are started early in childhood.
5. Inadequate development of jawbones due to consumption of more refined food which causes reduced functional stimulation for the growth of jaw bone.
6. Evolution theory.

Berger [7] listed the following local causes for impaction of teeth:

1. Irregularity in the position and pressure of an adjacent tooth.
2. The increased density of the overlying or surrounding bone.
3. Continued chronic inflammation with subsequent increase in density of the overlying mucous membrane.
4. Lack of space due to underdeveloped jaws.
5. Prolonged retention of the primary tooth.
6. Early loss of primary tooth.
7. Acquired diseases such as necrosis due to infection or abscess.

Impaction may also be found with no local predisposing conditions cited above.

According to Berger, the following are the systemic causes of impaction:

(a) Prenatal causes—Hereditary and miscegenation.
(b) Postnatal causes—Rickets, anemia, congenital syphilis, tuberculosis, endocrine dysfunction, and malnutrition.
(c) Rare conditions—Cleidocranial dysostosis, oxycephaly, progeria, achondroplasia, and cleft palate.

## 14.4 Indications for Removal

Despite the fact not all unerupted/impacted teeth cause problems, all have that potential. Based on extensive clinical studies, indications for removal have been identified.

1. *Pericoronitis and Pericoronal abscess* (Fig. 14.1a, b, c)—This is the most common cause for extraction of mandibular third molars (25–30%). Pericoronitis is frequently found to be associated with distoangular and

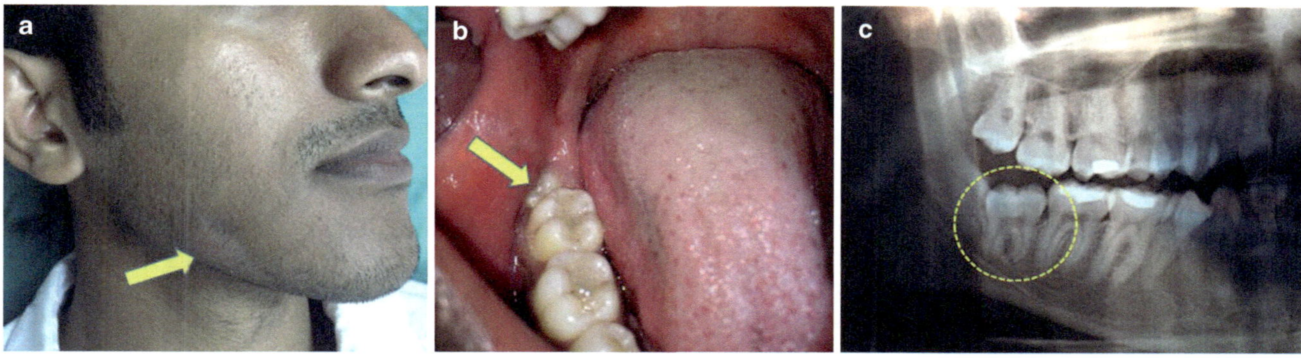




**Fig. 14.1** (**a**, **b**, **c**) Impacted right mandibular third molar with pericoronitis causing extraoral abscess (**a**) Extraoral abscess (Yellow arrow), (**b**) Impacted 48 with pericoronitis (yellow arrow), (**c**) OPG showing impacted 48 (Yellow circle)

vertical impaction. If treated inadequately, the infection may extent posteriorly resulting in submasseteric abscess.

2. *Dental Caries*—Incidence of caries of the second molar or third molar is about 15%. The reason for this high incidence is attributed to difficulty to perform oral hygiene measures in the third molar area (Fig. 14.2).
3. *Periodontal diseases*—Repeated food impaction and collection of food debris between the impacted third molar and the erupted second molar can lead to periodontal disease and subsequent bone loss. This weakens the bone support for the second molar and can cause pulpo-periodontal disease in the second molar (Fig. 14.3).
4. *Orthodontic reasons*
   (a) *Crowding of incisors:* Third molars has the potential to generate force in an anterior direction, which in turn can cause mandibular incisor crowding. Hence, removal of third molars has been recommended during or after orthodontic treatment. The hypothesis that the mesial pressure from the third molars is transferred through the contact points resulting in the narrow contacts of the lower incisors is slipping. Contemporary studies have questioned this hypothesis. However, it is still believed by certain clinicians, and third molars may be removed for these reasons.
   (b) *To facilitate orthodontic treatment*—Since the recent trends in orthodontics prefer non-extraction modalities of treatment, distalization of molars has become ever more popular, particularly with regard to Class II malocclusions. In such cases, in order to expedite the distal movement of maxillary molars, the impacted or erupted maxillary third molar tooth may be extracted.

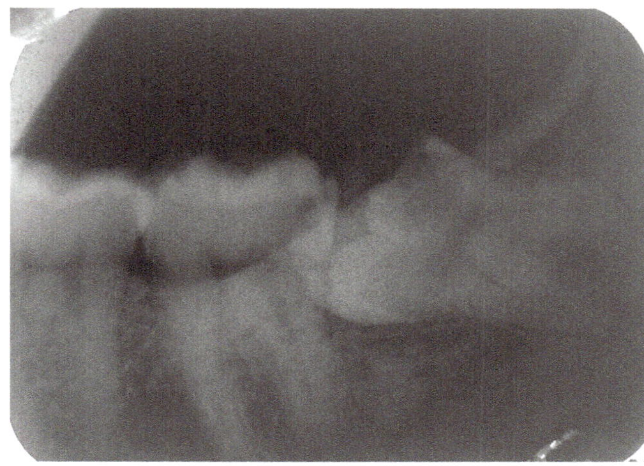



**Fig. 14.2** IOPA X-ray of Horizontally impacted tooth 38 with dental caries

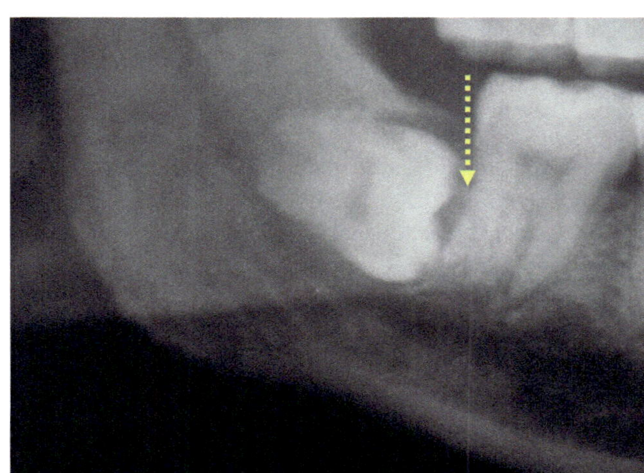



**Fig. 14.3** Horizontal impaction of 48 causing bone loss (yellow arrow) distal to 47

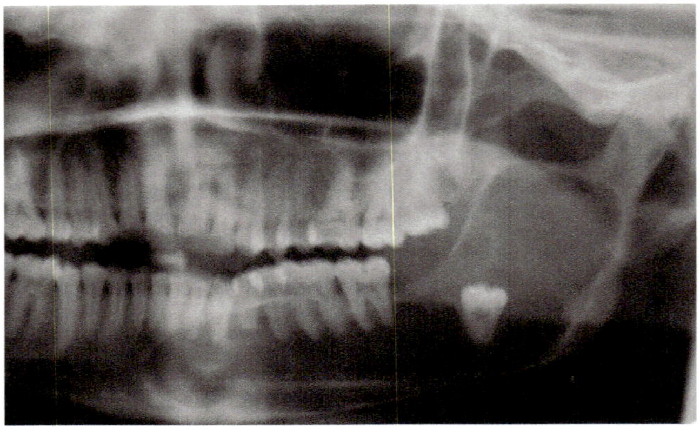



**Fig. 14.4** OPG showing impacted 38 associated with dentigerous cyst of mandible involving the left ramus, angle, and body

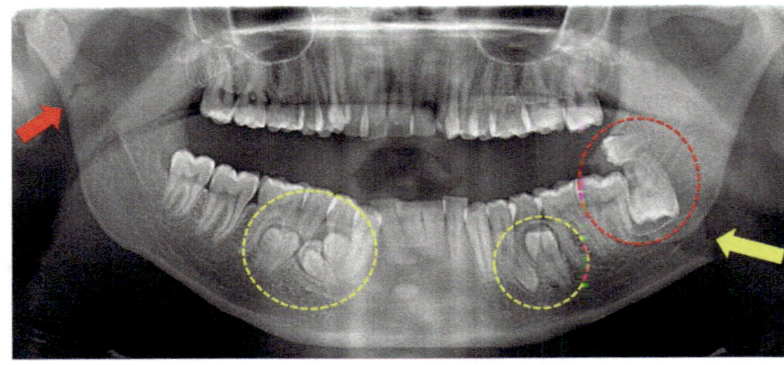



**Fig. 14.5** OPG showing impacted left mandibular third molar in inverted position associated with supernumerary (red circle) with fracture of left angle mandible (yellow arrow). Note multiple impacted supernumeraries (yellow circles) and fracture of right condyle (red arrow)

5. *To facilitate orthognathic surgery*—Removal of third molars should be considered in the presurgical preparation for orthognathic surgery. Making bone cuts in Bilateral sagittal split osteotomies (BSSO) is easier after third molars are removed. To ensure that adequate bone exists in this region, these must be extracted at least one year before the planned osteotomy.
6. *Odontogenic cysts and tumors*—Cysts and tumors may develop from the retained follicle around the impacted tooth (Fig. 14.4). To prevent this, extraction of asymptomatic third molars is recommended.
7. *Unexplained pain*—Sometimes, unexplained pain may be alleviated simply by removing impacted teeth, although the mechanism is still unclear. However, the pros and cons must be discussed with the patient.
8. *Resorption of the adjacent tooth root*—Pressure from the impacted tooth can cause the root of the second molar to resorb. When this is identified, the third molar must be removed as early as possible to avoid further damage.
9. *For placement of dental prosthesis*—The removal of impacted teeth under dental prosthesis must be assessed carefully, with the evaluation of risk versus benefits. Removal may be done for teeth that are superficial. However, sometimes the impacted tooth may lie deep within the mandible and in such cases, the tooth is better off left in situ.
10. *Prevention of jaw fracture*—For those engaged in contact games, it may be better to prophylactically remove the impacted third molars, as this area may be prone to fracture due to lowered bone resistance (Fig. 14.5).
11. *Infection of deep fascial spaces—When* pericoronitis is associated with impacted tooth, infection can track into deep fascial spaces.
12. *To remove a potential infection source* (e.g. prior to administration of radiotherapy)—Teeth which are at risk of infection like partially erupted third molar tooth may lead to local complications like osteoradionecrosis or systemic complications like endocarditis. Removal must be considered for these cases as well as other procedures such as chemotherapy, organ transplantation, or insertion of alloplastic implants.
13. *Removal for autogenous transplantation*—Even though this was a very popular procedure in the past, it fell into disrepute due to unpredictable results. However, it is worth considering when indicated for first molar replacements.

### 14.4.1 Relative Contraindications for Removal of Impacted Tooth

1. *Compromised systemic status*—It may not be advisable to undertake surgical removal of impacted third molars in patients with uncontrolled or poorly controlled systemic disease, as they can develop complications during or after the procedure. Hence, a proper history, physical examination, and, if needed, appropriate laboratory investigations must be performed.
2. *Advanced age*—Bone sclerosis increases with advancing age. This leads to poor healing, a larger defect size, and increased difficulty of the procedure. Risk of mandibular fracture is also high in these cases.
3. *Damage to any adjacent structures*—If the inferior alveolar canal is in close contact with the impacted tooth, inadvertent damage can result in paresthesia.
4. *Questionable status of the second molar*—If the second molar is badly decayed and unrestorable, removing it may allow the third molar to come into a

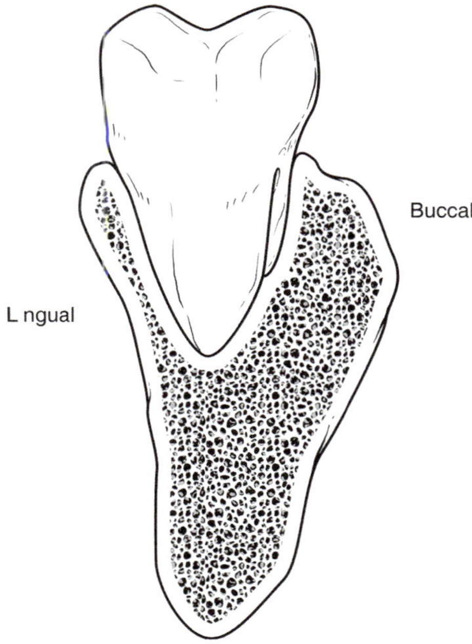


©Association of Oral and Maxillofacial Surgeons of India

**Fig. 14.6** Coronal section of mandible in the region of the third molar showing a thick buccal alveolar bone and a thin lingual plate

functional position. The third molar may also serve as a bridge abutment. Such cases require multidisciplinary evaluation with the prosthodontist and endodontist.

5. *Deeply impacted third molars* which do not appear to be associated with local or systemic pathology must not be removed.

## 14.5 Surgical Anatomy

The mandible comprises of a body which is horseshoe shaped and has the ramus on either side, which are flat and broad rami. Each ramus has two processes at the superior end—the coronoid process, which is more anterior, and condylar process, which is continuous with the posterior border.

The mandibular third molar tooth is usually present at the distal end of the mandibular body, which adjoins a thin ramus. The body-ramus junction is a weak area that can fracture if excessive force is employed during the elevation of the third molar. The tooth lies between the buccal cortical plate, which is thick, and the thin lingual cortical plate (Fig. 14.6). In most instances, the thickness of the lingual plate may be less than 1 mm, and the tooth may get displaced into the lingual pouch if untoward force is applied.

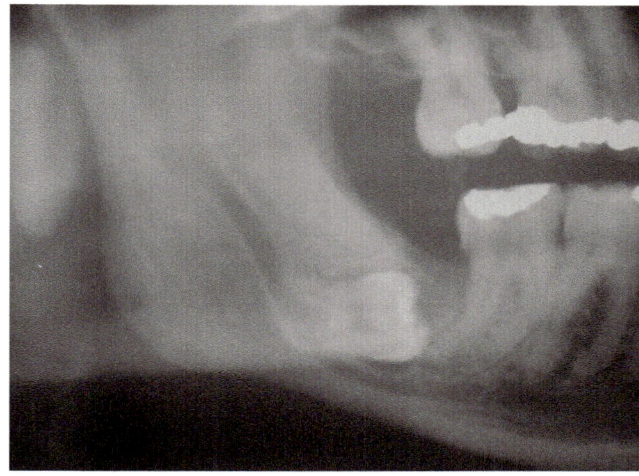

©Association of Oral and Maxillofacial Surgeons of India

**Fig. 14.7** Radiograph showing the proximity of impacted third molar roots to the mandibular canal

### 14.5.1 Neurovascular Bundle

The mandibular canal lies beside or below the third molar roots. Usually, the canal lies slightly buccal and apical to the third molar roots, but this varies frequently (Fig. 14.7). The canal contains the inferior alveolar neurovascular bundle including the artery, vein, and nerve within a sheath of fascia. The third molar roots may sometimes be indented by the canal, but actual penetration is rare. In these cases, attempting to elevate fractured root tips may result in the displacement of the tips into the mandibular canal. If the canal vessels get injured by instruments or forceful intrusion of the tooth roots, profuse hemorrhage may result.

### 14.5.2 Retromolar Triangle

This is a depressed roughened area behind the third molar bounded by the buccal and lingual alveolar ridge crests. The retromolar fossa is a shallow depression that occurs just lateral to the retromolar triangle. Mandibular vessel branches may emerge at the fossa or triangle and can be injured during surgical exposure of the third molar region if the incision is not taken laterally. This can result in brisk hemorrhage (Fig. 14.8).

### 14.5.3 Facial Artery and Vein

The facial artery and anterior facial vein are related to the mandibular body, anterior to the masseter muscle, where they cross the inferior border of the mandible. They lie below the second and third molar teeth and may be injured when a buccal incision is placed at an inferior level. To avoid this, it is best to start the incision at the sulcus depth and move upward toward the tooth.

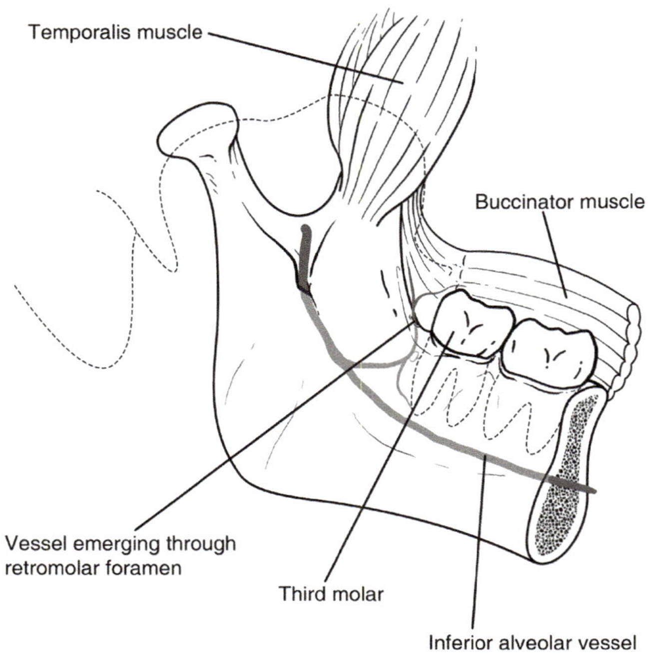




**Fig. 14.8** Schematic diagram showing the retromolar vessel emerging through retromolar foramen

### 14.5.4 Lingual Nerve

The lingual nerve often runs below and behind the third molar, and contacts the periosteum over the lingual cortex at a sublingual level. Cardinal anatomic studies have shown the close relation of the lingual nerve to the lower third molar region [8, 9].

> The lingual nerve usually lies 2.3 mm below the lingual alveolar crest, and 0.6 mm medial to the mandible, when viewed from a frontal plane.

Since the lingual nerve is close to the third molar, it is at risk of damage during surgical removal of the tooth. This may lead to anesthesia of the tongue in its anterior two-thirds, and also loss of taste sensation in this area.

The surgeon should also be aware of the course and direction of the mylohyoid and long buccal nerve to prevent inadvertent injuries to these nerves (Fig. 14.9).

### 14.5.5 Bone Trajectories of Mandible

The bone trajectories of the mandible, referred to as grains, course in a longitudinal direction. Even though the technique of chisel and mallet has almost become obsolete, it is important to know the bone trajectories. On the buccal side, a horizontal chisel cut that is oriented parallel to the superior border may cause extensive splitting till the first molar region due to the grain direction. To prevent this, the operator must make a “vertical stop cut” (Fig. 14.10), with the bevel ori-

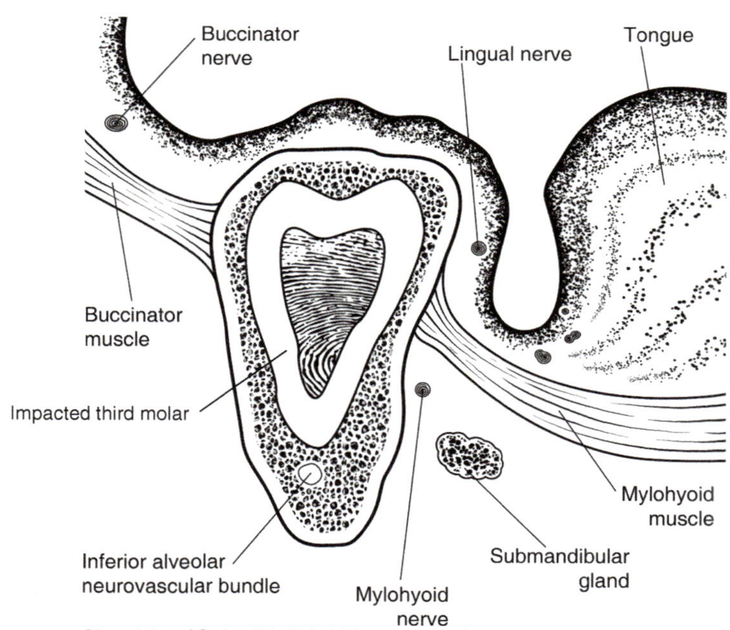




**Fig. 14.9** Schematic diagram showing coronal section through the third molar region and the relationship of important anatomical structures

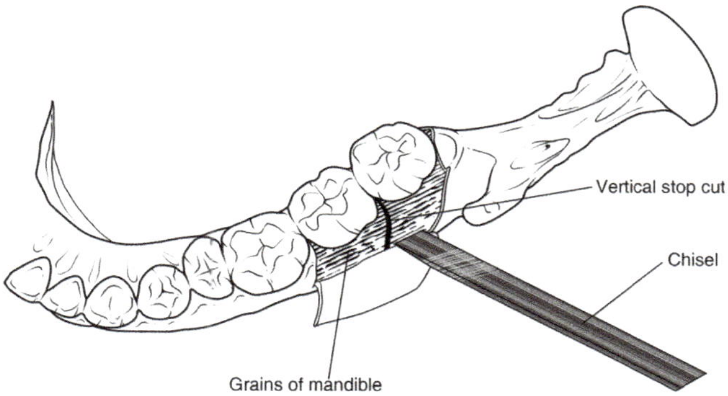




**Fig. 14.10** Bone trajectories of the mandible

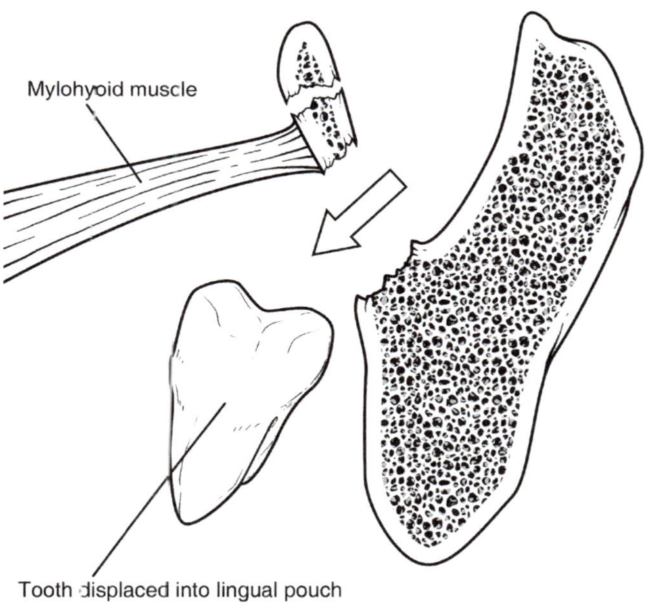




**Fig. 14.11** Whole tooth displaced into lingual pouch beneath the mylohyoid muscle

ented posteriorly, just distal to the second molar. The chisel must be angulated correctly at all times to avoid fracture of mandible distal to the third molar.

### 14.5.6 Lingual Plate

Since the lingual pate is very thin, it may be perforated by the apices of lower third molar roots. If the roots are fractured, attempting to elevate may cause them to be displaced into the "lingual pouch," from where it will be difficult to retrieve. The entire tooth also may rarely be pushed into the lingual pouch (Fig. 14.11).

## 14.6 Classification of Impacted Mandibular Third Molar

To assess surgical difficulty, several classifications have been proposed, which can help formulate a treatment plan that is efficient and has minimum morbidity. Either the periapical radiograph or the Orthopantomogram is used to analyze the impacted tooth for its classification.

The most commonly used are:-

1. *Angulation* [10] of the impacted tooth (Fig. 14.12) (George Winter classification).
   Vertical,
   Mesioangular,
   Horizontal,
   Distoangular,
   Buccoangular,
   Linguoangular,
   Inverted,
   Unusual
2. *Relationship* between the impacted tooth and the *anterior ramal border* [11]—This assesses the amount of space present between the anterior border of the ramus and the distal wall of the second molar. This indicates the effective space available for the tooth to erupt (Fig. 14.13).
   *Class I*—There is enough mesiodistal space between the anterior border of ramus and second molar to accommodate the third molar.
   *Class II*—Space between anterior border of the ramus and second molar is less than the mesiodistal width of the crown of the third molar.
   *Class III*—No mesiodistal space available and the third molar is almost completely within the ramus.
   Class III impactions present greater difficulty in removal.
3. *Depth of the impacted tooth* and tissue type that overlies the tooth (Pell and Gregory Classification based on occlusal level of the tooth)—i.e. soft tissue, partial bony, or complete bony impaction (Fig. 14.14).
   *Position A*—The highest point of the tooth is at the same level of the occlusal plane or above it.
   *Position B*—The highest point of the tooth is above the cervical line of the second molar but below the occlusal plane.
   *Position C*—The highest point of the tooth is well below the cervical line of the second molar (Figs. 14.15 and 14.16).
4. *Type of tissue that lies over the tooth*—i.e. soft tissue, partial bony, or complete bony impaction.
5. *Level of Eruption*
   (a) Erupted.
   (b) Partially erupted.
   (c) Unerupted.

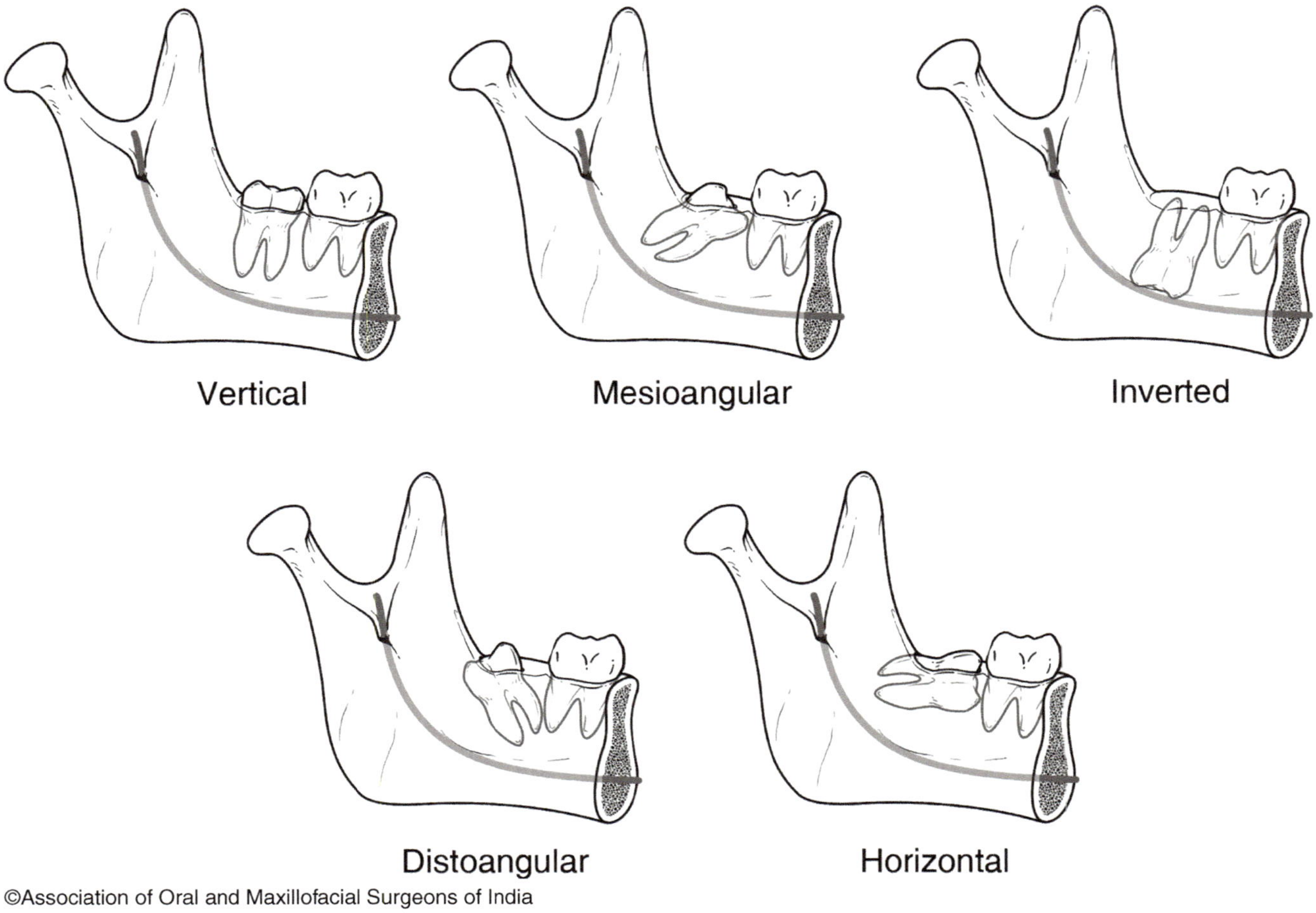


**Fig. 14.12** Classification based on angulation of tooth (Winter's classification)

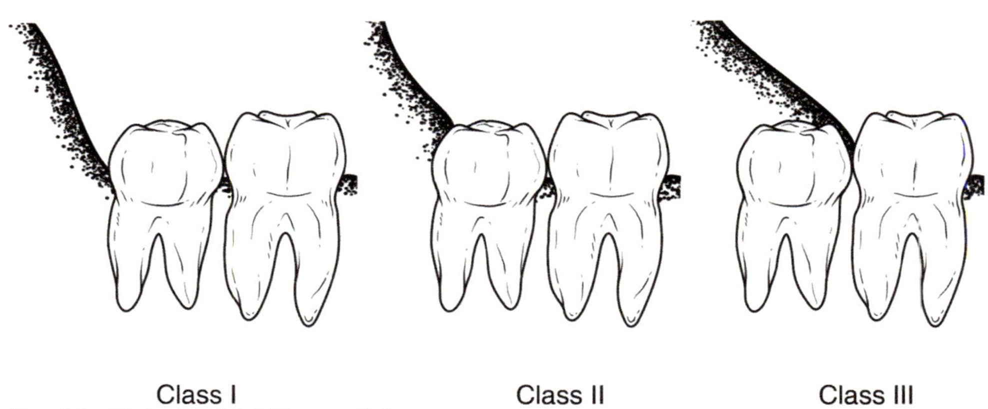


**Fig. 14.13** Pell and Gregory Classification based on relationship to the anterior border of ramus

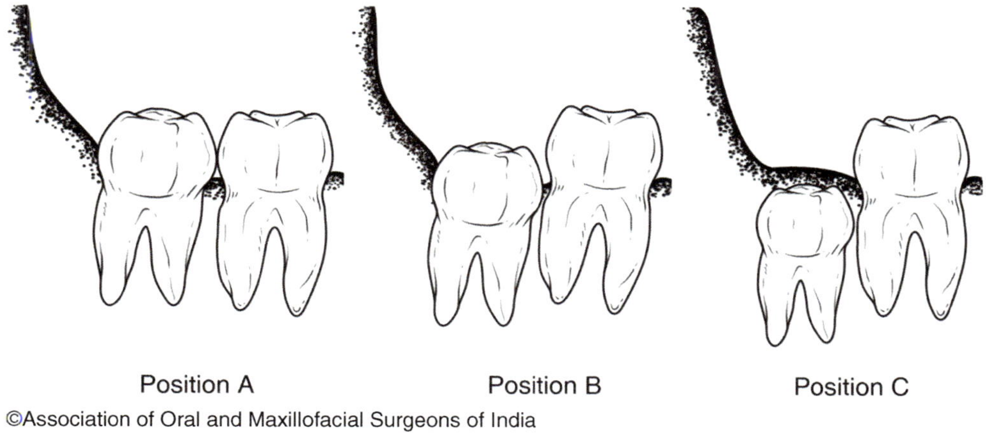


**Fig. 14.14** Pell and Gregory Classification based on relationship to the occlusal plane of the impacted tooth to that of the second molar

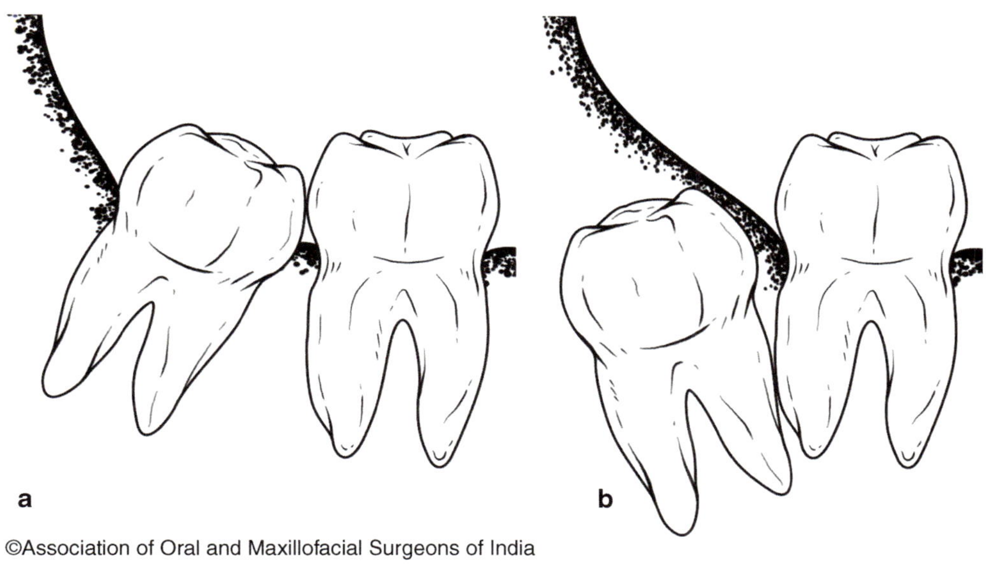


**Fig. 14.15** Examples of impaction showing combination of angulation of tooth. relationship to anterior border of ramus and depth of impaction. (**a**) Mesioangular impaction in Class I ramus relation and Position A depth—an impacted tooth easy for removal. (**b**) Distoangular impaction in Class III ramus relation and Position B depth—an impacted tooth difficult for removal

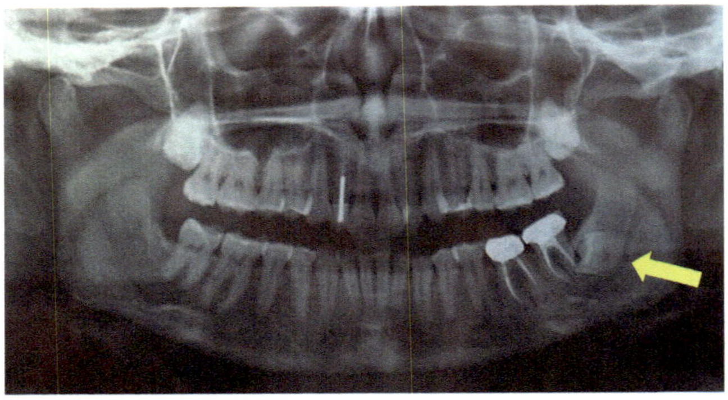

©Association of Oral and Maxillofacial Surgeons of India

**Fig. 14.16** OPG showing impacted mandibular third molar displaying only crown of the tooth with no roots visible (yellow arrow) with close proximity to inferior alveolar canal in a 52-year-old male. Surgical removal of 38 was attempted without taking CT or CBCT. During surgery, there was accidental fracture of left angle for which internal fixation has to be done. Note impacted 18 and 28

## 14.7 Preoperative Planning

Presence of an impacted third molar must be diagnosed systematically using the patient's chief complaint and history, clinical examination, and appropriate investigations.

The impacted third molar must be evaluated both clinically and radiographically prior to surgery for successful and speedy removal. Ideally, a periapical radiograph must be taken and an OPG must be added if the intraoral radiograph does not provide enough information about the tooth or adjacent structures.

Manuel et al. has [12] developed a simple format for evaluation of third molar impactions.

This comprehensive format is ideal for residents in oral surgery during their learning years. Using this format, third molar impactions may be analyzed, and difficulty level may be assessed and anticipated. Residents can judge problems that they may encounter during the procedure and can evaluate the patient better postoperatively.

### 14.7.1 Clinical Examination

This includes taking the patient's history, clinical examination extraorally and intraorally.

1. *History taking*
   *Complaints of the patient*—Impacted teeth are usually asymptomatic and patients are aware of their existence only when told by the dental practitioner. Symptoms, if any, are usually due to acute or chronic pericoronitis, or due to acute pulpitis secondary to dental caries.
2. *Extraoral examination*
   The clinician must examine the face and neck for redness and swelling related to infection. The lower lip is tested for anesthesia or paresthesia. The regional lymph nodes must be assessed by palpation for any tenderness or enlargement.
3. *Intraoral examination*—The following points are noted:
   (a) Mouth opening—The ability of the patient to open the mouth is analyzed, and any trismus, fibrosis, or hypermobility of the joint is noted. The size of the mouth (microsomia/macrosomia) is also checked. Third molar access may be restricted if the mandible is retrognathic, while a prognathic mandible offers good access.
   (b) General examination of oral cavity- oral mucosa, teeth, and oral hygiene.
   (c) Examination of the third molar area for signs of pericoronitis and state of eruption of the tooth.
   (d) Condition of the impacted tooth- presence of caries, dental fillings, and internal resorption (which may resemble caries). The angle of the tooth and locking beneath second molar must be noted and confirmed with appropriate radiographs.
   (e) Condition of first and second molars—presence of caries, fillings, or crowns; root canal treatment may put the second molar at risk of fracture and the patient must be warned of this. Distal periodontal pocketing, root resorption, and absence of the second molar must also be noted.
   (f) Space present between the second molar distal surface and the ascending ramus: A small distance makes access difficult, and a large distance makes the tooth more accessible. For maxillary teeth, the distance between the second molar and tuberosity must be considered. Access can also be decreased by distal tilting of second molar.
   (g) Adjacent bone may develop infection, which can spread along the mesial surface of the tooth and affect the second molar, which would then require extraction. Infection/osteomyelitis can spread to the ramus in the case of distoangular impacted third molars, through recurrent submasseteric abscesses in this region.
   (h) Systemic skeletal diseases may cause pathological complications which should be noted. For instance, conditions such as osteogenesis imperfecta and osteosclerosis may cause fractures during the procedure. In acromegaly, the mandibular bone is massive which makes the procedure difficult because the mandible consists of massive bone. In Paget's disease also tooth removal is difficult as the bone is affected by resorption and repair.

(i) Presence of cysts and tumors—The impacted tooth may be associated with eruption cysts or large odontogenic cysts can occur in relation to impacted tooth. By and large, they cause displacement of the tooth. Benign and malignant tumors such as ameloblastoma may also be found involving the tooth. Odontomes may also be present in relation to the third molar.

### 14.7.2 Radiography of Impacted Mandibular Third Molar

Any factor that increases the difficulty of third molar removal can be analyzed from the preoperative radiograph.

The following radiographs may be used for analysis:

1. Intraoral periapical radiograph.
2. Occlusal X-ray of mandible.
3. Lateral oblique view of mandible.
4. Panoramic radiograph (Orthopantomogram).

An essential criterion for a good film is that the buccal and lingual cusps of the second molar must be superimposed on each other in the same vertical and horizontal plane. This appearance of the second molar is referred to as 'enamel cap'.

1. *Periapical radiograph:* The radiograph should include the entire third molar tooth along with the investing bone. It should also show the anterior border of ramus, the second molar, and the inferior alveolar canal.
2. *Lateral oblique view of the mandible:* This radiograph is inevitably distorted because the opposite side of the mandible is rotated away from the beam during film exposure. Therefore, it is inferior to the periapical X-ray, but it has its use in certain clinical situations:
   - When periapical X-ray cannot be taken due to trismus or retching.
   - To provide supplementary information like height of mandible in the region of the third molar, or bone height beneath a deeply buried tooth. The latter is useful to assess the risk of pathological fracture in thin mandible, or in cases of cysts or tumors.

   Since the introduction of OPG, the use of lateral oblique view is limited and is only considered when an OPG is unavailable.
3. *Orthopantomogram (OPG):* This provides the same information as the lateral oblique view, with less distortion. The OPG is now used routinely to precisely the locate impacted teeth.

#### 14.7.2.1 Interpretation of Periapical X-ray

(a) Access. By observing the inclination of the radio-

The following points must be noted in the periapical radiograph:-

(a) Access.
(b) Depth and position of the tooth.
(c) Root pattern of impacted tooth.
(d) Shape of crown.
(e) Texture of investing bone.
(f) Relation to inferior alveolar canal.
(g) Root pattern and position of second molar.

is drawn distally over the third molar region. This line indicates the axial inclination of the impacted tooth. For example, the white line is parallel to the occlusal surface of the third molar if the tooth is vertically impacted, whereas, the "white" line converges with the occlusal surface in front of the tooth in distoangular impactions.

The "white" line also indicates the depth of the tooth as compared to the erupted second molar.

The second "amber" line extends from the bone surface distal to the third molar and is drawn to the interdental septum crest between the first and second molar. When drawing this line, it must be clearly differentiated from the external oblique ridge shadow, which can lie above and in front of the posterior end of the "amber" line. The posterior end is the shadow cast by the bone in the retromolar fossa and not the external oblique ridge. The "amber" line shows the margin of the alveolar bone enclosing the tooth. Hence, when soft tissues are reflected, the portion of the visible tooth will be the part that was lying above and in front of the "amber" line in the radiograph. The rest of the tooth will be covered by bone.

The third line or "red" line assesses how deep the impacted tooth is within the mandible. This is drawn by dropping a perpendicular from the "amber" line to the point at which the elevator will be applied to elevate the tooth (an imaginary point). This point usually lies on the mesial surface of the impacted tooth, at the cementoenamel junction, except in the case of distoangular impactions. The longer the red line, the more deep the tooth is impacted, and the surgical procedure will be more difficult.

(c) *Root pattern of impacted tooth*—The number, shape, and curvature of roots are noted. Hypercementosis is noted if present. If the root apex takes a sharp bend toward the X-ray beam, it may appear blunt and short on the image. This finding should therefore be investigated in more detail.

The type of root morphology dictates the difficulty of the surgical procedure. If root development is limited, it

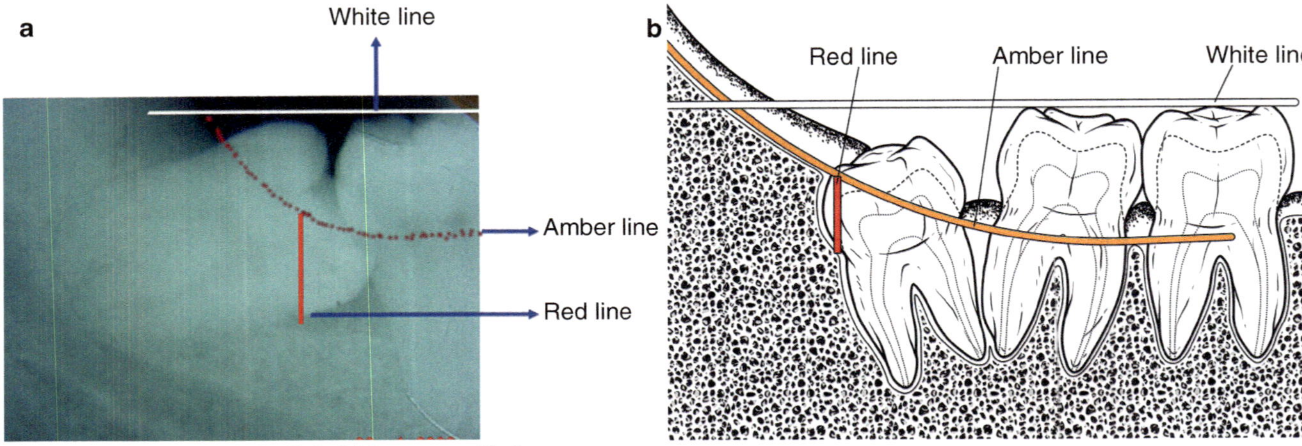




**Fig. 14.17** (**a**) White, amber, and red lines (Winter's WAR lines) marked in the periapical X-ray. (**b**) WAR lines drawn on a distoangularly impacted mandibular third molar. Note that in distoangular impactions, the perpendicular "red" line should be dropped to the cementoenamel junction on the distal side of the impacted tooth and not on the mesial side as in other angulations

can result in a "rolling" tooth, which is challenging to remove.

(d) *Shape of crown*—If the tooth has prominent cusps, or large, square crowns, the difficulty increases as compared to small crowns and flat cusps. The size and shape of the crown of third molar is particularly important with regard to the "line of withdrawal." Sometimes, the path of crown removal can be obstructed by the second molar crown (Fig. 14.18).

In these cases, the cusp of the third molar appears to be superimposed on the distal surface of the second molar in the radiograph. If elevation is attempted by applying force on the mesial surface of the impacted tooth, the second molar may get displaced from the socket, and there is a risk of mandible fracture. The risk is especially high for second molars with conical roots. In such cases, sectioning the third molar is advisable.

(e) *Texture of the investing bone*—As age advances, the bone undergoes sclerosis and becomes less elastic. The bone texture can be analyzed by visualizing the size of the cancellous spaces and the bone density. Bone that has large spaces and fine structure is generally elastic. On the contrary, sclerotic bone has small spaces and dense bone structure. Dense bone does not expand easily during luxation and more bone removal may be required.

(f) *Inferior alveolar canal*—Although radiographs often show the canal crossing the third molar roots, this is usually due to superimposition. Sometimes, however, this may indicate grooving or perforation of the root.. The classical papers by Howe and Poynton [13] and Rood and Shehab [14] have given predictable signs to assess the relationship between the nerve and the third molar roots.

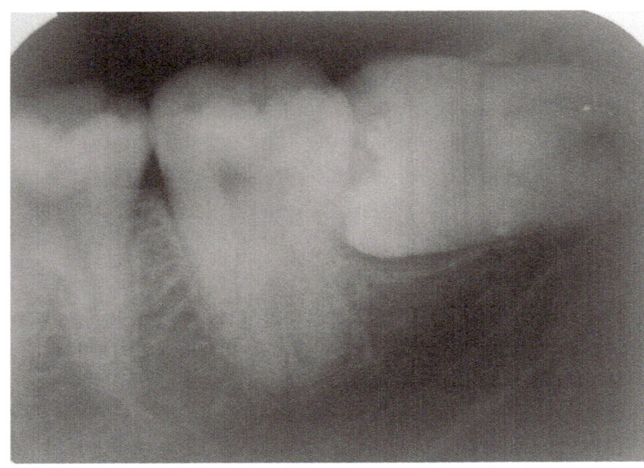



**Fig. 14.18** "Locking of the crown" of impacted third molar by the second molar. Note that the cusp of third molar is superimposed upon the distal surface of second molar

1. If there is a band of reduced radio-opacity that crosses the roots, and this band coincides with the outline of the inferior alveolar canal, this is a sign that the tooth root may be grooved by the canal. This sign reflects the lesser amount of tooth structure lying between the X-ray source and the film.
2. The roof and floor of the canals are formed of compact bone, which is indicated by continuous, parallel radio-opaque lines. If the lines lose continuity, it is an indication that the root is grooved by the inferior alveolar canal. These grooves usually form on the lingual side of the roots.

3. In cases where the radiolucent band crosses the apex of the root and if only the upper white line is broken, a notching of the root is present.
4. Characteristic narrowing of the radiolucent band with loss of white lines is suggestive of perforation of the root by the inferior alveolar canal.

   The following signs have been demonstrated to be associated with a significantly increased risk of nerve injury during third molar surgery: (Fig. 14.19a, b, c)

   - Diversion of the inferior alveolar canal (IAC).
   - Darkening of the root where crossed by the canal.
   - Interruption of the white lines of the canal.

In the presence of any of the above findings, great care should be taken in surgical exploration and the decision to treat is carefully reviewed. If on the initial panoramic radiograph there is an evidence of a close relationship between the roots of the lower third molar and the IAC, a second radiograph should be taken using different projection geometry.

If the third molar is found to be in close relationship with the inferior alveolar canal, the patient should be informed in advance regarding the likelihood of impairment of labial sensation following the surgical removal of the tooth. This should be recorded in the case record and in the consent form. In such cases, authors have recommended coronectomy (partial tooth removal, intentional root retention, partial odontectomy) as an option. However, this technique cannot be considered foolproof and long-term studies are required to know the success of coronectomies [15, 16]

(g) *Position, root pattern, and nature of crown of second molar.*

The space between the distal surface of the second molar and the mesial surface of the impacted third molar has an effect on the ease of removal of the third molar. The closer the third molar is to the second molar, the more challenging the surgery becomes. If the long axis of the second molar is tilted distally, it is more difficult to remove.

*Cone beam computed tomography* (CBCT) (Fig. 14.20a, b, c) CBCT is now available for dental use and offers low dose imaging in multiple planes.

Using this modality, accurate three-dimensional imaging can be done to determine the relationship between the roots of the third molar and the inferior alveolar nerve (IAN). The recent recommendation is that when the OPG suggests a close relationship between the roots of the lower third molar and IAN, cone beam CT scanning should be advised [17–19]. The effective dose from CBCT is comparatively less than the conventional CT scan and also at a lower expense.

### 14.7.3 Lingual Nerve Protection and Injury

Locating the lingual nerve clinically and by imaging is more challenging. Lingual nerve injury although less common than inferior alveolar nerve (IAN) injury is often more unbearable to the patient. Patients find it difficult to tolerate lingual nerve damage, including loss of taste and sensation of tongue, as compared to IAN damage. Unlike the IAN, the lingual nerve is not usually imaged prior to third molar surgery. In cases where

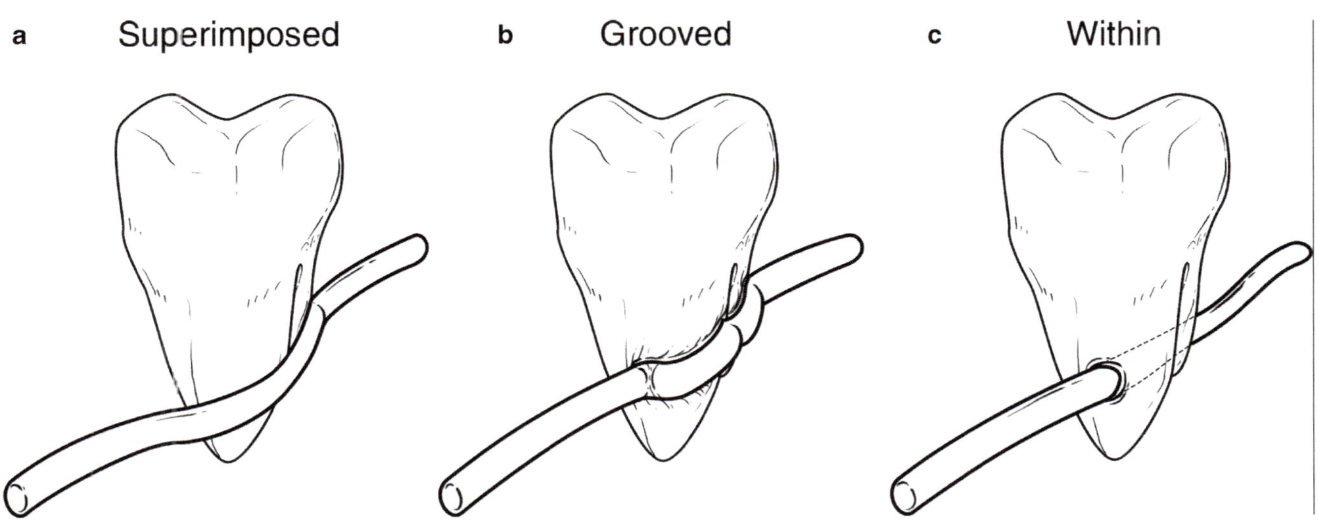




**Fig. 14.19** (**a–c**) Radiographic relationship of third molar root to inferior alveolar nerve (**a**) Cortical outline of the canal is intact. This probably represents superimposition only. (**b**) There is loss of cortical outline of the nerve canal. The nerve may be grooving the tooth. (**c**) There is loss of cortical outline as well as narrowing and deviation of the nerve canal, denoting an intimate relationship of the nerve with the tooth and possibly perforation of the tooth roots by the nerve

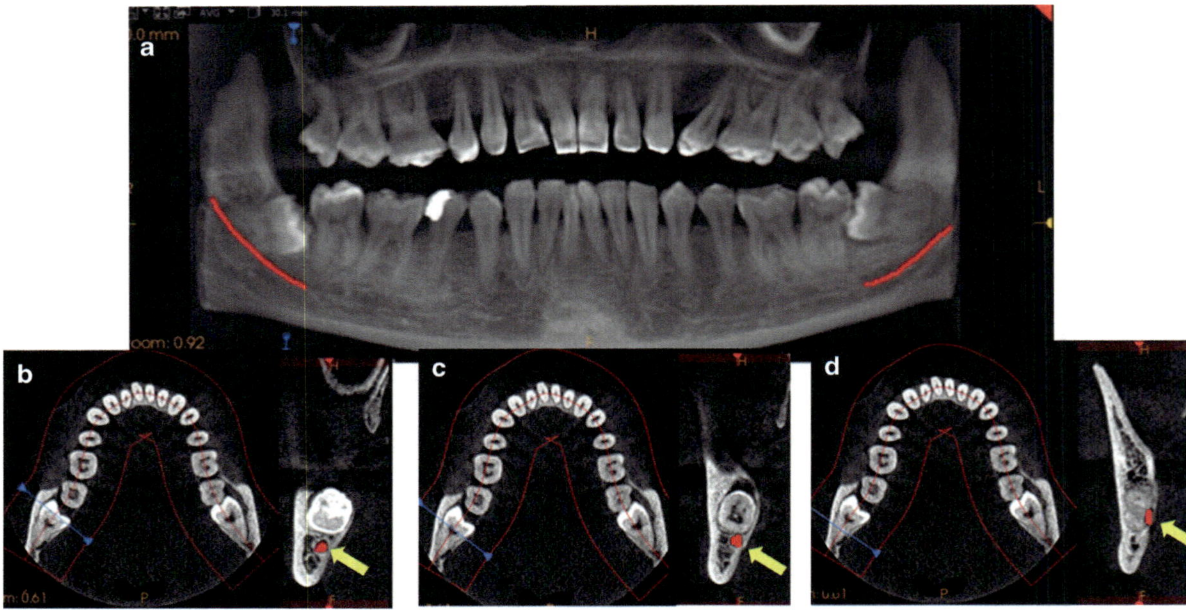




**Fig. 14.20** (**a**) CBCT Panoramic view showing the relationship of 38 and 48 to the inferior alveolar canal (IAC) [red line]. The changing relationship of the IAC to 48 can be noted in (**b–d**). Relationship of IAC (yellow arrow) at coronal level (**b**), at cervical level (**c**), and at apical one third level (**d**)

distal, distolingual, and lingual bone is to be removed, technique of raising the lingual flap and protecting the lingual nerve by a broad smooth lingual flap retractor in a subperiosteal plane has been advocated by certain authors and this technique is followed in certain parts of the world. Again, there are conflicting reports where the lingual flap retraction itself has caused an increase incidence of lingual nerve paresthesia [8, 20–22].

*To summarize, the difficulty of the surgical procedure is dictated by 3 major factors:- (1) Depth of impaction (2) Type of overlying tissues, and (3) Age of the patient.*

Any standard operative plan consists of the following stages:-

1. Placement of an incision to access the region of the impacted tooth.
2. Removal of enough bone to allow for delivery.
3. Sectioning the tooth and delivering it from the socket.
4. Debridement of the surgical site.
5. Wound closure.

as bone density, flexibility of the cheek, and mouth opening.

Surgical removal of impacted teeth may be easier in younger patients because of incompletely formed roots, large follicular space, incompletely formed roots separated from inferior alveolar canal, and greater elasticity of bone. In young patients, the bone texture is usually soft and resilient, but in older adults, the bone becomes progressively more dense, hard, and brittle. Therefore, the extraction of a partially erupted/impacted tooth in an elderly adult with sclerotic bone may cause great difficulty. While a tooth with adverse root morphology in soft, resilient bone of a young adult can be elevated expeditiously.

As a general rule, the more difficult and time-consuming the surgical procedure is, the more difficult and protracted is the postoperative recovery period.

## 14.8 Operative Procedure

Surgical removal impacted third molar becomes difficult with the following factors:-

1. Unfavorable root morphology- Excessive curvature, divergent roots, hypercementosis, proximity to canal
2. Third molar crown is locked beneath the second molar.
3. Condition of the impacted tooth (Carious or with

### 14.8.1 Incision and Designing the Flap

Envelope flap, which is commonly used, extends from the posterior margin of the impacted tooth, and runs forward till the level of the first molar. The posterior end of the incision is directed buccally along the external oblique ridge (Fig. 14.21a, b).

If greater access is required, the envelope flap will not be adequate. In such cases, a release incision is given on the anterior-most point of the incision, which creates a triangular flap (Fig. 14.22a, b). This incision must begin at a point that lies approximately 6 mm below the gingival margin in the buccal sulcus and then extend upward in an oblique fashion to the gingival margin. The incision ends on the margin at a point between posterior and middle thirds of the second molar.

The envelope incision has been associated with fewer complications, and healing occurs faster as compared to the triangular flap. A small artery, the buccal artery, may sometimes be encountered while placing the releasing incision, and mild bleeding can result if this is injured. If more exposure is needed, the vertical release incision can be brought forward, and placed between the second and first molar as shown in the Fig. 14.23a, b.

The incision is then continued along the cervical line of the second molar and reaches the middle of its posterior border. The incision continues in a posterior and lateral direction, along the anterior border of the ramus, depending on the exposure required. It is essential that this arm of the incision is oriented laterally, and not in a straight line, because the mandible diverges laterally. If the incision is extended straight, the knife may cause lingual nerve damage. The lateral extension will also preserve small vessels that emerge from retromolar fossa (Fig. 14.24).

The mucoperiosteal flap is then reflected laterally with a periosteal elevator. An Austin's retractor (third molar retractor) is used to hold the flap in position. The "Minnesota retractor" may also be used to hold the flap. This retractor must be placed just lateral to the external oblique ridge. Stability is achieved by resting against the lateral surface of the mandible. While holding the retractor, fingers must rest at its distal end so that the retractor can be moved laterally without blocking the vision of the operator.

The literature shows various flap designs with modifications for lower third molar impactions with each claiming its own merits [27, 28]. However, for the majority of the cases, the conventional flap designs will serve the purpose.

### 14.8.2 Bone Removal

After flap reflection, the next step is bone removal from around the impacted tooth. The amount of bone to be removed will depend on the depth of impaction. This can be done either by use of bur/rotary instruments or by chisel and mallet or ultrasonic devices/peizo surgery [29, 30] or laser devices [31]. The method used may depend on individual preference. Sufficient amount of bone must be removed, both to free the tooth from obstruction and to provide a point of application for the elevator.

The buccal cortex plays an important role in maintaining the strength of the mandible. Hence, the removal of buccal bone should be minimized, in order to prevent weakening and fracture of the mandible. The bone buccal to and distal to the impacted tooth must be removed until the cervical line of the tooth. Beyond this, bone removal must be done judiciously, in such a way that the strength of mandible is not affected, but, at the same time, the efficiency of surgery is maintained. To achieve this, a deep vertical gutter is drilled on the buccal side, and, if required on the distal side of the

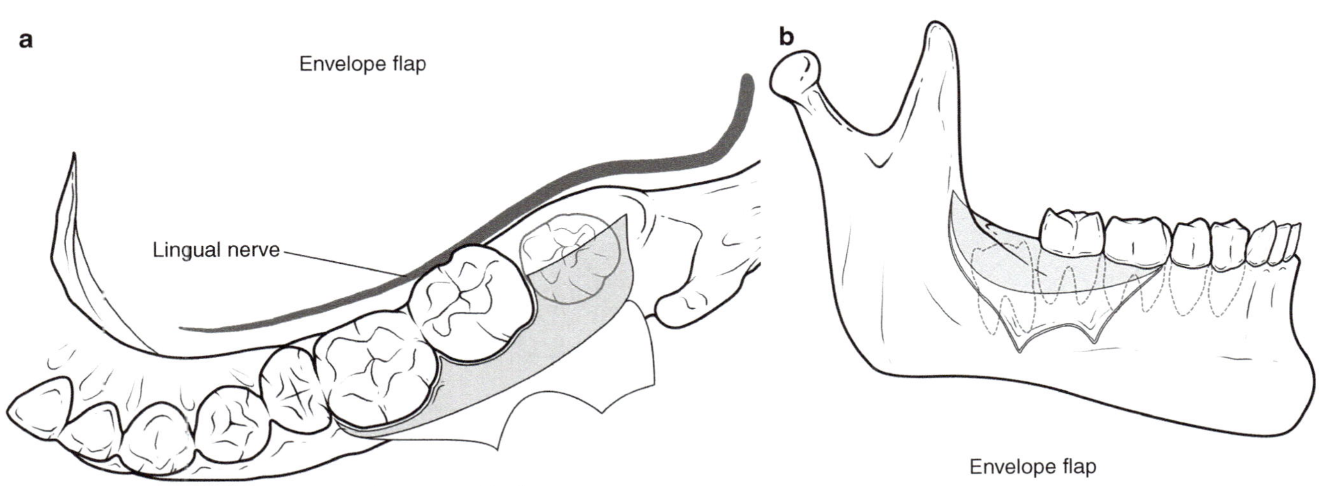




**Fig. 14.21** (**a**, **b**) Envelope flap design

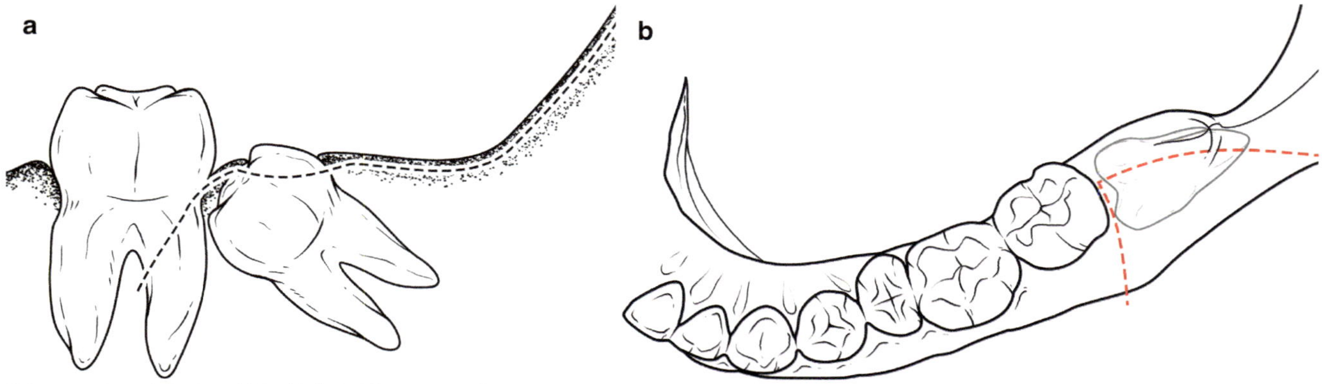




**Fig. 14.22** (**a**, **b**) Standard triangular flap with a release incision in the anterior aspect

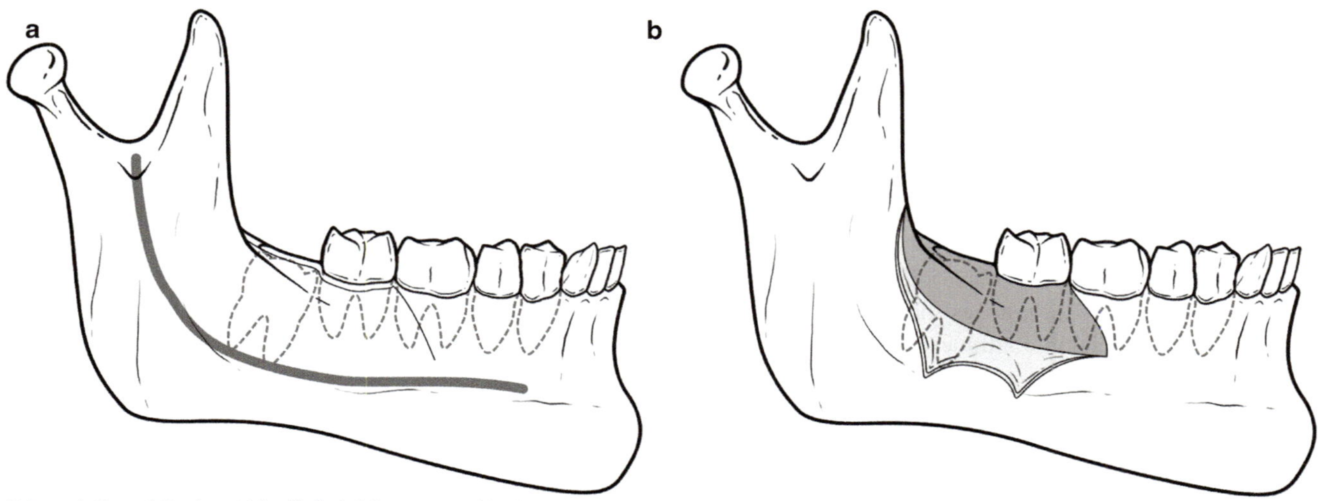




**Fig. 14.23** (**a**, **b**) Where more exposure is needed, the vertical release of the triangular flap is placed between the second and first molar

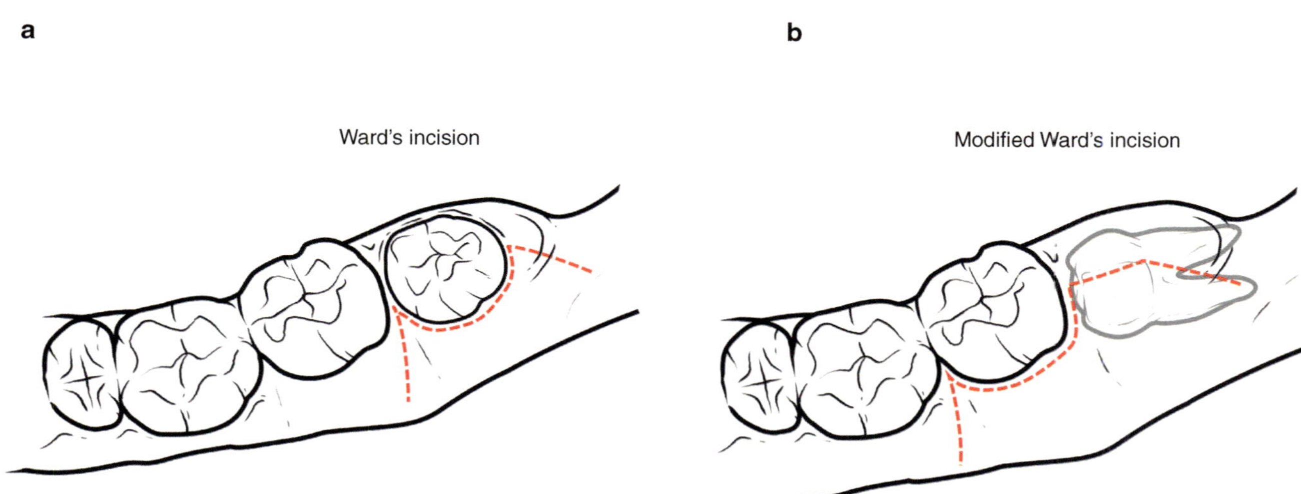




**Fig. 14.24** (**a**) Classical Terrence Ward's incision, (**b**) Modified ward's incision

tooth. This "guttering method" maintains the buccal plate height, does not weaken the mandible, and at the same time, creates adequate space around the tooth to permit its free movement (Fig. 14.25).

The "Postage stamp" method of bone removal used in transalveolar extractions can also be used to remove the buccal bone, but this method may be more time-consuming. The surgical removal of an impacted tooth is basically a transalveolar extraction and all the basic principles, right from the mucoperiosteal flap design to bone removal and closure has to be followed religiously to achieve good healing.

Bone can also be removed from the mesial aspect of the impacted tooth using this method. In this region, bone removal must be extremely conservative to avoid damage to the distal aspect of the adjacent second molar. Extreme care is taken while removing bone on the distolingual aspect, and proper retraction must be used to prevent lingual nerve damage from the bur. Due to the likelihood of damage to the lingual nerve, bone must not be removed on the lingual aspect. The commonly used burs for bone removal are the #8 round bur and a #703 fissure bur, although a wide variety may be used based on individual preference.

After the tooth is exposed, a point of application is created for the elevator. This allows the tooth to be displaced using only moderate force. If the tooth is resistant, further bone removal or tooth sectioning must be considered.

### 14.8.3 Elevation of Tooth from the Socket

Once bone removal is complete, tooth elevation can be attempted. Undue force should not be used for this purpose. Applying inappropriate amount of force, especially without sufficient bone removal, can cause the tooth to fracture, or can even cause fracture of the mandible. Because of the above risk, the use of instruments with high mechanical efficiency is contraindicated for third molar removal. These instruments include dental extraction forceps and cross bar elevators. Once the obstructing bone has been removed, only a small amount of force alone is needed to deliver the tooth. Elevators such as the Warwick James elevator (both straight and curved types) and Coupland elevator, which have lower mechanical efficiency, may be used for this purpose.

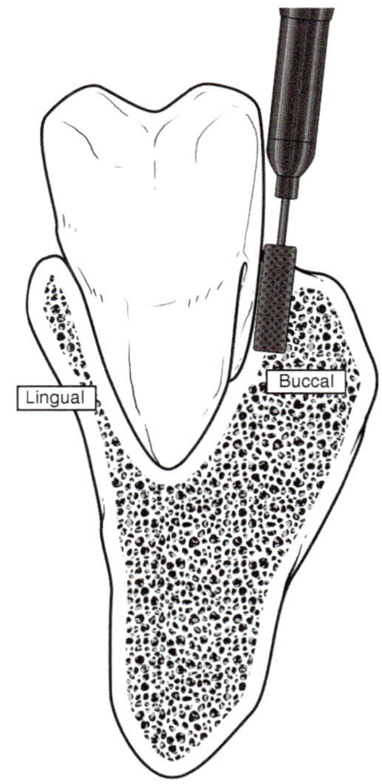




Fig. 14.25 "Guttering method"- A deep vertical gutter using bur is made alongside the buccal aspect and if required on the distal aspect of the tooth

### 14.8.4 Sectioning and Tooth Delivery

If the tooth has been sufficiently exposed but is still resistant to moderate force, tooth sectioning must be considered. The tooth is sectioned into appropriate pieces for easy delivery from the socket. Sectioning of the tooth not only avoids additional bone removal, but it also reduces operating time. Tooth sectioning can be carried out using a bur, which is preferred, or a chisel. In the standard technique, sectioning is carried out using the bur at the neck of the tooth, which facilitates crown removal first, followed by the roots in a single piece. Alternatively, the tooth may be divided horizontally also. Nevertheless, in cases of divergent roots, or where the path of withdrawal is complex, the roots may have to be divided and removed separately.

The manner of sectioning of crown and root must be decided individually for each case and the standard technique need not be followed exactly (Fig. 14.26).

### 14.8.5 Modifications of standard technique

Although the principles of third molar removal remain fundamentally the same, the angulation of the tooth may dictate certain modifications. Angulation dictates the site of application of the elevator, as the path of withdrawal of the third molar should be along the line of least resistance. Therefore, the angulation, in terms of mesioangular, horizontal, vertical, and distoangular impactions must be considered.

The *mesioangular* impaction (Fig. 14.27a, b, c) (Video 14.1) is generally considered to be the least difficult to remove. After elevating the mucoperiosteal flap and exposure of the crown, the buccal guttering is carried out till the mesial surface of impacted tooth, to a point below the cementoenamel junction. This allows the tip of the elevator to be introduced to engage beneath the cervical cementum on the mesial side of the tooth. When the elevator is rotated, the interdental bone is used as the fulcrum and the tooth rotates distally. Thus the tooth, which had an initial mesial angulation, now occupies a vertical position. When more force is applied using the elevator, the tooth is delivered. In some instances, although the tooth becomes vertical, further movement is prevented by the distal bone. This obstruction may be relieved by one of the following methods:

(a) Using a bur, distal bone may be removed and the tooth may be dislodged distally. Then the tooth is removed.
(b) The distal half of the crown may be sectioned by slicing from the buccal groove to a point just below the cervical line on the distal side of the tooth. This slice is removed, and then the remainder of the tooth is delivered using a straight elevator placed on the mesial aspect.
(c) The point of application of the elevator is changed from mesial to the buccal side and a firm upward force is exerted. A purchase point can be created with a bur and the toot can be delivered using a Cryer's elevator.

Sometimes, the mesioangular tooth may be entrapped beneath the distal convexity of the crown of the second molar. In such cases, the tooth may be divided at the cervical region to separate the crown, which is then removed by applying force beneath its inferior surface. The roots may then be delivered by engaging at the bifurcation.

If the tooth roots are in close contact with the mandibular canal, applying levering force can force the root apex downward which may damage the neurovascular bundle. Crown sectioning must be preferred in such cases, which will allow the roots to be delivered upward away from the canal. This would prevent damage to the canal.

The *horizontally impacted* (Fig. 14.28a, b, c, d) (Video 14.2) tooth may need more bone to be removed as compared to mesioangular impaction. A deeply impacted tooth tends to engage either the crown or root of the second molar. This makes its removal difficult. Adequate bone is removed superiorly to expose the entire crown width, as well as the upper third of the root. The point of application of elevator is procured below the mesiobuccal aspect of the impacted crown.

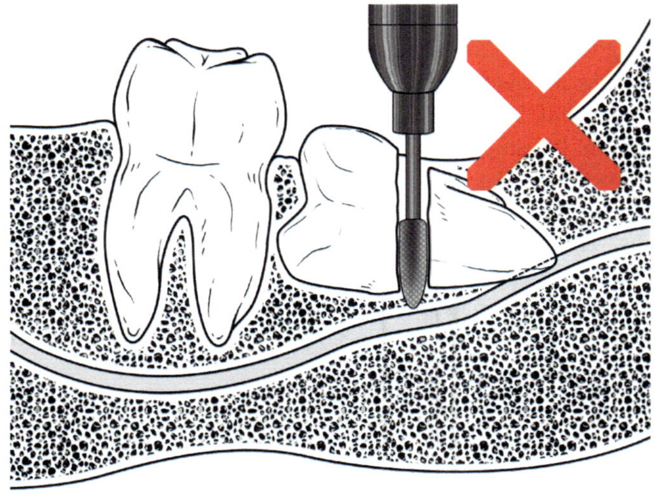



**Fig. 14.26** Possible damage to inferior alveolar neurovascular bundle if the bur is carried to the full width of the tooth inferiorly. Hence, bur is used to cut only three-fourth width of the tooth and the rest of the tooth is separated using a suitable instrument

The tooth is then sectioned at the cervical region and the crown is removed from the socket. The root is then brought forward into the vacant space previously occupied by the crown and it is then removed either in a single piece or after sectioning.

In cases where the impacted tooth is not locked beneath the distal convexity of the crown of the second molar and when an adequate amount of distal bone has been removed, it is possible to turn the tooth into a vertical position by application of force in the mesial aspect. This is similar to the procedure already described for the removal of mesioangular impactions. Use of further force with the elevator will expel the tooth out of the socket or force can be applied on the buccal side to remove the tooth.

Another method of removing horizontal impactions is to split the tooth horizontally into two by sectioning via the buccal groove into separate mesial and distal roots (technique shown in Fig. 14.29). The distal root with the attached crown part is elevated out first followed by the deeply lying mesial root and part of the crown. If there is difficulty in elevating the deeply placed mesial root segment, it can be again sectioned into two at the cervical region and the crown and the root parts may be removed separately.

The *vertical impaction* (Fig. 14.29a, b, c) is one of the more difficult ones to remove, especially if it is impacted very deeply. The procedure for bone removal and the sectioning is similar to that of a mesioangular impaction. Here also the bone is removed first from the occlusal, buccal, and distal aspect. The distal half of the crown is then sectioned and removed, and the tooth is elevated by applying a small straight elevator at the mesial aspect of the cervical line. Alternatively, similar to mesioangular impactions, a pur-

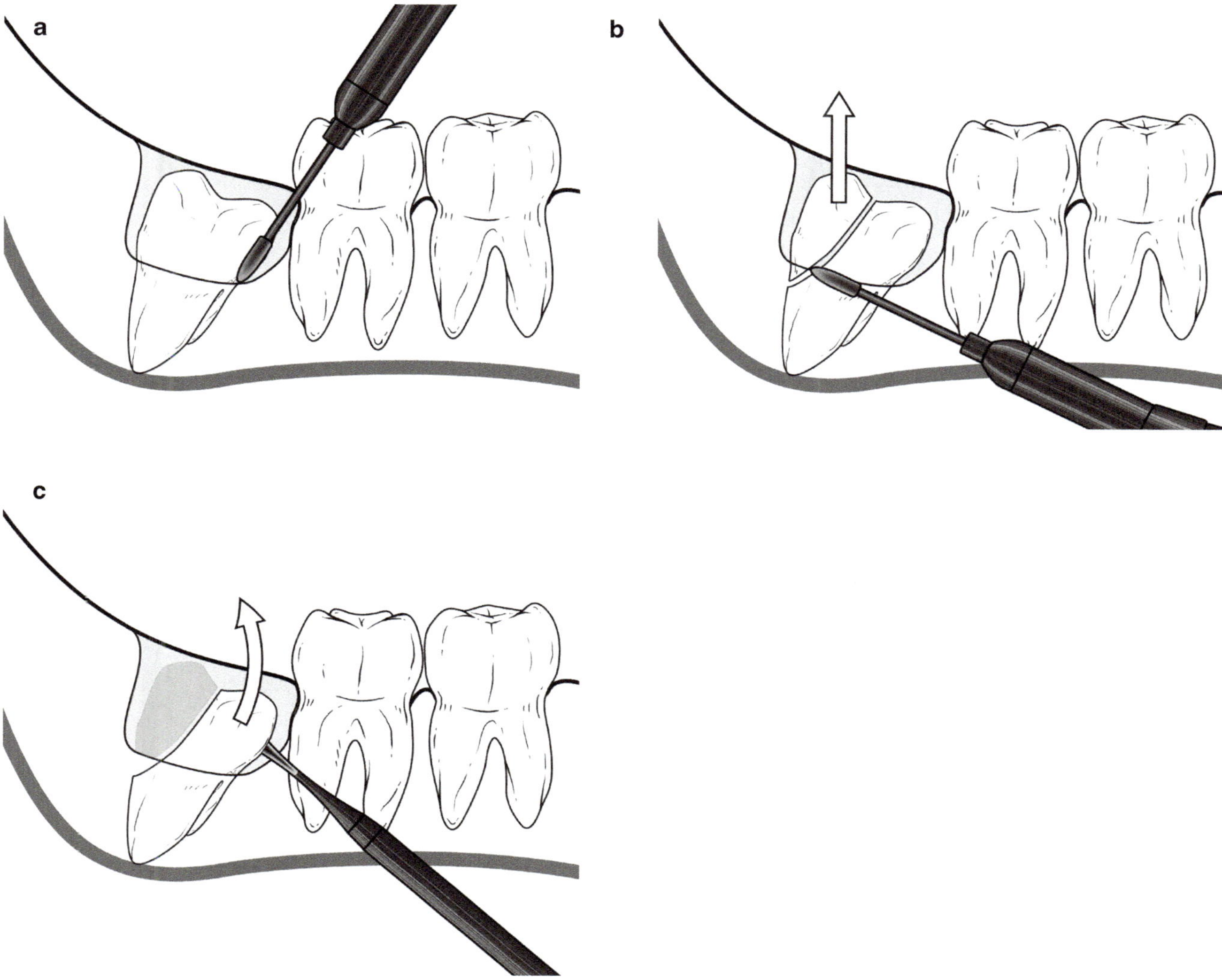




**Fig. 14.27** (**a**, **b**, **c**) (see text for details) Steps in the surgical removal of mesioangular impaction. (**a**) Bone removed up to cemento enamel junction using bur, (**b**) Sectioning of tooth, (**c**) Tooth delivery using elevator

chase point can be made on the buccal side of the tooth, and a Cryer's elevator may be used to deliver the tooth.

The *distoangular impaction* (Fig. 14.30a, b, c) is considered to be the most difficult tooth to remove. The goal of the technique for removal of these teeth is to create an adequate buccal and distal trough (guttering) around the crown of the tooth to a depth below the cervical line. This will permit to make a point of application of elevator on the buccal aspect of the tooth. Then, using the buccal cortical plate as the fulcrum, force is applied to elevate the tooth out of the socket upward and distally. If some movement is obtained, the distal portion of the crown or the complete crown can be sectioned in a horizontal fashion from the roots and removed. It is preferable in this case to section the tooth segments further as needed rather than to remove more bone. It would be wise to remember the adage that "Tooth belongs to the surgeon and Bone belongs to the patient". This will ensure preservation of the structural integrity of the mandible. The roots are then delivered together or sectioned and delivered independently with a Cryer's elevator.

In cases where tooth sectioning is required, the distal root should be elevated first followed by the mesial root.

### 14.8.6 Debridement

After tooth delivery, all bone debris and tissue must be removed from the socket. This is best accomplished by irrigation with saline and mechanically debriding the socket and the area under the flap with a cruet. A bone file or a large bur is used to smooth any rough and sharp edges of the bone. Any remaining dental follicle must be removed using a mosquito hemostat, to prevent cyst formation. An artery

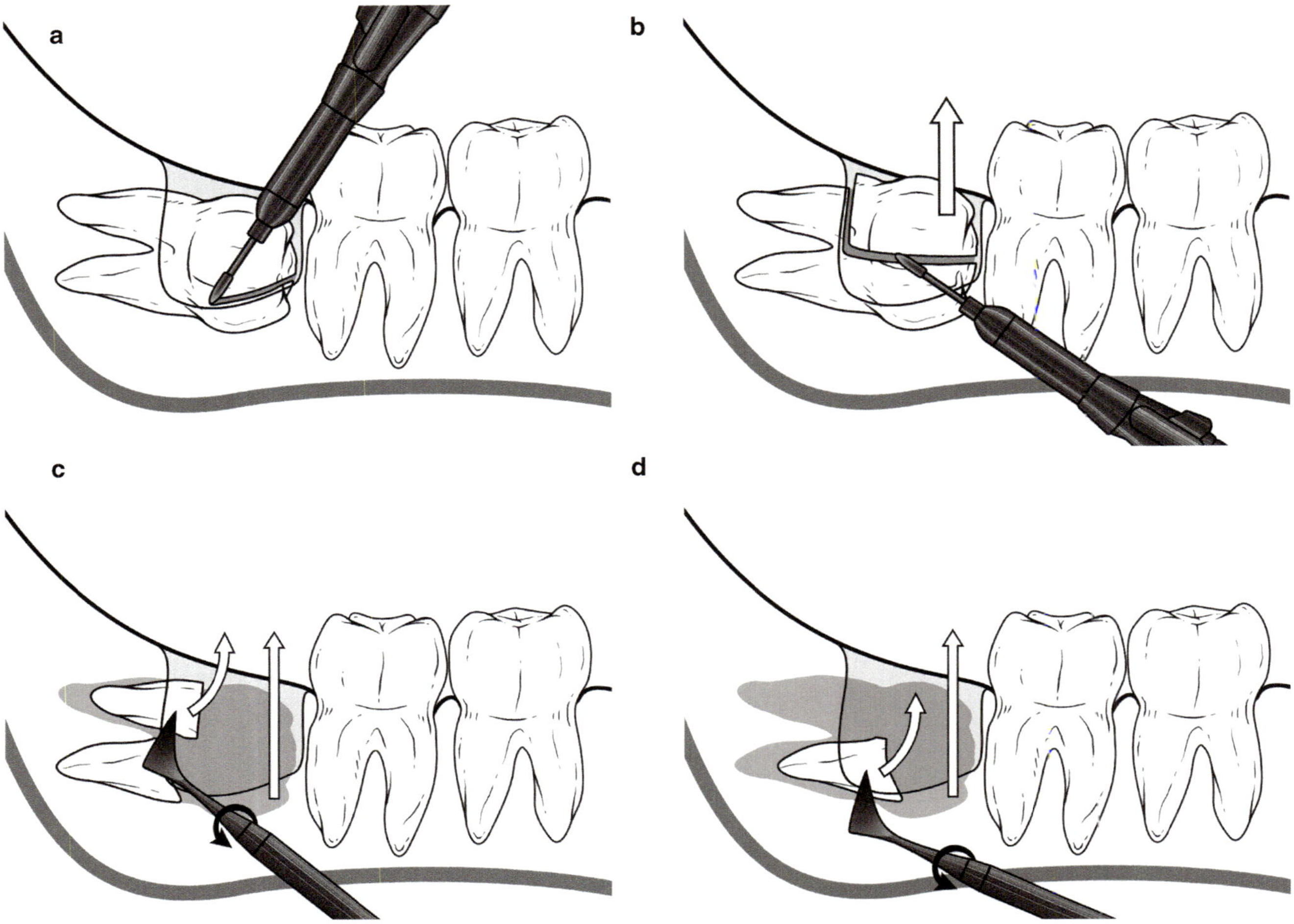


©Association of Oral and Maxillofacial Surgeons of India

**Fig. 14.28** (**a**, **b**, **c**, **d**) Steps in the surgical removal of a horizontally impacted mandibular third molar. (**a**) Bone removal to expose the width of the crown and the upper third of the root, (**b**) Crown may be sectioned into two as shown in the figure and elevated separately. Another technique is to divide the tooth at cemento enamel junction and elevate the crown as a single piece, (**c**) After removal of the crown, the distal root sectioned at the furcation is brought forward into the space occupied by the crown, (**d**) Removal of the mesial root. (the technique shown in Fig. 14.29 can also be used for horizontal imapctions where the tooth is sectioned via the bifurcation and distal crown and root is elevated out first, followed by the mesial crown and root)

forceps may be used to remove fractured interdental septum or large pieces of bone. The socket and the wound margins (including under surface of mucoperiosteum) is irrigated with saline or sterile water to remove bone and tooth debris.

### 14.8.7 Wound Closure

Before attempting closure, bleeding from the socket is completely arrested. Further bleeding from the socket can be controlled using bone wax, Surgicel, or Gelfoam. If there is bleeding from the socket underneath a tight suture, blood will accumulate in surrounding tissue spaces leading to buccal or lingual hematoma or ecchymosis. The flap is then replaced to its original position and the initial suture placed just distal to the second molar. This suture reduces the possibility of the development of periodontal pocket distal to the second molar. The needle is passed from the buccal to the lingual side. Additional sutures are then placed as necessary. The sutures should be just tight enough to hold the flap. Over tightening should be avoided. The vertical component of the incision is left unsutured since it will act as a wound toilet.

Following the procedure, oral and written postoperative instructions given to patient and bystander ensure better patient compliance.

The influence of lower third molar impactions on the periodontal health of the adjacent second molar and the influence of third molar removal on the periodontal attachment of the second molar is a very contentious topic and multiple studies have been done in this regard [32].

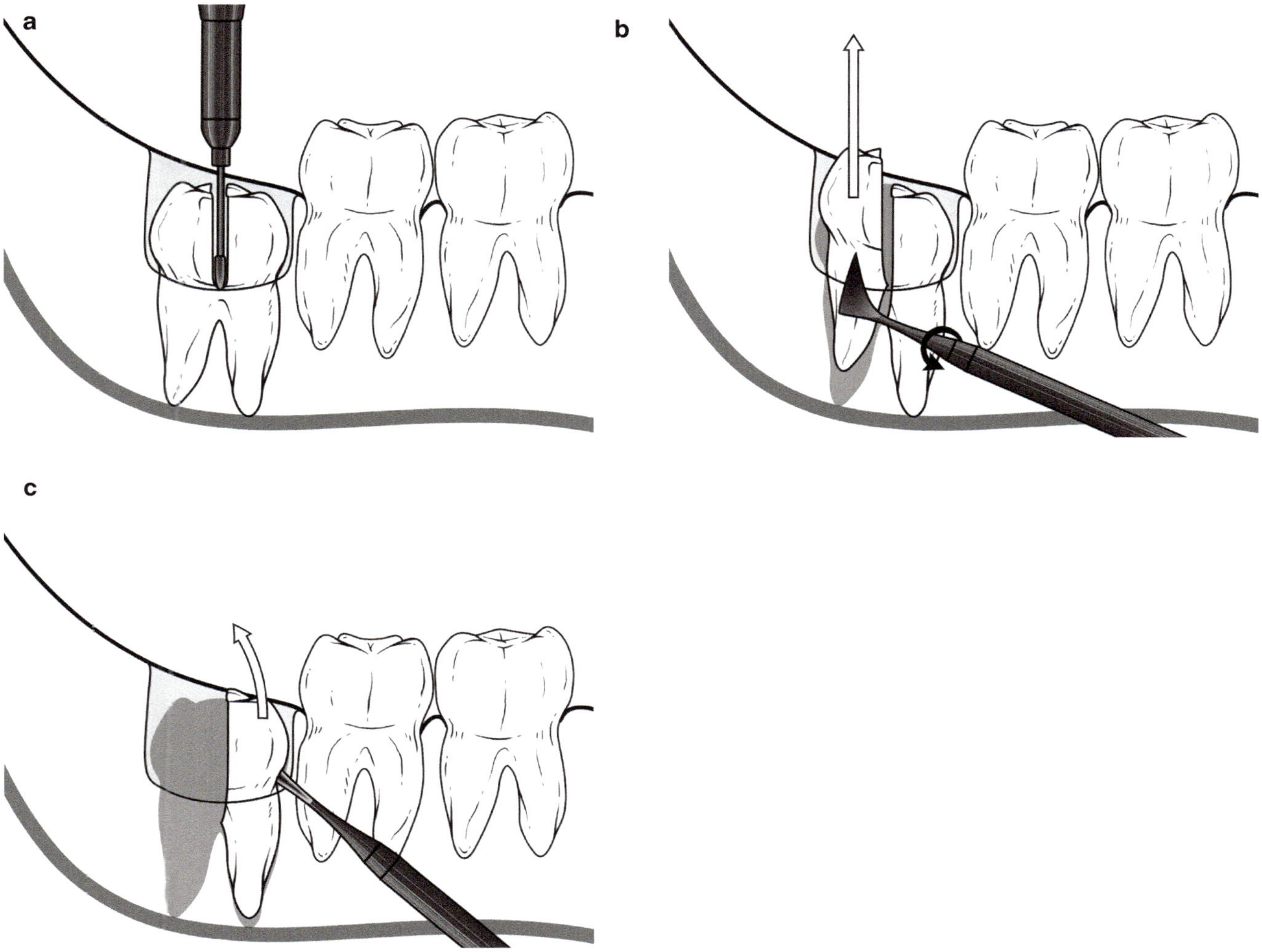




**Fig. 14.29** (**a**, **b**, **c**) Steps in the surgical removal of a vertically impacted mandibular third molar. (**a**) Bone removal to expose the width of the crown, (**b**) Distal half of the crown sectioned up to the furcation and it is removed along with the root, (**c**) Mesial half of the tooth is elevated by mesial application of force at the cervical line

### 14.8.8 Other Methods for Removal/Partial Removal of Impacted Lower Third Molar

In addition to the standard surgical technique described above, there may be occasions where other methods of surgical removal also have to be considered. This is because no technique is suited to every case and it will be ideal to learn the different methods and choose the suitable one depending upon the case. Readers are advised to refer the concerned publications to get more details.

## 14.9 Impacted Maxillary Third Molar (Video 14.3)

Surgical management of upper third molars in general is less complicated compared to lower third molars. They cause less discomfort, are more likely to erupt and are simpler to remove unless unerupted and encased in bone. Removal of upper third molars results in far less postoperative morbidity.

The commonest type of impaction in maxillary third molar is vertical [42].

*Classification of impacted maxillary third molars*—The system of classification of impacted upper wisdom tooth is basically the same as that for mandibular third molar. However, there are some additional parameters to be considered which will aid in preoperative assessment of the

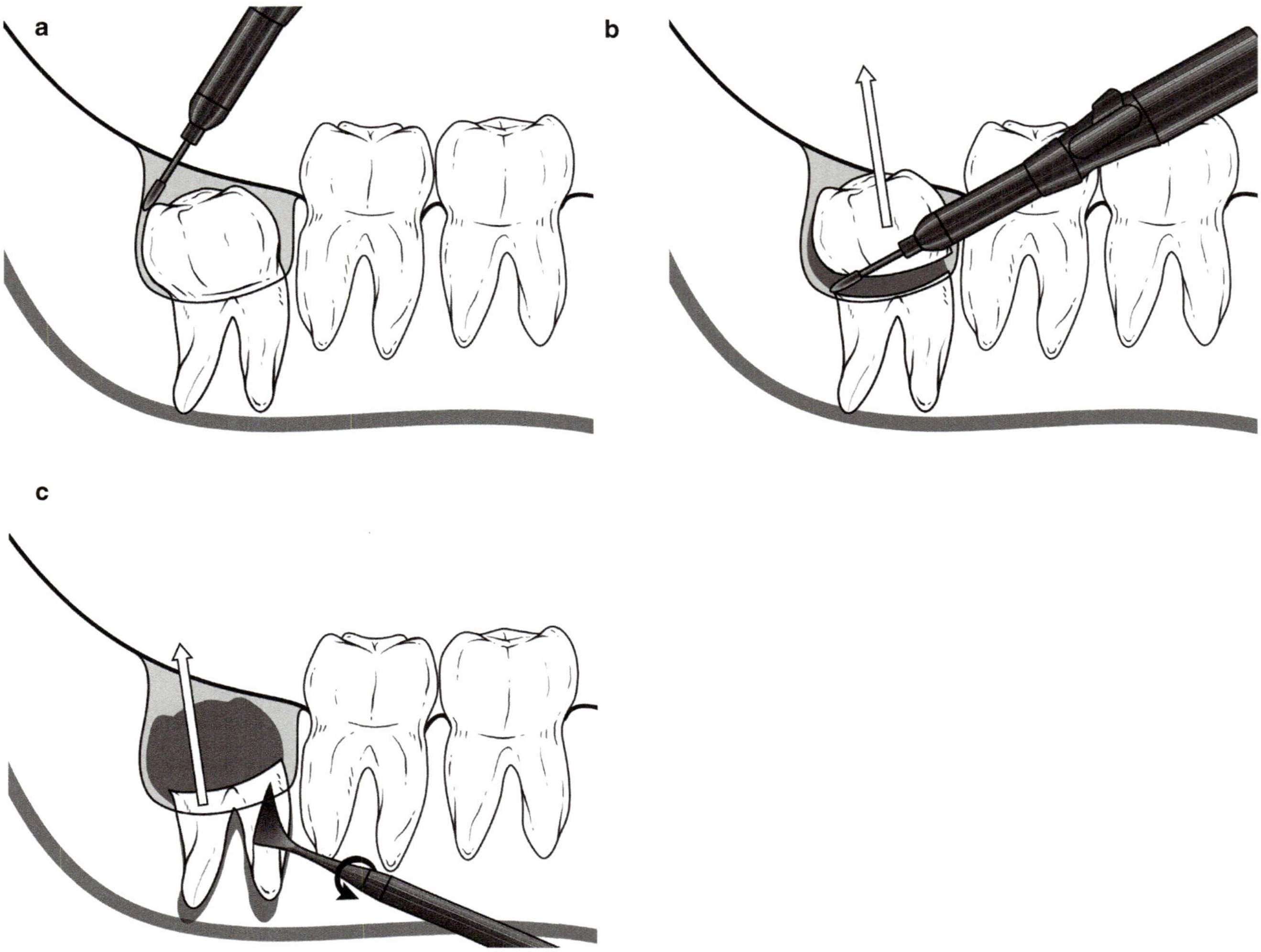




**Fig. 14.30** (**a**, **b**, **c**) Steps in the surgical removal of a distoangularly impacted mandibular third molar. (**a**) Bone removed to expose the full crown of the tooth to a depth below the cervical line, (**b**) Crown sectioned in a horizontal fashion from the roots and removed (some surgeons prefer to remove only the distal portion of the crown of third molar, so that a point of elevation is available distal to the second molar tooth), (**c**) Roots are then delivered together or sectioned and delivered independently with a Cryer's elevator

case and guide in planning the surgery for a successful outcome.

1. *State of eruption.*
   (a) Fully erupted.
   (b) Partially erupted.
   (c) Unerupted:
      - within the bone
      - immediately beneath the soft tissues

2. *Angulation of the tooth* (Fig. 14.31).
   (a) Vertical.

Some of the other methods seen in the literature are

1. Removal via sagittal split osteotomy [33].
2. Buccal corticotomy technique [34].
3. Lingual split bone technique [35, 36].
4. Lateral trephination technique [37, 38].
5. Partial odontectomy/Coronectomy [15, 16, 39].
6. Removal of the tooth after orthodontic extrusion [40, 41].

   (b) Mesioangular.
   (c) Distoangular.
   (d) Laterally displaced with the crown facing the cheek, horizontal, inverted, and transverse positions.
   (e) Aberrant position sometimes associated with pathological condition such as cyst.
3. *Pell and Gregory classification*—This is based on the relative depth of the impacted maxillary third molar, (Fig. 14.32).
   Position A—Occlusal surface of the third molar is at the same level as that of the second molar.
   Position B—Occlusal surface of the third molar is located between the occlusal plane and cervical line of the second molar.
   Position C—Occlusal surface of the third molar is at or above the cervical line of the second molar.
4. *Relationship of impacted maxillary third molar to the maxillary sinus.*
   (a) Sinus approximation (SA)—No bone or a thin partition of bone between the impacted maxillary third molar and maxillary sinus.
   (b) No sinus approximation (NSA)—2 mm or more bone between the impacted maxillary third molar and maxillary sinus.
5. *Nature of roots.*
   (a) Fused (conical).
   (b) Multiple—Favorable/Unfavorable.

### 14.9.1 Radiographic Examination

The following are the useful radiographs:

1. Periapical X-ray.
2. Orthopantomogram (OPG).
3. Occlusal X-ray.
4. True lateral view—occasionally helpful.
5. Paranasal sinus view: useful to view pathologies associated with the tooth.
6. CT scan—more useful for suspected pathologies in relation to the impacted tooth.

### 14.9.2 Indications for the Removal of Maxillary Third Molar

1. Unrestorable dental caries.
2. Recurrent pericoronitis.
3. A tooth that has erupted in a buccoverted or distal direction, which cause cheek bite, or abnormal bite patterns.
4. Tooth involved in pathological process such as cyst.
5. Overerupted and nonfunctional upper third molar.

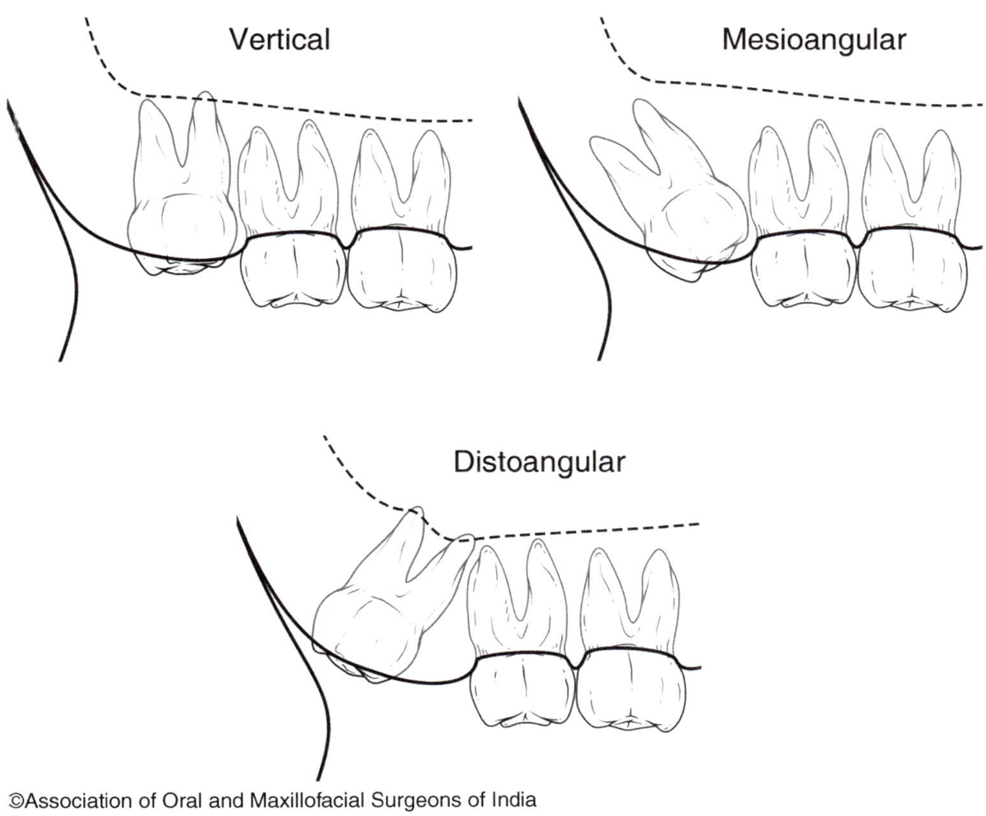


**Fig. 14.31** Classification of impacted maxillary third molar based on angulation

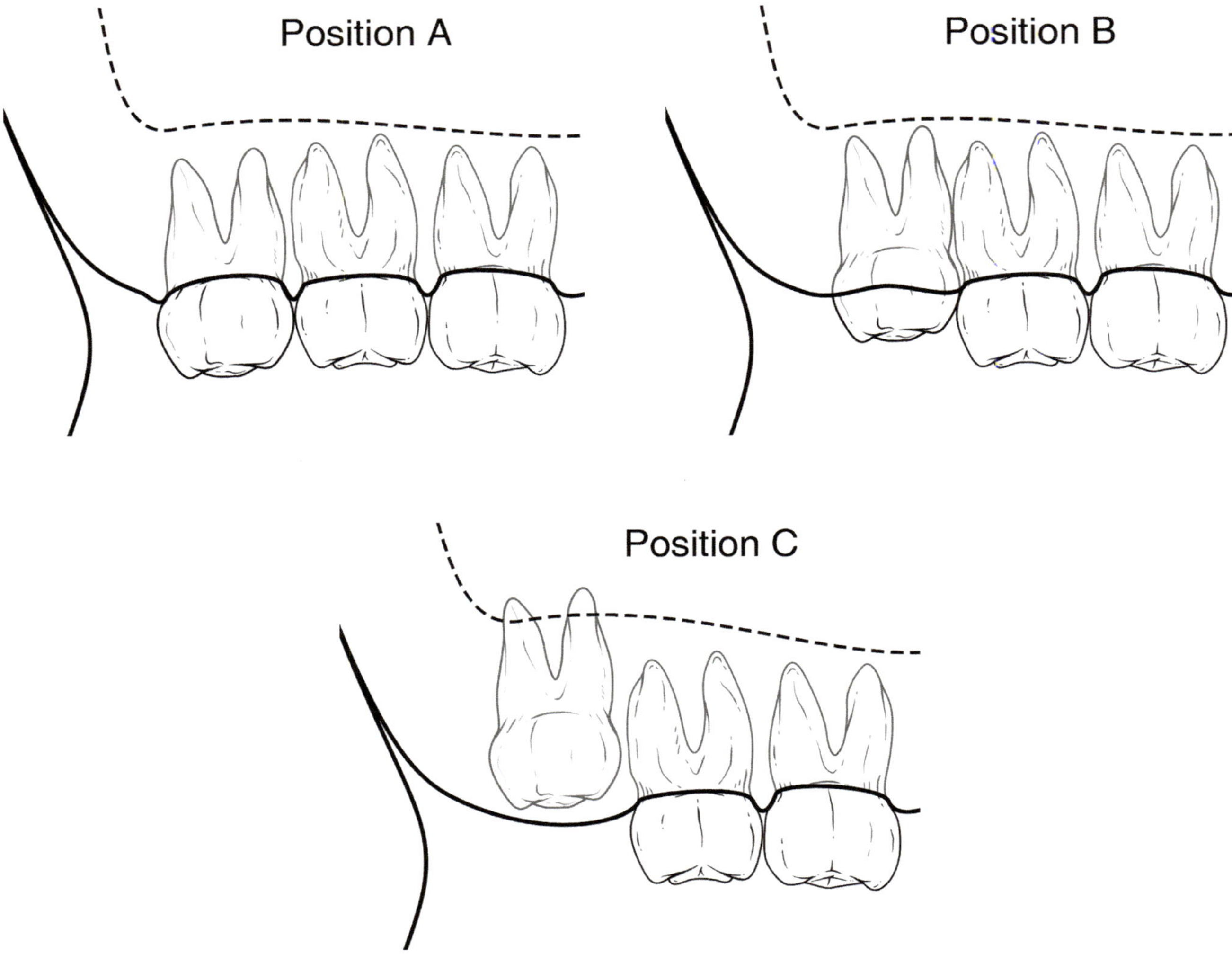




**Fig. 14.32** Pell and Gregory classification based on relative depth of impacted maxillary third molar

6. Interference with the placement of prosthesis.

### 14.9.3 Adjacent Anatomical Factors to be Considered: (Fig. 14.33a–d)

- Proximity to maxillary sinus (Fig. 14.34).
- Proximity to maxillary tuberosity.
- Buccal pad of fat.
- Pterygopalatine fossa.
- Infratemporal fossa.

### 14.9.4 Surgical Removal of Impacted Maxillary Third Molar (Figs. 14.35a–d and 14.36a, b)

The main difficulty here is that the coronoid process may block access to this region, which may be overcome by limiting the amount of mouth opening.

The procedure for maxillary third molar surgical removal is almost the same as that of the mandibular third molar.

#### 14.9.4.1 Incision

It starts from the mesial aspect of the first molar and extends distally beyond the distobuccal aspect of the second molar and is then continued into the tuberosity. In case of a deeply impacted tooth if greater access is required, a triangular flap may be raised by placing a release incision mesial to the second molar.

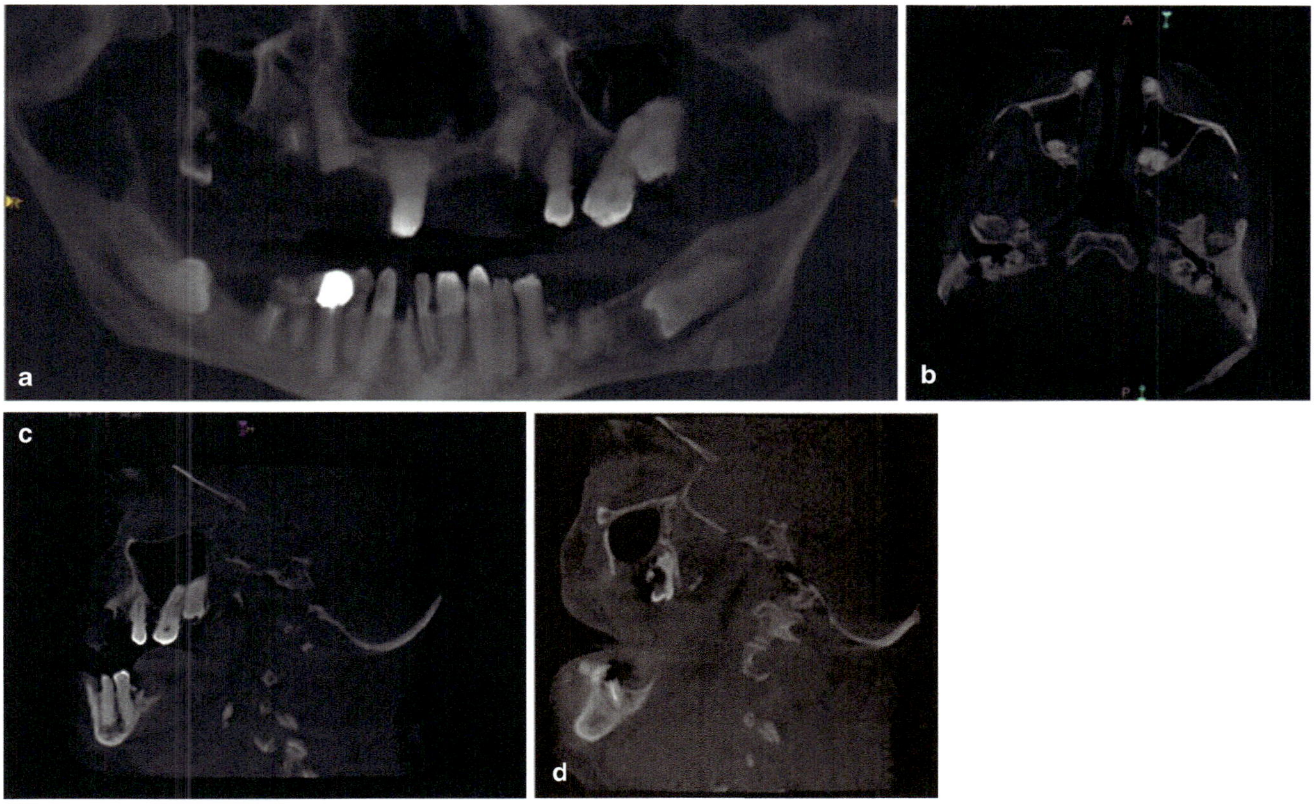




**Fig. 14.33** (**a–d**) Impacted third molars in a 75-year-old male. (**a**) OPG showing impacted 28, 38, and 48 with multiple root stumps and dental caries for 18. (**b**) Axial CBCT showing close relationship of 18 and 28 to maxillary sinus, (**c**) Sagittal view showing sinus approximation of roots of 27 and 28, (**d**) Sagittal view showing close relationship of 18 to sinus floor

The mucoperiosteum is then reflected using a Howarth's periosteal elevator, which may also be used to retract the flap.

#### 14.9.4.2 Removal of Overlying Bone

Bone removal is generally limited to the occlusal and the buccal aspect of the tooth down to the cervical line to expose the entire crown (Figs. 14.35b and 14.36a). This is done using bur. To create space for the elevator to be inserted, more bone may be removed from the mesial part of the tooth, at a point above the maximum bulge of the crown.

Unlike mandibular third molars, *maxillary third molars rarely need sectioning*, as maxillary bone expands easily, being thin and elastic. Instances where the bone is thicker, sclerotic and less elastic as in old patients, tooth removal is enabled by bone removal rather than tooth sectioning. Chisel is contraindicated to section the tooth due to the danger of displacement of the tooth into the maxillary antrum.

Maxillary third molar teeth must not be sectioned unless absolutely necessary, as displacement of small fragments into the sinus or infratemporal fossa may occur.

#### 14.9.4.3 Delivery of the Tooth

This is achieved using small straight elevators or angled elevators with force exerted in the distobuccal direction. If angled elevators are used, access may be easier. Angled elevators which can be used for this purpose are the Warwick James, Cryer, Pott's, and the Apex elevator. During surgical removal, placement of Laster retractor will help in better access and vision and may also prevent accidental displacement of the maxillary third molar into tissue space beyond the tuberosity.

During tooth elevation, one must remember the following points:-

1. Due to the proximity of the maxillary sinus and the infratemporal fossa, pressure should not be exerted in the superior direction during bone removal and delivery of the tooth.
2. Sufficient space is created between the height of contour of the crown (i.e. above the maximum bulge of the tooth) and surrounding bone so that the tip of the elevator can be placed above the height of contour of the tooth. Then pressure is exerted in a distobuccal direction.

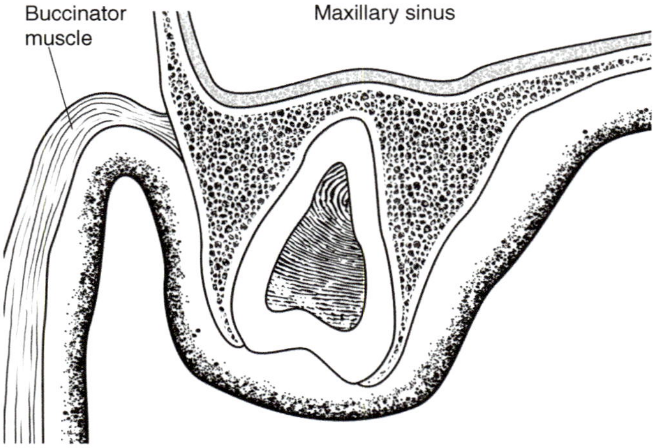




**Fig. 14.34** Schematic diagram showing the relationship of impacted maxillary third molar to the floor of the maxillary sinus

3. Moderate pressure is then exerted distally, buccally and occlusally (i.e. downward and outward) with the fore finger placed posterior to maxillary tuberosity to detect tuberosity fracture if it occurs.
4. In case an accidental opening into the sinus is suspected, every effort should be made to ensure proper closure and the patient is instructed appropriately to prevent the development of an oro-antral fistula.

### 14.9.5 Complications That Occur During Surgical Removal of Impacted Maxillary Third Molar

1. *Tooth displacement into maxillary sinus*—This usually occurs in cases of partially erupted maxillary third molars, which have conical roots and are located close to the floor

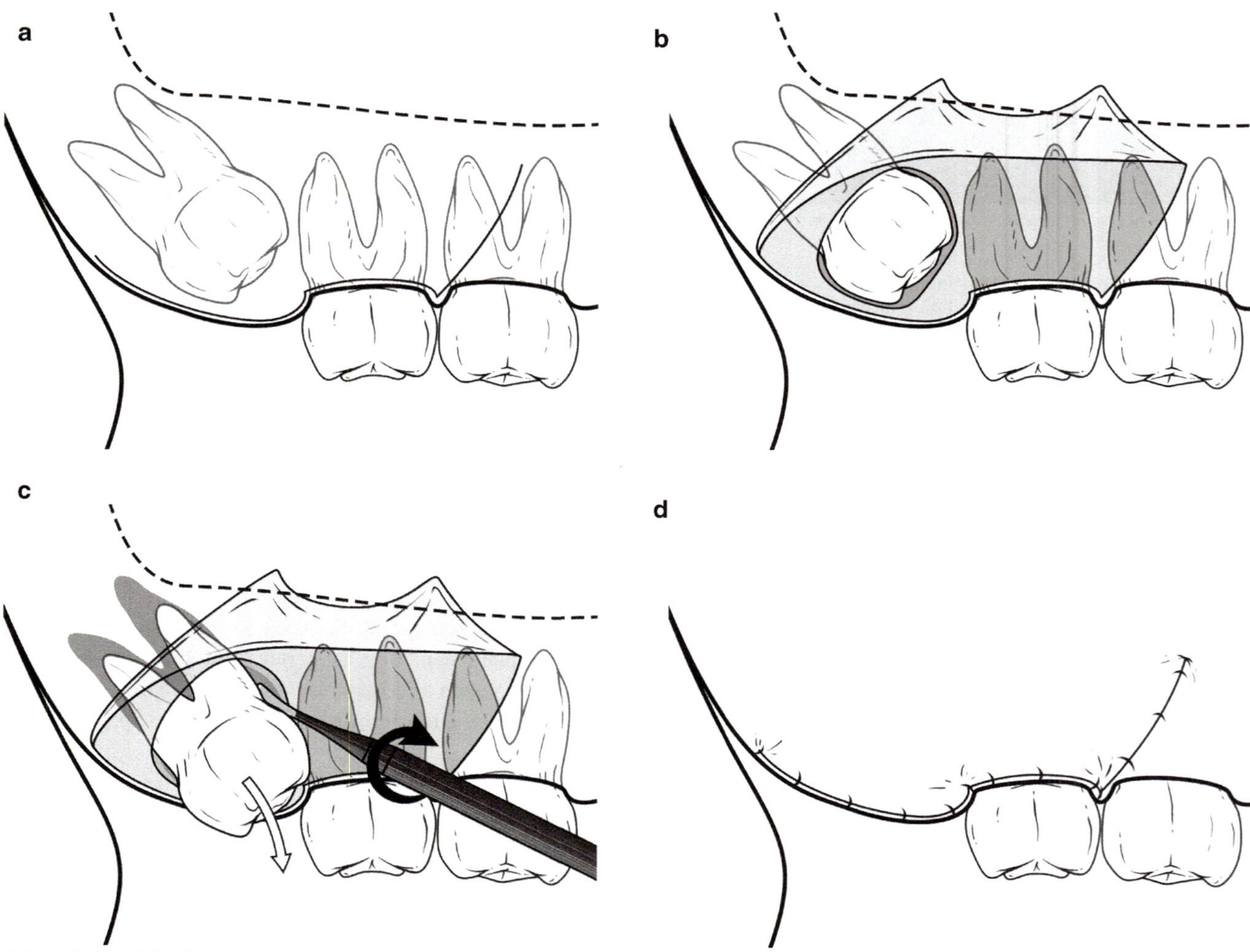




**Fig. 14.35** (**a–d**) Steps in the surgical removal of a mesioangularly impacted maxillary third molar. (**a**) Incision to raise a triangular flap, (**b**) Mucoperiosteal flap reflected, (**c**) Overlying bone removed from occlusal and buccal aspect up to the cervical line and elevation of tooth, (**d**) Suturing completed

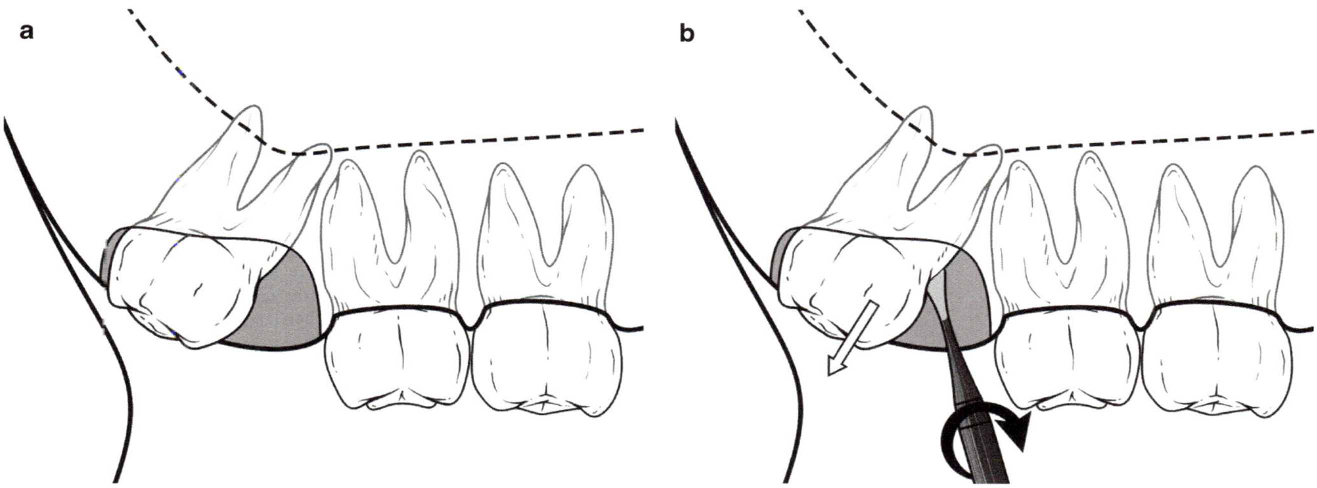




**Fig. 14.36** (**a**) Bone removal achieved on the occlusal and the buccal aspect of tooth down to the cervical line to expose the entire crown, in a disto angular maxillary third molar impaction (**b**) Delivery of the tooth using an elevator

of the sinus. The risk increases if the root apex is in contact with the floor of the sinus, and the initial position of the tooth is high.

If this complication occurs, the tooth may have to be removed from the sinus in order to avoid infection. Initially, a suction tip may be placed at the sinus opening to retrieve the tooth. Alternately, saline irrigation into the sinus may be followed by applying the suction tip. If these methods do not work, it is best to stop attempts and place the patient on antibiotics and nasal decongestants. The tooth may be retrieved later through Caldwell-Luc approach, and the oro-antral fistula may then be closed. The tooth may also be removed using endoscopic sinus surgery [43, 44]. Detailed sequential approach of dealing with root/tooth displaced into the sinus is mentioned in the Chap. 24 on Oro antral communication and fistula in this text book.

2. *Dislodgement into soft tissues*—The upper third molar can be inadvertently displaced into the buccal soft tissues [45] or into the infratemporal fossa [46]. Usually, this happens: (a) when the flap raised buccally is not adequate for access, (b) there is insufficient visibility during the procedure, (c) improper extraction technique, (d) disto-lingual angulation of tooth, and (e) the crown of the third molar is at a level above the root apices of the adjacent molar tooth.

   Dimitrakopoulos et al. [46] have discussed the various methods to remove a maxillary third molar that has been displaced into the infratemporal fossa.
3. *Damage to adjacent second molar.*
4. *Fracture of maxillary tuberosity.*
5. *Oro-antral communication/fistula.*

## 14.10 Complications of Impaction Surgery

Complications of removal of impacted tooth can happen during the procedure and late after the procedure. Mild post operative pain, swelling and trismus can be expected

**B. Postsurgical Sequelae and Complications**

1. Pain
2. Edema
3. Trismus
4. Haemorrhage
5. Infection
6. Alveolar osteitis (Dry socket)
7. Nerve Injury:
   (a) Lingual nerve injury
   (b) Inferior alveolar nerve injury
8. Surgical Emphysema
9. Hematoma
10. Pain during swallowing
11. Pyrexia
12. Osteomyelitis
13. Temporomandibular joint (TMJ) complications
14. Fracture of instruments
15. Periodontal pocket formation distal to second molar
16. Aspiration/Swallowing of tooth

The management of impacted third molars involves several considerations, and several controversies also exist in this area. Some of these are as follows:

- Whether to remove Asymptomatic/Disease-free tooth [4–6].
- Age of removal [47]

At present, the various evidence-based guidelines available should help the clinician in taking informed decisions regarding third molar impactions [55–57]. Efforts have been made to reach a consensus in various areas, which itself shows conflicting propositions, and only time will prove the best methods which can be used in the management of third molar impactions.

**A. Complications that can occur during the Surgical Procedure:**

These can happen at various steps in the procedure, including:

1. Placement of incision.
2. Removal of bone.
3. Sectioning of the tooth.
4. Tooth elevation and delivery.

1. *Complications during incision*:
   (a) Bleeding from retromolar vessels.
   (b) Bleeding from facial vessels.
   (c) Damage to lingual nerve.
2. *Complications during bone removal:*
   (a) *Use of bur.*
   - Accidental burns.
   - Laceration of soft tissues.
   - Injury to inferior alveolar neurovascular bundle.
   - Injury to adjacent tooth.
   - Injury to lingual nerve.
   - Necrosis of bone.
   - Emphysema.

   (b) *Use of chisel*
   - Splintering of bone.
   - Fracture of mandible.
   - Displacement of tooth into lingual pouch.
   - Injury to lingual nerve.
   - Injury to the soft tissues or second molar.
3. *Complications during sectioning of tooth.*
   *During bur usage*
   - Sectioning along an incorrect line.
   - Injury to mandibular canal.
   - Breakage of bur.
4. *Complications during elevation of tooth:*
   - Fracture of impacted tooth/root.
   - Injury to second molar.
   - Fracture of mandible.
   - Displacement of the entire tooth or crown alone into the lingual pouch or lateral pharyngeal space.

## References


1. Archer WH. Oral and maxillofacial surgery, vol. I. 5th ed. Philadelphia: W.B. Saunders; 1975.
2. Lytle JJ. Indications and contraindications for removal of impacted tooth. Dent Clin of North Amer. 1979;23(3):333–46.
3. Andreasen J.O, Petersen J.K, Laskin D.M. Textbook and color atlas of tooth impactions, 1, Copenhagen, Munksgaard 1997.
4. Dodson TB. The management of the asymptomatic, disease-free wisdom tooth: removal versus retention. Atlas Oral Maxillofac Surg Clin North Am. 2012 Sep;20(2):169–76.
5. Rafetto LK. Removal of asymptomatic third molars: a supporting view. J Oral Maxillofac Surg. 2006 Dec;64(12):1811–5.
6. Hill CM. Removal of asymptomatic third molars: an opposing view. J Oral Maxillofac Surg. 2006 Dec;64(12):1816–20.
7. Berger A. As cited by Archer, W. H., Oral and maxillofacial surgery, vol. I, 5th ed. Philadelphia: W.B. Saunders; 1975.
8. Pogrel MA, Renaut A, Schmidt B, et al. The relationship of the lingual nerve to the mandibular third molar region: an anatomic study. J Oral Maxillofac Surg. 1995;53:1178–81.
9. Behnia H, Kheradvar A, Shahrokhi M. An anatomic study of the lingual nerve in the third molar region. J Oral Maxillofac Surg. 2000;58:649–51.
10. Winter GB. Principles of exodontia as applied to the impacted third molar. St Louis: American Medical Books; 1926.
11. Pell GJ, Gregory BT. Impacted mandibular third molars: classification and modified techniques for removal. Dent Digest. 1933;39:330–8.
12. Suvy Manuel, Surej Kumar LK, Mathew P Varghese. A comprehensive proforma for evaluation of mandibular third molar impactions. J Maxillofac Oral Surg. 2014 Dec; 13(4):378–385.
13. Howe G, Poynton HG. Prevention of damage to the inferior alveolar nerve during the evaluation of mandibular third molars. Br Dent J. 1960;109:355–63.
14. Rood JP, Shehab BA. The radiological prediction of inferior alveolar nerve injury during third molar surgery. Br J Oral Maxillofac Surg. 1990 Feb;28(1):20–5.
15. Pogrel MA, Lee JS, Muff DF. Coronectomy: a technique to protect the inferior alveolar nerve. J Oral Maxillofac Surg. 2004;62:1447.
16. Renton T, Hankins M, Sproate C, McGurk M. A randomised controlled clinical trial to compare the incidence of injury to the inferior alveolar nerve as a result of coronectomy and removal of mandibular third molars. Br J Oral Maxillofac Surg. 2005;43:7.
17. Tantanapornkul W, Okouchi K, Fujiwara Y, et al. A comparative study of cone-beam computed tomography and conventional panoramic radiography in assessing the topographic relationship between the mandibular canal and impacted third molars. Oral Surg Oral Med Oral Pathol Oral Radiol Endod. 2007;103:253.
18. Ohman A, Kivijarvi K, Blomback U, Flygare L. Pre-operative radiographic evaluation of lower third molars with computed tomography. Dentomaxillofac Radiol. 2006;35:30.
19. Danforth RA, Peck J, Hall P. Cone beam volume tomography: an imaging option for diagnosis of complex mandibular third molar anatomical relationships. JCDA. 2003;31(11):847–52.

20. Gargallo-Albiol J, Buenechea-Imaz R, Gay-Escoda C. Lingual nerve protection during surgical removal of lower third molars. J Oral Maxillofac Surg. 2000;29:268.
21. Pichler JW, Beirne OR. Lingual flap retraction and prevention of lingual nerve damage associated with third molar surgery: a systematic review of the literature. Oral Surg Oral Med Oral Pathol Oral Radiol Endod. 2001;91:395.
22. Pogrel MA, K.E. Goldman: lingual flap retraction for third molar removal. J Oral Maxillofac Surg. 2004;62:1125.
23. Gulicher D, Gerlach KL. Sensory impairment of the lingual and inferior alveolar nerves following removal of impacted mandibular third molars. Int J Oral Maxillofac Surg. 2001;30:306.
24. Valmaseda-Castellon E, Berini-Aytes L, Gay-Escoda C. Inferior alveolar nerve damage after lower third molar surgical extraction: a prospective study of 1117 surgical extractions. Oral Surg Oral Med Oral Pathol Oral Radiol Endod. 2001;92:377.
25. Pederson GW. Oral surgery. Philadelphia: WB Saunders; 1988. (Cited in: Koerner KR. The removal of impacted third molars—principles and procedures. Dent Clin North Am. 1994; 38:255–78)
26. Yuasa H, Kawai T, Sugiura M. Classification of surgical difficulty in extracting impacted third molars. Br J Oral Maxillofac Surg. 2002 Feb;40(1):26–31.
27. Erdogan O, Tatlı U, Ustün Y, Damlar I. Influence of two different flap designs on the sequelae of mandibular third molar surgery. Oral Maxillofac Surg. 2011 Sep;15(3):147–52.
28. Goldsmith SM, De Silva RK, Tong DC, Love RM. Influence of a pedicle flap design on acute postoperative sequelae after lower third molar removal. Int J Oral Maxillofac Surg. 2012 Mar;41(3):371–5.
29. Rullo R, Addabbo F, Papaccio G, D'Aquino R, Festa VM. Piezoelectric device vs. conventional rotative instruments in impacted third molar surgery: relationships between surgical difficulty and postoperative pain with histological evaluations. J Craniomaxillofac Surg. 2013 Mar;41(2):e33–8.
30. Piersanti L, Dilorenzo M, Monaco G, Marchetti C. Piezosurgery or conventional rotatory instruments for inferior third molar extractions? J Oral Maxillofac Surg. 2014 Sep;72(9):1647–52.
31. Stübinger S, von Rechenberg vB, Zeilhofer HF, Sader R, Landes C. Er:YAG laser osteotomy for removal of impacted teeth: clinical comparison of two techniques. Lasers Surg Med. 2007 Aug;39(7):583–8.
32. Krausz A, Machtei E, Peled M. Effects of lower third molar extraction on attachment level and alveolar bone height on the adjacent second molar. Int J Oral Maxillofac Surg. 2005;34:756.
33. Amin M, Haria S, Bounds G. Surgical access to an impacted lower third molar by sagittal splitting of the mandible: a case report. Dent Update. 1995;22:206–8.
34. Tay Andrew BG. Buccal corticotomy for removal of deeply impacted mandibular molars. Br J Oral Maxillofac Surg. 2007;45:83–4.
35. Ward TG. The split bone technique for removal of lower third molars. Br Dent J. 1956;101:297.
36. Farish SE, Bouloux GF. General technique of third molar removal. Oral Maxillofacial Surg Clin N Am. 2007;19:23–43.
37. Henry CB. Excision of the developing mandibular third molar by lateral trepanation. Br Dent J. 1969;127:111–8.
38. Chiapasco M, Crescentini M, Romanoni G. Germectomy or delayed removal of mandibular impacted third molars: the relationship between age and incidence of complications. J Oral Maxillofac Surg. 1995;53(4):418–22.
39. Pogrel MA. Partial odontectomy. Oral Maxillofacial Surg Clin N Am. 2007;19:85–91.
40. Checchi I, Alessandri Bonetti G, Pelliccioni GA. Removing high risk impacted mandibular third molars: a surgical-orthodontic approach. J Am Dent Assoc. 1996;127:1214.
41. Alessandri Bonetti G, Bendandi M, Checchi V, Checchi I. Orthodontic extraction: riskless extraction of impacted lower third molars close to the mandibular canal. J Oral Maxillofac Surg. 2007;65(12):2580–6.
42. Peterson LJ, Ellis E, Hupp JR, Tucker MR. Contemporary oral and maxillofacial surgery. 4th ed. St. Louis: Mosby; 2003. p. 185–237.
43. Bouloux Gary F, Steed Martin B, Perciaccante VJ. Complications of third molar surgery. Oral Maxillofacial Surg Clin N Am. 2007;19:117–28.
44. Pogrel M. Complications of third molar surgery. Oral Maxillofac Surg Clin North Am. 1990;2:441.
45. Matthew I. What should I do if a maxillary third molar is inadvertently displaced into the adjacent soft tissues during surgical removal? [point of care]. J Can Dent Assoc. 2007;73(4):311–2.
46. Dimitrakopoulos I, Papadaki M. Displacement of a maxillary third molar into the infratemporal fossa: case report. Quintessence Int. 2007;38(7):607–10.
47. Haug RH, Perrott DH, Gonzalez ML, Talwar RM. The American association of oral and maxillofacial surgeons age-related third molar study. J Oral Maxillofac Surg. 2005;63(8):1106–14.
48. Pasqualini D, Cocero N, Castella A, Mela L, Bracco P. Primary and secondary closure of the surgical wound after removal of impacted mandibular third molars: a comparative study. Int J Oral Maxillofac Surg. 2005 Jan;34(1):52–7.
49. Rakprasitkul S, Pairuchvej V. Mandibular third molar surgery with primary closure and tube drain. Int J Oral Maxillofac Surg. 1997 Jun;26(3):187–90.
50. Simon D, Manuel S, Geetha V, Naik BR. Potential for osseous regeneration of platelet-rich plasma--a comparative study in mandibular third molar sockets. Indian J Dent Res. 2004 Oct-Dec;15(4):133–6.
51. Varghese MP, Manuel S, Kumar LKS. Potential for osseous regeneration of platelet-rich fibrin-a comparative study in mandibular third molar impaction sockets. J Oral Maxillofac Surg. 2017 Jul;75(7):1322–9.
52. Canellas JVDS, Medeiros PJD, Figueredo CMDS, Fischer RG, Ritto FG. Platelet-rich fibrin in oral surgical procedures: a systematic review and meta-analysis. Int J Oral Maxillofac Surg. 2019 Mar;48(3):395–414.
53. Al-Hamed FS, Tawfik MA, Abdelfadil E, Al-Saleh MAQ. Efficacy of platelet-rich fibrin after mandibular third molar extraction: a systematic review and meta-analysis. J Oral Maxillofac Surg. 2017 Jun;75(6):1124–35.
54. Dodson T. Is there a role for reconstructive techniques to prevent periodontal defects after third molar surgery. J Oral Maxillofac Surg. 2005;63:891.
55. Task Force for Third Molar Summary. Summary of the third molar clinical trials: report of the AAOMS task force for third molar summary. J Oral Maxillofac Surg. 2012 Sep;70(9):2238–48.
56. https://www.nice.org.uk/guidance/ta1
57. https://www.aaoms.org/docs/govt_affairs/advocacy_white_papers/white_paper_third_molar_data.pdf

# 15 Management of Impacted Canines

George Varghese

Impacted canines are one of the common problems encountered by the oral surgeon. Patients may present at different ages and many cases will be incidental findings. Close interaction with the paedodontist and orthodontist is required to get an optimal out come. Surgical removal may not be the best treatment in all the cases and particular treatement plan will have to be tailored for the needs of the patient. Localising the impacted canine seems not a challenge any more with the advent of CBCT, in indicated cases. This chapter elaborates on canine impaction, keeping in mind the basic principles mentioned in the chapter on third molar impactions. Premolars, incisors and other teeth may be impacted but most of the surgical principles and approaches mentioned for canine can be applied to them as well.

## 15.1 Introduction

Maxillary canine is the second most commonly impacted tooth, after the mandibular third molar. The permanent maxillary canine may be considered as impacted when the eruption of the tooth lags behind as compared to the eruption sequences of other teeth in the dentition. Diagnosis of maxillary canine impaction may be made by clinical examination and by radiography.

The normal path through which maxillary canines erupt may be altered due to changes in the eruption sequence in the maxilla, and also by space limitations due to crowding. It is essential to diagnose and treat this condition early, to prevent the development of complications. An ideal management protocol for impacted permanent maxillary canines should involve an interdisciplinary approach linking the specialties of oral and maxillofacial surgery, periodontology and orthodontics.

## 15.2 Aetiology of Canine Impaction

Although the exact cause of impacted maxillary canines remains unknown, multiple factors may play a role. Primary causes that have been linked to impacted maxillary canines include the rate at which roots resorb in the deciduous teeth, any trauma to the deciduous tooth bud, disruption of the normal eruption sequence, lack of space, rotation of tooth buds, premature root closure and canine eruption into a cleft. Secondary reasons include febrile diseases, endocrine disturbances and Vitamin D deficiency. Impacted canine can be concomitant with other conditions.

Except the third molars, maxillary canines are among the last teeth to erupt. They usually develop high in the maxilla and need to travel a considerable distance before they erupt.

Local factors may also play a role in canine impaction, and these include:

1. A longer eruption path that the tooth has to traverse from its point of development to normal occlusion [1].
2. Thick palatal bone and mucoperiosteum, which can obstruct eruption of palatally oriented canines.
3. More developed root at the time of eruption, which may minimize the eruptive force.
4. Disorder of the primary canine can affect the position of the permanent one. This is because the crown of the developing permanent canine lies just palatal to the apex of the primary canine root.

**Electronic Supplementary Material** The online version of this chapter (https://doi.org/10.1007/978-981-15-1346-6_15) contains supplementary material, which is available to authorized users.

G. Varghese (✉)
Principal, Professor and Head, Department of Oral and Maxillofacial Surgery, Pushpagiri College of Dental Sciences, Tiruvalla, Kerala, India


K. Bonanthaya et al. (eds.), *Oral and Maxillofacial Surgery for the Clinician*, https://doi.org/10.1007/978-981-15-1346-6_15

5. Canines are more susceptible to environmental influences as they are among the last teeth to erupt (except the third molars).
6. Limited space for eruption as the canines erupt between teeth which are already in occlusion. The second molar may further reduce the space.
7. The permanent canine has a greater mesiodistal width than the primary canine.

## 15.3 Classification of Impacted Maxillary Canines

### 15.3.1 The Following Classification Suggested by Archer (1975) [2] is Very Practical

*Class I: Impacted canines in the palate.*
1. Horizontal
2. Vertical
3. Semivertical

- *Class II: Impacted canines located on the labial surface.*
  1. Horizontal
  2. Vertical
  3. Semivertical
- *Class III: Impacted canine located labially and palatally*—crown on one side and the root on the other side.
- *Class IV: Impacted canine located within the alveolar process*—usually vertically between the incisor and first premolar.
- *Class V: Impacted canine in edentulous maxilla*—Impacted canine can be in unusual positions like inverted position.

### 15.3.2 Field and Ackerman (1935) Classification [3]

*Maxillary Canines*
1. Labial position
   - Crown in intimate relation with incisors.
   - Crown well above apices of incisors.
2. Palatal position
   - Crown near surface.
   - Crown deeply embedded in close relation to apices of incisors.
3. Intermediate position
   - Crown between lateral incisor and first premolar roots.
   - Crown above these teeth with crown labially placed and root palatally placed or vice versa.
4. Unusual position
   - In nasal or antral wall.
   - In infraorbital region.

*Mandibular Canines*
1. Labial
   - Vertical
   - Oblique
   - Horizontal
2. Aberrant
   - At inferior border.
   - On the opposite side.
   - Mental protuberance.

**Complications that Can Occur Due to Canine Impaction**

1. Adjacent teeth may undergo internal or external resorption.
2. Change in alignment or proclination of lateral incisor (Fig. 15.1).
3. Odontogenic Cyst formation.
4. Development of Odontogenic Tumour.

The clinical signs that indicate an impacted maxillary canine include:

1. Prolonged retention of the primary canine [4] and or delayed eruption of the permanent canine.
2. Lack of a bulge on the labial side of the alveolus in the canine region.
3. Delayed eruption of the lateral incisor, or an incisor that is tipped distally or migrated.
4. Loss of vitality or increased mobility of the permanent incisors.

## 15.4 Radiographic Localization of Impacted Canine

The position of the impacted canine may be determined by visual inspection, palpating intraorally or by radiography.

Radiographic examinations may include periapical X-ray with cone shift technique, occlusal radiography, anteroposterior and lateral radiographic views of maxilla, OPG, CBCT, CT scan.

### 15.4.1 Radiographic Features to Consider

- Labiopalatal position of the canine relative to the erupted teeth—either labial, palatal or directly above the teeth.
- Orientation of the long axis of the canine in relation to the adjacent teeth.
- Size and shape of the canine, and its root pattern.
- Status and health of the adjacent teeth.

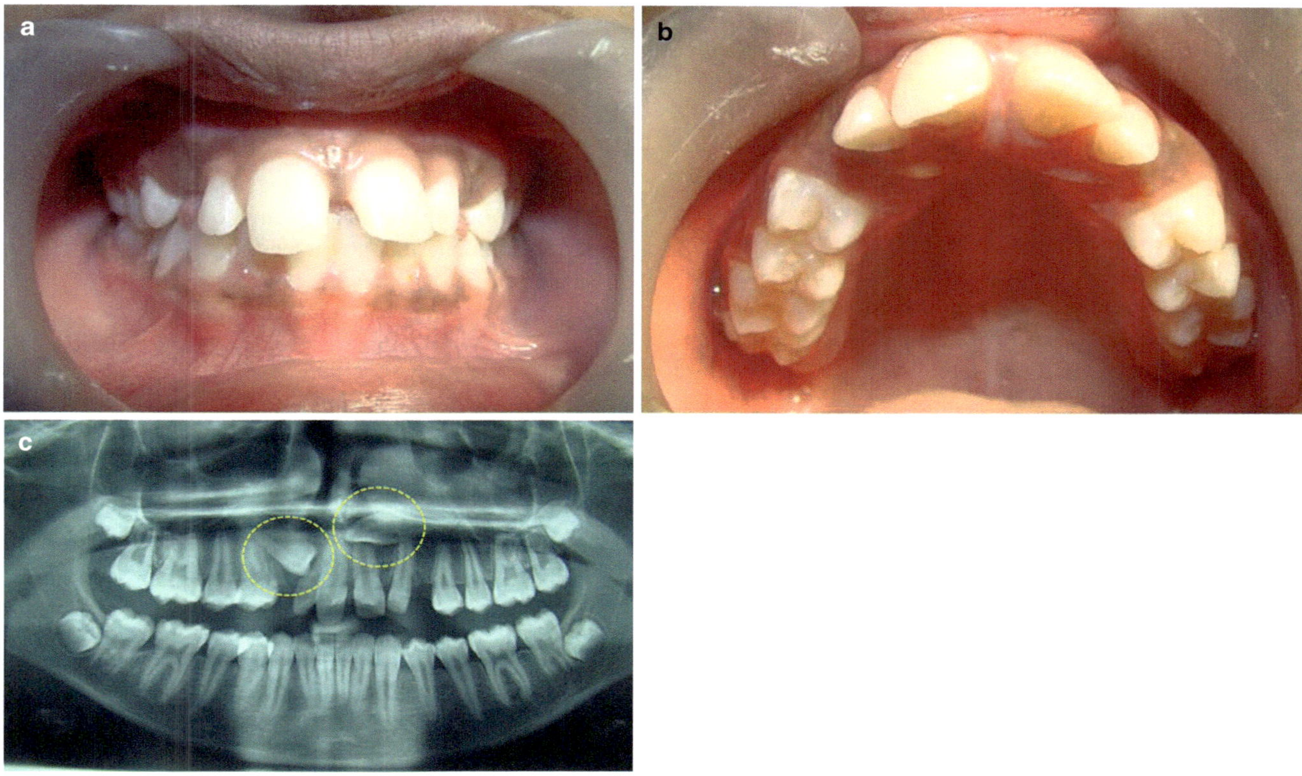



**Fig. 15.1** Bilaterally impacted maxillary canine causing proclination and spacing of incisors. (**a**) Frontal view, (**b**) Occlusal view, (**c**) OPG showing impacted canines (yellow circle)

- Location and orientation of the crown and root in relation to the adjacent teeth, in three dimensions (vertical, mesiodistal and labiopalatal).
- Presence of associated cyst, odontomas or supernumerary teeth.
- Curvature of the root of impacted tooth.

Going into the fine details of localization of canine is beyond the purview of this chapter. It is an area which has been extensively studied with regard to the various imaging modalities and their advantages.

Various radiographic methods are considered routinely by practitioners for localization. A few of them are mentioned below.

#### 15.4.1.1 Parallax

This was first introduced by Clark [5], and involves two radiographs taken at two different horizontal angles, but using the same vertical angulation. Owing to parallax error, the object that is further away appears to travel in the same direction as the direction in which the tube was shifted. The object nearer to the tube appears to move in the opposite direction [Same Lingual Opposite Buccal (SLOB) rule]. This technique can also be performed with differing vertical angulations (vertical parallax). There are different combinations of parallax techniques:

1. Clark technique: Two intra-oral periapical radiographs are taken using different horizontal angulations [5].
2. Southall and Gravely technique: One maxillary anterior occlusal radiograph and one maxillary lateral occlusal radiograph are taken [6].
3. Rayne technique: This involves differing vertical angulations, with one periapical and one maxillary anterior occlusal radiograph being taken [7].
4. Keur technique: This is also a vertical parallax method, in which one panoramic and one maxillary anterior occlusal radiograph are taken [8].

#### 15.4.1.2 OPG

1. Magnification

   The magnification technique depends on a principle known as 'image size distortion'. According to this, for a given 'focal spot'—film distance, objects that are far away from the film will appear more magnified than those that are closer to the film. This has been applied using

OPGs for the impacted canine. (Wolf and Matilla [9]; Fox et al. [10]). In the OPG, if a canine looks bigger as compared to the adjacent teeth in the arch or the contralateral canine, it is probably located closer to the tube (palatal). If it is relatively small, it is located further away from the tube (labial). This method can be applied effectively only when the canine is not rotated, does not touch the incisor root and the incisor is not tipped [11].

Kuftinec [12, 13] asserts that if the canine's cusp is mesially at the root of the lateral incisor, the impaction is probably palatal but if the cuspid is found overlapping the distal half, a labial impaction is more probable.

2. Chaushu et al. [14] stated that a single panoramic radiograph could be used to assess the mesiodistal dimensions of the canine and the ipsilateral central incisors. The canine would be palatally placed if the ratio of the sizes between the canine and the central incisors is 1.15 or greater.
3. Katsnelson [15] et al. suggested a technique that used a horizontal line that extended from the mesiobuccal cusp tip of the right and left maxillary first molars, along the long axis of the impacted canines. The degree of inclination of the canine as compared to the midline is recorded. If the inclination is greater than 65°, the canine is 26.6 times more likely to be buccally placed than palatal.

#### 15.4.1.3 Computed Tomography

Computed Tomography readily provides excellent tissue contrast and eliminates blurring and overlapping of adjacent teeth [16]. However, since CT exposes the patient to a high dose of radiation, the unfavourable relationship between cost and benefit to the patient determines its use only in particular cases, such as in the presence of craniofacial deformities. CT makes it possible to easily identify the position of impacted teeth and evaluate precisely the location of nearby anatomical structures and identify any root resorption in the adjacent teeth.

#### 15.4.1.4 Cone Beam CT

Conventional CT imaging is associated with high radiation dose and high cost. Cone Beam Computed Tomography (CBCT) have been used instead for localization of the impacted canine. As CBCT uses cone-shaped radiation, the radiation dose is significantly reduced, and a high spatial resolution is achieved [17, 18].

**Reason for Surgical Removal of Impacted Canines**

- Associated cyst/tumour with the impacted tooth.
- Development of caries.
- For prosthetic replacement.
- For orthodontic reasons.
- Resorption of roots in adjacent tooth.
- Malalignment of adjacent teeth.
- Pain referred to other regions.

**Treatment Options for Impacted Canines**

1. Observation.
2. Surgical exposure.
3. Surgical exposure and orthodontic traction.
4. Surgical removal.

## 15.5 Modalities of Management of Impacted Canine

The impacted maxillary canine may be managed by several different techniques. The chosen method would depend on the degree of impaction, age of the patient, stage of root formation, presence of any associated pathology, dental condition of the adjacent teeth, position of the tooth, patient's willingness to undergo orthodontic treatment, available facilities for specialized treatment and patient's general physical condition.

1. *Extraction of primary canine.*
   This method is as an interceptive form of management. Extraction of the deciduous tooth may be considered when the maxillary permanent canine is not palpable in its normal position and the radiographic examination confirms the presence of an impacted canine. However, this treatment will not necessarily correct the problem. Surgical intervention may be required if the permanent canine fails to erupt within one year of the deciduous extraction.
2. *No treatment—Leave the tooth in situ.*
   In some asymptomatic cases, no treatment may be required apart from regular clinical and radiographic follow-up. There is a small risk of follicular cystic degeneration, although the incidence of this is unknown. Rarely, odontogenic tumours may develop in relation to the impacted tooth.

3. *Surgical exposure of the tooth.*
   This technique may be used in cases where there is enough space for the canine to erupt, and where the root formation is incomplete. Surgically exposing the crown of the canine may allow it to come into position by normal eruptive forces.
4. *Surgical exposure and orthodontically assisted eruption.*
   This is the most appropriate approach for an impacted canine. For attempting this technique, the case must fulfil the following criteria:
   (a) The impacted canine must be favourably positioned.
   (b) The patient must be compliant with both surgery and long term orthodontics.
   (c) The patient must not have associated medical problems.
5. *Surgical removal of the impacted tooth.*
   This technique is preferred for teeth that are in an unfavourable position, and which are likely to cause problems in the future. It may also be considered when a patient is not willing for orthodontic treatment or cannot afford it, even if the impacted tooth is in a favourable position.
6. *Surgical repositioning/Autotransplantation.*
   Impacted canines that are malpositioned, but have a favourable root pattern (without hooks or sharp curves) may be considered for autotransplantation into the dental arch. This may be done by utilizing the socket of deciduous canine or first premolar, depending on the amount of space needed and available.

### 15.5.1 Surgical Exposure of Impacted Canines

**Surgical Exposure Techniques**

- Gingivectomy and exposure of crown/ surgical window.
- Closed eruption method (Repositioned flap) [19, 20].
- Apically repositioned flap technique (window flap) [19, 20].
- Tunnel Technique [21].

Various studies have compared the effects of the different exposure techniques in the periodontium; however, a consensus is yet to be reached [22–24].

Chapokas et al. in 2012 have brought out a useful classification of maxillary canine impactions based on which the exposure technique may be decided [25].

#### 15.5.1.1 Procedure

1. Palatally positioned canine
   The location of the crown of the impacted canine may be determined by radiographs. The possible position of the crown is determined, and a cruciform incision made over this. Along the incision arms, flaps are elevated on four sides so that the crown is uncovered. The flaps may be excised. If there is haemorrhage, it can usually be controlled by pressure application. If there is any bone overlying the crown, it is removed and sharp edges are smoothened so that the crown lies in a saucer-shaped bony cavity. To prevent soft tissue regrowth over the exposed crown, a pack (such as a perio pack or roller gauze impregnated with iodoform or antibiotics) may be inserted or sutured in place. Another alternative technique is to use a crevicular incision, expose palatally and place orthodontic brackets as shown in Fig. 15.2.
2. Labially positioned canines
   Any one of the following techniques may be employed depending on the depth and position of the impacted tooth:
   (a) *Creating a surgical window/Gingivectomy:* This is done if the tooth lies just underneath the gingiva. The overlying soft tissue is simply excised to expose the crown.

   If the impacted canine is close to the alveolar crest, or if a broad band of keratinized tissue covers the tooth, a surgical window may be created. Gingivectomy may be done when it is possible to uncover at least one

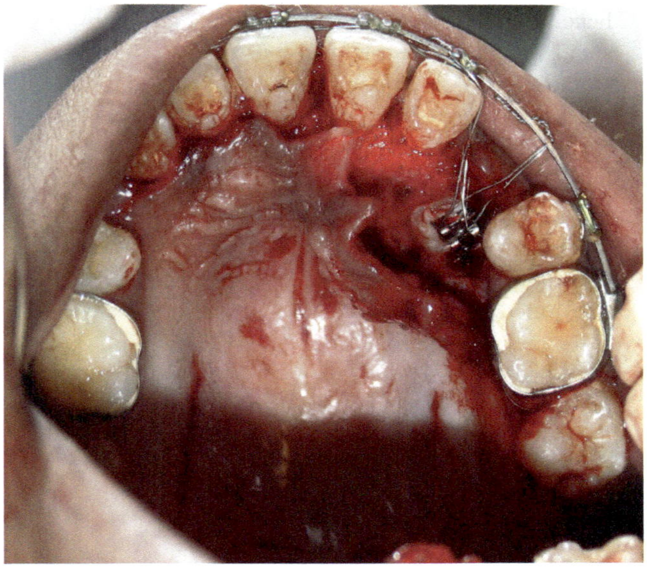



**Fig. 15.2** Exposure of a palatally impacted canine

half to 2/3 of the crown, leaving at least 3 mm of gingival collar. Usually in these cases, the tip of the impacted tooth lies near the cemento-enamel junction of the adjacent tooth (Fig. 15.3).

(b) *Closed eruption technique:* If the impacted canine lies in the middle of the alveolus, near the nasal spine, or high in the buccal vestibule or the palate, this technique may be indicated (Vermette et al., 1995) [19]. A flap is first elevated over the area of the impacted tooth. If necessary, the crown is then exposed after removal of the overlying bone. An orthodontic bracket may be bonded to the crown and to the bracket, a traction wire is affixed. The flap is then sutured, with the traction wire left exposed to the oral cavity. Sufficient time is given for the flap to undergo initial healing. Later on, the traction wire may be connected to an archwire and optimal force may be applied as needed for the tooth to erupt. Drawback of this technique is that the tooth cannot be inspected directly once the flap has been sutured (Fig. 15.4).

(c) *Apically positioned flap:* In cases where the cervical portion of the crown does not lie within the attached gingiva, removal of the soft tissue may cause the attached gingiva to be lost. Later on, this can lead to periodontal problems. In such a case, it may be better to use an apically repositioned flap.

The flap is designed in such a way that vertical incisions are placed on the soft tissue at the distal side of the lateral incisor and at the mesial side of the first premolar. Then a horizontal incision is made that links the two vertical incisions. Subsequently, after locating the crown of the impacted tooth, the flap may be sutured back into at the apical end, while the crown is exposed to the oral cavity (Fig. 15.5a, b).

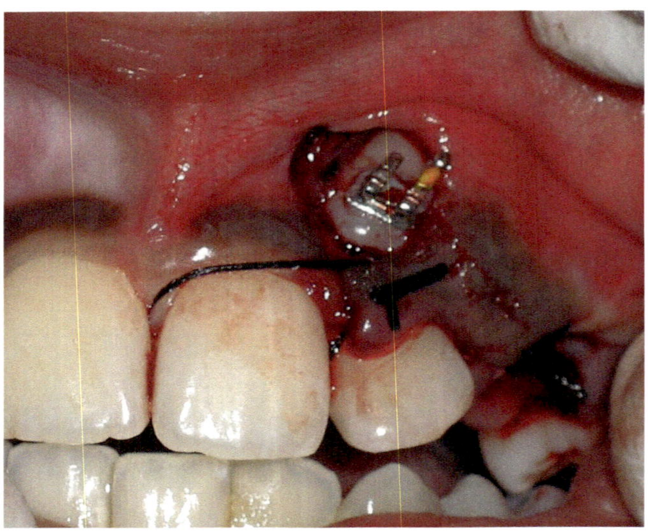



**Fig. 15.3** Exposure of labially impacted canine by surgical window technique

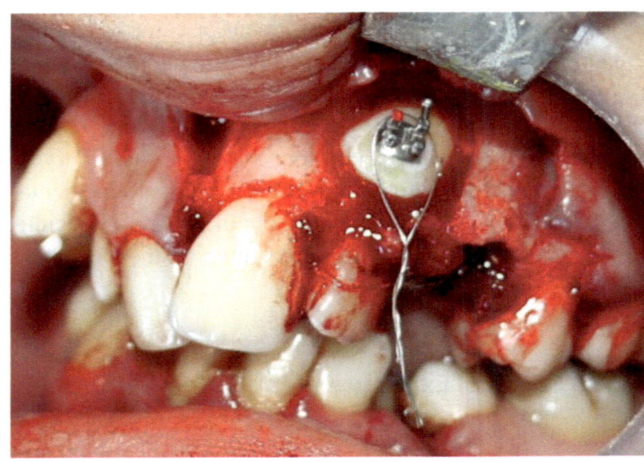



**Fig. 15.4** Closed eruption technique for labially impacted canine

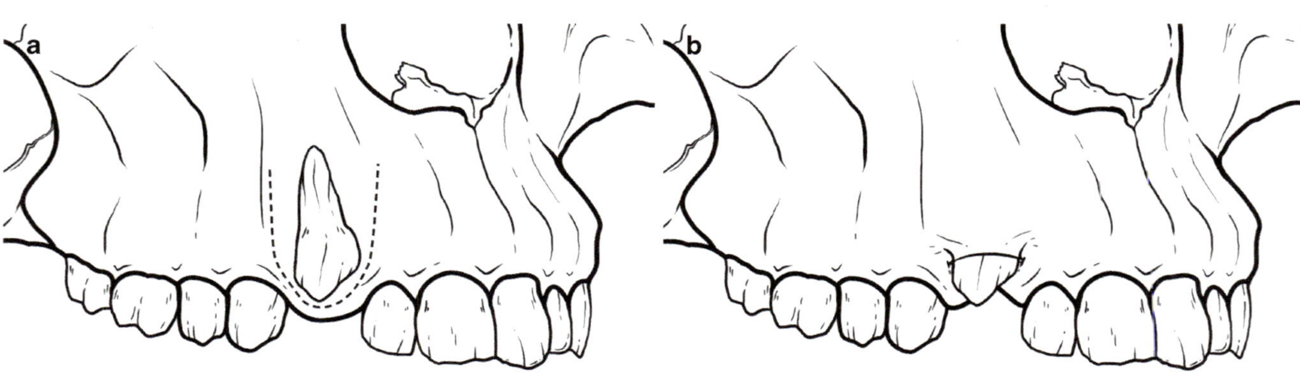




**Fig. 15.5** (**a**, **b**) Schematic diagram of apically positioned flap for exposure of a labially positioned crown. (**a**) Incision, (**b**) Suturing

### 15.5.2 Surgical Removal of Palatally Impacted Maxillary Canines

If the impacted maxillary canine is in an unfavourable position, and cannot be brought into normal occlusion, it should be removed earlier rather than later. This is because increasing age increases the difficulty of the procedure, and by removing early, damage to the adjacent structures may be minimized.

#### 15.5.2.1 Surgical Anatomy

The impacted canine is separated by a thin layer of the bone from the maxillary sinus and nasal cavity (Fig. 15.6). Infrequently, this bone may be absent. In these cases, the risk of tooth or root displacement into the maxillary sinus is high. It is also not uncommon to have the likelihood of creating a communication between the oral cavity and antrum, which may lead to post-operative nasal bleeding.

#### 15.5.2.2 Procedure (Fig. 15.7a–d) (Fig. 15.8a, b)

The incision is initiated in the gingival margin on the palatal side from the ipsilateral first premolar and, depending on the position of the impacted tooth, is extended up to the contralateral lateral incisor or premolar.

In cases of unilateral impaction, instead of extending the incision to the contralateral side, a vertical incision may be given in the mid palatal region. In situations where there is bilateral canine impaction and both teeth are close to the midline, the incision should always extend between the first or second premolars of both sides (Fig. 15.8). Elevation of a single palatal flap not only avoids sloughing but also provides adequate visualization. This method may pose a risk of haemorrhage from the nasopalatine vessels which can, however, be controlled by pressure pack or by electrocautery.

The mucoperiosteal flap is then reflected to reveal the palatal bone and the tooth. Division of the nasopalatine vessels and nerve may be done for further exposure.

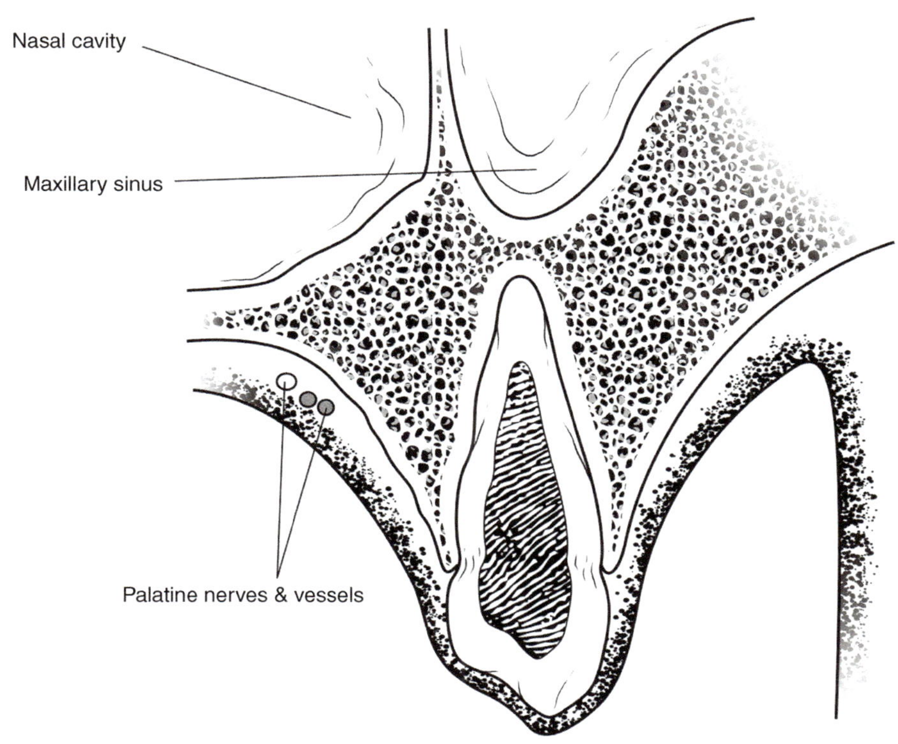


Fig. 15.6 Surgical anatomy of maxillary canine area. Note the close relationship of the root of the impacted canine to the floor of the maxillary sinus and nose

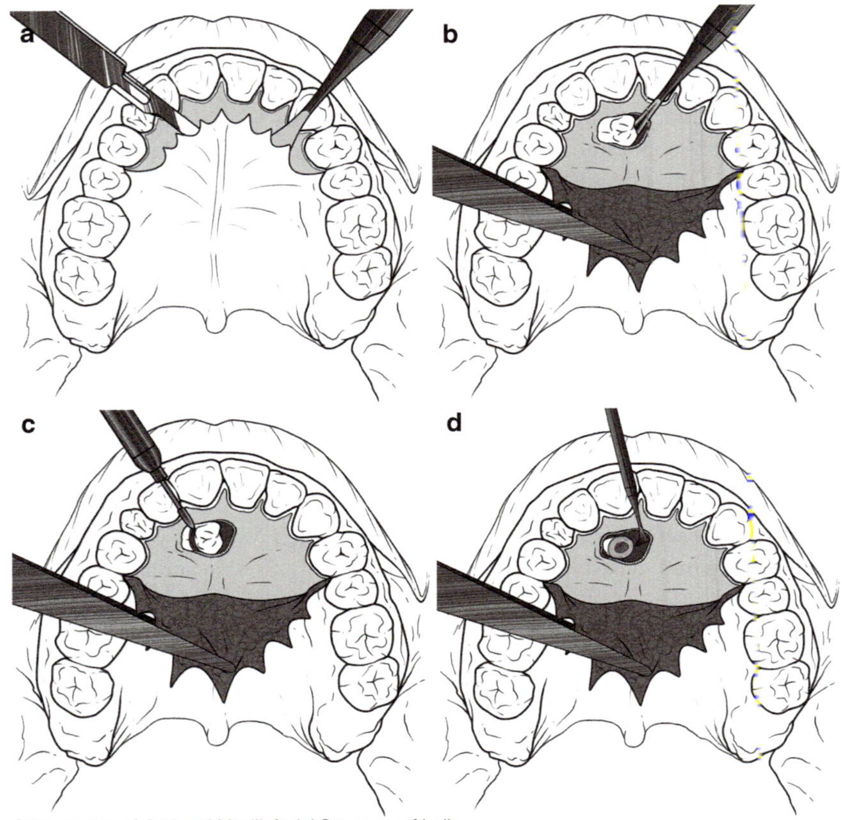


**Fig. 15.7** (**a–d**) Schematic diagram showing steps in the surgical removal of palatally positioned impacted maxillary canine (**a**) Reflection of the flap, (**b**) Removal of bone to expose the crown, (**c**) Sectioning of the crown, (**d**) Removal of the root

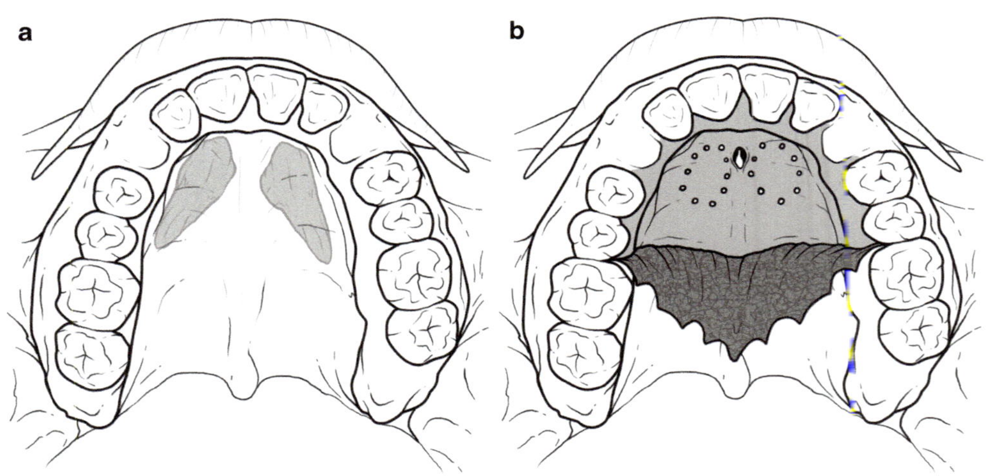


**Fig. 15.8** (**a**, **b**) Palatal flap elevation for exposure of bilaterally impacted palatally positioned canine. (**a**) Flap outlined from the second premolar on one side to the second premolar of the opposite side, (**b**) Following reflection of the mucoperiosteal flap, multiple drill holes are placed in the bone overlying the crown. These drill holes are then connected together to remove the bone thereby exposing the crown

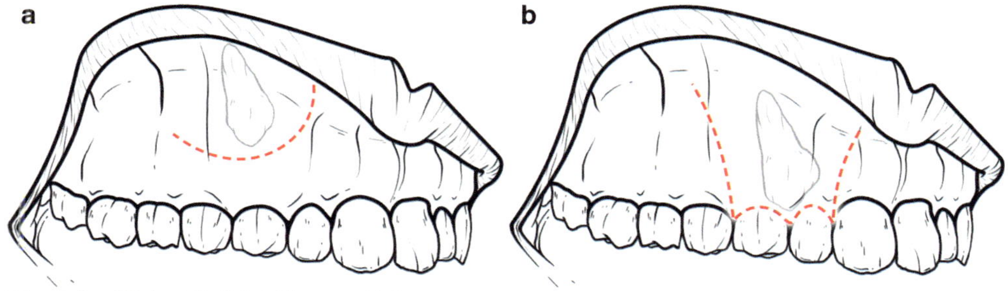


**Fig. 15.9** (**a**, **b**) Incisions for removal of labially placed canine. (**a**) Semilunar incision, (**b**) Trapezoidal (3 sided) incision

The crown of the tooth may be visible occasionally, or a bulge may be felt. Bone around the area is removed with bur, taking care to protect the roots of the adjacent teeth from damage. Once adequate bone is removed, a groove is prepared on the mesial side and an elevator may be inserted into it. An attempt is made to luxate the tooth. Once the crown is moved out, it may be grasped using an upper anterior or premolar forceps. Dislodgement of the root apex may require a certain amount of torsion, as this is often curved.

If the tooth is resistant to elevation, more bone removal is done to enlarge the opening. Tooth sectioning (odontotomy) may be carried out using a straight fissure bur if there is any obstruction to movement (Fig. 15.7c, d). The crown portion is removed first. A portion of the root may then be visualized. If not, bone is removed to expose the root. A hole is created in the root and an elevator is used to engage this and remove the root.

Meticulous debridement and curettage is done to remove the tooth follicle. Saline irrigation is used to clear out bone debris. The flap is replaced and sutured into position. It is held in close contact with the palatal bone by pressing a gauze pack with the dorsum of the tongue, for an hour or two. Healing follows without any complications.

To decrease chances of hematoma formation, a prefabricated clear acrylic plate may be used to cover the palate post-operatively.

### 15.5.3 Surgical Removal of Labially Positioned Impacted Maxillary Canine (Fig. 15.9a, b) (Video 15.1)

#### 15.5.3.1 Incision

A semilunar incision (Fig. 15.9a) is usually used, and it provides good exposure. The lower part of the incision must lie at least 0.5 cm away from the gingival margin.

For cases that are deeply impacted, triangular flaps (2 sided) or trapezoidal flaps (3 sided) may be used, with incisions along the gingival margin and relieving incisions. (Fig. 15.9b).

#### 15.5.3.2 Operative Procedure (Fig. 15.10a–f) (Fig. 15.11a–i)

The mucoperiosteal flap is elevated and the bone with the tooth bulge is exposed. Using a bur, a window is created over the crown prominence. The window is enlarged so that the entire crown is exposed, taking care not to cause damage to the adjacent tooth roots. The tooth is then luxated using an elevator.

If there is any resistance during elevation, the tooth must be sectioned, so that the fragments can be removed easily. If three fragments are created, the middle one may be removed first, and the remaining two fragments may be elevate using the resultant space (Fig. 15.10a–f).

The area is carefully debrided and checked for a residual follicle, which must be removed. The mucoperiosteal flap is repositioned and sutured (Fig. 15.11a–i) shows the localisation and surgical removal of a labially positioned impacted maxillary canine.

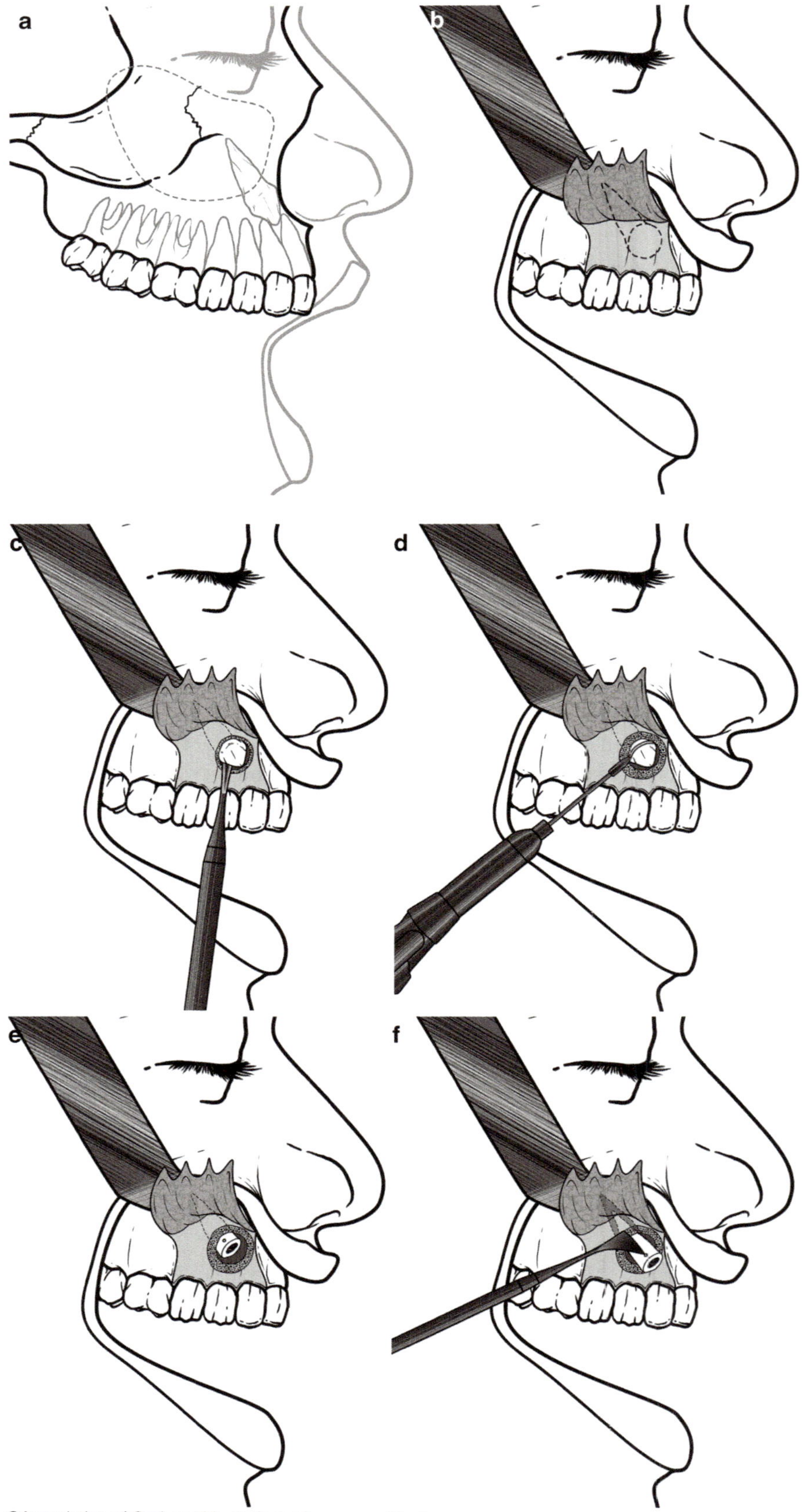


**Fig. 15.10** (**a**–**f**): Schematic diagram showing surgical removal of labially impacted maxillary canine. (**a**) Impacted maxillary canine. Note the relationship of the cuspid to the roots of the adjacent teeth, nasal cavity and maxillary sinus. (**b**) trapezoidal mucoperiosteal flap reflected. (**c**) Drill holes placed in the cortical plate overlying the crown so as to expose the crown, after the full exposure of the crown, elevator is applied beneath the crown to mobilize the tooth, (**d**) If the tooth is resistant to elevation, the crown is sectioned using bur and it is removed, (**e**) Cavity created following removal of crown, (**f**) The root is moved into the space created by the removal of the crown and it is then removed

### 15.5.4 Removal of Maxillary Canine in an Intermediate Position (Fig. 15.12a–h)

The impacted maxillary canine may be located in an intermediate position, with the root oriented labially and the crown palatally, or vice versa. Removing a maxillary canine in the intermediate position may be challenging and may take more time as it may require a labial and palatal approach. The risk of damaging adjacent teeth is also higher with teeth in an intermediate position. CBCT or CT scan is very useful to locate the exact position of such a tooth. Figure 15.12a–h illustrates the steps involved in removing an impacted canine that has its root oriented labially and crown palatally.

**Complications of removal of maxillary canines:**

- Perforation through the nasal or antral mucosa.
- Tooth or root displacement into the maxillary sinus
- Haemorrhage
- Adjacent tooth root damage
- Fracture of apical third of the root of the impacted tooth.

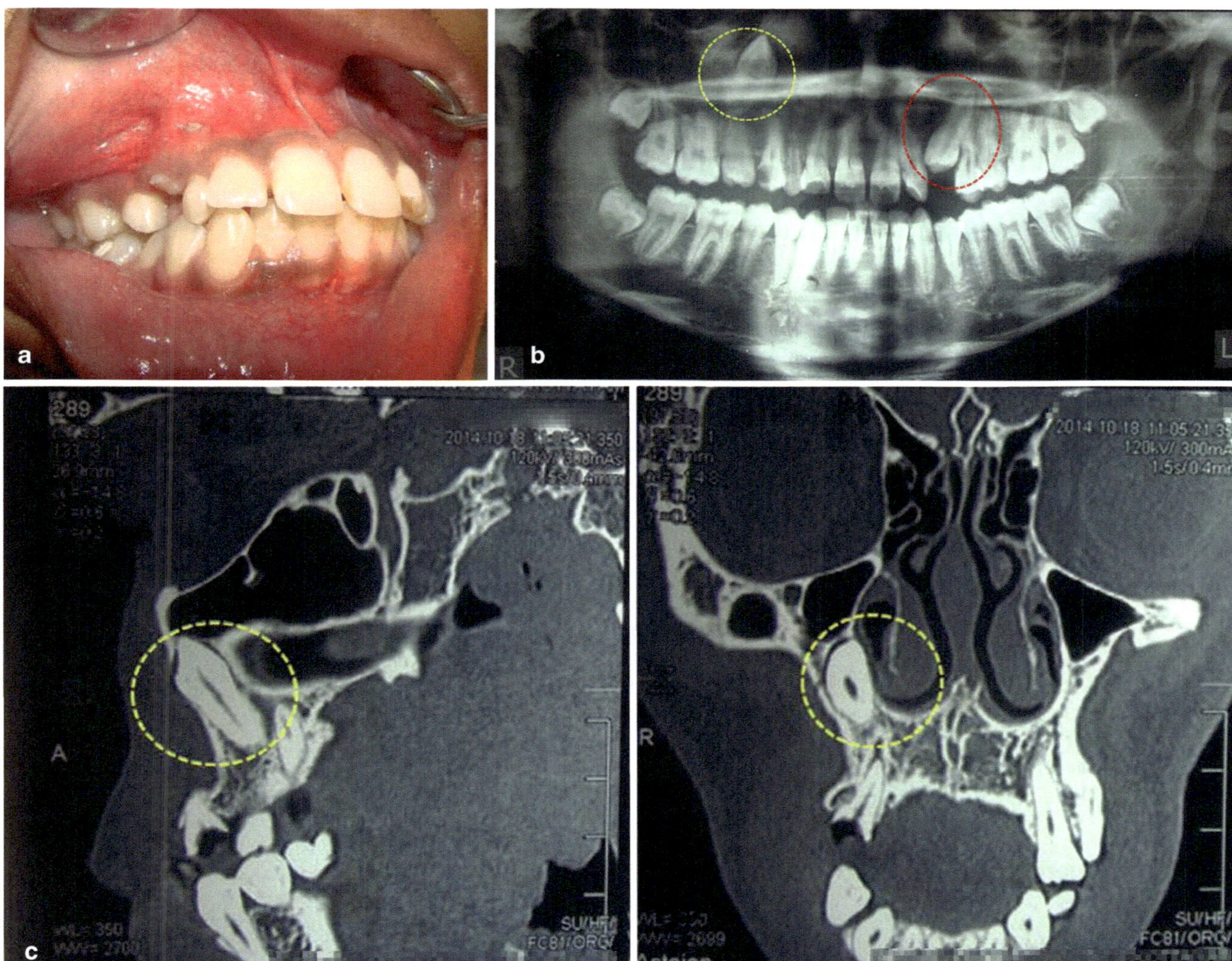


Fig. 15.11 (a–l) show the clinical and radiographic images of the steps in removing a labially impacted canine by odontectomy. Bilaterally impacted maxillary canines (**a**) Intra-oral right lateral view, (**b**) OPG showing 13 in inverted position (yellow circle) with close proximity to maxillary sinus and impacted 23 (in red circle). CT of the same patient showing the relationship of the inverted 13 (yellow circle) to adjacent structures such as maxillary antrum, nasal floor and nearby teeth. (**c**) Sagittal view, (**d**) Coronal view, (**e**) Axial view, (**f**) 3-D view. Steps in the surgical removal of impacted 13. (**g**) Incision marked, (**h**) Mucoperiosteal flap reflected, (**i**) Tooth division done, (**j**) Tooth removed and debridement (**k**) Suturing completed, (**l**) Specimen

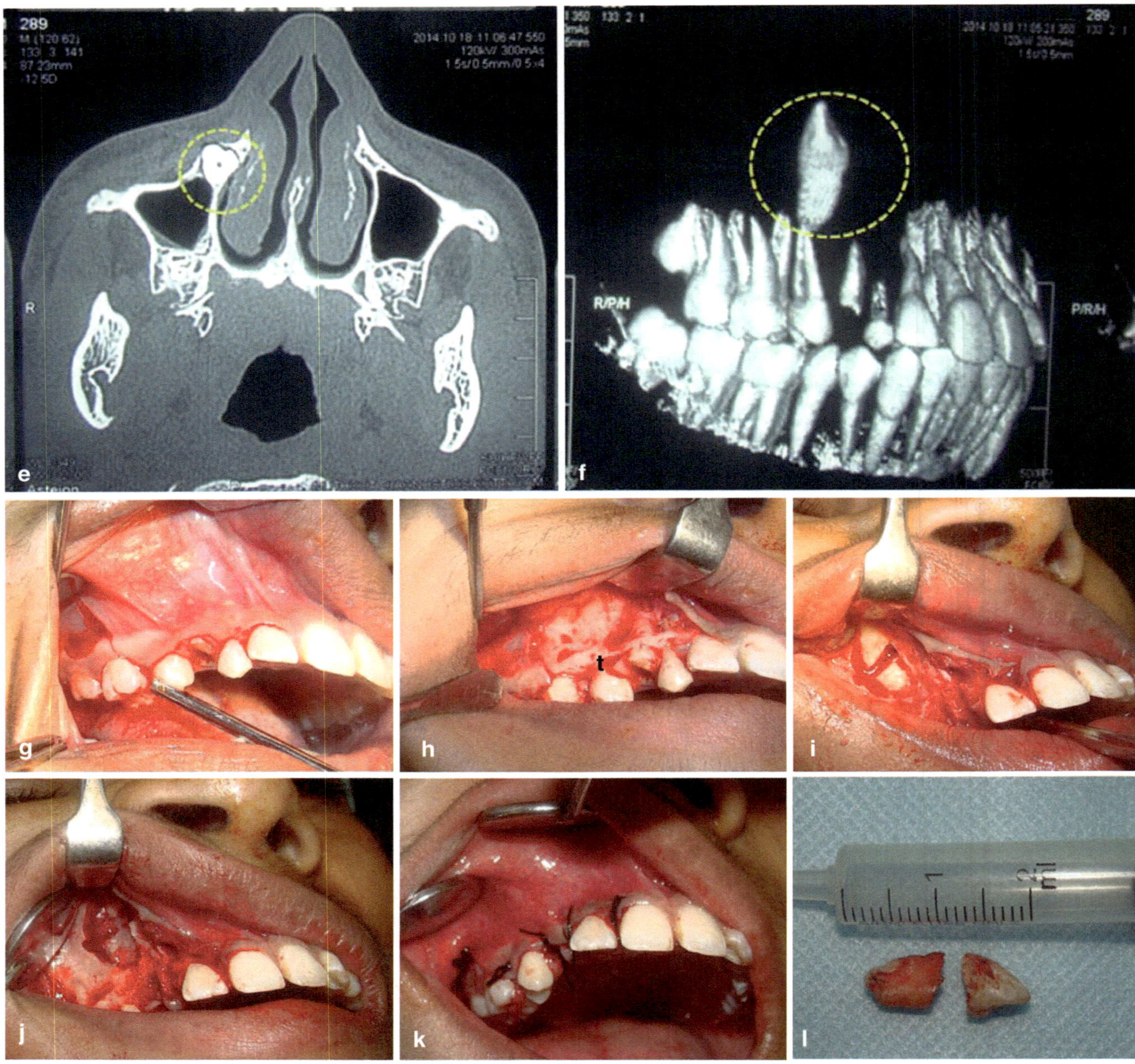




**Fig. 15.11** (continued)

### 15.5.5 Management of Impacted Mandibular Canines

Impacted mandibular canines are not as frequent as maxillary canines, and are usually found in a labial position. However, they may occasionally migrate to the mental protuberance or even the lower border of mandible, where they can lie in a transverse position. They can also drift to the opposite side of the mandible, referred to as transposition/transmigration of the canine. It must be noted that these teeth retain their original innervation, which is important to consider while administering local anaesthesia.

The diagnosis of an impacted mandibular canine is similar to that of the impacted maxillary canine, and it presents with similar features. These include retained primary teeth, proclination/displacement of adjacent incisors or clinical features associated with cyst formation. Impacted canines may not be associated with any symptoms, and may be accidentally discovered during the routine radiographic exami-

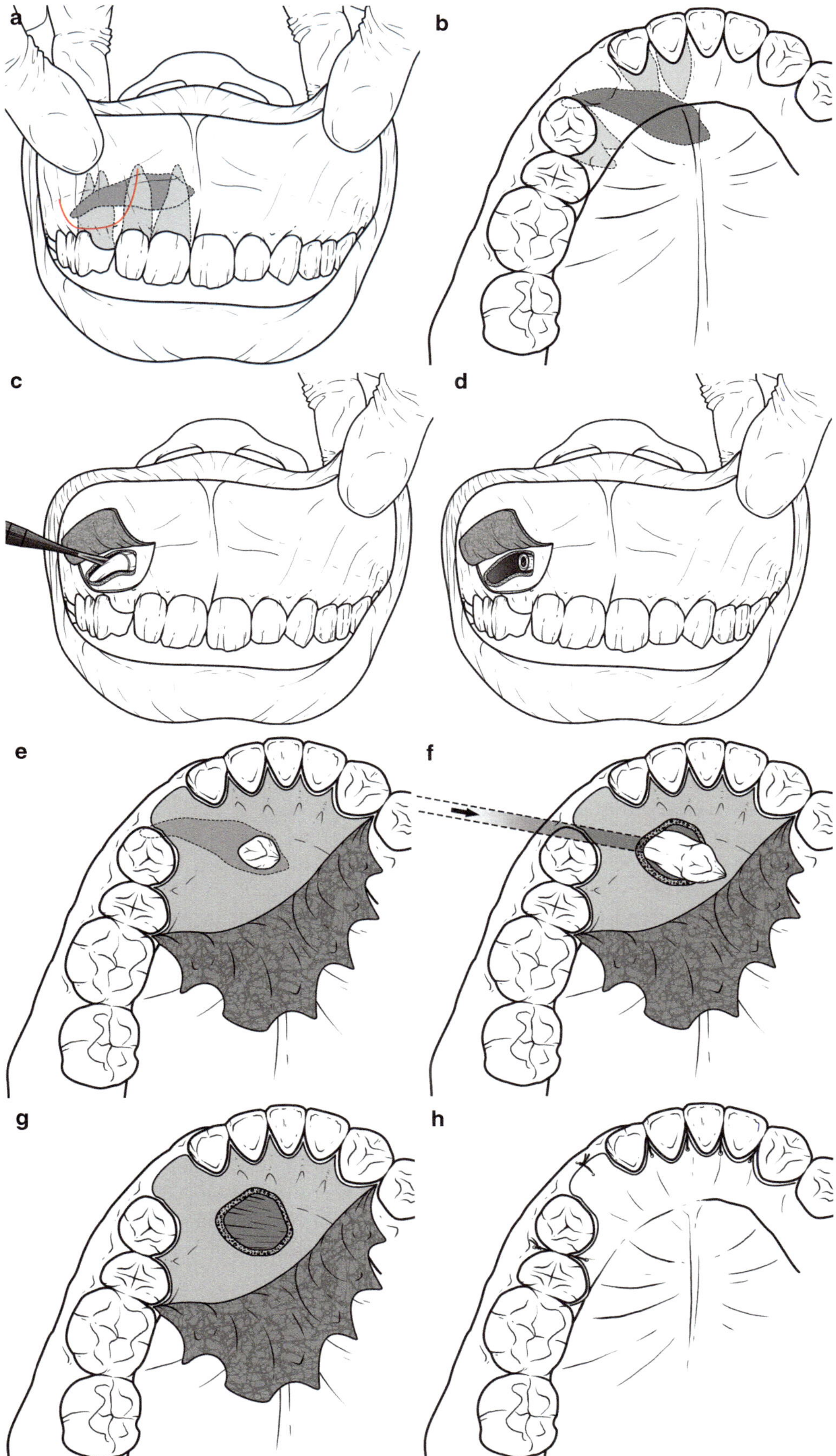


**Fig. 15.12** (**a**–**h**) Schematic diagram showing the steps in the surgical removal of impacted maxillary canine with root on the labial side and crown on the palatal side. (**a**) Outline of the impacted canine and its relation to the roots of the adjacent tooth. Note the semilunar incision marked, (**b**) Outline of the crown of the impacted canine on the palatal aspect, (**c**) Mucoperiosteum reflected on the buccal side overlying the bone to be removed and the root of the impacted tooth sectioned. An elevator is being used to dislodge the root, (**d**) Empty socket after removal of the root. (**e**) Palatal flap is outlined and reflected. Bone covering the crown of the impacted tooth is removed using bur. (**f**) Using a blunt instrument placed in the socket of the tooth on the buccal side, pressure is exerted on the cut end of the crown (see black arrow) to push the crown palatally, (**g**) Empty socket on the palatal side after removal of the crown, (**h**) Flap is replaced back and suturing completed

nation, or during the investigation of other dental conditions. Sometimes, however, these teeth can cause recurrent pain and infection.

Dalessandri et al. in 2017 opined that the most common treatment strategies for the treatment of mandibular canine impactions are surgical extraction and orthodontic traction. Surgical extraction and radiographic monitoring were suggested for transmigrant mandibular canines: The authors proposed a decision tree in order to guide practitioners through the treatment plan of impacted mandibular canines [26].

#### 15.5.5.1 Treatment Options

The impacted mandibular canine may be treated using one of the following strategies:

1. *Observation*
2. *Exposure and orthodontic repositioning*
3. *Surgical repositioning*
4. *Surgical removal of the tooth*—The impacted mandibular canine may be removed if one of the following conditions is present:
   (a) Pathology such as follicular cyst or tumour in relation to the impacted tooth.
   (b) Orthodontic reasons, such as the need to move an adjacent tooth into the area of impaction.

#### 15.5.5.2 Surgical Anatomy (Fig. 15.13)

The bone in the mandibular canine region consists of a thick lingual cortex and a thin buccal cortex. The impacted tooth usually lies mesial or distal to the actual canine region. A buccal flap must ideally be used for surgical access, as a lingual flap may not provide adequate access, and is associated with increased post-operative morbidity. While raising the buccal flap, the mentalis muscle insertion (at the mental fossa) and incisive muscle insertion (at the height of the canine alveolus) are divided.

#### 15.5.5.3 Removal of Mandibular Canine (Figs. 15.14 and 15.15)

For tooth exposure, a trapezoidal (3 sided) flap is used. Alternately, a horizontal incision may be made below the attached gingiva. If the tooth lies close to the lower border of the mandible, an additional incision may be needed extra-orally for proper exposure. As in the case of maxillary canine in the labial position, bone removal is done with bur. The tooth may be elevated in toto, or may require sectioning if resistance is met (Figs. 15.14a–h and 15.15).

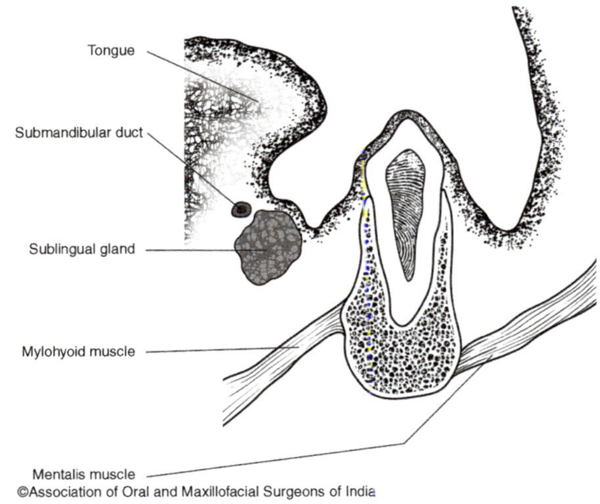


**Fig. 15.13** Surgical anatomy of mandibular canine area

#### 15.5.5.4 Complications of Surgical Removal

These Include the Following

1. *Injury/mobility of the adjacent tooth*—This can occur during bone removal, if the supporting bone of the lateral incisor is removed accidentally. This is managed by splinting the lateral incisor to the adjacent tooth.
2. *Mental nerve injury*—If the distal vertical incision is extended too far backwards and inferiorly, the mental nerve may accidentally be severed.

## 15.6 Summary

The management of impacted canine teeth requires skilful handling and careful observation on the part of an oral and maxillofacial surgeon. If any tooth is absent in the dental arch after the normal time of eruption has lapsed, the surgeon must investigate. The management of an impacted tooth is simple if the basic principles of surgery are followed appropriately for all the teeth. The case must be evaluated carefully for proper diagnosis and treatment planning. Treatment planning requires a multidisciplinary approach, and the general dental surgeon must consult with the oral and maxillofacial surgeon, orthodontist and paedodontist for achieving optimal results.

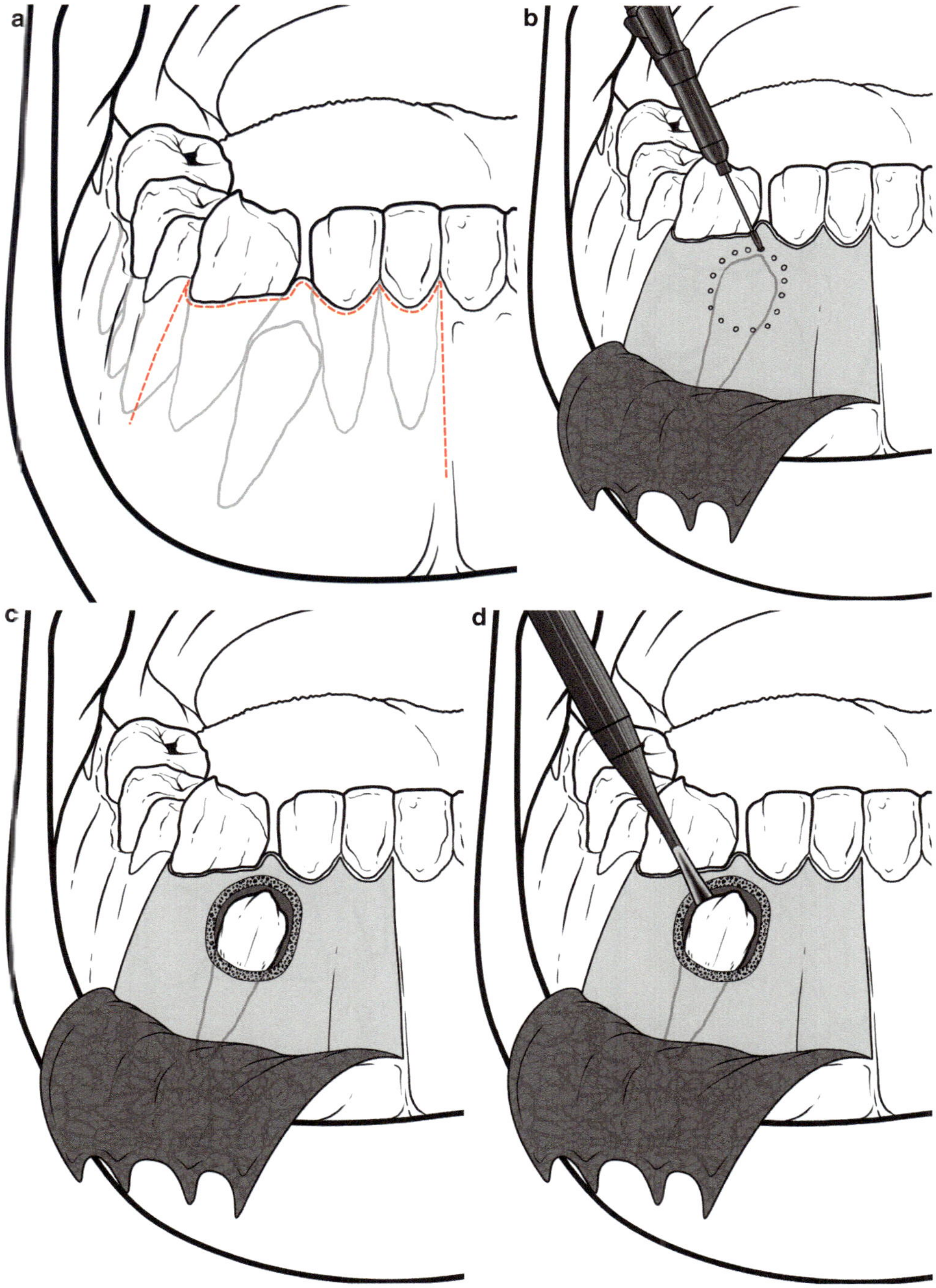


**Fig. 15.14** (**a**-**h**) Schematic diagram showing steps in the surgical removal of impacted mandibular canine. (**a**) Incision to raise a trapezoidal flap, (**b**) Mucoperiosteal flap reflected and the bone overlying the crown removed using bur and chisel, (**c**) Crown of impacted canine exposed, (**d**) Elevator is applied in an attempt to luxate the tooth. (**e**) if elevation unsuccessful tooth division is performed using bur, (**f**) Crown removed and more of the root exposed to create a purchase point on the root using bur, (**g**) Root removed using an elevator applied at the purchase point, (**h**) Closure of the incision

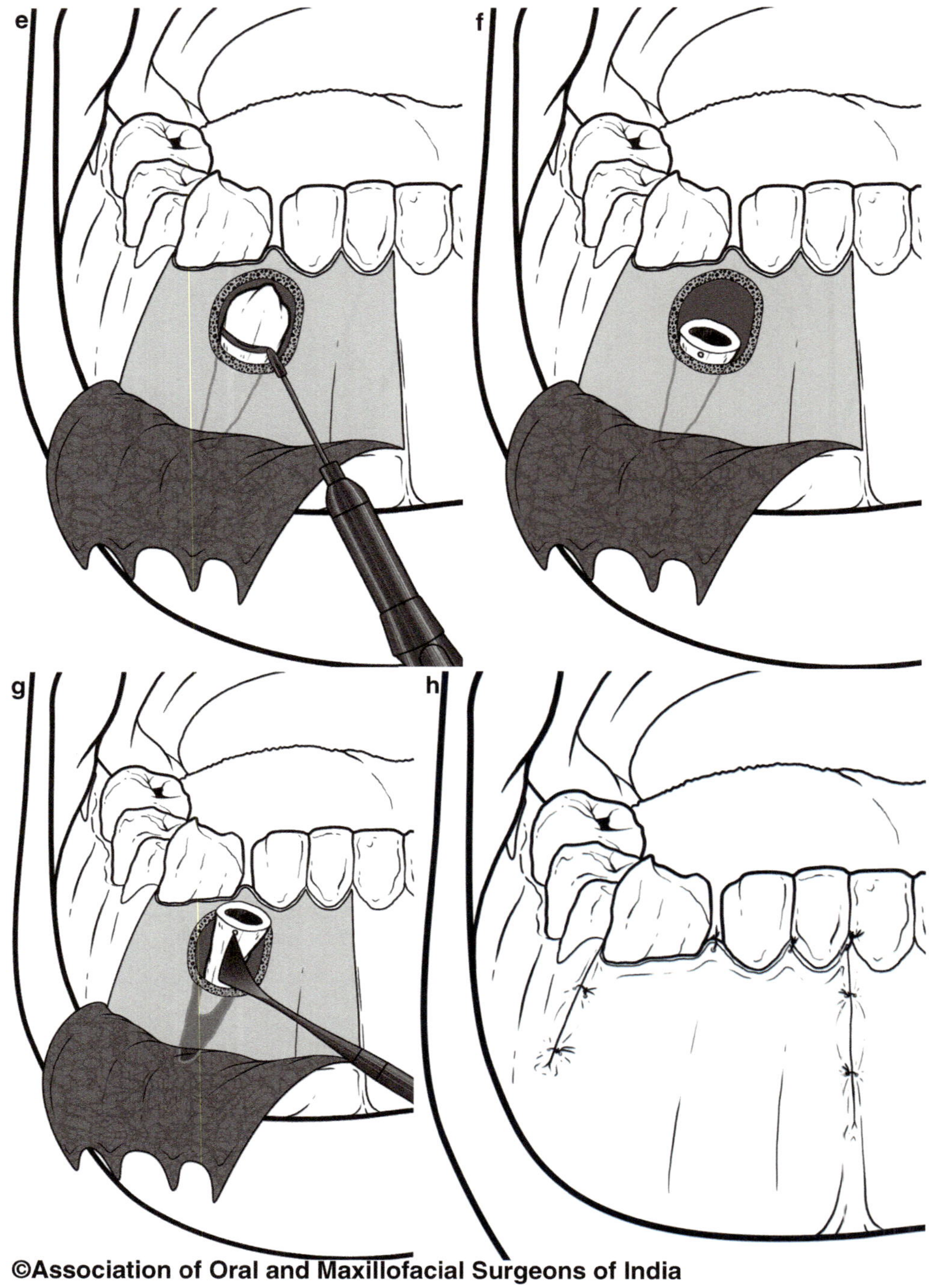


Fig. 15.14 (continued)

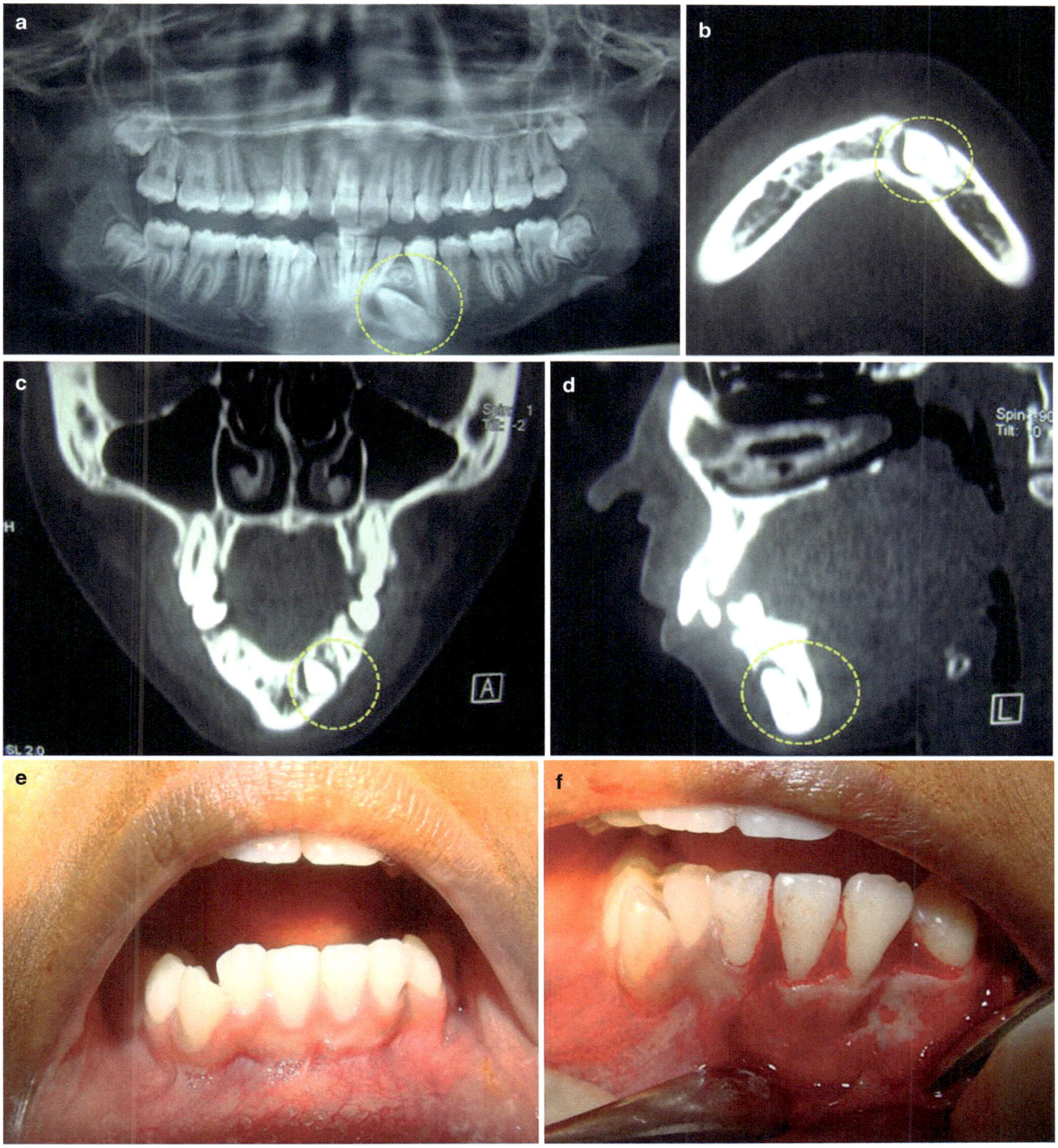


**Fig. 15.15** (**a**–**m**) Shows the clinical and radiographic images of the steps in removing a labially impacted canine by odontectomy. Impacted left mandibular canine (yellow circle) with an associated odontome (**a**) OPG showing impacted 33, (**b**) CT Axial view, (**c**) Coronal view, (**d**) Sagittal view. (**e**) Intra-oral view, (**f**) Mucoperiosteal flap reflected, (**g**) Overlying odontome exposed, (**h**) Odontome removed and crown of 33 exposed. (**i**) Sectioning of crown of 33, (**j**) Removal of crown and root of 33 followed by debridement, (**k**) Suturing completed (**l**) Specimen of 33 with follicle and odontome, (**m**) Pressure dressing applied to reduce oedema

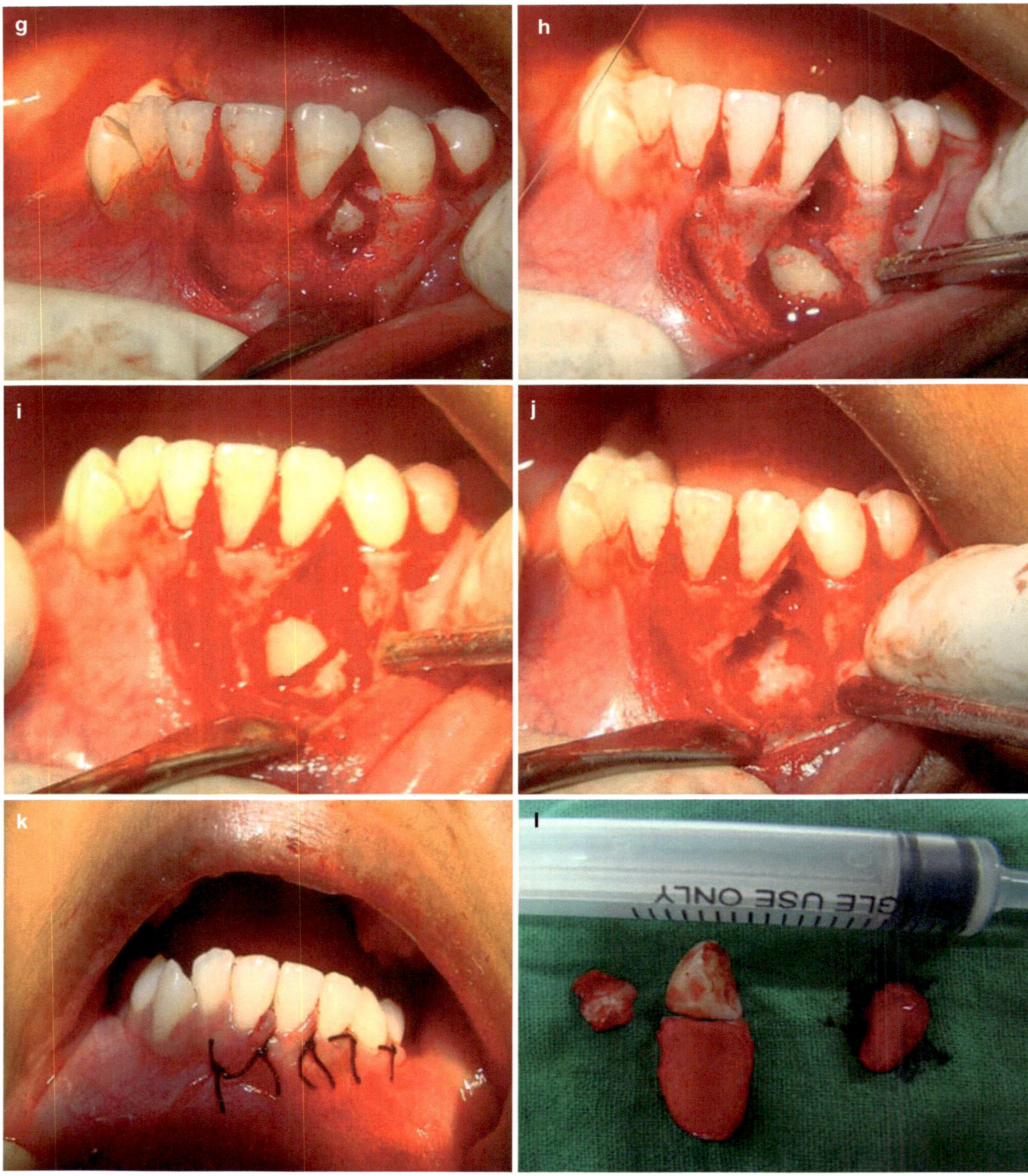


**Fig. 15.15** (continued)

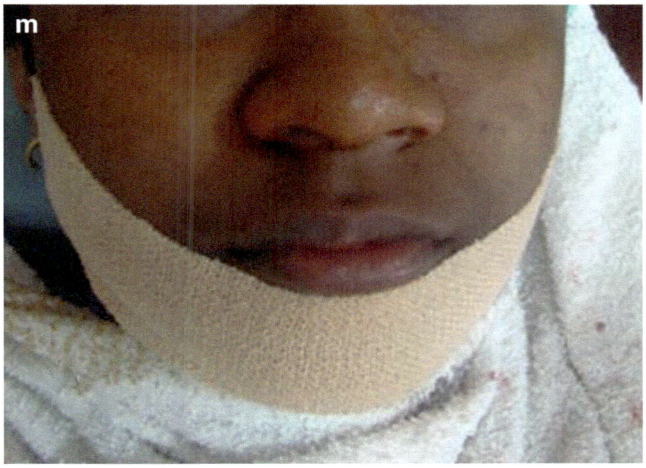


©Association of Oral and Maxillofacial Surgeons of India

**Fig. 15.15** (continued)

## References


1. Dewel B. The upper cuspid: its development and impaction. Angle Orthod. 1949;19:79–90.
2. Archer WH. Chapter 5, Oral and maxillofacial surgery, vol. 1. 5th ed. Philadelphia, PA: WB Saunders; 1975. p. 325.
3. Field HJ, Ackerman AA. The impacted upper Cuspid. Dent Cosmos. 1935;77:378.
4. Thilander B, Jakobsson SO. Local factors in impaction of maxillary canines. Acta Odontol Scand. 1968;26(2):145–68.
5. Clark C. A method of ascertaining the position of unerupted teeth by means of film radiographs. Proc R Soc Med. 1909;3:87–90.
6. Southall PJ, Gravely JF. Vertical parallax radiology to localize an object in the anterior part of the maxilla. Br J Orthod. 1989;16:79C.
7. Rayne J. The unerupted maxillary canine. Dent Pract. 1969;19:194Ñ.
8. Keur JJ. Radiographic localization techniques. Aust Dent J. 1986;31:86H.
9. Wolf JE, Mattila K. Localization of impacted maxillary canines by panoramic tomography. Dentomaxillofac Radiol. 1979;8:85–9.
10. Fox NA, Fletcher GA, Horner K. Localizing maxillary canines using dental panoramic tomography. Br Dent J. 1995;179:416.
11. Mason C, Papadakou P, Roberts GJ. The radiographic localization of impacted maxillary canines: a comparison of methods. Eur J Orthod. 2001;23:25.
12. Kuftinec MM, Shapira Y. The impacted maxillary canine: I. review of concepts. II. Clinical approaches and solution. J Dent Child. 1995 62:317–34.
13. Maverna R, Gracco A. Different diagnostic tools for the localization of impacted maxillary canines: clinical considerations. Prog Orthod. 2007;8(1):28–44.
14. Chaushu S, Chaushu G, Becker A. Reliability of a method for the localization of displaced maxillary canines using a single panoramic radiograph. Clin Orthod Res. 1999;2:194.
15. Alexander Katsnelson A, Flic WG, Susarla S, Tartakovsky JV, Miloro M. Use of panoramic X-ray to determine position of impacted maxillary canines. J Oral Maxillofac Surg. 2010;68:996–1000.
16. Preda L, La Fianza A, Di Maggio EM, Dore R, Schifino MR, Campani R, et al. The use of spiral computed tomography in the localization of impacted maxillary canines. Dentomaxillofac Radiol. 1997;26:236–41.
17. Liu D, Zhang W, Zhang Z, Wu Y, et al. Localization of impacted maxillary canines and observation of adjacent incisor resorption with cone-beam computed tomography. Oral Surg Oral Med Oral Pathol Oral Radiol Endod. 2008;105:91–8.
18. Walker L, Enciso R, Mah J. Three-dimensional localization of maxillary canines with cone-beam computed tomography. Am J Orthod Dentofacial Orthop. 2005;128(4):418.
19. Vermette ME, Kokich VG, Kennedy DB. Uncovering labially impacted teeth: apically positioned flap and closed-eruption techniques. Angle Orthod. 1995;65(1):23–32.
20. Chaushu S, Becker A, Zeltser R, Branski S, Vasker N, Chaushu G. Patients perception of recovery after exposure of impacted teeth: a comparison of closed-versus open-eruption techniques. J Oral Maxillofac Surg. 2005 Mar;63(3):323–9.
21. Crescini A, Clauser C, Giorgetti R, Cortellini P, Pini Prato GP. Tunnel traction of infraosseous impacted maxillary canines. A three-year periodontal follow-up. Am J Orthod Dentofac Orthop. 1994 Jan;105(1):61–72.
22. Incerti-Parenti S, Checchi V, Ippolito DR, Gracco A, Alessandri-Bonetti G. Periodontal status after surgical-orthodontic treatment of labially impacted canines with different surgical techniques: a systematic review. Am J Orthod Dentofacial Orthop 2016 Apr;149(4):463–472. Review.
23. Schmidt AD, Kokich VG. Periodontal response to early uncovering, autonomous eruption, and orthodontic alignment of palatally impacted maxillary canines. Am J Orthod Dentofac Orthop. 2007;131:449–55.
24. Quirynen M, Op Heij DG, Adriansens A, Opdebeeck HM, van Steenberghe D. Periodontal health of orthodontically extruded impacted teeth. A split-mouth, long-term clinical evaluation. J Periodontol. 2000 Nov;71(11):1708–14.
25. Chapokas AR, Almas K, Schincaglia GP. The impacted maxillary canine: a proposed classification for surgical exposure. Oral Surg Oral Med Oral Pathol Oral Radiol. 2012 Feb;113(2):222–8.
26. Dalessandri D, Parrini S, Rubiano R, Gallone D, Migliorati M. Impacted and transmigrant mandibular canines incidence, aetiology, and treatment: a systematic review. Eur J Orthod 2017 Apr 1;39(2):161–169. Review. (Open Access).

# Endodontic Surgery

# 16

Deepti Simon

## 16.1 Definition

Endodontic surgery is a dental procedure to treat apical periodontitis in cases that did not heal after nonsurgical retreatment or, in certain instances, primary root canal therapy [1]. It is the branch of dentistry that deals with the diagnosis and treatment of lesions of endodontic origin, which cannot be treated by or do not respond to conventional root canal therapy.

## 16.2 Historical Frame of Reference

Guerini documented the first endodontic surgery as incision and drainage of an acute endodontic abscess, approximately 1500 years ago [2]. Infected root sections were removed, and the healthy tooth portion was retained in attempting to cure infected teeth for about 200 years. Histological bone regeneration was demonstrated in treated cases of infected periapical lesions in 1930 [3]. For a long time, pulpless teeth were implicated in a plethora of systemic disorders like nephritis and arthritis by the exponents of the focal theory of infection [4].

The terms apicoectomy, periapical surgery, periapical endodontics, root end surgery, apical microsurgery, and surgical endodontics have been used in the literature. Apicoectomy, which means cutting the root apex, limits the understanding of the procedure, which includes removal of the irritants in the root canal system and the periapical pathology as well. Today, endodontic surgery is one of the most puissant branches of dentistry and falls in the twilight zone among surgery, dentistry, and endodontics. Recent advances in techniques and materials have resulted in a paradigm shift toward a more judicious strategy for treating periapical pathologies. The new benchmark for success is tissue regeneration. Nonsurgical retreatment for endodontic failures and surgical endodontics has been radically revolutionized by the introduction of the "microscope".

A periapical lesion is defined as any radiolucent image exceeding 1 mm in the periapical vicinity of the tooth. Lesions with a mean diameter > 5 mm are classified as large lesions, and those less than or equal to 5 mm are classified as small lesions [5]. In lesions greater than 10 mm, tooth extraction may or may not be done after considering factors like tooth mobility, pain, and the periodontal condition [6]. A periapical lesion may be noticed clinically or radiographically at a dimension of 5 mm [7].

## 16.3 Indications for Endodontic Surgery [8]

1. Failures of nonsurgical treatment (treatment should have been done at least twice)
2. Failure of nonsurgical treatment and retreatment is not feasible or impractical due to calcified canals, silver point filling, apical perforation, severely curved roots, and the presence of post and core or if the tooth is fractured at its apical one third
3. To obtain a biopsy from the periapical region
4. To retrieve broken instruments

### 16.3.1 Updated Indications (The European Society of Endodontology) (2006) [9]

1. Radiological findings of apical periodontitis and/or symptoms associated with an obstructed canal (the obstruction proved not to be removable, displacement of the obstruction did not seem to be feasible, or the risk of damage was too great)

D. Simon (✉)
Department of OMFS, Government Dental College, Trivandrum, Kerala, India

Kerala University of Health Sciences, Thrissur, Kerala, India


K. Bonanthaya et al. (eds.), *Oral and Maxillofacial Surgery for the Clinician*, https://doi.org/10.1007/978-981-15-1346-6_16

2. Extruded material with clinical or radiological findings of apical periodontitis and/or symptoms continuing over a prolonged period
3. Persisting or emerging disease following root canal treatment when root canal retreatment is inappropriate
4. Perforation of the root or the floor of the pulp chamber and when it is impossible to treat from within the pulp cavity

## 16.4 Relative Contraindications

1. Compromised medical status of the patient
2. Anatomical considerations
3. Surgeon's skill and clinical expertise
4. Vertically fractured tooth
5. Unrestorable tooth
6. Tooth with compromised periodontal support
7. Nonfunctional tooth
8. Tooth with short roots

**Principles of Endodontic Surgery**

1. Preoperative assessment and planning
2. Achieving adequate anesthesia and hemostasis
3. Appropriate surgical access through overlying soft and hard tissues
4. Periapical curettage and root end preparation
5. Would closure and care
6. Postoperative management of the local surgical site

**Classification of Endodontic Surgery [8]**

1. Fistulative Surgery
   (a) Incision and drainage
   (b) Cortical trephination
   (c) Decompression procedures
2. Periapical Surgery
   (a) Curettage
   (b) Root end resection
   (c) Root end preparation
   (d) Root end filling
3. Corrective Surgery
   (a) Perforation repair
      (i) Mechanical (iatrogenic)
      (ii) Resorptive
   (b) Periodontal management
      (i) Root resection
      (ii) Tooth resection
      (iii) Intentional replantation

## 16.5 Preoperative Assessment and Planning

### 16.5.1 Anatomical Reflections

The nasal floor, maxillary sinus, inferior alveolar, and mental and greater palatine neurovascular bundles offer potential road blocks to the surgeon.

### 16.5.2 Important Considerations in the Maxilla and Maxillary Sinus

If the roots of the maxillary anteriors are very long and the lesion extends superiorly, proximity to the nasal floor should be borne in mind. Eberhardt et al. have commented that the mesiobuccal root apex of the maxillary second molar is closest to the sinus floor and the buccal root apex of the maxillary first premolar is the farthest [10]. The greater palatine neurovascular bundle presents a risk while working on the palatal roots of maxillary molars. If the vessel is severed, pressure must be applied by packs or bone wax and the eventuality of external carotid artery ligation should not be precluded. Vertical releasing incisions on the palate are to be eschewed, and if these are unavoidable, it is prudent to place the same between the maxillary canine and first premolar, where the artery has a narrow caliber. Palatal roots can be accessed buccally or across the sinus or palatally (direct approach). The contour and depth of the palatal vault greatly determine the surgeon's accoutrement; greater the depth, greater the comfort.

Inadvertent loss of root tips into the maxillary sinus should be avoided and retrieved endoscopically if such a situation arises. Sinus communications, if they occur seldom, pose an impediment to healing neither are they implicated in sinustis [11]. The sinus membrane usually regenerates, and a thin bone forms at the apex [12]. Shallow vestibule, palatally or lingually inclined roots, compounds the surgeon's difficulties.

### 16.5.3 Important Considerations in the Mandible

In the mandible, the facial artery, mental nerve, and inferior alveolar neurovascular bundle should be reckoned with. The facial artery can be safeguarded if incisions placed in the vicinity of the mandibular first molar are not extended beyond the vestibular depth. The route taken by the inferior alveolar neurovascular bundle is of particular significance. It winds buccal (second molar) to lingual (first molar) and then again buccal (the second premolar) before it exits the mental foramen [12]. In the vertical dimension, the mandibular sec-

**Table 16.1** Anthropometric measurements of significance in endodontic surgery [10, 12]

| Sl. No | Landmarks | Distance in mm |
|---|---|---|
| 1. | Apex of mesiobuccal root of the maxillary second molar and sinus | 0.83 |
| 2. | Apex of buccal root of the maxillary first premolar and sinus | 7.05 |
| 3. | Apex of the maxillary second premolar and sinus | 2.8 |
| 4. | Apex of mesiobuccal and distobuccal root of the maxillary first molar and sinus | 2.8 |
| 5. | Apex of the mandibular second molar and mandibular canal | 3.7 |
| 6. | Apex of mesial root of the mandibular first molar and mandibular canal | 6.9 |
| 7. | Apex of the mandibular second premolar and mandibular canal | 4.7 |
| 8. | Buccal cortical plate and distal root of the mandibular second molar | 8.5 |
| 9. | Apex of maxillary canine and buccal cortical plate | 1.64 |

ond molar is closest to the canal as when compared to the mandibular first molar or second premolar. For all practical purposes, the mandibular second molar is not conducive to endodontic surgery and should be attempted bearing in mind these encumbrances. The mandibular anteriors offer a particular challenge while performing perpendicular root resection [12].

Excessive salivation, shallow vestibule, thick alveolus, and small rima oris are other determinants. A comprehensive assessment of all these variables is mandatory prior to embarking upon endodontic surgery (Table 16.1).

## 16.6 Investigations

Until recently, periapical radiographs were the workhorse of endodontic surgery. Their obvious shortcomings were due to compression of three-dimensional structures into a two-dimensional image and geometric distortion of anatomy. In the year 2000, Cone Beam Computer Tomography (CBCT) was introduced to dentistry. The limited CBCT offers higher resolution, and images are displayed in three planes: axial, coronal, and sagittal. Simultaneously, radiation dose is comparable to panoramic x-rays, and superimposition of neighboring structures is obviated [12]. The relationship between the teeth apices and anatomic structures, variations in root morphology, additional canals, and external root resorption are just a few of the diagnostic conundrums that can be assessed via CBCT.

Surgical workup also includes complete blood count, routine urine examination, viral markers, and a thorough medical history. Appropriate regulation of insulin, anticoagulants, and other drugs should be undertaken in liaison with the attending physician.

A well-informed patient is the best patient. The importance of informed consent cannot be overdrawn, and the patient is entitled to know about the prognosis, benefits, and surgical complications, anticipate damage to vital structures, and follow up. Communication regarding the above details is mandatory, and the patient should be made aware of alternate treatment modalities like extraction followed by implant placement.

## 16.7 Anesthesia and Hemostasis

### 16.7.1 Premedication

Nonsteroidal anti-inflammatory drugs (NSAIDs) in conflation with a long-acting local anesthetic can scale down postoperative pain. Ainsworth surmised that routine use of prophylactic antibiotics in periapical surgery is unwarranted [12]. A presurgical mouth rinse with chlorhexidine gluconate (0.12%) will reduce the salivary bacteria significantly, especially their growth on sutures and wound margins, but may obtrude with fibroblast reattachment to the root [12].

Most patients tolerate the surgical procedure under local anesthesia but for the apprehensive, conscious oral sedation with benzodiazepines or nitrous oxide/oxygen inhalation should be opted for. Diazepam 10 mg can be started on the night before the surgery, and another dose can be administered 1 hour before the procedure [13].

### 16.7.2 Local Anesthesia and Sedation

The merits and demerits of various local anesthetics have been elaborated in detail elsewhere in this book. Conventional nerve blocks are augmented by local infiltration. Of equal momentousness is the preference for the vasoconstrictor. Adrenaline in concentrations ranging from 1:50,000, 1: 100,000, and 1:200,000 have performed commendably.

## 16.8 Surgical Access

### 16.8.1 Armamentarium

Incisions can be placed with no.11, no. 12, no 15, or no. 15-C blades (Fig. 16.1). Sharp, blunt dissection and elevation of the mucoperiosteal flap are accomplished by a Molts' or Howarths' periosteal elevator (Fig. 16.2). Endodontic tissue retractors like Austin, Seldon, or Minnesota should be judiciously selected in order to minimize trauma to the mucoperiosteal flap and neurovascular bundles (Fig. 16.3). Overlying bone is cut with No.4/6/8 round burs or 701/702 fissure burs (Fig. 16.4). These can be used to resect the root apex as well. Surgical handpiece with 45 ° angle head and rear air exhaust is advocated. Sharp surgical curettes like Lucas curette, angled periodontal curettes, and spoon excavators help to remove the inflamed soft tissue from the bony cavity (Fig. 16.5).

Root end resections can be done either with conventional burs or lasers (Er-YAG or Ho-YAG lasers) [14, 15].

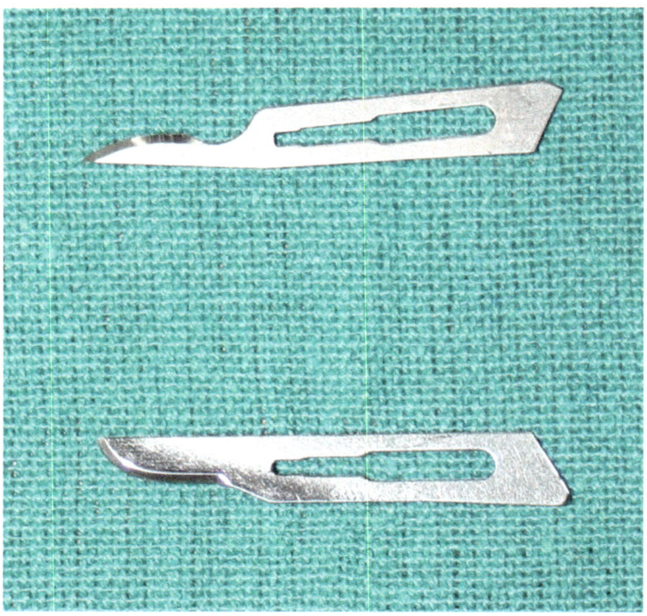



Fig. 16.1 No. 15 and No. 15 C Blades

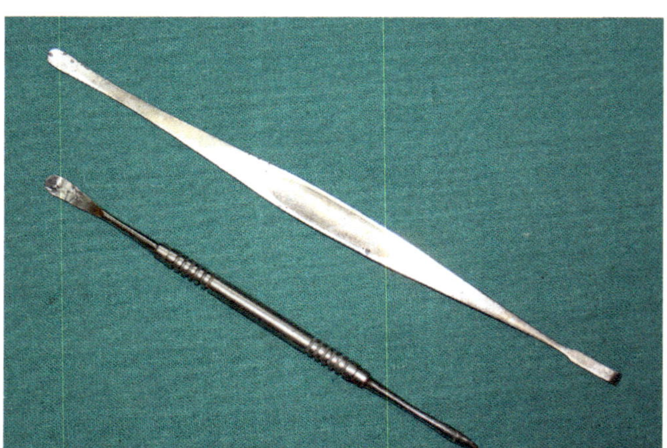



Fig. 16.2 Molt's Periosteal Elevator and Howarth's Elevator

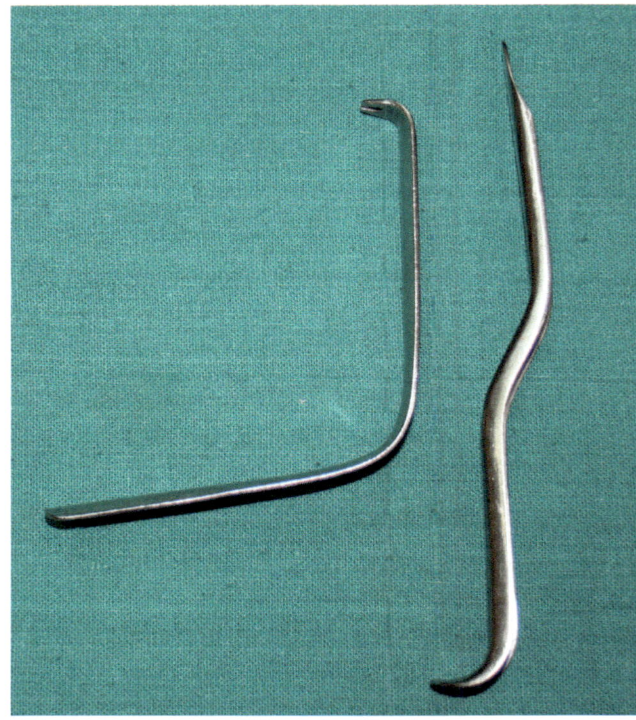



Fig. 16.3 Austin retractor and Minnesota retractor

The advantages of lasers include greater patient comfort, decreased vibrations, lesser surgical site contamination, and minimal trauma to the juxtaposed tissues.

Ultrasonic microsurgical tips are invaluable for root end preparation. Earlier, hand files and rotary burs were used. Teflon sleeves, pluggers, and Messing gun-type syringes can be used to place various root-end filling materials like MTA (Fig. 16.6). Review of literature validates the superiority of microsurgical techniques over conventional surgery (97% to 59%) [1]. The dental operating microscope, ultrasonic tips, and diamond coated micromirrors (Fig. 16.7) have found their niche in the surgeon's armamentarium. Micromirrors (Fig. 16.8) can be used to inspect the buccal and lingual walls of the retrocavity. Microsurgical scalpels are useful for incising the intrasulcular areas and dissection of the interproximal papillae.

### 16.8.2 Surgical Management

The aims of periapical surgery are to visualize and debride the affected area and provide hermetic seal at the root end that aids in periodontal regeneration (Figs. 16.9, 16.10 and 16.11). Gutmann and Harrison [4] have categorized flaps as

1. Full mucoperiosteal flaps
2. Limited mucoperiosteal flaps

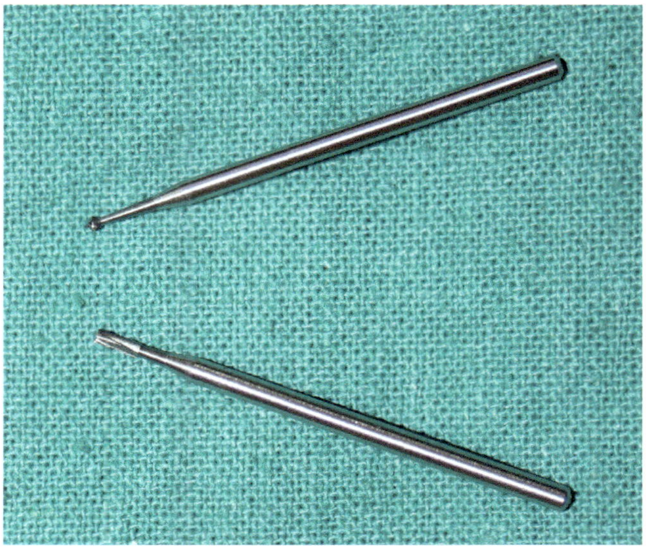



**Fig. 16.4** No.701 bur and No.4 bur

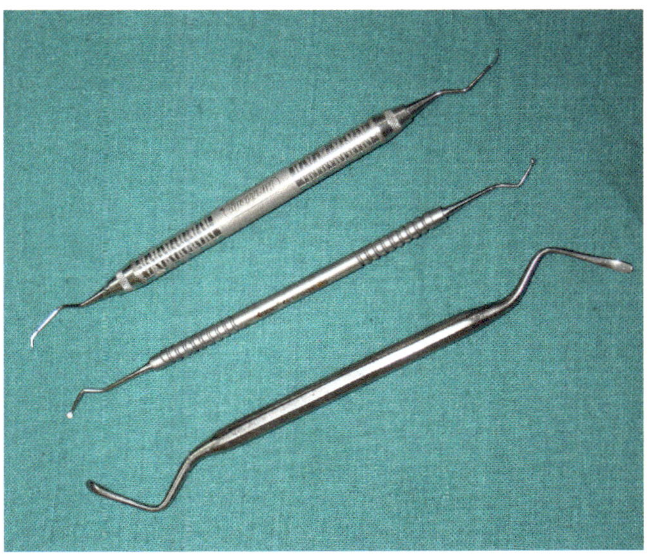



**Fig. 16.5** Lucas curette, Spoon excavator, and Periodontal curette

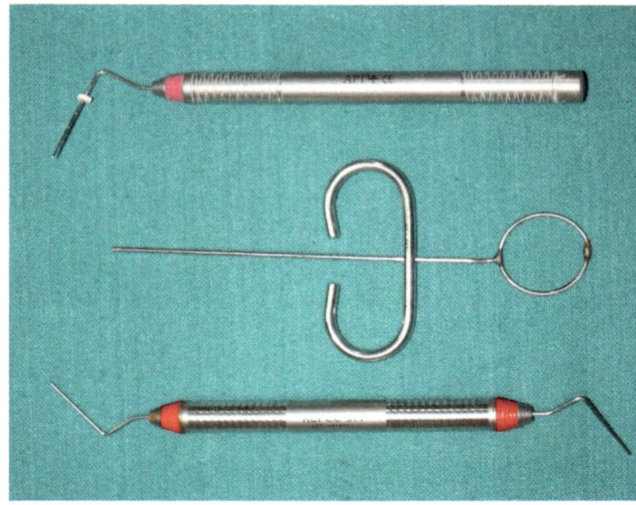



**Fig. 16.6** Pluggers and Messing gun syringe

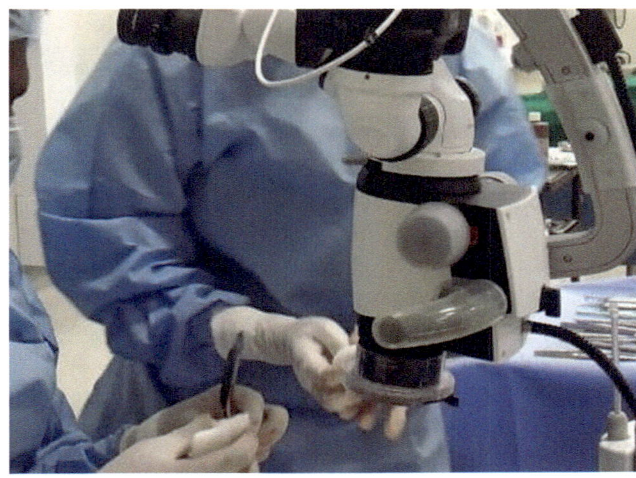



**Fig. 16.7** Microsurgical root end surgery

The main difference is that marginal interdental tissues are included in the full flaps, whereas the latter conserves them. Researchers opine that limited flaps prevent loss of papilla height, but careful adaptation of the reflected soft tissues rarely causes changes in gingival attachment level. It is vital to preserve the root attached tissues. In the absence of periodontal pathology, anatomic and functional status quo can be maintained via full mucoperiosteal flaps. Elevating palatal flaps is by and large a cumbersome affair. If the clinical situation demands a palatal approach, the envelope and triangular flaps can be considered. Contrary to popular teaching, vertical incisions can be placed on the palate, rather than stretching and renting a flap, which may impede healing. This approach is best reserved for palatal roots for posteriors. Anterior palatal cysts can be accessed labially or palatally, according to the surgeon's discretion. To aid in surgical access, it is prudent to pass a long suture through

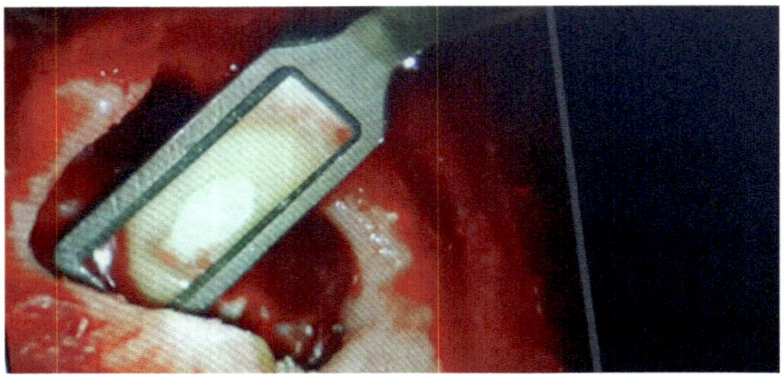



**Fig. 16.8** Diamond-coated mirror

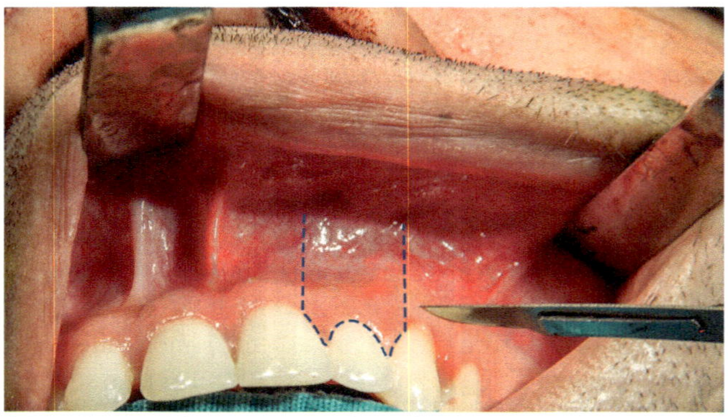



**Fig. 16.9** Trapezoidal flap

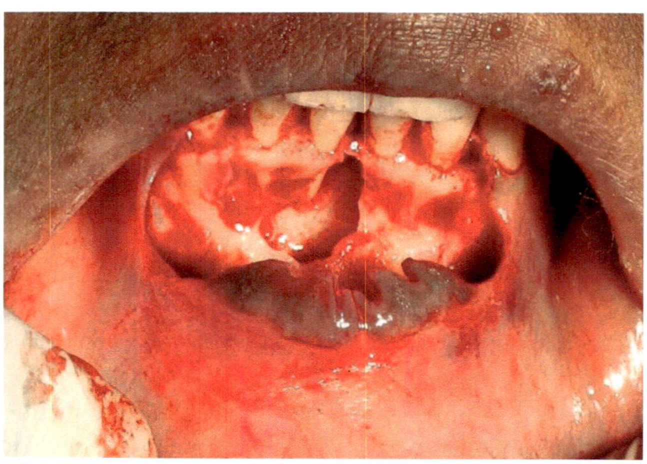



**Fig. 16.10** Clinical image of a trapezoidal flap for periapical lesion in lower anterior region

the palatal flap and have the assistant retract the tissue. Table 16.2 details the advantages and disadvantages of various types of flaps that can be used for endodontic surgery.

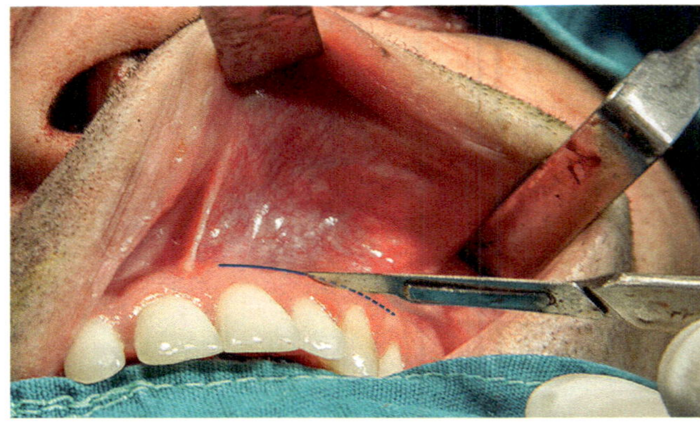



**Fig. 16.11** Submarginal incision

### 16.8.3 Basic Principles of Flap Design

1. Straight or parallel incisions are preferred over severely angled ones, in order to preserve the supraperiosteal blood supply of the attached gingiva and submucosa. Fewer vessels and collagen fibers are transected with parallel incisions, resulting in less hemorrhage and flap shrinkage
2. Root eminences of canines and maxillary premolars are covered by thin bone with a poor blood supply and should be spared. Incisions should be placed between adjacent teeth on interdental bone
3. Flaps should lie on solid healthy bone. At least 5 mm of bone should be present between the defect and incision line
4. Do not incise frena and muscle attachments as it compromises the healing
5. Do not incise through the dental papilla
6. The entire mucoperiosteum should be included in the flap; this is imperative for uneventful healing
7. Retractors should rest on solid bone
8. The horizontal incision should extend at least one tooth beyond the pathologic area of interest

The position of the tooth in the arch, the dimensions of the periapical pathology, gingival recession, and the presence of artificial crowns also determine the choice of the incision that is placed.

### 16.8.4 Flap Elevation

The horizontal element of a full mucoperiosteal flap commences in the gingival sulcus and severs the gingival attachment fibers to the crestal bone. The interdental papilla should be incised at the midcol level. While incising a limited flap, the horizontal component must conform to the contour of the marginal gingiva and should be 2 mm apical to the depth of

**Table 16.2** Various flap designs used in endodontic surgery [4, 12]

| Name and description | Recommended | Advantages | Disadvantages |
|---|---|---|---|
| Triangular flap (full)horizontal, intrasulcular incision, one vertical releasing incision | Maxillary incisors and posteriors | Rapid wound healing due to good vascular supply<br>Facilitates in bone graft placement | Limited access |
| Rectangular flap (full) horizontal, intrasulcular incision, two vertical releasing incisions | Mandibular anteriors and Maxillary canines | Extensive surgical access<br>Facilitates in bone graft placement | Difficult wound closure and more sutures |
| Trapezoidal flap (full) horizontal, intrasulcular incisions, two divergent angled, vertical incisions | Not recommended | Base is wider than apex | Damage to supraperiosteal vessels and hence more bleeding and flap shrinkage |
| Horizontal /envelope flap (full). No vertical releasing incision | Limited use<br>Only in repair of cervical defects, hemisections, and root amputations | Rapid healing | Limited access |
| Papilla based flap (full)<br>Shallow first incision at the base of the papilla second incision directed to crestal bone | Esthetically important regions | Conserves the papilla | Technically challenging |
| Submarginal curved/semilunar flap (limited). Curved incision in alveolar mucosa and attached gingiva | Not recommended | – | Limited access and poor healing unaesthetic scarring<br>Exact location of the root should be known |
| Submarginal scalloped rectangular /Luebke-Ochsenbein (limited). Scalloped horizontal incision follows the shape of the marginal gingiva on the attached gingival<br>At least 2 mm of attached gingiva is retained<br>Also called freeform rectilinear | Maxillary teeth where esthetics of crown margins are important | No exposure of crestal bone<br>Prevents papillary recession and clefting | Unaesthetic scarring. More bleeding and flap shrinkage<br>Depth of gingival sulcus should be measured |

the gingival sulcus. The vertical incision should begin in the alveolar mucosa and proceed toward the crown till it abuts the horizontal incision. To achieve the above objectives fresh, sharp blades should be opted for.

Hemostasis and healing are enhanced if the entire mucoperiosteal flap is elevated as a single unit, due to adherence of the flap with its microvasculature. The broad end of the elevator can be maneuvered beneath the vertical incision, a few millimeters from the junction of the horizontal and vertical incision in the attached gingiva. This preserves the supracrestal root-attached fibers. This is followed by coronal dissection, and forces are directed toward the periosteum and bone. This technique is termed undermining elevation and should be continued throughout the length of the horizontal incision and apically to the alveolar mucosa [4]. An approximate distance of 1 cm from the apex should be exposed for adequate access. The bleeding tags seen on the bone contain periosteum that aids in healing and reattachment of the flap.

### 16.8.5 Flap Retraction

The soft tissues must be gently retracted to preclude the possibility of inadvertent crushing. This may lead to flap hypoxia, swelling, ecchymosis, and/or delayed healing. The retractor of a correct size should be selected and placed on cortical bone in such a way that the tissue is prevented from engaging with rotary instruments.

The periosteal surface of the flap should be irrigated with sterile, cool, and physiologic saline to keep it hydrated. The superficial surface is more resistant to dehydration due to the stratified squamous epithelium [16, 17].

### 16.8.6 Hard Tissue Management

Once the flap is raised, the surgeon encounters either intact cortical bone over the lesion or the lesion sans cortical bone. In the former scenario, it is imperative to localize the lesion and remove bone in the adjacent periapical area. Well-angled radiographs can aid in this aspect. Sounding the bone with the sharp end of the periosteal elevator can also be useful, as there is a change in resonance when one approaches the diseased area. It is also prudent to identify the root by calculating twice the crown length and then shave the thin bone at the apex. If digital technology is used, the distance from the alveolar crest to the root apex can be measured using the ruler function [3]. The root is smooth, hard, and yellow in color, surrounded by a periodontal ligament, and does not bleed on probing. Methylene blue dye staining can aid in locating the periodontal ligament.

Bone is vulnerable to thermal damage at any temperature above the normal body temperature. This is the crucial aspect of periapical surgery and influences the choice of burs, coolants, and handpieces. Bone when subject to temperatures between 40 °C and 50 ° C undergoes a spectrum of irreversible changes. These include reduction in microcirculation, tissue necrosis, fatty cell infiltration, and decrease in alkaline phosphatase.

While selecting bone cutting burs, sharp ones with wide spaces between the flutes are preferred. Round burs meeting these criteria promote excellent healing. Chilled saline effectively reduces the heat produced and flushes out the debris, thus enhancing efficiency. Excess pressure applied to the bone is detrimental to the tissues and handpiece. Gentle shaving or brushing motion must be used in short, multiple phases.

Hirsch et al. have used a piezoelectric device to create a bony aperture while performing apicoectomies in maxillary anteriors. The buccal bone was removed, preserved in Hank's Balanced Salt Solution (HBSS), and later replaced in the bony crypt after the procedure, thus acting as an autologous bone graft. This is feasible in cases where there is minimal bone loss or in the presence of intact bone over the lesion [18].

The bony aperture should be wide enough to permit visual and surgical access into the lesion, enabling the insertion of bone curettes and excavators. In traditional root surgery, the size of the aperture is approximately 8–10 mm and 3-4 mm in microsurgery. The rate of healing is faster when the size of osteotomy is smaller. Granulomas and granulation tissues exhibit a propensity to bleed profusely, hindering the surgery. To circumvent this, local anesthetic with a vasoconstrictor can be injected within. Using a curette of appropriate dimension, the surgeon works from the periphery toward the center. The instrument is inserted between the tissue and the lateral edge of the cavity with its concave face toward the bone. This is continued all around the circumference of the cavity and slowly progresses toward the depth of the crypt in a scraping manner. After freeing all the tissue, it is gently grasped with a pair of tissue forceps and immersed in 10% buffered formalin solution. The specimen should not be left to dry. Lin et al. opine that complete curettage is not mandatory, if the irritant is eliminated [19]. Though a majority of periapical lesions have been diagnosed histopathologically as granulomas or cysts, there have been documented reports of perfectly innocuous looking periapical lesions diagnosed as odontogenic keratocysts, central giant cell granulomas, or squamous cell carcinoma [20, 21].

### 16.8.7 Root end Preparation

#### 16.8.7.1 Root end Resection (Fig. 16.12)

Regeneration of alveolar bone, periodontal ligament, and cementum in the periapical area can be encouraged by removing the diseased root end tissues and placing a root end seal to stop the recontamination of the periapical region. Resection of apical 3 mm of the root apex will eliminate 78% of apical ramifications and 93% of lateral canals, which could contain material that would contribute to the periradicular disease [12]. The isthmus area should be included in the resection in roots with multiple canals. Anatomical obstructions, broken instruments, and perforations can be removed, orthograde sealing can be assessed, and trapped lingual tissue can be curetted out. In the case of apical fenestration, the apex can be reduced below the surrounding cortex to enable bone formation over the apex. The resection should enable the surgeon to prepare a root end cavity and place a restoration within.

A smooth, flat resected surface is considered ideal. This should be assessed for cracks, anatomical variations, and orthograde obturating material by means of an operating microscope at high power magnification and methylene blue staining [2]. The resection is made in order to surround the filling by normal dentin. Conventionally, a 30–45° bevel was placed, but the advent of the microscope has enabled a resection perpendicular to the long axis of the tooth. This substantially decreases the number of exposed dentinal tubules. Cohen opines that this aids in root end cavity preparation beyond the

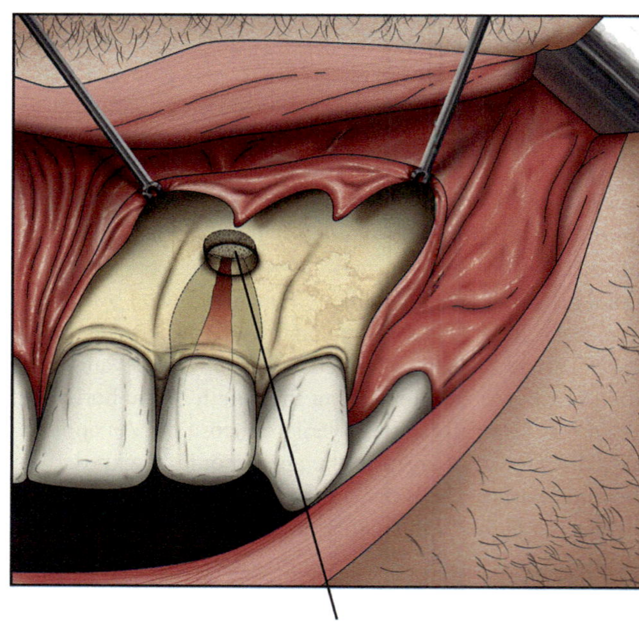



Fig. 16.12 2 to 3 mm root tip resection

coronal extent of the root surface and apical stresses are well distributed, thus reducing apical fractures [11].

After the perpendicular root resection, the root must be conditioned to remove the smear layer produced. This exposes the collagen matrix of dentin and promotes growth. 5% aqueous citric acid has been used for this purpose. EDTA and tetracycline have also been studied, but have not found clinical popularity.

#### 16.8.7.2 Root end Cavity Preparation

A 3 mm-deep Class I cavity is prepared along the long axis of the tooth, in order to place the filling material [22]. Ultrasonic tips have been specifically designed for this purpose. The tips produce less smear layer, need less beveling, and can be inserted through a smaller aperture. However, the ultrasonic vibrations can predispose to root fractures. This can be minimized when it is used at the lowest setting and with water coolant. Ultrasonic tips coated with stainless steel, diamond, or zirconium nitride are superior to uncoated tips. If the tips have a curvature of 70° or more, they are prone to fracture [23]. The root end filling is placed into the prepared cavity. When bonded materials like Retroplast are used, no root end preparation is needed; the filling is placed like a dome onto the resected root. This is termed bonded cap approach.

It is imperative to have a dry bloodless field prior to placement of the root end filling regardless of the setting properties of individual filling materials. To achieve this, adrenaline-saturated pellets, bone wax, Gelfoam, surgical, calcium sulfate, thrombin, collagen, or ferric sulfate may be used. Electrocautery may also be used, but this may delay bone healing.

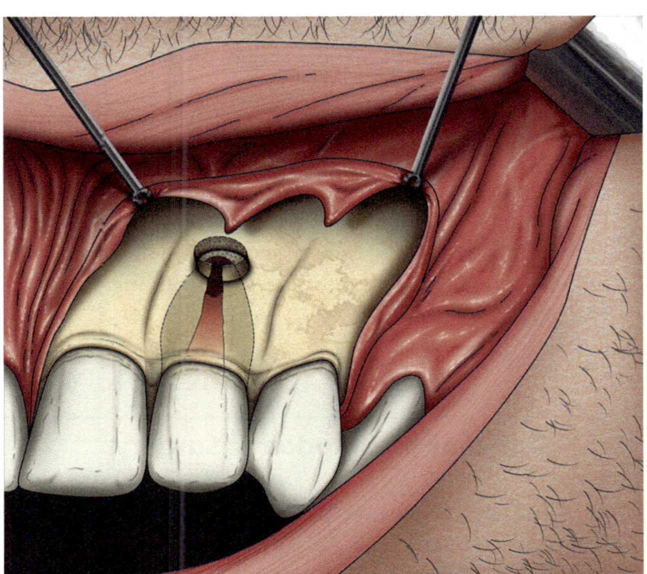

©Association of Oral and Maxillofacial Surgeons of India

**Fig. 16.13** Root end filling

#### 16.8.7.3 Root end Filling (Fig. 16.13)

Amalgam used to be the quintessential retrograde filling material as it is cheap, easy to use, and radio opaque. However, it may stain the tissues and is sensitive to moisture [3]. Research has yielded a plethora of retrofilling materials, which has enhanced the outcome of endodontic surgery (Table 16.3).

**Table 16.3** Synopsis of root-end filling materials [4, 12]

| Sl. No | Material | Composition | Characteristics |
|---|---|---|---|
| 1. | Zinc oxide eugenol | Zinc oxide powder eugenol liquid | Affected by powder-liquid ratio. Eugenol can inhibit prostaglandins and cause fibroblast toxicity; final compound has high solubility |
| 2. | Intermediate restorative material (IRM) | Zinc oxide, polymethyl methacrylate powder, eugenol, and acetic acid—Liquid | Not affected by powder liquid ratio. No evidence of cementogenesis |
| 3. | Super EBA (epoxy benzoic acid) | Zinc oxide, aluminum oxide, natural resins-powder, eugenol, and o-methoxybenzoic acid-liquid | No evidence of cementogenesis |
| 4. | Glass ionomer | Calcium alumino silicate—powder and polyacrylic acid liquid | Moisture sensitive. Risk of detachment from teeth |
| 5. | Retroplast | Paste A- Bis-GMA/TEGDMA 1:1, benzoyl peroxide N,N-di-(2-hydroxyethyl)-p-toluidine, and butylated hydroxytoluene; Paste-B ytterbium fluoride aerosil ferric oxide | Dentin bonding composite resin. Hard tissue formation seen, probably cementum. Evidence of PDL regeneration seen. Biocompatible. Adequate setting time and compressive strength. Strict control of hemorrhage is mandatory |
| 6. | Mineral trioxide aggregate (MTA) | Calcium silicate, calcium carbonate, bismuth sulfate, calcium sulfate, and calcium aluminate | Evidence of cementogenesis seen. Long setting time ≈ 3 h, unaffected by blood and moisture. Gray MTA can cause tooth discoloration. Least amount of microleakage. Less marginal gap formation. Better adaptation |
| 7. | Bioceramics | Calcium silicate, monobasic calcium phosphate, and zirconium oxide | Newer material. Biocompatible. Antimicrobial activity present. Needs more clinical evaluation. |

After placing the root end filling, a radiograph must be obtained to assess its quality. If the radiograph reveals an incomplete root resection or an inadequate retrofill, the surgeon must rectify the above-said deficiencies. These are the most common surgical pitfalls that contribute to endodontic surgical failures.

The surgical site is gently cleaned and irrigated with sterile saline to remove debris of hemostatic agents and filling materials. Bone grafts or guided regeneration barriers can be placed into the crypt if indicated, but sterile technique should be adhered to, at all times to obviate infection. Calcium phosphate bioceramics, bioactive glass composite, and bioactive self-setting cements have been evaluated in vitro as well as in vivo [24, 25]. The flap is repositioned and delicately compressed with a moist gauze to vent out the excess blood, and tissue fluids 4–0 Silk or 6–0 monofilament suture materials are used. Tissue adhesives like cyanoacrylate and fibrin may be used as alternatives in the future. Suturing commences at the corners, approximately 2–3 mm from the wound margins. Interrupted sutures and sling sutures work well for closure of full mucoperiosteal flaps. Continuous locked suturing can also be done in marginal flaps as it reduces the time taken for suturing.

Following wound closure, moist gauze is placed on the flap for 5 min to stabilize clot formation and hemostasis. Compressing the flap with sterile ice packs in the immediate postoperative period minimizes the thickness of the fibrin clot and enhances wound healing. Intermittent cold compresses for 20 min on the day of surgery aids in patient comfort. Analgesics are prescribed, and verbal and written instructions are given to the patient and primary care provider. The wound must be cleaned gently with cotton. Chlorhexidine mouthwash is beneficial and can be continued till sutures are removed, i.e., on the fifth day postoperatively. Sutures can be removed after 3 days in microsurgical procedures.

## 16.9 Biology of Wound Healing [12]

The dynamics of healing in endodontic surgery involve various mechanisms germane to the nature of the individual tissues. The soft tissue incision heals by primary intention, whereas the bone defect and resected root surface heal via secondary intention. The endpoint of surgery should be regeneration, rather than repair where the normal tissue architecture and function are restored instead of a fibrous scar tissue.

The soft tissue healing progresses through three phases, i.e., inflammatory, proliferative, and maturation. The inflammatory phase begins with clot formation. The local microvasculature contracts, the platelets release serotonin, and a protein-rich exudate enters the wound site. Intravascular aggregation of platelets forms a platelet plug, and the extrinsic and intrinsic pathways are activated. This results in a randomly arranged thick fibrin clot. Within 6 hours of clot formation, polymorphonuclear leukocytes enter the wound and decontaminate the area by phagocytosis of bacteria. Their activity tapers off by 96 hours; monocytes and macrophages continue the phagocytic activity. A reduction in macrophages hampers the next phase of wound healing, especially in the older population where there is a step down of estrogen regulation of macrophages. The proliferative phase is dominated by fibroplasia and angiogenesis. The granulomatous nature of the wound transforms into granulation tissue by the activity of cytokines like platelet derived growth factor (PDGF), fibroblast growth factor (FGF), and insulin-like growth factor (IGF-1). By the third day, fibroblasts lay down Type III collagen, which matures to Type I. Myofibroblasts orient themselves parallel to the wound surface and contract, thus drawing the wound edges together. Concurrently, capillary networks form within the wound stimulated by proangiogenic factors like vascular endothelial growth factor (VEGF), FGF, transforming growth factor $\alpha$, $\beta$ (TGF-$\alpha$, $\beta$), and interleukin-1 (IL-1). An epithelial seal is formed on the surface of the fibrin clot by the first day. In the next 5–7 days, the wound matures by the formation of larger collagen bundles.

In the osseous crypt, there is a hematoma and proliferation of granulation tissue, callus formation, and woven bone deposition, which is converted to lamellar bone. These events are regulated by TGF-$\beta$, PDGF, FGF, IGF, and bone morphogenic protein (BMP). At the root end, cementum forms over the resected surface. Cells responsible for cementogenesis are believed to originate from the ectomesenchymal cells in the tooth germ. By 28 days, the root end is covered by cementum.

## 16.10 Postoperative Complications

1. Flap necrosis and breakdown, due to poor design and careless handling
2. Transient paresthesia of mental and inferior alveolar nerves
3. Exposure of the maxillary sinus, which heals in a majority of cases
4. Perforation or Fracture of tooth roots
5. Gingival recession and Scar tissue formation
6. Staining of gingival tissues due to retrofilling materials like amalgam

## 16.11 Outcome of Endodontic Surgery

Clinical and radiographic assessments are made to determine the outcome of periapical surgery. The Periapical Index (PAI) has been used for radiographic assessment in both surgical and nonsurgical series [26]. Ingle opines that the terms 'healed', 'healing', 'disease,' and 'asymptomatic' can be used to describe the outcome.

1. Healed cases show complete clinical and radiographic normalcy with no signs and symptoms or residual radiolucency
2. Healing cases show a decrease in the size of the radiolucency and clinical normally within 4 years of surgery
3. Diseased cases show radiolucency, new, increased, unchanged, or decreased after 4 years, regardless of radiographic appearance
4. Asymptomatically functional teeth show clinical normalcy with or without persistent radiolucency, decreased or unchanged

## 16.12 Aids to Endodontic Surgery

Loupes, endoscopes, and the operating microscope have enhanced visualization of the operating field and thereby the quality of surgery.

### 16.12.1 Endoscopes

It has a rod lens system, camera head, and control unit with a monitor and light source placed on a mobile rack. The depth of perception is comparable with the naked eye. Tactile perception is excellent; diseased tissue behind and between roots can be visualized. Irrigation fluids can be used without clouding the visual field. Fabbro and Taschiere have reported success rates of 91.1 and 90.7% using the endoscope [27]. They offer rapid and easy adjustment of the viewing angle, direct viewing sans micromirrors, which is versatile and transportable.

### 16.12.2 Dental Operating Microscope

The resolution of the human eye is 0.2 mm. The power can be increased by moving closer to the surgical field, but can pose strain to the eye. Hence, magnifying lenses and illumination are used to bypass this problem.

The operating microscope offers up to 30 times magnification, coaxial light supply, and shadow free illumination. 200 mm objective lenses and 180° inclinable binoculars are optimum configurations. Light can be sourced from either xenon or quartz halogen bulbs. Digital camera, video camera, and co-observation tube are included in the setup. Endodontic microsurgery amalgamates magnification, illumination, and microinstrumentation, leading to predictable treatment outcomes. Deeper root end cavities can be prepared, which follow the contour of the root, hence minimizing lateral perforation [28]. The high cost of the equipment and need for specialized training deter many from adopting this tool on a routine basis, but the high success rates should be sufficient encouragement for clinicians and patients to adopt this new tool.

## 16.13 Future Perspectives

The role of mesenchymal stem cells in regeneration of periapical tissues has been explored with great enthusiasm. Dental pulp stem cells (DPSCs) and those from exfoliated deciduous teeth are multipotent in capacity and can be used along with scaffolds and signaling molecules [29]. These entities, when combined in the ideal proportion, aim to recreate the embryonic milieu, hence augmenting the biological concepts of wound healing. The future may usher in radical changes in our approach to endodontic surgery in terms of materials and techniques with respect to regenerative medicine.

**Acknowledgments** Dr. Khaleel Ahamed Thaha, Assistant Professor, Department of Conservative Dentistry and Endodontics, Government Dental College, Kozhikode, Kerala.

## References


1. Frank CS, Sweta BS, Meetu RK, Bekir K, Syngcuk K. Outcome of endodontic surgery: a meta analysis of the literature – part I: comparison of traditional root end surgery and endodontic microsurgery. JOE. 2010 Nov;36(11):1757–65.
2. Guerini VA. History of dentistry. Philadelphia: Lea and Febiger; 1909. p. 117.
3. Franco PB, Karlis V. In: Kademani D, Tiwana PS, editors. Apicoectomy in atlas of oral and maxillofacial surgery. St. Louis, MO: Elsevier; 2016.
4. Gutmann JL, Harrison JW. Surgical endodontics. St. Louis, MO: Ishiyaku euro America; 1994.
5. Quality assurance guidelines. Chicago: American Association of Endodontists; 1987, p. 1–27.
6. Simsek-Kaya G, Saruhan N, Yapia-Yavuz G, Ertas U. A decision analysis for periapical surgery: retrospective study. J Clin Exp Dent. 2018 Sep;10(9):e914–20.
7. El-Swiah JM, Walker RT. Reasons for apicoectomies: a retrospective study. Endod Dent Trauma. 1996;12:185–91.
8. Glickman GN, Hartwell GR. Endodontic surgery in ingle's endodotnics. 6th ed. Hamilton, ON: BC Decker Inc; 2008.
9. European Society of Endodontology. Quality guidelines for endodontic treatment: consensus report of European society of endodontology. Int Endod J. 2006;39:921–30.
10. Eberhardt JA, Torabinejad M, Christiansen EL. A computed tomographic study of the distances between the maxillary sinus floor and apices of the maxillary posterior teeth. Oral Surg Oral Med Oral Pathol Oral Radiol Endod. 1992;73:345.
11. Benninger MS, Sebak BA, Levine HL. Mucosal regeneration of the maxillary sinus after surgery. Otolaryngol Head Neck Surgery. 1989;101:33.

12. Johnson BR, Fayad MI. Hargreaves KM, Berman LH, editors. Periradicular surgery in Cohen's pathways of the pulp. 9th ed. St. Louis, MO: Elsevier.
13. Jastak JT, Yagiela JA. Regional anesthesia of the oral cavity. St. Louis, MO: Mosby; 1981.
14. Nedderman TA, Hartwell GR, Portell FR. A comparison of root surfaces following apical root resection with various burs: scanning electron microscope evaluation. J Endod. 1988;14:423.
15. Komori T, Yokoyama K, Matsumoto Y. YAG laser root resection of extracted human teeth. J Clin Laser Med Surg. 1997;15:9.
16. Harrison JW, Jurosky KA. Wound healing in the tissues of the periodontium following periradicular surgery. I. The incisional wound. J Endod. 1991;17:425.
17. Harrison JW, Jurosky KA. Wound healing in the tissues of the periodontium following perpendicular surgery. II. The dissectinal wound. J Endod. 1991;17:544.
18. Hirsch V, Meetu RK, Kim S. Apicoectomy of maxillary anterior teeth through a piezoelectric bony window osteotomy: two case reports introducing a new technique to preserve cortical bone. Restor Dent Endod. 2016 Nov;41(4):310–5.
19. Lin LM, Gaengler P, Langeland K. Periradicular curettage. Int Endod J. 1996;29:220.
20. Garlock JA, Pringle GA, Hicks ML. The odontogenic keratocyst: a potential endodontic misdiagnosis. Oral Surg Oral Med Oral Pathol Oral Radiol Endod. 1998;85:452.
21. Jeevanand D, Ratika S, Rachappa M. Giant radicular cyst of the maxilla. BMJ Case Rep. 2014; https://doi.org/10.1136/bcr-2014-203678.
22. de Lange J, Putters T, Baas EM, van Ingen JM. Ultrasonic root end preparation in apical surgery: a prospective randomized study. Oral Surg Oral Med Oral Pathol Oral Radiol Endod. 2007;104:84.
23. Walmsley AD, Lumley PJ, Johnson WT, Walton RE. Breakage of ultrasonic root-end preparation tips. J Endod. 1996;22:287.
24. Komath M, Varma HK, Annie J, Vinod K, Simon D, Ramanathan M, Bhuvaneshwar GS. Designing bioactive scaffolds for dental tissue engineering in regenerative medicine: laborotary to clinic. Berlin: Springer; 2017.
25. Simon D, Manuel S, Varma HK. Novel nanoporous bioceramic spheres for drug delivery application: a preliminary in vitro investigation. Oral Surg Oral Med Oral Pathol Oral Radiol. 2013 Mar;115(3):e7–14.
26. Friedman S. Treatment outcome: the potential for healing and retained function in Ingle's endodontics. 6th ed. Hamilton: BC Decker Inc; 2008.
27. Del Fabbro M, Taschieri S. Endodontic therapy using magnification devices: a systematic review. J Dent. 2010 Apr;38(4):269–75.
28. von Arx T. Failed root canals: the case for apicoectomy (periradicular surgery). J Oral Maxillofac Surg. 2005;63:832–7.
29. Shiehzadeh V, Aghmasheh F, Shiehzadeh F, Joulae M, Kosarieh E, Shiehzadeh F. Healing of large periapical lesions following delivery of dental stem cells with an injectable scaffold: new method and three case reports. Indian J Dent Res. 2014 Mar–Apr;25(2):248–53.

## Additional Reading (Algorithm for Periapical Surgery)

Lieblich SE. Periapical surgery: clinical decision making. Oral Maxillofac Surg Clin N Am. 2002;14:181.
Leiblich S. Current concepts of periapical surgery. Oral Maxillofacial Surg Clin N Am. 2015;27(3):383–2.

# Preprosthetic Surgery

# 17

Bobby John

*The human mandible has no one design for life. Rather it adapts and remodels through the seven stages of life, from the slim arbiter of things to come in the infant, through a powerful dentate machine and even weapon in the full flesh of maturity, to the pencil-thin, porcelain like problem that we struggle to repair in the adversity of old age.*

Poswillo

## 17.1 History

The management of discontented denture patients by the act of preprosthetic surgical procedures to enhance the denture-bearing areas of the intraoral cavity is a daunting task, which has been performed by the oral and maxillofacial surgeon from time immemorial. Preprosthetic surgery encompasses a distinguished and evolving category of soft and hard tissue procedures.

Pre-prosthetic surgery has emerged from being virtually unknown, passed through a period of opposition and into a state of venerability, and has ultimately made a powerful impact on oral surgery and prosthetic dentistry alike.

A meticulously nurtured and evolved repertoire of ingenious salvage procedures is now alarmingly threatened by a populist 'implants-first' belief that usurps, rather than expands, the traditional prosthodontic treatment spectrum.

Willard [1] is honoured to be the first American dentist to call attention to proper preparation of the mouth for full dentures. Beers [2] in 1876 advocated excision of the alveolus after extraction of teeth, especially if the alveolar process is unusually exhibiting protuberance. Surgery has always been an integral part of the preparation of alveolar ridges for dentures. The last few decades have witnessed an escalating interest in preprosthetic surgery, which has harboured the development of many new techniques.

## 17.2 Pattern of Resorption

Immediately after extraction, the socket will suffer a reduction in the dimensions both in buccolingual and apicocoronal aspects. This catabolic process can be counteracted by the placement of implants. The resorption of the walls occurs in two phases, which are overlapping in nature. The first phase is characterised by the resorption of bundle bone and replacement with woven bone. The second phase involves the outer surfaces. The exact aetiology for this bone loss is unknown. Roux [3] opined the loss of alveolar bone occurring after tooth loss in the old age is an illustration of disuse atrophy. According to studies by Wolff [4], the mass and structure of the bone can get adapted to the mechanical demands. The resorption is a multifactorial, biomechanical process that results from a combination of anatomic, metabolic, and mechanical determinants. Since all of these factors vary from one patient to the next, these different cofactors may combine in infinite variety of ways, thus explaining the variations in resorption between patients. So ridge resorption is a chronic, progressive, irreversible, and cumulative phenomenon resulting from physiologic, environmental and pathologic components.

Mercier [5] illustrated the general resorptive changes that take place in an edentulous ridge. He summarised the stages as follows:

1. The ridge is wide enough at its crest to accommodate the recently extracted teeth.
2. The ridge becomes thin and pointed.
3. The pointed ridge flattens to the level of the basal bone.
4. The flattened ridge becomes concave as the basal bone resorbs.

**Electronic Supplementary Material** The online version of this chapter (https://doi.org/10.1007/978-981-15-1346-6_17) contains supplementary material, which is available to authorized users.

B. John (✉)
Department of Oral and Maxillofacial Surgery, Government Dental College, Kottayam, Kerala, India


K. Bonanthaya et al. (eds.), *Oral and Maxillofacial Surgery for the Clinician*, https://doi.org/10.1007/978-981-15-1346-6_17

Based on these stages, he grouped the residual ridges as

Group 1—minor ridge remodelling.
Group 2—sharp atrophic residual ridge.
Group 3—basal bone ridge.
Group 4—basal bone resorption.

The pattern of resorption in maxilla differs from that of the mandible. Also, the pattern varies with the site in maxilla and mandible. The extensive study by Cawood and Howell [6] depicts the following conclusions.

Basal bone does not change shape significantly. But if subjected to harmful local effects, it undergoes change.

Alveolar bone exhibits significant changes in shape in both horizontal and vertical axes.

In anterior mandible, the bone loss is vertical and horizontal, but in posterior mandible, the bone loss is mainly vertical.

In anterior maxilla, the bone loss is both vertical and horizontal. The same pattern is exhibited in the posterior maxilla. To summarise, the stage of bone loss varies anteriorly and posteriorly and between the jaws.

**Box 17.1 Effects of Edentulism**

- Typical overclosed appearance.
- Neurosensory disturbances.
- Encroachment of muscle tissues leading to instability.
- Prolonged effects of edentulism culminates in pathological fracture.

**Box 17.2 Goals of Preprosthetic Surgery**

- Rehabilitation of tissues.
- Relieving of interferences.
- Repositioning of attachments.
- Restoration of alveolar ridge dimensions.
- Re-establishing maxillomandibular relationships in all spatial dimensions.
- Satisfying aesthetics and function.

### 17.2.1 Types of Ridges

Ridges can be classified by their shape. There are V–shaped, U–shaped and knife edged types. The U shaped is the ideal while the V shaped, though successfully distribute the stress but may be unable to retain the peripheral seal during the jaw movements. Knife edged ones are a constant source of soreness under the stress.

A more scientific categorisation is made by Cawood and Howell [6].

Cawood and Howell [6] classification of edentulous jaws:

- Class I—dentate.
- Class II—Immediately post-extraction.
- Class III—well-rounded ridge form, with adequate height and width of the alveolar process.
- Class IV—knife-edge form with adequate height but inadequate width of the alveolar process.
- Class V—flat-ridge form with inadequate height and width.
- Class VI—depressed ridge form with evident basal bone loss.

## 17.3 Treatment Planning

The preliminary step is the assessment of the patient, which commences from the history taking to the physical examination. The role of radiograph is relevant especially the panoramic view to reveal the deep-seated disorders. Storer [7] found 32% of edentulous patients had an asymptomatic pathologic condition, which warrants the need for radiographic examination. Crandell and Trueblood [8] also advised radiographic examination to rule out the presence of pathologies, root remnants, and even impacted tooth. Radiographic assessment is one of the parameters in detecting bone quality.

Lekholm and Zarb [9] categorise bone quality as follows

Type 1: bone in which almost the entirety is composed of homogeneous compact bone.
Type 2: bone in which a thick layer of compact bone surrounds a core of dense trabecular bone.
Type 3: bone in which a thin layer of cortical bone surrounds a core of dense trabecular bone.
Type 4: bone characterised as a thin layer of cortical bone surrounding a core of low-density trabecular bone of poor strength.

**Box 17.3 Preprosthetic Surgical Procedures can be Classified**

**Ridge correction procedures**
***Hard-tissue correction***
Alveoloplasty
Alveolectomy
• Reduction of,
  Genial tubercles
  Mylohyoid ridge,
  Maxillary tuberosity.
• Correction of tori, exostoses.
***Soft-tissue correction***
• Frenectomy
  Labial
  Lingual
  Excision of hypertrophic tissues

**Ridge extension procedures**
Vestibuloplasty
***Ridge augmentation procedures***
Superior border
Inferior border
Interpositional grafting
Visor osteotomy
Combined with orthognathic surgery

## 17.4 Ridge Correction Procedures

### 17.4.1 Alveoloplasty

The term refers to the restructuring or resurfacing of the alveolar process bone to provide a functional skeletal relationship. Simple plasty insists on the reshaping of the alveolar bone during the extraction procedure. The sharp edges of the alveolus will impede the healing process with symptoms of pain and discomfort. The shape of the ridges with sufficient width and height should be able to distribute the forces properly.

Preservation of alveolar bone is of utmost importance in the extraction procedure. Simple alveolar contouring includes compression and infracture of the socket, but overcompression and reduction should be avoided. If extractions are carried out before the prosthesis fabrication, attempts are made to preserve the alveolus. In multiple extractions, postextraction irregularity exists, which warrants the need for extended alveoloplasty. Here, mucoperiosteal flap may be raised by a crestal incision to get adequate access for the bone reshaping. Extreme care has to be taken during flap elevation since the soft tissues are tightly adhered to the bony irregularities. The use of bone rongeur or file is needed to smooth the edges, but large irregularities may be rectified by rotary instruments. Ensure saline irrigation to keep the temperature below 47 degrees to prevent necrosis. Once the hard tissue is removed, the excess soft tissue is trimmed to prevent the instability of the prosthesis. Closure with absorbable sutures in running or lock stitch fashion is achieved.

### 17.4.2 Intercortical Alveoloplasty

In situations where the alveolar process is prominent but regular, the need for alveoloplasty by the removal of interseptal bone and collapsing the buccal or labial cortical plates to meet the palatal or lingual plates is warranted. This method was propagated by Dean and Mackay [10]. This is an ideal procedure in case of immediate denture placement and usually carried out in the anterior region (Fig. 17.1a and b). This is done by the placement of vertical bone cuts in the canine region through subperiosteal tunnels. Apply the digital pressure to infracture the bone. If unsuccessful, the labial plate can be fractured with an osteotome inserted through a horizontal subperiosteal tunnel made through the vertical lateral incision. The bone distal to the canine is rounded off to maintain the contour. Mucosa is sutured appropriately to retain the new position of the cortices and if needed an acrylic splint may be used to stabilise it.

### 17.4.3 Genial Tubercle Reduction

Genioglossus muscle is one which is adhered to the lingual aspect of the anterior mandible and when the resorption continues, the genial tubercle becomes more prominent and along with the attached muscles creating a displacement of prosthesis. In this case, the pronounced tubercle may be trimmed and released. This procedure may be done alone or in combination with procedures suggestive of lowering the floor of the mouth.

#### 17.4.3.1 Procedure

A crestal incision from the midline to the midbody of mandible is made to get adequate access, followed by dissection in subperiosteal fashion, thus exposing the tubercle and the attached muscle. Muscle may be excised from the bony attachment by using a monoplanar electrocautery with care to be taken to achieve haemostasis or else chance of airway embarrassment by the occurrence of expanding hematoma. The exposed genial tubercle is trimmed by round or fissure bur. Further smoothening is made by bone file. The flap is returned to the original position and closed by nonresorbable

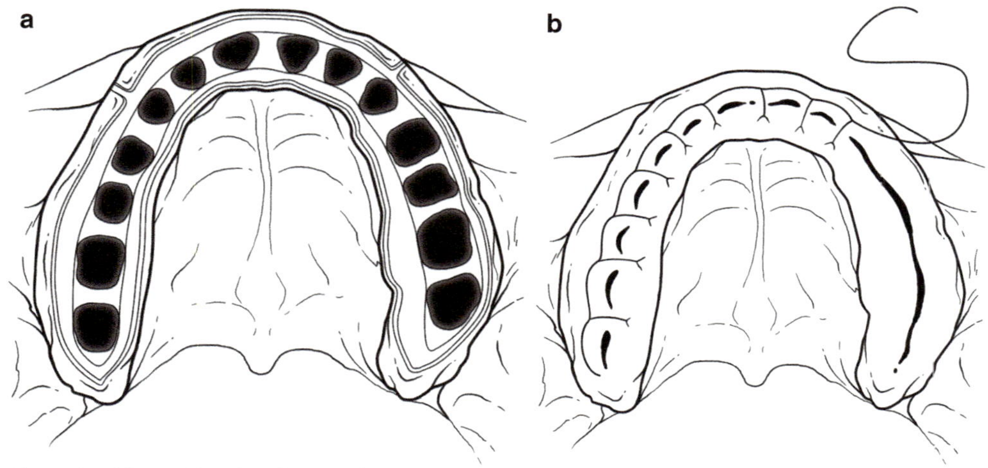


**Fig. 17.1** (**a**) Incision for intercortical alveoloplasty (**b**) closure of wound

sutures. Anderson [11] proposed reattaching the genioglosus and geniohyoid muscles at a lower level. Here, he advocated using a sagittal incision in the midline in the periosteum and exposing the genial shelf. The tubercle is reduced and the incision is closed with absorbable sutures.

### 17.4.4 Mylohyoid Ridge Reduction

In cases of extensive resorption, the ridge becomes prominent and creates hurdle for the smooth placement of denture; hence, the need for ridge reduction occurs. The denture flanges impinge on the sharp mylohyoid ridge and patient experiences pain and discomfort. The advent of implants may obviate the need for such a surgical procedure, yet in many cases where implant placement is not feasible, the dentures become a necessity and the mylohyoid ridge reduction needs to be accomplished.

#### 17.4.4.1 Procedure

The procedure can be carried out under local anaesthesia or sedation. After successful nerve block, the incision is carried out along the crest of the ridge in the posterior mandible area followed by subperiosteal dissection and exposure of the mylohyoid ridge and the attached muscle (Fig. 17.2a and b). The muscle is detached and relieved. The residual ridge is smoothed with file, flap returned, and closed with sutures (Fig. 17.2c). Care is ensured to obtain haemostasis.

## 17.5 Maxillary Tuberosity Reduction

Maxillary tuberosity may be enlarged in size and it engorges the intermaxillary space and interferes with denture placement. The reduction of the tuberosity may be needed to create space for the placement of dentures. Generally, the intermaxillary distance should be at least 1 cm when patients are placed into the correct or planned vertical dimension of occlusion. The excessiveness of the tuberosity and the need for its reduction can be assessed by some clinical manoeuvres. An instrument like a dental mirror can be used to assess the vertical clearance by passing it between the tuberosity and retomolar tissues. The mirror may be positioned in the lateral aspect and the patient is instructed to open and close mouth so as to determine the need for reduction of tuberosity in the horizontal plane. The pneumatisation status should be ascertained before the reduction procedure is undertaken since the maxillary sinus may descend into the tuberosity. So a radiographic examination is essential prior to surgical management. An elliptical incision is made followed by subperiosteal dissection. The engorged tuberosity is trimmed to the desired level and excessive tissue is removed from both buccal and palatal side. The amount of bone removal can be dictated by a surgical guide that was created from study models. Rotary instrumentation, rongeur and a bone file may be used to remove the bone. The flaps are trimmed to leave the excess redundant tissue and sutured in place (Fig. 17.3a–f). Guernsey [12] proposed a different technique for the reduction of the tuberosity. He advised placing a horizontal incision superiorly in the vestibule from the premolar area to the posterior aspect of the tuberosity and a mucoperiosteal flap is released inferiorly to get access to the tuberosity region. Any excessive soft tissue of fibrous nature is removed from within the flap and excessive bone is also removed by using suitable instruments. To correct the redundancy of tissues, soft tissue may be removed from the superior aspect of the incision and flap is sutured back to the periosteum and a stent is placed. This method claims to increase the vestibular depth to some extent (Fig. 17.4a–d). Antral communication should be checked and if present managed accordingly.

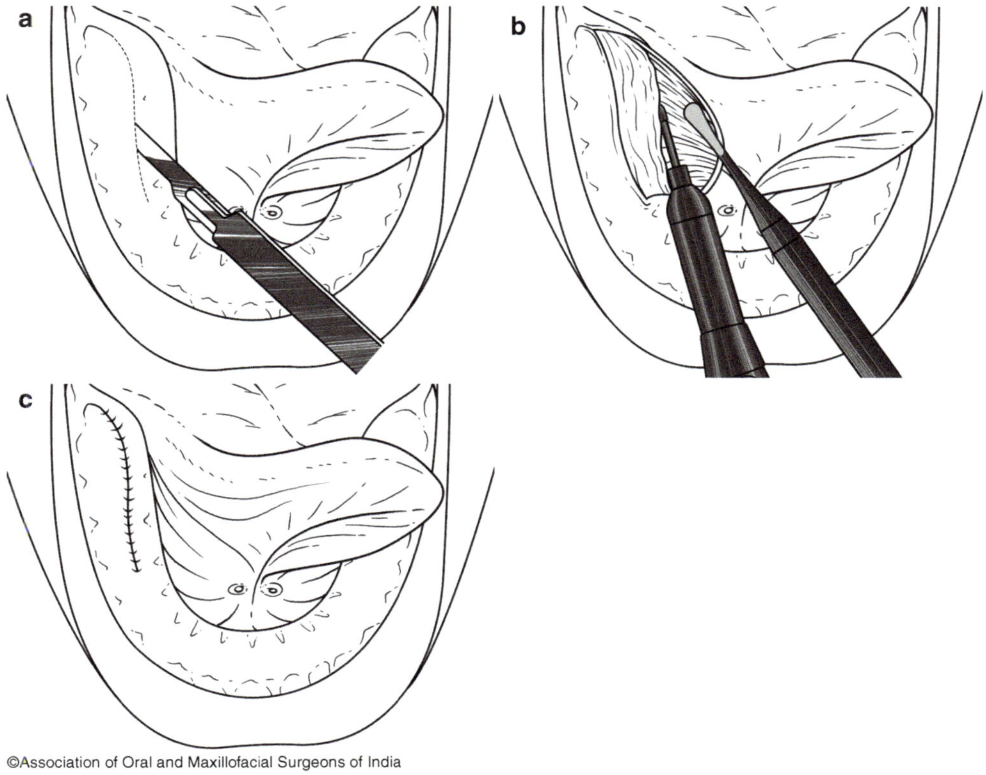


**Fig. 17.2** (**a**) Incision along the crest of the ridge (**b**) flap raised and bone trimmed (**c**) sutured the incision

## 17.6 Torus Removal

*Tori,* meaning 'to stand out' or 'lump in Latin, refer to innocuous bony outgrowths. The aetiology of the occurrence is unclear. Early description of the occurrence of tori is found in the Proceedings of the Royal Society of Medicine by Rickman Godlee [13], which was followed by the reports from various authors and later beautifully summarised by Garcia Garcia [14]. In dentate individuals, the removal of torus may not be needed unless it impedes with functions or it generates discomfort. But in edentulous, the presence of tori precludes the smooth placement of denture, so the removal becomes mandatory. Other indications include mucosal surface getting traumatised with frequent episodes of ulceration, presenting with deep undercuts and multiple nodules and psychological issues. Literature also suggests tori as donor sources of autogenous bone for intraoral grafting procedures. Morraes et al. [15] and Hassan et al. [16] describe the versatility of the grafts from torus for reconstructive methods.

Classification of tori was initially proposed by Kolas [17], who classified them according to number of nodes and their placement as bilateral single, bilateral multiple, unilateral single, and unilateral multiple [18].

Haugen [19] formulated the categorisation of torus based on the size. It is illustrated as.

Type A—small tori into less than 2 mm in their largest diameter.
Type B—medium—2–4 mm in their largest diameter.
Type C—large- and more than 4 mm in their largest diameter.

Reichart [20] in his modification of Haugen's classification suggested few changes:

Grade I—Tori up to 3 mm in their largest dimension,
Grade II—Tori up to 6 mm in their largest dimension and.
Grade III—Tori above 6 mm belong to this group.

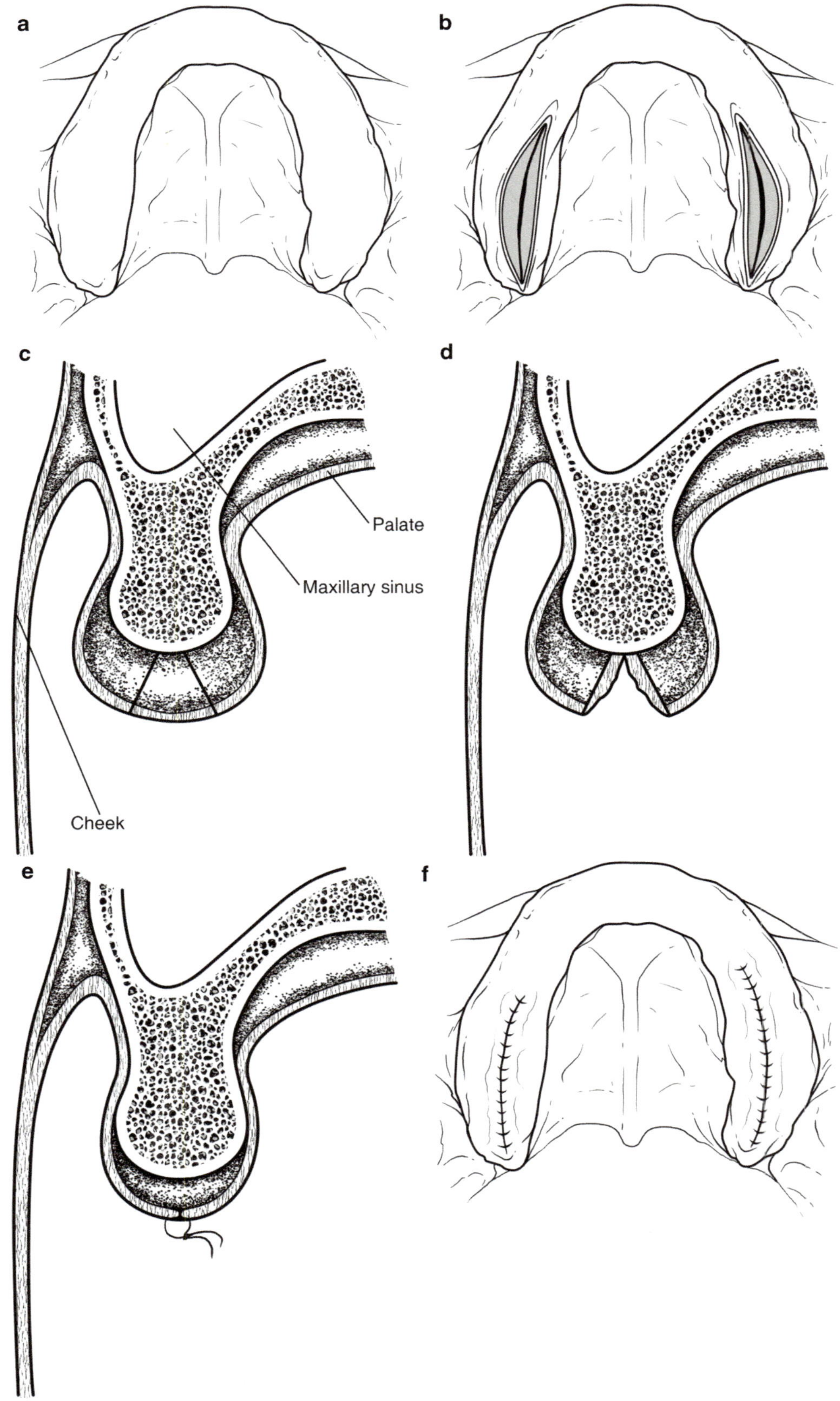




**Fig. 17.3** (**a**) Bulbous tuberosity, (**b**) incision placed and flap raised (**c** and **d**) reduction, (**e** and **f**) sutured incision

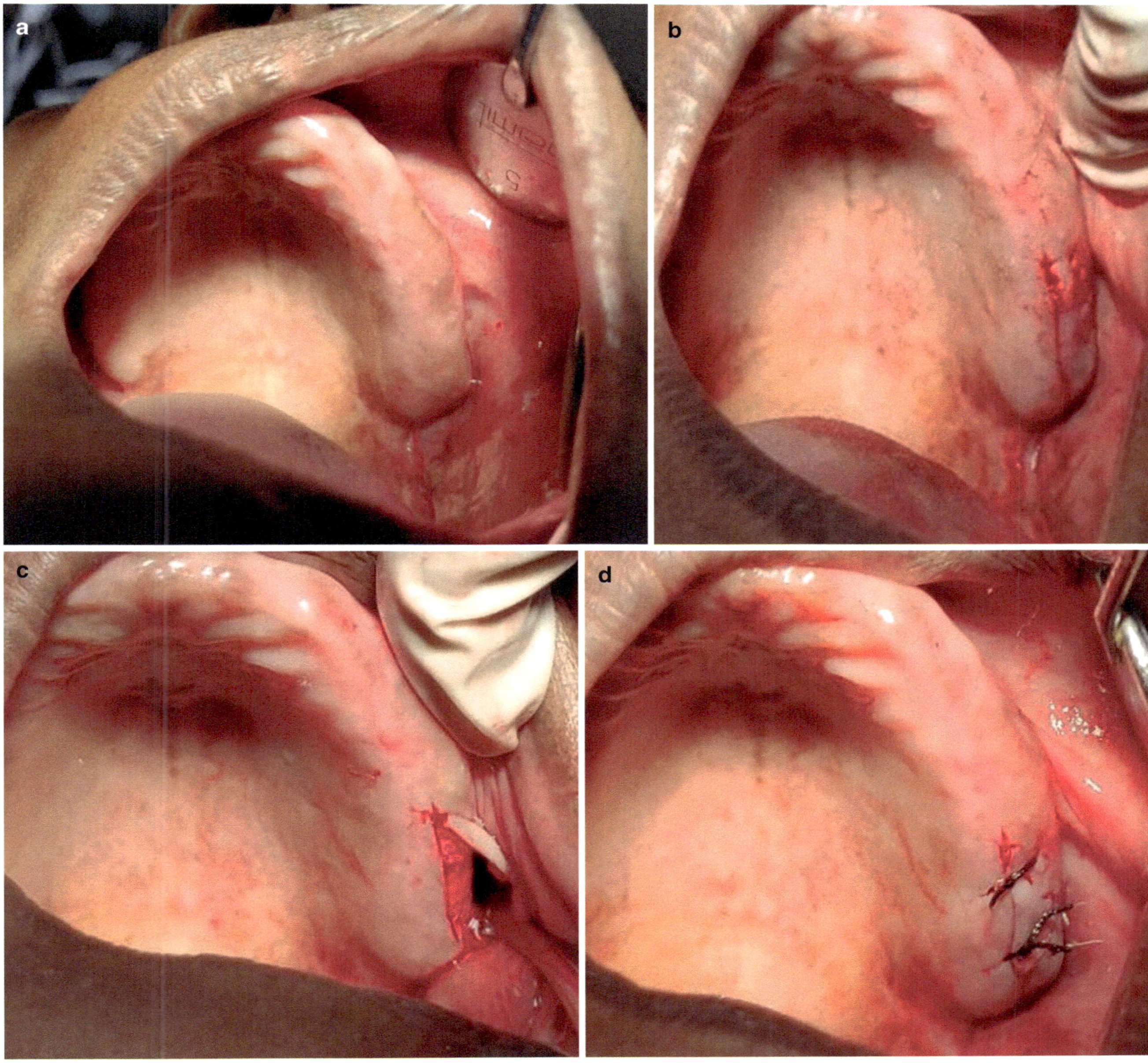


©Associat on of Oral and Maxillofacial Surgeons of India

**Fig. 17.4** Clinical photograph showing (**a**) bulbous tuberosity (**b**) incision (**c**) flap reflection (**d**) sutured wound

### 17.6.1 Palatal Tori Removal

As in any surgical procedures, here also the general systemic condition of the patient may be ascertained and the patient should be warned of the potential complications like the perforations leading to oronasal communication and wound dehiscence. To overcome this problem, preoperatively an impression may be made and cast is fabricated and splint is prepared. Palatal tori may be of different shapes, like lobulated or nodular. The morphology of the torus dictates the incisions required to expose it. Surgical access is accomplished by various types of incisions, "C-" or "U-" shaped incision, palatal incision or double "Y" incision also known as open-door technique. Most commonly used is double Y incision (Fig. 17.5a–f). After successful anaesthesia, a midline incision in anteroposterior direction is made from a few

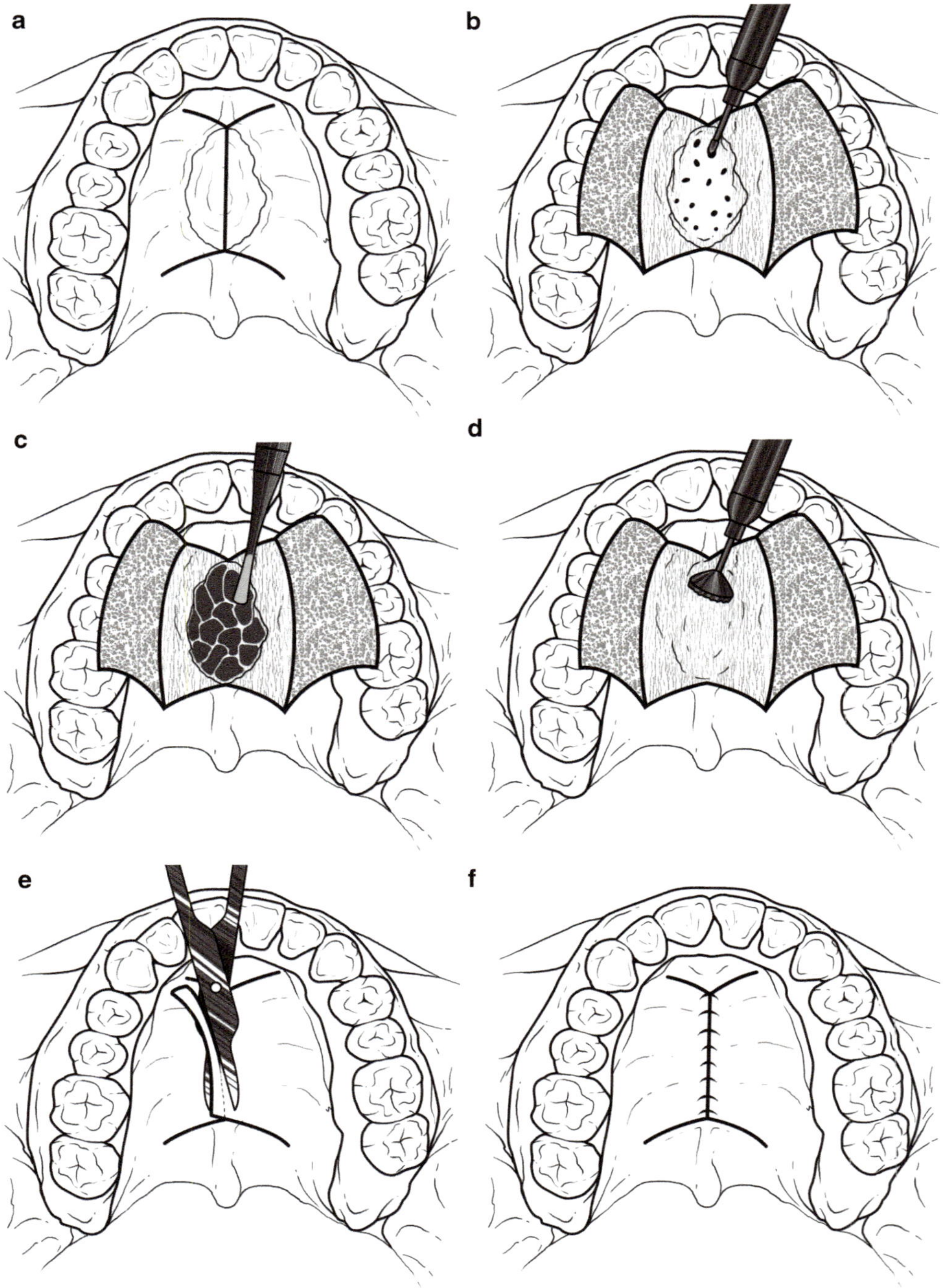


**Fig. 17.5** (**a**) Incision, (**b**) flap raised, (**c**) multiple grooves made, (**d**) final trimming by acrylic trimmer, (**e**) excess soft tissue trimmed, (**f**) closure

mm ahead of the anterior margin of the torus and continued posteriorly to the most posterior visible point of the torus. Oblique-releasing incisions may be placed at the anterior end of the midline incision and may be extended laterally and anteriorly to end lateral to the lateral margins of the torus. From the posterior end of the midline incision without violating the soft palate, posterior releasing incisions may be placed to extend obliquely in a lateral and posterior direction. Thus, a fair access is obtained. The subperiosteal flap is raised. The small torus can be easily removed by round. But in case of large ones, grooves are created and separated into discrete segments with bur and then by osteotome (Fig. 17.6).

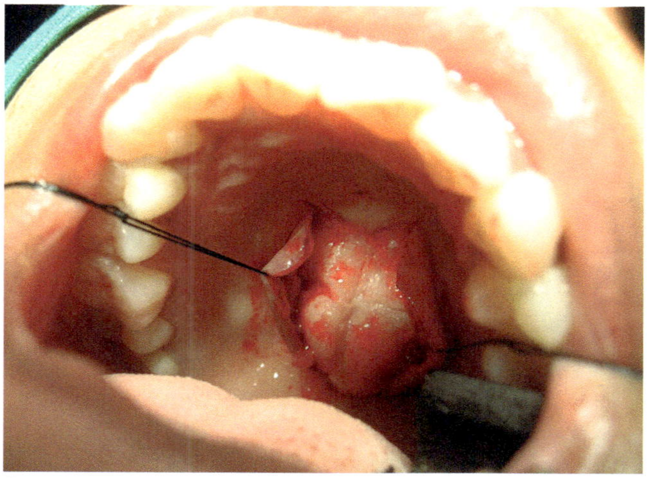



**Fig. 17.6** Clinical photograph showing palatal tori and surgical exposure, double Y-incision used

Copious irrigation is done to clear the debris and flap repositioned in primary fashion. The fabricated stent may be placed to avoid the haematoma and the dead space formation.

#### 17.6.2 Lingual Torus

The lingual tori are found in the lingual aspect of the alveolar ridge in the canine and premolar regions. They vary in size and shape; some are pedicled, while others are broad based. An intrasulcular incision without releasing is made from the lingual midline to a point beyond the posterior limit of the tori. In edentulous case, the incision may be placed in the crest of the alveolar ridge. A full-thickness flap is raised to expose the tori and if needed local anaesthetic may be injected in the area to balloon the tissues for easy elevation of the flap. The vertical-releasing incision should be avoided to prevent the vascularity compromise.

The lingual torus may be removed by bur or osteotome. Smaller ones can be easily removed by bur, but the larger require cleavage plane created by bur and later completed by osteotomes. After the removal of the tori, it is essential to check the surface and clear of the irregularities by the use of rongeur and bone files. The flap repositioned and sutured.

## 17.7 Exostosis

It is a benign osseous hypertrophic formation with more predilections to the maxilla. A mucoperiosteal flap is elevated after adequate infiltration of the mucosa. The bone is resected and smoothed with an osteotome or a bur. The smooth placement of the prosthesis is achieved by the facilitation of the errorless foundation, constituted by both hard and soft tissues. In many cases, the hard-tissue framework may be normal, but the soft-tissue impediments affect the stability of the prosthesis. So, the correction of the interferences by the abnormal soft tissues is needed.

Apart from hard tissues, sometimes soft-tissue interferences inhibit the smooth placement of the prosthesis. The unfavourable soft-tissue framework affects the stability of the prosthesis and needs correction by various procedures.

## 17.8 Excision of Reactive Inflammatory Papillary Hyperplasia

This is commonly associated with prolonged wearing of an ill-fitting denture. The condition is recognised as reddened, nodular, or papillary excrescences arising from the palatal mucosa. It can be seen in areas where the denture flanges rest. Removal is accomplished by local anaesthesia or sedation (Fig. 17.7).

## 17.9 Frenectomy

Active and strong frenal attachments interfere with the placement of dentures and the relief of attachments are needed. Various incisions like v-y, z plasty, and diamond-shaped incisions are used in frenectomy procedures.

#### 17.9.1 Labial Frenectomy (Video 17.1)

In the edentulous state, the abnormal frenal attachment gets irritated by the denture flanges leading to instability. The denture area can be relieved but it may be unaesthetic, so the need for frenectomy arises. Z plasty is used to eliminate the abnormal attachment. Another method is the V- Y procedure but has a disadvantage of creating excessive bulk of tissue at the depth of vestibule. The operative procedure is as follows (Fig. 17.8a, b and c). It is carried under local anaesthesia, but the tissue should not be overdistended. The lip is extended and everted to tense the frenum. The V-shaped piece of tissue is held by tissue forceps or Allis clamp, and an incision is made down to the periosteum on either side of the frenum. Resorbable sutures are preferred since the removal is difficult in this area. The first suture should be placed at the depth of the vestibule and should engage the periosteum to prevent the loss of the vestibular depth (Fig. 17.9a–e).

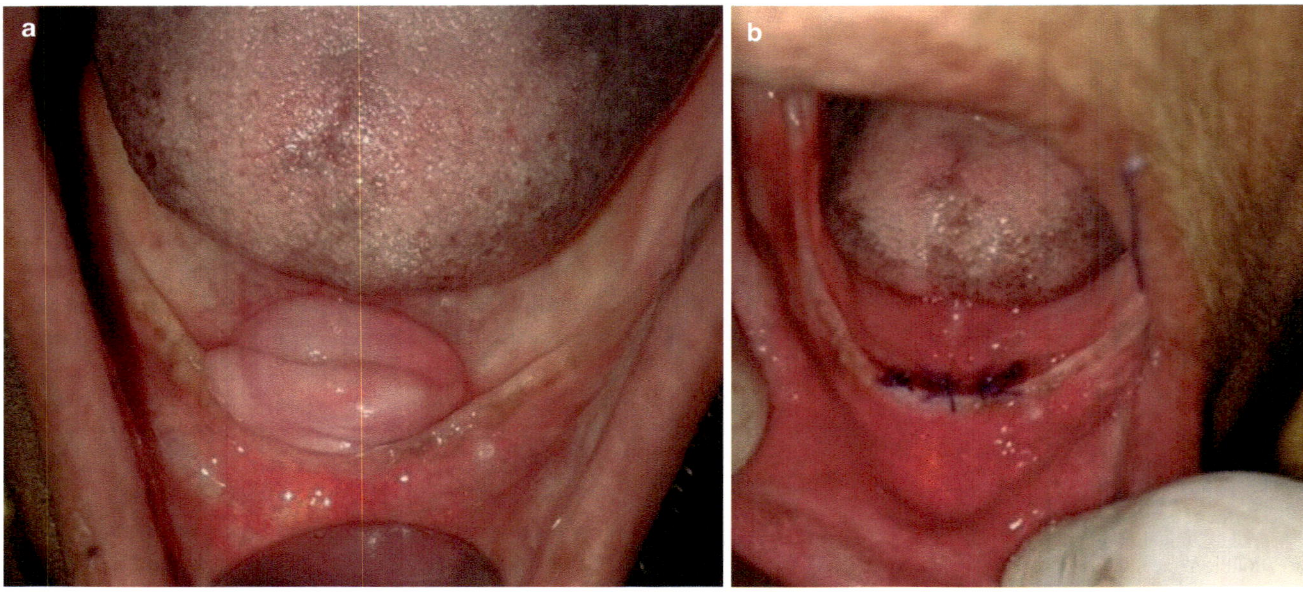



**Fig. 17.7** Clinical photographs showing (**a**) lingual papillary hyperplasia (**b**) suturing after excision

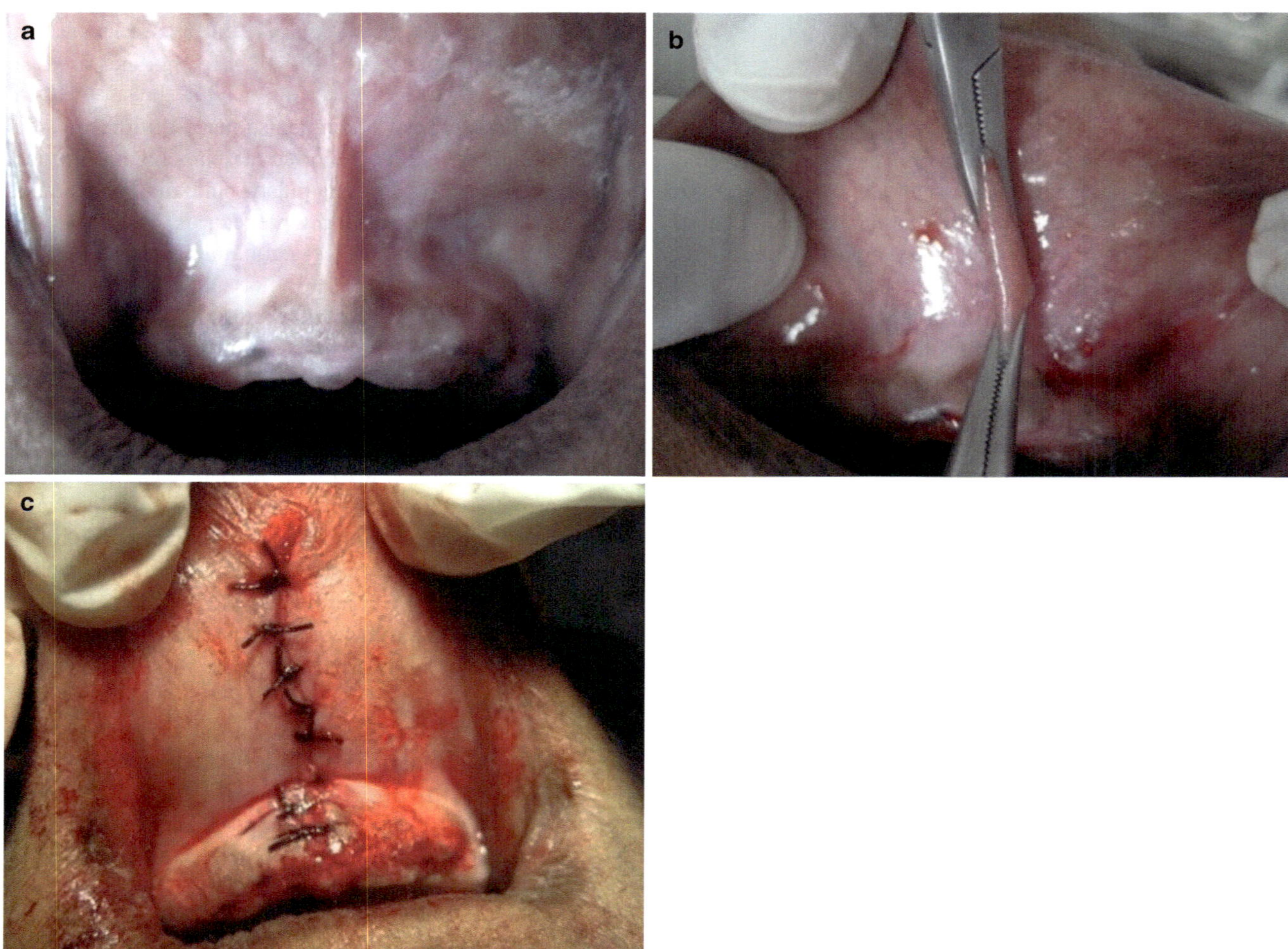



**Fig. 17.8** Clinical photographs showing (**a**) abnormal attachment of frenum (**b**) tissue held with mosquito forceps (**c**) suturing

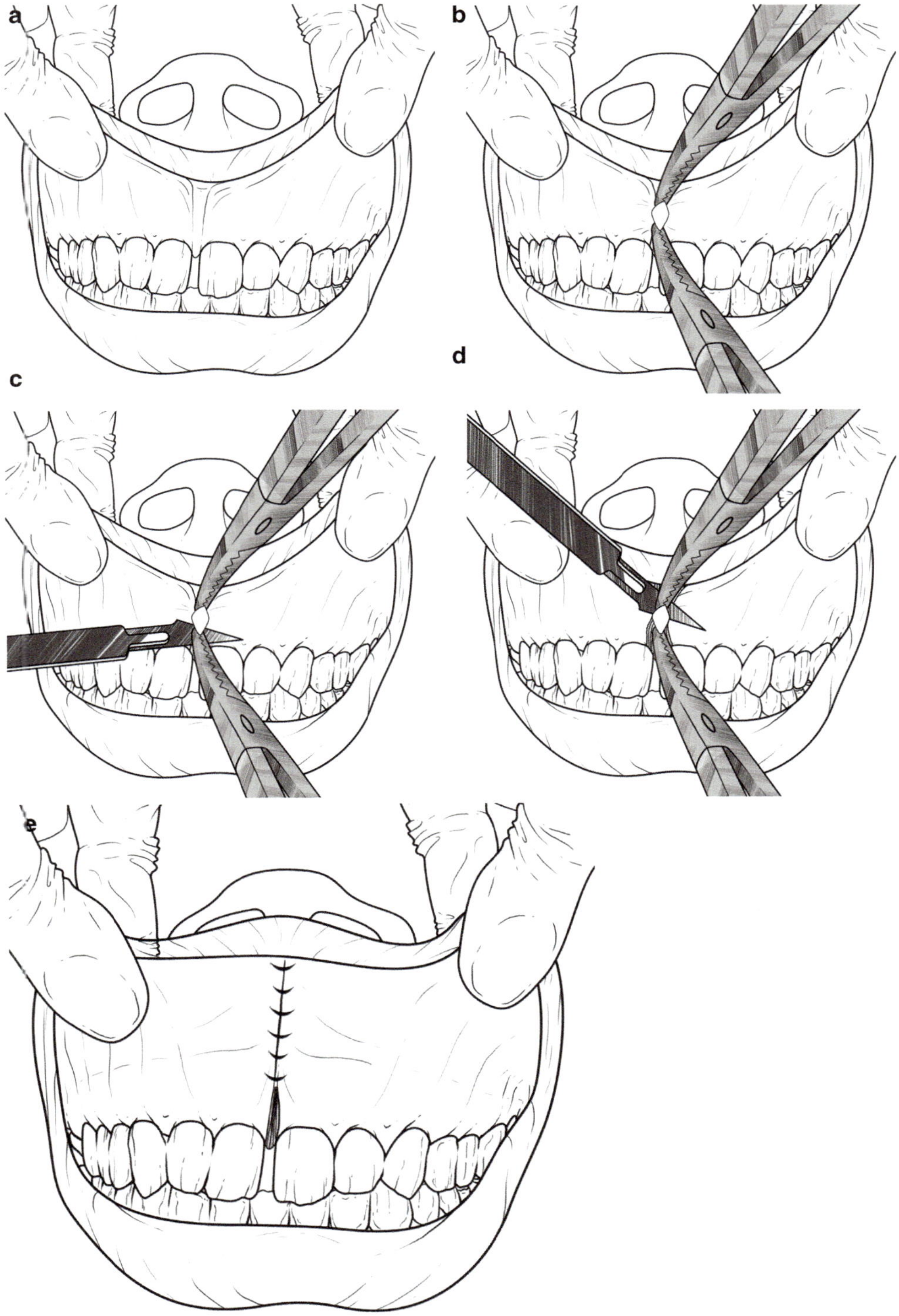




**Fig. 17.9** (**a**) low attached frenum, (**b**) frenal tissue grasped by forceps, (**c** and **d**) diamond-shaped tissue removal, (**e**) closure

### 17.9.2 Lingual Frenectomy (Video 17.2)

If the frenal attachment is near the crest of the lingual aspect, it will displace the denture. So the need for relief of the high attached frenum is needed. This procedure can be done under local anaesthesia or general anaesthesia (Fig. 17.10a–d). When local anaesthesia is used, bilateral lingual nerve block and infiltration are used. The tongue is grasped with traction sutures or forceps and the attachment of frenum to the ridge is cut and the wound is closed with sutures. In

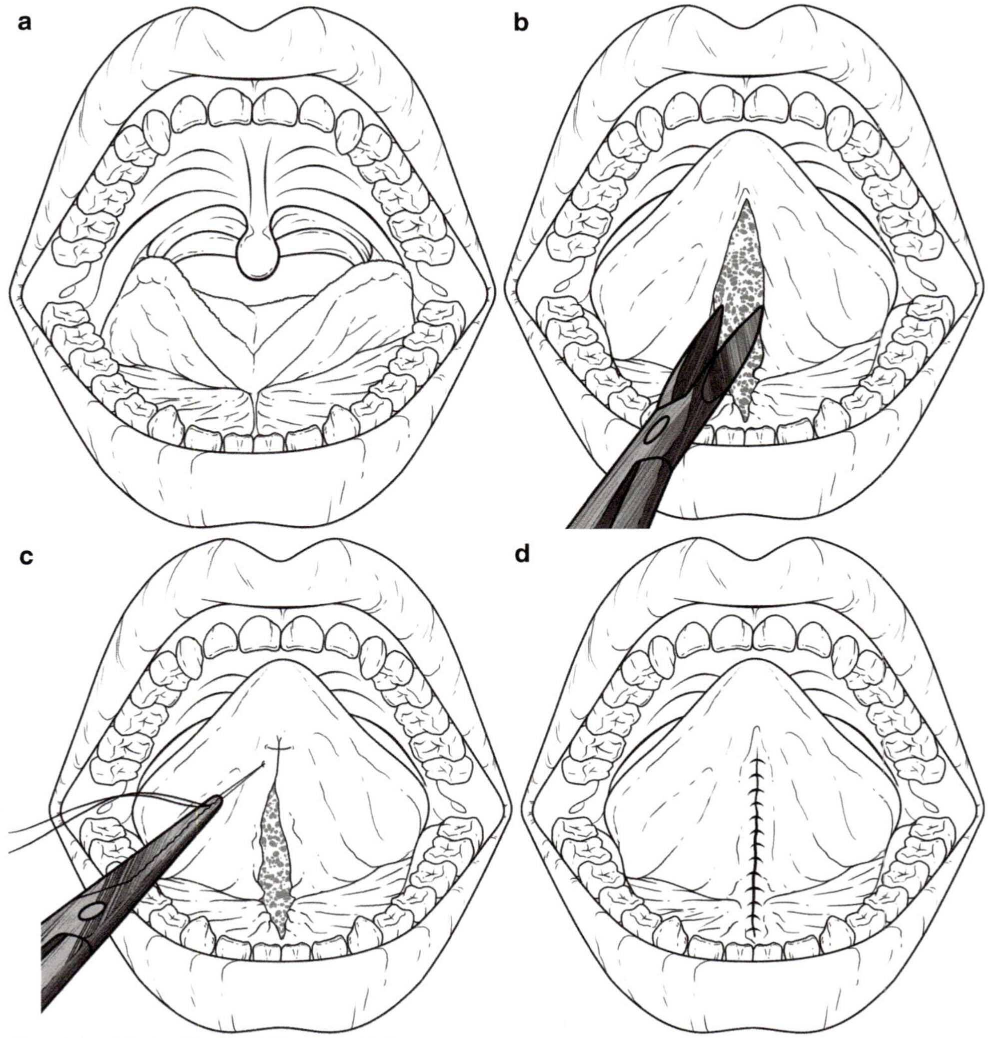




**Fig. 17.10** (**a**) High attached lingual frenum, (**b**) excision of frenum, (**c** and **d**) closure

some, a more extensive procedure is needed. Here, a transverse incision is made between ventral aspect of tongue and caruncle of submandibular duct. Sectioning of some fibres of the genioglosus muscle may yield greater degree of freedom. Diamond-shaped defect is closed with interrupted sutures. Postoperative pain is managed by analgesics and oedema controlled by steroids. There may be some ecchymosis in the floor of the mouth.

## 17.10 Ridge Extension Procedure

They are defined as the procedures surgically designed to uncover the existing basal bone of the jaw by repositioning the overlying mucosa and muscle attachments to an inferior position in mandible or to a superior position in maxilla. This will enable to accommodate the larger denture flanges, thus contributing to stability and retention (Tables 17.1 and 17.2).

### 17.10.1 Vestibuloplasty [Sulcoplasty, Sulcus Extension] (Box 17.4)

The reduction or obliteration of the sulcus is caused by [1] resorption of the alveolar process, [2] abnormally high muscle attachment in mandible or low on the maxilla, [3] scar tissue resulting from trauma or infection from the contiguous soft tissue.

Vestibuloplasties are carried out in mandible and maxilla. In mandible, both labial and lingual vestibuloplasties are performed. Stability of a denture can be improved by deepening the mandibularsulcus, generating more attached tissues over the functional ridge, and permanently maintaining the

**Table 17.1** Mandibular ridge extension procedures

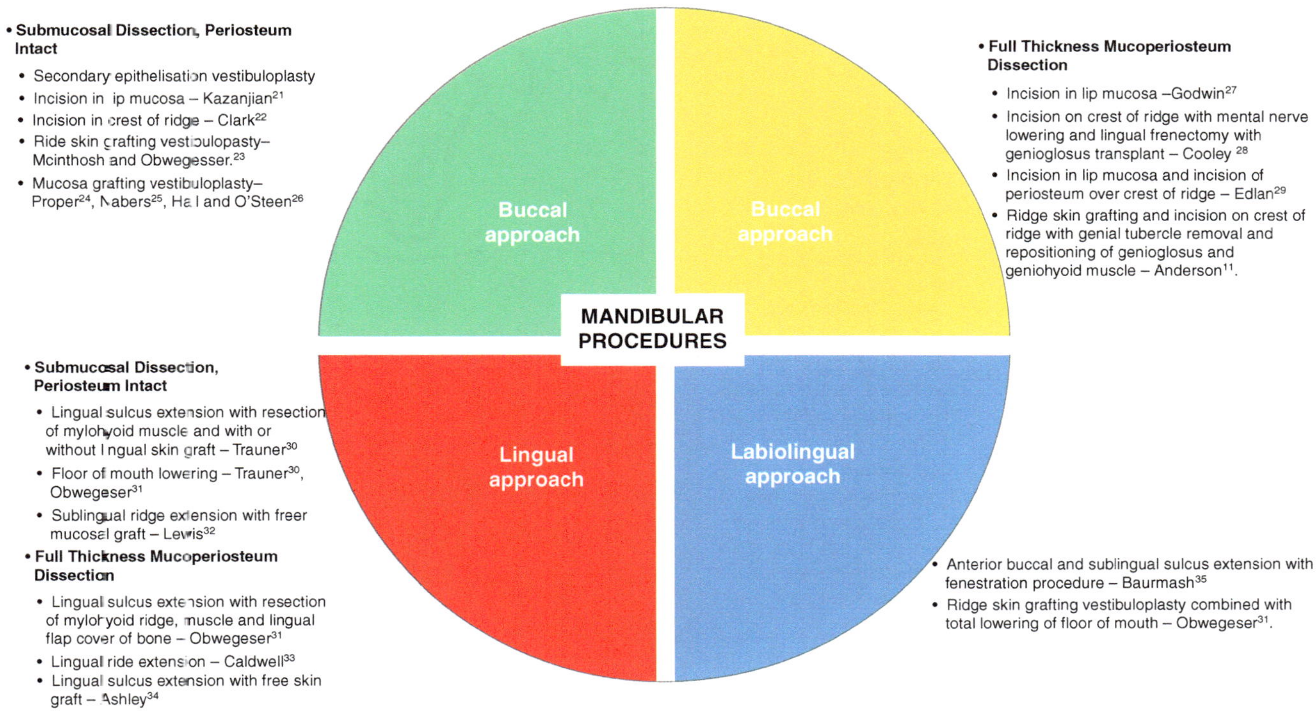


**Table 17.2** Maxillary ridge extension procedures

| Maxillary procedure | Buccal approach |
| --- | --- |
| | 1.Secondary epithelization vestibuloplasty<br>a.Full thickness mucoperiosteal dissection-Collett[36]<br>b.Submucosal dissection,periosteum intact-Szaba[37] |
| | 2.Submucosal vestibuloplasty-Obwegesser[31],Yrastorza[38]<br>3.Ridge skin grafting vestibuloplasty-Weiser[39], Schuchardt[40]<br>4.Buccal sulcus skin grafting-Esser[41],Gilles[42] |
| | 5.Ridge mucosa grafting vestibuloplasty-Obwegesser[31],Steinhauser[43],Maloney and associates[44] |

improved vestibular depth. Mandibular vestibuloplasty is carried out to predictably increase and maintain the functional alveolar ridge.

Preoperative preparation of the vestibuloplasty patients includes history, clinical examination, and suitable radiographs. Radiographs, especially orthopantomograph, help to evaluate the ridge height. The commonly performed ones are discussed in this section.

### 17.10.2 Transpositional Flap Vestibuloplasty [Lip-Switch Procedure]

The credit of this procedure goes to Kazanjian [21], later modified by many in the literature. Kethley and Gamble [45] modification finds more acceptance in the literature. The selection criteria for this procedure are the minimum bone height of 15 mm between the mental foramen areas.

**Box 17.4 Other Historically Relevant Vestibuloplasty Methods**

| Kazanjian's [21] | Clark's [23] |
|---|---|
| Flap is raised supraperiosteally from the lower lip.<br>Mobilised to the new vestibule and positioned<br>Stabilised by stent or dentures<br>The raw area in the lower lip is allowed to heal by secondary epithelisation | The facial surface of the ridge is chosen to raise the flap<br>The dissection in supraperiosteal fashion is done.<br>The raw area is in the ridge surface |
| *Godwin* [27] *modification*<br>A similar technique, except subperiosteal stripping, was performed | *Obwegessor* [31] *modification*<br>The use of skin grafts over the denuded surface to facilitate healing. |
| *Kethley and Gamble* [45] *modification of Kazanjian*—the lip switch technique<br>A labial mucosal flap is raised and extended to the crest of the ridge from the lip incision placed initially | *Tortoerlli* [46] *modification*<br>Fenestrations are made in the periosteum along the base of the newly created vestibule in a horizontal fashion. |

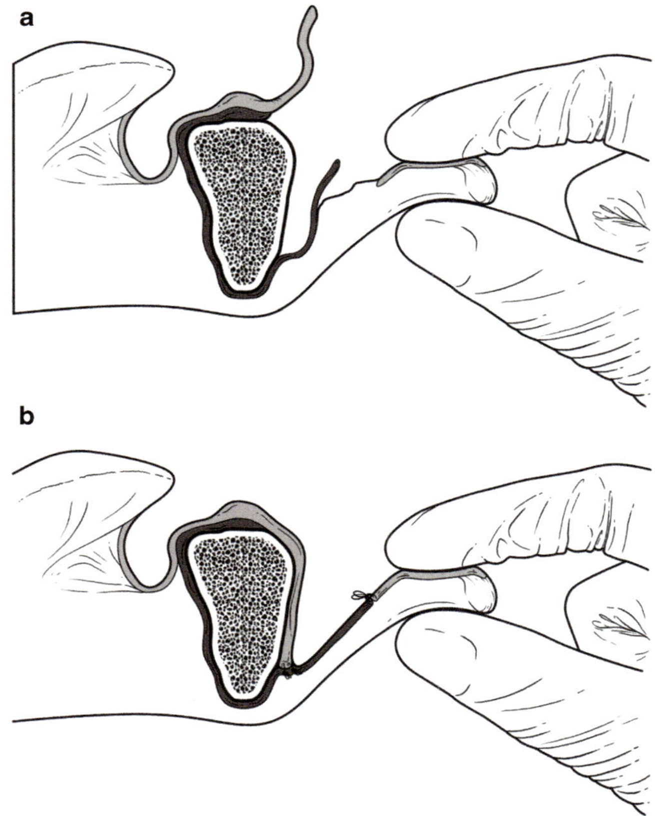




**Fig. 17.11** Lip switch vestibuloplasty (**a**) Labial mucosa pedicled near the crest of the ridge (**b**) pedicled flap sutured to the depth of the vestibule

#### 17.10.2.1 Procedure

The technique involves the administration of local anaesthesia followed by mucosal incision. The mucosal flap is elevated and pedicled near the crest of the ridge (Fig. 17.11a and b). An incision is placed near the superior portion of the periosteum. A supraperiosteal dissection is carried in the inferior direction, thereby removing the attachments of the muscular and connective tissues to the indicated vestibular depth. The labial periosteal margin is sutured to the incised lip mucosa. This is followed by the suturing of the pedicled flap to the periosteum at the depth of the vestibule.

### 17.10.3 Mandibular Vestibuloplasty with Grafting

Indicated in cases where the lip switch procedure is not possible due to the inadequate tissue availability. The options permissible in such cases were either secondary epithelisation or covering the denuded areas with grafts. The former became less popular because of wound contraction leading to the loss of vestibular depth. Here, the desired alveolar height between the mental foramina is not less than 10 mm in contrast to the minimum of 15 mm in lip switch.

#### 17.10.3.1 Procedure

An incision is placed at the mucogingival junction and a supraperiosteal dissection carried out to the desired vestibular depth. During the dissection, care is taken not to dissect more than half of the mentalis muscle to avoid the chance of the ptosis of the submental tissues referred as 'witch chin'. The margin of the incision is now sutured to the periosteum in the depths of the vestibule. The harvested graft is now placed over the recipient bed after ensuring adequate haemostasis. The graft is contoured to the correct shape, fenestrated, placed, and fixed on the periosteum with the help of stent or by sutures.

The grafts may be harvested from cutaneous or mucosal areas or allogenic in nature. The best sites for skin graft harvesting are medial thigh or caudal to the iliac crest, where fewer adnexal structures are present in the skin. Areas where smaller grafts are needed, mucosal grafts may be considered, which may be taken from the palate or buccal mucosa. Cultured skin grafts are also becoming popular but lack the mechanical and functional elements of the autogenous grafts. The narration of techniques of grafting is beyond the scope of this chapter.

### 17.10.4 Lingual Vestibuloplasty: Anterior Region

The severe atrophy of the mandible in the anterior region makes the genial tubercles prominent and affects the stability of the denture by the attached muscles. The exposure of the tubercles and the detachment of the genial muscles are accomplished by the procedure of lingual vestibuloplasty. Initially proposed by Kazanjian [21] and later modified by Lewis [32], the disadvantage of this procedure may be the loss of tongue function and difficulty in swallowing, which is encountered if more than half of the muscle is removed.

#### 17.10.4.1 Procedure

Incision is made in the anterior aspect of the crest of the alveolar ridge and subperiosteal flap is elevated. Dissection continued till the prominent genial tubercle with the attached muscle is encountered. The genial muscles are separated from the ridge and the tubercle is trimmed with bur and smoothed with bone file. The flap along with the muscle is lowered to the desired depth and it is maintained in the new position by stent and extraoral sutures. The exposed area is allowed for secondary re-epithelisation.

#### 17.10.4.2 Lingual Vestibuloplasty: Posterior Region

If the amount of the resorption is severe that it results in the displacement of the denture by the action of mylohyoid, then lowering of the mylohyoid muscle should be considered. This can be done alone or in combination with labial vestibuloplasty. The amount of the available depth can be assessed by a clinical manoeuvre, by placing a gloved finger along the lingual side of the mandible and asking the patient to touch the palate with the tip of the tongue. If this action displaces the finger, lowering the floor of mouth should be considered.

**Trauner's Technique** [30]

Incision is made from the retromolar area to the premolar area of the lingual aspect of the alveolar crest. Mucoperiosteal flap is raised and exposes the mylohyoid and the overlying periosteum. Dissection in the supraperiosteal plane is preferred to avoid the chance of the damage of the lingual nerve. The muscle with the flap is lowered to the desired depth. Sutures are passed through the mylohyoid and mucosa and secured to the skin extraorally. The exposed area is allowed for secondary re-epithelisation (Fig. 17.12a–f).

#### 17.10.4.3 Other Variations Include (Box 17.5)

*Brown* [47]—incision similar to Trauner's but a full-thickness mucoperiosteal flap is reflected to reveal the mylohyoid ridge. Here, the muscle is detached and the ridge is smoothed. The difference here is the sulcus is not deepened, but the problem with the ridge prominence is solved.

*Caldwell* [33]—here a crestal incision is employed and a supraperiosteal approach to access the mylohyoid ridge and the attached muscle. The flap is sutured to the original position. The new position is secured by a stent or a modified denture. Instead a polyethylene tubing can be also used to maintain the position.

*Edlan* [29]—here, a combination of the lip switch vestibuloplasty and lowering the floor of mouth is accomplished. Incision is made in the buccal sulcus instead of the crest of alveolar ridge. Plastic tubes are used to maintain the depth of the sulcus.

*Hopkin* [48]—mentioned as Hopkin's operation in the literature, it uses the combined modalities like labial vestibuloplasty, submucous sulcoplasty to remove the buccinator insertion and bilateral mylohyoid ridge reduction.

## 17.11 Ridge Augmentation Procedures

In atrophic maxilla, the alveolus may be accentuated by different options; earlier, vestibuloplasty was the choice of procedure. But the results achieved were not long lasting because of the continued resorptive process. So, the advent of augmentation came into action. In severe resorbed and atrophic ridges of Cawood and Howell [6] classes IV—VI, augmentation became mandatory. Unfortunately, this area of preprosthetic surgery has gained little attention, possibly there seemed to be no effective operation for ridge augmentation using an extraoral method; moreover, the penetration into the oral cavity during the procedure was deemed tantamounting to failure, as the surgeons are reluctant to perform the elective augmentation of mandible (Table 17.3).

Classification of alveolar ridge deficiency by Kent et al. [49] acts as a yardstick to identify the ridge nature and the grafting options.

Class 1—alveolar ridge is adequate in height but inadequate in width, usually with lateral deficiencies or undercut areas. Patient receives hydroxyapatite alone.

Class 2—alveolar ridge is deficient in both height and width and presents a knife-edge appearance. Patient receives hydroxyapatite alone.

Class 3—alveolar ridge has been resorbed to the level of the basilar bone producing a concave form in the posterior areas of mandible and a sharp bony ridge form with bulbous mobile soft tissues in the maxilla. Patient receives hydroxyapatite with or without autogenous cancellous bone.

Class 4—there is resorption of the basilar bone producing pencil-thin flat mandible or maxilla. Patient receives both hydroxyapatite with autogenous bone.

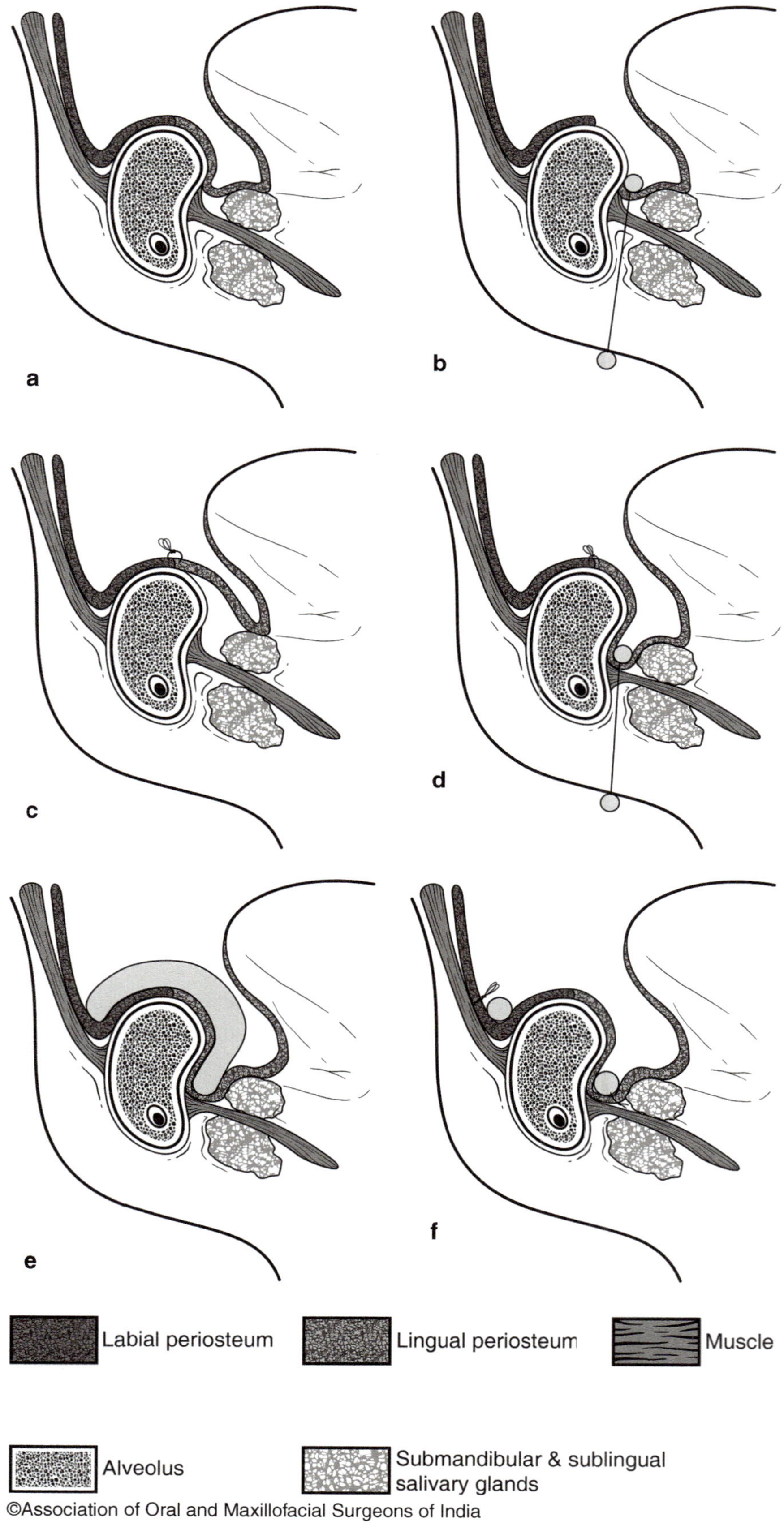


**Fig. 17.12** Lingual vestibuloplasty methods (**a**) Normal, (**b**) Trauner, (**c**) Brown, (**d**) Caldwell, (**e**) Hopkins, (**f**) Edlan

**Box 17.5 Lingual Vestibuloplasty Techniques**

| Trauner [30] | Brown [47] | Caldwell [33] | Edlan [29] |
|---|---|---|---|
| Carried over the posterior areas from retromolar pad to the premolar region with supraperiosteal dissection | Full thickness mucoperiosteal flap reflected | Carried over both posterior and anterior areas | Combination of lip switch vestibuloplasty with floor of mouth procedure |
| Mylohyoid muscle lowering is performed | Ridge is smoothened after the mylohyoid muscle is released<br>Not used alone but is combined with other vestibuloplasties | Detachment of mylohyoid and genioglosus muscle is done | |

**Table 17.3** Ridge augmentation procedures

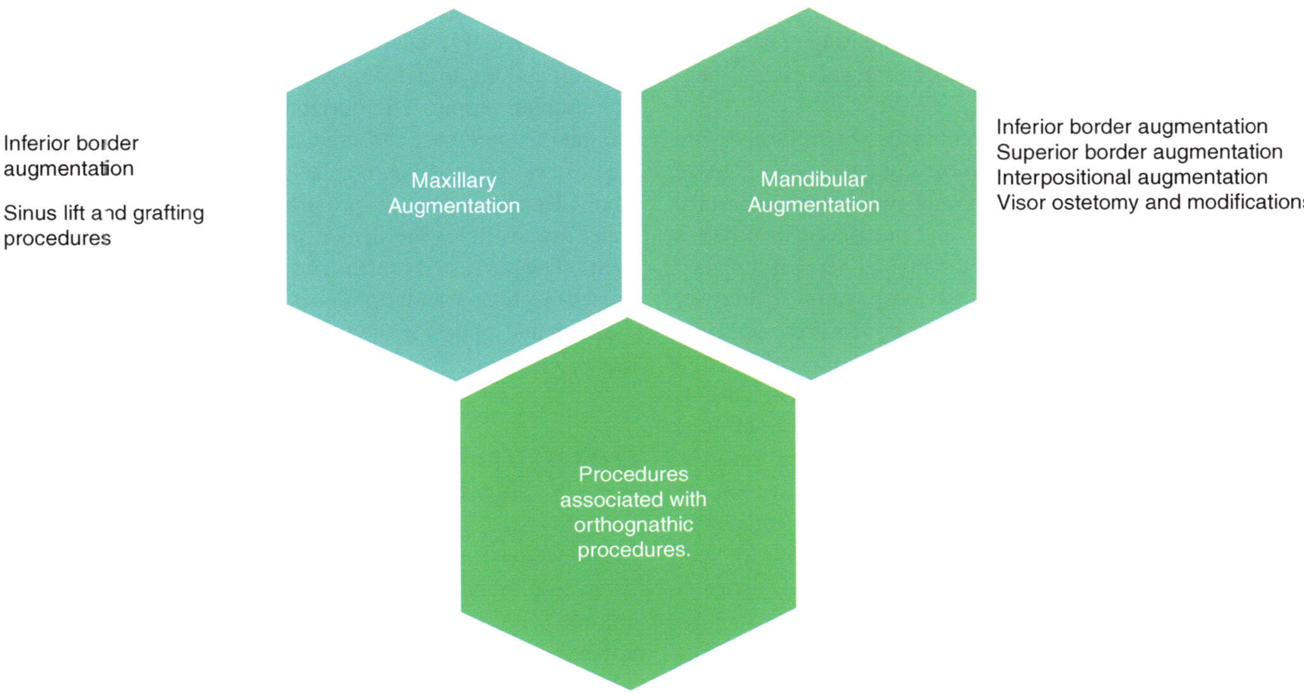


Autogenous bone grafting remains the ideal option to rectify the deficiency but accompanied by disadvantages like the need for hospitalisation and general anaesthesia, donor site morbidity, extensive surgical procedure, professional expertise and patient compliance.

### 17.11.1 Inferior Border Augmentation

The resorption of the mandible has been so extensive that it results in the severely atrophic condition and liable for a pathological fracture. In such a case, augmentation has to be achieved in the inferior border. The procedure was originally proposed by Marx and Sanders [50] and later modified by Quinn [51]. The procedure carries the advantages of non-obliteration of the sulcus, allowing the placement of the interim denture and making the secondary vestibuloplasty easier. But the procedure carries the burden of an extraoral scar and the chance of altering the facial appearance. Access to the lower border is gained by different ways by different authors. Some literature supports the use of incision used in the neck dissection, viz. a supraclavicular incision. It extends from the anterior border of sternocleidomastoid to the opposite counterpart. According to Sanders [50], a continuous submandibular incision from angle to angle is sufficient. Ridley and Mason [52] proposed the use of three small submandibular incisions connected by subperiosteal tunnels. The latter is opposed by Sanders [50] for the high chance of resorption by the pressure on the graft. Dissection is carried out to expose the inferior border of mandible. Two ribs of 15 to 20 cm long are harvested and bent to adapt the shape. Three or four transosseous holes are drilled in the lower border of mandible and wires are passed through these holes. One rib is placed against the lingual aspect and the other abutted against the buccal aspect. The space between the ribs is packed with available cortical chips. Ribs are secured in place by interosseous wires in circumferential pattern. Closure is achieved in layers and pressure dressing is applied. The narration of the technique of graft harvesting is beyond the limit of this chapter.

### 17.11.2 Superior Border Augmentation

The superior border enhancement is needed [53] in cases where the resorption is so severe that the height of the mandible is insufficient to accommodate the prosthesis or in cases where the patient suffers from pain during mastication, secondary to the pressure on the mental neurovascular bundle (Fig. 17.13a and b).

Recipient site is prepared and the mucosa is infiltrated with local anaesthetic solution containing epinephrine to achieve haemostasis. Crestal incision from the retromolar area to the opposite retromolar area is made and mucoperiosteal flap is raised. Care to be taken to avoid the mental nerve if it is near the superior border. Depending on the position, it may be lowered or freed. The existing superior border is exposed and prepared to receive the graft. The lingual flap is reflected to the level of the mylohyoid muscle. Davis and colleagues [54] described the technique of ridge augmentation, which uses two rib grafts of 15 cm. The ribs may be adjacent or alternate. One rib may be contoured by vertical scoring on the inner surface or by bending. Leake [55] recommends splitting the rib longitudinally and then bending it with forceps. The second rib is cut into pieces and packed against the solid rib. Before the placement of the rib, the superior aspect of the mandible is already prepared and suited to receive it. The posterior aspect of the rib should be in contact with mylohyoid shelf, slightly on the lingual aspect of the ramus. The ribs are fixed by three interosseous wires, one placed through each mylohyoid shelf and the other in the anterior region in the midline. Flaps returned to cover the graft.

### 17.11.3 Interpositional Grafting

Concept of placing bone grafts between the osteotomised segments of the mandible was initially proposed by Barros saint and Pasteur [56] and later experimentally proved by Danielson and Nemarich [57]. The horizontal osteotomy is achieved by an incision made inferior to the crest of the ridge. The length of the incision is determined by the area to be augmented. Incision is designed from the retromolar area to the other. A buccolabial mucoperiosteal flap is raised and the flap is greatly undermined to get adequate coverage of the graft. Issues are left untouched to ensure the patency of the vascular supply. The horizontal osteotomy is made by burs and osteotomes, and precise osteotomy is obtained by use of saws. The cut may be placed either above or below the canal, depending on the proximity to the inferior border. Transosseous holes are drilled in the lower and upper segments. The harvested graft is interposed between the osteotomised segments and stabilised by the wires. The flap is returned and approximated with sutures (Fig. 17.13c and Table 17.4).

### 17.11.4 The Visor Osteotomy and Modified Visor

The procedures of vestibuloplasty and floor of the mouth lowering may not be always successful to provide a stable and adequate basis for the prosthesis. The situation of the reduced vertical height needs to get addressed. Harle [58] published a report of an original and promising method to augment the alveolar ridge by means of a pedicled bone

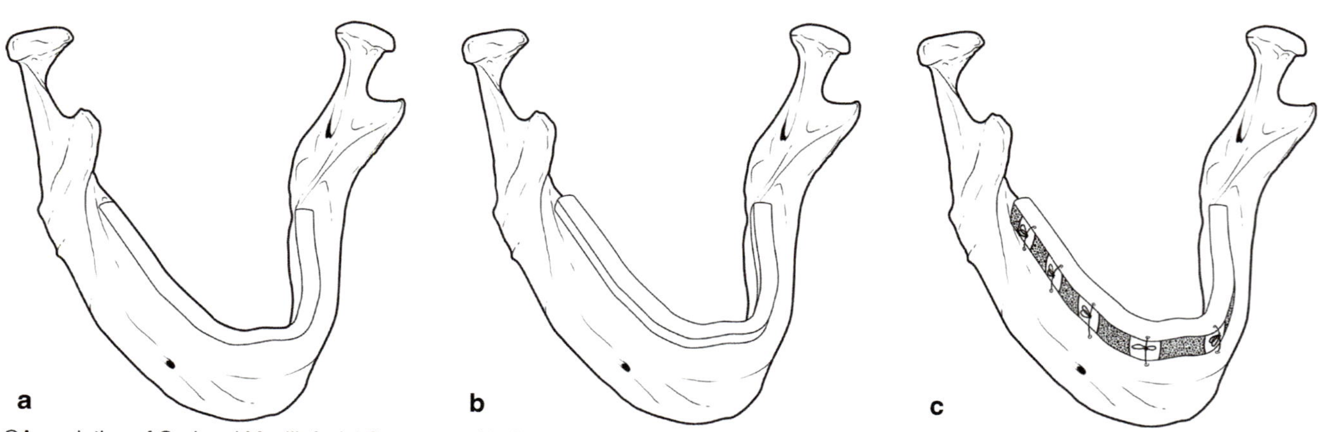



**Fig. 17.13** (**a** and **b**) Superior border augmentation, (**c**) Interpositional grafting

**Table 17.4** Mandibular ridge augmentation procedures

| Superior border augmentation | Interpositional grafting | Visor osteotomy |
|---|---|---|
| Two rib grafts of 15cm- Davis[54] | Bone graft between the osteotomized segments of the mandible- Barrors Saint and Pasteur[56] | Mandible in frontal region osteotomised and lingual fragment slided upwards- Harle[58] |
| Splitting rib longitudinally and then bending with forceps- Leake[55] | | Combination of osteotomy and vestibuloplasty along with lowering of FOM- Bosker[59] |

graft. This procedure possesses less danger of infection and rejection of the transplant and of resorption by remodelling processes. The muscles and periosteum in the labial side are reflected and the mandible in the frontal region is osteotomised and split in the length. The mobile lingual fragment is slid upwards, together with the adherent soft tissue, and fixed to the basal part of the mandible by intraosseous and perimandibular wiring. Bosker [59] improved this method by combining the osteotomy and the vestibuloplasty and lowering of the floor of the mouth in a one-stage procedure.

The advantage of this modified technique of Bosker [59] is it needs only single operation and hospitalisation of the patient, the prosthesis can be made in 4–6 weeks sooner, and the operative procedure is simpler.

Sladen and peterson [60] describe the body sagittal osteotomy and raising the lingual cortical portion of the mandible without detaching the lingual soft tissues for the intact vascular pattern. The raised lingual ridge is positioned in the new place, while the buccal counterpart is augmented with cancellous marrow. This procedure is now referred to as visor osteotomy in the literature.

The incision and the mode of raising the mucoperiosteal flap is essentially the same as that used in the horizontal osteotomy as described earlier. Sagittal cut is made between the buccal and lingual cortical plates from the third molar to the opposite third molar area. Precise cutting is achieved by the use of oscillating and reciprocating saws. The lingual segment, which is pedicled to the mylohyoid, digastrics and genial musculature and the soft tissues, is elevated vertically and fixed in the preplanned position with wires through the transosseous holes. The lateral aspect of the elevated segment may be filled with the cancellous bone to compensate the height deficiency created by the vertical repositioning. The flap is returned and wound is closed by sutures.

### 17.11.5 Graft Materials

Iliac bone crest and rib have traditionally been applied to augment the jaws. Boyne [61] suggested a bone regeneration method, which employs a vitalium mesh tray containing haematopoietic bone marrow encased in a nylon-reinforced Millipore filter. The filter prevents the connective tissue elements accessing the defect and thereby enhances the osseous regeneration. The concern regarding the graft material is the resorption shrinkage in the future. Many attempts are done by surgeons to minimise the resorption shrinkage of the grafted bone. Danielson and Nemarich [57] advocated the subcortical insertion of bone graft. Farell [62] and associates went ahead with interpositional bone graft with simultaneous vestibuloplasty. Sanders and Cox [50] proposed the use of inferior border rib grafting for augmentation. Notched rib can be contoured to the arc of the mandible, but 50% loss by shrinkage is a great disadvantage with rib. The literature suggests the use of pure cancellous iliac graft, iliac cortical—cancellous sectional grafts with appropriate immobilisation showing excellent healing even in the event of occasional incision dehiscence.

### 17.11.6 Augmentation with Synthetic Graft Materials

A myriad of materials is used for the augmentation of the atrophied ridge. It consists of resorbable and nonresorbable materials. The former finds its application in periodontal pockets, while the latter is extensively used in the management of alveolar atrophy. Hydroxyapatite, a calcium phosphate material with physical and chemical attributes, is nearly similar to dental enamel and cortical bone has been successfully using for decades. Studies by Kent et al. [49] and Drobeck et al. [63] illustrate the usage. Kent et al. [49] used hydroxyapatite in combination with corticocancellous autogenous bone for augmentation. This combination provides additional strength to the mandible as advised by Jarcho et al. [64]. Though block forms are used by Frame and Brady [65], the granular forms also get used in the augmentation process as guided by Kent et al. [51]. When anterior mandible needs augmentation, a single midline vertical incision is used, while for the complete augmentation of mandible, bilateral vertical incisions anterior to mental foramen are used. A subperiosteal tunnel is formed, which can be assessed by a dental mirror and the syringe loaded with graft material is inserted through the tunnel and delivered in place. After the tunnel is filled with graft material, the incision is closed with interrupted or horizontal sutures.

In maxilla, a single vertical incision in midline may be sufficient, but in many cases bilateral incisions in the canine regions may accommodate more amount of graft material. It is similar to the procedure in mandible except for the palatal dissection, where the ridge width is needed. Denture can be placed at about 1 month in cases where augmentation is carried out by hydroxyapatite alone or 6–8 weeks in which both hydroxyapatite and bone are used together. If vestibuloplasty is planned, Kent [49] advocated a waiting period of 8 weeks after graft placement.

## 17.12 Conclusion

The art of designing the soft- and hard-tissue framework for the smooth placement of the prosthesis is a challenging task. This task is achieved by the meticulous planning and execution of the planned presurgical procedures in a systematic manner. The intimidating impressive trends of implantology might have downsized the charm of preprosthetic surgery, yet in certain avenues the preprosthetic surgical manoeuvres become inevitable. The magnitude of vestibuloplasty and ridge augmentation procedures associated with the anticipated patient discomfort should not demote the benefits of preprosthetic surgery in deserving patients, where they suffer from pain or embarrassment by a juggling ill-fitting denture. Such corrections may alter their present situations and successful denture wearing is ensured. So it is not possible to completely thwart or baffle the procedures belonging to the preprosthetic surgery as an obsolete one.

**Acknowledgments** Fig. 17.6 - Suvy Manuel.

## References


1. Willard AT. Preparing the mouth for full sets of artificial teeth. Dent News Letter. 1853;6:238.
2. Beers WG. Notes from practice. Mo Dent J. 1876;8:294.
3. Roux W. Der Kampf der Teile im Organismus. Ein Beitrag zur Vervollständigung der mechanischen Zweckmässigkeitslehre. Leipzig: Verlag von Wilhelm Engelmann; 1881.
4. Wolff J. Das Gesetz der Transformation der Knochen. Berlin: August Hirschwald; 1892.
5. Mercier P. Residual alveolar ridge atrophy: classification and influence of facial morphology. J Prosthet Dent. 1979;8:24.
6. Cawood JI, Howell RA. A classification of the edentulous jaws. Int J Oral Maxillofac Surg. 1988;17:232–5.
7. Storer R. A radiographic survey of edentulous mouth. Br Dent J. 1957;102:344.
8. Crandell CE, Trueblood SN. Roentgenographic findings in edentulous areas. Oral Surg Oral Med Oral Pathol. 1960;13:1343.
9. Lekholm U, Zarb GA, Albrektsson T. Patient selection and preparation in Per-Ingvar Branemark et al Tissue-Integrated Prostheses. Chicago: Quintessence; 1985. p. 199–209.
10. Dean OT. Surgery for the denture patient. J Am Dent Assoc. 1936;23:2124.
11. Anderson JO. Intra oral skin grafts-an aid to alveolar ridge extension. J Oral Surg. 1969;27:427.
12. Guernsey L. Preprosthetic surgery. In: Kruger GO, editor. Oral and maxillofacial surgery. 6th ed. St. Louis: C V Mosby.
13. Godlee RJ. The torus palatinus. Proc R Soc Med. 1909;2:175.
14. García García AS, Martínez González JM, GómezFont R. Current status of the torus palatines and torus mandibularis. Med Oral Patol Oral Cir Bucal. 2010;15:e353.
15. Moraes Junior EF, Damante CA, Araujo SR. Torus palatinus: a graft option for alveolar ridge reconstruction. Int J Periodontics Restorative Dent. 2010;30:283.
16. Hassan KS, Alagl AS, Abdel H. A Torus mandibularis bone chips combinedwith platelet rich plasma gel for treatment of intrabony osseous defects: clinical andradiographic evaluation. Int J Oral Maxillofac Surg. 2012;41:1519.
17. Kolas S, Halperin V, Jefferis K, Huddleston S, Robinson HB. The occurrence of torus palatinus and torus mandibularis in 2478 dental patients. Oral Surg Oral Med Oral Pathol. 1953;6:44.
18. Kalaignan P, Mohan JS, Jayakumar A. Determination of grading for maxillary and mandibular Tori- an in vivo study. Biomed Pharmacol J. June 2018;11(2):679–88.
19. Haugen LK. Palatine and mandibular tori: a morphologic study in the current Norwegian population. Acta Odontol Scand. 1992;50:65.
20. Reichart PA, Neuhaus F, Sookasem M. Prevalence of torus Palatinus and torus mandibularis in Germans and Thai. Community Dent Oral Epidemiol. 1988;16:61–4.
21. Kazanjian VH. Surgery as an aid to more efficient service with prosthetic dentures. JADA. 1935;22:566–81.
22. Clark HB Jr. Deepening the labial sulcus by mucosal flap advancement: report of a case. J Oral Surg. 1953;11:165.
23. Mcinthosh RB, Obwegeser H. Preprosthetic surgery: a scheme for its effective employment. J Oral Surg. 1969;27:427.
24. Propper RH. Simplified ridge extension using free mucosal grafts. J Oral Surg. 1964;22:469.
25. Nabers JM. Free gingival grafts. Periodontics. 1966;4:243.
26. Hall RD, Steen O. Free grafts of palatal mucosa in mandibular vestibuloplasty. J Oral Surg. 1970;28:565.
27. Godwin JG. Submucous surgery for better denture service. J Am Dent Assocn. 1947;34:678.
28. Cooley DO. Method of deepening maxillary and mandibular sulci to correct deficient edentulous ridges. J Oral Surg. 1952;10:27.
29. Edlan A, Mejchar B. Plastic surgery of the vestibulum inperiodontal therapy. Int Dent J. 1963;13:593.
30. Trauner R. Alveoplasty with ridge extensions on the lingual side of the lower jaw to solve the problem of a lower dental prosthesis. Oral Surg. 1952;5:340.
31. Obwegeser H. Surgical preparation of the maxilla for the prosthesis. J Oral Surg. 1964;22:127.
32. Lewis ET. Surgical correction to the sublingual region. J Am Dent Assoc. 1963;67:364.
33. Caldwell J. Lingual ridge extension. J Oral Surg. 1955;13:287.
34. Ashley FN, Schwartz AN, Dryden MF. A modified technique for creating a lower lingual sulcus. Plast Reconstr Surg. 1953;22:204.
35. Baurmash H, Mandel L, Strelioff M. Mandibular sulcus extension – a new technique:preliminary report. J Oral Surg. 1962;20:390.
36. Collett HA. Immediate maxillary ridge extension. Dent Dig. 1954;60:104.
37. Szaba, Garner, Rumpel. Surgical preparation of the maxilla for prosthesis. J Oral Surg. 1964;22:127.

38. Yrastorza JA. Mandibular sulcus deepening: a modified technique. J Am Dent Assoc. 1963;67:859.
39. Weiser R. Ein Fall von ankylose, verlust des alveolar forsatzes under. Zahnheilk. 1918;34:147.
40. Schuchardt K. Die epidermis transplantation bie der mund vorhofplastik. Dtsch Zannarztl Z. 1952;7:364.
41. Esser JF. Studies in plastic surgery of the face. Ann Surg. 1917;65:297.
42. Gillies HD, Millard DR. Principles and art of the plastic surgery. Boston: Little Brown; 1957.
43. Steinhäuser EW. Vestibuloplasty- skin grafts. J Oral Surg. 1971;29:777–85.
44. Maloney PL. Mucosal grafts in oral reconstructive surgery. J Oral Surg. 1974;32:705.
45. Ketheley J, Gamble J. The lipswitch – a modification of Kazanjian's labial vestibuloplasty. J Oral Surg. 1978;36:705.
46. Tortoerelli AF. A technique for vestibular sulcus extension. J Prosthet Dent. 1968;20(1):14–20.
47. Brown LJ. A surgical solution to a lower denture problem. Br Dent J. 1953;95:215.
48. Hopkins R, Staford GD. Pre prosthetic surgery of the edentulous mandible. Br Dent J. 1980;148(7):183–8.
49. Kent JN, et al. Alveolar ridge augmentation using nonresorbable hydroxylapatite with or without autogenous cancellous bone. J Oral Maxillofac Surg. 1983;41:629.
50. Sanders B, Cox R. Inferior border rib grafting for augmentation of the atrophic edentulous mandible. J Oral Surg. 1976;34:897.
51. Kent JN, Quinn JH. Correction of alveolar ridge deficiencies with nonresorbable hydroxylapatite. J Am Dent Assoc. 1982;105:993.
52. Ridley MT, Manson KG. Resorption of rib graft to inferior border of mandible. J Oral Surg. 1978;36:46.
53. Blackstone CH, Parker ML. Rebuilding the resorbed alveolar ridge. J Oral Surg. 1956;14:45.
54. Davis WH. Rib graft augmentation to the superior border of the mandible. In: Preprosthetic oral and maxillofacial surgery. Saint Louis: C V Mosby; 1980.
55. Leake D. Contouring split ribs for the correction of severe mandibular atrophy. J Oral Surg. 1976;34:940.
56. Barros saint- pasteure: plastia reconstructive del rebord alveolar: neustra investigacion clinicoquirugica. Acta Odont Venez 1970;8:168.
57. Danielson PA, Nemarich AN. Subcortical bone grafting for ridge augmentation. J Oral Surg. 1976;34:887.
58. Harle F. Visor osteotomy to increase the absolute height of the atrophied mandible- a preliminary report. J Maxillofac Surg. 1975;3:257.
59. Bosker, et al. Visor osteotomy and vestibuloplasty – A one-stage procedure. Int J Oral Surg. 1977;6:127–30.
60. Slade E. Text book of maxillofacial surgery. In: Kruger GO, editor. Personal communication. 6th ed. Saint Louis: C V Mosby; 1977, July.
61. Boyne PJ. Restoration of the alveolar ridge by intramandibular transposition osseous grafting. J Oral Surg. 1968;26:569.
62. Farrell CD. One stage interpositional bone grafting and vestibuloplasty of the atrophic maxilla. J Oral Surg. 1976;34:901.
63. Drobeck HP, et al. Histologic observation of soft tissue responses to implanted, multifaceted particle and discs of hydroxylapatite. J Oral Maxillofac Surg. 1984;42:143.
64. Jarcho M, et al. Hydroxylapaptite synthesis and characterization in polycrystalline form. J Mater Sci. 1976;11:2027.
65. Frame JW, Brady CH. Augmentation of an atrophic edentulous mandible by interpositional grafting with hydroxylapatite. J Oral Maxillofac Surg. 1984;42:89.

# Part VII

# Dental Implantology

# 18 Basics of Dental Implantology for the Oral Surgeon

Supriya Ebenezer, Vinay V. Kumar, and Andreas Thor

## 18.1 History and Evolution of Dental Implants

Modern implant dentistry started more than 50 years ago when Dr. P.I. Brånemark, a Professor from the University of Gothenburg (Sweden), discovered in rabbit studies that titanium chambers placed in the fibula became firmly anchored in bone and could not be removed. Later, this direct bone-to-implant contact was termed osseointegration [1]. He demonstrated that titanium was structurally integrated into living bone with a high degree of predictability and without long-term soft-tissue inflammation or fixture rejection. He introduced a two-stage threaded root form pure titanium implant that was placed in patients in 1965. Therefore, Prof. P.I. Brånemark is recognized as the most important pioneer in modern implant dentistry.

The second pioneer is Prof. Andre Schroeder from the University of Bern (Switzerland) experimented with prototype dental implants in the early 1970s and could demonstrate first osseointegration in nondecalcified histologic sections [1]. Both pioneers with their teams, independent of each other, performed several preclinical and clinical studies to establish the current scientific basis for dental implantology. This was the start to successful osseointegration in dentistry.

Between the 1970s and the 1980s, companies presented different implant designs such as the Tübingen implants made of aluminum oxide, the IMZ titanium plasma-sprayed surface, and the American Core vent implants made of titanium aluminum vanadium alloy [1]. However, based on the research from Albrektsson, commercially pure titanium became the material of choice. One-piece implants slowly evolved to two-piece implants to provide prosthetic flexibility.

Over the next 15 years, implantology shifted from the treatment of fully edentulous patients to the treatment of partially edentulous patients as well. Prosthetic components for the rehabilitation of different edentulous situations emerged, and different surgical techniques and regenerative materials were developed to improve the hard and soft tissues around implants. Concepts of implant placement, loading, occlusion, and maintenance evolved. Progress was made in implant surface technology, which permitted the use of shorter and narrower implants and reduced loading time [2]. Over the last decade, development has included strategies to provide long-term stability with optimum functional, esthetic, and phonetic results along with reduced complications. Advanced diagnostic aids, such as cone beam computed tomography (CBCT), enabled proper assessment of the surgical site and surgical planning to provide better outcomes. Devices to examine implant stability objectively, using resonance frequency analysis, improved the quality of treatment provided. Digital technology is increasingly being incorporated to improve accuracy, minimize invasiveness, and fulfill esthetic demands. On the material front, ceramic implants and implants using alloys of increased strength have been introduced [2]. The field of implantology is a fast-evolving one where the clinician has to be constantly updated to keep pace.

## 18.2 The Concept of Osseointegration

Titanium implants could become permanently incorporated within bone, such that the two could not be separated without fracture [3]. Osseointegration was the term given to this con-

**Electronic Supplementary Material** The online version of this chapter (https://doi.org/10.1007/978-981-15-1346-6_18) contains supplementary material, which is available to authorized users.

S. Ebenezer (✉)
Department of Oral Surgery and Stomatology, University of Bern, Bern, Switzerland

V. V. Kumar · A. Thor
Department of Maxillofacial and Plastic Surgery, Uppsala University Academic Hospital, Uppsala, Sweden


K. Bonanthaya et al. (eds.), *Oral and Maxillofacial Surgery for the Clinician*, https://doi.org/10.1007/978-981-15-1346-6_18

tact and refers to a direct bone to metal interface without interposition of soft tissue seen at the optical microscope level. Osseointegration is defined as "a direct structural and functional connection between ordered living bone and the surface of a load-carrying implant." [4]

### 18.2.1 The Biological Process of Osseointegration

The cellular response after implantation depends on implant surface characteristics, the stability, and heating injuries of the host bone. Bone healing around implants involves a cascade of cellular and extracellular biological events (similar to fracture healing) until the entire implant surface is embedded in bone.

The first biological component to contact the implant surface is blood and blood cells from the surrounding vasculature. These blood cells are activated and release cytokines and other growth and differentiation factors on and around the implant. Platelets undergo biochemical and morphological changes due to contact with the implant surface and undergo adhesion, spreading, and aggregation. They induce phosphotyrosine, increase intracellular calcium, and cause hydrolysis of phospholipids to form a fibrin matrix that regulates cell adhesion and binding of minerals. This matrix is a calcified afibrillar layer consisting of osteoid and lamina limitans (organic layer) that is rich in calcium, phosphorus, osteopontin, and bone sialoprotein [5]. This matrix acts as a scaffold for osteogenic cells to migrate and differentiate to form osteoid and trabecular bone (osteoconduction), which will ultimately remodel to form lamellar bone around the implant surface. The ability of the implant surface to retain fibrin attachment during the initial phase is critical in determining if the migrating cells reach the fibrin clot. Roughened surfaces promote osteoconduction. The chemistry of the implant surface also influences osteoconduction, and for example, hydrophilic implant surfaces have increased osteoconduction as compared to hydrophobic surfaces.

Peri-implant osteogenesis occurs in two ways with the native bone as described by Osborn and Newesley in 1980.

1. Distance osteogenesis is a phenomenon that occurs from the native bone toward the implant surface. The existing bone surface provides a population of osteogenic cells, which lay down matrix, slowly encroach on the fibrin-meshwork-covered implant surface, and connect to this network as osteogenesis progresses. Osteoclasts, derived from mononuclear cells from the surrounding marrow spaces, remodel the old bony surface before new bone is laid down [5].
2. Contact osteogenesis occurs from the surface of the implant toward the healing bone. The fibrin-covered implant surface that has attracted osteogenic cells slowly has calcified afibrillar tissue forming into it. Blood vessels and mesenchymal cells fill up the spaces in between. Cement lines of poorly mineralized osteoid separate the areas of resorption and initiation. Woven and trabecular bone fill the initial gap and provide biological fixation to the implant at about 10–14 days postsurgery. However, the random orientation of the collagen fibers gives it reduced mechanical properties as compared to lamellar bone. This biological fixation differs from primary stability obtained at implant placement and is commonly seen with rough implant surfaces. Woven bone is slowly remodeled in response to stress and mechanical loading and replaced by lamellar bone until it reaches a high degree of mineralization. At approximately 3 months postimplant placement, the bone is a mixture of both woven and lamellar matrix [6].

(Figure 18.1: histology showing adequate osseointegration)

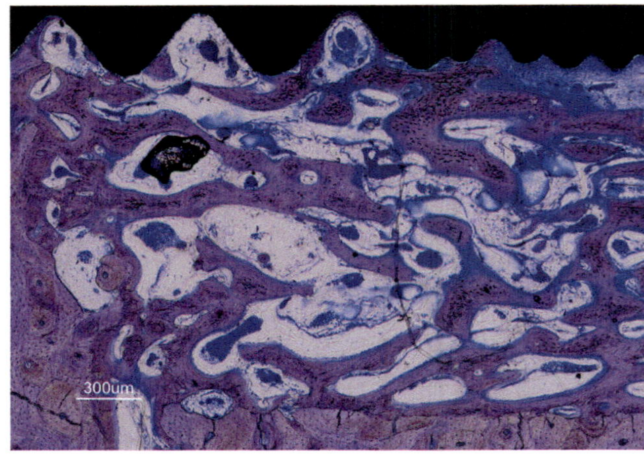




**Fig. 18.1** Histology of osseointegration. Osseointegration is defined as the direct apposition of bone onto the titanium implant surface as seen in this histology section

### 18.2.2 Assessment of Osseointegration

An implant is considered to be osseointegrated when an implant is in direct contact with the bone, and there is no relative movement between the implant and the bone. In other words, osseointegration is expressed clinically as long-term state of stability of the implant in the vital bone. According to Albrektsson (1985), a loaded implant is considered osseointegrated if the average surface contact with bone is a minimum of 50% [7]. Initially, the strength of the interface (initial stability) between bone and implant is high due to mechanical stability; however, it decreases over the next few weeks due to bone remodeling and then increases again due to new bone formation (secondary stability). The stability also depends on biophysical stimulation and the healing time. To clinically evaluate osseointegration mobility tests, standardized radiographs and Resonance Frequency Analysis (RFA) are used [6].

### 18.2.3 Factors that Determine Osseointegration

There are many factors that influence the formation and maintenance of bone at the implant surface [3, 6].

1. *Biocompatibility of the implant material* - Commercially pure titanium (CpTi) is widely used as an implant material as it is highly biocompatible, it has good resistance to corrosion and no toxicity on macrophages or fibroblasts and lacks inflammatory response in peri-implant tissues, and it is composed of an oxide layer and has the ability to repair itself by re-oxidation when damaged. Alloys of titanium such as Ti-6Al-4 V (Aluminum 6% and Vanadium 4%) and other Aluminum and Vanadium-free alloys of Titanium have been popularly used. Currently, a Ti-Zr alloy (Titanium 83–87% and Zirconium 13–17%) has been introduced, which has mechanical properties superior to those of CpTi and Ti-6Al-4 V [8].
2. *Implant geometry* - The shape of the implant determines the surface area available for stress transfer and the initial stability of the implant. Implants were previously available as cylinders, but currently, most implants come in screw-shaped (threaded) designs. Threaded implants with a circular cross section provide easy surgical placement and provide a greater functional surface area. These implants provide initial rigid fixation and limit micromovement during wound healing. The shape of the thread alters the force transmitted to the bone; it can be square, V, or reverse buttress shaped. The thread depth increases the surface area of the implant. Length of the implant contributes to the overall surface area. Increasing the length within limits increases the bone to implant contact for an implant, which is essential for osseointegration. Shorter implants are recommended today only with strict selection criteria and preferably work well only when splinted with other implants. Considering the width of an implant, although a wider implant increases the surface area for osseointegration, width depends on factors related to the surgical site. Overall, the shorter and smaller diameter implants have lower survival rates than their longer or wider counterparts. Longer implants have been suggested to provide greater stability under lateral loading conditions [9].
3. *Surface characteristics* –With exposure to air, Ti and its alloys form an oxide layer on the surface ($TiO_2$). The oxide layer protects against corrosion and also helps in calcium and phosphate ion exchange at the surface. Surfaces were modified to increase microroughness and hence the surface area for osseointegration. The additive processes are Ti plasma spraying, hydroxyapatite coating, discrete crystalline deposition (DCD), and electrochemical anodization (to increase the $TiO_2$ layer). These processes increased the surface area for bone contact with the implant surface, which increases the osseointegration. Subtractive processes to increase microroughness were also utilized in several implants to increase the microroughness, which also contributed to better osseointegration. Sandblasting, acid etching, and laser modification are some of the subtractive processes. Sandblasting produces a macrotexture, which is converted to a microtexture by acid etching. This surface promotes greater osseous contact at earlier time points compared to plasma-sprayed coated implants. Titanium surfaces were treated with fluoride, and this roughened the surface and demonstrated better bone anchorage, as compared to unmodified titanium surfaces [10]. Research is currently oriented toward making biomimetic implant surfaces that shorten healing times and provide better bone to implant contact [11].
4. *Systemic factors* – Irradiation of the region, osteoporosis, smoking, and diabetes although not absolute contraindications for implant placement can interfere with the normal healing process and osseointegration. Heavy smoking results in significantly lower success rates with oral implants [12]. The local site anatomy such as the amount of residual ridge for successful implant placement can also affect the outcome [13].
5. *Surgical technique* – The extent of tissue manipulation, thermal irritation by use of rotary instruments, and protocols for a surgical procedure can affect the outcome of osseointegration [14].
6. *Occlusal load* – During the initial healing phase, the absence of micromotion is critical for implant osseointegration. Based on the primary stability achieved, different protocols for loading are selected. The amount of force and timing of loading are critical for osseointegration [15].

## 18.3 Comparison Between Implant and Tooth Surface [16]

Figure 18.2a, b, and c show the differences between implants and tooth.

Implant prosthetics provide highly esthetic results that mimic the natural tooth; however, certain critical differences in the structure of the peri-implant tissues and periodontal structures exist. The lack of a periodontal ligament is the most striking difference; this absence means that the connec-

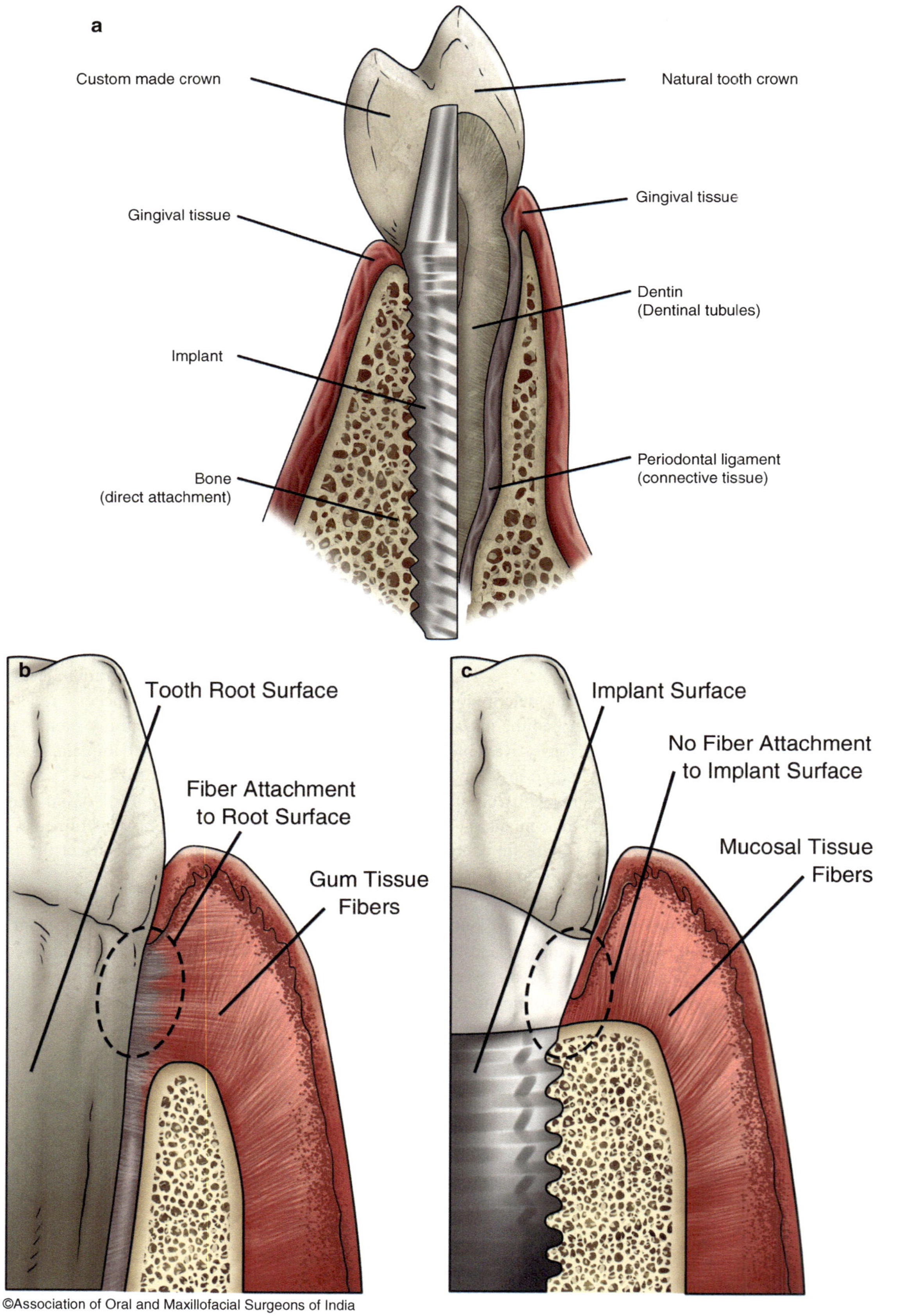


**Fig. 18.2** (**a**, **b**, and **c**) show diagrammatic representation of the biological differences between an implant and a tooth in longitudinal section

tion between the implant and the surrounding bone is not as resilient as that around the tooth. Implants, unlike teeth, do not intrude or migrate to compensate for premature contacts, and hence, the repercussions of occlusal disharmony can be detrimental. Implants lack proprioception and reflex function due to the absence of the periodontal ligament. This is critical when implant-supported prosthesis opposes each other. Implants do not supraerupt with time and hence lead to occlusal disharmonies when used as replacements for young and growing individuals. Hence, any form of overload on an implant causes fracture in the prosthesis, the implant structure, or bone loss surrounding the implant.

## 18.4 Types of implants

(a) Based on the type of material:

(i) Pure titanium and titanium alloys:

Commercially pure titanium(CpTi) was the material of choice due to its high biocompatibility and resistance to corrosion. CpTi is available in Grades I to IV; however, to improve the mechanical properties, alloys of titanium such as Ti-6Al-4 V have been used. Several alloys with Ti, such as Ti-Au, Ti-In, Ti-Sn, Ti-Pb, Ti-Cu, and Ti-Nb, have been tested. A Ti-Zr alloy (Titanium 83–87% and Zirconium 13–17%) is presently very popular as it has mechanical properties superior to those of the previously used alloys as well as high corrosion resistance.

(ii) Zirconia implants:

These implants are made from the oxide form of Zirconia ($ZnO_2$) and are "ceramic" implants that have high biocompatibility and ability to osseointegrate. In addition to the high mechanical properties, they were introduced especially for esthetic areas and in patients who maybe potentially allergic to titanium. The drawback of these implants is that most of the designs are one piece and only a few systems have two-piece implants. The idea of zirconia implants seems to be potential; however, no long-term evidence for its success exists at this time.

(b) Based on the shape:

(i) Screw-type implants:

Threads in screw-type implants increase the surface area for osseointegration. Threads help in stabilization by improving bone to implant contact and in stress distribution. There are several differences in thread shape, thickness, pitch, thread-face angle, etc. based on the manufacturers. These are the most widely used and documented form of implants.

(ii) Cylindrical and tapered implants:

Based on the shape of the implant body, implants are considered cylindrical (with parallel walls) or tapered. When the endosseous part of a cylindrical implant narrows in diameter toward the apex, an implant is considered tapered. The taper can be in the cervical, middle, or apical parts only or continuously taper from the cervical to the apex. Tapered implants were introduced to improve initial stability in less dense bone.

(iii) Platform switch implants:

When a smaller-diameter abutment is used on a larger-diameter implant collar, the implant-abutment junction shifts inward toward the central axis of the implant. This is considered to be a major factor in limiting crestal bone resorption especially in esthetic sites.

(iv) Bone-level and tissue-level implants:

Tissue-level implants have a butt joint transition from the smooth collar to the rough portion, and this transition zone is placed almost level with the bony crest. This design is generally used for non-submerged healing; here, the implant-abutment microgap is away from the bony tissues. Bone-level implants have minimal/no smooth collar and are completely microrough, and they are inserted almost level with the bone. This is meant for submerged healing, and here, the implant-abutment microgap is adjacent to the bone crest. In these implants, platform switch is used to limit crestal bone resorption.

(c) Based on implant surface.

(i) Machined (Brånemark surface):

These are the minimally rough implant surfaces made of turned CpTi, which were not further treated. These were used earlier and are also well documented. However, with a need to increase the surface area for bone attachment especially in less dense bone and to reduce time for osseointegration, these surfaces were modified. Smooth surfaces had an advantage of reduced attachment of plaque biofilms.

(ii) Textured/rough surfaces:

The smooth surfaces of the implants were altered to a textured surface to increase the surface area for osseointegration. They were classified as macro-, micro-, and nano-sized topologies based on the scale of roughness [17, 18]. Macrotopographic profiles of dental implants had a surface roughness in the range of millimeters to microns. This roughness was directly related to geometry of the implant, threaded screw, and macroporous surface treatment. Microrough topographies were in the range of 1 and 10 μm. A profile roughness average of 1–2 μm is optimal for osseointegration [19]. The surfaces were altered by different processes. Additive processes resulted in these popular types—sintered porous surfaces, titanium plasma sprayed, and hydroxyapatite plasma sprayed. Subtractive processes also created a rough texture, and they were sandblasting, acid etching, and laser alteration. Rough surfaces were demonstrated to have better bone to implant contact, which resulted in better osseointegration [20, 21]. Over the years, nanotopographies have been explored. Compaction of nanoparticles (such as titanium dioxide), molecular self-assembly method, and acid/alkali treatments or peroxidation for nanoparticle deposition have been advocated to increase nanoroughness.

(iii) Hydrophobic and hydrophilic implant surfaces [22]:

Initially, modification of implant surfaces concentrated on surface topography, and hence, the surfaces were hydrophobic. It was observed that porous devices should have a hydrophilic surface to induce the adsorption of bodily fluids into small pores and cavities of the structure. The surface chemistry of implants was altered to allow for hydrophilicity, and these surfaces have enhanced bone apposition during the initial phases of healing [23].

(d) Based on length (Al-Johany 2017) [24].
  (i) Extra-short: 6 mm in length or less.
  (ii) Short: From more than 6 mm to less than 10 mm.
  (iii) Standard: From 10 mm to less than 13 mm.
  (iv) Long: More than 13 mm.

Although traditionally, the concept was to get implants "as long as possible" for good osseointegration, the current trend with improved surfaces is "as long as needed". The introduction of shorter implants is to reduce the invasiveness and reduce morbidity.

(e) Based on diameter (Al-Johany 2017) [24].
  (i) Extra narrow: Less than 3.0 mm.
  (ii) Narrow: From 3.0 mm to less than 3.75 mm.
  (iii) Standard: From 3.75 mm to less than 5 mm.
  (iv) Wide: 5.0 mm or more.

Earlier, implants with diameters as wide as the tooth being replaced were used. Changing concepts of jumping gap, preserving the buccal cortical plate, and optimal 3-dimensional position coupled with improved surfaces encouraged slightly narrow diameters as compared to previous trends. Extra-narrow and narrow-diameter implants are used in deficient sites to minimize invasiveness and morbidity.

**Box 18.1 Types of Implants**

*Implants can be classified as follows:*

(a) Implant Material
  (i) Titanium and titanium alloys
  (ii) Zirconia
(b) Shape:
  (i) Screw type implants
  (ii) Cylindrical, apically tapered, and fully tapered
  (iii) Platform-switch implants
  (iv) Bone level vs. tissue level implants
(c) Implant surface
  (i) Machined (Brånemark surface)
  (ii) Textured/rough surfaces
  (iii) Hydrophobic/Hydrophilic surfaces
(d) Implant length
(e) Implant diameter

## 18.5 Preoperative Examination of Potential Implant Patients

### 18.5.1 Clinical Examination

Before implant treatment, a careful analysis should be conducted. This includes patient's current health status and medications and details of past medical history and medical treatments.

Patients should be questioned about parafunctional habits, oral hygiene, and personal habits such as tobacco, alcohol, and drugs. The compliance, motivation, attitude, understanding, and expectations of the patient are important for optimal treatment outcome.

Clinical examination should include extra-oral examination, i.e., lip line, lip competence, and temporomandibular joint. Intraoral assessment should include assessment of the edentulous space, occlusion, status of adjacent and opposing teeth, overall periodontal status, presence of other implants and restorations, shape of the teeth, gingival biotype, and any other local factor that may impact the success of the treatment.

Diagnostic study models and intraoral clinical photographs are essential for documentation as well as for the further assessment of spatial and occlusal relationships.

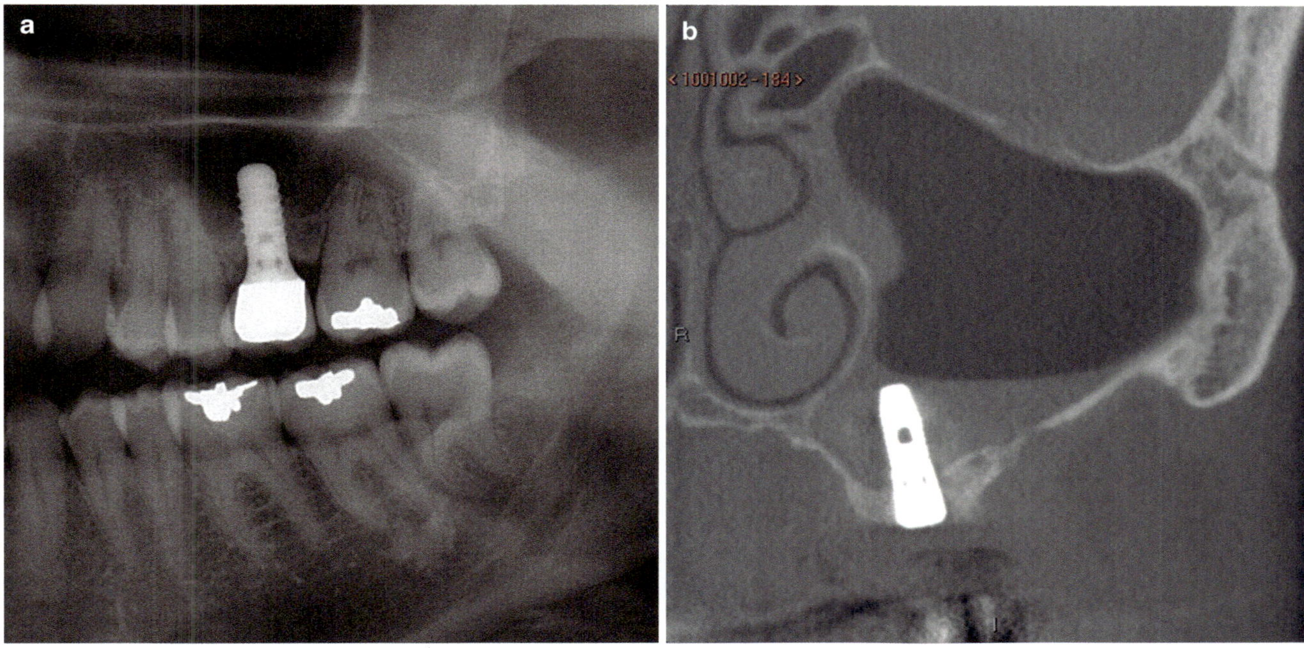




**Fig. 18.3** (**a** and **b**) show examples of two-dimensional and 3-dimensional examination of an implant placed with sinus floor elevation

### 18.5.2 Radiographic Examination

Figure 18.3a and b show examples of two-dimensional and 3-dimensional examination of the maxillary sinus.

Radiographic examination should be done in the evaluation phase to determine the status and anatomy of the underlying bone, if implant placement is possible and if any other surgical procedures are required before implant placement. A 2-dimensional radiograph of the area is desired; however, this is insufficient to provide a detailed 3-dimensional assessment of the site. Hence, the radiograph of choice is the Cone Beam Computerized Tomography (CBCT) as it provides a detailed three-dimensional analysis of the edentulous area along with the neighboring anatomical structures. With the software for CBCT, it is possible to measure accurately the dimension of the site and distances from critical structures and accurately plan which implant dimension would be appropriate. CBCT imaging also gives us information on which sites require augmentation and if so the location and extent required.

### 18.5.3 Correct 3-Dimensional Position for an Implant

For the site of implant placement, the available space should be evaluated in three dimensions, i.e., mesiodistal, buccolingual, and apicocoronal dimensions. A graduated periodontal probe can be used for clinical measurements; however, this information is best recorded from imaging techniques such as CBCT. While evaluating the available space, factors such as proximity to adjacent anatomical structures such as maxillary sinus, mandibular nerve, nasal floor, adjacent tooth roots, etc. should be considered.

The minimal space required for an implant depends on the size of the implant to be used (in terms of length and diameter), whether the implant is placed adjacent to two natural teeth or adjacent to an implant and the apicocoronal distance in the bone.

1. Implant adjacent to a natural tooth: Buser et al. (2004) suggested a concept for correct 3-dimensional implant placement [25]. They designated zones called as comfort zones (which is the ideal position for an implant) and danger zones (in which implants should not be placed). This was defined in three directions mesiodistally, coronoapically, and orofacially. (Figure 18.4 a, b, and c show diagrammatic representation of the correct positioning of implants in a 3-dimensional manner). The ideal mesiodistal distance between a natural tooth and the shoulder of an implant is 1.5 mm [25]. The zone up to 1–1.5 mm from the adjacent teeth on either side was the danger zone. Between the danger zone was the comfort zone that is safe for implant placement [25]. For

example, if an implant of 4.1 mm in diameter is placed between two natural teeth, the minimum mesiodistal distance available should be 7 mm (to allow 1.5 mm between the implant and the natural teeth on either side). If placed too close to the adjacent teeth, it causes bone loss. In the orofacial dimension, the implant shoulder is positioned palatal to the incisal edge of the future restoration (or 1 mm palatal to the point of emergence of the

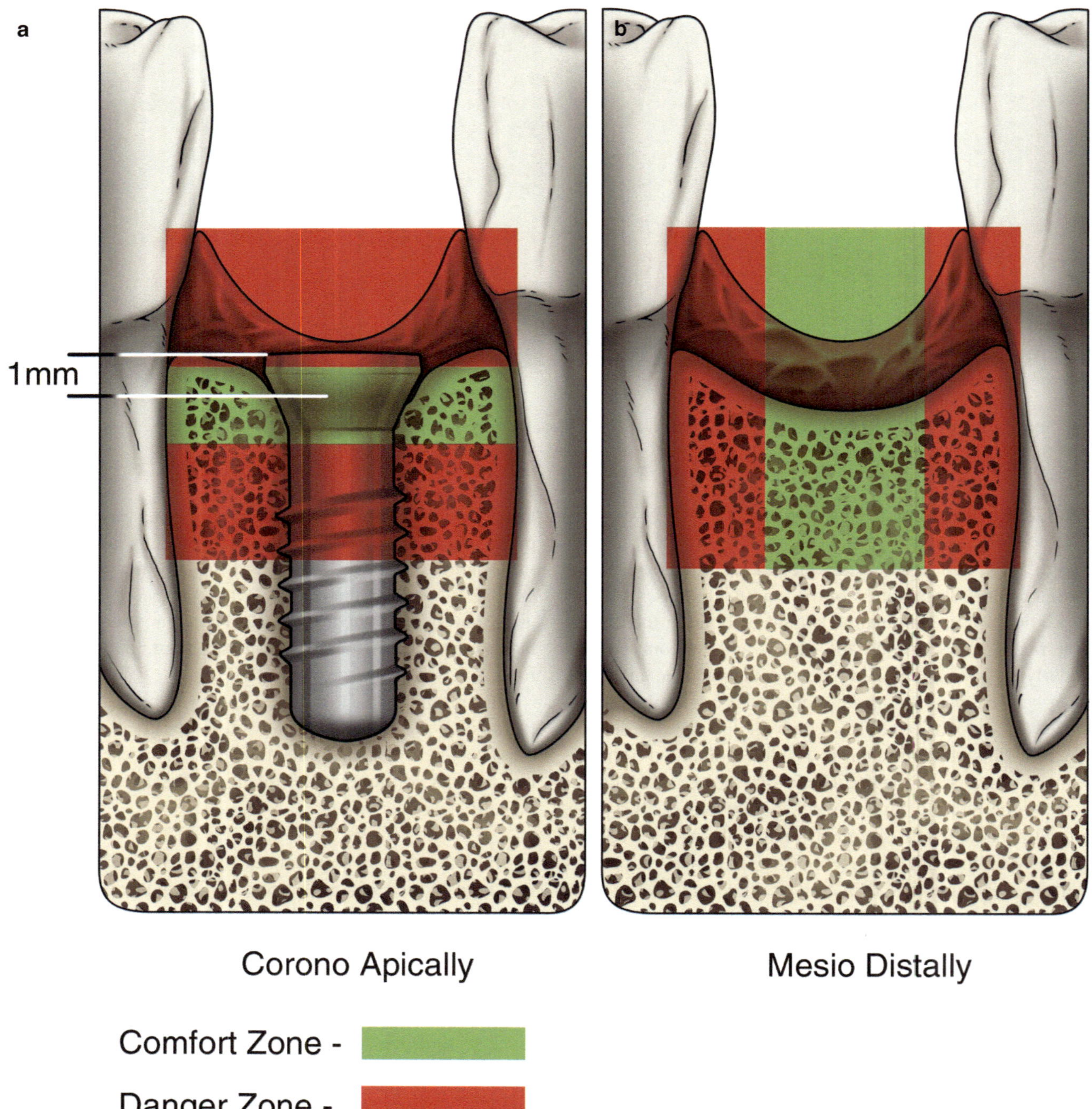


**Fig. 18.4** (**a**, **b**, and **c**) diagrammatic representation of ideal placement of a single implant in green shadow and unideal positions that could lead to complications (in red shadow). (**a**) ideal coronoapical position, (**b**) ideal mesiodistal position, and (**c**) ideal orofacial position

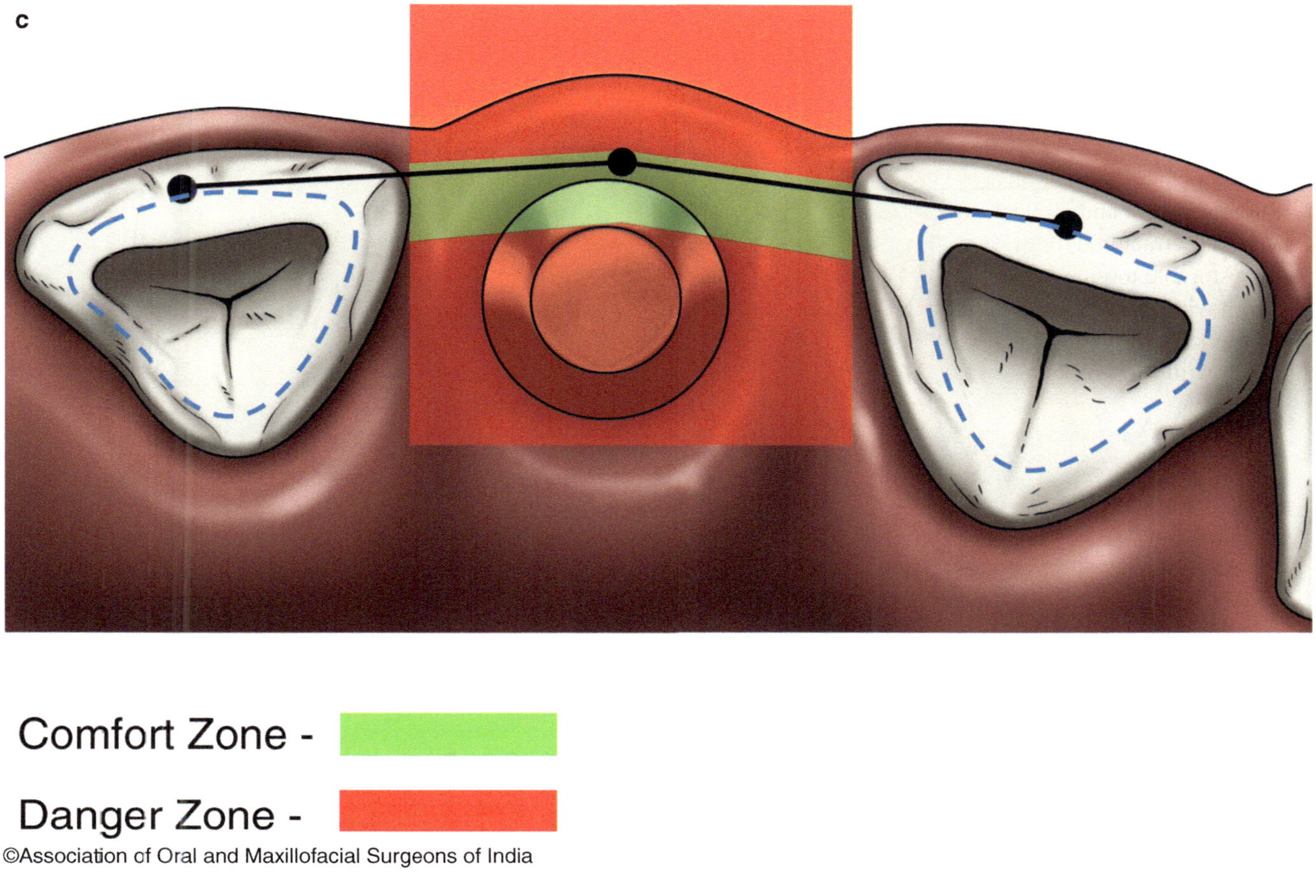


Fig. 18.4 (continued)

adjacent teeth). The oral aspect has a danger zone as well, indicating that an implant should not be placed too far orally to prevent the use of a ridge lap restoration. Too far facially will result in increased mucosal recession. In the apicocoronal direction, the apex of the implant should be at least 1-2 mm away from any anatomical structure such as nerve, sinus, or tooth roots. Also, in the shoulder of the future implant should be at least 1 mm apical to the cementoenamel junction of the adjacent teeth to allow for a proper emergence profile [25]. Placing an implant too deep will result in too much countersinking, difficult handling, and facial mucosal recession. Placing an implant too superficially will cause the metal margin to be visible and improper emergence profile. In addition to this, the ideal facial bone thickness should be 2 mm [26] and the lingual bone thickness should be 1.5 mm. Hence, for a 4.1 mm implant, minimum orofacial distance should be approximately 7.5 mm. Also, to prevent the appearance of black triangles, the apicocoronal distance from the interdental contact point to the crest of bone should not exceed 5 mm. (Figure 18.5a shows diagrammatic representation of the distance between interdental contact point and the crest of bone, for adequate papilla preservation).

2. Implants adjacent to each other: The mesiodistal distance between the implants should be at least 3 mm [25, 26]. This is critical to allow adequate interimplant bone and hence the formation of a soft tissue papilla overlying the bone. The other requisites for mesiodistal, orofacial, and apicocoronal dimensions, as previously mentioned, apply in addition. (Figure 18.5b shows diagrammatic representation of the distance between interdental contact point and the crest of bone, for adequate papilla preservation).

When the space for an implant of a particular diameter is less than ideal, a decision should be made either to augment the site with bone or to choose an implant of smaller diameter. However, this decision requires clinical expertise as augmentation procedures are technique sensitive and using smaller diameter implants depends on evaluation of the occlusal forces in the area. The interocclusal distance also needs to be evaluated prior to implant placement as it determines the choice of prosthetic rehabilitation of the implant. If the interocclusal distance is reduced,

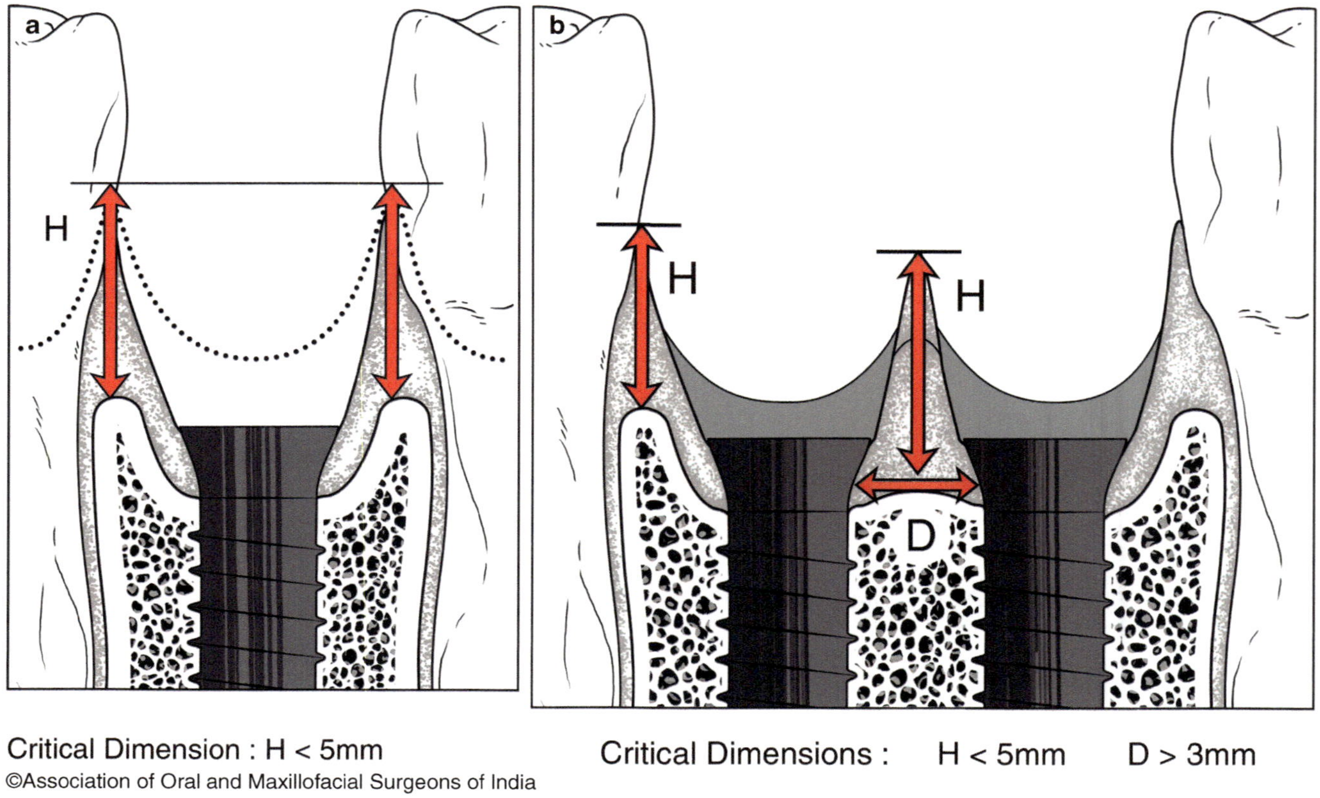


**Fig. 18.5** (**a** and **b**) diagrammatic representation of the critical dimensions in implant placement in relation to interdental papilla. (**a**) The height (H) of the interdental contact from the crest of the interdental alveolar bone should not be more than 5 mm for obtaining adequate interdental papillary morphology. (**b**) The interimplant distance (D) should be at least 3 mm for obtaining adequate interdental papillary morphology

the choice would be to use a screw-retained prosthesis over a cement-retained one. Screw-retained prosthesis, however, is the more preferred technique due to ease in retrievability and cleansability.

The amount of keratinized tissue in the site should also be evaluated before surgery as this determines the location of the incision. Ideally, a band of at least 2 mm (minimum 1 mm) keratinized tissue should surround the implant, and this is critical to the long-term success of the implant. If this is not achievable, procedures to augment the keratinized mucosa should be planned. Keratinized mucosa is necessary as it provides a physical barrier to oral plaque and to the forces of mastication as compared to nonkeratinized mucosa [27].

## 18.6 SAC Classification

The International Team for Implantology (ITI) proposed a classification of sites for implant placement based on the analysis of several factors [28].

Based on these factors, sites for implant surgery could be classified as straightforward (S), advanced (A), and complex (C).

This provides the clinician an assessment of the site for implant placement before the surgery is planned and is based on the level of expertise of the clinician who can either treat or refer to a specialist.

The determinants of the classification are.

1. Esthetic or nonesthetic site: Any case in the esthetic zone or has an esthetic risk should be considered as advanced or complex.
2. Complexity of the process: The level of complexity can be assessed by considering the number of steps and the number of areas in which an acceptable outcome has to be achieved.
3. Risk of complications: The SAC Classification can be used to identify and quantify risks for complications. This allows pretreatment planning to control and minimize risks.

The general modifying factors are.

1. Clinical competence and expertise: The SAC Classification for a case type is independent of the clinician's skill and competence. A Straightforward case is an uncomplicated

procedure, and a Complex case is the one that is difficult to manage.

2. Compromised patient's health: Patients with risk factors such as smoking, diabetes, irradiated bone, history of periodontal disease, poor oral hygiene, and bruxism need to be monitored as they have a higher risk for complications.
3. Growth considerations: Implants placed in the jaws of growing individuals are modifying factors as they present esthetic and functional issues.
4. Iatrogenic factors: Suboptimal planning and treatment outcomes increase the difficulty in the implant treatment phase. For example, incorrect three-dimensional implant placement will complicate the restorative process.

Tables 18.1, 18.2, and 18.3 show the esthetic, surgical, and restorative modifying factors to be considered during implant treatment planning and execution.

**Table 18.1** The esthetic modifying factors are determined by the Esthetic Risk Assessment (ERA)

| Esthetic factors | Level of risk | | |
|---|---|---|---|
| | Low | Medium | High |
| Medical status | Healthy and co-operative patient with an intact immune system. | – | Reduced immune system |
| Patients' esthetic expectation | Low | Medium | High |
| Smoking habit | Nonsmoker | Light smoker (<10 cigs/day) | Heavy smoker (>10 cigs/day) |
| Lip line | Low | Medium | High |
| Shape of tooth crowns | Rectangular | | Triangular |
| Gingival biotype | Low scalloped and thick | Medium scalloped and medium thick | High scalloped and thin |
| Bone anatomy of alveolar crest | Alveolar crest without bone deficiency | Horizontal bone deficiency | Vertical bone deficiency |
| Bone level at adjacent teeth | ≤5 mm to contact point | 5.5 to 6.5 mm to contact point | ≥7 mm to contact point |
| Soft tissue anatomy | Intact soft tissue | | Soft tissue defects |
| Width of edentulous span | 1 tooth (≥7 mm) | 1 tooth (≤7 mm) | 2 teeth or more |
| Restorative status of neighboring teeth | Virgin | | Restored |
| Infection at implant site | None | Chronic | Acute |

Adapted with permission from Dawson A, Chen S, Buser D, Cordaro L, Martin W. Belser U. The SAC Classification in Implant Dentistry. Editors: Dawson A, Chen S. Quintessence Publishing Co. Ltd. 2009

The above-mentioned modifiers have to be considered for every implant case during the assessment and planning phase of treatment. Risks can be identified prior to treatment, thus minimizing complications. To classify as Straightforward, Advanced, or Complex for a specific case, the specific features of the case can be matched with the descriptions in the tables. The level that best matches the factors of the individual case will provide the SAC Classification for that case.

The final treatment plan including additional surgical procedures (if required) should be formulated after accurate diagnosis and consideration of the patient's systemic and local factors, bearing in mind the requirements of the patient.

**Table 18.2** Surgical modifying factors

| Site factors | Risk or degree of difficulty | | |
|---|---|---|---|
| | Low | Moderate | High |
| Anatomic risk | | | |
| Proximity to vital anatomic structures | Minimal risk of involvement | Moderate risk of involvement | High risk of involvement |
| Bone volume | | | |
| Horizontal | Adequate | Deficient, but allowing simultaneous augmentation | Deficient, requiring prior augmentation |
| Vertical | Adequate | Small deficiency crestally, requiring slightly deeper coronoapical implant position. Small deficiency apically due to proximity to anatomical structures, requiring shorter than standard implant lengths. | Deficient, requiring prior augmentation |
| Esthetic risk | | | |
| Esthetic zone | No | | Yes |
| Biotype | Thick | | Thin |
| Thickness of facial bone wall | Sufficient ≥1 mm | | Insufficient <1 mm |
| Complexity | | | |
| Number of prior or simultaneous procedures | Implant placement without adjunctive procedures | Implant placement with simultaneous procedures | Implant placement with staged procedures |
| Complications | | | |
| Risk of surgical complications | Minimal | Moderate | High |
| Consequences of complications | No adverse effect | Suboptimal outcome | Severely compromised outcome |

Adapted with permission from Dawson A, Chen S, Buser D, Cordaro L, Martin W, Belser U. The SAC Classification in Implant Dentistry. Editors: Dawson A, Chen S. Quintessence Publishing Co. Ltd. 2009

**Table 18.3** *Restorative modifiers*: These are the restorative factors that influence the SAC classification

| | | Degree of difficulty | | |
|---|---|---|---|---|
| Issue | Notes | Low | Moderate | High |
| Oral environment | | | | |
| General oral health | | No active disease | | Active disease |
| Condition of adjacent teeth | | Restored teeth | | Virgin teeth |
| Reason for tooth loss | | Caries/trauma | | Periodontal disease or occlusal parafunction |
| Occlusion | | | | |
| Occlusal scheme | | Anterior guidance | | No guidance |
| Involvement in occlusion | The degree to which the implant prosthesis is involved in the patient's occlusal scheme | Minimal involvement | | Implant restoration is involved in guidance |
| Occlusal parafunction | Risk of complication to the restoration, but not to implant survival | Absent | | |
| Restorative volume | | | | |
| Interarch distance | Refers to the distance from the proposed implant restorative margin to the opposing occlusion | Adequate for planned restoration | Restricted space, but can be managed | Adjunctive therapy will be necessary to gain sufficient space for the planned restoration |
| Mesiodistal space | The arch length available to fit tooth replacements | Sufficient to fit replacements for missing teeth | Some reduction in size or number of teeth will be necessary | Adjunctive therapy will be needed to achieve a satisfactory result |
| Span of restoration | | Missing tooth | Extended edentulous space | Full arch |
| Volume and characteristics of the edentulous saddle | Refers to whether there is sufficient tissue volume to support the final restoration, or some prosthetic replacement of soft tissues will be necessary | No prosthetic soft-tissue replacement will be necessary | | Prosthetic replacement of soft tissue will be needed for esthetics or phonetics |
| *Provisional restorations* | | | | Present |
| During implant healing | | Not required | | Fixed |
| Implant supported provisionals needed | Provisional restorations will be needed to develop esthetics and soft tissue transition zones | Not required | Restorative margin <3 mm apical to mucosal crest | Restorative margin >3 mm apical to mucosal crest |
| *Materials/ manufacture* | Materials and techniques used in the manufacture of definitive prostheses | Resin-based materials ± metal reinforcement | Porcelain fused to metal | |
| *Loading protocols* | To date, immediate restoration and loading procedures are lacking scientific documentation | Conventional or early loading | | Immediate loading |
| *Maintenance needs* | Anticipated maintenance needs based on patient presentation and the planned prosthesis | Low | Moderate | High |

Adapted with permission from Dawson A, Chen S, Buser D, Cordaro L, Martin W, Belser U. The SAC Classification in Implant Dentistry. Editors: Dawson A, Chen S. Quintessence Publishing Co. Ltd. 2009

## 18.7 Implant Solutions for Different Edentulous Situations

Implants can be used as replacement options for all kinds of edentulous situations varying from single tooth gaps to completely edentulous jaws (Figure 18.6 shows an example where an implant has been used for the restoration of single tooth, and 7b shows an example where implants have been used for the replacement of the edentulous upper and lower jaws). The treatment plan varies in complexity as the number of teeth replacements increases, if it is an esthetic site or not and if the opposing dentition is implant-supported or not and depending on the occlusal load. As few as possible but as many as needed should be the key when placing implants. The selection of the size of the implant (length and width) and the number of implants especially in areas of poor bone quality is important for providing the correct solution.

For large edentulous spans, it is preferable to use as many implants as required, to support the occlusal forces in that area. Cantilever prosthesis on implants has to be used with discretion and is limited to areas of low occlusal demand. It is not preferable to splint implant with natural teeth as

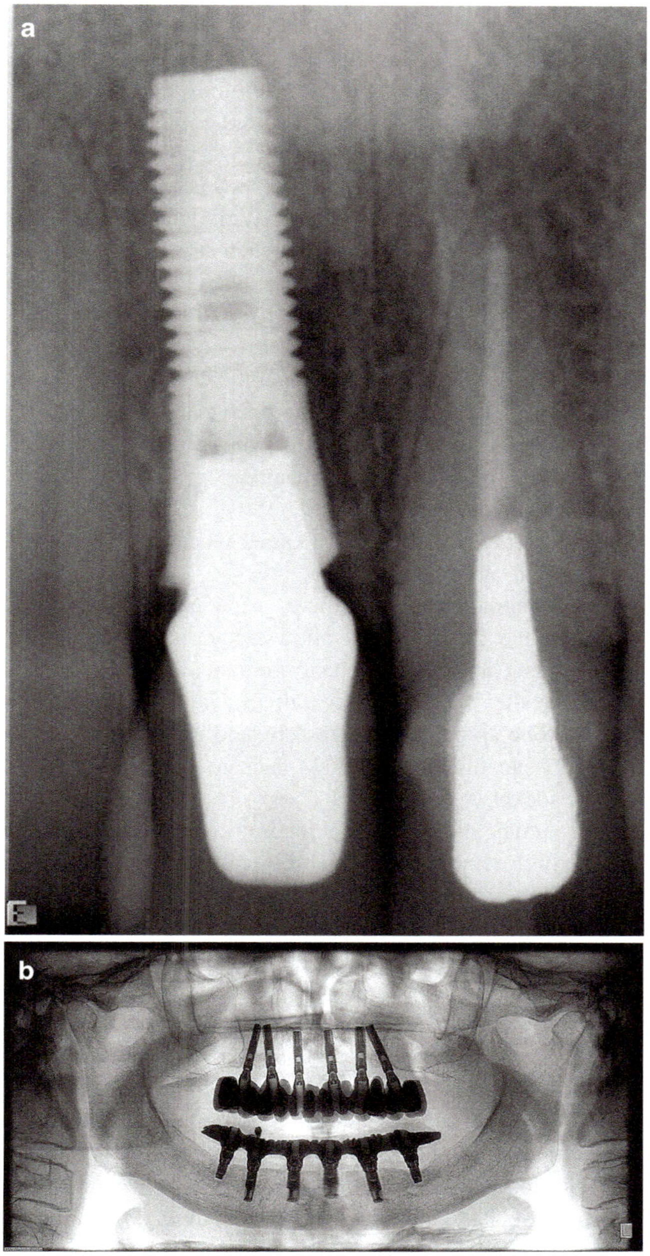



**Fig. 18.6** (**a**) shows an example where an implant has been used for the restoration of single tooth, and (**b**) shows an example where implants have been used for the replacement of the edentulous upper and lower jaws

implants cannot intrude with force like natural teeth. Long-span bridges on implants are not advisable in soft bone, e.g., in the completely edentulous maxilla, a fixed prosthesis can be given on six implants, while in the mandible, the same can be achieved with only four implants. For removable prosthesis, in an edentulous maxilla, four to six are sufficient, while in the edentulous mandible, the similar prosthetic solution can be achieved with two to four implants. There are several concepts of implant replacement for long edentulous spans and several designs of implants indicated for specific types of sites; however, the details of these are beyond the scope of this chapter.

## 18.8 Timing of Implant Placement Postextraction

### 18.8.1 Hard and Soft Tissue Alterations Postextraction

Studies in beagle dog revealed that postextraction, the bundle bone resorbs as the blood supply to this bone is compromised due to tooth extraction [29, 30]. This results in vertical bone loss in both facial and lingual walls of the socket, but it is more pronounced on the facial aspect as most often it is thinner in width than the lingual wall [30]. In human studies, ridge width reduction of up to 50% occurred during the first year after tooth loss in premolar and molar sites, and two-thirds of the total change took place within the first 3 months following extraction [31]. Dimensional alterations occurred in both height and width, with approximately 2.6–4.5 mm in width and 0.4–3.9 mm in height being lost in the healed sockets [32]. Histologically, the density of vascular structures and macrophages reduced from 2 to 4 weeks, the osteoclastic activity slowly decreased over a 4-week period, and osteoblasts peaked at 6–8 weeks remaining almost stable thereafter [33]. Thin facial walls seem to be prone for resorption, and sites with facial bone wall thickness of 1 mm or less had vertical bone loss of 7.5 mm (62%) of the original bone height after an 8 week healing period. Patients with thick wall phenotype, having facial bone wall thickness of more than 1 mm, had only about 1.1 mm (9%) vertical bone loss [34]. Also, for single extraction sites, the dimensional alteration occurred mainly in the central mid-facial area of the socket wall, while the proximal areas that had viable periodontal ligament of the adjacent teeth remained nearly unchanged after flapless tooth extraction at 8 weeks of healing [35]. With this pattern of resorption, a thin wall phenotype will develop a two-wall defect, while a thick-wall phenotype will result in a three-wall defect after initial remodeling [34]. Thus, the evaluation of facial wall thickness is critical to predict the future of bone loss prior to extraction [13]. With the above findings related to the pattern of bone remodeling and the timing of the cellular activity, in thin bone wall phenotypes, it is recommended to allow the initial postextraction remodeling to take place before initiating regenerative procedures. An early implant placement would be recommended for thin bone phenotypes. Immediate implant placement would be recommended only for thick wall phenotypes and thick gingival biotypes where minimal remodeling would be expected.

The soft tissue thickness in maxillary anterior teeth is thin in most patients, ranging from 0.5 mm to 1 mm. This soft tissue thickness has not shown significant correlation to the underlying facial bone wall thickness [36]. For single extraction sites, 50% of the soft tissue change occurs within the first 2 weeks postextraction. The increase in soft tissue thickness significantly depends on the underlying bone dimensions. In thick wall phenotypes, the soft tissue dimensions do not significantly change. In these defects, the alveolus acts as a self-contained bony defect and favors the growth of bone-forming cells from the adjacent socket walls. In thin wall phenotypes, the facial bone wall resorbs rapidly and the highly proliferative soft tissue occupies its position. There is a sevenfold increase in soft tissue occupying the crestal area of the socket defect, and this is termed as spontaneous soft tissue thickening [13]. The tissue formed is highly vascularized granulation tissue with fibroblasts migrating into it, some of which differentiate into myofibroblasts that are involved in the thickening phenomenon. At 8 weeks, there is a peak in endothelial cell density, BMP-7, and osteocalcin expression, indicating that the molecular and cellular mechanisms that regulate new bone formation also influence the soft tissue thickening. The clinical implications of this soft tissue thickening are that, after an 8 week healing period, the soft tissues are sufficiently thickened and provide increased keratinized tissue in the site that allows for primary closure favoring bone regeneration. With this thickened soft tissue, there is no requirement for additional soft tissue grafts. However, this soft tissue thickening can mask the underlying bone defect, often misleading the clinician while selecting the appropriate treatment protocol [37].

### 18.8.2 Concept of Timing for Implant Placement

Implant placement can be classified based on the timing of implant placement. According to the ITI Consensus Conferences in 2003 and 2008, it is classified as Type 1, Type 2, Type 3, and Type 4 implant placement [38].

**Box 18.2 Concept of Timing for Implant Placement**

Type 1: When placed immediately after tooth extraction, it is called immediate implant placement.

Type 2: When placed 4–8 weeks after tooth extraction, it is an early implant placement with only soft tissue healing

Type 3: When placed 12–16 weeks after tooth extraction, it is an early implant healing with partial bone healing

Type 4: When placed after 6 months after tooth extraction, there is complete bone healing, and this is called delayed implant placement.

The choice of timing of implant placement depends on several factors. The four options are available to the clinician, who can select the option based on the following criteria, provided that they have the required clinical expertise.

- *Immediate implant placement (type I)* is recommended to be performed only by experienced clinicians in sites that have ideal anatomic conditions, such as:
  - (i) a completely intact, thick wall phenotype (i.e., >1mm) facial bone wall at the extraction site
  - (ii) thick gingival biotype,
  - (iii) absence of acute infection at the extraction site, and
  - (iv) adequate volume of bone apical and palatal of the extraction site to allow sufficient primary stability of the implant while placing it in the correct 3-dimensional position.
- *Type 2 placement* is recommended when the above ideal conditions are not met.
  - (i) In situations where there is inadequate keratinized tissue, this technique allows an additional 3-5 mm of tissue as the tissues heal spontaneously.
  - (ii) In sites where there is a thin facial bone, the bundle bone spontaneously resorbs and a spontaneous soft tissue thickening takes place to fill the extraction socket.
  - (iii) Acute and chronic infections resolve leaving the future implant site free of infections.
  - (iv) Bone forms in the apical portion of the socket, thus allowing primary stability from the apical bone during implant placement. At the stage of implant placement, a guided bone regeneration procedure with bone graft and membrane is most often required.
- *Type 3 implant placement* is recommended in cases where either primary stability cannot be achieved even after 4–8 weeks of healing postextraction or where the proper 3-dimensional position for implant placement cannot be achieved. The healing time in these cases is extended to 12–16 weeks to allow partial bone healing. This is generally ideal for multirooted teeth such as mandibular molars. In this case also, guided bone regeneration with bone graft and membrane is often required.
- *Type 4 implant placement* is often not a preferred treatment by the patient. However, the indications for this type of implant placement are determined by certain patient-related factors or site-specific factors. Patient related factors include.
  - (i) patients with systemic conditions that require treatment to be deferred, e.g., pregnant patients,
  - (ii) adolescent patients who are too young to receive implants and require the treatment to be deferred, and
  - (iii) patients who are unable to make an early appointment due to personal reasons.

Site-related factors include.

(a) Large Apical Lesions

(b) Impacted or ankylosed teeth that cause a lot of bone removal in the apical aspect of the site. In all these cases, it is recommended that socket grafting with a low substitution filler is used to reduce ridge alterations and ridge atrophy. The crestal bone resorption is inevitable; however, the use of socket grafting minimizes the need for ridge augmentation at a later date.

### 18.8.3 Healing Modality: Concept of Submerged and NonSubmerged Healing

When an implant is placed, the operator can choose to either submerge the implant (completely enclose it within the healing tissues) or keep it nonsubmerged (implant is visible through the healing soft tissue). (Figure 18.7 shows diagrammatic representation of submerged and nonsubmerged healing).

In the nonsubmerged/one-stage approach, the healing cap/abutment of the implant emerges through the mucosal tissues at the time of flap closure after implant placement. Nonsubmerged implants can be one-piece or two-piece implants. In one-piece implants, there is no micromovement and no microgap between the implant and the abutment. In the two-piece nonsubmerged implants, there is no need for a second surgical procedure to expose the implant for prosthetics; however, the potential of the microgap between the two components exists. This technique is generally preferred for standard implant placement procedures where there is no need to augment the site.

In the submerged/two-stage approach, the healing cap/cover screw is completely covered with the soft tissue flap after implant placement surgery. The implants are allowed to osseointegrate in a closed environment without loading or any form of micromovement, for a period of time. The submerged protocol is used for implant placement with simultaneous bone augmentation. Following this healing period, the implant is surgically exposed to place the abutment. Both these techniques are well accepted and can be selected based on the treatment plan.

## 18.9 Surgical Procedure for Conventional Implant Placement

As mentioned before, the most important step before implant surgery is the analysis of the general patient factors and then the local edentulous site factors. Depending on whether it is an implant replacement for a single tooth, multiple teeth, or a completely edentulous ridge, the planning differs. The

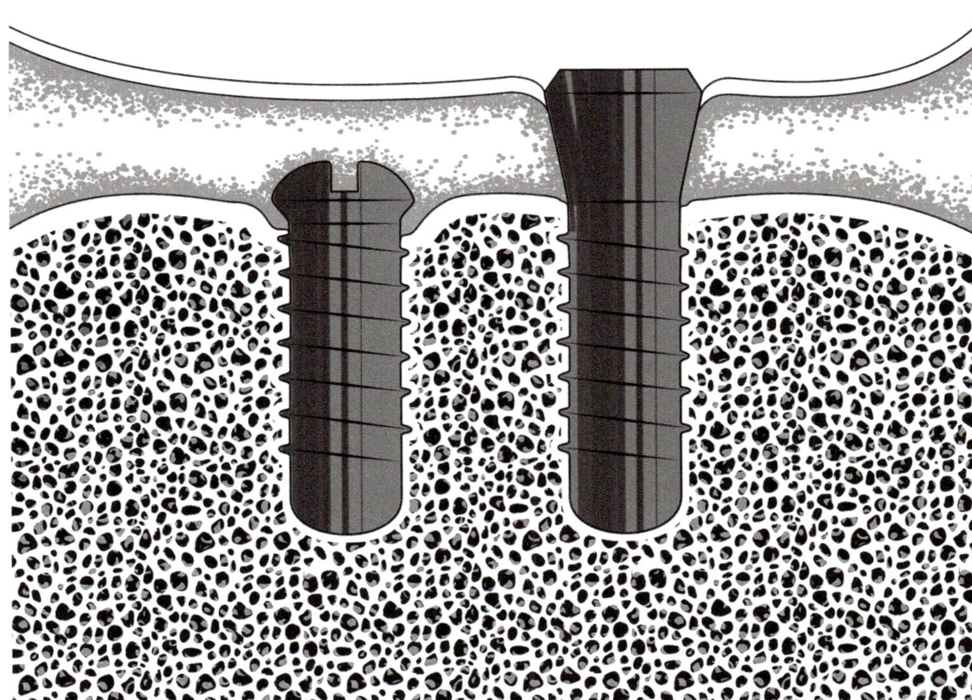

Fig. 18.7 Diagrammatic representation of submerged and nonsubmerged healing

treatment protocol also differs depending on whether it is an esthetic site or not. Single tooth replacements in a nonesthetic site are simpler as compared to multiple teeth replacements in an esthetic site.

For standard implant placement:

1. Local anesthesia: the area of surgery including at least two teeth mesial and distal should be well-anesthetized.
2. Incision: a scalpel blade no 15 is used to make a horizontal paracrestal incision. This bisects the existing zone of keratinized mucosa with at least 2 mm on the buccal aspect of the future implant. The incision extends to one tooth mesially and distally with a papilla sparing incision. If required, a vertical release incision can be given on the distal aspect to create a triangular flap.
3. Flap elevation: A full thickness mucoperiosteal flap is elevated on the buccal and on the lingual aspect. A retraction suture can be placed in the buccal and lingual flaps if required. The crestal bone should be exposed sufficiently so as to get visible access to the implant site as well to check the palatal and buccal curvature of the ridge.
4. Flattening of the ridge: A large round rose bur is used to flatten the ridge, thus removing any bony slopes in the crestal area. This also allows removal of the narrower portions from the crest of the ridge; however, extensive removal in short ridges should be done judiciously.
5. Drilling of the osteotomy: all drilling should be done along with copious amounts of cold saline irrigation with the speed as specified by the manufacture for each particular bur/drill (generally in the range of 800–1500 rpm). It is important to keep an eye for the correct positioning and the neighboring anatomic structures during each stage of drilling.
   (a) Initially, a small diamond bur is used to mark the site. The mark created corresponds to the center of the osteotomy and should be in the correct mesiodistal and buccolingual position. This bur is used to make a hole of 1–2 mm deep to create a start point for the pilot drill.
   (b) The pilot drill is the first twist drill used to create the osteotomy up to the desired length. Ideally, the length of the osteotomy should be slightly more than the implant so that the implant can be placed slightly subcrestal (to compensate for future crestal bone resorption). Also, the shoulder of the future implant should be 1 mm apical to the cementoenamel junction of the adjacent teeth in esthetic areas to allow for a proper emergence profile. While drilling, the correct axis should be maintained. The drills should be repeatedly pumped in and out of the osteotomy to expose the bone debris to the water coolants for clearing. If multiple implants are to be placed, a guide pin is used in the first osteotomy to align the second implant before commencing the second osteotomy preparation.
   (c) Subsequent drills are used in the same way as the pilot drill to enlarge the osteotomy to the desired depth.
   (d) Profile drills or countersink drills are used between the sequential drills to widen the crestal part of the osteotomy to allow the next drill into the osteotomy. The countersink drill also flares the preparation to allow the placement of the cover screw over the implant without any bony interference.
   (e) Bone tapping is an optional step that is required only in very dense bone. This is done at very slow speeds (20–40 rpm) without water irrigation.
6. Implant placement: implants are placed with a handpiece at slow speeds (18–25 rpm) or by hand using a torque wrench. Implant insertion should follow the same path of insertion as that of the osteotomy. For multiple implants, guide pins serve as a direction indicator to obtain parallelism. Care is taken to insert the implant such that the microrough surface of the implant is 1–1.5 mm subcrestal. This prevents exposure of the rough surface of the implant to the environment during the eventual crestal bone remodeling. The implant should also be placed such that the shoulder of the implant should be at least 3–4 mm apical to the cementoenamel junction of the adjacent teeth. It is also important that primary stability is achieved at placement and the average insertion torque should be 35 $Ncm^2$; however, ISQ values are a more accurate recording as they can be measured from time to time and a comparison can be obtained unlike insertion torque, which is only a one-time measurement. Once the desired position and stability are achieved, the cover screw (for submerged healing)/healing abutment (nonsubmerged healing) should be fitted over.
7. Flap closure and suturing: the flap should be approximated so as to provide tension-free closure. If required, a periosteal release incision can be done. If a submerged healing is planned, the flap should be completely closed over the implant by primary closure. If a nonsubmerged healing is intended, then the flap is closed around the healing abutment. Although any technique of suturing is acceptable, it is preferable that for long horizontal spaces, horizontal mattress sutures along with interrupted sutures

are placed in 4–0 or 5–0 nonresorbable sutures. Suturing of vertical incisions and papillae is generally done with 5–0 or 6–0 nonresorbable sutures.

8. Postoperative care: Simple implant surgery in a healthy patient does not require antibiotic coverage; however, if the patient has any systemic complications or at risk of infection, it is advisable to put the patient on postoperative antibiotic coverage. Analgesics are recommended for the first few days after surgery. Patient is given routine postsurgical instructions such as use of ice packs for the first 24 h, soft diet, no vigorous rinsing, no brushing on the surgical site, no tobacco smoking, and no vigorous exercise. Provisional replacements should not transmit direct forces to the underlying implant and should be adequately relieved from the surgical site, particularly in the early healing period (4–8 weeks). Patient is recalled on the second postsurgical day and after that 1 week postoperatively to check for healing.
9. Prosthetic phase: depending on the choice of timing to load the implant, the reopening phase can be planned. For nonsubmerged implants, often, no second surgery is required as the healing abutment is exposed. For submerged implants, the healing cap/abutment can be exposed by a small surgical procedure and a taller healing abutment can be inserted so as to allow the mucosal tissue to heal around and create an emergence profile.

(Figure 18.8 shows an example of the surgical phase of single implant placement)

## 18.10 Concepts of Implant Loading

An implant loading protocol is the time period between implant placement and the attachment of the prosthesis. The loading protocols have changed over the years, and the ITI Consensus Conferences in 2003, 2008, and 2013 had slight variations in defining them. The current definition as per the ITI Consensus Conference 2018 is as follows [39]:

- immediate loading,
- early loading,
- and conventional loading.

**Box 18.3 Concepts of Implant Loading**

(a) *Immediate loading:* Loading of dental implants earlier than 1 week after implant placement. This can be done with either a provisional prosthesis or a final prosthesis. The provisional prosthesis is used to reshape the peri-implant soft tissues for better esthetic outcomes, modify the occlusion, or evaluate a planned implant prosthesis. A final prosthesis can be directly given in cases with low esthetic risk and in areas of stable occlusion. This protocol significantly reduces the treatment time, and both soft tissue and bony healing occurs under functional loading.

(b) *Early loading:* Loading of dental implants between 1 week and 2 months after implant placement. In this treatment approach, functional forces are exerted on the implants during the later stages of bone healing. Soft tissues are still healing, and by two months, they are almost completely healed. Here also, the time between placement and loading is reduced.

(c) *Conventional loading:* Loading of dental implants more than 2 months after implant placement [40, 41]. This allows for a complete healing of bone and peri-implant soft tissue and requires a longer treatment time between implant placement and loading. This protocol is selected in cases when there are medical or risk factors, low implant stability at surgery, and extensive augmentation in the implant site and with short or narrow diameter implants.

Patient-related factors such as medical and systemic risk factors, surgical site factors (augmented site), and implant stability as assessed by insertion torque (20–50 $Ncm^2$) and resonance frequency analysis (>55 ISQ) are determinants for selecting the loading protocol. Implant design and characteristics also affect the loading protocol, surface modification of implants has added to faster healing rates of bone around implants, and hence, the healing period before loading has reduced [23]. Hence, selection of a correct loading protocol is case specific.

a

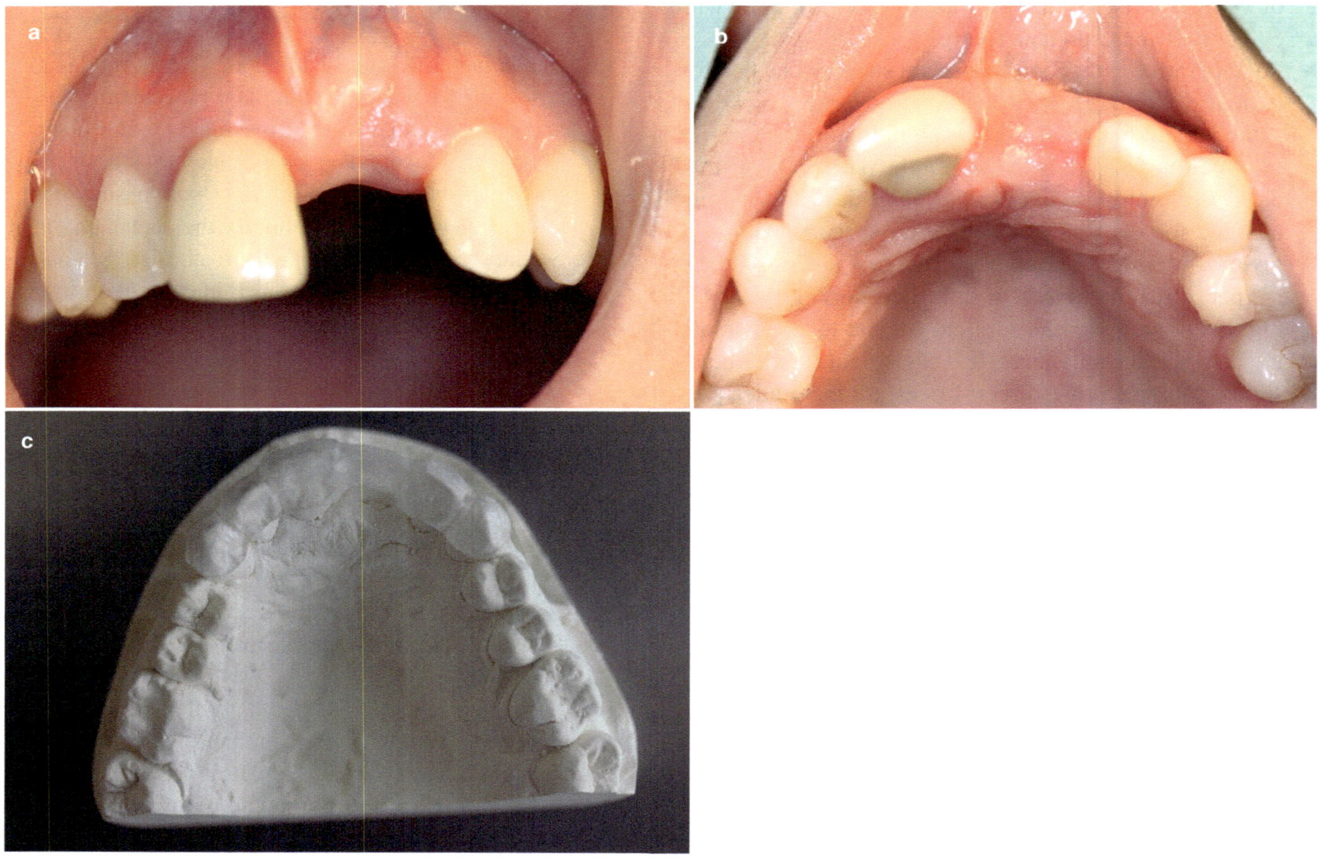


b

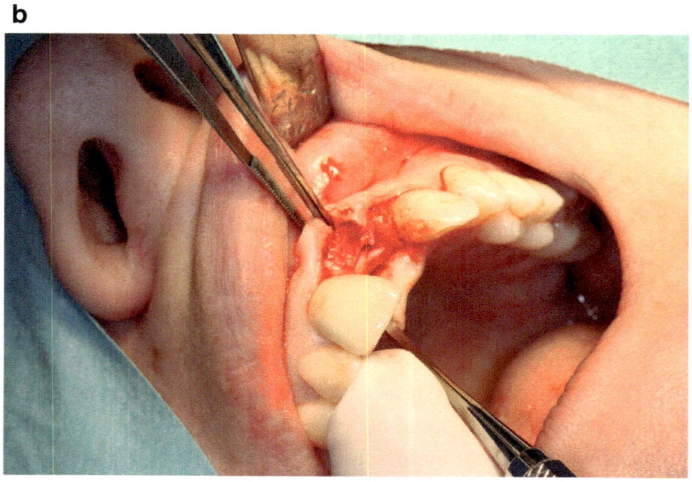

**Fig. 18.8** These series of figures show steps in implant placement with restoration of a single tooth edentulous space. (**aa**) Preoperative facial view of edentulous space. (**ab**) Preoperative occlusal view of edentulous space. (**ac**) Preoperative master cast with surgical splint. (**b**) Incision and reflection of mucoperiosteal flap. (**ca**) Initial drilling. (**cb**) Checking for ideal placement of initial drill with surgical guide, which would lead to *prosthodontically* driven implant placement and a favorable emergence profile. (**cc**) Checking for the depth of implant osteotomy using a depth gauge. (**da**) Subsequent drilling to accommodate the chosen dimension of the implant. (**db**) Subsequent drilling to accommodate the chosen dimension of the implant. (**e**) Implant insertion. (**f**) Placement of healing abutment for transmucosal/ non submerged healing. (**g**) Suturing and wound closure

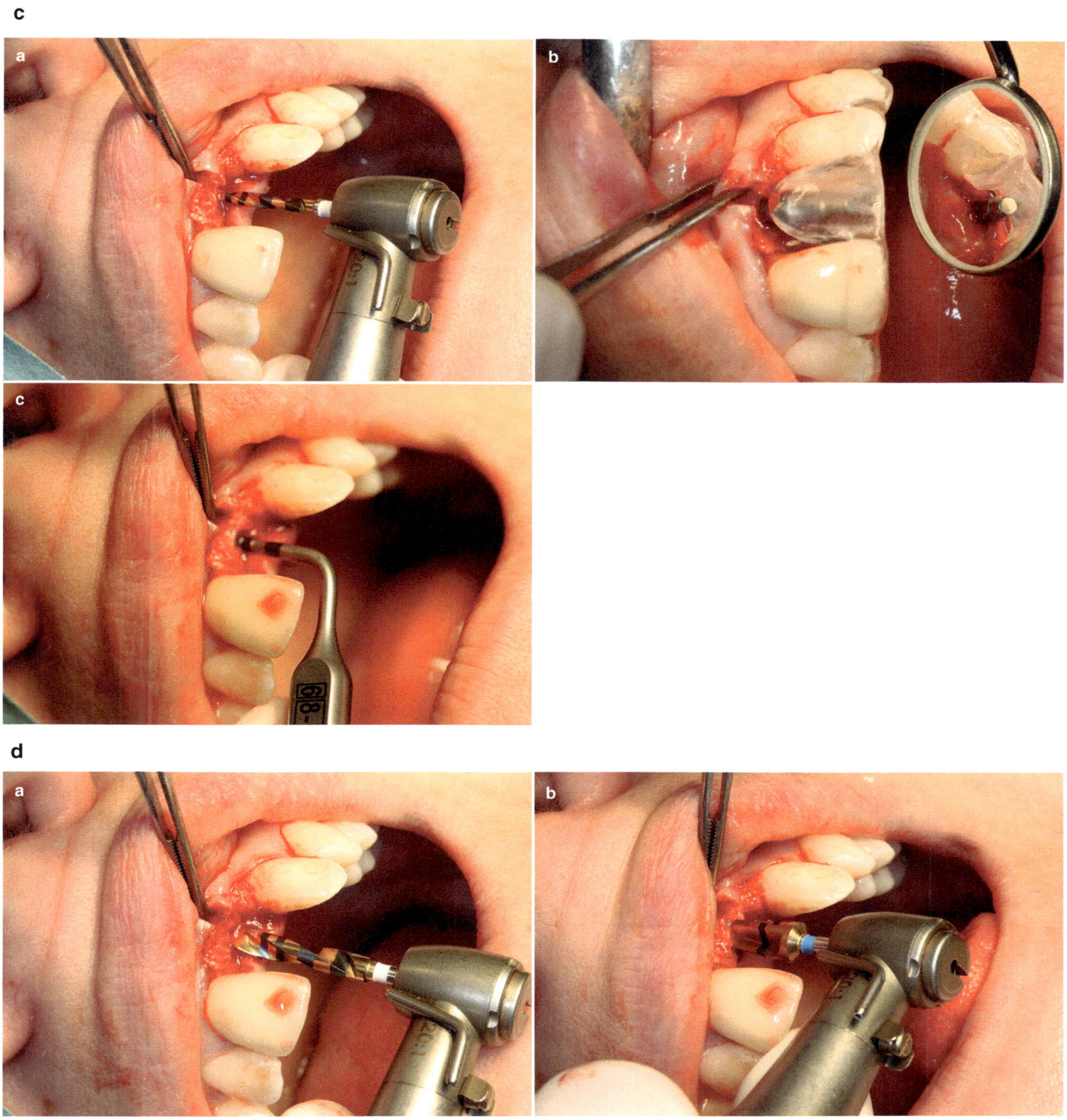


Fig. 18.8 (continued)

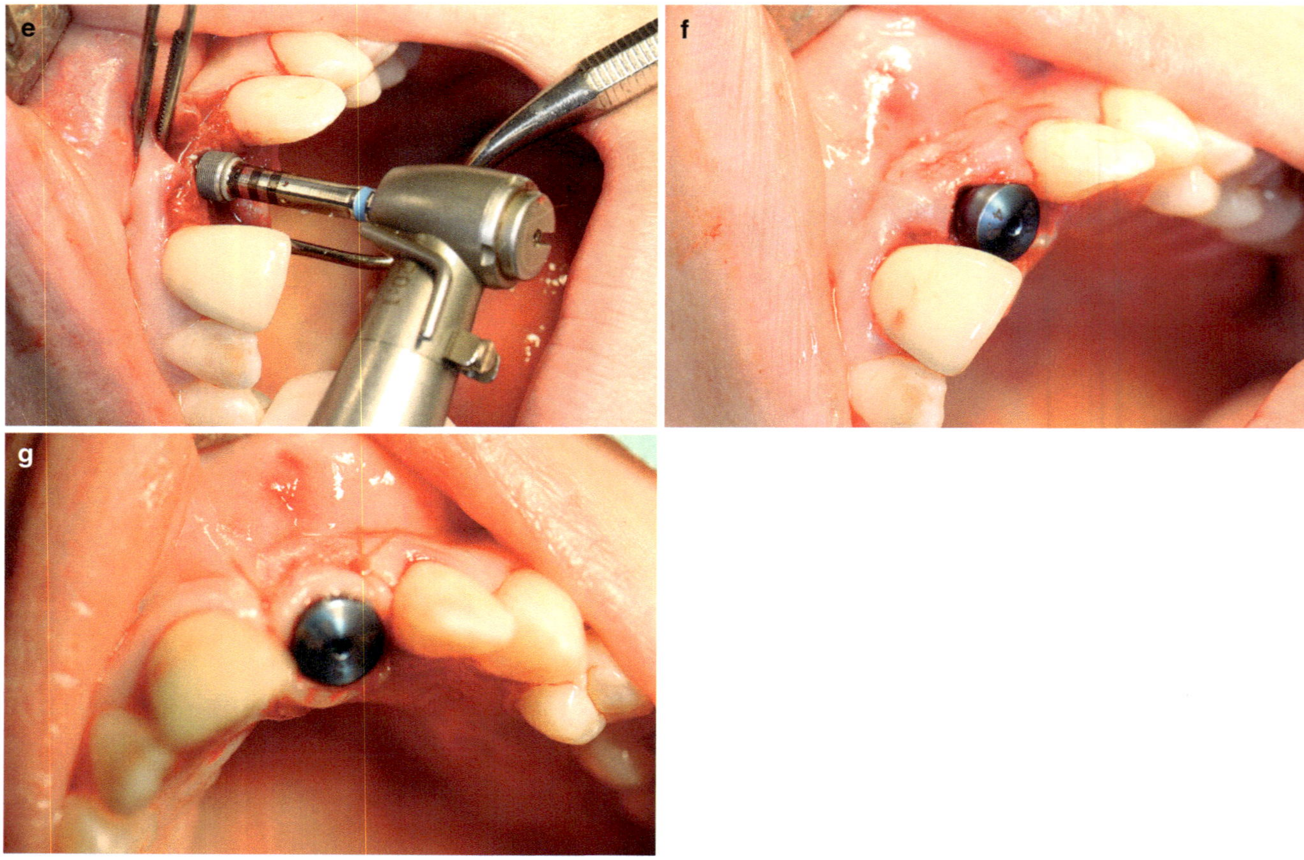




**Fig. 18.8** (continued)

## 18.11 Suggested Reading

ITI Treatment guides 1–10.

## References

1. Abraham CM. A brief historical perspective of dental implants, their surface coatings and treatment. Open Dent J. 2014;8(Suppl 1-M2):50–5.
2. Buser D, Sennerby L, De Bruyn H. Modern implant dentistry based on osseointegration: 50 years of progress, current trends and open questions. Periodontol 2000. 2017;73(1):7–21.
3. Mavrogenis AF, Dimitriou R, Parvizi J, Babis GC. Biology of implant osseointegration. J Musculoskelet Neuronal Interact. 2009;9(2):61–71.
4. BrånEmark PI. Introduction to osseointegration. In: BråNemark PI, Zarb G, Albrektsson T, editors. Tissue integrated protheses. Osseointegration in clinical dentistry. Chicago and Tokyo: Quintessence; 1985. p. 350.
5. Stanford CM, Keller JC. The concept of osseointegration and bone matrix expression. Crit Rev Oral Biol Med. 1991;2(1):83–101.
6. Reddy VK. Osseointegration. Int Dent Med J Adv Res. 2015;1:1–7.
7. Albrektsson T, Albrektsson B. Osseointegration of bone implants. A review of an alternative mode of fixation. Acta Orthop Scand. 1987;58(5):567–77.
8. Osman RB, Swain MV. A critical review of dental implant materials with an emphasis on titanium versus Zirconia. Materials (1996–1944). 2015;8(3):932–58.
9. Vootla NR, Reddy KV. Osseointegration- key factors affecting its success-an overview. IOSR J Dent Med Sci (IOSR-JDMS). 2017;16(4):62–8. e-issn: 2279-0853, p-issn: 2279-0861
10. Ellingsen JE, Johansson CB, Wennerberg A, Holmen A. Improved retention and bone-to-implant contact with fluoride-modified titanium implants. Int J Oral Maxillofac Implants. 2004;19:659–66.
11. Novaes AB Jr, de Souza SL, de Barros RR, Pereira KK, Iezzi G, Piattelli A. Influence of implant surfaces on osseointegration. Braz Dent J. 2010;21(6):471–81.
12. Moraschini V, E dS P B. Success of dental implants in smokers and non-smokers: a systematic review and meta-analysis. Int J Oral Maxillofac Surg. 2016;45(2):205–15.
13. Chappuis V, Araujo MG, Buser D. Clinical relevance of dimensional bone and soft tissue alterations post-extraction in esthetic sites. Periodontology 2000. 2017;73:73–83.
14. Eriksson AR, Albrektsson T. Temperature threshold levels for heat-induced bone tissue injury: a vital-microscopic study in the rabbit. J Prosthet Dent. 1983 Jul;50(1):101–7.

15. Parithimarkalaignan S, Padmanabhan TV. Osseointegration: An update. J Indian Prosthodont Soc. 2013;13(1):2–6.
16. Fiorellini J, Wada K, Stathopoulou P, Klokkevold PR. Chapter 71: periimplant anatomy, biology, and function in carranza's clinical periodontology. 12th ed. Amsterdam: Saunders, Elsevier Inc; 2015.
17. Stanford CM. Surface modifications of dental implants. Aus Dent J. 2008;53(1 Suppl):s26–33.
18. Le Guehennec L, Soueidan A, Layrolle P, Amouriq Y. Surface treatments of titanium dental implants for rapid osseointegration. Dent Mater. 2007;23:844–54.
19. Albrektsson T, Wennerberg A. Oral implant surfaces: part 1--review focusing on topographic and chemical properties of different surfaces and in vivo responses to them. Int J Prosthodont. 2004 Sep–Oct;17(5):536–43.
20. Buser D, Schenk RK, Steinemann S, Fiorellini JP, Fox CH, Stich H. Influence of surface characteris- tics on bone integration of titanium implants. A histo- morphometric study in miniature. J Biomed Mater Res. 1991;25:889–902.
21. Wennerberg A. The role of surface roughness for implant incorporation in Bone. Cells Mater. 1999;9(1):1–19.
22. Lang NP, Salvi GE, Huynh-Ba G, Ivanovski S, Donos N, Bosshardt DD. Early osseointegration to hydrophilic and hydrophobic implant surfaces in humans. Clin Oral Implants Res. 2011 Apr;22(4):349–56.
23. Buser D, Broggini N, Wieland M, Schenk RK, Denzer AJ, Cochran DL, Hoffmann B, Lussi A, Steinemann SG. Enhanced bone apposition to a chemically modified SLA titanium sur- face. J Dent Res. 2004;83(7):529–33.
24. Al-Johany SS, Al Amri MD, Alsaeed S, Alalola B. Dental implant length and diameter: a proposed classification scheme. J Prosthodont. 2017 Apr;26(3):252–60.
25. Buser D, Martin W, Belser UC. Optimizing esthetics for implant restorations in the anterior maxilla: anatomic and surgical considerations. Int J Oral Maxillofac Im- plants. 2004;19(suppl):43–61.
26. Grunder U, Gracis S, Capelli M. Influence of the 3-D bone-to-implant relationship on esthetics. Int J Periodon Restor Dent. 2005;25:113–9.
27. Klokkevold PR, Cochran DL. Clinical evaluation of the implant patient. Chapter 72, carranzas clincical periodontology. 12th ed. Amsterdam: Elsevier. p. 693–705.
28. Dawson A, Chen S, Buser D, Cordaro L, Martin W, Belser U. In: Dawson A, Chen S, editors. The SAC classification in implant dentistry. Chicago, IL: Quintessence Publishing; 2009.
29. Cardaropoli G, Araujo M, Lindhe J. Dynamics of bone tissue formation in tooth extraction sites. An experimental study in dogs. J Clin Periodontol. 2003;30:809–18.
30. Araujo MG, Lindhe J. Dimensional ridge alterations following tooth extraction: an experimental study in the dog. J Clin Periodontol. 2005;32:212–8.
31. Schropp L, Wenzel A, Kostopoulos L, Karring T. Bone healing and soft tissue contour changes following single-tooth extraction: a clinical and radiographic 12-month prospective study. Int J Periodontics Restorative Dent. 2003;23:313–23.
32. Ten Heggeler JM, Slot DE, Van der Weijden GA. Effect of socket preservation therapies following tooth extraction in non-molar regions in humans: a systematic review. Clin Oral Implants Res. 2011;22:779–88.
33. Trombelli L, Farina R, Marzola A, Bozzi L, Liljenberg B, Lindhe J. Modeling and remodeling of human extraction sockets. J Clin Periodontol. 2008 Jul;35(7):630–9.
34. Chappuis V, Engel O, Reyes M, Shahim K, Nolte LP, Buser D. Ridge alterations post-extraction in the esthetic zone: a 3D analysis with CBCT. J Dent Res. 2013;92:195S–201S.
35. Chen ST, Buser D. Clinical and esthetic outcomes of implants placed in postextraction sites. Int J Oral Maxillofac Implants. 2009;24(Suppl):186–217. Review
36. Chappuis V, Engel O, Shahim K, Reyes M, Katsaros C, Buser D. Soft tissue alterations in esthetic postextraction sites: a 3-dimensional analysis. J Dent Res. 2015 Sep;94(9 Suppl):187S–93S.
37. Morton D, Chen ST, Martin WC, Levine RA, Buser D. Consensus statements and recommended clinical procedures regarding optimizing esthetic outcomes in implant dentistry. Int J Oral Maxillofac Implants. 2014;29(Suppl):216–20.
38. Buser D, Chappuis V, Belser U, Chen S. Implant placement post extraction in esthetic single tooth sites: when immediate, when early, when late? Periodontology 2000. 2017;73:84–102.
39. Gallucci GO, Hamilton A, Zhou W, Buser D, Chen S. Implant placement and loading protocols in partially edentulous patients: a systematic review. Clin Oral Implants Res. 2018;29(Suppl. 16):106–34.
40. Gallucci GO, Benic GI, Eckert SE, Papaspyridakos P, Schimmel M, Schrott A, Weber HP. Consensus statements and clinical recommendations for implant loading protocols. Int J Oral Maxillofac Implants. 2014;29(Suppl):287–90.
41. Weber HP, Morton D, Gallucci GO, Roccuzzo M, Cordaro L, Grutter L. Consensus statements and recommended clinical procedures regarding loading protocols. Int J Oral Maxillofac Implants. 2009;24(Suppl):180–3.

# Bone Augmentation Procedures in Implantology

19

Vinay V. Kumar, Supriya Ebenezer, and Andreas Thor

## 19.1 Introduction

Dental implants have been used successfully to rehabilitate patients with edentulousness. For implant dentistry to be successful, the implants have to be placed in an appropriate three-dimensional manner that supports the prosthesis adequately. This means that implants have to be placed in a prosthodontically driven predetermined position. This requirement often results in a clinical situation where there is a lack of bone volume to completely embed the implant in an ideal position.

Implants that do not have an adequate amount of bone covering them in all aspects (at least 1.5 mm bone buccal and lingual to the implant shoulder or about 2 mm in aesthetic zones) are at high risk for crestal bone loss with concomitant inflammation and infection of the surrounding soft tissues due to exposure and colonisation of the implant surfaces by bacterial biofilms [1]. This in turn results in soft-tissue recession, which leads to further loss of bone and eventually failure of the implant. Hence, bone augmentation is often necessary to ensure adequate bony housing around implants [2].

The most commonly used bone-augmentation surgical procedures are guided bone regeneration (GBR), block bone grafting and maxillary sinus floor elevation (SFE). When deciding to augment, there are multiple sources of bone-augmentation materials ranging from autogenous, allogenic, xenogenic and synthetic materials. A knowledge of these materials is essential prior to undertaking augmentation procedures. Knowledge of bone biology and bone physiology is also important.

**Electronic Supplementary Material** The online version of this chapter (https://doi.org/10.1007/978-981-15-1346-6_19) contains supplementary material, which is available to authorized users.

V. V. Kumar (✉) · A. Thor
Department of Maxillofacial and Plastic Surgery, Uppsala University Hospital, Uppsala, Sweden

S. Ebenezer
Department of Oral Surgery and Stomatology, University of Bern, Bern, Switzerland

It is obvious that a thorough medical history should be obtained before implant treatment and prior to augmentation procedures. Patients should be evaluated regarding their general health status, medical history, history of any medication, allergies, the use of tobacco and compliance to oral hygiene methods. Patients with conditions that affect bone healing would be poor candidates for augmentation procedures. Patients with a history of head and neck radiotherapy, uncontrolled diabetes, transplant patients undergoing prolonged immunotherapy, patients undergoing bisphosphonate therapy or medications that could induce osteonecrosis of the jaws, heavy smokers and patients with neuropsychiatric disorders are high-risk patients to undergo augmentation.

It is also obvious that prior to undertaking augmentation procedures, adequate radiographic assessment of the region should be performed. In most situations, Cone Beam Computed Tomography (CBCT) is the imaging of choice.

The use of tilted or angulated implants, narrow implants, zygomatic implants, short implants or the use of non-implant-supported prosthesis can avoid the need for augmentations, and this should be discussed with the patient prior to undertaking augmentation surgery [3, 4].

## 19.2 The Alveolar Bone-Resorption Pattern and the Need for Augmentation

The alveolar bone is functionally and macroscopically unique. It is that functional area of the maxilla and mandible that is responsible for the anchorage of teeth. Both the mandible and the maxilla are irregular bones and are of mesenchymal origin. The maxilla consists for the most part of cancellous bone with a thin cortex layer, whereas the mandible has more cortical bone and is denser. As the alveolar process of the maxilla and mandible are basically functional components to support the teeth, after tooth loss, the alveolar bone starts to resorb. However, the pattern of bone resorption in the two bones is different. The maxillary alveolar bone



K. Bonanthaya et al. (eds.), *Oral and Maxillofacial Surgery for the Clinician*, https://doi.org/10.1007/978-981-15-1346-6_19

resorbs from the labial plate inwards and the mandibular alveolar bone from the lingual plate outwards. Therefore, in the cases of long-standing edentulousness, this resorption pattern results in a narrower maxilla and mandible. The bone height is also reduced in a vertical direction in areas of tooth loss, leading to a reduced alveolar bone height in the maxillary posterior area (beneath the sinuses) and a reduced distance from the crest to the mandibular canal in the posterior mandible. The sagittal relation is also affected due to jaw atrophy, leading to an often retrognathic maxilla in relation to the wider mandible. In short, both the width of the bone (also called the volume of bone) and the quality of bone (described by Lekholm & Zarb and Cawood & Howell), [5, 6] must be taken into consideration before implant placement. Additionally, due to ridge resorption, the vertical and sagittal bone relations between the upper and lower jawbones and the toothless space must be taken into consideration before implant placement and bone augmentation, when treatment is planned from a prosthodontic point of view. Figure 19.1 shows the changes in edentulous jaws and the classification of bone quality and bone quantity as described by Lekholm and Zarb, 1985.

Also, in patients with tooth loss secondary to other reasons of bone loss such as trauma, pathologies, etc.; bone should be replaced to reconstruct the lost tissue as well as to support placement of implants in the best prosthetically driven position.

## 19.3 Bone Biology

Depending on the macroscopic form and mechanical function, bone can be designated as cancellous bone (also called spongiosa or trabecular bone) and cortical bone (also called compact bone). Cortical bone is the dense outer aspect of bone that is responsible for the mechanical strength. The inner cancellous part of the bone that predominantly consists of bone marrow and provides nutrition to the bone [7].

Microscopically cortical bone consists of concentric circles of osteons (also known as Haversian systems) (Fig. 19.2). Each osteon consists of a central canal of nerves and blood vessels that is surrounded by layers of compact bone. Microscopically, cancellous bone architecture consists of bone organised into a three-dimensional lattice framework called trabeculae. The trabecular spaces are filled with blood vessels and marrow. Bone marrow is a specialised connective tissue that produces erythrocytes, leucocytes, platelets and osteoblasts. Depending on age and location, bone marrow additionally contains fat cells and other connective tissue elements [8].

Under higher magnification, bone can be further designated as woven or lamellar bone. Woven bone is immature bone that forms following injury to mature bone (such as fractures or tooth extraction) or during the foetal growth period. After an injury to mature bone that causes a break in its continuity such as tooth extraction, a haematoma results and following this woven bone is formed rapidly to fill the defect in the bone. This bone is mechanically weak and its collagen fibrils have a random orientation. Woven bone is then replaced by mature and mechanically strong lamellar bone that has collagen fibrils arranged parallelly and regularly into distinct layers.

Bones of the human body are in a constant state of renewal, the process known as bone remodelling. Bone remodelling is essential to regulate mineral balance in the bone and circulatory system, as well as to maintain bone strength. Regular day stress and strain causes microdamage in bone, which is repaired and replaced by new bone by the

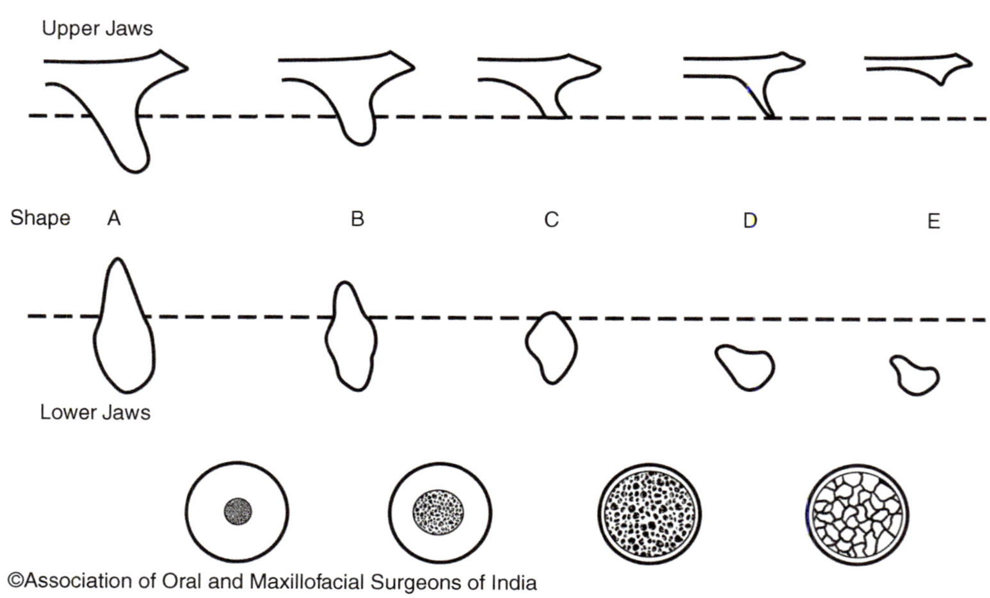


Fig. 19.1 Classification of bone for implant placement by Lekholm and Zarb, 1985. Adapted from Lekholm and Zarb, 1985 [6]

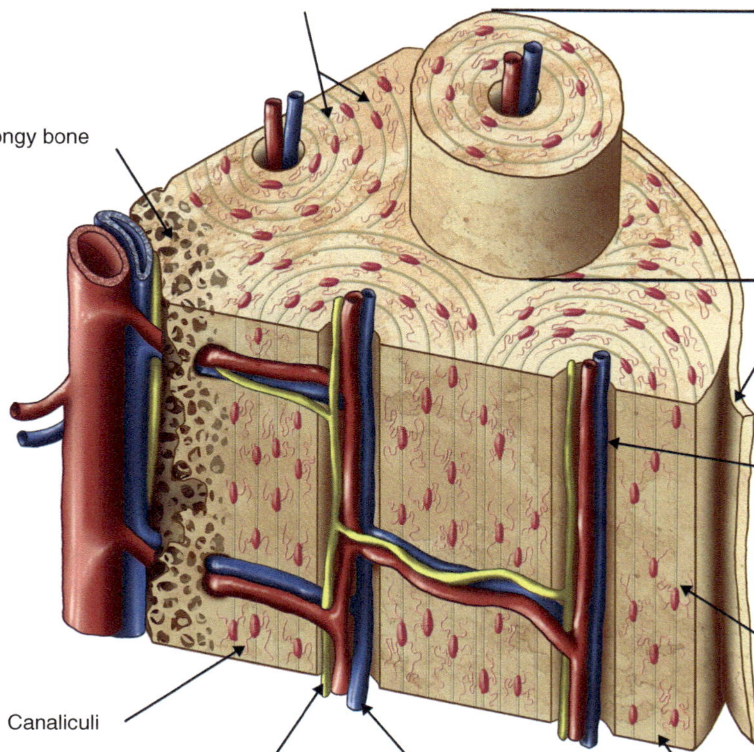


**Fig. 19.2** Cross-section of bone showing a cortical bone and spongy/cancellous bone. Please note the osteon containing a central canal with blood vessels and nerves surrounded by concentric lamellae with osteocytes and lacunae

process of bone remodelling. Therefore, the process of bone remodelling helps the bone to adapt to changing mechanical and biologic needs during the lifetime of the individual. For the ease of description, bone remodelling can be divided as consisting of four continuous stages:

bone resorption,
reversal phase,
mineralisation phase
and resting phase (Fig. 19.3).

During the resorption phase, specialised cells called osteoblasts are activated, which eat away old bone. In the reversal phase, bone-forming cells known as osteoblasts begin to appear on the surface of the resorbed bone. In the bone-formation phase, the osteoblasts lay down osteoid, which is the unmineralised organic portion of bone and bone mineralisation occurs when calcium hydroxyapatite and other minerals are incorporated into the organic unmineralised osteoid, thereby providing mechanical strength. Bone remodelling occurs all throughout life and consists of a closely coupled phenomenon of bone apposition and resorption. Under normal healthy conditions in adults, bone resorption and apposition during remodelling are balanced in time, space and amount so that the bone mass of the body remains more or less constant.

### 19.3.1 Composition of Bone

Bone is a connective tissue that consists of bone cells (approximately 10%) in a connective tissue matrix (approximately 90%). Cells of the bone are the osteoblasts, the osteocytes and osteoclasts. The osteoblasts are large uninucleate cells that form bone. They work in groups and predominantly lay down the collagen matrix known as osteoid. Osteoblasts also produce proteins such as bone morphogenetic proteins that stimulate bone healing and mineralisation. About 10% of the osteoblasts become entrapped inside the calcified bone matrix and are known as Osteocytes. Osteocytes reside in small bone cavities known as lacunae and are interconnected with each other and with osteoblasts and lining cells on the bone surface. Osteoclasts, on the other hand, are multinucleated cells that line the surface of the bone where resorption takes place.

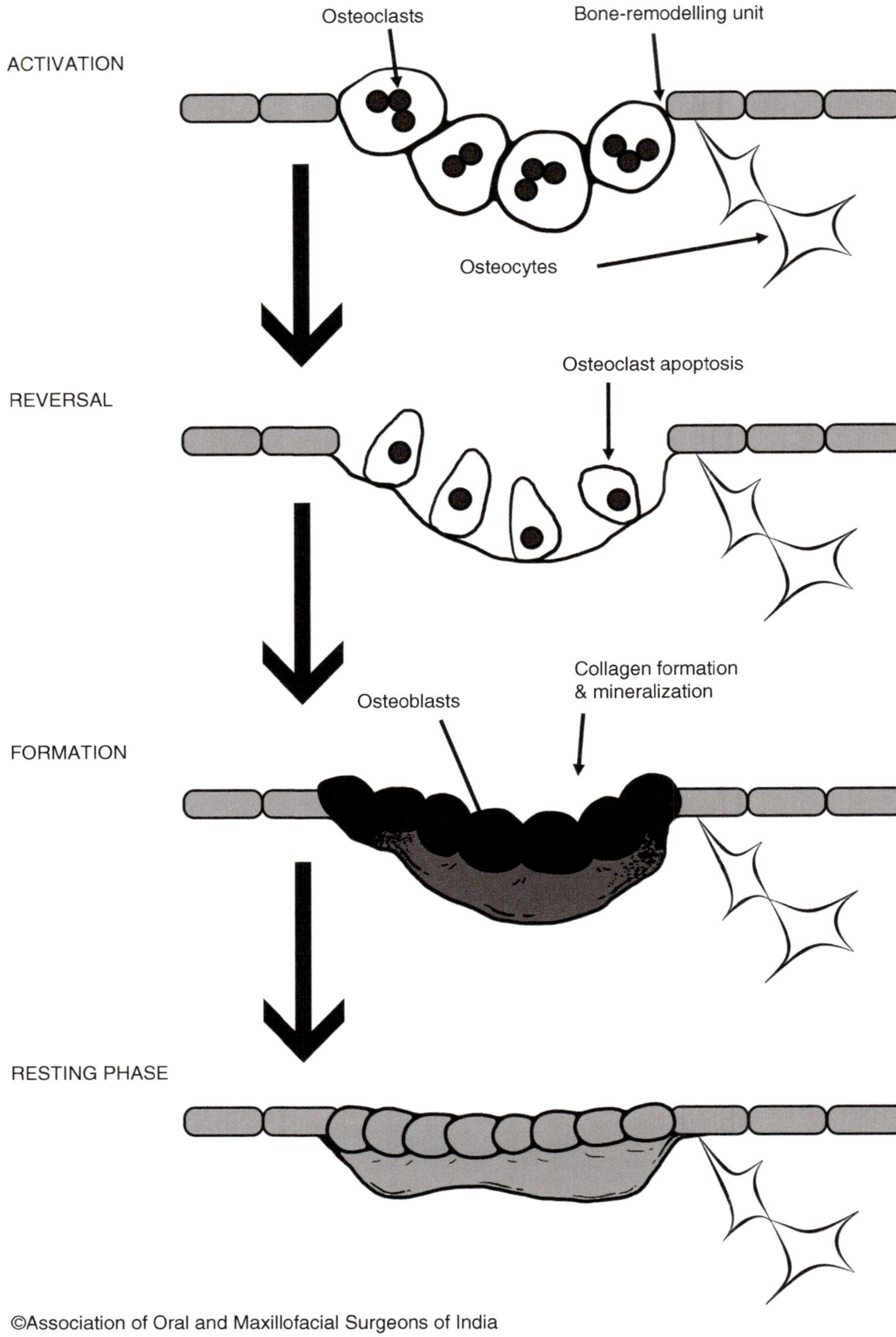


**Fig. 19.3** describes the four phases of bone remodelling

These cells release powerful degrading enzymatic proteins that are responsible for the removal of bone minerals.

The extracellular bone matrix consists of about 35% organic and 65% inorganic materials. About 90% of the organic phase is collagen type I fibres, while the remaining 10% consists of various non-collagenous proteins. The bone matrix also contains growth factors such as the bone morphogenetic proteins important for bone healing. The inorganic phase of the bone matrix consists of low-crystallinity carbonated hydroxyapatite [9].

## 19.4 Bone Grafts and Bone Substitutes

Currently, there are a wide variety of biomaterials that can be used for bony augmentation [10].

Table 19.1 describes the classification of bone grafts [11] (Adapted from Katsuyama H., Jensen S.S. Treatment Options for Sinus Floor Elevation).

Most commonly, bone grafts and bone substitutes are classified according to their source of origin in relation to the intended recipient. Autogenous or autologous bone grafts are obtained from the same individual. Allogeneic bone grafts or allografts are obtained from a genetically distinct individual of the same species. In contrast, xenogeneic bone grafts or xenografts are obtained from a different species than the intended recipient. Alloplastic bone substitutes are synthetically produced materials.

*Autogenous bone graft or autograft* refers to bone originating from the same patient, and it can be harvested from intra-oral or extra-oral sites. It is preferred to harvest the bone as close to the surgical defect as possible in order to avoid donor-site morbidities. However, of course this decision is dependent on the amount of bone required. For smaller augmentations and guided bone regeneration, bone is commonly harvested from the bone tissue neighbouring the defect site. In this case, donor-site access can be gained from the same incision that is used to access the recipient site. In cases where slightly larger amounts are needed, bone can be harvested from the anterior mandibular ramus or the mandibular symphysis. These are the most common intra-oral bone donor sites. Although one may need an additional incision to harvest bone in intra-oral sites, these can be obtained in the same surgical area. When even larger amounts of bone are needed, harvesting from extra-oral sites is needed. The most commonly used donor sites are the iliac bone, the calvarium and the tibia. In most of these cases with the need of an extraoral donor-site harvest, the surgical time as well as hospital stay is often prolonged. A more detailed explanation of different donor sites is provided in the section on onlay bone grafting. In the case of very large bony reconstructions where the defect size is more than 6 centimetres, vascularised bone containing free flaps are used, such as the free fibula flap [12, 13]. These procedures are commonly carried out for benign and malignant tumours, and are not described in this chapter, but described in detail in the relevant chapter of this textbook.

*Allogeneic bone graft* or allograft refers to bone originating from another human, either a living donor or following the death of an organ donor. Usually, the allogeneic bone is harvested from the iliac bone or tibia and can be fresh-frozen, freeze-dried or processed as demineralised freeze-dried bone.

*Xenogeneic bone substitute or xenograft* is bone-substitute material originating from another species. These could be sea algae, corals, equine (originating from horses), porcine (originating from pigs) or most commonly, bovine (originating from cows).

Bone-substitute materials can also be manufactured purely by synthetic means, produced in the laboratory. These are called *alloplastic graft materials* examples of these are hydroxyapatite, beta-tricalcium phosphate, calcium silicophosphate, bioglasses, polymers, titanium particles or a combination of these.

**Table 19.1** Classification of bone-grafting materials

| Autogenous bone Origin: the same person | Allogenic bone Origin: another human | Xenogenic bone Origin: another species | Alloplastic bone Origin: synthetic |
|---|---|---|---|
| Block graft | Fresh frozen bone | Bone from another animal such as bovine, porcine | Calcium phosphates |
| Particulate bone | Freeze-dried bone allograft | Materials from corals | Glass ceramics |
| | Demineralised freeze-dried bone allograft | Materials derived from calcifying algae | Polymers |
| | Deproteinised bone allograft | | Metals |

Adapted from Katsuyama H and Jensen S.S: 2011 [11]

**Box 19.1**

*Block bone grafts/Particulate bone grafts:* Depending upon the shape and constitution of the bone graft, they can be described as block bone grafts or particulate bone grafts or a combination of these. Bone blocks are large pieces of autogenous bone. Autogenous bone that has been harvested by bone scrapers and chisels is in the form of small chips and is referred to as a particulate graft. Particulate grafts can also be made from block grafts by using special milling machines to break down the block (Fig. 19.4a, b).

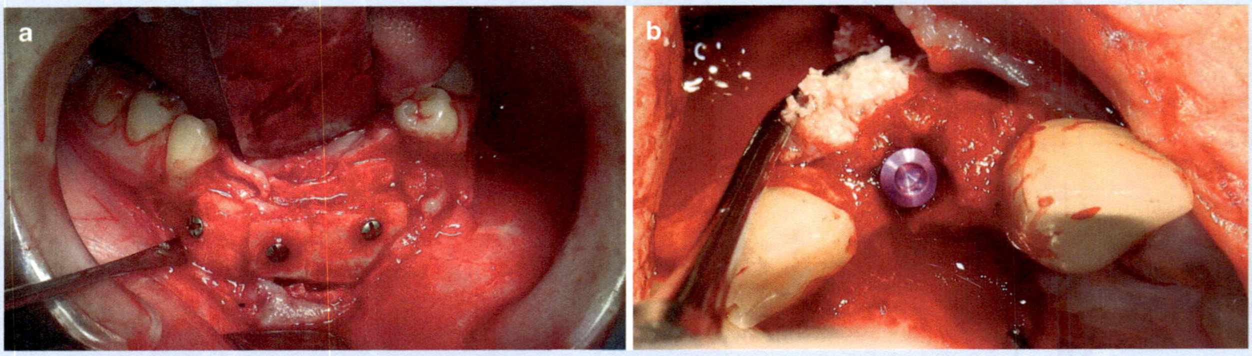



**Fig. 19.4** (**a**) an example of block bone graft (**b**) an example of a particulate bone graft

### 19.4.1 Classification of Bone Grafts Based on the Mechanism of Action

Bone grafts can also be described and classified based on the mechanism of action and biological activity into *osteogenic, osteoinductive and osteoconductive*.

**Box 19.2**

*Osteogenic grafts* provide a source of new bone formation by the osteoblasts that are present in the graft material. At present, this can only be seen in the cases of autogenous bone grafts, where the donor bone is from the same subject and the transplantation procedure has preserved the viability and vitality of osteoblasts in them. Developments using stem cell harvesting may enable development of osteogenic bone grafts without the use of the subject's own bone tissue.

*Osteoinduction* is defined as the mechanism whereby a bone-substitute material induces bone formation by stimulating undifferentiated mesenchymal cells to turn into osteoblasts, which in turn produce new bone. Many proteins such as bone morphogenetic proteins are being investigated for their osteoinductive properties.

*Osteoconduction* is the mechanism whereby bone formation is enhanced by providing a scaffold for osteogenic cells that are present in the local environment of the host. Osteoconductive materials form a passive support for cells to migrate and colonise the scaffold and then produce new bone.

In spite of the large number of products available in the market, the gold standard in bone augmentation is autogenous bone. Depending on the indication for grafting and the amount of graft needed, autogenous bone can be used in a particulate form that is used either stand alone, or mixed with a bone-substitute material, used encased in titanium meshes or membranes, as a block graft, or as combination of any of these. Vascularised autogenous bone grafts such as the free fibula flap, the iliac crest and scapula free flap can be used not only as bone flaps but also as composite tissue to reconstruct complete jaws.

Bone augmentation and healing of the graft occurs in the following stages [14]: The surgical intervention gives rise to a haematoma and an acute inflammatory reaction, which is similar to the most cases of tissue trauma. This inflammatory reaction invokes a migration of inflammatory cells into the region, along with osteoblasts and osteoblast precursor cells. In a day's time, proliferation of blood vessels and the beginning of granulation tissue formation occur. This phase is followed by the resorption of the graft by osteoclast precursor cells, and in the case of autogenous bone, this releases bone morphogenetic proteins from the bone matrix, marking the start of the osteoinductive activity. At the same time, osteoblasts from the host bone start to migrate into the grafted region and begin to produce new bone, marking the phenomenon of osteoconduction. The graft is over time incorporated into the regional host bone by undergoing varying degrees of resorption and remodelling.

Although the procedure is largely similar regardless of the origin of the bone graft, the properties of osteoinduction and osteoconduction as well as biocompatibility can vary depending upon the particular bone-substitute material in use. Most bone-substitute materials are osteoconductive and vary in the resorption and bone turn-over rates. As a result, certain materials are shown to completely resorb within a period of a few months, whereas certain bone-substitute materials are present after many years.

*Autogenous bone* is the only type of graft that contributes to bone regeneration via all three mechanisms. A limited number of osteoblasts survive the procedure of grafting and these cells contribute towards osteogenesis; the graft itself provides a scaffold for osteoblasts from the host site to migrate into, facilitating osteoconduction; finally, the growth factors included within the graft matrix and released during graft resorption facilitate osteoinduction. Autogenous bone also has a high rate of resorption.

*Allogeneic bone* grafts are classified as mineralised and demineralised. Mineralised allografts—such as fresh frozen bone allograft and freeze-dried bone allograft—contribute to bone regeneration primarily through osteoconduction, but they may also possess some potential for osteoinduction. On the other hand, demineralised freeze-dried bone allograft is said to contribute to bone regeneration primarily through osteoinduction, and only secondarily by osteoconduction. However, it should be noted that variations in the processing of allogenic bone grafts from different tissue banks using different methodologies result in a large variation in the composition as well as osteoconductive potential of demineralised freeze-dried bone.

The choice of a commercially available bone-substitute material is most commonly based on the preference of the recipient patient (some patients would not like bone substitutes from an animal source or a cadaveric source), the available product information and documentation of clinical success, product availability, the ease of use and the preference of the clinician.

## 19.5 Barrier Membranes

Barrier membranes are an important component for the success of the GBR procedure. Ideally, the barrier membranes must be non-toxic, biocompatible, cell occlusive with a certain degree of permeability for diffusion of nutrients, permit bonding and ingrowth of connective tissue during healing, should be of sufficient rigidity to maintain the space created and not collapse into the defect, it should be easy to handle clinically and should be able to be trimmed to tailor the material as per the size of the defect [15].

Although traditionally many materials such as PTFE had been developed as membranes, currently most membranes being used are made up of collagen (type I, type III or a combination of these) [16]. These collagen membranes are derived from porcine or bovine sources [17]. Collagen membranes resorb as a result of enzymatic action of macrophages and polymorphonuclear leukocytes. Some manufacturers cross-link collagen membranes with glutaraldehyde to reduce the rate of membrane resorption, thereby prolonging the barrier function. However, crosslinking with glutaraldehyde can result in cytotoxic residues in the membrane following its manufacture. Resorbable membranes have a less likelihood to cause early membrane exposure, and that additionally due to the property of being resorbable, they do not need to be removed at a second surgical procedure.

Clinically, the main advantage of resorbable membranes is their decreased susceptibility to infective complication. If premature membrane exposure occurs, secondary soft tissue healing takes place within 4 weeks, and the bone-regenerative outcome remains favourable. Collagen membranes are also easier to handle clinically and adapt well to the surgical site once they are wet with blood or saline. Significantly, the membranes do not need to be removed via a second surgical procedure because they biodegrade. The main disadvantage is that non-cross-linked collagen membranes collapse easily because they do not have space-maintaining properties.

When a membrane with insufficient stiffness and rigidity is used in larger defects, there is a high likelihood of membrane collapse. Collapse of the membrane would lead to a situation where there would be no space for guided bone regeneration. Hence, clinically this problem is solved by using a bone graft or a bone-substitute material that fills the bone defect and provides support to the membrane. Other methods to support the barrier membranes include the incorporation of bendable titanium frameworks into PTFE material, tenting screws to support the membrane and titanium mesh that can be shaped and adapted to the site. However, these procedures would require an additional surgical procedure to remove the hardware [18].

### 19.5.1 Success Parameters of Autogenous Bone Graft Healing

The success of bone augmentation is dependent on the ability of the augmented bone to support an implant fixture at the desired position. However, in biological terms the extent of graft incorporation, turnover, replacement, the volume stability and the time taken for healing are dependent on many factors such as surgical factors, patient-related factors and material-related factors. It has been shown in multiple systematic reviews and innumerable clinical studies that there is no one single superior bone-substitute material [14]. Bone augmentation, although having well-documented success rates, depends upon surgical as well as patient-related factors. Amongst the surgeon-related factors are the training of the surgeon, their surgical expertise, the adherence to protocol and treatment of the graft material as well as the recipient site, adequate fixation of the graft to prevent movement between the graft and recipient bone and so on.

Patient-related factors that contribute to healing include underlying systemic diseases such as immunodeficiency, diabetes; local factors and habits such as oral hygiene and oral health, smoking and use of tobacco and defect-related factors such as the size of the defect and the morphology of the defect. It should be noted that smaller augmentations in a three-walled defect are more successful than large only vertical bone augmentation.

Regarding the influence of the grafted material used, it has been shown that particulated autogenous bone has the advantage of relatively fast incorporation in comparison with autogenous bone blocks [19]. However, particulate bone lacks structural stability and is prone to undergo unpredictable and extensive resorption. In contrast, autogenous bone blocks provide structural stability leading to better dimensional stability. However, block grafting requires a longer healing period of at least 6 months with about 50% (half the initial augmented volume) resorption at the end of the healing period.

Regarding the influence of bone-substitute materials, there exists a large variation in the physicochemical characteristics of the various bone substitutes available in the market, including their composition, particle size and form and surface properties. These differences can result in varying outcomes following augmentation.

Differences in the amount of new bone formation can be due to true differences in the osteoconductive potential of the biomaterial, but may also partly be explained by differences in resorption capacity amongst the various bone substitutes, which in turn determine the space available for new bone tissue formation within the defect site. For example, beta-tricalcium phosphate is replaced rather quickly, while sintered bovine bone is resistant to resorption and will be present in the augmented site for decades.

## 19.6 Commonly Carried Out Augmentation Procedures

Currently implantology has developed rapidly. Newer techniques and materials are constantly being introduced. The choice of procedure depends mainly upon the surgeon. Based upon the amount of bone augmentation required, the commonly carried out procedures are:

GBR (guided bone regeneration)
Onlay bone grafting
Sinus floor elevation
These procedures are described in detail below.

## 19.7 Guided Bone Regeneration

Guided bone regeneration is a bone-augmentation technique that uses the principle of space maintenance within a bony defect with the use of a barrier membrane. The barrier membrane excludes rapidly proliferating epithelial cells and connective tissue fibroblasts, thus allowing the ingrowth of slower-growing bone cells and blood vessels into the blood clot within the defect.

The concept of guided bone regeneration was introduced and developed first by Nyman and colleagues; Dahlin and colleagues in the early 1980s [20, 21]. Multiple animal studies showed that bone defects protected by a barrier membrane, which did not permit ingress of cells, had increased bone fill as compared to defects that were not protected by a barrier membrane. Although the technique was first described for periodontal defects around natural teeth, later studies showed that GBR was also predictable in forming bone around implant defects.

Clinically, GBR is performed by raising a mucoperiosteal flap and exposing the bony defect. This defect is filled with a bone substitute and then covered with a barrier membrane. The bone defect with the bone substitute is filled with blood, which later clots and forms a haematoma. Over a period of time, the haematoma is ingressed by blood vessels and osteoprogenitor cells from the surrounding environment, which over a period of time forms bone tissue by resorbing the existing substitute and replacing it or growing into the substitute that acts as a scaffold. The barrier membrane prevents the ingress of fast proliferating fibroblasts and epithelial cells into the bone defect, thereby creating a space for bone to form and mature.

However, GBR does not produce similar successful outcomes in all morphology of defects [22]. The more the bone walls the defect contains, the better the bone fill following GBR. Bone walls provide an exposed surface of bone-recruiting cells. With more bone walls, an increased number of osteogenic cells are able to migrate along newly proliferating blood vessels into the haematoma in the defect. When two or three walls are present, the blood clot is less likely to be moved and better protected during the healing phase.

Guided bone regeneration can be applied for the correction of minor requirements of bone augmentation. They are documented to be successful in the following clinical situations:

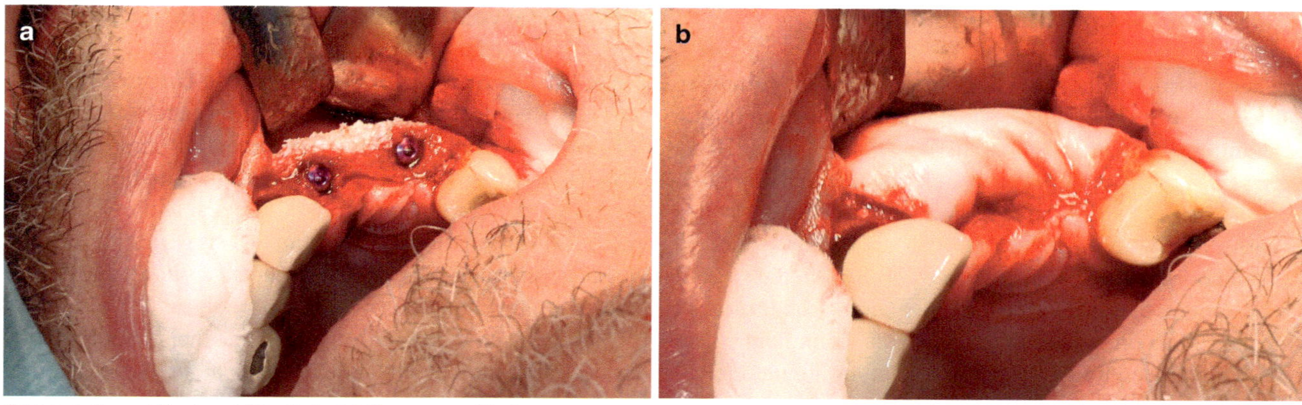




**Fig. 19.5** (**a**, **b**) Shows a clinical case of GBR for a 2 walled defect

1. Used to augment 2- or 3-walled crestal bone defects when implants are placed into extraction sites.
2. Used for augmenting bone when there is an apical fenestration following implant placement.
3. GBR can be used for ridge preservation.
4. GBR can be performed as a combination to other larger augmentation procedures.
5. GBR can be used for contour augmentation to increase the thickness of the facial bone for aesthetic reasons.

### 19.7.1 Augmentation of 2 and 3 Walled Defects

Guided bone regeneration can be successfully used in cases with crestal bone defects that are seen while placement of implants into extraction sites. If an implant can be placed with sufficient primary stability and results in a 2 or 3 walled defect, or if the defect is well contained in the bony envelope, GBR can be successfully performed at the time of implant placement. If these factors are not present, the augmentation must be performed prior to implant placement as a staged approach. In these cases, depending on the size and morphology of the defect, augmentation can be performed either by GBR, or by other augmentation methods described later in the chapter.

Figure 19.5a, b shows a case of GBR augmentation of 2 walled defect.

### 19.7.2 For Augmenting Apical Fenestrations

Often when implants are placed in the correct prosthetic position, with the correct angulation in order to provide screw retained restorations, the ideal angulation of placement would result in an apical fenestration, with the apical part of the implant threads being exposed. In these situations, the fenestration defects can be covered by using particulate bone/substitute material, covered with a membrane, as per the principles of GBR.

### 19.7.3 GBR for Ridge Preservation

During preoperative assessment and after extraction of a hopeless tooth that is planned to be restored with an implant, it is essential to inspect the shape of the resulting socket. In many situations, either due to trauma or chronic infection, the facial bone wall is missing. In these cases, it is important to augment the ridge/preserve the ridge at the time of tooth extraction. GBR can be well employed for this procedure known as ridge preservation/alveolar ridge preservation. In cases of acute infection in the sockets, ridge preservation can be carried out at a later stage after the infection has subsided.

### 19.7.4 GBR in Combination with Other Larger Augmentation Procedures

In the cases of localised prolonged ridge atrophy, GBR can be combined with other methods of augmentation such as with block grafts or ridge split techniques. In the cases of prolonged ridge atrophy affecting a complete segment of the jaws, the bone defects would often contain a single wall or two walls with a requirement for larger volumes of grafting. GBR alone will not provide a sufficient amount of bone augmentation. In these situations, it is advisable to augment using block grafting, and in addition use particulate bone graft around the blocks and protect the augmented particulate material with a membrane. Implant placement can then be carried out after a period of around 6 months.

### 19.7.5 GBR for Contour Augmentation

One successful method of placing implants is following 4–8 weeks of healing. In this situation, in contrast to immediate implant placement, soft tissue healing would have taken place, thereby permitting the clinician with better quality of soft tissues while placing implants. However, in this scenario, especially in the aesthetic zone, the resorption of the facial bone would produce crater-like bone defects. GBR can be done in these situations, to over correct the lost facial bone as well as provide bulk to the region of implant placement. This procedure is also called 'contour augmentation' [23]. By doing this procedure, the buccal bone wall is intentionally overbulked so as to provide long-term stable aesthetic results as shown by multiple studies [24].

## 19.8 Onlay Bone Grafting

Onlay bone grafting is a predictable procedure carried out for the correction of cases with severe ridge resorption, either horizontally or vertically [25]. Autogenous bone grafts are the most documented and commonly used donor bone, although recently other allogenic and xenogenic materials are being clinically investigated. For augmentation of severe ridge defects (less than 2 walls and require more than 3 mm of augmentation), augmentation utilising autogenous bone blocks results in increased success rates as compared to guided bone regeneration alone. However, irrespective of the augmentation technique, vertical-ridge augmentation is less predictable as compared to horizontal-ridge augmentation [26].

Donor sites for autogenous onlay bone augmentation may be intra-oral or extra-oral. Most common intra-oral donor sites are the mandibular symphysis and the ramus of the mandible. Most common extra-oral donor sites for harvesting non-vascularised bone grafts are the iliac crest, the calvarium and the tibial bone. Most common vascularised bone containing free flap donor sites are the free fibula flap, the DCIA-free flap and scapula-free flap.

Once the bone graft is harvested, they should be trimmed and shaped to fit into the recipient site defect, stabilisation with osteosynthesis screws followed by adequate soft tissue mobilisation and tension-free primary closure of the grafted site. It is advisable to over-augment the defect in order to compensate for the eventual resorption. A mixture of particulate bone, slow-resorbing xenografts either alone or in combination is used to fill up the area between a corticocancellous block and the recipient site. The augmented material may be protected with a barrier membrane prior to being enveloped by the soft-tissue closure.

### 19.8.1 Harvesting Bone from the Donor Site

#### 19.8.1.1 Mandibular Ramus as the Donor Site

The outer cortical plate of the ascending ramus of the mandible is a popular choice for the harvest of intra-oral bone. This is probably because many oral and maxillofacial surgeons are well accustomed to the approach to the ramus during routine mandibular third molar surgeries or routine orthognathic surgeries. (Fig. 19.6a, b, c shows harvest of bone from the mandibular ramus).

The incision starts with a crevicular incision around the last standing molar teeth and continues along the ridge curving buccally upwards along the external oblique ridge. After elevation of the mucoperiosteal flap, and gaining adequate access to the anterior and lateral border of the ascending ramus of the mandible and the angle region, bone harvesting can begin. Usually, a block graft of approximately 30 mm × 15 mm can be harvested. The block thickness depends on the thickness of the lateral cortical bone plate of the ascending ramus and can vary from about 3 to 4 mm. The outline of the graft is usually made with two parallel anterior and posterior osteotomy cuts of about 3 mm in depth, on the lateral surface of the ramus of the mandible till the cortical bone is penetrated completely. Round bur points can also be made outlining the bone graft prior to making parallel cuts. Use of piezosurgery is advantageous in the cases of bone grafting. The two horizontal osteotomies are then joined by the sagittal bone cut superiorly. This cut corresponds to the thickness of the cortical bone. Once the sagittal bone cut is complete, the bone graft can be gently fractured and mobilised by the introduction of an osteotome or a periosteal elevator. Some surgeons prefer to make a cortical cut at the inferior end of the bone block prior to introducing the periosteal elevator to prevent unfavourable fractures of the block graft. After bone harvest, the surgical area is irrigated well and a haemostatic agent is applied if necessary and the wound is closed in layers. Some surgeons prefer to insert a glove drain that will be removed after 3 days.

#### 19.8.1.2 Chin (Anterior Mandible) as the Donor Site

The chin is also a popular donor site, predominantly because of the ease of access to the donor site. However, block grafts from the chin have shown an increased risk towards complications, especially neurosensory and vascularity disturbances to the mandibular incisors. Bone grafts of 50 mm in length and about 8 mm of width can be harvested. The cortical portion of the anterior mandible is thicker (around 3–11 mm) and hence the chin would provide a thicker area of bone and would be a choice for thick bone grafts. It is also popular to harvest bone grafts from the chin using trephine

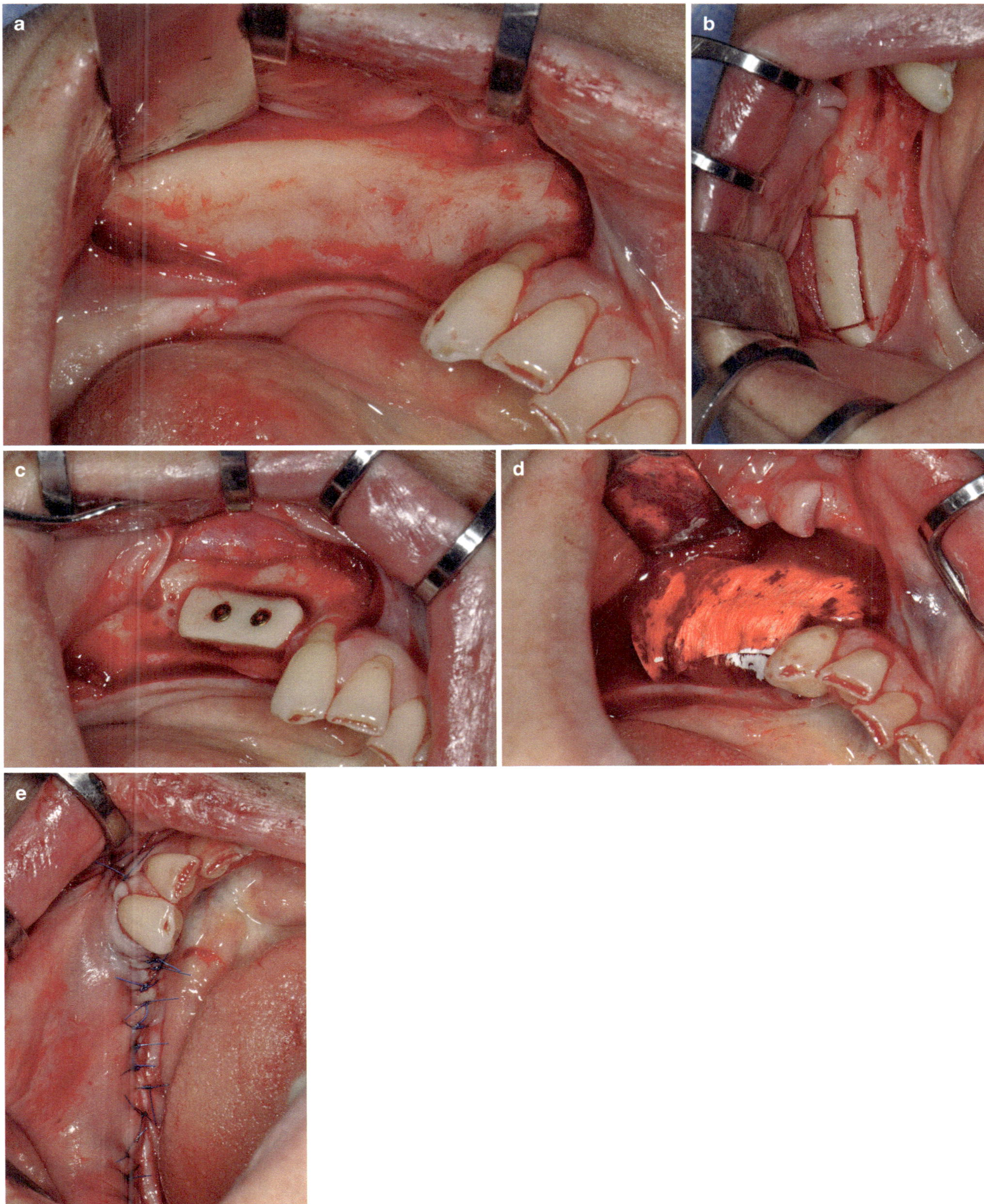




**Fig. 19.6** Shows harvest of bone from the mandibular ramus. (Picture courtesy PD Dr.med.dent. Simone Janner, Department of Oral Surgery and Stomatology, University of Bern, Switzerland). (**a**) Incision for access to ascending ramus. (**b**) Outline of the osteotomy. (**c**) Graft fixed at recipient site. (**d**) Coverage with membrane following additional particulate augmentation. (**e**) Closure

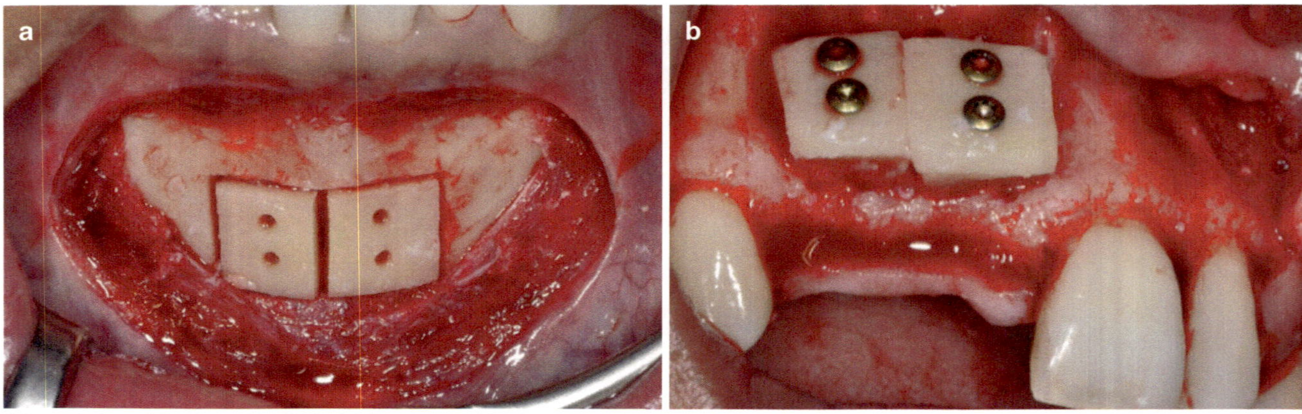




**Fig. 19.7** (**a**, **b**) Shows harvest of bone from mandibular symphysis. (Picture courtesy PD Dr.med.dent. Simone Janner, Department of Oral Surgery and Stomatology, University of Bern, Switzerland). (**a**) Harvest of bone from symphysis. (**b**) Graft secured at recipient site

burs of varying diameters (7–12 mm), and using upto 4 trephine harvests. (Fig. 19.7a and b shows harvest of bone from mandibular symphysis).

The access to the chin is by a standard vestibular incision from one canine to another with approximately 15 mm away from the mucogingival margin. Once the mucosa is incised, the underlying mentalis muscle is seen, which is incised obliquely to reach the symphysis of the mandible. Full thickness flap is elevated and the donor site inspected. For harvesting larger grafts, it is advisable to expose both the mental foraminae. Once the donor site is exposed as per the requirement, the boundaries of bone harvesting are carefully noted. An intact area of 5 mm must be preserved inferior to the root ends of the anterior teeth and 5 mm above the lower border of the mandible. Bone graft can be outlined within these borders, either using piezo surgical device or round burs or fissure burs or most popularly, trephine burs. After the outline of the bone graft is made, osteotomy of the cortical portion is done and connected. An osteotome or a periosteal elevator is then gently introduced to tease out the graft.

After harvesting of the bone graft, haemostasis is achieved and the wound closed in layers. It is important to close the periosteal layer and approximate the mentalis muscle prior to mucosal closure. A compressive chin dressing is provided to apply pressure to the donor-site region.

#### 19.8.1.3 Iliac Crest as the Donor Site

Iliac bone provides a large quantity of bone and is the preferred donor site for large bone augmentation as it is an excellent source for cortical and cancellous as well as corticocancellous bone. Both the anterior and posterior iliac crest can be used as a donor site. Anterior iliac crest grafts are associated with higher complication rates of sensory disturbances, gait problems and untoward ilium fracture. Posterior crest grafts are associated with lesser complications but increased post-operative pain. Additionally, posterior crest grafts require the patient to be repositioned and hence many surgeons prefer the anterior iliac crest. (Fig. 19.8a, b, c shows a case of harvest of bone from iliac crest).

The harvest of bone from the anterior iliac crest is generally performed with the patient under general anaesthesia. The patient is positioned supine and the side of the pelvis to be operated on is raised by placing surgical towels or sandbag towels underneath the hip. The skin over the crest is made taut by placing a fist above the iliac crest and only pushing the abdominal wall medially. The skin incision is made generally about 2 cm larger than the intended length of the bone harvest, running parallel to the iliac crest, so that after relaxation of the taut skin, it lies lateral to the iliac crest thereby avoiding mechanical irritation of the scar. After skin is incised, blunt dissection of the subcutaneous tissue is made until the periosteum of the iliac crest is seen. Bleeding should be controlled during dissection. The periosteum of the iliac crest is incised and the periosteal layer with the attached muscle is elevated and reflected medially. The iliac fossa is dissected to the desired depth. Care should be taken to avoid injury to the lateral femoral cutaneous nerve. Bone can be harvested using an oscillating saw or a piezosurgical device as per the preference of the surgeon by splitting the outer cortex of the iliac crest and transverse bone cuts. The two transverse cuts are then joined by a cortical osteotomy at the inner table paralleling the crestal cut. An osteotome is used to gently fracture the bone graft. This results in a cortico cancellous bone graft. Additional cancellous bone

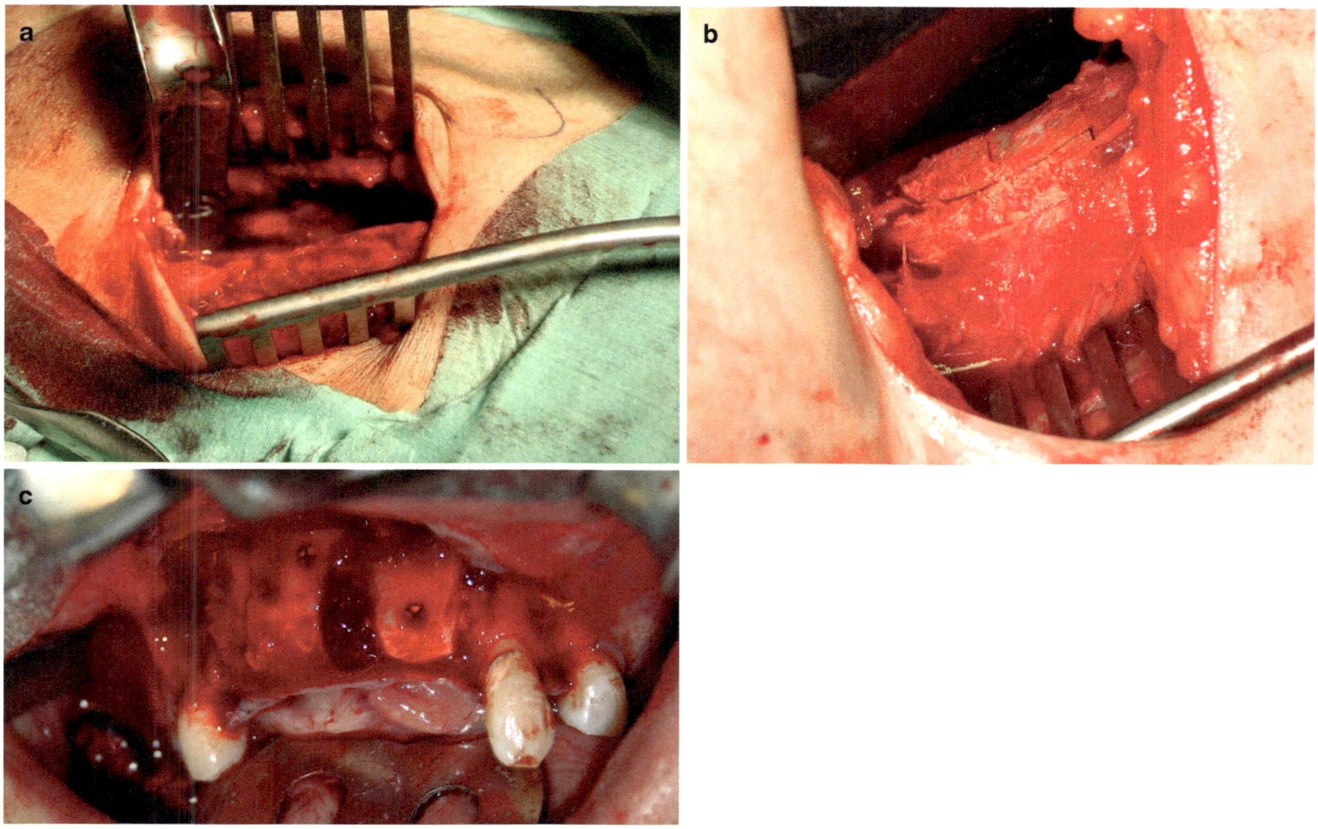



**Fig. 19.8** (**a**, **b**, **c**) Shows a case of harvest of bone from iliac crest used to augment anterior maxilla. (**a**) Shows the exposure of the anterior iliac crest for bone harvesting. (**b**) Shows the osteotomy of iliac crest for harvest of bone. (**c**) Shows the harvested bone fixed at recipient site

can be taken with a large curette if needed. The wound is meticulously closed in layers and a pressure dressing is applied.

#### 19.8.1.4 Calvarium as a Donor Site

Calvarium is a good source of cortical bone graft due to its high density and is opined by some surgeons as being the most resistant to resorption [27]. The location of the donor site is at the parietal bone lateral to the sagittal suture. The bone has distinct outer and inner table at this region separated by a diploic layer. A typical situation where calvarial bone grafts are harvested is in the cases of residual deformities following trauma, where a bicoronal flap and exposure of the parietal bone are already planned. (Fig. 19.9a, b, c shows a case of calvarial bone harvest used for bone augmentation of the anterior mandible).

The harvest is performed under general anaesthesia and the parietal bone exposed as part of the bicoronal flap. The outline of the bone graft is first made with round burs and then joined with straight fissure burs. The outline of the graft is broadened to permit placement of a chisel that would fracture the outer cortical plate at the diploic space. Haemostasis is achieved and the wound is closed.

### 19.8.2 Recipient Site Preparation and Completion of the Procedure

The preparation of the recipient site is done by a crestal incision with adequate releasing incisions as required. The surface of the bone is cleared of soft tissue and the cortical bone plate of the recipient site is perforated with a small round bur to produce bleeding and gain access to the cancellous part of the recipient bone. The harvested bone is then placed onto the recipient site and fixed with osteosynthesis screws. Some surgeons prefer to use lag screws for additional compression. The spaces between the block graft and recipient bone can be filled with particulate bone, especially at the borders. A resorbable membrane may be used to cover the augmentation. Adequate soft tissue release must be performed prior to

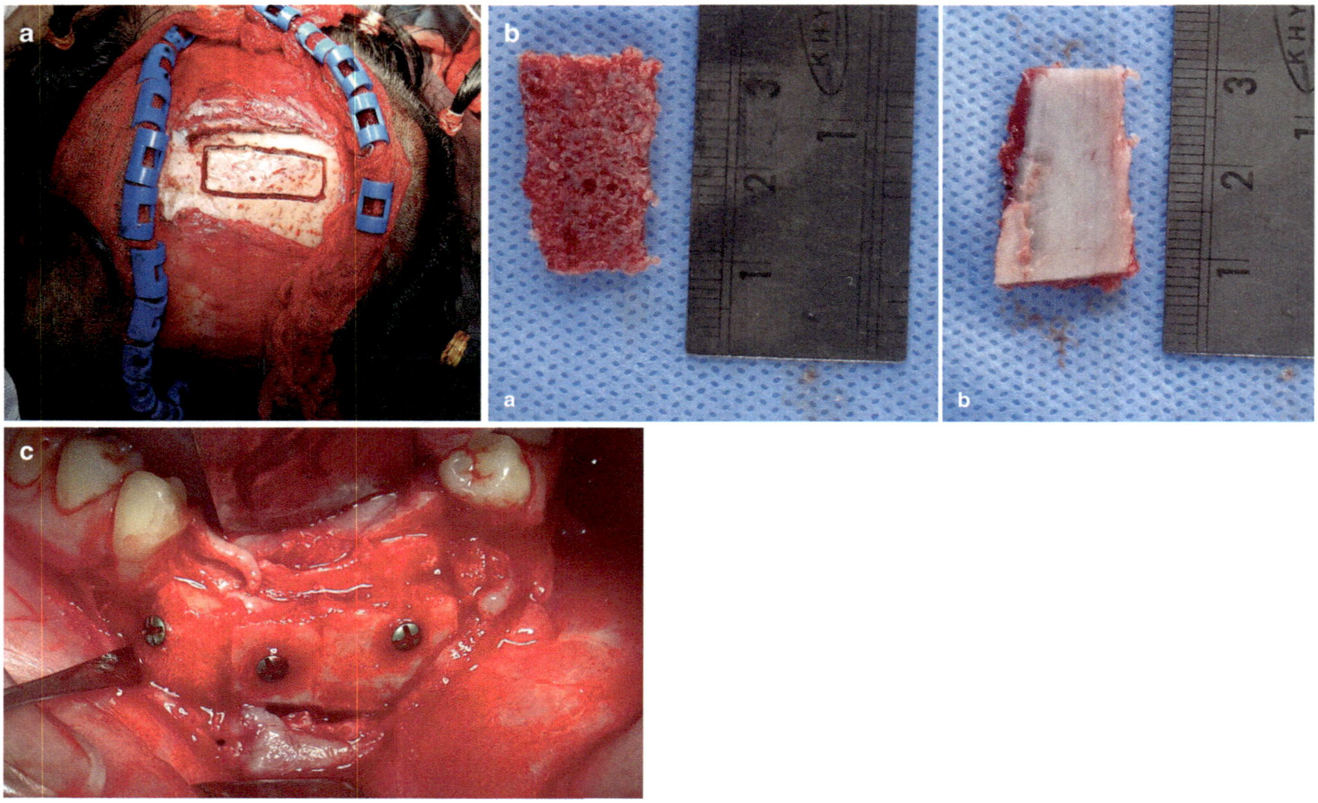



**Fig. 19.9** (**a**, **b**, **c**) shows a case of calvarial bone harvest used for bone augmentation of the anterior mandible. (**a**) Shows the exposure of the donor site with the outline of bone to be harvested. (**ba**) Shows the cancellous side of the harvested bone. (**bb**) Shows the cortical side of the harvested bone. (**c**) Shows the harvested bone further shaped and fixed at the recipient site

closure, so as to provide a tension-free watertight closure. Onlay grafts are usually left to heal for at least 6 months, after which implant placement can be carried out as another surgical procedure.

Another variation of onlay bone grafting is to use the cortical shell technique, where a thin cortical shell of bone is harvested and cancellous bone marrow placed in between the cortical shell and the recipient bone wall.

Other methods of bone augmentation include ridge split for lateral augmentation, alveolar distraction osteogenesis for vertical augmentation, interpositional bone grafting and free flap reconstruction of extremely resorbed ridges [28, 29]. These procedures will not be described in detail as they are not the most commonly carried out procedures.

## 19.9 Sinus Floor Elevation

Sinus floor elevation, also known as sinus augmentation or sinus lift is a bone-augmentation procedure to gain an increased bone volume to support in the maxillary sinus following sinus pneumatisation. The bone augmentation is done to provide an adequate quantity of bone that would permit dental rehabilitation with implants.

Maxillary sinus floor elevation can be performed by either as a transcrestal technique (also known as indirect sinus floor elevation) or a lateral window technique (also known as direct sinus floor elevation).

Irrespective of the individual techniques, the principle is to elevate the Schneiderian membrane and to create space for bone to fill up between the elevated Schneiderian membrane and residual maxillary bone. Although most clinician commonly use bone grafts to fill the space between the membrane and the floor, it has also been shown that bone fill occurs irrespective of using a bone substitute or leaving the elevated area to be occupied by a blood clot that eventually forms bone [30–32]. (Fig. 19.10a, b, c, d shows a clinical case of sinus floor elevation with blood clot and no additional biomaterial).

The maxillary sinus is a pyramidal-shaped cavity in the posterior region of each of the maxillary bones. The base of this pyramid is the lateral nasal wall and the tip of the pyramid is within the zygomatic buttress. The infraorbital floor, the posterior maxillary wall and the alveolar process form the walls of the pyramid. The maxillary sinus communicates

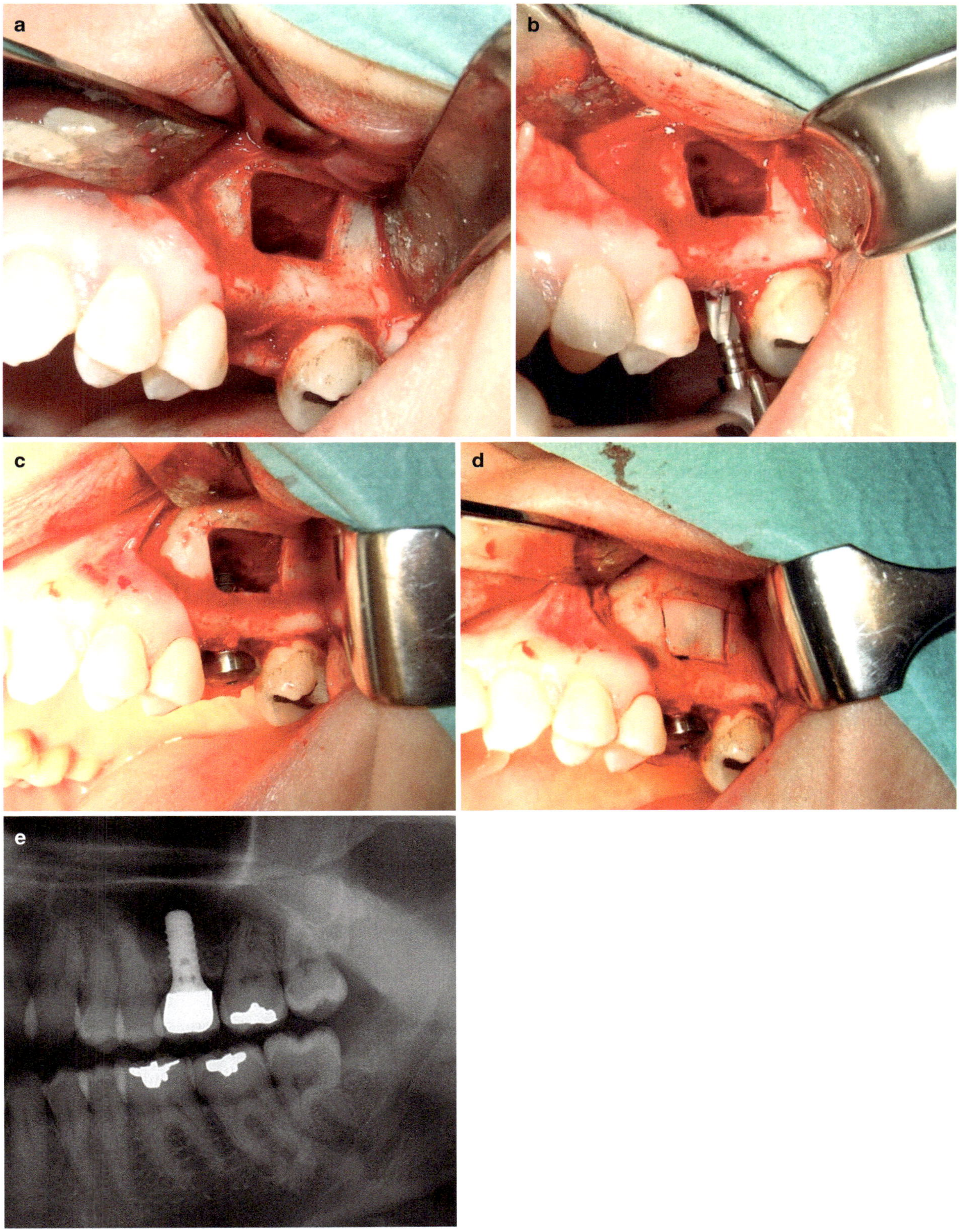



**Fig. 19.10** (**a**, **b**, **c**, **d**, **e**) shows a clinical case of sinus floor elevation with blood clot and no additional biomaterial. (**a**) Preparation of lateral window and elevation of the sinus membrane. (**b**) Implant osteotomy taking care to protect the membrane. (**c**) Implant placed (note the space between the implant and membrane that will eventually fill with blood clot). (**d**) Closure of the lateral window. (**e**) Long-term follow-up radiograph showing successful implant placement and restoration

to the lateral nasal wall through the semilunar hiatus at the posterosuperior aspect below the medial nasal concha. At birth, the maxillary sinus is very small and underdeveloped. As the permanent teeth begin to erupt, the maxillary sinus increases in size and continues to grow along with age. The sinus floor (the alveolar bone) is concave in shape with the lowest dip corresponding to the maxillary molar region. However, after the loss of maxillary posterior teeth, the sinus usually dips into this region. Over a period of time due to the increasing pneumatisation of the sinus, the sinus may surround the roots of the maxillary posterior teeth. In the case of the loss of maxillary posterior teeth, the maxillary sinus expands thinning the floor of the alveolar process that may result in a thin shell of bone. In many situations, this expansion of the maxillary sinus leaves an inadequate amount of bone to support successful implant placement. In these situations, maxillary sinus floor elevation is the procedure of choice to augment bone. However, it is also important to bear in mind that alveolar bone resorption may give rise to vertical and horizontal deficiencies in the posterior maxillary sinus. In prolonged cases, this might give rise to a situation where along with sinus floor elevation, it would also be necessary to augment bone both horizontally and vertically by onlay bone augmentation.

The morphology of the maxillary sinus floor can vary. Maxillary sinus floors are often irregular corresponding to the elevations and depressions of the teeth roots. The floor of the sinus also may be divided by septae. Some maxillary floors are broad and flat whereas others may be irregular and narrow. The lateral wall of the maxillary sinus can also vary in thickness, from being paper thin to being about 3 mm in thickness. The thicker the lateral wall, the more difficult would be the lateral sinus floor-augmentation procedure.

The blood supply of the maxillary sinus arises from the branches of the maxillary artery namely: the posterosuperior alveolar artery and the greater palatine artery as well as the infraorbital artery. Care must be taken to look out for the posterosuperior alveolar artery that may be encountered while preparation of the lateral sinus floor augmentation, although it is unlikely to cause excessive bleeding.

As required for all surgical procedures, a thorough preoperative assessment must be carried out prior to sinus floor elevation. Acute sinusitis, oro-antral communications, chronic periodontitis and poor oral hygiene pose a high risk for sinus floor elevation. Moderate risk factors include smoking, chronic sinusitis and extremely poor bone density, amongst others.

### 19.9.1 Classification and Treatment Options for the Posterior Edentulous Maxilla

According to the International Team for Implantology, the edentulous posterior maxilla can be classified into 4 types [11]:

Group 1: where there is an insufficient sub-antral bone height to place implants, however with an adequate width of the alveolar ridge with acceptable vertical and horizontal interarch relations. These cases can be treated with a sinus floor elevation procedure alone.

Group 2: where there is an insufficient subantral bone height, and an inadequate width of the alveolar ridge with acceptable vertical interarch relation. In these cases, sinus floor elevation should be performed along with horizontal-bone augmentation.

Group 3: where there exists an insufficient subantral bone height, and an adequate width of alveolar ridge with acceptable horizontal interarch relations but with unfavourable vertical interarch relationship. In these cases, sinus floor augmentation should be performed along with vertical-ridge augmentation.

Group 4: There exists insufficient subantral bone height, and unfavourable interarch relations in addition to advanced horizontal and vertical crestal resorption. These cases must be treated with sinus floor elevation along with horizontal and vertical-ridge augmentation.

Misch 1987 [33] classified the edentulous posterior maxilla based on the amount of subantral bone available into:

SA1: more than 12 mm of the subantral bone height.
SA2: 0–2 mm less than the ideal bone height (10–12 mm).
SA3: 5–10 mm of the subantral bone height.
SA4: less than 5 mm subantral bone height.

### 19.9.2 Decision-Making: Lateral Versus Transcrestal Technique

Transcrestal technique avoids the use of a large surgical flap and an osteotomy for a lateral window and hence is much reduced in invasiveness and decreased post-operative morbidity to the patient. However, the transcrestal technique can predictively increase bone height to about 4–5 mm and, therefore, cannot be used for severely atrophic cases. Additionally, in situations where the sinus floor is not uniform (or at oblique angles), there is an increased tendency to perforate the sinus mucosa. In such cases, it is preferable to perform lateral sinus floor elevation. It must be remembered that the transcrestal technique is in essence a blind procedure and it is not possible to inspect the sinus mucosa for perforations or pathologies using this technique, hence in the cases of intra-operative perforation, a lateral sinus floor elevation procedure must be performed. Hence, it is wise to always obtain a consent for the lateral technique prior to undertaking the transcrestal procedure.

### 19.9.3 Decision-Making: Simultaneous Versus Staged Approach

The prerequisite of simultaneous implant placement is the possibility to obtain sufficient primary implant stability [33, 34]. In cases where primary implant stability cannot be obtained, implants should be placed at a second surgical procedure 2–6 months following sinus floor elevation. Decreased residual bone volume and poor bone density are factors that predispose towards poor primary implant stability. Traditionally, less than 5 mm was considered as the minimum amount of sub-antral bone height required for simultaneous implant placement. This has. However. been challenged and many recent studies have shown sufficient primary stability in cases with lesser sub-antral bone height. Implant stability has been achieved in these cases by using a tapered implant design, implants with engaging threads, by using the underdimensional drilling protocol and by using bone-condensing drills. Conventionally, it is understood that while undertaking a transcrestal procedure, implants would be placed simultaneously.

*Armamentarium* for sinus floor elevation consists in addition to the regular minor surgical kit and the implant kit, hand and rotary instruments that are specifically designed for sinus floor elevation. Many companies have introduced kits specifically for this procedure. Some surgeons prefer the use of piezosurgery for access to the lateral window. Additionally, implant companies have also introduced specific burs and elevation kits that reportedly make sinus floor elevation easier to perform. It is ultimately the preference of the surgeon in choosing the armamentarium.

### 19.9.4 Transcrestal Surgical Technique

After local anaesthesia, a crestal incision is made and the implant osteotomy is performed according to the instructions of the respective implant manufacturer. The osteotomy is made 2 mm short of the sinus floor. A periapical radiograph can be taken to confirm this. After the depth has been defined, remainder of the implant preparation is done as per the respective manufacturers protocol. Following preparation of the implant bed of appropriate dimension (it is recommended to use an implant of at least 4.0 mm diameter till further evidence suggests otherwise), an osteotome is introduced into the implant bed and with the help of a mallet, gentle tapping is performed till the sinus floor is fractured. Care should be taken that the osteotome does not perforate the sinus mucosa and enter the sinus cavity. Once the sinus floor has been fractured, a part of the membrane can be visualised to be intact. A careful Valsalva procedure can also be performed to test the patency of the sinus floor. An appropriate graft material is introduced through the implant preparation onto the sinus mucosa. Incremental introduction of the graft material is done, which will push the sinus membrane upwards creating a space between the sub-antral bone and the sinus mucosa. After introducing the appropriate amount of graft material, an implant is inserted to the desired three-dimensional position. Following implant installation, the crestal incision is closed with either a transmucosal or submerged healing protocol. Implant loading is done as per the instructions of the manufacturer, generally within 3 month time. (Fig. 19.11a, b, c, d shows a digrammatic representation of transcrestal sinus floor elevation).

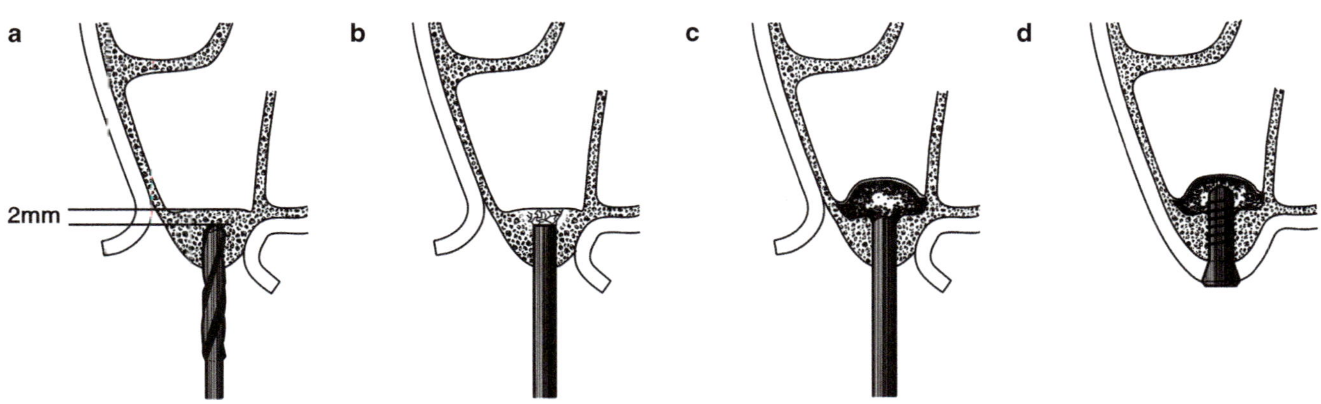




**Fig. 19.11** (**a**, **b**, **c**, **d**) shows a diagrammatic representation of transcrestal sinus floor elevation. (**a**) Implant osteotomy made 2 mm short of the sinus floor. (**b**) Osteotome introduced through the implant osteotomy to fracture the sinus floor. (**c**) Biomaterial introduced to elevate the sinus membrane. (**d**) Implant placement completed

A periapical radiograph must be taken at the end of the procedure to confirm no breach of the sinus floor. A well-circumscribed dome-shaped elevation around the apex of the implant confirms no breach of the sinus membrane. In contrast, if the bone graft is seen around the sinus floor and poorly localised, it denotes a perforation of the sinus floor membrane and in this case, a lateral window approach should be immediately done to clean the sinus cavity.

### 19.9.5 Lateral Window Technique

The lateral window technique can be done alongside lateral and vertical augmentation of the ridge, and with or without simultaneous implant placement. After adequate local anaesthesia, a crestal incision is made with releasing incisions well away from the planned window. A mucoperiosteal flap is elevated and the lateral wall of the maxillary sinus is exposed. A bony window is made according to the local bone anatomy. If vertical septae are present, two bony windows are made on either side of the bony septae. The bony window should be large enough to introduce the graft materials, as well as big enough to permit exploration of the floor, the anteroposterior aspect of the floor to the medial aspect of the maxillary sinus. When the lateral window is made, care should be taken to avoid perforation of the sinus membrane. The lateral window can either be removed from the underlying sinus mucosa or be attached to the to it and pushed inwards. The sinus floor is then slowly teased and reflected away from the floor of the maxillary sinus and elevated using special instruments that resemble a curette to create space for the graft material. It is important to elevate the membrane medially and anteriorly in the areas where augmentation is planned.

(Fig. 19.12a, b, c, d shows diagrammatic representation of the procedure for sinus floor elevation using a lateral window).

If simultaneous implant placement is planned, implant osteotomies should be carried out with the elevated mucosa well protected with an instrument in such a way that the implant drills do not come in contact with the sinus mucosa. Bone graft material is now introduced into the space created by elevation of the membrane. After adequate filling of the space with augmentation material, implants can be placed if planned. The lateral window bone wall (if preserved) can be replaced, or the window can be covered with a barrier membrane. The mucoperiosteal flap is then closed and tension-free suturing should be placed.

Although, bone graft materials and membranes are commonly used it is not mandatory for the success of sinus floor elevation. Some suggest, elevation of the sinus mucosa and placement of the implant that tents the membrane up, the blood clot that is formed into the space eventually forms bone to surround the implant.

### 19.9.6 Complications Following Sinus Floor Elevation

Sinus perforation is the most common complication following sinus floor elevation. Other complications include (but not limited to) poor primary implant stability, implant migration into the sinus, graft migration into the sinus and intra-operative and post-operative bleeding, wound dehiscence and infection.

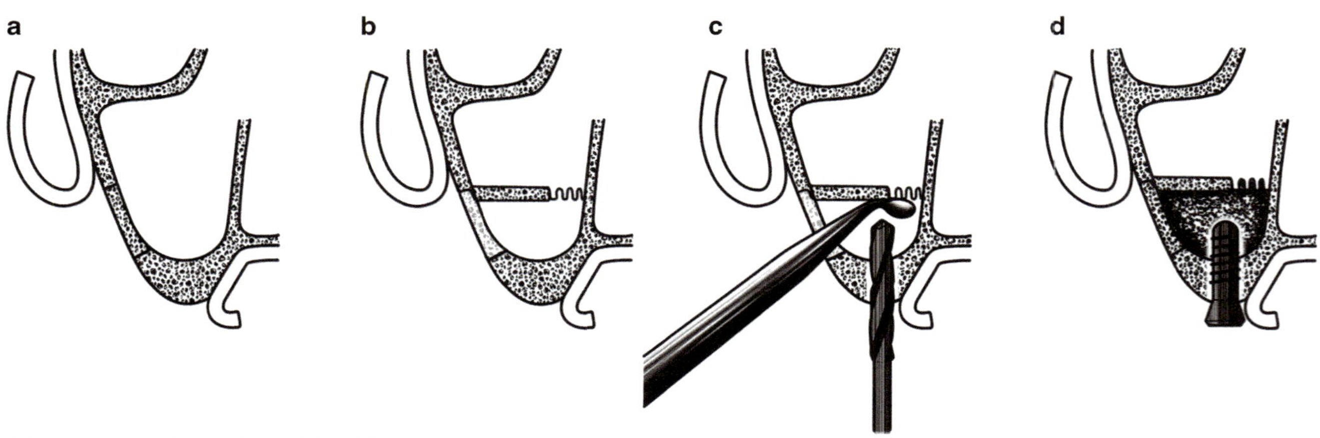




Fig. 19.12 (**a**, **b**, **c**, **d** shows diagrammatic representation of the procedure for sinus floor elevation using a lateral window). (**a**) Mucoperiosteal flap elevated to access the lateral wall of the maxillary sinus. (**b**) Lateral wall bony window made and in-fractured. (**c**) Implant osteotomy done. (**d**) Placement of biomaterial and implant

Alternatives to sinus floor elevation: The use of short implants [35], angled or tilted implants [3], zygomatic or pterygoid implants [36] are treatment alternatives that may avoid the need for maxillary sinus floor elevation.

## 19.10 Suggested Reading

ITI Treatment guides Volume 5: Sinus floor elevation
ITI Treatment guide Volume 7
ITI Treatment guide series Volume 1–10
ITI Online Academy
Contemporary implant dentistry: Carl Misch

## References


1. Chappuis V, Rahman L, Buser R, Janner SFM, Belser UC, Buser D. Effectiveness of contour augmentation with guided bone regeneration: 10-year results. J Dent Res. 2018;97(3):266–74.
2. Chappuis V, Araujo MG, Buser D. Clinical relevance of dimensional bone and soft tissue alterations post-extraction in esthetic sites. Periodontol 2000. 2017;73(1):73–83.
3. Toljanic JA, Ekstrand K, Baer RA, Thor A. Immediate loading of implants in the edentulous maxilla with a fixed provisional restoration without bone augmentation: a report on 5-year outcomes data obtained from a prospective clinical trial. Int J Oral Maxillofac Implants. 2016;31(5):1164–70.
4. Trbakovic A, Bongenhielm U, Thor A. A clinical and radiological long-term follow-up study of narrow diameter implants in the aesthetic area. Clin Implant Dent Relat Res. 2018;20(4):598–605.
5. Cawood JI, Howell RA. A classification of the edentulous jaws. Int J Oral Maxillofac Surg. 1988;17(4):232–6.
6. Lekholm U, Zarb GA. Patient selection and preparation. In: Branemark PIZG, Albrektsson T, editors. Tissue integrated prosthesis: osseointegration in clinical dentistry. Chicago IL: Quintessence; 1985. p. 199–209.
7. Kumar VV, Sagheb K, Klein MO, Al-Nawas B, Kann PH, Kammerer PW. Relation between bone quality values from ultrasound transmission velocity and implant stability parameters--an ex vivo study. Clin Oral Implants Res. 2012;23(8):975–80.
8. Lindhe J, Bressan E, Cecchinato D, Corra E, Toia M, Liljenberg B. Bone tissue in different parts of the edentulous maxilla and mandible. Clin Oral Implants Res. 2013;24(4):372–7.
9. Mackiewicz Z, Niklinska WE, Kowalewska J, Chyczewski L. Bone as a source of organism vitality and regeneration. Folia Histochem Cytobiol. 2011;49(4):558–69.
10. Jensen SS, Terheyden H. Bone augmentation procedures in localized defects in the alveolar ridge: clinical results with different bone grafts and bone-substitute materials. Int J Oral Maxillofac Implants. 2009;24(Suppl):218–36.
11. Katsuyama H, Jensen SS. Treatment options for sinus floor elevation. In: Chen S, Buser D, Wismeijer D, editors. ITI treatment guide sinus floor elevation procedures. ITI treatment guide. Berlin: Quintessence Publishing; 2011. p. 34–59.
12. Kumar VV, Jacob PC, Ebenezer S, Kuriakose MA, Kekatpure V, Baliarsing AS, et al. Implant supported dental rehabilitation following segmental mandibular reconstruction- quality of life outcomes of a prospective randomized trial. J Craniomaxillofac Surg. 2016;44(7):800–10.
13. Kumar VV, Ebenezer S, Kammerer PW, Jacob PC, Kuriakose MA, Hedne N, et al. Implants in free fibula flap supporting dental rehabilitation – implant and peri-implant related outcomes of a randomized clinical trial. J Craniomaxillofac Surg. 2016;44(11):1849–58.
14. Bosshardt D, Schenk RK. Bone regeneration: biologic basis. In: Buser D, editor. 20 Years of guided bone regeneration in implant dentistry. 2nd ed. Chicago, IL: Quintessenz; 2009. p. 15–45.
15. Caballe-Serrano J, Munar-Frau A, Ortiz-Puigpelat O, Soto-Penaloza D, Penarrocha M, Hernandez-Alfaro F. On the search of the ideal barrier membrane for guided bone regeneration. J Clin Exp Dent. 2018;10(5):e477–e83.
16. Caballe-Serrano J, Munar-Frau A, Delgado L, Perez R, Hernandez-Alfaro F. Physicochemical characterization of barrier membranes for bone regeneration. J Mech Behav Biomed Mater. 2019;97:13–20.
17. Gruber R, Stadlinger B, Terheyden H. Cell-to-cell communication in guided bone regeneration: molecular and cellular mechanisms. Clin Oral Implants Res. 2017;28(9):1139–46.
18. Caballe-Serrano J, Abdeslam-Mohamed Y, Munar-Frau A, Fujioka-Kobayashi M, Hernandez-Alfaro F, Miron R. Adsorption and release kinetics of growth factors on barrier membranes for guided tissue/bone regeneration: a systematic review. Arch Oral Biol. 2019;100:57–68.
19. Maestre-Ferrin L, Boronat-Lopez A, Penarrocha-Diago M, Penarrocha-Diago M. Augmentation procedures for deficient edentulous ridges, using onlay autologous grafts: an update. Med Oral Patol Oral Cir Bucal. 2009;14(8):e402–7.
20. Nyman S. Bone regeneration using the principle of guided tissue regeneration. J Clin Periodontol. 1991;18(6):494–8.
21. Dahlin C, Linde A, Gottlow J, Nyman S. Healing of bone defects by guided tissue regeneration. Plast Reconstr Surg. 1988;81(5):672–6.
22. Urban IA, Monje A. Guided bone regeneration in alveolar bone reconstruction. Oral Maxillofac Surg Clin North Am. 2019;31(2):331–8.
23. Buser D, Chappuis V, Kuchler U, Bornstein MM, Wittneben JG, Buser R, et al. Long-term stability of early implant placement with contour augmentation. J Dent Res. 2013;92(12 Suppl):176S–82S.
24. Buser D, Chappuis V, Bornstein MM, Wittneben JG, Frei M, Belser UC. Long-term stability of contour augmentation with early implant placement following single tooth extraction in the esthetic zone: a prospective, cross-sectional study in 41 patients with a 5- to 9-year follow-up. J Periodontol. 2013;84(11):1517–27.
25. Thor A, Wannfors K, Sennerby L, Rasmusson L. Reconstruction of the severely resorbed maxilla with autogenous bone, platelet-rich plasma, and implants: 1-year results of a controlled prospective 5-year study. Clin Implant Dent Relat Res. 2005;7(4):209–20.
26. Dasmah A, Thor A, Ekestubbe A, Sennerby L, Rasmusson L. Marginal bone-level alterations at implants installed in block versus particulate onlay bone grafts mixed with platelet-rich plasma in atrophic maxilla. A prospective 5-year follow-up study of 15 patients. Clin Implant Dent Relat Res. 2013;15(1):7–14.
27. Smolka W. Calvarial grafts for alveolar ridge reconstruction prior to dental implant placement: an update. Oral Maxillofac Surg. 2014;18(4):381–5.
28. Chiapasco M, Casentini P, Zaniboni M. Bone augmentation procedures in implant dentistry. Int J Oral Maxillofac Implants. 2009;24(Suppl):237–59.
29. Milinkovic I, Cordaro L. Are there specific indications for the different alveolar bone augmentation procedures for implant placement? A systematic review. Int J Oral Maxillofac Surg. 2014;43(5):606–25.
30. Riben C, Thor A. Follow-up of the sinus membrane elevation technique for maxillary sinus implants without the use of graft material. Clin Implant Dent Relat Res. 2016;18(5):895–905.
31. Riben C, Thor A. The maxillary sinus membrane elevation procedure: augmentation of bone around dental implants without grafts-a review of a surgical technique. Int J Dent. 2012;2012:105483.

32. Duan DH, Fu JH, Qi W, Du Y, Pan J, Wang HL. Graft-free maxillary sinus floor elevation: a systematic review and meta-analysis. J Periodontol. 2017;88(6):550–64.
33. Misch CE. Contemporary implant dentistry. St. Louis: Mosby; 1987.
34. Stefanski S, Svensson B, Thor A. Implant survival following sinus membrane elevation without grafting and immediate implant installation with a one-stage technique: an up-to-40-month evaluation. Clin Oral Implants Res. 2017;28(11):1354–9.
35. Srinivasan M, Vazquez L, Rieder P, Moraguez O, Bernard JP, Belser UC. Survival rates of short (6 mm) micro-rough surface implants: a review of literature and meta-analysis. Clin Oral Implants Res. 2014;25(5):539–45.
36. Tuminelli FJ, Walter LR, Neugarten J, Bedrossian E. Immediate loading of zygomatic implants: a systematic review of implant survival, prosthesis survival and potential complications. Eur J Oral Implantol. 2017;10(Suppl 1):79–87.

# Part VIII

# Odontogenic Infections

# 20 Odontogenic Infections: General Principles

Anand Shukla and Divya Mehrotra

## 20.1 Introduction

Relationships like symbiosis, commensalism, ectoparasitism, and endoparasitism exist between various species in the biological world. An infection is a classic example of either ectoparasitism or endoparasitism. All infections occurring in the human body are usually of microbial origin and odontogenic infections are no exception.

This relationship is based on discordance in the delicate balance between the host defense mechanism and pathogenicity or the virulence of the infecting microbes depending upon their potentially harmful biomolecules viz. exotoxin, endotoxin, enzymes, and others that disrupt the host defense. Essentially, the environment also seems to play an important role in the overall pathogenic behavior of the microorganism. This interrelationship can be expressed by a simple triangle.

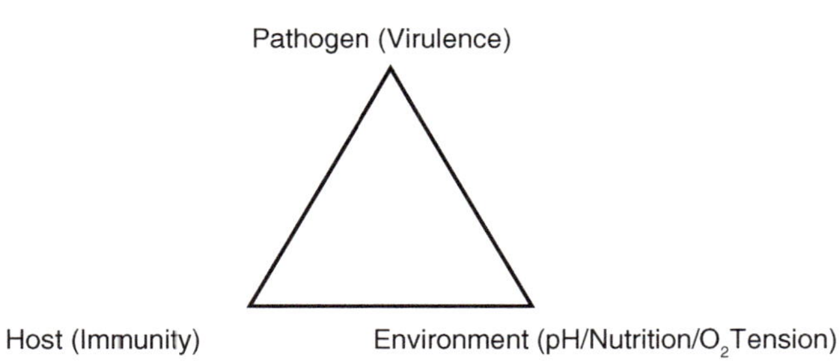


In short, when a low host resistance, pathogen-friendly environment, and a pathogen of high virulence are seen in states of physical being, we refer to as Infections

A. Shukla · D. Mehrotra (✉)
Department of Oral and Maxillofacial Surgery, King George's Medical University, Lucknow, India

## 20.2 Host Defense Mechanisms

As a generalization, host defense mechanisms may be studied as

1. Local.
2. Systemic

- Local Mechanisms:
  1. Oral Mucosa:

     The oral mucosa forms the first line of defense against the pathogens with an epithelialization rate of 4–5 days wherein the entire oral mucous membrane is replaced by newer more equipped cells take its place. The cells that are infected or otherwise worn out are replaced. As both the skin and oral mucosa are keratinized structures, water and along with it the microbes cannot naturally percolate into the deeper tissues. The oral mucosa is water resistant and relatively dry and does not form a congenial niche for microbial adherence and growth.
  2. Natural spillways:

     Human dentition has evolved to chew the food we eat. The surface anatomy of the occlusal surfaces is such that with a fibrous diet, the food automatically spills off the occlusal table into the labio-lingual vestibule. The interdental contacts are also evolved and provide natural spillways for masticated food.
  3. Dental Histology:

     The microscopic structures of our dentition reveal the hardest substance of the human body (the dental enamel) to cap its relatively softer structures (dentin and pulp). Thus, even if microbes are able to hold onto the enamel layer, the sheer density and mineralization of this layer are sufficient enough to handle most of the microbial attacks.


K. Bonanthaya et al. (eds.), *Oral and Maxillofacial Surgery for the Clinician*, https://doi.org/10.1007/978-981-15-1346-6_20

4. Saliva:

By virtue of evolution, the human race has been privileged with 3 pairs of major salivary glands and numerous minor salivary glands. Their secretions, on the one hand, keep the oral environment moist to avoid inadvertent trauma and, on the other hand, help transform the chewed food into a bolus to be swallowed. Salivary secretion continues throughout the awake state, so even if one is not eating, the salivary secretions flush out the food debris deposited on the hard and soft surfaces of the mouth, in conjunction with the movements of the muscular elements of oral region such as lips, cheek, tongue, etc. Other physiological properties of the human saliva such as pH (6.5–8.5) and the presence of immunoglobulins (IgG and IgA) makes saliva a biological bacteriostatic fluid.

5. Oral sub mucosal immune system (OSMIS):

A large number of immunocompetent cells, such as the mononuclear leukocytes, T cells, and B cells, are present between the oral mucous membrane and are responsible for the production of antibodies as well as offering a direct cellular immune response to the host and oral environment. The cell concentrations of IgG, IgA, and IgM may remarkably reach 85, 72, and 75%, respectively, with respect to plasma concentration, in the gingival sulcular fluid. However, generally only IgA levels are high in the oral mucosa, while the concentrations of IgG may rise dramatically during infectious states. Also, the true ponderance of mast cells in the submucosal layer and the presence of IgE explain the immediate hypersensitivity (type I) reaction. The role of these immunoglobulins is to neutralize the microbial toxins and maintain hemostasis in the oral environment.

6. Dentinal reparative mechanisms:

If the bacterial attack breaks the enamel barrier, the toxins reach the dentinal tubules and through them irritate the pulp. This may or may not be symptomatic but pulpal reaction is evident with the formation of reparative dentin to seal off the breach as part of the defense mechanism. When this occurs, we know it as arrested caries and the dentin so formed is the affected dentin. If due measures are not taken at this stage, an advanced carious lesion may result.

7. Waldayer's Ring:

The OSMIS, lingual tonsil, palatine tonsil, all other lymphoid structures in the naso-oropharyngeal region together make a ring-like primary defense mechanism against microbes in the oro-digestive tract and are constitutionally known as the Waldayer's ring.

- *Systemic Mechanisms*: Broadly speaking, the systemic host immunity may be classified as.
  1. Cellular.
  2. Humoral.

Both these immune systems may be either innate (natural) or acquired (adaptive). Majority of pathogens are dealt with by the innate component of the host systemic immunity. However, when the innate response is overwhelmed, the adaptive or active immunity comes into play.

Components of Innate Immunity:

- Physical barriers/skin/mucosa.
- Neutrophils.
- Macrophages.
- Dendritic cells.
- Natural killer cells.
- Lymphoid cells.
- Complement system.

Components of Acquired Immunity:

- B-lymphocytes.
- Dendritic cells.
- T-lymphocytes.
  - Helper.
  - Cytotoxic.
  - Regulatory.

Innate immunity is basically a receptor-pattern recognition mechanism, where about 100 intracellular and extracellular receptors (e.g., toll-like receptors, NOD-like receptors, KIG like receptors, etc.) recognize over 1000 different cell injury-related patterns generated from bacterial, viral, or fungal inflictions [1]. These receptors generate a response mediated by cytokines and antiviral interferon and stimulate the most proactive immune response.

Acquired immunity is of two types, viz. humoral immunity, mediated by soluble proteins known as antibodies (produced by B lymphocytes) and cell-mediated immunity effected by T lymphocytes (T cells). While antibodies provide protection against extracellular pathogens in blood, mucosa, and tissues, T lymphocytes work to defend against intracellular microbes to kill ingested microbes by production of soluble proteins mediators, the cytokines (produced by helper T cells).

## 20.3 The Infectious Microbes

The concept of an infectious agent was established by Robert Koch. Koch's postulates became the standard for defining infectious agents, but they do not apply to uncultivable organisms (e.g. M. leprae) or members of normal humoral flora (e.g. *E. coli*).

Koch's postulates:

1. The same organism must be present in every case of that disease but not in any healthy individual.
2. The organism must be isolated from the diseased individual and cultured.
3. The isolate must cause the disease, when inoculated in a healthy individual.
4. The organisms must be re-isolated from inoculated diseased individual.

Odontogenic infections arise within or around the dentition, initiating from simple dental caries, periodontal diseases, and pulpitis, and may spread way beyond their loco-regional origin, invading deeper structures of the face, oral cavity, head and neck, and even mediastinum or the vertebral column.

These infections are principally bacterial in nature Tables 20.1 and 20.2. These bacteria are a part of normal oral flora found in the dental plaque, mucosal surfaces, and the gingival sulcus. These primarily are aerobic gram positive cocci, anaerobic gram positive cocci, and gram negative rods [3].

**Table 20.1** Types of bacteria in periapical abscess [4]

| Types of bacterial infections | Percentage |
|---|---|
| Anaerobic only | 50% |
| Mixed anaerobsic and aerobic | 44% |
| Anaerobic only | 6% |

**Table 20.2** Common bacterial species in periapical abscess

| Endodontic | Periodontal [2] |
|---|---|
| 1. Anaerobic gram negative bacteria | (a) Aggregatibacter actinomycetemcomitans |
| (a) Treponema | (b) Treponema denticola |
| (b) Dialister | (c) Campylobacter rectus |
| (c) Porphyromonas | (d) Prevotella intermedia |
| 2. Facultative gram negative bacteria | (e) Tannerella forsythia |
| (a) Neisseria | (f) Porphyromonas gingivalis |
| (b) Capnocytophaga | |
| (c) Haemophilus | |
| 3. Anaerobic gram positive bacteria | |
| (a) Actinomycetes | |
| (b) Peptostreptococcus | |
| 4. Facultative gram positive | |
| (a) Enterococcus | |
| (b) Streptococcus | |

## 20.4 Pathways of Odontogenic Infection

Odontogenic infections have two major origins (Fig. 20.1).

(a) Periodontal- due to bacterial inoculations into underlying tissues via deep periodontal pockets and
(b) Periapical-, more common, and occur subsequent to pulpal necrosis, reaching the periapical structures (Fig. 20.2).

Once the periodontal or periapical tissues get inoculated with bacteria, the infection may spread equally in all directions but mostly follows the path of least resistance. It travels through the cancellous bone to reach the cortical plate. If the cortical plate is thin, infection easily perforates it to enter the surrounding soft tissue. Periapical enzymes that help the bacteria in doing so include collagenase, hyaluronidase, and streptokinase, which dissolve through the organic matrix of the bone, while the acids produced by the bacteria eliminate the mineral content.

At this stage, if an intervention such as an endodontic or periodontal procedure or dental extraction is done, the further spread may be arrested or even abolished with judicious antibiotics. Antimicrobials alone may not cure the condition as the focus of infection from necrotic pulp or periapical tissues still remains and may cause recurrence of the infection, if the therapy is stopped [5].

When left untreated, the infection continues to spread depending principally on the thickness of bone and the type of muscle attachment. For example, if maxillary anterior tooth gets involved in the periapical region and the inclination of the root is such that the apex is closer to the labial cortical plate, the soft tissue reaction would present as swelling on the labial side (Fig. 20.3a) and if the apex is closer to the palatal cortical plate, swelling would be palatal. (Fig. 20.3b). Similarly, in case of carious involvement of maxillary first molar: if the apices of the buccal roots lie above the attachment of the buccinator, swelling is likely to occur facially (Fig. 20.4a) and if apices are below, a vestibular swelling is more likely to occur (Figs. 20.4b and 20.5).

Apart from these factors, the angulation of root apex is also important. For example, in periapical abscess with respect to maxillary lateral incisor, swelling is likely to occur on the hard palate rather than labial vestibule as its root apex is slightly palato-distally curved. (Fig. 20.6).

Muscle attachment is another influencing factor. Supposing a mandibular second molar gets apically infected and the apices lie above the external oblique ridge, infection following the path of least resistance and assisted with gravity, may manifest as swelling in a more anterior region of the jaw, buccally than the relative position of the first mandibular molar. Similarly, in the mandibular posterior region, the lingual cortex is closer to the root apices and relatively thinner

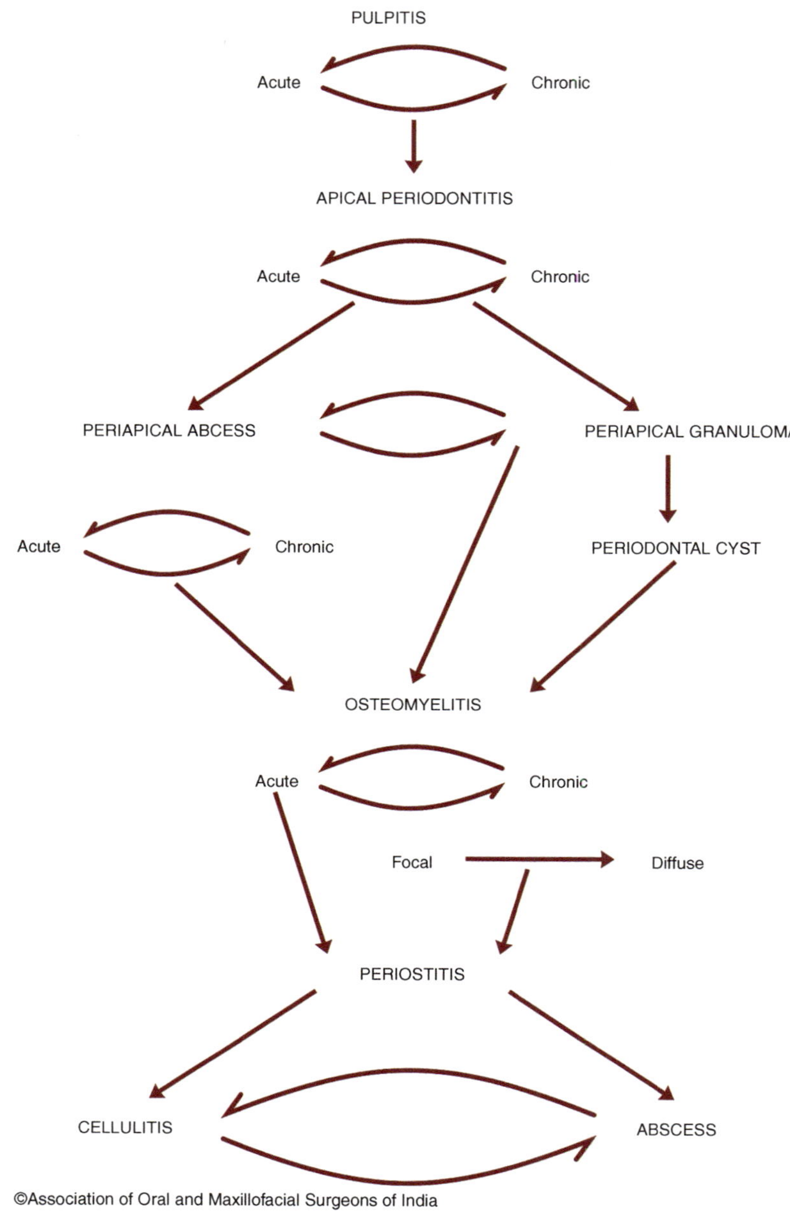


**Fig. 20.1** Natural progression of odontogenic infection

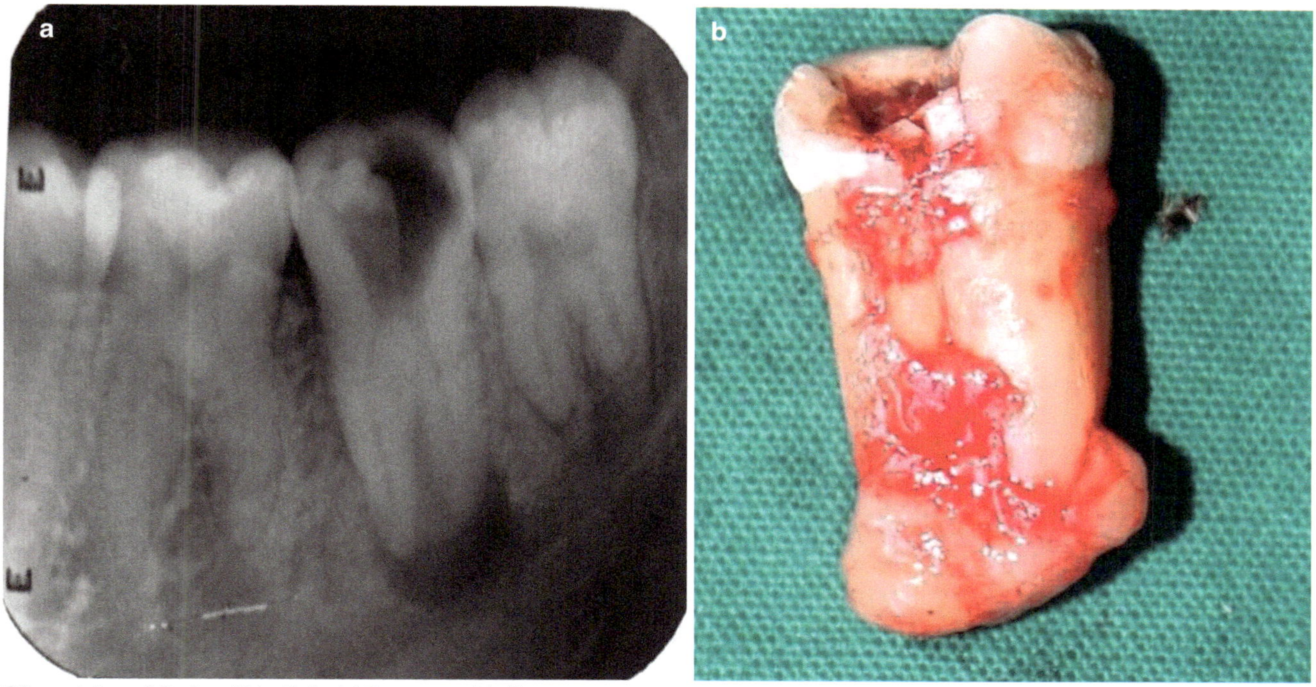




Fig. 20.2 (**a**, **b**) shows a lower left second molar with a periapical radiolucency. On extraction, the periapical granuloma can be seen attached to the root. If this tooth was not extracted, the infection would have progressed in any of the pathways as shown in Fig. 20.1

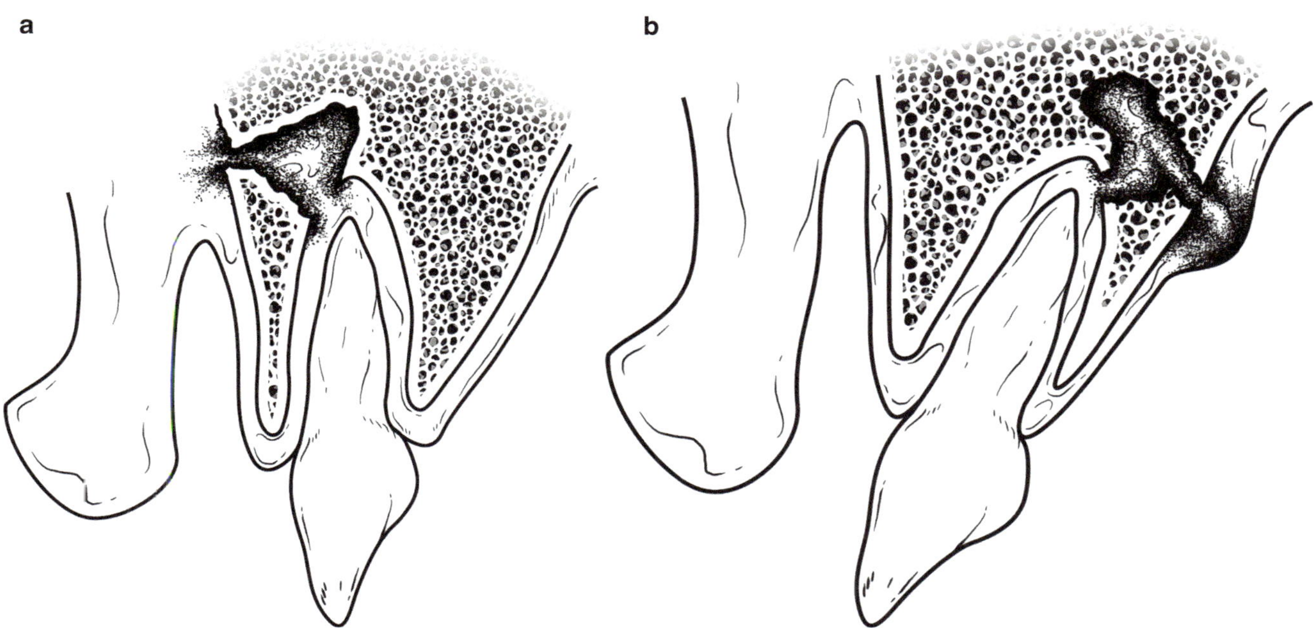




Fig. 20.3 (**a**, **b**) Infection following the path of least resistance in case of maxillary incisors based on angulation of root

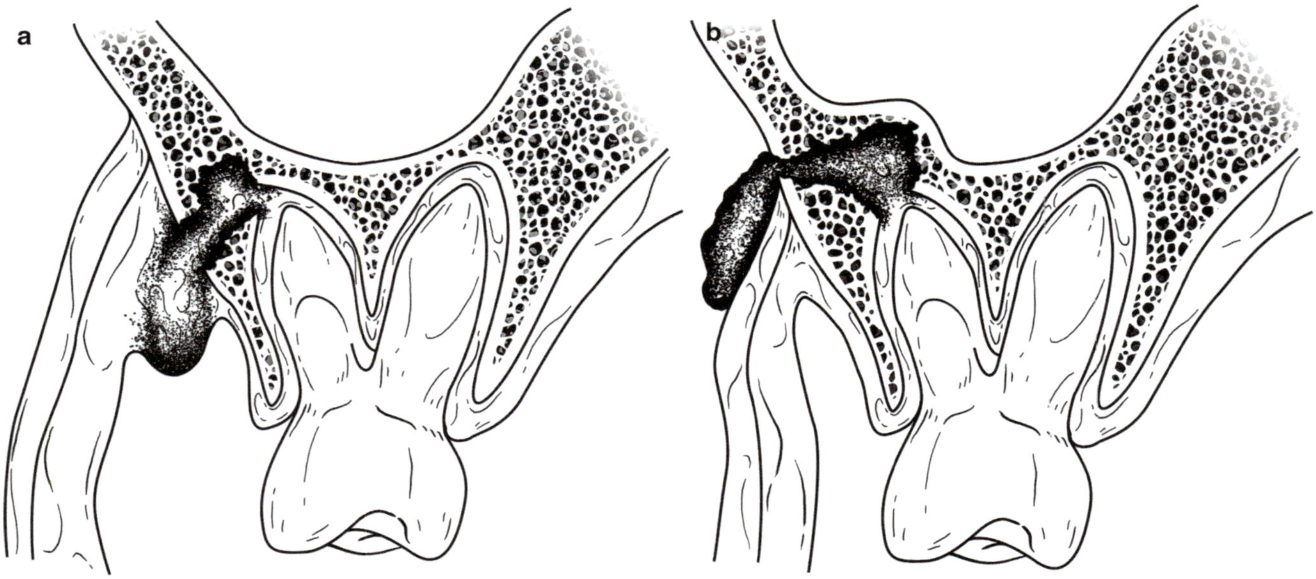


©Association of Oral and Maxillofacial Surgeons of India

**Fig. 20.4** (**a**, **b**) Effect of buccinator muscle attachment on the site of appearance of swelling in case of maxillary molars. In (**a**) the infection has localised to the vestibule while in (**b**) the infection has spread to the buccal space, as the root apex is situated above the attachment of the buccinator muscle

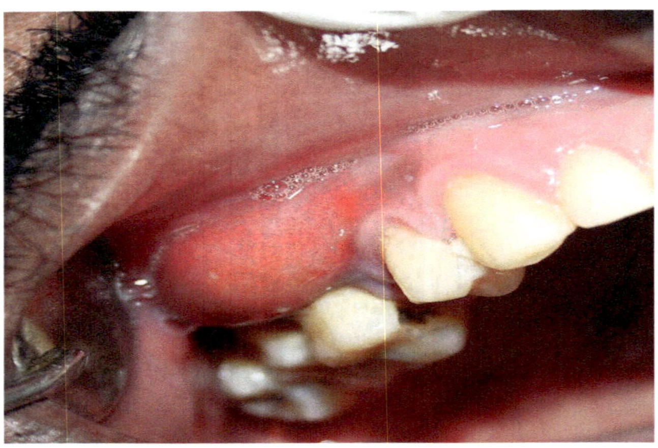

©Association of Oral and Maxillofacial Surgeons of India

**Fig. 20.5** Shows the clinical picture of a vestibular abscess arising from an infected upper right first molar

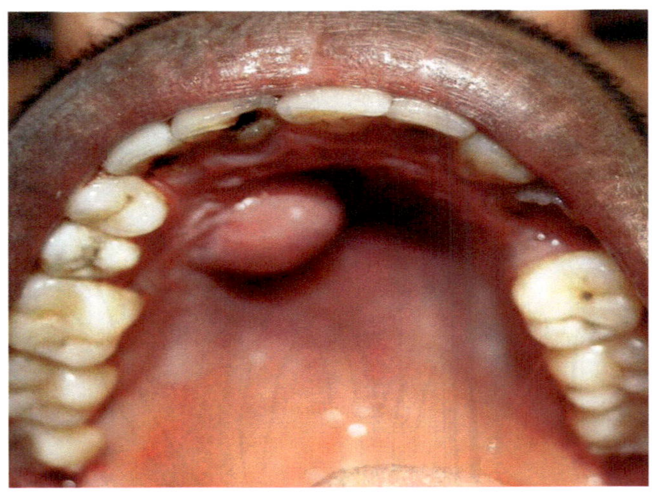

©Association of Oral and Maxillofacial Surgeons of India

**Fig. 20.6** Palatal abscess arising from upper incisors

as compared to the buccal cortical plate. If this gets perforated above the mylohyoid line, a sublingual swelling occurs and if below it, a submandibular swelling occurs.

The commonest manifestation of odontogenic infections is either a palatal or a vestibular abscess. When untreated, it may lead to an intraoral or extraoral drainage, in due course establishing a sinus tract. The treatment involves removing the cause (endodontically or via exodontia) and management of the sinus tract. In certain cases, the sinus tract resolves by itself, following the treatment of the offending cause (Fig. 20.7).

## 20.5 Pathways of Spread of Periapical Infections

An odontogenic infection follows the path of least resistance. A periapical infection may perforate the nearest or the weakest cortex and travel along the soft tissue, initially as cellulitis and eventually resulting in abscess formation. This abscess may drain spontaneously, extraorally or intraorally and may involve one or more anatomically potential spaces. When this happens, it is known as a space infection.

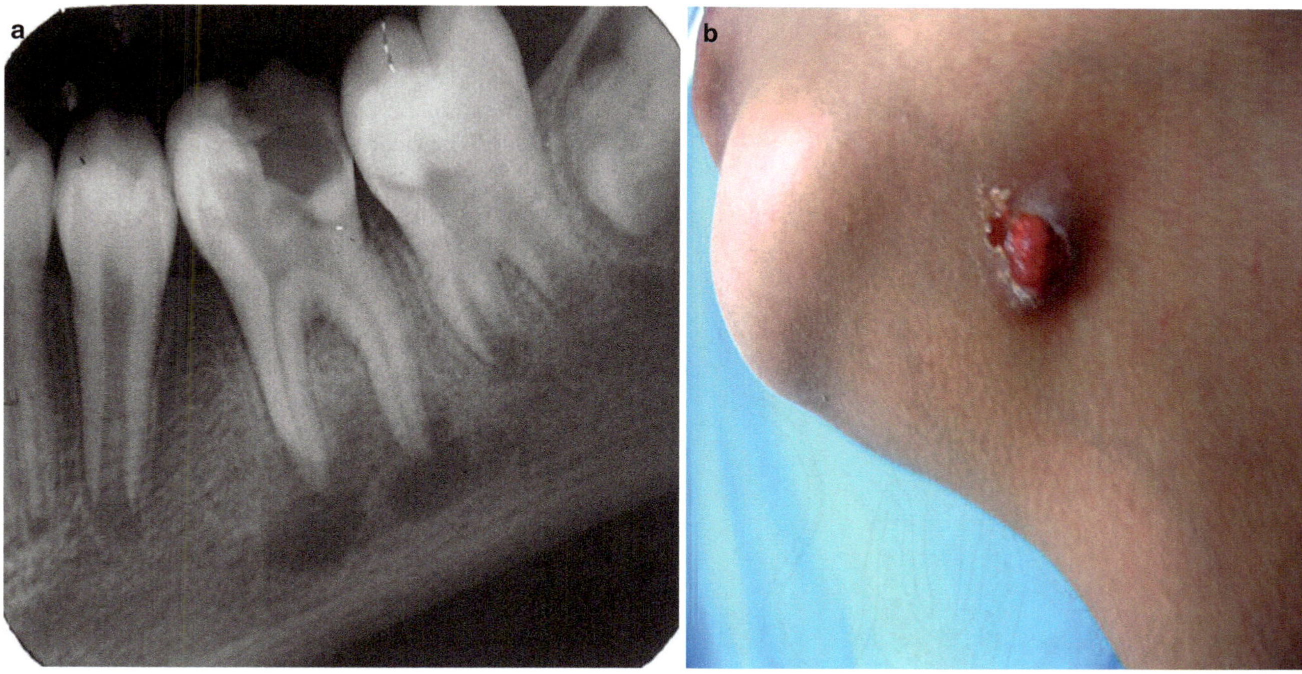




**Fig. 20.7** (**a**, **b**) Shows the periapical lesion in lower left first molar in a 14-year-old patient causing extraoral sinus at the left lower border mandible region

Following are frequently affected anatomic spaces, (Fig. 20.8):

1. With any tooth.
   - Subcutaneous.
   - Vestibular.
   - Buccal.
2. With any offending maxillary tooth.
   - Buccal.
   - Maxillary along with other para nasal sinuses.
   - Infraorbital.
   - Infratemporal.
   - Temporal.
3. With any offending mandibular tooth.
   - Medullary space of mandibular body.
   - Submandibular.
   - Sublingual.
   - Submental.
   - Masticator.
     - *Submasseteric.*
     - *Pterygomandibular.*
     - *Superficial temporal.*
     - *Deep temporal.*
4. Deep fascial spaces.
   - Lateral pharyngeal.
   - Retropharyngeal.
   - Pretracheal.
   - Danger (Alar space).
   - Prevertebral.

Various spaces involved in an infection differ in their relative severity depending upon the proximity of the vital anatomic structures in their vicinity. This may be seen as follows.

## 20.6 Various Space Infections and Their Relative Severity

MILD—Vital structures and airway may be mildly threatened

- Subperiosteal.
- Infraorbital.
- Buccal.
- Vestibular.
- Osteomyelitis of the mandible.

MODERATE—Airway may be compromised

- Pterygomandibular.
- Superficial temporal.
- Submandibular.
- Sublingual.
- Submental.

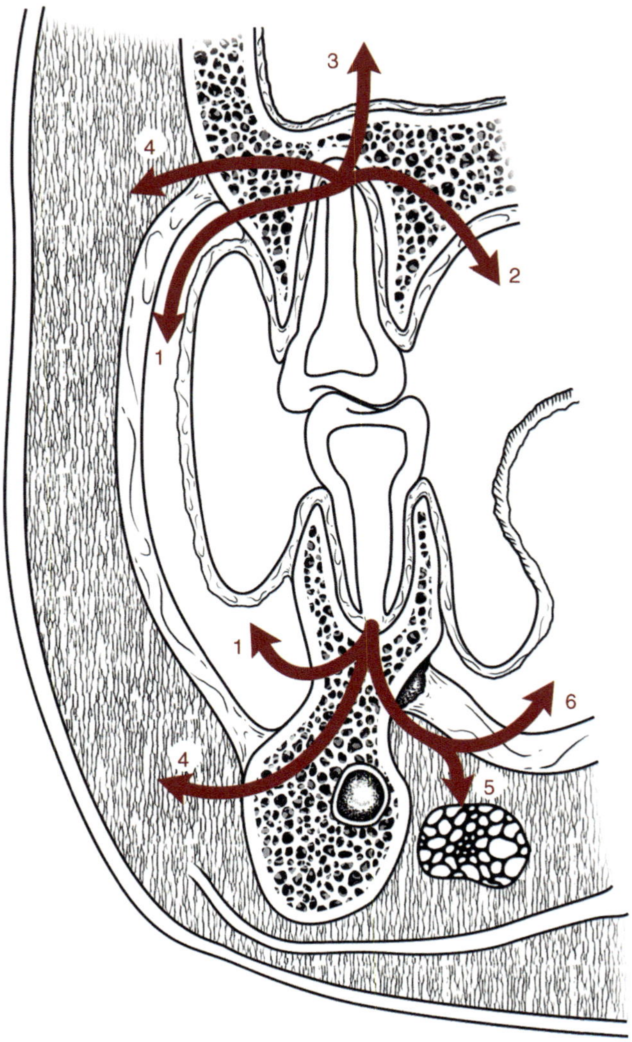


**Fig. 20.8** Pathways of spread of periapical infection. (1) Vestibular space. (2) Palatal abscess. (3) Maxillary sinus/odontogenic sinusitis. (4) Buccal space. (5) Submandibular space. (6) Sublingual space

- Submasseteric.
- Infratemporal.
- Deep temporal.
- Masticator.

HIGH—Vital structures or airway under direct threat

- Lateral pharyngeal.
- Retropharyngeal.
- Danger space (Alar space).
- Pretracheal.
- Cavernous sinus thrombosis.
- Intracranial infections (brain abscess).
- Mediastinal.
- Prevertebral.

## 20.7 Basic Therapeutic Principles

1. Delineation of cause and severity.
2. Assessment of host's immune response.
3. Role of specialist.
4. Surgical intervention.
5. Pharmacotherapeutics.
6. Follow-ups.

1. *Delineation of cause and severity:* As a standard protocol, a proper history should be recorded in chronological order stating the patients' chief complaints in his/her own words.

   Once the chief complaint is noted, history of present illness is determined with an estimation of how long back the patient was absolutely symptom free. Usually, infections have a short history of onset as compared to tumors in their acute state [6].

   Next thing to be noted is any change in the patients' state of physical well-being since the symptoms first appeared, i.e. if they have been the same, improved, or worsened with time. Since the response to an infection is essentially an inflammatory one, classic sign of inflammation are always looked for (tumor, rubor, dolor, color, and loss of function). Principal presenting feature is pain, so the nature of pain, site, and diurnal variation should be noted. A sharp, piercing, and lancinating type of pain is generated by Aδ nerve fibers that usually awake the patient at night (in accordance with the hydrodynamic theory of pulpal pain by Brannstrom [7]); however, a dull, aching, and gnawing kind of pain arises due to stimulation of slowly firing "c" type nerve fibers.

   Swelling, redness, and rise of temperature should be inquired for and inspected even during history taking if these are apparent. Loss of function may manifest in the form of dyspnea, dysphagia, difficulty in chewing, or trismus [8]. A feeling of general malaise usually indicates a physical or physiological response against moderate to severe infection [9].

   At this point, an enquiry into any previous treatments by another dentist, specialist, and/or self-treatment should be made and recorded. After carefully listening to the chief complaints and history of present illness, a comprehensive medical history should be recorded. The most efficient means of doing so is either by personal structured interview or by means of a questionnaire along with a discussion with the patient for any positive findings.

History taking is followed by a physical examination that begins with the recording of patients' vitals as temperature, pulse rate, respiratory rate, and blood pressure. Patients with infections usually have elevated body temperature, and increased pulse and respiratory rates [10]. If the pain is significant, patient's blood pressure may be elevated. However, hypotension is seen in septicemic states. Since odontogenic infections are inflammatory states, a partial or complete upper airway compromise may occur owing to an extension of the current infection to the deep facial spaces of the neck [11]. The patients may present with fatigue, fever, and malaise or so-called toxic appearance (Table 20.3) [12].

Palpation of swellings should be done to know the tenderness and consistency of the swelling. Consistency of a swelling may vary from normal, firm, fleshy (dough like) to indurated (consistency of a taught muscle/wooden like/brawny hard), or fluctuant (feel of a fluid-filled balloon). Fluctuation almost always indicates presence of pus in the center.

Intraoral examination gives a fair amount of idea as to the cause of the infection, i.e. the offending tooth. A careful look may reveal a grossly carious tooth/teeth, periodontal diseases, and/or a fractured tooth.

Investigative phase begins with a radiograph; intraoral periapical (IOPA) or orthopantomogram (OPG) depending on the symptomatology and clinical examination. CT scan may be required in severe cases to assess the pathway of the spread of infection [13].

If any surgical intervention is required, a routine blood assessment is always helpful in deciding the type of procedure to be followed.

A decision has to be made as to the stage of the infection, i.e. inoculation, cellulitis, or abscess stage. Usual attributes are as follows.

2. *Assessment of Immune response:* General medical history is the guide to detect any interfering systemic conditions that may compromise the host defense mechanism and may worsen patient's condition rapidly. Conditions of compromised host defense mechanism are as under:

**Table 20.3** Stages of infection

| Stage of infection | Clinical features |
|---|---|
| Inoculation | Edema/Inflammation |
| Cellulitis | Acute pain |
| | Firm to borderline swelling/induration |
| | Diffuse borders |
| | All cardinal features of inflammation |
| Abscess | Localized pain (acute abscess) |
| | Fever (more often than not) |
| | Fluctuant swelling |

(a) Diabetes Mellitus (type I and II): When uncontrolled, it results in an overall decrease in the immunity owing to decreased phagocytosis, chemotaxis, and generalized decrease in leukocyte function. However, in patients with moderate to severe infection, an increased random blood sugar cannot be a diagnostic criteria for underlying diabetes. Since these are high-stress states, the body gluconeogenic mechanisms are upregulated to meet the increased BMR. So, a more comprehensive analysis like $HBA_1C$ is performed to know the long-term glycemic status.

(b) Leukocytic upsurge is expected in infection. The baseline leukocyte/neutrophil count serves as a marker to track the response of the patient to medical and surgical intervention in a case of severe odontogenic infection.

(c) Immuno-deficient states: HIV infection principally affects the T lymphocytes, meaning that the humoral immune system is still intact. Odontogenic infections are generally bacterial and usually well defended by the patients' immune system, but in immunocompromised states, the basic host defense mechanism no longer functions. When the disease advances to involve even the B-cells, then, even simple infections may become serious life-threatening issues in such patients. It is hence important to know that such immunocompromised HIV-positive individuals need more intensive therapy than a normally infected individual.

(d) Another example of systemic immuno-deficient states may be prolonged corticosteroid therapy. Here the inflammatory cascade itself gets modulated, and affects the immune system as a whole, resulting in decreased production of the cell adhesive molecules, deficient leukocyte chemotaxis, and decreased cytokines production (IL-1, TN $\alpha$, IL-6, etc.). No apoptotic activity results in generalized lymphocytopenia along with IL-2 mediated cyto-proliferative responses. When used long enough or in high doses, delayed-type hypersensitivity (type IV) response is inhibited along with decreased antibody formation. Such patients soon develop oral thrush and other superimposed bacterial or viral infections of the oral cavity, worsening of an existing odontogenic infection being no exception.

(e) End Stage Renal Diseases (ESRD): End stage renal diseases affect almost all aspects of the innate and acquired immunity, and many such patients will be on maintenance hemodialysis. ESRD patients having odontogenic infections also may have to be managed comprehensively where adequate support from the allied speciality is available.

(f) Drug-induced immuno-incompetence: While blood counts less than 1000 cells/ml are typically seen in patients on anti-cancer chemotherapy, patients who undergo organ transplants have to be on immune-suppressive therapy (IST). Drugs like corticosteroids and cyclosporins have decreased B and T lymphocyte function and consequently deficient immunoglobulin production. As such, patients are likely to have exaggerated manifestation for even mild odontogenic infections.

(g) Alcoholism and/or Hepatic insufficiency: Alcoholics are usually malnourished and have pending hepatic damage that leads to poor qualitative and quantitative immunoglobulin supply.

Above discussion reinforces that while assessing a patient, a through medical history as well as a history of habits provides vital clues for the action to be adopted for his/her management.

3. *Role of Specialist:* Role for patient care should shift from a general dentist to a maxillofacial surgeon. Antibiotics should be started if indicated as in Table 20.4. When the situation demands, either a hospital admission or immediate surgical care under regional or general anesthesia is required. The following criteria may be adopted for making this vital discussion in patient's interest:
   (a) Failed earlier management.
   (b) Medically compromised patients.
   (c) Toxic appearance patients.
   (d) Febrile patient: temperature greater than 101 °F.
   (e) Signs of dehydration.
   (f) Dyspnea.
   (g) Difficulty swallowing (dysphagia).
   (h) Moderate to severe trismus (with mouth-opening between 10 and 20 mm).
   (i) Need for general anesthesia.
   (j) Airway compromise.
   (k) Signs of ascending or descending facial infections (cavernous sinus thrombosis/deep neck infections/mediastinitis).

**Table 20.4** Indications for antimicrobial therapy

1. Trismus (mouth opening between 10 and 20 mm).
2. Cellulitis (infection may not have drained completely).
3. Lymphadenopathy (lymph nodes may harbor residual infection).
4. Temperature > 101 °F (bacteremia).
5. Osteomyelitis.
6. Severe soft tissue involvement (e.g. necrotizing fasciitis).
7. Swelling extends beyond alveolar anatomy.
8. Systemically compromised patient.

4. *Surgical Intervention:* Surgical drainage and removal of the course of infection is the mainstay of surgical management of odontogenic infection [14]. This may be as simple as endodontic therapy to wide incision in the submandibular/neck region that may require mediastinal exploration. The removal of the cause is the primary goal and drainage of the accumulated pus and necrotic debris is the secondary goal.

Incision and drainage principally includes insertion of a drain in the abscess cavity to prevent premature closure of the mucosal/skin incision. Purpose of this procedure is to achieve adequate drainage, if it is not possible by endodontic means (especially in mandibular teeth) (refer Chap. 21 for details on incision and drainage).

*Pus culture and Sensitivity Tests:* This must be done before the incision and drainage procedure if possible. The site is prepared with antiseptics and a thick needle is used to aspirate pus, may be in multiple directions, under negative pressure of syringe, and taking due care to prevent relevant anatomic structures. In case of complex space infections involving the digastric/carotid triangle, ultrasound-guided aspiration must be done. This culture when obtained from sites of cellulitis (Ludwig's Angina) usually contains serosanguinous fluid but harbors sufficient bacteria for culture. This aspirate is inoculated into both anaerobic and aerobic cultures (sterile tubes having sterile swabs and bacterial transport medium) with viable shelf life [15].

## 20.8 Antimicrobial Therapy

Once the culture and sensitivity reports are available, specific antimicrobial therapy may be installed but meanwhile empirical antibiotics should be started immediately [16]. The choice of antibiotic should be carefully thought off to prevent unnecessary disturbance of the essential microflora of the gut and development of cross resistance (Also refer Chap. 10 of this book).

Cases of moderate to severe infection generally need postoperative antibiotics, where the host defense cannot be solely relied upon to fight the residual infection. Since the antibiotic sensitivity of usual causative organisms of odontogenic infections is fairly well known and consistent, an empirical therapy may include clindamycin, metronidazole, and penicillin. Metronidazole being narrow spectrum covers only obligate anaerobic population and the rest may be covered by other drugs dealing with facultative microbes.

Odontogenic infections are complex entities, both, on the basis of the plethora of flora associated and mechanism of their spread to the adjacent as well as distant anatomic

Following principles should be additionally borne in mind before prescribing antibiotics [17]:

1. Use of narrowest possible spectrum- prevents bacterial resistance.
2. Use of antimicrobial with least toxicity and side effects- prevents vital organ damage.
3. Use of bactericidal rather than bacteriostatic drug- prevents residual infection.
4. Weigh cost to benefit ratio- prevents over expenditure.
5. Use only in prescribed dose and duration- restricts side effects and maintains efficacy.
6. Use the appropriate route of administration- restricts side effects and maintains efficacy.

sites. Fortunately, culture and sensitivity behaviors of the causative microbes are fairly consistent and well understood. As such timely management should alleviate most of the dangerous outcomes but still these infections remain one of the leading cause of maxillofacial morbidity and at times mortality.

## 20.9 Conclusion

Odontogenic infection can be severe enough and become life threatening, hence should be dealt with very carefully. Proper evaluation of the signs and symptoms guide the clinician to make the diagnosis. Radiographic assessment may suggest the involvement of one or more teeth. Surgical intervention includes drainage of abscess, and pus be sent for culture and sensitivity to help choose the right antibiotic regime.

## References


1. Chinen J, William T. Secondary immunodeficiencies. Am Acad Allerg Asth Immunodef. 2010;125(2 Suppl 2):S195–203.
2. Socransky SS, Haffajee AD. Periodontal microbial ecology. Periodontol 2000. 2005;38:135–87.
3. Newman M, Takei H, Klokkevold P, Carranza F. Carranza' clinical periodontology. 12th ed. Saunders: Elsevier; 2014.
4. Brook I, Frazier EH, Gher ME. Aerobic and anaerobic microbiology of periapical abscess. Oral Microbiol Immunol. 1991;6(2):123–25.
5. Chandra S. Grossmann's endodontic practice. 13th ed. South Holland: Wolters Kluwer; 2014.
6. Walker B, Colledge NR, Ralston S, Penman I. Davidson's medicine. 22nd ed. Edinburgh: Churchill Livingstone; 2014.
7. Brännström M. The hydrodynamic theory of dentinal pain: Sensation in preparations, caries, and the dentinal crack syndrome. J Endod. 1986;12(10):453–7.
8. Mathew GC, Ranganathan LR, Gandhi S, Jacob ME, Singh I, Solanki M, et al. Odontogenic maxillofacial space infections at a tertiary care center in North India: a five-year retrospective study. Int J Inf Dis. 2012;16:e296–302.
9. Hupp JR, Ellis E III, Tucker MR. Contemporary oral and maxillofacial surgery. 6th ed. St Louis Mosby: Elsevier; 2014.
10. Al-Malik M, Al-Sarheed M. Pattern of management of orofacial infection in children: a retrospective. Saudi J Biol Sc. 2017;24:1375–9.
11. Kuo J, Lin Y, Lin YT. Odontogenic cellulitis in children requiring hospitalization. J Dent Sc. 2013;8:129–32.
12. Alotaibi N, Cloutier L, Khaldoun E, Bois E, Chirat M, Salvan D. Criteria for admission of odontogenic infections at high risk of deep neck space infection. Eur Ann Otorhinolaryngol Head Neck Dis. 2015;132:261–4.
13. Yonetsu K, Izumi M, Nakamura T. Deep facial infections of odontogenic origin: CT assessment of pathways of space involvement. Am J Neuroradiol. 1998;19:123–8.
14. Sánchez R, Mirada E, Arias J, Paño JR, Burgueño M. Severe odontogenic infections: epidemiological, microbiological and therapeutic factors. Med Oral Patol Oral Cir Bucal. 2011;16(5):e670–6.
15. Kumar V, Abbas A, Aster J. Robin's pathological basis of disease. 10th ed. Philadelphia, PA: Elsevier; 2017.
16. Kuriyama T, Karasawa T, Nakagawa K, Nakamura S, Yamamoto E, et al. Antibiotic susceptibility of major pathogens of orofacial odontogenic infections to 11 β lactam antibiotics. Oral Microbiol Immunol. 2002;17:285–9.
17. Topazian RG, Goldberg MH, Hupp JR. Oral and maxillofacial infections. 4th ed. Philadelphia: WB Saunders Company; 2002.

# 21 Fascial Space Infections

Rajasekhar Gaddipati

## 21.1 Introduction

There is considerable amount of change in the behavior of infections for the past one decade. The severity of infection is far greater than before which may be due to increased co-morbid conditions, demanding swift action and aggressive treatment.

Fascial spaces do not exist in a normal healthy individual. These are latent spaces created by distention of tissues secondary to infection from the dental pulp, periodontal tissues and bone, where the infection perforates the cortical plate and discharge into the surrounding spaces.

The infections range from simple superficial periapical abscess to deep infections in the neck region; some resolving with little consequences and some lead to life-threatening conditions.

Shapiro states that "The fascial planes are potential areas between layers of fascia. These areas are normally filled with loose connective tissue, which readily breakdown when invaded by infection". The infection started in any area is automatically limited by tough fascial layers. If the infection becomes massive, it breaks through a nearby fascial barrier into the next fascial space [1].

## 21.2 Definition of Fascial Space

The fascial spaces in the Head and Neck are the potential spaces between the various fascia normally filled with loose connective tissue and bounded by the anatomical barriers usually of bone, muscle, or fascial layers [2].

Facial planes offer anatomic highways for infection to spread superficially to deep planes. Antibiotic availability in fascial spaces is limited due to poor vascularity.

R. Gaddipati (✉)
Mamata Dental College, Khammam, Telangana, India

## 21.3 Spread of Infection

The spread of the infections could be either through tissues, blood, or lymphatics leading to fatal consequences like Airway obstruction, Meningitis, and Septicemia; however, various factors influence the spread of infection.

They are as follows:

- Virulence of the organism.
- Pathogenicity of the organisms.
- Immune status of the patient.
- Malnutrition.
- Thickness of bone adjacent to the offending tooth.
- Position of muscle attachment in relation to root tip.

In the Oral and Maxillofacial region, fascial spaces are almost always of relevance due to the spread of odontogenic infections. As such, the spaces can be classified according to their relation to the upper and lower teeth, and whether infection may directly spread into the space called primary space, or must spread via a primary space to the secondary space [3].

## 21.4 Classification of Spaces

### 21.4.1 Primary Spaces and Secondary Spaces

Failure to adequately treat a primary space infection or a compromised host results in secondary space involvement (Table 21.1).

#### 21.4.1.1 Cervical Spaces

Since hyoid bone is the most important anatomic structure in the neck that limits the spread of infection, the spaces can be classified according to their relation to the hyoid bone:


K. Bonanthaya et al. (eds.), *Oral and Maxillofacial Surgery for the Clinician*, https://doi.org/10.1007/978-981-15-1346-6_21

Table 21.1 Classification of spaces in odontogenic infections based on mode of involvement

| Mode of Involvement |
|---|
| **Primary spaces (Direct)** |
| ***Primary maxillary spaces*** |
| • Canine space |
| • Buccal space |
| • Infratemporal space |
| ***Primary mandibular space*** |
| • Buccal space |
| • Sub-mental space |
| • Sub-mandibular space |
| • Sub-lingual space |
| **Secondary spaces (Indirect)** |
| • Masseteric space |
| • Pterygomandibular space |
| • Temporal (Superficial & Deep) spaces |
| • Temporal (Superficial & Deep) spaces |
| • Para-pharyngeal (Lateral & Retro) spaces |
| • Pre-vertebral space |

Table 21.2 Severity score for spaces [4]

| Severity score | Risk | Spaces involved |
|---|---|---|
| 1 | Low risk | Subperiosteal space<br>Vestibular space<br>Buccal and<br>Infraorbital space |
| 2 | Moderate risk | Submandibular space<br>Submental space<br>Sublingual space<br>Pterygomandibular space<br>Submasseteric space and<br>Temporal spaces |
| 3 | High risk | Lateral pharyngeal space<br>Retropharyngeal space and pretracheal space |
| 4 | Extreme severe | Danger space<br>Mediastinum<br>Intracranial infection |

- Suprahyoid (above the hyoid).
- Infrahyoid (below the hyoid).
- Fascial spaces traversing the length of the neck.

#### 21.4.1.2 Severity Score Anatomic Space [4]

The severity score for a given patient is the sum of the severity scores for all of the spaces involved by cellulitis or abscess, based on clinical and radiological examination (Table 21.2).

The fascial spaces are divided into:

- Spaces around the Maxilla.
- Spaces around the Mandible.

The infections arising from the maxillary anterior teeth spread to Canine space, while the infection from molars spread to Buccal space, Infratemporal space, or cause palatal abscess. Likewise, the infection from the mandibular anterior teeth spread to Submental space or cause gingival abscess. Infection from mandibular molars spread to the Sublingual space or the Submandibular space. While the infection from mandibular third molars spread to Submasseteric space, Pterygomandibular space and Lateral Pharyngeal space.

However, it is not a "rule of thumb" for the involvement of a particular space with a specific tooth infection.

Table 21.3 Characteristic features of cellulitis and abscess

| Clinical feature | Cellulitis | Abscess |
|---|---|---|
| Duration | Acute | Chronic |
| Pain | Severe and generalized | Localized |
| Size | Large | Small |
| Localization | Diffuse borders | Well defined |
| Palpation | Doughy to indurated | Fluctuant |
| Pus formation | No | Yes |
| Seriousness | Greater | Lesser |
| Bacteria | Aerobic | Anaerobic |

## 21.5 General Priciples of Management of Infection

1. Remove the cause.
2. Establish drainage.
3. Institute antibiotic therapy.
4. Supportive care, including proper rest and nutrition.

Pyogenic infections are primarily managed by surgical intervention comprising decompression or drainage. It is better to proceed with decompression at the earliest, without waiting for the localization of the infection (abcess formation), thereby preventing the spread of infection in tissue planes and mounting of pressure under the skin (Table 21.3).

Early decompression has the following benefits:

1. Prevents the spread of infection.
2. Prevents ischemic necrosis of the tissues.
3. Prevents pressure in the tissues.
4. To get rid of toxic purulent discharge.
5. Improves the drainage, by opening the lymphatic and venous channels, which were blocked by the edema and congestion.
6. To allow better perfusion of blood thereby improving the delivery of antibiotics and defensive elements to the required site.
7. Prevents further complications.

## 21.6 Hilton's Method of Abscess Drainage (Figs. 21.1a and 21.1b)

This is a method of abscess drainage which ensures that no blood vessel or nerve in the vicinity of the incision is damaged.

1. Topical anesthesia is achieved by ethyl chloride spray.
2. Stab incision with the help of 11 number blade is made at the most dependent area along the skin crease.
3. Sinus forceps is inserted through the incision and all the locules in the abscess are explored.
4. Purulent discharge, toxic material, gases, and necrotic tissue drained through the incision.
5. Pus collected and sent for culture and sensitivity test.
6. Abscess cavity is irrigated with antiseptic solution.
7. Corrugated rubber drain is inserted deep into the abscess cavity and secured to the edge of the incision and the drain is removed once there are no active exudates.
8. Dressing placed over the incision.

**Fig. 21.1a** Hilton's method of transoral incision and drainage. (a) Abscess associated with tooth. (b) Stab incision given with blade. (c) sinus forceps is entered into the cavity and opened. (d) Drain entered into the cavity. (e) Drain secured with suture

a

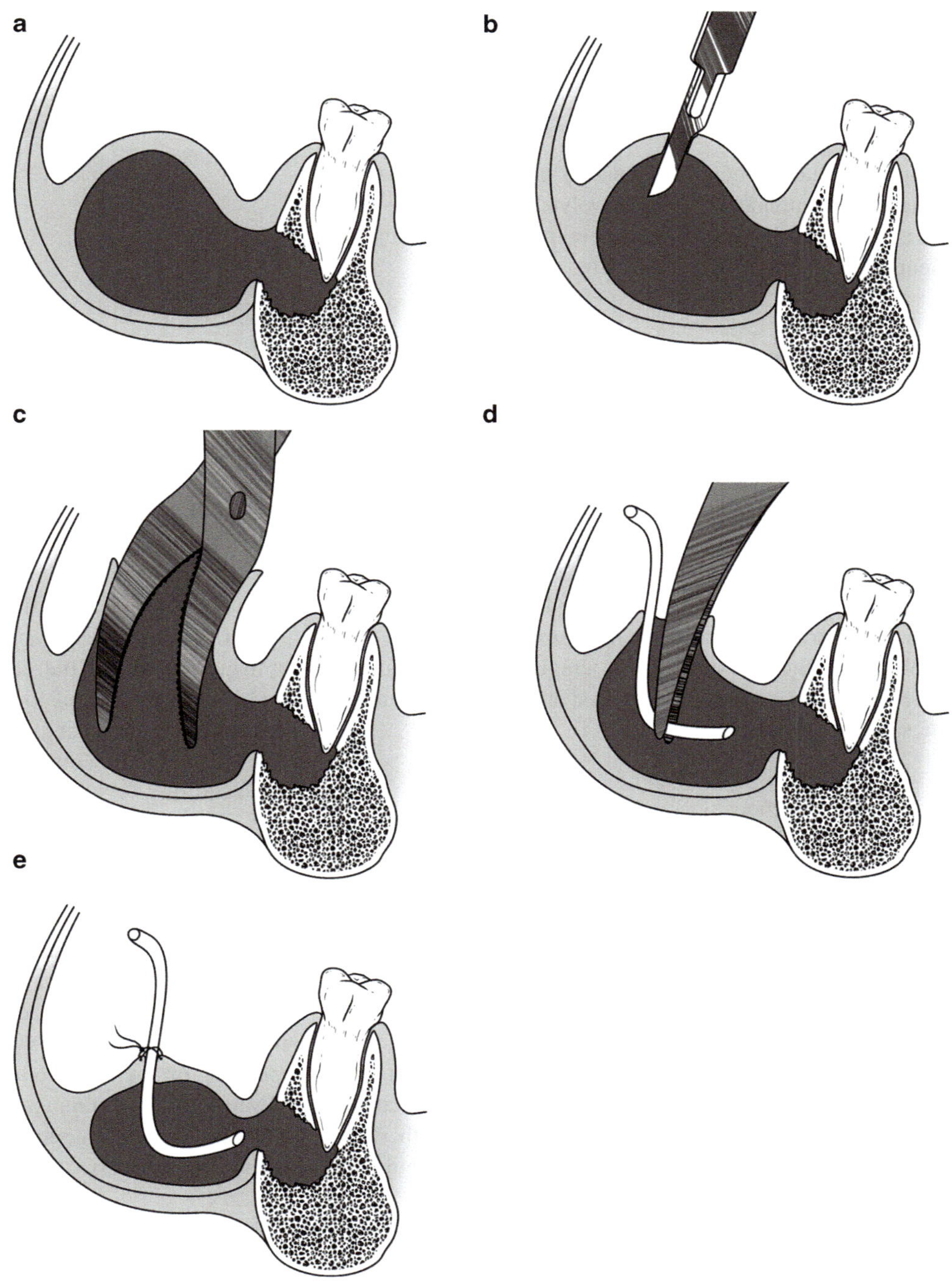

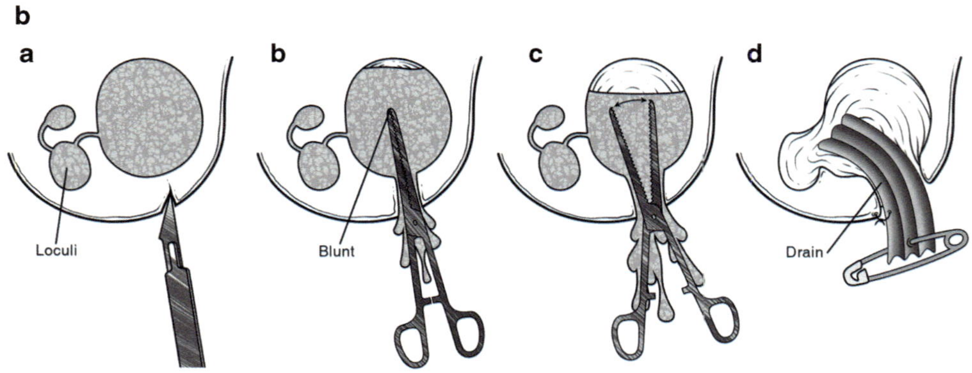


**Fig. 21.1b** Hilton's method of incision and drainage (extra oral site). (a) Incision given at the dependent site of the abscess. (b) Sinus forceps entered into the abscess cavity. (c) Sinus forceps opened in the cavity and removed. (d) Drain entered into the cavity and secured with suture

*Removal of the source of the infection is mandatory apart from drainage.*

## 21.7 Medical Management

Supportive management is mandatory in the form of antibiotics, anti-inflammatory, and electrolytes. The reader is also advised to refer the chapter on general principles of management of facial infections (Chap. 20).

### 21.7.1 Antibiotic Therapy

Antibiotics are advised depending upon the patient's systemic condition; initially, after pus collection, empirical antibiotic is given; later, after the culture and sensitivity is performed, -specific antibiotics are advised.

Route of administration depends upon the general condition and severity of the infection. Para-enteral route is preferred when the infection is acute and severe or when the patient is nutritionally or medically compromised.

With evidence of slough, gas, crepitus, and foul smell, anaerobic infection may be suspected and appropriate antibiotics have to be given.

Principles of choosing appropriate antibiotic

- Causative organism,
- Sensitivity,
- Specific, narrow-spectrum antibiotic,
- Least toxic antibiotic,
- Drug history (success, allergic, and toxic).

Flynn TR [5] in their systemic review concluded that antibiotics should be chosen which are safe and cost effective, because no one antibiotic is clearly superior to all others. In otherwise healthy patient, a 3–4-day regimen of antibiotic therapy should be adequate. The primary importance should be given to the surgical treatment consisting of incision and drainage, extraction, or endodontic therapy of the involved tooth. According to their review, the choice of empiric antibiotics for odontogenic infections is listed in Table 21.4.

**Table 21.4** Choice of empirical antibiotics (also refer Chap. 10)

| Severity/Penicillin allergy | Antibiotics of choice |
|---|---|
| In patient | Ampicillin/Sulbactam<br>Clindamycin<br>Penicillin + metronidazole<br>Ceftriaxone |
| Penicillin allergy | Clindamycin<br>Moxifloxacin<br>Vancomycin + metronidazole |
| Out patient | Amoxicillin<br>Clindamycin<br>Azithromycin |
| Penicillin allergy | Clindamycin<br>Azithromycin<br>Metronidazole<br>Moxifloxacin |

Martins JR et al. [6] suggests that after incision and drainage/removal of the cause is mandatory. Antibiotics should be administered for the shortest duration possible duration and should act as an adjuvant for the primary surgical treatment in countering any regional or systemic co-morbidities.

## 21.8 Fluid and Electrolytes

Apart from antibiotics and anti-inflammatory drugs, administration of fluids and electrolytes is mandatory, as there is a loss of fluids due to infection and fever. In non-ambulatory patients, intravenous fluids are administered depending on their systemic status.

Daily calorie requirement also increases by up to 13% for each degree rise in temperature, which needs to be addressed for a speedy recovery.

Supportive therapy.

It involves those modalities which aid the patient's own body defenses. It consists of the following:

1. Administration of antibiotics.
2. Hydration of patient through IV route, maintain adequate nutritional status-high protein intake.
3. Analgesic.
4. Bed rest.
5. Application of heat in the form of moist pack, advice mouth rinses.
6. Dental management by extraction or root-canal treatment for drainage.

## 21.9 Selection of Anesthesia

A simple and superficial abscess can be drained comfortably under local anesthesia, while deep-seated, multi-loculated abcesses may not be amenable for treatment under local anesthesia and may be managed under procedural sedation provided the patient has adequate mouth-opening and patent airway.

Fiber-optic intubation or tracheostomy may be considered in; patients with limited mouth opening (trismus) or in patients having intra-oral and pharyngeal infections (sub-lingual, lateral/retropharyngeal spaces) where the chances of aspiration is high in the event of oro/naso-tracheal intubations.

## 21.10 Spaces Around the Maxilla

### 21.10.1 Canine Space/Infraorbital Space

The canine space, synonymous with Infraorbital space, is situated in the anterior surface of the maxilla at the infraorbital region above canine fossa.

#### 21.10.1.1 Source of Infection

- From upper canine and bicuspids.
- Skin infections of upper lip [7].

#### 21.10.1.2 Boundaries (Fig. 21.2)

- Anterior—Elevator muscles of upper lip (Orbicularis oris).
- Posterior—Anterior surface of Maxilla.
- Medial—Levator Labii Alaeque nasi.
- Lateral—Zygomaticus major.

#### 21.10.1.3 Contents

- Angular artery and vein.
- Infraorbital nerve.

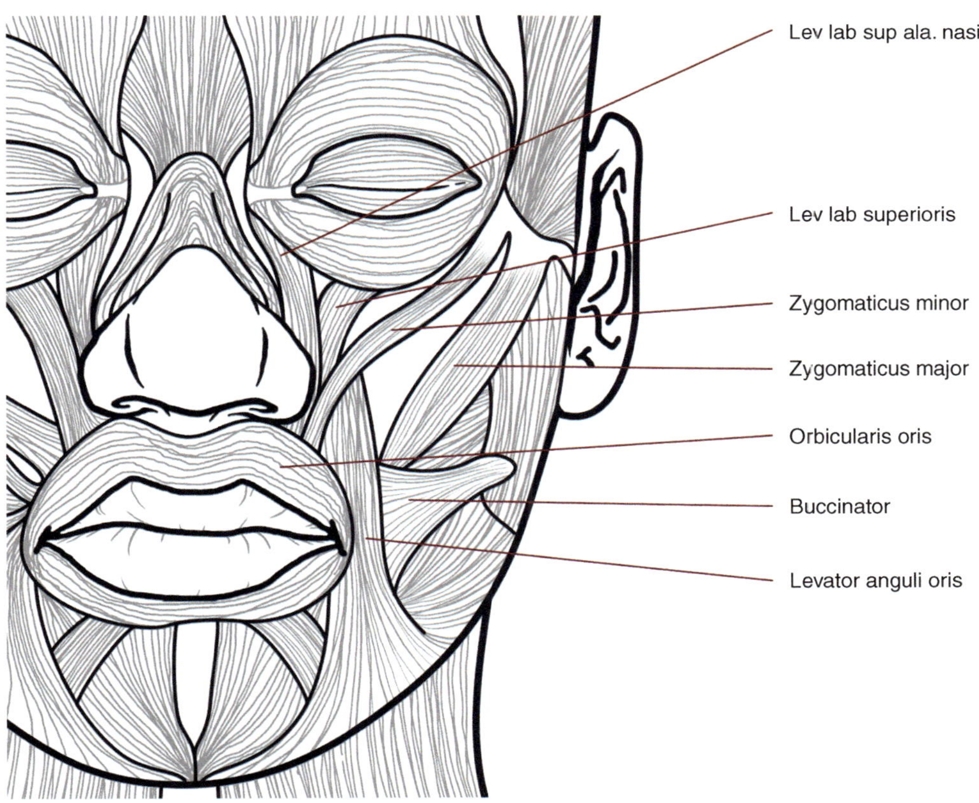




**Fig. 21.2** Shows boundaries of canine (infraorbital) space

#### 21.10.1.4 Clinical Features

1. Pain and tenderness.
2. Swelling in the anterior cheek region.
3. Obliteration of Nasolabial folds.
4. Edema of lower eyelid and upper lip.
5. Obliteration of labial vestibule.

#### 21.10.1.5 Management

Drainage of the space infection either intraorally or percutaneously is done; intraoral incision and drainage are preferred as these will not produce a facial scar. Drainage is made by making an in-depth incision of the maxillary vestibule near canine fossa. Sinus forceps is inserted superiorly, laterally, and medially for complete breakage of locules and drainage. Care is taken while using sinus forceps, so as to not damage the infraorbital nerve and its branches.

Aggressive antibiotic therapy is mandatory to prevent the spread as it lies in the danger area of the face and also to prevent Cavernous sinus thrombosis from septic thrombi entering into angular vein.

The involved tooth is either removed or subjected to root canal treatment with multiple dressings. Patient is advised good hydration and rest.

### 21.10.2 Buccal Space

The buccal space occupies the portion of the subcutaneous space present between the fascial skin, buccinator muscle, and masseter muscle [8].

Source of infection—From maxillary premolar and molar teeth root apices above buccinator attachment.

From mandibular premolar and molar teeth root apices below the buccinator attachment.

#### 21.10.2.1 Boundaries

- Medial: Buccinator muscle, buccopharyngeal fascia, and mucosa.
- Lateral: Skin of cheek and subcutaneous tissue.
- Anterior: Posterior border of zygomaticus major above and depressor anguli oris below.
- Posterior: Edge of masseter muscle.
- Superior: Zygomatic arch.
- Inferior: Lower border of mandible.

#### 21.10.2.2 Contents

- Buccal pad of fat.
- Stenson's duct.
- Facial artery.

#### 21.10.2.3 Clinical Features

1. Pain and tenderness.
2. Diffuse swelling on the side of the cheek.
3. Obliteration of buccal vestibule.
4. Swelling of upper/lower lip (Fig. 21.3).

#### 21.10.2.4 Management

Drainage of the space infection either intraorally or percutaneously is done; intraoral incision and drainage are preferred as these may not produce a facial scar. Drainage is made by making an in-depth incision of the maxillary vestibule near the involved tooth. Sinus forceps is inserted superiorly, laterally, and medially for complete breakage of locules and drainage. Care is taken while using sinus forceps, so as to not to damage duct and artery (Fig. 21.4a, b, c).

For mandibular buccal space infection, intraoral drainage may not achieve the desired result, hence extraoral drainage at the lower border of mandible is made taking care of the facial artery and marginal mandibular nerve.

The involved tooth is either removed or subjected to root canal treatment as required. Literature advocates early extraction of the involved tooth/teeth. According to Igoumenakis D et al. [9], extraction of the involved tooth shortens the hospital stay and provides faster recovery on a biological level.

### 21.10.3 Temporal Pouches

Infections in this region are relatively rare to occur when involved swelling occurs at the temporal region above zygomatic arch and behind the lateral orbital rim [10]. They are two in number—*Superficial temporal space* and *Deep temporal space* (Fig. 21.5).

#### 21.10.3.1 Superficial Temporal Space

This space lies between the temporal fascia and temporalis muscle.

Source of infection—From upper third molars and infection from other spaces.

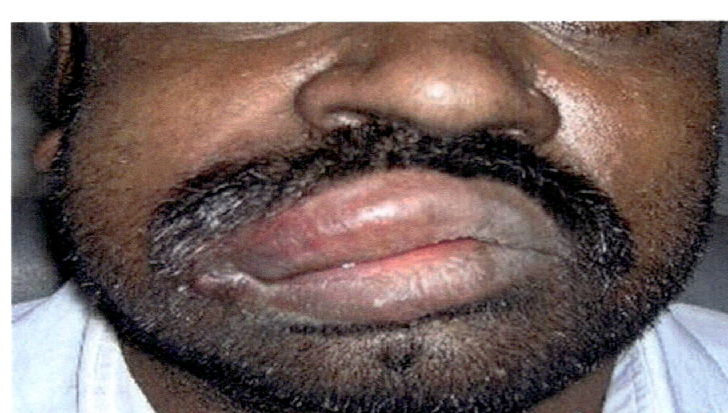



**Fig. 21.3** Clinical picture showing the buccal space infection

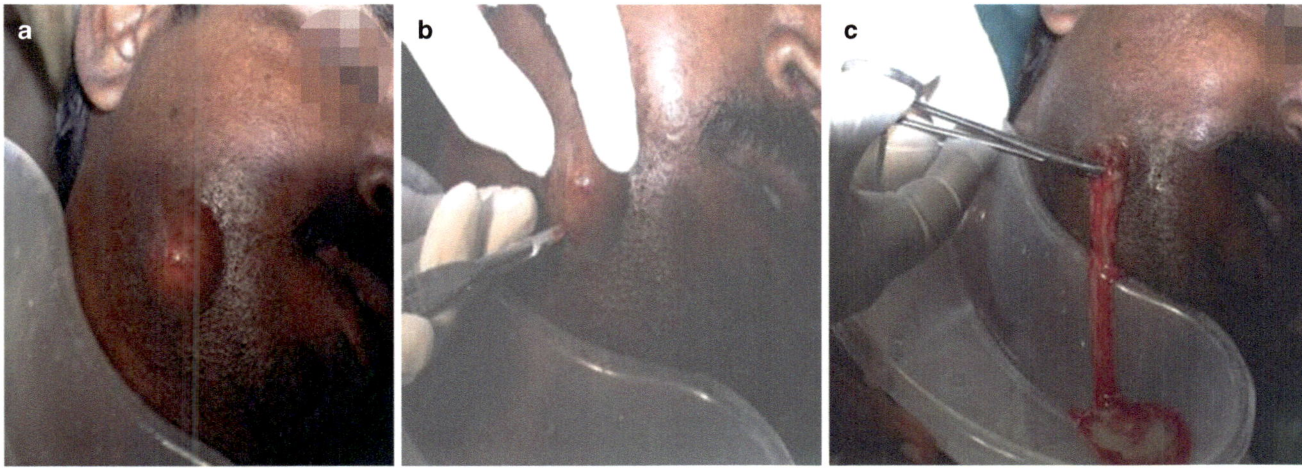




**Fig. 21.4** (**a**, **b**, **c**) Clinical pictures showing the procedure of incision and drainage for buccal space infection (also see Fig. 21.1B)

**Fig. 21.5** Shows the superficial and deep temporal spaces

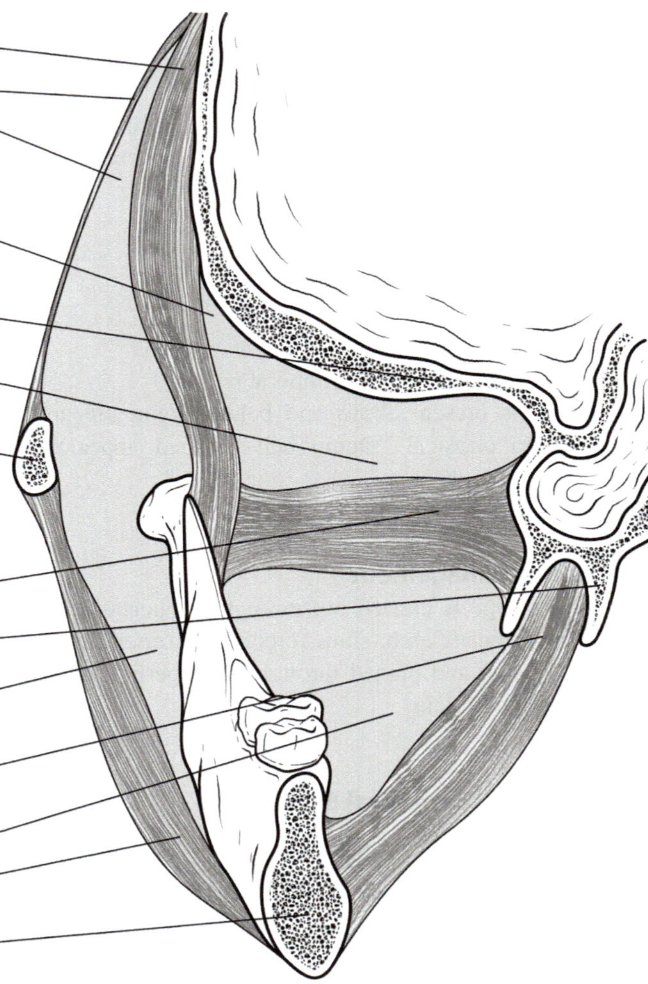

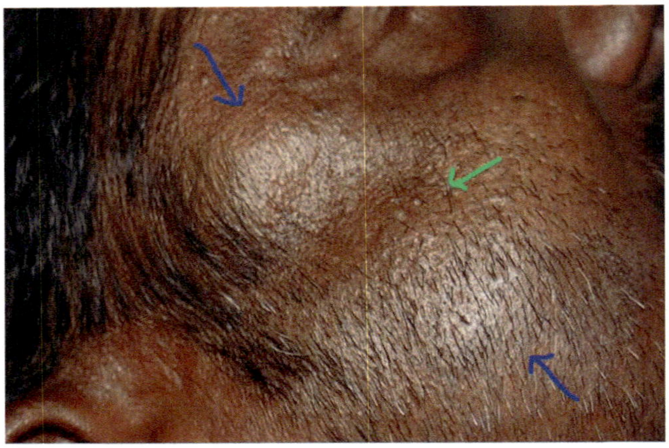



**Fig. 21.6** Clinical image of the classical dumb bell swelling (blue arrows). The isthmus of the swelling at the zygomatic arch is shown by the green arrow

#### 21.10.3.2 Boundaries

- Superior—superior temporal lines.
- Inferior—zygomatic arch.
- Lateral—superficial temporal fascia.
- Medial—temporalis muscle.
- Anterior—posterior surface of lateral orbital rim.
- Posterior—fusion of temporal fascia with pericranium.

#### 21.10.3.3 Contents

- Temporal fat pad.
- Temporal branch of Facial nerve.

#### 21.10.3.4 Clinical Features

1. Pain and tenderness at the temporal region.
2. Swelling is present above and below zygomatic arch, leading to classical "Dumb bell" shaped appearance (Fig. 21.6).
3. Trismus may be present.

#### 21.10.3.5 Management

Surgical drainage is carried out through an incision made above the zygomatic arch; sinus forceps is inserted through the skin incision and passed through the superficial fascia and the temporal fascia.

### 21.10.4 Deep Temporal Space

This space lies between the temporalis muscle and the skull. Slightly below the level of zygomatic arch; both the superficial and deep temporal spaces communicate with each other.

Source of Infection—Upper third molar and spread from other spaces.

#### 21.10.4.1 Boundaries

- Superior—Attachment of temporal fascia to the cranium.
- Inferior—Lateral pterygoid muscle.
- Medial—Medial pterygoid plate and lower part of infratemporal fossa.
- Lateral—Medial surface of the temporalis muscle.

#### 21.10.4.2 Contents

Branches of Internal maxillary artery.
Mandibular division of trigeminal nerve.

#### 21.10.4.3 Clinical Features

1. Pain.
2. Swelling at the infratemporal region and lateral aspect of the eye.
3. Obliteration of buccal sulcus at tuberosity area.
4. Trismus due to proximity of masticatory muscles.
5. Infection may extend to the infratemporal and pterygomandibular region.

#### 21.10.4.4 Management

If the trismus is not severe, intraoral incision is given in the buccal sulcus at the second and third molar region. With the sinus forceps, the space is entered medial to coronoid process superiorly and the pus is drained. Corrugated rubber tube is placed and secured with a suture.

In case of severe trismus, extraoral incision is made above the zygomatic arch at the junction of frontal and temporal process of zygoma, sinus forceps is inserted and directed inferiorly and medially to enter the space and drain the pus. The disadvantage of this approach is that it cannot produce dependent drainage.

## 21.11 Spaces Around the Mandible

### 21.11.1 Submental Space

The infection from any of the six anterior teeth in the mandible may perforate the labial bone inferior to the mentalis muscle attachment and the pus may present at the anterior and lower border of the mandible and below the mylohyoid muscle lingually [11].

#### 21.11.1.1 Source of Infection

- Infection from lower anterior teeth.
- Infected symphyseal or parasymphyseal fractures.
- Suppuration of submental lymphnodes.

#### 21.11.1.2 Boundaries (Fig. 21.7)

- Lateral: Skin, superficial fascia, platysma, superficial layer of deep cervical fascia.
- Medial: Mylohyoid, hyoglossus, and styloglossus.
- Inferior: Anterior and posterior belly of digastric muscles.
- Posterior: Hyoid bone.
- Superior: Medial aspect of mandible and the attachment of mylohyoid muscle.

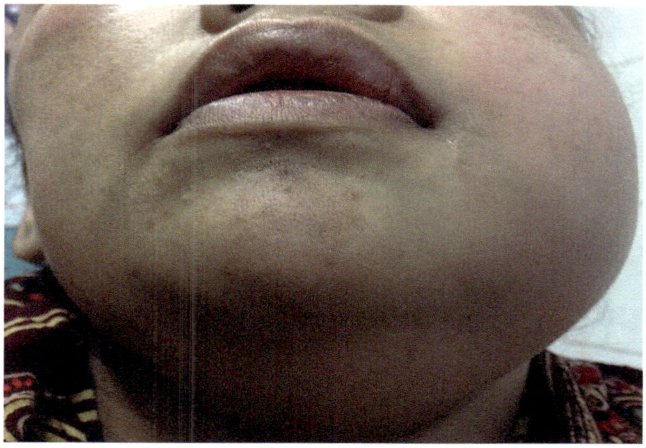



**Fig. 21.7** Clinical picture showing spread of infection to the submental space and buccal space

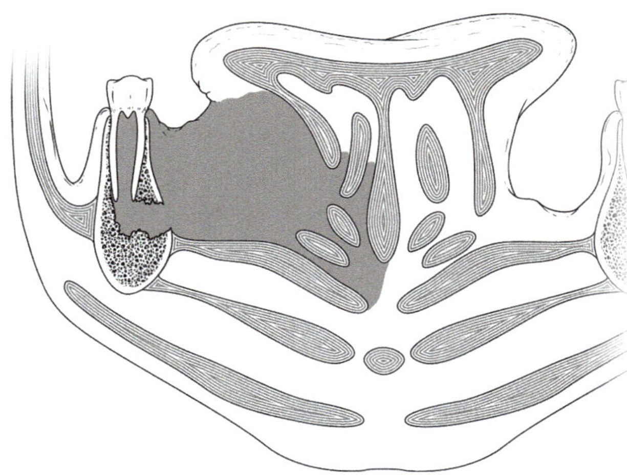



**Fig. 21.8** Shows the spread of infection to the sublingual space (grey shaded area)

#### 21.11.1.3 Contents

- Submental nodes.
- Anterior jugular vein.

#### 21.11.1.4 Clinical Features

1. Pain and tenderness in the chin region.
2. Firm swelling at the chin.
3. Difficulty in swallowing.
4. Tenderness of lower anterior teeth.

#### 21.11.1.5 Management

Transcutaneous approach in the chin region is the most effective drainage; incision is made below the symphysis menti to produce dependent drainage. Sinus forceps is inserted upward and backward to break the locules and the pus is drained. A corrugated rubber drain is inserted and secured with a suture. Intraoral approach is cumbersome as we need to pierce mentalis muscle to reach the submental space and also drainage against gravity is not possible.

### 21.11.2 Sublingual Space

The space is V-shaped lying lateral to the muscles of the tongue and in the lingual aspect of the body of the mandible. Anteriorly communicates with submental space and posteriorly communicates with the submandibular space at the edge of the mylohyoid muscle [12].

#### 21.11.2.1 Source of Infection

- Periapical infection from mandibular teeth is situated above mylohyoid muscle.
- Infection from sublingual gland.

#### 21.11.2.2 Boundaries (Fig. 21.8)

- Anterior: Lingual aspect of mandible.
- Posterior: The body of hyoid bone.
- Superior: Mucosa of oral cavity.
- Inferior: Mylohyoid muscle.
- Medial: Geniohyoid, genioglossus, and styloglossus muscle.

#### 21.11.2.3 Contents

- Lingual nerve and Hypoglossal nerve.
- Deep part submandibular gland and duct.

#### 21.11.2.4 Clinical Features

1. Pain and discomfort during deglutition.
2. Due to edema, there is elevation and protrusion of the tongue.
3. In case of laryngeal edema, there may be breathlessness.
4. Speech may be affected.
5. Enlarged and tender submandibular nodes.

#### 21.11.2.5 Management

- An intraoral incision is made close to lingual cortical plate, near premolar region taking care of lingual nerve and the Wharton's duct. Sinus forceps or a thin mosquito forceps is inserted and the pus is drained.
- If an extraoral approach is planned, then incision is placed at the submandibular region, taking care of the facial artery and marginal mandibular nerve; a sinus forceps is inserted piercing the mylohyoid muscle to drain the pus and a corrugated rubber drain is inserted and secured with a suture, as this approach provides gravity-dependent drainage.

### 21.11.3 Submandibular Space

- The submandibular space is present at the inferior border of the mandible between the anterior and posterior bellies of digastric muscles [13].

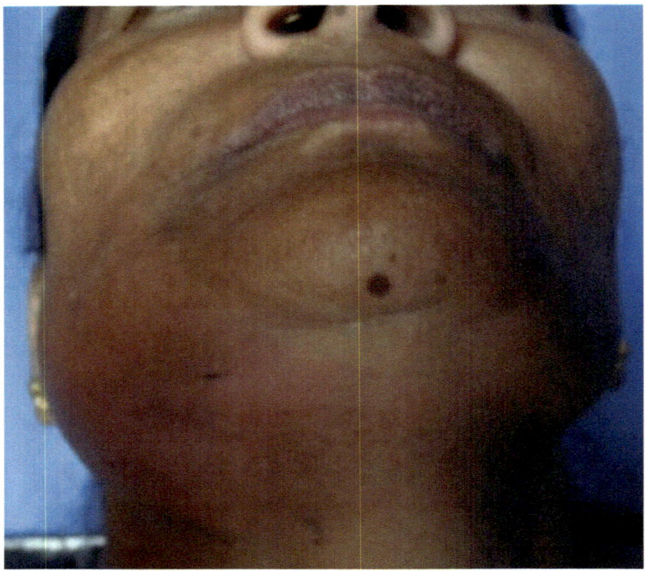



**Fig. 21.9** Clinical picture showing the submandibular space infection

#### 21.11.3.1 Source of Infection

- Infection from the periapical region of molar teeth below mylohyoid muscle.
- Septic fractures of the mandible body region.
- Infections from submandibular salivary gland.
- Infections from submental and sublingual.
- Infection from other space.

#### 21.11.3.2 Boundaries

- Laterally: Skin, superficial fascia, platysma, and superficial layer of deep cervical fascia.
- Medially: Mylohyoid, hyoglossus, and styloglossus.
- Inferiorly: Anterior and posterior belly of digastric muscles.
- Posteriorly: Hyoid bone.
- Superiorly: Medial aspect of mandible and the attachment of mylohyoid muscle.

#### 21.11.3.3 Contents

- Submandibular salivary gland.
- Submandibular nodes.
- Facial artery and vein.

#### 21.11.3.4 Clinical Features (Fig. 21.9)

1. Pain and tenderness.
2. Swelling is situated at the submandibular region, inferior to the lower of the mandible.
3. Swelling is firm to soft in consistency.
4. Submandibular nodes are palpable and tender.
5. Intraoral—the involved teeth are sensitive.
6. Mild trismus may be noticed.

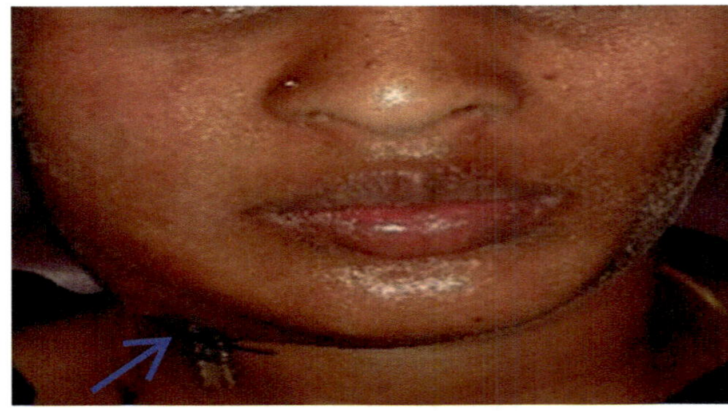



**Fig. 21.10** Clinical pictures showing drain inserted for submandibular space infection

#### 21.11.3.5 Management

It is managed through an extraoral approach; incision is placed at the submandibular region in the most dependent area to facilitate gravitational drainage, taking care of the facial artery and marginal mandibular nerve; a sinus forceps is inserted superiorly, medially, and laterally piercing through the superficial fascia. A drain is inserted and secured with a suture to facilitate dependent drainage (Fig. 21.10).

## 21.12 Masticator Space

Masticator space is formed by splitting of the investing fascia into superficial and deep layers. The superficial layer lies along the lateral surface of the masseter and lower half of the temporalis. Deep layer passes along the medial surface of the pterygoid muscles before attaching to the base of the skull superiorly.

The masticator spaces comprise the following four spaces:

- *Submasseteric space.*
- *Pterygomandibular space.*
- *Temporal space.*
- *Infratemporal space.*

### 21.12.1 Submasseteric Space

Masseter consists of three layers which are firmly attached anteriorly and loose posteriorly. The space is present lateral to ascending ramus of the mandible.

#### 21.12.1.1 Source of Infection

- Infection from buccally placed lower third molar.
- Septic foci from infected angle fracture.
- Infection from other space.

#### 21.12.1.2 Boundaries

- Anterior: Facial extension of parotidomasseteric fascia.
- Posterior: Parotid fascia and deep portion of parotid gland.
- Superiorly: Level of zygomatic arch.
- Lateral: Medial surface of the Masseter muscle.
- Medial: Lateral surface of the ramus.

#### 21.12.1.3 Clinical Features

1. Pain and tenderness at angle mandible.
2. Moderate size swelling at the angle region.
3. Firm consistency swelling.
4. Severe trismus.

#### 21.12.1.4 Management

The drainage of the infection is done through two approaches.

In intraoral approach, incision is placed at the retromolar area along the anterior border of the ramus of mandible. The sinus forceps is inserted through the incision laterally between the mandibular ramus and the masseter muscle to explore the Submasseteric space. The disadvantage of intraoral technique is that incision and drainage is not gravity dependent.

In extraoral approach, the incision is placed on the skin at the angle and inferior border of the mandible; sinus forceps is inserted directing superiorly piercing the subcutaneous tissue and masseter muscle. Abscess drained corrugated rubber tube is placed and secured with a suture. Precautions are taken not to damage the marginal mandibular nerve (Figs. 21.11 and 21.12).

### 21.12.2 Pterygomandibular Space

One of the most frequently encountered space in dental office is pterygomandibular space [14].

#### 21.12.2.1 Source of Infection

- From lower third molar.
- Contaminated needle used during inferior alveolar nerve block.

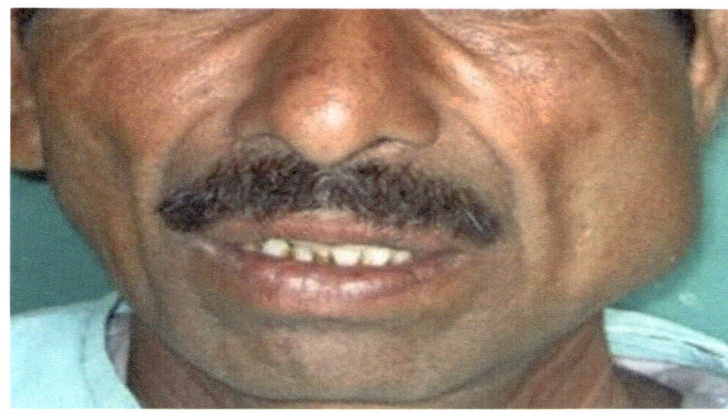



Fig. 21.12 Clinical picture showing submasseteric space infection left side, pus was drained extraorally

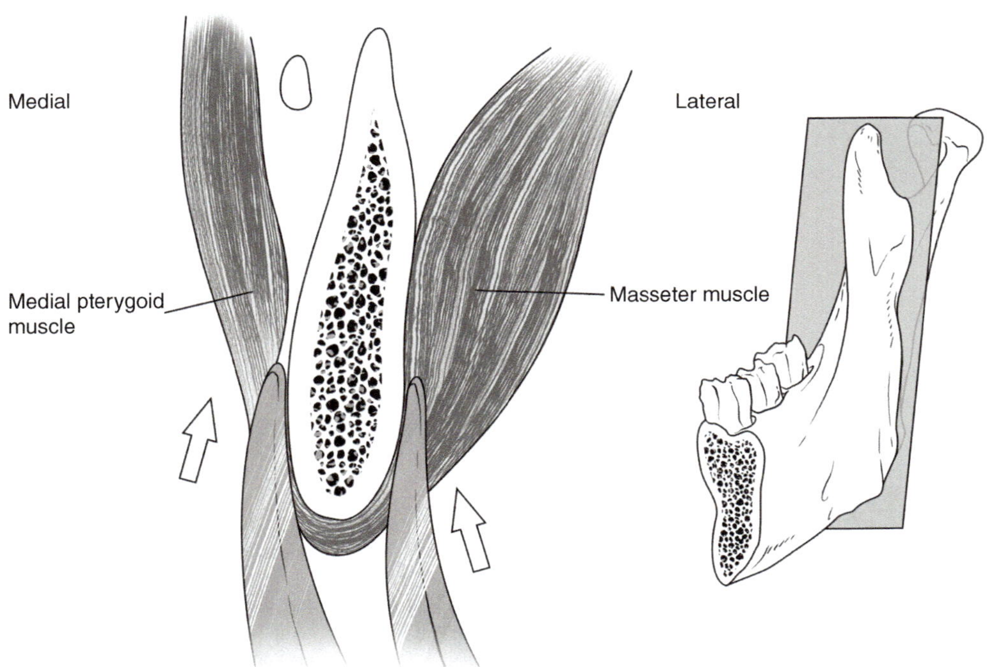




Fig. 21.11 Schematic representation of approaches to the masticator spaces

- Septic fractures of the mandibular angle.
- Infection from other spaces (Superficial temporal).

### 21.12.2.2 Boundaries

- Lateral: Medial surface of mandible.
- Medial: Lateral aspect of medial pterygoid muscle.
- Anterior: Pterygomandibular raphe.
- Posterior: Deep part of parotid gland.
- Superior: Lateral pterygoid muscle and infratemporal surface of greater wing of sphenoid bone.

### 21.12.2.3 Contents

- Inferior Alveolar Nerve and artery.
- Lingual Nerve.
- Long Buccal Nerve.
- Nerve to Mylohyoid.

### 21.12.2.4 Clinical Features (Fig. 21.13)

1. Pain at the retromolar region.
2. Dysphagia.
3. Trismus.
4. No obvious swelling extraorally.
5. Swelling near anterior tonsillar pillar.
6. Deviation of Uvula.

### 21.12.2.5 Management

Generally, incision and drainage are done through intraoral approach; however, in case of severe trismus, extraoral approach may be indicated. Drainage is done either under general anesthesia or by giving mandibular nerve block.

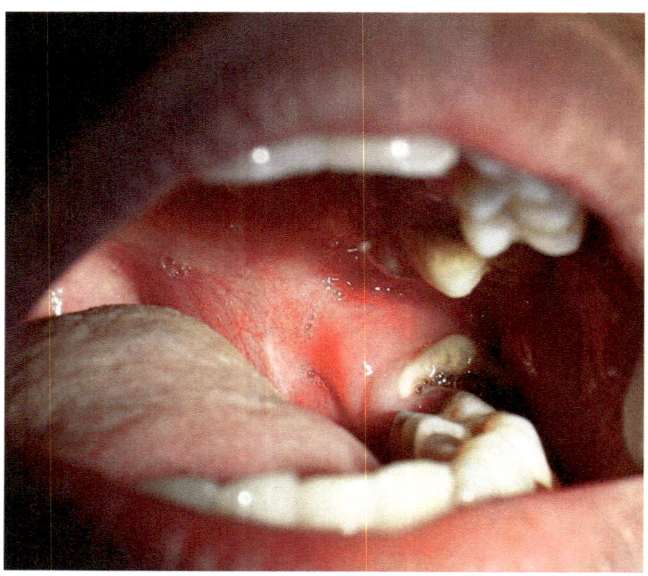



**Fig. 21.13** Clinical picture of left pterygomandibular space infection forming a decayed impacted lower left third molar. Note the limited mouth opening

#### Intraoral Approach

A vertical incision of 1.5 cm is made at the anterior and medial aspect of the mandible, sinus forceps is inserted into the abscess cavity, and pus is evacuated. Corrugated rubber drain is inserted and sutured to the margins of the incision to prevent dislodgement.

#### Extraoral Approach

In case of severe trismus, this approach is advised, an incision of 1.5 cm is made on the skin, toward the inner aspect of the angle region. Sinus forceps is inserted toward the medial aspect of the mandible directing superiorly close to the bone. Pus is evacuated and rubber drain is inserted and sutured to the margins of the incision.

Figure 21.14 shows various approaches which can be used for fascial space infections and Fig. 21.15 shows submandibular approach to the medial and lateral masticator spaces.

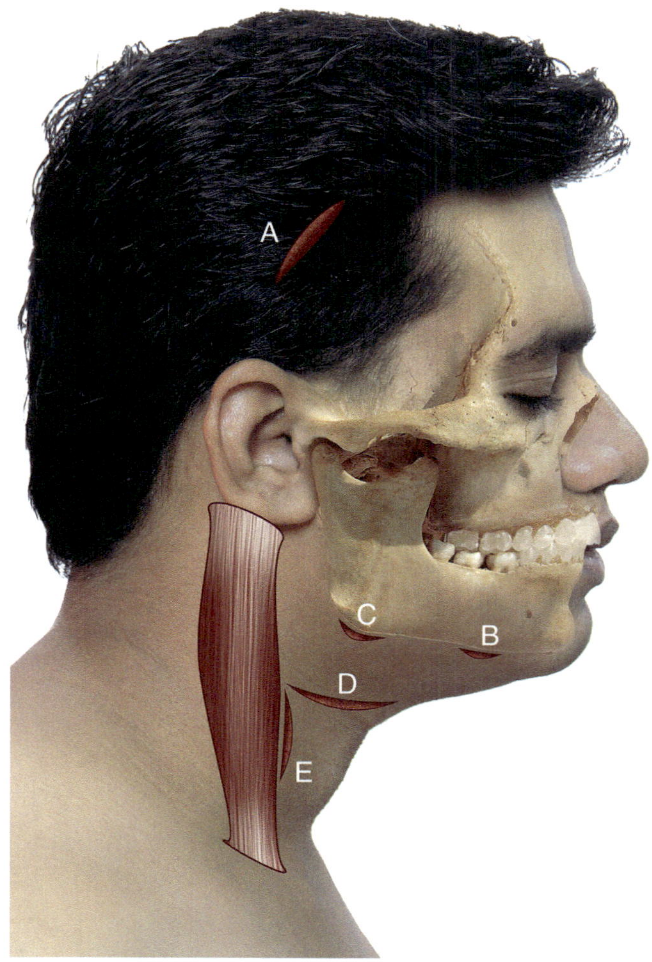




**Fig. 21.14** Shows the extraoral incisions for the space infections, (**a**) temporal space, (**b**) submental space, (**c**) submandibular space, (**d**) lateral pharyngeal space, (**e**) retropharyngeal space

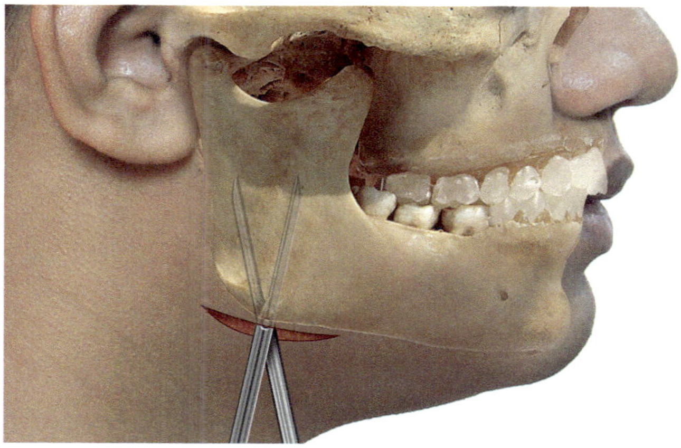



**Fig. 21.15** Diagrammatic representation of the approach to the pterygoid space (medial) or massetric space (lateral) via submandibular incision

## 21.13 Spaces of Neck

### 21.13.1 Parapharyngeal Spaces

The spaces around the pharynx form a 'Ring' and a pathway for spread of infections from the orofacial region to the neck and mediastinum. The Parapharyngeal space includes Lateral Pharyngeal space and Retropharyngeal space.

### 21.13.2 Lateral Pharnygeal Space

It is a potential space lying lateral to the pharynx, extending from base of the skull to the hyoid bone. The space is conical in shape, base being toward the base of the skull and apex toward the hyoid bone.

#### 21.13.2.1 Source of Infection

- From other spaces which includes.
- Pterygomandibular space.
- Submandibular space.
- From Tonsils.
- From the lower third molar region.

#### 21.13.2.2 Boundaries

- Superior: Base of the skull.
- Inferior: Hyoid bone.
- Anterior: Pterygomandibular raphe, Superior and middle pharyngeal constrictor.
- Posterior: Carotid sheath, Stylohyoid, Styloglossus, and Stylopharyngeus.
- Medial: Superior constrictor of Pharynx and Retropharyngeal space.
- Lateral: Medial pterygoid muscle, Deep lobe of the parotid gland.

#### 21.13.2.3 Contents

- Lymph nodes.
- Ascending Pharyngeal artery and Facial artery.
- Carotid sheath.
- Glossopharyngeal nerve, Spinal Accessory nerve, Hypoglossal nerve.

#### 21.13.2.4 Clinical Features

1. No or minimal external swelling on the lateral aspect of the neck.
2. Moderate limitation of mouth opening.
3. Rotation of neck to contralateral side is painful.
4. Dysphagia.
5. Uvula is pushed to opposite side.
6. Pharyngeal bulging is seen (Swelling over pillars of fauces and superior constrictor).

#### 21.13.2.5 Management

A combination of intra-oral and extra-oral approaches are advised for the managment of infections of the lateral pharyngeal space. They are preferably done under general anesthesia with care taken to secure the airway.

*Intraoral approach*—A 1.5 cm incision is made on the Pterygomandibular raphe, sinus forceps is passed through the raphe on the medial surface of the mandible, medial aspect of the medial pterygoid muscle, and lateral aspect of the superior constrictor muscle.

*Extraoral approach*—An incision of 2.5 cm is made in the submandibular region, blunt dissection is then carried through the fascia just anterior to the sternocleidomastoid muscle, and digital palpation can enter and dissect the lateral pharyngeal space bluntly (Fig. 21.16). The landmarks to be palpated are the angle of the mandible anterolaterally, the carotid sheath posterolaterally, the transverse processes of the cervical vertebrae posteromedially, and the endotracheal tube, if present, anteromedially. Caution must be taken not to perforate the posterior oropharyngeal wall by aggressive finger dissection toward the oropharynx [15].

*Combined approach*—Intraoral incision is made on the mucosa at the medial aspect of the ramus of the mandible, curved hemostasis is inserted lateral to superior constrictor muscle and medial to medial pterygoid muscle and the blunt dissection is carried out posterio-inferiorly below the angle of the mandible. The tip of the instrument is palpated at the anterior border of the sternocleidomastoid muscle extraorally and cutaneous incision is made over the tip. A drain is inserted and sutured to the wound margin to allow drainage.

Maintaining the endo-tracheal tube or tracheostomy may be considered depending on the severity of infection and the success of drainage.

### 21.13.3 Retropharyngeal Space

It is also called as prevertebral space, which is a potential space present in the midline between the pharyngobasilar

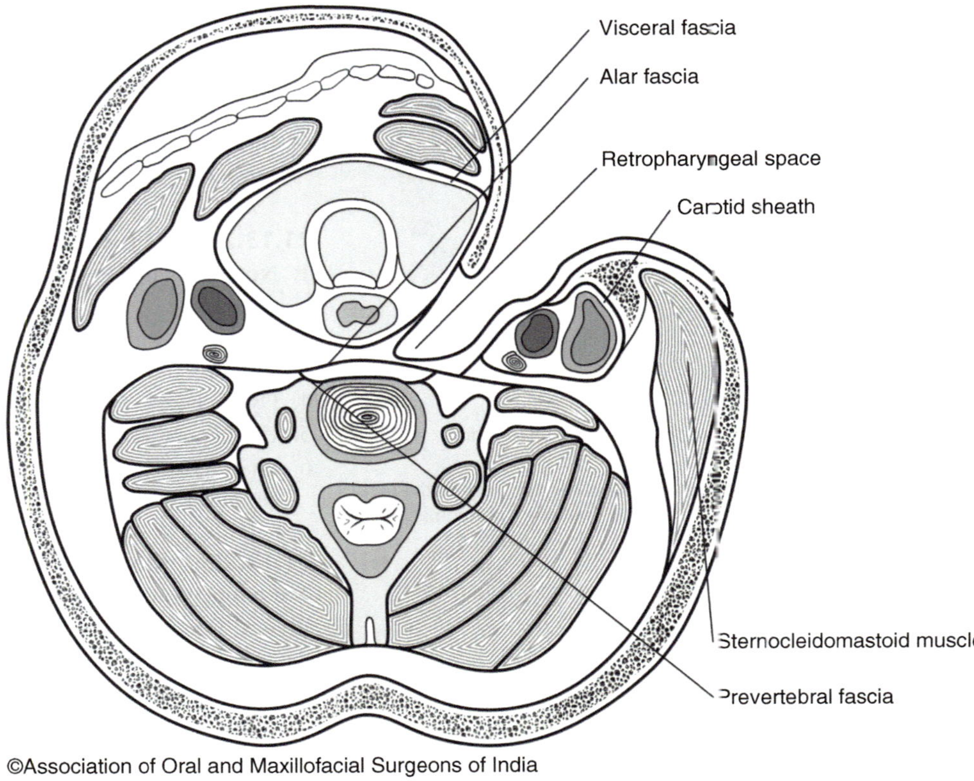


**Fig. 21.16** Shows the approach for the retropharyngeal space infection

fascia and prevertebral fascia. This space is continuous with retropharyngeal space into the posterior mediastinum.

#### 21.13.3.1 Source of Infection

- From Lateral pharyngeal space.
- From the lymph nodes that drain into Waldeyer's ring.
- Rarely from upper respiratory infections.

#### 21.13.3.2 Boundaries

- Superior—Base of the skull.
- Inferior—Fusion of alar and Prevertebral fascia.
- Anterior—Superior and Medial constrictors.
- Posterior—Alar fascia.
- Lateral—Carotid sheath and Lateral pharyngeal space.

#### 21.13.3.3 Contents of the Space

- Lymph nodes.

#### 21.13.3.4 Clinical Features

1. Stiff neck.
2. Sore throat.
3. Dysphagia.
4. Lateral neck swelling and occasional erythema.
5. Fever.
6. Dyspnea.
7. Mediastinitis is the most feared complication of this space.

#### 21.13.3.5 Management

Most important is to secure airway. may be an elective tracheostomy or fiber optic intubation is considered for airway maintenance.

Intraoral approach is generally done for the suprahyoid part of the retropharyngeal infection, procedure is similar to the one done for lateral pharyngeal space infection. Intraoral incision is made on the mucosa at the medial aspect of the ramus of the mandible, curved hemostat is inserted lateral to superior constrictor muscle and medial to medial pterygoid muscle, and the blunt dissection is carried out further inferiorly.

Extraoral approach is better for the infection at the infrahyoid region, incision is made transcutaneously anterior to the sternocleidomastoid muscle at the level of the angle of the mandible to the level of the hyoid bone. Both sternocleidomastoid muscle and Carotid sheath are identified, and retracted. Blunt dissection is carried out into lateral and retropharyngeal spaces, later being verified by the palpation of anterior process of the cervical spine posteriorly and the endotracheal tube anteriorly [16]. Drain is placed and secured to the edges of the cutaneous incision.

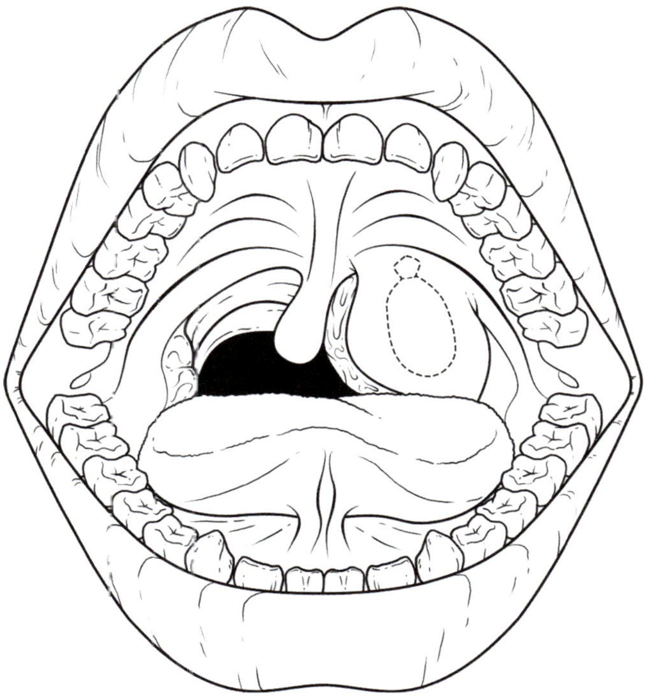

©Association of Oral and Maxillofacial Surgeons of India

Fig. 21.17 Shows the boundaries of peritonsillar abscess

### 21.13.4 Peritonsillar Abscess: (Quincy)

It is a localized infection near the tonsils, usually occurring as a secondary infection from the local sites.

#### 21.13.4.1 Source of Infection

- From tonsillitis.
- Rarely from Pericoronitis.
- From Lateral pharyngeal space.

#### 21.13.4.2 Boundaries

- Anterior—Anterior pillar of fauces.
- Posterior—Posterior pillar of fauces.
- Medially—Tonsil.
- Laterally—Superior constrictor muscle (Fig. 21.17).

#### 21.13.4.3 Clinical Features

1. Pain in the throat radiating to ear.
2. Fever.
3. Dehydration.
4. Dysphagia.
5. Swelling visible at anterior pillar of tonsillar fauces.
6. Redness and edema may be extended to soft palate.
7. Drooling of saliva.
8. Change of voice and speech difficulty in case of bilateral involvement.
9. Mouth opening difficulty may not be present.

#### 21.13.4.4 Management

Intraoral approach, superficial incision made at the most prominent area of the swelling near anterior pillar and the soft palate, sinus forceps is inserted deep into the tissues to break all the locules and drain the pus [17].

## 21.14 Sequelae of Space Infections, if Ignored

Possible life-threatening complications may be developed if the space infections of the jaws are not addressed adequately; for ease of understanding, the complications are classified as follows (Table 21.5).

**Specific warning signs in space infections include:**

- Dyspnea (difficulty breathing).
- Dysphagia (difficulty/pain with swallowing).
- Severe trismus.
- Rapidly progressive swelling.
- Edema of eyelids and abnormal eye signs.
- Impaired vision or eye movement or both.
- Change in voice quality.
- Lethargy.
- Agitation, restlessness due to hypoxia.
- Evidence of meningeal irritation-severe headache, stiff neck, vomiting.
- Decreased level of consciousness.

### 21.14.1 Ludwig's Angina

It was first described by Wilhelm Friedreich Von Ludwig in 1836, and the term Ludwig's Angina was coined by Camerer in 1937. The word Angina is derived from Latin language meaning suffocation or choking.

Ludwig's Angina is defined as an acute, firm, non-suppurating, necrotizing cellulitis involving bilateral Submandibular, Sublingual, and Submental spaces. The condition has been described by medical practitioners, by three unique features, starting with the alphabet 'F'—Feared, Fluctuant rarely, Fatal often.

Many terminologies were used for this condition like Marbus Strangularis, Angina Maligna, and Garotillo.

Table 21.5 Sequelae of space infections if ignored

| Complications from spaces around mandible | Comlications from spaces around maxilla |
|---|---|
| Ludwig's angina | Cavernous sinus thrombosis |
| Necrotizing fasciitis | Meningitis |

#### 21.14.1.1 Source

Predominantly (90%) odontogenic in origin, from the lower jaw.

Infection from 2nd and 3rd molar teeth may be Acute dentoalveolar abscess, Periodontal Abscess.

- Pericoronal Abscess. Infected cyst at the body and the angle of the mandible.
- Traumatic injuries especially to the mandible, either ignored or not managed well leading to sepsis.
- Salivary gland infections.
- Iatrogenic reasons.
- Hematogenous infections.

#### 21.14.1.2 Predisposing Factors

- Immunosuppression.
- Uncontrolled Diabetes.
- Steroid therapy.
- Debilitating conditions.

#### 21.14.1.3 Clinical Features (Table 21.6)

The infection of the sublingual space rapidly spreads along to its base which is present at the hyoid bone. A characteristic feature is edema of the epiglottis and the vocal cords, due to the spread of infection in a postero-inferior direction from the sub-lingual space to the laryngeal inlet. This may produce acute respiratory obstruction and death [18].

**Table 21.6** Clinical features of Ludwig's angina

| General/Systemic | Regional/Local |
|---|---|
| Patient appears toxic | Firm to hard swelling |
| Fever | Tense, nonfluctuant, non-pitting, and wood like/brawny |
| Dehydrated | Tender |
| Anorexia | Trismus |
| Malaise | Mouth open appearance |
| Difficulty in swallowing | Fetid odor |
| Hoarseness of voice | Raised floor of the mouth |
| | Shallow breathing |

#### 21.14.1.4 Management

It should be treated as life-threatening situation and intervened aggressively

The treatment of Ludwig's Angina is primarily surgical. The first priority in the management is always the life-saving measure. If the patient shows any signs of dyspnea, Tracheostomy should be performed promptly

Treatment protocol is as follows:

- Early diagnosis.
- Maintenance of airway.
- Intravenous broad spectrum antibiotics and fluids.
- Necessary investigations.
- Removal of the cause and surgical drainage and decompression of fascial spaces.

Endotracheal intubation is nearly impossible due to trismus, tongue elevation, and laryngeal edema. A skilled anesthetist with fiber optic laryngoscope may try Nasoendotracheal intubation, while the patient is conscious and awake, while the tracheostomy kit is kept on standby, in case of emergency (please refer Chap. 7 to read about anesthesia procedures in patients with space infections).

Once the airway is secure, the next step is surgical decompression of spaces and tissue planes; this is achieved by giving multiple cutaneous incisions in the submandibular and submental regions. Decompression of sublingual space is very important, which is achieved by piercing the mylohyoid muscle. This can also be achieved by placing an incision in the floor of the mouth, parallel to the lingual vestibule. There may not be much pus to drain as the condition is usually non-supperative (Fig. 21.18a, b, c). Corrugated rubber drain may be left in situ to keep the incisions patient and to drain the exudates [19]

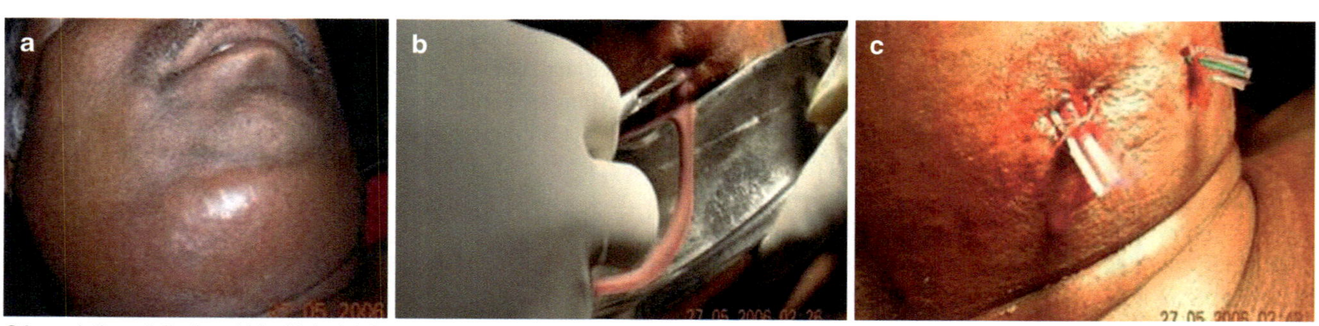




**Fig. 21.18** (**a**, **b**, **c**) Clinical pictures showing the drainage of Ludwig's angina

Purpose of decompression is threefold:

1. Reduces tension within the tissue planes and prevents further spread of infection.
2. As the pressure in the tissue drops, circulation improves and facilitates the reduction of the edema.
3. Drains septic material and prevents bacteremia.

After decompression, simultaneous removal of the cause is important, as this is the source of the condition.

Intravenous fluids are administered to maintain proper fluid and electrolyte balance and to fulfill the nutritional requirement of the patient. Definitive antibiotics are given intravenously based on the culture and sensitivity reports. Other symptomatic medicines like anti-inflammatory and analgesics may be prescribed. Local wound care is taken care of by irrigation and dressings. Drains to be changed every 48 hrs and maintained until the condition resolves.

### 21.14.2 Necrotizing Fasciitis

Necrotizing fasciitis is an uncommon soft tissue infection, occurs due to polymicrobes and spreads rapidly in the subcutaneous tissue and above superficial fascia, and as the disease progresses, muscle and skin involve giving rise to myonecrosis. The other name for this condition is Hospital Gangrene given by Brooks in 1966 and Hemolytic streptococcal gangrene. Necrotizing fasciitis may affect any part of the body; however, it most commonly affects the extremities, abdominal wall, and the perineum following trauma or surgery.

The condition shows no clear boundaries or palpable limits, mainly occurs with immunocompromised patients and those suffering from systemic illnesses (Fig. 21.19).

#### 21.14.2.1 Source

The causative organisms in this condition are multiple like Aerobic Group A—hemolytic Streptococcus and Staphylococcus and later identified microbes are Bacteroids, Proteus, coliforms, and peptostreptococcus. In most cases, the pathogens gain entry through disruption of the skin caused by trauma or surgery. Continuous bacterial overgrowth and synergy cause a decrease in oxygen tension and develop local ischemia and proliferation of anaerobic bacteria. The fulminating nature of the necrotic process is the result of the symbiotic relationship between the bacteria.

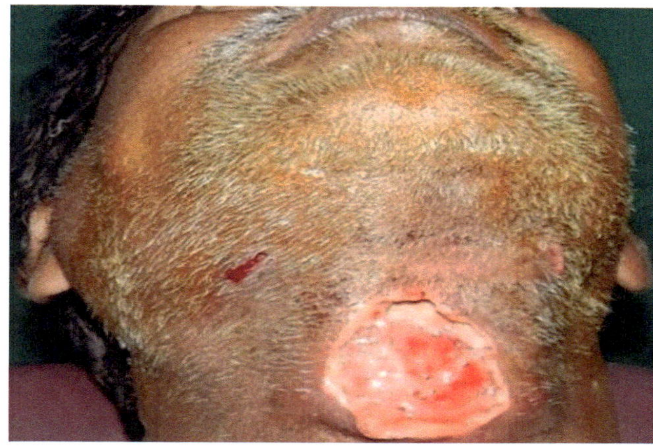



**Fig. 21.19** Clinical picture showing the necrotizing fasciitis

**Table 21.7** Clinical features of necrotizing fasciitis

| Systemic | Local |
|---|---|
| High fever | Involved area is swollen and erythematous |
| Weakness | Change of overlying skin color to dusky with purple mottling |
| Dehydration | Visible slough on the surface with underlying necrotic fascia |
| Toxic appearance | Paraesthesia of the affected area |
| Tachycardia | Foul smell |
| Sepsis | |
| Hemolysis | |

#### 21.14.2.2 Clinical Features (Table 21.7)

#### 21.14.2.3 Investigations

- Complete blood picture (Leukocytosis, Band cells, and Toxic granules in Leukocytes).
- Ultrasonography of the neck—Shows the collection in the superficial planes.
- CT Scans are useful in detecting the deep-seated collections and the necrosis.

#### 21.14.2.4 Management

Early recognition and aggressive surgical intervention is mandatory; taking the medical parameters into consideration and airway maintenance, general anesthesia is preferred in most cases.

Initially, intravenous broad spectrum antibiotics are administered to control the spread of the infection; these antibiotics may be changed once the culture report is obtained.

Surgical treatment is obligatory with incision and drainage, in addition to vigorous debridement of the necrotic fascia, subcutaneous tissue, muscle, and skin. Excision of tissue to the point of fresh bleeding is advised. Multiple and regular change of dressings are needed till the condition is resolved.

Some centers may follow Hyperbaric oxygen therapy for this condition.

### 21.14.3 Cavernous Sinus Thrombosis

Cavernous sinuses are the venous sinuses situated on either side of the sella tursica. The cavernous sinus on either side communicates freely with each other by anterior and posterior intracavernous sinuses they also communicate with sagittal sinus, transverse, sinus and sigmoid sinus. The cavernous sinus communicates extra cranially with veins of the head and neck.

1. The ophthalmic vein and angular veins into the anterior facial vein.
2. Through emissary veins from the pterygoid plexus of veins.

*External route*—Infection from face and lips carried by facial and angular veins and nasofrontal veins to the superior ophthalmic vein passes through the superior orbital fissure and enters the cavernous sinus.

*Internal route*—Infection from the posterior maxillary region to the pterygoid plexus to the inferior ophthalmic vein through the inferior orbital fissure and then through the superior orbital fissure to the cavernous sinus.

#### 21.14.3.1 Source

The area of the face between the inner canthus of the eyes and the corners of the mouth is called `Danger Triangle` of the face and any kind of severe sepsis in this area can spread in a retrograde manner and can extend to the cavernous sinus through the angular vein and ophthalmic vein.

Causative agents identified are Streptococcus, Staphylococcus, and Gram negative microbes.

#### 21.14.3.2 Clinical Features

- High fever.
- Sweating.
- Swelling (cellulitis) of the face.
- Edema, congestion, and tenderness of the eyelids.
- Ptosis.
- Exopthalmus.
- Diplopia due to involvement of 3rd, 4th, and 6th cranial nerves.
- Increased intracranial pressure due to venous congestion and cerebral edema.
- Altered level of consciousness.
- Pyogenic meningitis leading to brain abscess.
- Erosion of the internal carotid artery leading to fatal intracranial hemorrhage.

#### 21.14.3.3 Eagleton Criteria

Diagnostic criteria were suggested by Eagleton, prior to modern investigative methods.

1. Known site of infection or septicaemia.
2. Evidence of blood stream infection.
3. Early signs of venous obstruction in the retina, conjunctiva, or eyelid.
4. Paresis of the third, fourth, and sixth cranial nerve.
5. Abscess formation in the neighboring soft tissue.
6. Evidence of meningeal irritation.

#### 21.14.3.4 Management

The patient should be given broad spectrum intra venous antibiotics preferably those which cross the blood brain barrier. Aminoglycosides and Clindamycin are started in high therapeutic doses. IV Mannitol is given to decrease the intra cranial pressure. Anticoagulant Heparin 20,000 units in 1500 ml of 5% Dextrose is advised to reduce thrombosis.

Neurosurgical intervention is mandatory.

### 21.14.4 Meningitis

It is one of the neurological complications resulting from the infection of oro-facial region. It may develop from metastatic spread or may be due to nearby thrombophlebitis.

#### 21.14.4.1 Clinical Features

1. High fever with chills
2. Irritability and mental confusion
3. Head ache
4. Vomiting
5. Stiff neck—Brudzinski's sign
6. Positive Kernig's sign
7. Convulsions

#### 21.14.4.2 Diagnosis

Diagnosis is based on cerebrospinal fluid analysis. In CSF polymorpho-nuclear leukocytes, elevated protein levels and decreased glucose levels are noticed.

#### 21.14.4.3 Treatment

- Initially with Chloramphenicol 4 g/day-IV associated with Penicillin G 24 million units per day IV

– Mandatory neurosurgical consultation.
– For raised intracranial pressure IV Manniotol is given.

Maintenance of hydro-electrolyte balance is recommended. Change of antibiotics if required after culture and sensitivity report.

## 21.15 Conclusion

Odontogenic infections are typically polymicrobial. The pathogenesis of odontogenic infections depend on a synergistic relationship between aerobic and anaerobic bacteria.

The last decade showed a notable change in the behavior of odontogenic infections. The severity of these infections is far greater than in the past, demanding swift recognition of the disease followed by prompt and more aggressive treatment. Failing to identify and treat these infections promptly may result in disastrous outcomes.

Definitive treatment includes airway management, adequate resuscitation and optimization of pre-existing medical conditions prior to removal of the source of infection, and drainage of pus.

Oral and high-dose intravenous antibiotics should be administered as required depending on the severity of infection and based on the decision whether the patient is treated on an outpatient or inpatient basis, with the initial choice of antibiotics modified in the light of subsequent bacteriological reports. The treatment of all odontogenic infections must include removal of the focus of infection and drainage of pus.

## References


1. Shapiro DS, Schwartz DR. Exposure of laboratory workers to Francisella tularensis despite a bioterrorism procedure. J Clin Microbiol. 2002:40(6):2278–81.
2. Standring S, editor. Gray's anatomy: the anatomical basis of clinical practice. Philadelphia: Elsevier Churchill Livingstone; 2005.
3. Guidera AK, Dawes PJD, Fong A, Stringer MD. Head and neck fascia and compartments: no space for spaces. Head Neck. 2014;35(7):1058–68.
4. Mirochnik R, Araidy S, Yaffe V. Imad Abu El-Naaj severity score as a prognostic factor for Management of Infections of odontogenic origin, a study of 100 cases. Open J Stomatol. 2017;7:25–34.
5. Flynn TR. What are the antibiotics of choice for odontogenic infections, and how long should the treatment course last? Oral Maxillofac Surg Clin N Am. 2011;23:519–36.
6. Martins JR, et al. The use of antibiotics in odontogenic infections: what is the best choice? A systematic review. J Oral Maxillofac Surg. 2017;75:2606.e1–2606.e11.
7. Grodinsky M, Holyoke E. The fascial and fascial spaces of the head and neck and adjacent regions. Am J Anat. 1938;63:367–407.
8. Ansari MK, et al. Management of Odontogenic Buccal Space Infection in patient with severe hemophilia A-case report. Int Arch Oral Maxillofac Surg. 2008;2:1–4.
9. Igoumenakis D, et al. Effect of causative tooth extraction on clinical and biological parameters of odontogenic infection: a prospective clinical trial. J Oral Maxillofac Surg. 2015;73:1254–8.
10. Fiscaletti D, Sorli A. A-temporal physical space and introduction to the theory of everything. Sci Inq. 2007;8:65–80.
11. Carter LM, Layton S. Cervicofacial infection of dental origin presenting to maxillofacial surgery units in the United Kingdom: a national audit. Br Dent J. 2009;206:73–8.
12. Kao S, Jo C, Oral and Maxillofacial Infections. Clinical review of oral and maxillofacial surgery. Mosby. 2014:95–118.
13. Rizzo PB, Da Mosto MC. Submandibular space infection: a potentially lethal infection. Int J Infect Dis. 2009;13:327–33.
14. Khoury JN, Mihailidis S. Applied anatomy of the pterygomandibular space: improving the success of inferior alveolar nerve blocks. Aust Dent J. 2011;56:112–21.
15. Qureshi FG, Newman KD. Pediatric surgery. 7th ed; 2012. p. 737–43. Lymph Node Disorders
16. Albert T, Balderston R, Northrup B. Surgical approaches to the spine. Philadelphia: Saunders; 1997.
17. Scott GM, Fung K, Roth KE. Novel high-fidelity peritonsillar abscess simulator. Otolaryngol Head Neck Surg. 2016;154:634–7.
18. Farr J, Stanhope ED. Ludwigs angina. Br Med J. 1945;3:295–6.
19. Ramadhan A, et al. One incision approach to multiple facial spaces: technical note incision approach to multiple facial space. Int J Oral Care Res. 2017;5:9–14.


## Additional Suggested Reading


Flynn TR. Oral and maxillofacial infections: 15 unanswered questions. Oral Maxillofac Surg Clin North Am. 2011 Nov;23(4):ix–x.

# Osteomyelitis, Osteoradionecrosis, and Medication-Related Osteonecrosis of Jaws

# 22

Christian Walter and Christoph Renné

## 22.1 Introduction

Bones belong to the connective tissue. Their main function is the internal support and source of inorganic ions. Bones have an organic matrix that is secondarily calcified with calcium salts, mainly hydroxyapatite. The organic matrix consists of a huge extent of type I collagen. Only 5% are other proteoglycans and non-collagenous proteins [1].

There are two major bone parts: The outer compact and the interior cancellous part. In the compact bone, the collagen fibrils form concentric lamellae around a central canal that is called the Haversian canal. These canals harbor vessels which are interconnected by further vessels lying in the Volkmann's canals. The fibrils in neighboring lamellae have a perpendicular orientation resulting in higher stability of the bone. In between the calcified lamellae are therefore concentric orientated osteocytes. Their main function seems to be the mineralization of the bone [1]. The compact bone is responsible for approximately 80% of the entire bone weight [2]. The main function of the compact bone is mechanical stability whereas the cancellous bone mainly has a metabolic function [1]. The cancellous bone consists of small lamellae and has a surface 10 times bigger than the compact bone [2]. On the outside of the compact bone is the periosteum, on the inside the endosteum.

There are three kinds of bone cells: The osteoblasts, the osteocytes, and the osteoclasts.

C. Walter (✉)
Oral and Maxillofacial Surgery – Plastic Surgery, Mediplus Clinic Mainz, Mainz, Germany
e-mail: walter@mainz-mkg.de

C. Renné
Group Practice for Pathology Wiesbaden, Wiesbaden, Germany

### 22.1.1 Osteoblasts

Osteoblasts derive from a multipotential stem cell that differentiates via an osteoprogenitor cell into osteoblasts. Osteoblasts form new bone by the production of the inorganic matrix that mineralizes eventually. After a cycle of bone resorption and consecutive bone formation, most osteoblasts become lining cells covering the surface of the bone [1].

### 22.1.2 Osteocyte

During the course of bone formation, approximately 10% of the osteoblasts build themselves into the bony structure and become osteocytes [2]. It is assumed that the number of osteocytes is 10 times higher than the number of osteoblasts in the adult human body. The osteocytes are stellate cells that have lots of slim processes that are connected to surrounding cells. Osteocytes with their three-dimensional network seem to play the key role in bone remodeling [1].

### 22.1.3 Osteoclast

From all bone cells osteoclasts represent the smallest fraction. Osteoclasts are multinucleated giant cells that resorb bone. They derive from the monocyte macrophage line. Their only function is to resorb mineralized tissue as it is necessary for bone growth, remodeling, and tooth eruption. Most bone diseases are associated with an increased function of the osteoclasts. Therefore, osteoclasts are often the pharmaceutical target in the therapy of bone diseases such as malignancies or metabolic diseases as osteoporosis. Osteoclasts are regulated by the RANK RANKL OPG system [1, 3].


K. Bonanthaya et al. (eds.), *Oral and Maxillofacial Surgery for the Clinician*, https://doi.org/10.1007/978-981-15-1346-6_22

### 22.1.4 RANK RANKL OPG

The receptor activator of nuclear factor κB ligand (RANKL) is an osteoclast differentiating factor mainly expressed by osteoblasts. Secretion of RANKL leads to the differentiation of osteoclasts out of precursor cells, and the activation of osteoclasts to resorb bone by binding on RANK that is expressed on both the precursor cells and the mature osteoclasts. Osteoprotegerin (OPG) is the osteoclastogenesis inhibitor factor and functions as a decoy receptor for RANKL so that the osteoclasts cannot be activated. The RANK RANKL OPG system seems to be the most important part in the communication between the bone cells.

This system is not exclusively organizing the communication between osteoblasts and osteoclasts. This system has been proven to be responsible for the formation of the mammary gland and lymph nodes. RANK and RANKL are also expressed in the kidney, spleen, thymus, and brain, where it might influence the thermoregulation [3].

## 22.2 Osteomyelitis

The clinical picture of the different kinds of osteomyelitis is very inhomogeneous so that there are many definitions and classifications. In textbooks, the osteoradionecrosis and medication-associated osteonecrosis of the jaws are often subentities of the osteomyelitis. In this book, these entities are described in their own subheadings (Sects. 22.3 and 22.4 of the chapter).

### 22.2.1 Definition

The actual term "osteomyelitis" refers to an inflammation ("itis") of the bone marrow ("osteomyel") only but means an inflammation of the entire bone including the periosteum, the cortical, and cancellous bone as well as the bone marrow.

### 22.2.2 Classification

There are many different classifications that are either based on the etiology, pathogenesis, pathologic or anatomic differences, the clinical course of the disease, or radiologic patterns. This makes a comparison between different studies very complicated or impossible.

The Zürich classification [4] differs between three different kinds of osteomyelitis: The *acute osteomyelitis*, the *secondary chronic osteomyelitis,* and the *primary chronic osteomyelitis* (Table 22.1). The secondary chronic osteomyelitis results from the acute osteomyelitis and therefore is the same disease at a different time stage. Once the osteomyelitis persists for more than 4 weeks, it is defined as chronic [4].

**Table 22.1** The table describes the Zürich classification of osteomyelitis on the left-hand side. In the right column are the different kinds of osteomyelitis that are included in the respective group of the Zürich classification [4]

| Zürich classification [4] | Different types of osteomyelitis |
|---|---|
| Acute osteomyelitis<br>Secondary chronic osteomyelitis | Neonatal osteomyelitis |
| | Trauma-associated osteomyelitis |
| | Odontogenic osteomyelitis |
| | Foreign body-induced osteomyelitis |
| | Osteomyelitis based on a bone disease |
| | Osteomyelitis based on a systemic condition<br>• Diabetes<br>• Autoimmune diseases/ immunosuppression<br>• AIDS<br>• Agranulocytosis<br>• Anemia<br>• Leukemia<br>• Syphilis<br>• Malnutrition<br>• Cancer/chemotherapy<br>• Alcohol/tobacco/drugs<br>• Herpes zoster/Cytomegaly |
| Primary chronic osteomyelitis | Juvenile chronic osteomyelitis |
| | Adult onset osteomyelitis |
| | Syndrome associated<br>• SAPHO<br>• CRMO |

### 22.2.3 Epidemiology

Due to the different classifications and terms used for the entire group of osteomyelitis, it is hard to give general data regarding its epidemiology. Approximately 17% of all osteomyelitis cases belong to the group of the acute osteomyelitis, 70% to the secondary chronic osteomyelitis, and 10% to the primary chronic osteomyelitis [4]. The average age at the time of diagnosis is a little bit over 40 years for the acute and the secondary chronic osteomyelitis [4]. Because of the inhomogeneity of the secondary chronic osteomyelitis, a general age group cannot be given.

### 22.2.4 Etiology

In the etiology of the *acute osteomyelitis* and the *secondary chronic osteomyelitis,* usually an odontogenic infection can be identified such as a dead tooth, a periodontal disease, or conditions after dentoalveolar surgery. A hematogenic spread from a different primary location into the region of the jaws is extremely rare [4].

The etiology of the *primary chronic osteomyelitis* is an infection of unknown origin [4].

### 22.2.5 Pathogenesis

The acute osteomyelitis and secondary chronic osteomyelitis are caused by a local infection due to bacteria from the oral cavity. The likelihood of the development of the infection depends on the virulence and number of bacteria and the quality of the local immune response and the blood flow [4].

Therefore, general diseases affecting the immune system are risk factors in the development of osteomyelitis, e.g., diabetes, autoimmune diseases, or anemia.

A typical course of the acute and secondary chronic osteomyelitis is the contamination of the bone with bacteria. The bacteria proliferate and colonize the bone marrow and reach via the Haversian and Volkmann canals the periosteum. The edema under and in the periosteum disturbs the blood flow resulting in ischemic bone parts and potentially sequestrum building.

### 22.2.6 Histology

The *acute osteomyelitis* and the *secondary chronic osteomyelitis* are characterized by an inflammatory exudate, primary in the medullary spaces with fibrin, leucocytes, and macrophages that replace the fatty tissue and hematopoietic marrow (Fig. 22.1). In addition, necrotic debris and bacteria can be found [4, 5]. The most common bacteria being detected is *Staphylococcus aureus* (85%) [4]. Due to the blood flow disturbances (see pathogenesis), parts of the bone die so that empty osteocytic lacunae can be observed. Sequestrae may be present. New bone formation under the periosteum is not uncommon.

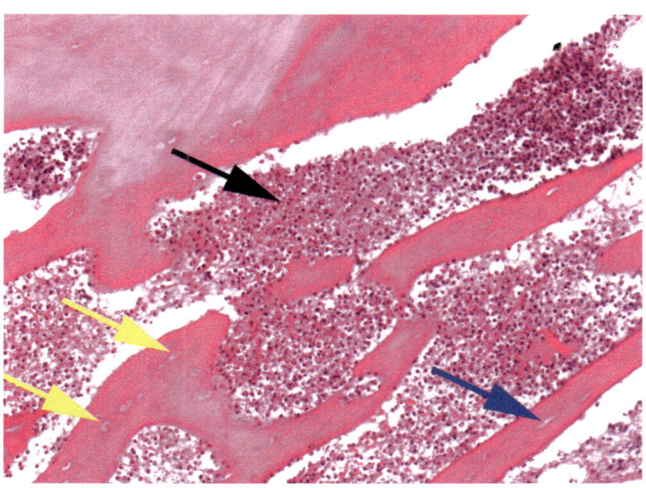



**Fig. 22.1** In this case of acute osteomyelitis, the medullary hematopoietic cells and the fatty tissue are completely replaced by cell debris, fibrin, and an inflammatory infiltrate mainly composed of neutrophil granulocytes (black arrow). Besides the vital bone with filled lacunes of osteocytes (yellow arrow), necrotic bone can be seen with loss of osteocytes (blue arrow)

In cases of secondary chronic osteomyelitis, sequestrum formation is more common than in the acute osteomyelitis. The more chronic the course is, the more likely is the development of bone marrow fibrosis and sclerosis of the bone. Bacteria might be present. Actinomyces drusen are typical.

In the *primary chronic osteomyelitis,* plasma cells are predominant in the inflammatory infiltrate. The proportion of neutrophils, lymphocytes, and macrophages is rather small. The bone marrow is altered due to fibrosis. New bone formation is a common sign. Osteoclastic activity leads to repeated bone remodeling without a distinct histological bone formation pattern. Microabscesses might be observed [4].

### 22.2.7 Symptoms

In cases of *acute osteomyelitis,* patients present with high fever and are listless. Local swelling can be observed with pain on palpation. The affected area is reddish, a trismus might be present, and quite often the teeth have higher mobility with pus coming out of the periodontium. If the inferior alveolar nerve is affected, patients report paresthesia of the lips (Vincent symptom [4]). There are cases in which the symptoms are not very distinctive.

Symptoms of the *secondary chronic osteomyelitis* are the painful swellings that are usually not as prominent as in the acute osteomyelitis. A common finding is a periosteal reaction causing a solid swelling. Further symptoms are sequester formation and fistulas.

The *primary chronic osteomyelitis* is characterized by a nonsuppurative inflammation and sometimes only barely noticeable symptoms. In active periods, the patients notice pain, swelling, and mouth-opening limitations. Due to the bone formation, permanent swelling will develop eventually [4].

### 22.2.8 Complications

A typical complication of the acute osteomyelitis is a shift into the chronic osteomyelitis that is very hard to treat sufficiently.

Further complications are the development of the Vincent syndrome, fistula, abscess and sequester formation, and potentially fractures [4].

### 22.2.9 Diagnosis

The diagnosis is based on the clinical course. This is completed by radiology: panoramic radiograph, cone beam CT, CT, or MRI. Changes in the bone can only be seen after a 30 to 40% reduction of the mineralized part of the bone. Therefore, the changes in the acute osteomyelitis are marginal at the beginning. In complex cases of osteomyelitis, a bone scintigraphy might be used to detect further active spots in the skeleton, e.g., in the diagnosis of chronic recurrent multifocal osteomyelitis or the SAPHO syndrome (SAPHO: Synovitis, acne, pustulosis, hyperostosis, osteitis) [6].

Radiological signs of *acute osteomyelitis* are: Bone resorption with increased radiolucency, loss of spongious structure of the bone, potentially sequester formation.

Radiological signs of the *secondary chronic osteomyelitis* are: Bone resorption with increased radiolucency, sequester formation, periosteal reaction, and pathological fractures.

Radiological signs of the *primary chronic osteomyelitis* are: Increased radiopacity with loss of trabecular bone, bone resorption, and periosteal reaction (Fig. 22.2) [4].

### 22.2.10 Differential Diagnoses

In the differential diagnosis, one should rule out malignancies in unclear cases so that biopsies should be performed.

### 22.2.11 Therapy

The therapy of the acute and secondary chronic osteomyelitis mainly consists of the therapy of the infection and of the improvement of the local blood flow. This is achieved via antibiotics and removing of the infected parts of the bone. A decortication supports this and helps to get well-vascularized tissue onto the bone.

*Acute osteomyelitis* is immediately treated with antibiotics. If an antibiogram suggests different antibiotics, an adaptation should be performed after the initial antimicrobiological therapy. Mouth rinses, hygiene, and cold application can be applied. In general, the highly mobile teeth should not be extracted since they will gain stability again after the acute stadium of the osteomyelitis is over.

The therapy of the *secondary chronic osteomyelitis* aims at sufficient pain management, limitation of the spread of the affected areas, fracture prevention, and the prevention of the onset of further active periods. Secondary diseases such as diabetes need to be treated as well.

The therapy of the *primary chronic osteomyelitis* consists of a surgical intervention to remove the necrotic bone parts and a potential disfigurement can be corrected. But recurrences of the symptoms are very common. Therefore, other treatment options should be used as well including antibiotics, nonsteroidal anti-inflammatory drugs (NSAIDS), steroids, and bisphosphonates (mainly pamidronate).

### 22.2.12 Prognosis

The therapeutic success is higher in patients with acute and secondary chronic osteomyelitis than in patients with primary chronic osteomyelitis. Approximately 75% of the acute and secondary chronic osteomyelitis are symptom-free after intervention whereas only about 25% are symptom-free of the patients with primary chronic osteomyelitis [4].

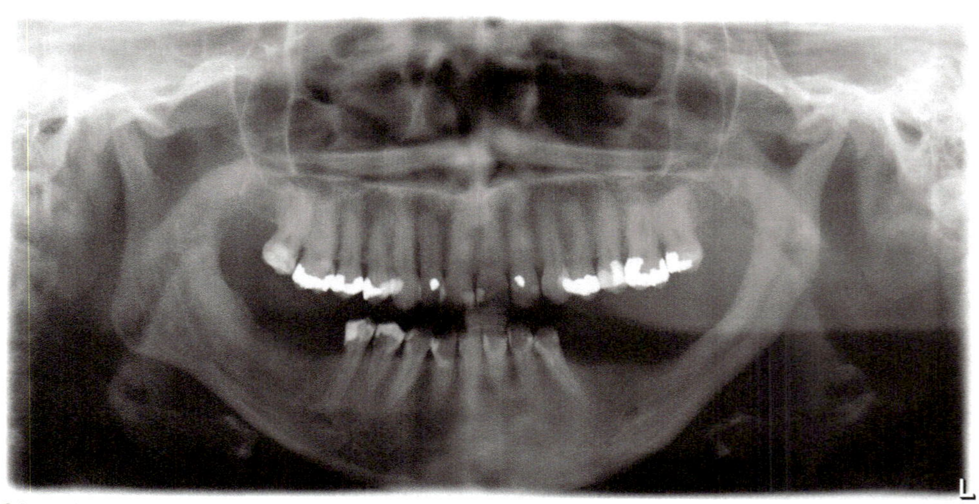




Fig. 22.2 Panoramic radiograph of a patient with primary chronic osteomyelitis after several surgeries have been performed. Several infusions of pamidronate prevented the occurrence of further active periods. In the left mandible, typical sclerosis can be seen with a prominent nerve canal

## 22.3 Osteoradionecrosis

The osteoradionecrosis is a side effect in the therapy of malignant diseases to the head and neck area with ionizing radiation.

### 22.3.1 Definition

Osteoradionecrosis describes the exposed necrotic bone due to radiation. The infected osteoradionecrosis describes the additional infection of the necrotic bone [7].

### 22.3.2 Epidemiology

The prevalence of osteoradionecrosis ranges from 0 to 23% of the patients with head and neck radiation [8]. Usually, older patients are affected (60 years ±10 years) since the primary disease causing the head and neck radiation are diseases in patients with advanced age [9]. Men are affected more than twice as often [9].

### 22.3.3 Etiology

The etiology of the osteoradionecrosis is radiation therapy to the head and neck area. Usually, another trigger is required in the development of the osteoradionecrosis (see pathogenesis).

### 22.3.4 Pathogenesis

Due to the radiation therapy, the vessels of the bone change and become hyalinized. It results in a lack of nutrition and hypoxia with the subsequent death of osteocytes [7]. This seems to be more likely in radiation doses above 40–50 Gy [10]. The radiation has additional side effects to all tissues being in the radiation field including the skin, the muscles, and the salivary glands. Due to the resulting xerostomia radiation, caries develops so that an osteoradionecrosis might develop.

The osteonecrosis occurs more often in the mandible most probably to the greater extent of cortical bone and the more critical vascularization of the mandible. And the mandible most probably is more often in the radiation field due to the location of the primary tumor [10].

There are several risk factors that are associated with a more frequent occurrence of the osteoradionecrosis. Those are male gender, insufficient oral hygiene, pressure denture sores, a tumor localized in the tongue, alveolar process of the mandible, the floor of the mouth, and retromolar as well as persisting alcohol and nicotine consumption. Next to these, there are therapy-linked risk factors, namely a tumor resection including resection of the bone and dentoalveolar surgery performed in timely proximity to the radiation therapy [10].

### 22.3.5 Classification

It is mainly differed between the aseptic osteoradionecrosis and the infected osteoradionecrosis. Another very common staging system uses the potential benefit of a rather controversially discussed therapy option the hyperbaric oxygen treatment and therefore won't be discussed in further detail.

### 22.3.6 Histology

The lacunae of the osteocytes in osteoradionecrotic bone are empty (Fig. 22.3). There is a lack of osteoblastic rimming and the Haversian and Volkmann canals do not harbor any blood vessels. The marrow of the bone shows acellular collagen. The periosteum is acellular and avascular [5].

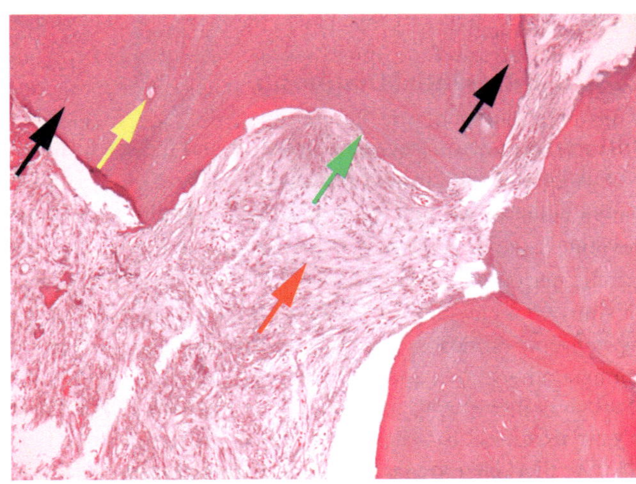



**Fig. 22.3** The examination of the osteoradionecrosis under the microscope shows avital bone with irregular fissured borders. The lacunae of the osteocytes are empty without osteocyte cell nuclei (black arrows) and also the blood vessels in the Haversian canals have undergone necrosis, so that only empty spaces are the visible remnants (yellow arrow). The necrotic bone is missing the osteoblastic rimming (green arrow). The bone marrow is replaced by a collagen fiber-rich scar like connective tissue (red arrow)

### 22.3.7 Symptoms

Symptoms are the exposed necrotic bone that can be visible or palpable with a probe. Further symptoms are pain, swelling, the development of granulation tissue, foetor ex ore, oral and extraoral fistulas, potentially increased mobility of the adjacent teeth, altered sensibility, and occlusion [10].

### 22.3.8 Complications

Main complications are extended infections of the site, the development of fistulas, and pathological fractures. This might result in resections of the altered bone including the loss of the continuity of the bone or the opening of the nasal cavity or sinus. This results in a reduced masticatory function. Due to the fibrosis of the soft tissues, trismus might occur. All these factors lead to a reduced quality of life [10].

### 22.3.9 Diagnosis

The diagnosis is a clinical one. There needs to be a mandatory head and neck radiation and the exposed necrotic bone.

Typical radiologic findings are bone destruction, altered bone density, the occurrence of sequestra, and pathological fractures.

### 22.3.10 Differential Diagnoses

Differential diagnoses are osteomyelitis and the medication-associated osteonecrosis of the jaws as well as the existence of malignancy so that a histological sample should be assessed.

### 22.3.11 Therapy

As already mentioned, the evidence of the use of hyperbaric oxygen treatment is rather low and is not recommended [11, 12]. Smaller necrotic areas can be treated conservatively using antiseptic mouth rinses, antibiotics, and pain killers. In some cases, a wait and see strategy is reasonable. Sometimes circumscribed debridement might be performed. Extended necrotic areas should be surgically removed [13]. The aim is to preserve damage to the alveolar nerve and to avoid a continuity defect of the mandible. The operation should be as atraumatic as possible. The periosteum should not be removed if possible. The necrotic areas should be removed, sharp edges need to be smoothened, and the bone should be covered with soft tissue. The surgery should be performed with perioperative antimicrobial therapy.

### 22.3.12 Prognosis

The risk for a recurrence of an osteoradionecrosis is high. Pressure denture sores, wound healing deficiencies, and mucositis are risk factors for a recurrence.

### 22.3.13 Prevention

A 3D-planning of radiation therapy might help to reduce the radiation doses in the bone. In addition, a splint inserted in the patient's mouth during the radiation might help to reduce the burst of the local mucosal membranes due to secondary radiation that might occur due to metallic dental restorations. An additional splint to provide fluorides to strengthen the teeth might help prevent the development of radiation caries.

It is feasible to reduce the existence of risk factors that might later on trigger the development of an osteoradionecrosis. Therefore, an initial dental checkup and therapy preceding the radiation therapy should be performed including the extraction of all non-restorable teeth. The patient should be motivated for exceptional good oral hygiene [10].

## 22.4 Medication-Associated Osteonecrosis of the Jaws

There are several pharmaceutical agents that cause osteonecrosis of the jaws. In the following, the main focus will be on the bisphosphonate-associated osteonecrosis.

### 22.4.1 Bisphosphonate-Associated Osteonecrosis of the Jaws

#### 22.4.1.1 Bisphosphonates

Bisphosphonates are used in patients with an increased osteoclastic activity due to malignancy such as solid tumors with osseous metastases or the multiple myeloma or due to metabolic bone diseases such as osteoporosis. The main target of bisphosphonates that can be administered orally of IV is the osteoclasts.

Bisphosphonates are classified into nitrogen- and non-nitrogen-containing bisphosphonates. The non-nitrogen-containing bisphosphonates are built into ATP and can no longer be used as a source of energy in the cells. The nitrogen-containing bisphosphonates inhibit the farnesyl pyrophosphate synthase in the mevalonate pathway leading to decreased osteoclastic function [14]. In 2003, the bisphosphonate-associated osteonecrosis was first mentioned in a scientific paper [15].

#### 22.4.1.2 Definition

The bisphosphonate-associated osteonecrosis is defined as the occurrence of the necrotic bone of the jaws that has been persistent for at least 8 weeks with a current or previous history of bisphosphonate use (Fig. 22.4). Furthermore, it is demanded that the patient had had no former head and neck radiation [16].

The last demand seems arbitrary since the coexistence of a further risk factor simply increases the risk of osteonecrosis development so that there is a special risk constellation. There is evidence that it is even possible to histologically distinguish an osteonecrosis derived from bisphosphonates compared to osteoradionecrosis [17].

#### 22.4.1.3 Epidemiology

The prevalence and incidence of the bisphosphonate-associated osteonecrosis of the jaws depend on the primary disease, comedication, and the existence of local trigger factors. The highest risk is present in oncologic patients with further compromising medications. Incidences for patients with malignant diseases range from 1 to 20% [18–20]. The prevalence of secondary osteoporosis is about 1% and for primary osteoporosis 0.1% [21]. There is only a small difference between the genders. Women are affected a little bit more often than men. Most probably due to the osteoporosis and breast cancer cases vs. the prostate cancer cases that exclusively occur in men. The average age is approximately 60 years ±10 years (standard deviation) [9].

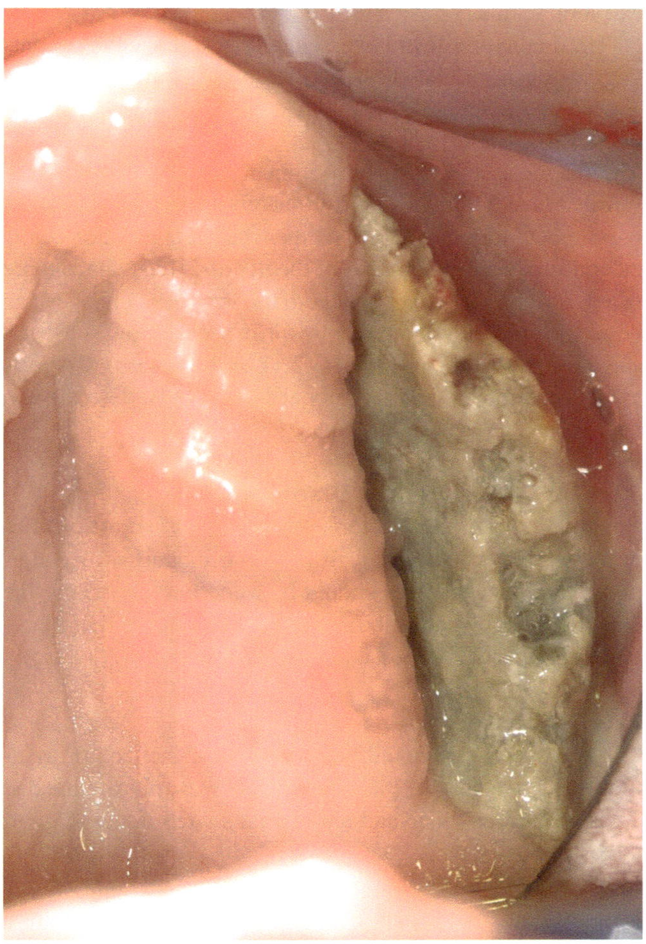



**Fig. 22.4** Huge bisphosphonate-associated osteonecrosis of the left maxilla in a patient with non-Hodgkin lymphoma and a zoledronate treatment for 2.5 years before a pressure denture sore triggered the osteonecrosis

#### 22.4.1.4 Etiology

The main factor is the use of nitrogen-containing bisphosphonates. Administered bisphosphonates will be incorporated in the bone. It is unclear if and how long these bisphosphonates are active. The development of bisphosphonate-associated osteonecrosis can be triggered by oral factors—this is usually a wound in the oral cavity: periodontal disease, surgical procedures, etc. [9, 22].

#### 22.4.1.5 Pathogenesis

The main target of the bisphosphonates is the osteoclast, thereby inducing reduced bone remodeling. Due to the unspecific interaction with cells, not only the osteoclasts are affected, but also, in lower concentrations, osteoblasts are stimulated [23]. The effect is an increase in total bone. Other affected cell lines are blood vessel cells, fibroblasts, and keratinocytes. The antiangiogenic function of bisphosphonates [24, 25] leads to decreased vascular exploitation [26]. This results in fewer potentially less potent vessels that have to support more bone. In addition, the soft tissues covering the bone are affected by the bisphosphonates so that potential wounds are less prone to heal [24]. In older articles, it is often described that tooth extractions are responsible for the development of the bisphosphonate-associated osteonecrosis of the jaws. This theory might not be right. It is more likely that these teeth have been extracted too late since they were extracted out of an already-existing, altered, infected, or necrotic bone [27].

#### 22.4.1.6 Classification

The bisphosphonate-associated osteonecrosis of the jaws is classified into several different stages. At-risk patients are all those receiving bisphosphonates.

> Stage 0 patients are patients that do have some symptoms without any visible uncovered bone.
> Stage I, the necrotic bone becomes visible. Patients in this stage usually do not have any symptoms.
> Stage II, an additive infection is existent.
> Stage III, further complications occur such as necrotic areas involving the base of the mandible or the sinus or pathologic fractures are existent [16].

### 22.4.1.7 Histology

Usually, there is a mucosal damage above the necrosis, perhaps some granulation tissue (Fig. 22.5). The necrotic bone is often avascular and covered in bacteria, especially Actinomyces (Fig. 22.6) [28]. The osteonecrotic bone has parts with empty osteocytic lacunae next to viable osteocytes so that there are necrotic areas of the bone that harbor parts of the viable bone. Inflammatory infiltrates are seen in nearly all cases consisting of granulocytes and lymphocytes. The obliteration of mainly the segmental arteries is not existent in every case [28]. The periosteum is usually viable [5].

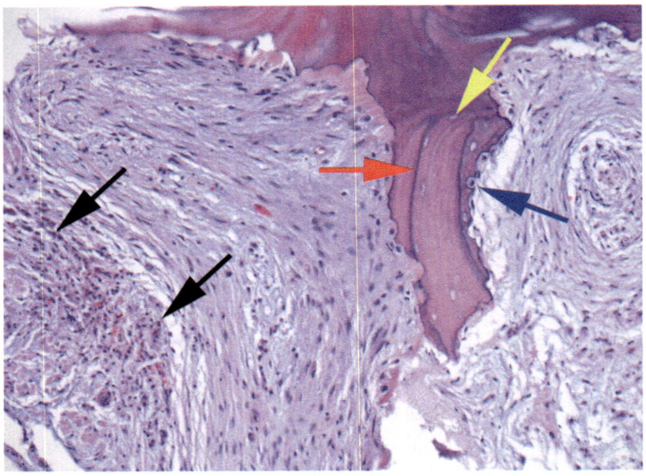



**Fig. 22.5** In this case, the bone necrosis is induced by bisphosphonates. Besides necrotic bone showing empty osteocyte lacunes (yellow arrow), inflammatory cellular infiltrate can be seen in the medullary cavity (black arrows). It is mainly composed of lymphocytes, neutrophil granulocytes, and also plasma cells. Here, signs of the bone remodeling are also visible. The dark line within the bone, the border of the periosteum before necrosis (red arrow) separates necrotic bone in the center from the new-built bone with a lining of active osteoblasts (blue arrow) on the outside

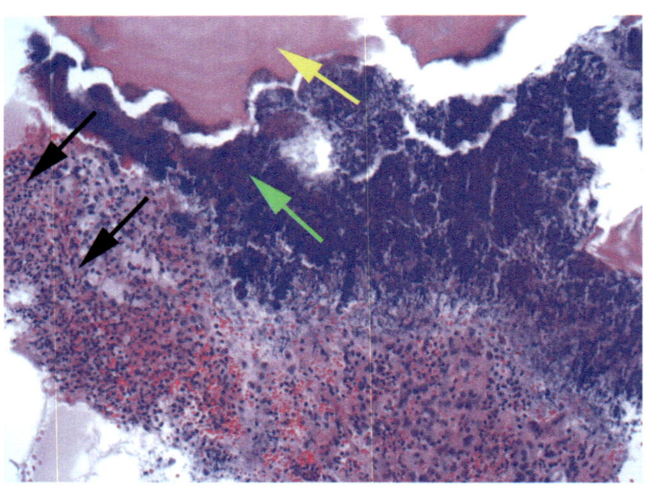



**Fig. 22.6** Actinomyces species (green arrow) frequently can be found next to necrotic bone (yellow arrow) in the jaws. Dense clouds of bacteria affecting the bone leading to deep excavations of the necrotic bone. An inflammatory infiltrate of neutrophil granulocytes and macrophages in fibrin-rich exudate fills the bone marrow (black arrows) as a border which limits bacterial growth

### 22.4.1.8 Symptoms

The classical symptoms are the visible necrotic bone and pain in case of an additional infection of the bone so that the symptoms are very unspecific.

### 22.4.1.9 Complications

The typical complications are the progress of the initial small necrosis so that big parts of the bone might be affected by the osteonecrosis. Since the bone is no longer covered with soft tissue, an additive infection can cause typical symptoms and leads to a shift to a different stage of the osteonecrosis. Major complications are the loss of the integrity of the bone and extraoral fistulas or abscesses.

The quality of life might essentially get affected in patients with medication-related osteonecrosis of the jaws [29].

### 22.4.1.10 Diagnosis

The diagnosis is primarily a clinical one if all criteria are fulfilled (see definition). Unfortunately, there is no sensitive radiological tool that shows neither the exact location of the osteonecrosis nor the extent of the necrosis [30]. Once there is a destruction of the bone due to the infection, changes can be seen in the radiologic pictures. But these changes are not specific for the changes (Figs. 22.7 and 22.8a, b). There is evidence that the potential osteonecrosis can be detected at a very early stage via scintigraphs [31].

### 22.4.1.11 Differential Diagnosis

Regarding the clinical picture, osteomyelitis and osteoradionecrosis are the other typical potential diagnoses. In addition, malignant diseases should be ruled out, especially the ones why the bisphosphonates were given in the first place, e.g., breast cancer or prostate cancer.

### 22.4.1.12 Therapy

The osteonecroses should be treated since the lack of treatment usually ends in the progression with more extended areas of necrotic bone and a potential switch in the stage of the osteonecrosis.

There are several approaches in the therapy of the bisphosphonate-associated osteonecrosis of the jaws. Smaller osteonecroses can be treated conservatively or with a moderate surgical intervention. Perioperative antibiotic treatment should be initiated. After the debridement or resection of the necrotic bone, a plastic coverage of the bone should be performed.

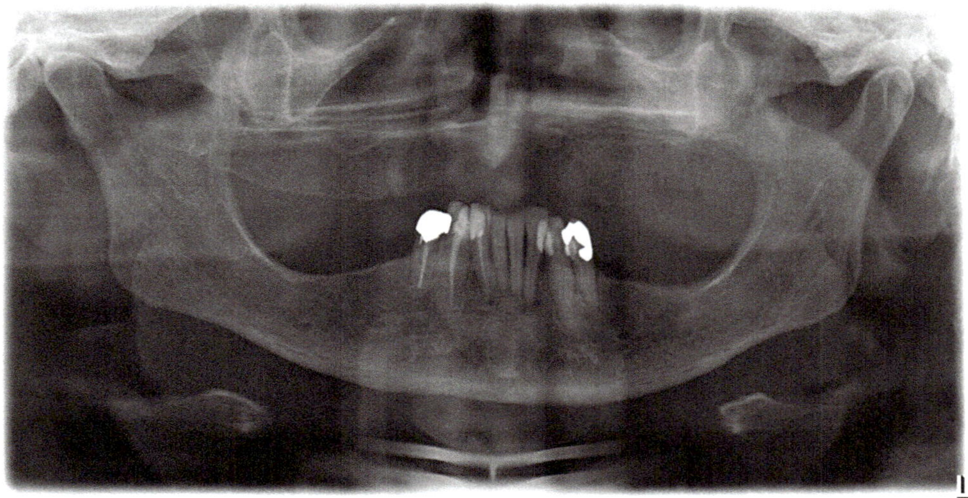

©Association of Oral and Maxillofacial Surgeons of India

**Fig. 22.7** This is the same patient as seen in picture 4. There are nearly no changes visible that indicate the existence of osteonecrosis. A very typical change that can be seen is the thickened and sclerotic lamina dura in the mandible and the honeycomb pattern of the bone due to the sclerotic trabeculae of the bone

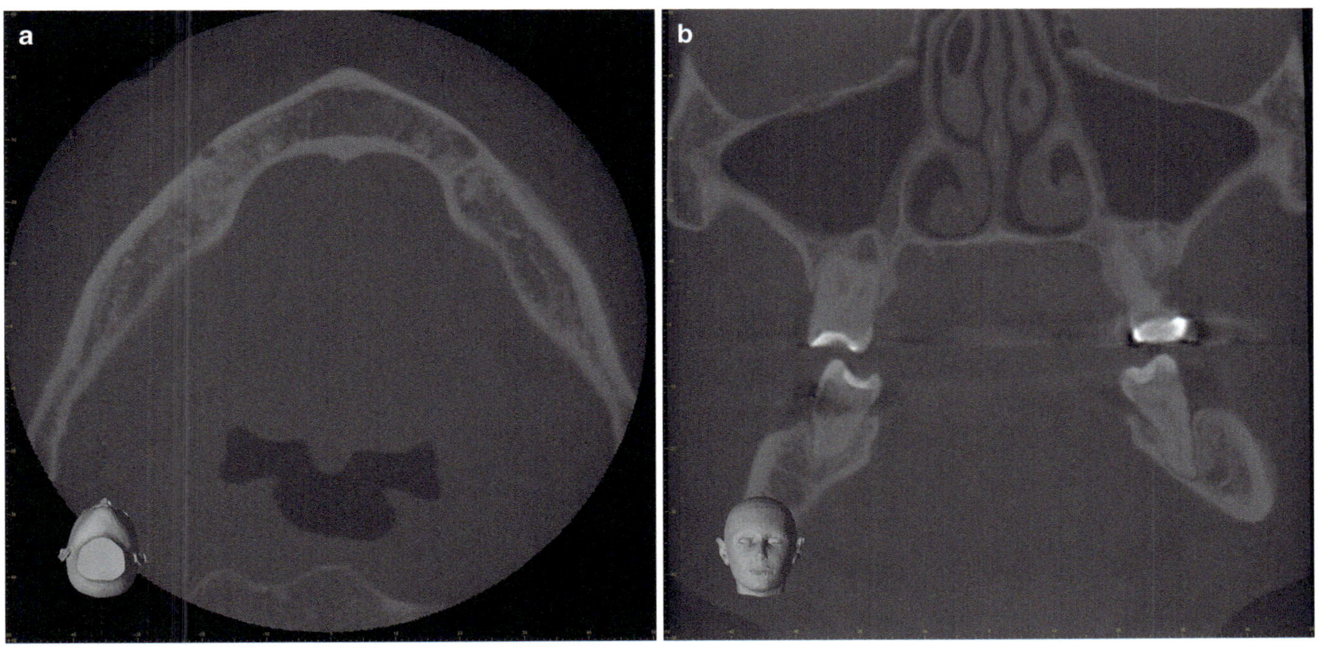


©Association of Oral and Maxillofacial Surgeons of India

**Fig. 22.8** Two slices from a cone beam CT from a patient with a malignant primary disease and bisphosphonate intake. (**a**) Axial slice from a patient with osteonecrosis of the left and the right mandible. On the right-hand side, a thickening of the cortical bone can be observed and sclerosis of the cancellous bone. On the left-hand side, the periosteal reaction is visible. (**b**) Coronal slice with a periapical translucency of the molar on the right-hand side as a potential trigger of the osteonecrosis that reached the level of the alveolar nerve canal. On the vestibular side of the left mandible the periosteal reaction can be seen

Extended or multiple osteonecrotic areas should be resected. This might include an inpatient setting with the postoperative use of a nasogastric tube and antibiotic iv treatment [32].

#### 22.4.1.13 Prognosis

The recurrence rate of the osteonecrosis depends on the mode of therapy and is the lowest for surgical interventions and the highest for purely conservative treatments. In the latter case, complete closure of the mucosal membrane cannot always be achieved [32].

#### 22.4.1.14 Prevention

It should be differed between preventive measures before initiating a bisphosphonate therapy and measures during or after the course of bisphosphonate therapy. Since the bisphosphonate-associated osteonecrosis of the jaws is usually triggered by an oral wound, potential dental foci should be eliminated before the start of bisphosphonate therapy [32].

If surgery needs to be performed in patients with bisphosphonate therapy, anti-microbiological prophylaxis should be performed [32].

### 22.4.2 Osteonecrosis of the Jaws Due to Other Medications but Bisphosphonates

There are other medications that can cause osteonecrosis of the jaws. The definition is the same compared to the osteonecrosis due to bisphosphonates.

#### 22.4.2.1 Denosumab

The most frequent osteonecroses can be observed in patients with denosumab that is administered in the same patients that receive bisphosphonates. The definition, etiology, classification, symptoms, complications, diagnoses, differential diagnoses, therapy, prognosis, and prevention are the same or similar to the ones of the bisphosphonate-associated osteonecrosis of the jaws.

The pathogenesis might be different since denosumab only affects the RANK/RANKL/OPG mechanism that is predominant in the communication between osteoblasts and osteoclasts. Therefore, an impact on the soft tissues including the vessels seems unlikely so that the likewise reduced bone remodeling seems to be the major component in the development of the denosumab-associated osteonecrosis of the jaws.

#### 22.4.2.2 Sunitinib

Sunitinib is an inhibitor of a tyrosine kinase and therefore has a less specific mode of action. It is given in patients with gastrointestinal cancers, renal cell carcinoma, and pancreatic neuroendocrine tumors [33]. A side effect in the use of sunitinib is the development of osteonecroses of the jaws [34].

#### 22.4.2.3 Imatinib

Imatinib is another tyrosine kinase inhibitor. Osteonecrosis in imatinib-only use has been described [35].

#### 22.4.2.4 Bevazicumab

Bevazicumab is a vascular endothelial growth factor- (VEGF-) inhibitor and is used in several oncologic treatment concepts, e.g., breast cancer, colorectal cancer, and lung cancer. Several cases of osteonecroses of the jaws have been described [36, 37].

#### 22.4.2.5 Ziv-aflibercept

Ziv-aflibercept is a recombinant vascular endothelial growth factor- (VEGF-) receptor. Several cases of the development of osteonecroses of the jaws have been described in patients that did not receive any of the other typical medications causing osteonecrosis [38]. In the pathogenesis, the antiangiogenic factor might be the reason for the development of the osteonecrosis.

#### 22.4.2.6 Everolimus

Everolimus is a mammalian Target of Rapamycin (mTOR) inhibitor. It is used in several oncologic diseases and was associated with the development of osteonecroses in the jaws [39].

#### 22.4.2.7 Corticosteroids

There is evidence that the use of corticosteroids increases the risk of osteonecrosis development of the jaws [40]. The femoral head osteonecrosis has been described in patients with long-term corticosteroid use [41].

It should be stated that the use of several of these agents in combination might further increase the risk of osteonecrosis development.

#### 22.4.2.8 Crystal Meth

Next to therapeutically used agents, some drugs are responsible for the development of osteonecroses. Crystal Meth is the crystalline form of methamphetamine hydrochloride. It functions as a sympathomimetic and has a very high potential for abuse and dependency. One side effect is the meth mouth with serious tooth and damage to the oral cavity including the development of osteonecroses [42]. The exact mechanism of osteonecrosis development is unclear. Methamphetamine causes the release of noradrenaline which increases the blood pressure by the increase of the peripheral blood vessel resistance.

## References


1. Bilezikian JP, Raisz LG, Rodan GA. Principles of bone biology. San Diego: Academic Press; 2002.
2. Bartl R, von Tresckow E, Bartl C. Bisphosphonat-manual. Berlin: Springer; 2006.
3. Liu W, Zhang X. Receptor activator of nuclear factor-kappaB ligand (RANKL)/RANK/osteoprotegerin system in bone and other tissues (review). Mol Med Rep. 2015;11(5):3212–8.
4. Baltensperger MM, Eyrich GK. Osteomyelitis of the jaws. Berlin: Springer; 2009.
5. Marx RE, Tursun R. Suppurative osteomyelitis, bisphosphonate induced osteonecrosis, osteoradionecrosis: a blinded histopathologic comparison and its implications for the mechanism of each disease. Int J Oral Maxillofac Surg. 2012;41(3):283–9.

6. Muller-Richter UD, Roldan JC, Mortl M, Behr M, Reichert TE, Driemel O. SAPHO syndrome with ankylosis of the temporomandibular joint. Int J Oral Maxillofac Surg. 2009;38(12):1335–41.
7. Marx RE. Osteoradionecrosis: a new concept of its pathophysiology. J Oral Maxillofac Surg. 1983;41(5):283–8.
8. Schuurhuis JM, Stokman MA, Witjes MJ, Dijkstra PU, Vissink A, Spijkervet FK. Evidence supporting pre-radiation elimination of oral foci of infection in head and neck cancer patients to prevent oral sequelae. A systematic review. Oral Oncol. 2015;51(3):212–20.
9. Walter C, Sagheb K, Bitzer J, Rahimi-Nedjat R, Taylor KJ. Analysis of reasons for osteonecrosis of the jaws. Clin Oral Investig. 2014;18(9):2221–6.
10. Krüger M, Hautmann M, Bartella A, Al-Nawas B, Grötz KA. S2k-Leitlinie: Infizierte Osteoradionekrose (IORN) der Kiefer. AWMF Online 2018.
11. Annane D, Depondt J, Aubert P, Villart M, Gehanno P, Gajdos P, et al. Hyperbaric oxygen therapy for radionecrosis of the jaw: a randomized, placebo-controlled, double-blind trial from the ORN96 study group. J Clin Oncol. 2004;22(24):4893–900.
12. Sultan A, Hanna GJ, Margalit DN, Chau N, Goguen LA, Marty FM, et al. The use of hyperbaric oxygen for the prevention and Management of Osteoradionecrosis of the jaw: a Dana-Farber/Brigham and Women's Cancer center multidisciplinary guideline. Oncologist. 2017;22(3):343–50.
13. Pitak-Arnnop P, Sader R, Dhanuthai K, Masaratana P, Bertolus C, Chaine A, et al. Management of osteoradionecrosis of the jaws: an analysis of evidence. Eur J Surg Oncol. 2008;34(10):1123–34.
14. Hagelauer N, Ziebart T, Pabst AM, Walter C. Bisphosphonates inhibit cell functions of HUVECs, fibroblasts and osteogenic cells via inhibition of protein geranylgeranylation. Clin Oral Investig. 2015;19(5):1079–91.
15. Marx RE. Pamidronate (Aredia) and zoledronate (Zometa) induced avascular necrosis of the jaws: a growing epidemic. J Oral Maxillofac Surg. 2003;61(9):1115–7.
16. Ruggiero SL, Dodson TB, Fantasia J, Goodday R, Aghaloo T, Mehrotra B, et al. American association of oral and maxillofacial surgeons position paper on medication-related osteonecrosis of the jaw--2014 update. J Oral Maxillofac Surg. 2014;72(10):1938–56.
17. Hansen T, Kirkpatrick CJ, Walter C, Kunkel M. Increased numbers of osteoclasts expressing cysteine proteinase cathepsin K in patients with infected osteoradionecrosis and bisphosphonate-associated osteonecrosis--a paradoxical observation? Virchows Arch. 2006;449(4):448–54.
18. Rugani P, Walter C, Kirnbauer B, Acham S, Begus-Nahrman Y, Jakse N. Prevalence of medication-related osteonecrosis of the jaw in patients with breast cancer, prostate cancer, and multiple myeloma. Dent J (Basel). 2016;4(4):32.
19. Walter C, Al-Nawas B, Frickhofen N, Gamm H, Beck J, Reinsch L, et al. Prevalence of bisphosphonate associated osteonecrosis of the jaws in multiple myeloma patients. Head Face Med. 2010;6:11.
20. Walter C, Al-Nawas B, Grotz KA, Thomas C, Thuroff JW, Zinser V, et al. Prevalence and risk factors of bisphosphonate-associated osteonecrosis of the jaw in prostate cancer patients with advanced disease treated with zoledronate. Eur Urol. 2008;54(5):1066–72.
21. Grötz KA, Piesold U, Al-Nawas B. Bisphosphonate-assoziierte Osteonekrose (BP-ONJ) und andere Medikamenten-assoziierte Kiefernekrosen. AWMF [Internet]. 2012; (007/091):1–18.
22. Walter C, Grotz KA, Kunkel M, Al-Nawas B. Prevalence of bisphosphonate associated osteonecrosis of the jaw within the field of osteonecrosis. Support Care Cancer. 2007;15(2):197–202.
23. Koch FP, Merkel C, Ziebart T, Smeets R, Walter C, Al-Nawas B. Influence of bisphosphonates on the osteoblast RANKL and OPG gene expression in vitro. Clin Oral Investig. 2012;16(1):79–86.
24. Walter C, Klein MO, Pabst A, Al-Nawas B, Duschner H, Ziebart T. Influence of bisphosphonates on endothelial cells, fibroblasts, and osteogenic cells. Clin Oral Investig. 2010;14(1):35–41.
25. Ziebart T, Pabst A, Klein MO, Kammerer P, Gauss L, Brullmann D, et al. Bisphosphonates: restrictions for vasculogenesis and angiogenesis: inhibition of cell function of endothelial progenitor cells and mature endothelial cells in vitro. Clin Oral Investig. 2011;15(1):105–11.
26. Pabst AM, Ziebart T, Ackermann M, Konerding MA, Walter C. Bisphosphonates' antiangiogenic potency in the development of bisphosphonate-associated osteonecrosis of the jaws: influence on microvessel sprouting in an in vivo 3D Matrigel assay. Clin Oral Investig. 2014;18(3):1015–22.
27. Saia G, Blandamura S, Bettini G, Tronchet A, Totola A, Bedogni G, et al. Occurrence of bisphosphonate-related osteonecrosis of the jaw after surgical tooth extraction. J Oral Maxillofac Surg. 2010;68(4):797–804.
28. Hansen T, Kunkel M, Springer E, Walter C, Weber A, Siegel E, et al. Actinomycosis of the jaws--histopathological study of 45 patients shows significant involvement in bisphosphonate-associated osteonecrosis and infected osteoradionecrosis. Virchows Arch. 2007;451(6):1009–17.
29. Kyrgidis A, Triaridis S, Kontos K, Patrikidou A, Andreadis C, Constantinidis J, et al. Quality of life in breast cancer patients with bisphosphonate-related osteonecrosis of the jaws and patients with head and neck cancer: a comparative study using the EORTC QLQ-C30 and QLQ-HN35 questionnaires. Anticancer Res. 2012;32(8):3527–34.
30. Berg BI, Mueller AA, Augello M, Berg S, Jaquiery C. Imaging in patients with bisphosphonate-associated osteonecrosis of the jaws (MRONJ). Dent J (Basel). 2016;4(3):E29.
31. Thomas C, Spanidis M, Engel C, Roos FC, Frees S, Neisius A, et al. Bone scintigraphy predicts bisphosphonate-induced osteonecrosis of the jaw (BRONJ) in patients with metastatic castration-resistant prostate cancer (mCRPC). Clin Oral Investig. 2016;20(4):753–8.
32. Otto S, Pautke C, Van den Wyngaert T, Niepel D, Schiodt M. Medication-related osteonecrosis of the jaw: prevention, diagnosis and management in patients with cancer and bone metastases. Cancer Treat Rev. 2018;69:177–87.
33. Imbulgoda A, Heng DY, Kollmannsberger C. Sunitinib in the treatment of advanced solid tumors. Recent Results Cancer Res. 2014;201:165–84.
34. Koch FP, Walter C, Hansen T, Jager E, Wagner W. Osteonecrosis of the jaw related to sunitinib. Oral Maxillofac Surg. 2011;15(1):63–6.
35. Viviano M, Rossi M, Cocca S. A rare case of osteonecrosis of the jaw related to imatinib. J Korean Assoc Oral Maxillofac Surg. 2017;43(2):120–4.
36. Estilo CL, Fornier M, Farooki A, Carlson D, Bohle G 3rd, Huryn JM. Osteonecrosis of the jaw related to bevacizumab. J Clin Oncol. 2008;26(24):4037–8.
37. Santos-Silva AR, Belizario Rosa GA, Castro Junior G, Dias RB, Prado Ribeiro AC, Brandao TB. Osteonecrosis of the mandible associated with bevacizumab therapy. Oral Surg Oral Med Oral Pathol Oral Radiol. 2013;115(6):e32–6.
38. Mawardi H, Enzinger P, McCleary N, Manon R, Villa A, Treister N, et al. Osteonecrosis of the jaw associated with ziv-aflibercept. J Gastrointest Oncol. 2016;7(6):E81–E7.
39. Yamamoto D, Tsubota Y, Utsunomiya T, Sueoka N, Ueda A, Endo K, et al. Osteonecrosis of the jaw associated with everolimus: a case report. Mol Clin Oncol. 2017;6(2):255–7.

40. Saad F, Brown JE, Van Poznak C, Ibrahim T, Stemmer SM, Stopeck AT, et al. Incidence, risk factors, and outcomes of osteonecrosis of the jaw: integrated analysis from three blinded active-controlled phase III trials in cancer patients with bone metastases. Ann Oncol. 2012;23(5):1341–7.
41. Drescher W, Bunger MH, Weigert K, Bunger C, Hansen ES. Methylprednisolone enhances contraction of porcine femoral head epiphyseal arteries. Clin Orthop Relat Res. 2004;423:112–7.
42. Pabst A, Castillo-Duque JC, Mayer A, Klinghuber M, Werkmeister R. Meth mouth-a growing epidemic in dentistry? Dent J (Basel). 2017;5(4):E29.

# Part IX

# Maxillary Sinus and the Oral Surgeon

# 23 Maxillary Sinusitis

Kandasamy Ganesan and Neelam Rathod

## 23.1 Introduction

Sinusitis, also known as rhinosinusitis with the association of rhinitis, is a common presentation within the primary care setting, due to the effect it can have on individuals' quality of life. It is defined as the inflammation of the mucosal lining in at least one of the paranasal sinuses with an acute presentation lasting for less than 12 weeks and chronic extending to durations greater than this. The maxillary sinus is the largest of four paranasal sinuses and, with its close relationship to the underlying dentition, it is often susceptible to inflammatory processes. This chapter explores the anatomy, physiology of the maxillary sinus, the aetiology, assessment and management of maxillary sinusitis.

## 23.2 Anatomy of Maxillary Sinus

The maxillary sinus is the largest of the paranasal sinuses and develops during day 65–75 of gestation, with a volume of approximately 1 $cm^3$ at birth. Up untill an average age of 12, pneumatisation of the maxillary sinus continues as the space occupied by tooth germs is freed through their eruption [1]. In the latter stages of development, it pneumatises inferiorly, guided by the eruption pathway of the permanent dentition.

The main function of the maxillary sinus is involved in the humidification and warming of inspired air as well as prevention of microorganism ingress through mucociliary action. In addition to this, the paranasal sinus contributes to voice resonance. A possible evolutionary function may also be as a 'crumple zone' during trauma, thus protecting the brain (Fig. 23.1).

In an adult, the maxillary sinus takes the form of a quadrangle pyramidal shape, with the base adjacent to the nasal cavity and the peak extending towards the zygomatic process, and a volume in the region of 15 $cm^3$. The roof of the sinus is formed of the orbital floor in the centre of which runs the infraorbital neurovascular bundle. The anterior wall of the maxillary sinus is the weakest of the walls, with the thinnest section superior to the canine resulting in the canine fossa. It is also perforated by the infraorbital nerve that supplies the maxillary sinus, along with the greater palatine nerve. The posterior wall of the sinus lies in front of and shelters the internal maxillary artery, sphenopalatine artery, Vidian canal and the greater palatine nerve. The inferior wall is the most varying in shape, with invaginations corresponding to the alveolar bone of the maxilla; the anatomical root structures of maxillary molars and the hard palate. The bone separating the dental roots can be varying

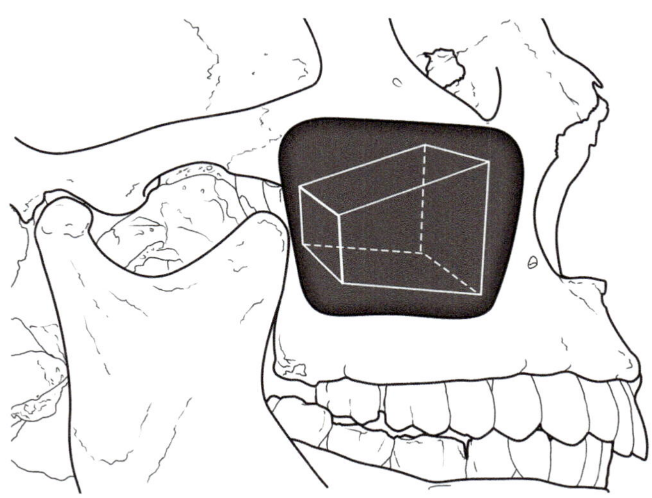

©Association of Oral and Maxillofacial Surgeons of India

**Fig. 23.1** Schematic diagram of the maxillary sinus with representation of the geometric shape of the cavity

K. Ganesan (✉)
Department of Oral and Maxillofacial Surgery, Southend University Hospitals NHS Trust, Southend-on-Sea, UK

University of Leeds, Leeds, UK
e-mail: mailme@kandyganesan.com

N. Rathod
Department of OMFS, Southend University Hospital NHS Trust, Southend-on-Sea, UK
e-mail: n.rathod@nhs.net


K. Bonanthaya et al. (eds.), *Oral and Maxillofacial Surgery for the Clinician*, https://doi.org/10.1007/978-981-15-1346-6_23

in its quantity; from complete absence to thicknesses of up to 12 mm [2]. This close proximity is a contributing factor towards the likelihood of dental iatrogenic and inflammatory pathology presenting in the maxillary sinus. The medial wall that is parallel to the nasal cavity communicates with it through the natural sinus ostium at the postero-superior aspect of sinus. This ostium opens in to a triangular space of approximately 15 $mm^2$ diameter formed by the uncinate process medially, the lamina papyracea laterally and the ethmoidal bulla posteriorly before communicating with the nasal cavity through a semilunar hiatus in the middle meatus. This is an area of common drainage from the maxillary, anterior ethmoidal and frontal sinuses. Some individuals may exhibit anterior/posterior fontanelles; bony dehiscences inferior to this, covered with mucosa. These can act as accessory ostia, points of drainage when the main osteomeatal complex is blocked or there is a change in sinus pressure. An osteomeatal complex (OMC) is an important functional unit and is also a key area for the pathogenesis of chronic rhinosinusitis. It consists of multiple bony structures, air spaces and ostia. The bony structures include the middle turbinate, uncinate process of the ethmoid and bulla of the ethmoid. Air spaces are formed by the frontal recess, infundibulum of the ethmoid and the middle meatus. Ostia consists of anterior ethmoid, maxillary and frontal sinuses. The classic OMC as mentioned above has been described as the anterior osteomeatal unit. The sphenoethmoidal recess and the superior meatus are referred to as the posterior meatal unit (Fig. 23.2).

Maxillry sinus septa, present in approximately 28.4% of cases [3], are thin projections of cortical bone that divide the sinus into more than one compartment either in the transverse, sagittal or horizontal plane, usually in the region of the first or second molar.

Smaller air-filled compartments in the periphery of the maxillary sinus can include Haler cells and Concha bullosa. Haller cells are air cavities encompassed in the ethmoidal capsule and are located below the inferomedial aspect of the orbital floor, and lateral to the ethmoidal cells. These can be present in a range of sizes as well as unilaterally or bilaterally. Concha bullosa is another variant air-filled cavity pneumatised in to the middle turbinate. These particular anatomical (Fig. 23.3) varia-

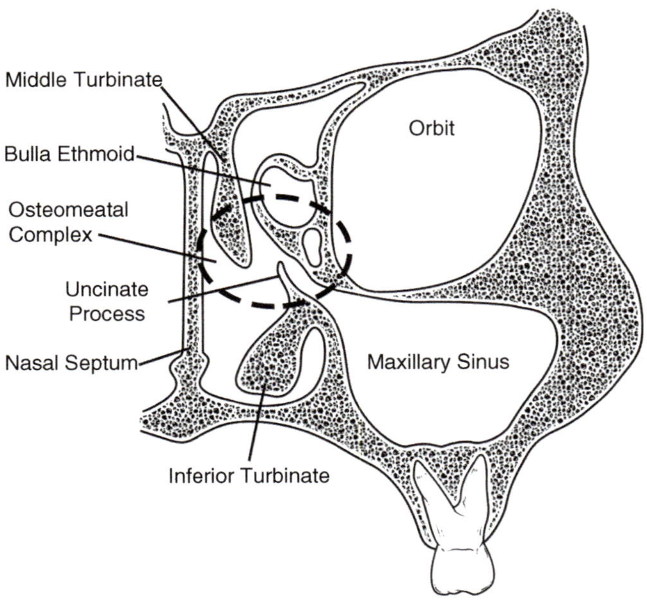




Fig. 23.2 Schematic diagram showing a coronal cross section of the maxillary sinus and the osteomeatal complex

Fig. 23.3 Schematic diagram with a sagittal cross section of the nasal cavity and the respective openings in to it

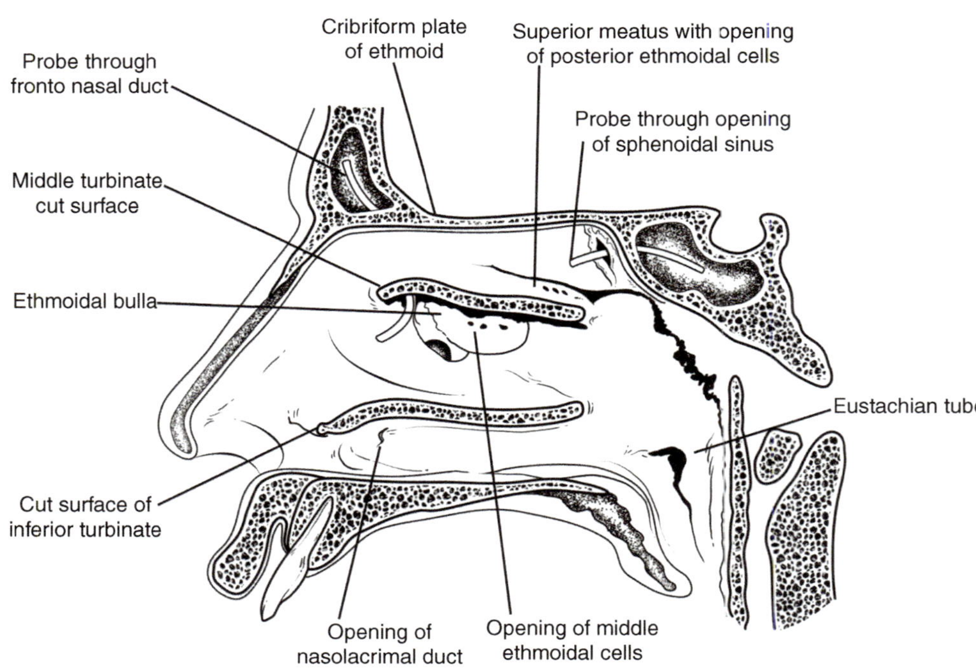

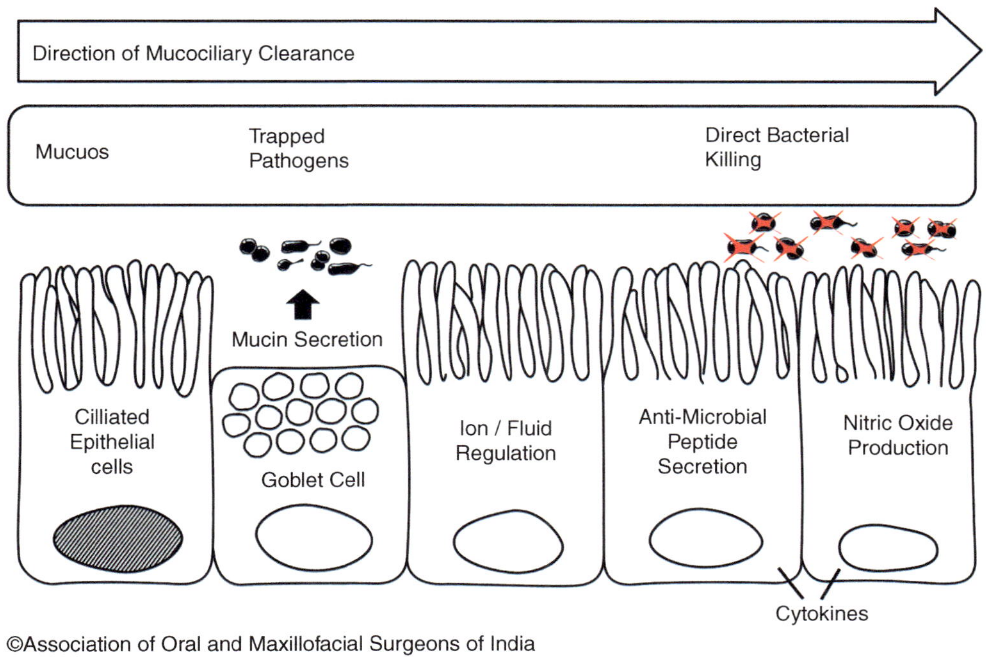


**Fig. 23.4** Schematic diagram of the secretary and clearance of the mucous via the mucociliary cells

tions have the potential to influence the dimensions of the osteomeatal complex, increasing the likelihood of sinus disease [4] .

## 23.3 Maxillary Sinus Physiology

At a histological level, the maxillary sinus consists of ciliated columnar cells, basal cells and goblet cells and thus forming respiratory epithelium architecture. Unlike the rest of the respiratory pathway, the sinuses have fewer ciliated and goblet cells; friable epithelium and fewer seromucous cells, making them prone to microorganism ingress and related pathology.

The clearance of secretions from the sinuses is through a combination of ciliary and mucous action. The mucous secreted by the goblet cells consists of 96% water, with the rest consisting of glycoproteins, immunoglobulins, histamines, lactoferrin, prostaglandins and lysozymes [5]. It functions to trap foreign body and defend against bacterial ingress. This is combined with the ciliary action that promotes a spiral action of movement of the mucous through active transport from the base of the sinus towards the natural ostium in the supero-posterior aspect of the medial sinus wall and thus working against the forces of gravity.

Normal flora within the maxillary sinus is usually a combination of sterile aerobic and anaerobic organisms including bacteria organised in a complex biofilm within the sinus mucus layer. These usually include mainly aerobic B-hemolytic streptococci, staphylococci and *haemophilus spp*. The anaerobic organisms, that are fewer in quantity, include peptostreptococcus, *fusobacterium sp* and bacteroides. Whether these organisms are present in normal physiology or transiently is poorly understood. Host specific and non-specific defence against these bacterial species is also part of normal physiology with the sinus mucosa producing secretion including antimicrobial peptides, proteins, neutrophils, macrophages coupled with the mucociliary transport towards the ostium (Fig. 23.4).

## 23.4 Sinusitis Pathophysiology

Due to the narrow size of the ostium opening, occlusion and related pathology of the maxillary sinus space are very likely possibilities. Obstruction of the sinus ostium can either be primary to the sinusitis process or secondary inflammation originating from elsewhere in the sinus.

With obstruction of the natural ostium, there is reduced oxygenation and gas exchange within the maxillary sinus, alongside reduced mucociliary action and mucous stasis. In the most common acute form of sinusitis, viral upper respiratory tract infections result in significant nasal congestion that results in maxillary sinus blockage and stasis. Anatomical differences such as large middle turbinates, deviated nasal septums or concha bullosa can increase the likelihood of ostium occlusion. Polyps, in particular those originating from the ethmoid, may also obstruct the maxillary sinus opening (Table 23.1).

Any form of obstruction and subsequent stasis in the maxillary sinus produce a favourable environment for the flourishing of an anaerobic environment, encouraging the formation of purulent secretions. In addition to this, changes in the sinus pressure, coupled with local mucosal inflammation, contribute to the symptoms of pain and pressure in the region [6]. The initial lower sinus pressure is caused by the

**Table 23.1** Membrane swelling leading to sinus infection

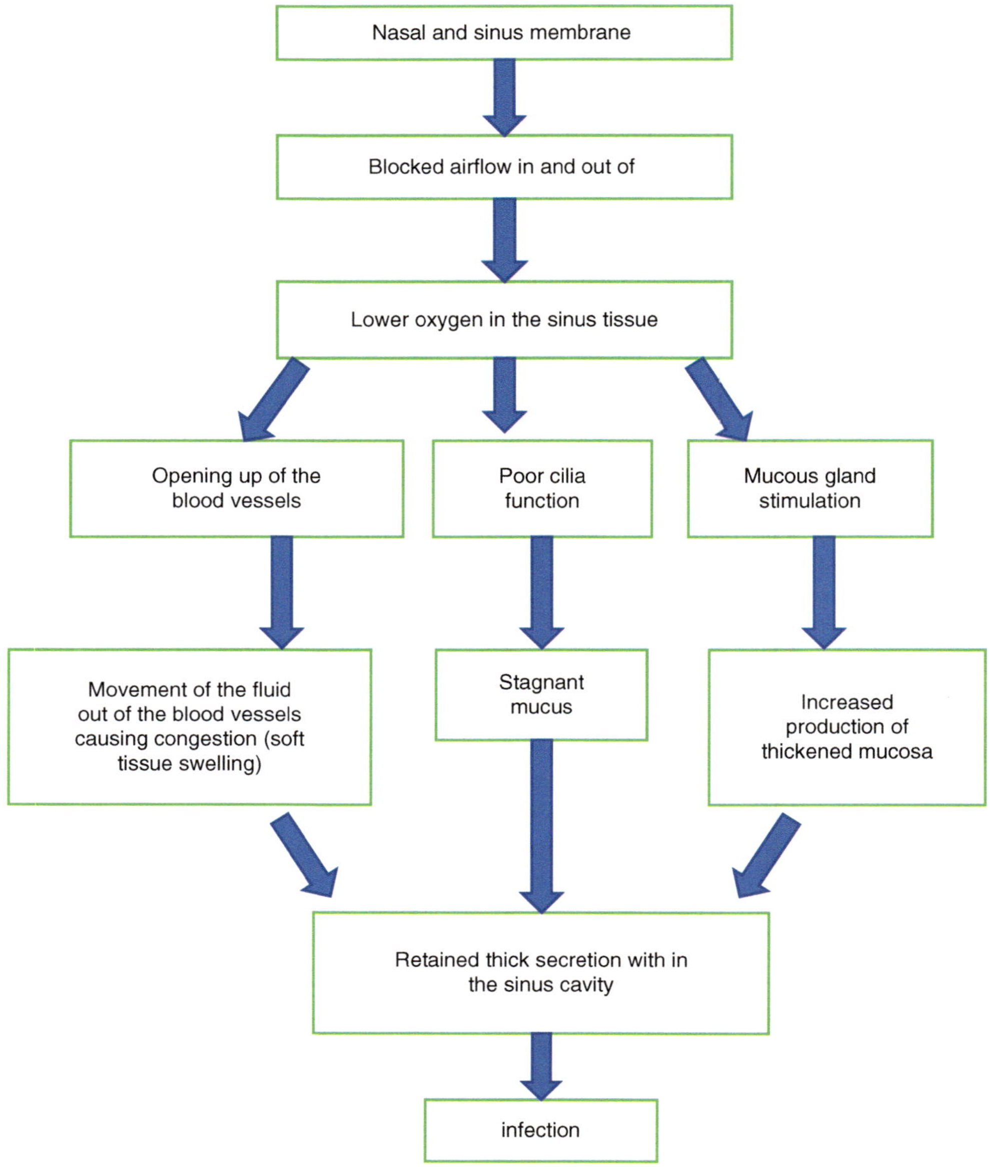


consumption of the finite oxygen within the blocked and confined maxillary sinus cavity. This is followed by a transient increase in pressure where there is a greater production of carbon dioxide and sinus secretion.

Chronic rhinosinusitis has features of long-term inflammation, rather than primary infection, of the nasal passages and paranasal sinuses with an unknown underlying cause. It is likely to be part of a cycle involving inflammation, infection and subsequent obstruction of the ostium [7]. Without the presence of polyps, chronic sinusitis may be multi-factorial in nature, with one or several predisposing factors as outlined below.

Nasal polyps are oedematous masses of the mucosal membrane found in the nasal passages and paranasal sinuses. Histologically, they show squamous epithelial proliferation, a thickened basement membrane, absence of neurosensory filaments and inflammatory cell infiltrate with high numbers of oesinophils [8]. The pathogenesis in the formation of polyps and its contribution towards chronic rhinosinusitis is poorly understood. One in vivo study involving rabbits with stimulated maxillary sinusitis observed the formation of inflammatory-type polyps in subjects with purulent infection and granulation based polyps in both purulent and non-purulent infections. In both infective processes, epithelial damage to the mucosal lining appeared to be a significant factor in the initiation of polyp formation [9]. Other evidence shows that high levels of interleukin 5, 13 and histamines in the polypoid tissue may also have a contributing role [10]. The general consensus of studies shows a high level of inflammatory mediators in the initiation and presence of nasal polyps, suggesting chronic inflammation to be a key factor.

### 23.4.1 Microorganisms of Sinusitis

The polymicrobial nature of maxillary sinusitis has been well documented. The initial aerobic bacterial infective organisms often include *Streptococcus pneumoniae*, Haemophilus influenzae and Moraxella catarrhalis in acute sinusitis [11]. Chronic sinusitis has found to harbour the aforementioned organisms in addition to Prevotella species, Fusobacterium species and anaerobic streptococci [12]. More recent studies have cultured *Staphylococcus aureus*, in particular methicillin resistant-type from sinus mucosal samples [13].

## 23.5 Predisposing Factors

### 23.5.1 Anatomical Variation

Any variation deemed to alter the volume or the size of the maxillary ostium may contribute to an increase risk of sinusitis. This includes [14]:

- Haller cells.
- Concha bullosa.
- Reduced infundibular width.
- Septal deviation.
- Choanal atresia.
- Nasal polyps.
- Hypoplasia of the sinus.
- Maxillary dentition roots in the sinus.

### 23.5.2 Atopy (Allergy)

The distinct relationship between the allergy and inflammation remains unclear. Current hypothesis predicts that with the ventilation passage in continuum with the nasal mucosa, inflammation along the rest of the airway can affect the nasal passages, thus causing narrowing of the ostium. This is supported by the high incidence of chronic rhinosinusitis with allergies driven by IgE mediators.

### 23.5.3 Asthma

The association between chronic sinusitis, mainly with nasal polyps, and asthma has been well documented. Several studies have shown radiographic sinus mucosal abnormalities in individuals with asthma, in particular with those suffering from severe steroid-dependent asthma [15]. Similar studies show a trend in the severity of sinusitis correlating to the severity of asthma experienced, supporting the theory of inflammation of a unified mucosal airway concept of the disease process. The association between asthma and sinusitis is further indicated with studies showing individuals reporting improvement in their asthma symptoms subsequent to medical and/or surgical treatment of their sinusitis [16].

### 23.5.4 Aspirin

Aspirin/NSAID hypersensitivity has been found to have an association with a persistent form of chronic sinusitis, usually with the presence of nasal polyps. Along with severe asthma, this disease process has been named the 'Aspirin-triad'. The mechanism of pathogenicity is thought to be linked to cyclooxygenase inhibition and inhibition of arachnoid acid metabolism rather than an underlying immunological process. The presence of hyperplastic sinus mucosa contributes to a high level of recurrence in nasal polyps subsequent to sinus surgery for removal [14].

### 23.5.5 Environmental

Several environmental factors have been associated with an increased incidence of sinusitis with changes in air quality acting as suggestive stimulants. Greater prevalence has been identified in patients exposed to chemical air pollutants including pharmaceutical products, photocopying ink by-products, smoke and dampness [14, 17].

### 23.5.6 Ciliary Impairment

This may be present in the form of reduced cilia or ciliary cells, causing impairment of mucociliary flow and thus creating environments favourable for bacterial or viral sinusitis.

### 23.5.7 Smoking

Smoking is likely to diminish the presence of normal microbiological flora in the nasal and paranasal spaces, allowing for the growth of pathogenic microorganisms and thus eliciting a hypersensitivity reaction in the sinonasal mucosa [14].

### 23.5.8 Gastro-Oesophageal Reflux

It has been suggested that inflammation may be elicited when the oro- and nasopharynx comes in contact with gastric acids during reflux and subsequently contributing to sinusitis [18].

### 23.5.9 Odontogenic Maxillary Sinusitis

As part of the examination process, this should be evaluated at the early stages and could prevent prolonged periods of investigations and symptomatic management (Fig. 23.5). Approximately 15–24% of unilateral maxillary sinusitis cases are believed to be of odontogenic origin [19], with some studies indicating this figure to be as high as 40% [20]. In a meta-analysis of 15 observational review studies consisting 770 cases, the first molars were found to be the most common tooth to be causative for odontogenic sinusitis (22.51%), followed by third molars (17.21%), second molars (3.97%), premolars (5.96%) and lastly canines (0.66%). The etiological contribution to the sinusitis was found most commonly to be from iatrogenic factors (55.97%), periodontal disease (40.38%) and odontogenic cysts (6.66%) [21]. Figure 23.6 outlines the distribution of the iatrogenic processes leading to sinusitis [21].

The disruption in maxillary sinus floor, from whichever odontogenic source, causes localised inflammation that remains persistent in that area or spreads along the sinomucosal surface with subsequent obstruction of the sinus ostium. Bacterial colonisation have been shown to consist of both aerobic and anaerobic species in 75% of cases, with the other 25% predominantly anaerobic in nature. *Staphylococcus aureus* and streptococcus pneumonia were the predominant aerobic bacteria isolated. When looking at the anaerobic bacteria distribution, Peptococcus and Prevotella species dominated and haemophilus and Moraxella species were absent in cases of odontogenic maxillary sinusitis [20].

## 23.6 Classification of Sinusitis

Sinusitis is defined as an inflammation of the paranasal sinus mucosal lining; however, it rarely presents in isolation and is usually coupled with the inflammation of the nasal mucosa, thus being termed as rhinosinusitis. The cardinal features, of which two are required for a suggestive diagnosis of a rhinosinusitis, are outlined in the 2012 European position paper by the International Rhinology Society (Table 23.2). The condition is broadly classified based upon the chronicity of the condition as well as whether there is presence of polyps.

### 23.6.1 Acute Rhinosinusitis

Acute rhinosinusitis (ARS) is defined as persistent sinusitis that resolves within a 12-week period. It is a common presentation within the populations globally, with prevalence rates between 6 and 15% [14].

### 23.6.2 Chronic Rhinosinusitis

Chronic rhinosinusitis is defined by the persistence of sinusitis symptoms for greater than 12 weeks, with no resolution after initial sinusitis treatment. It is further subdivided into whether there is a clinical and radiographic presentation of nasal polyps.

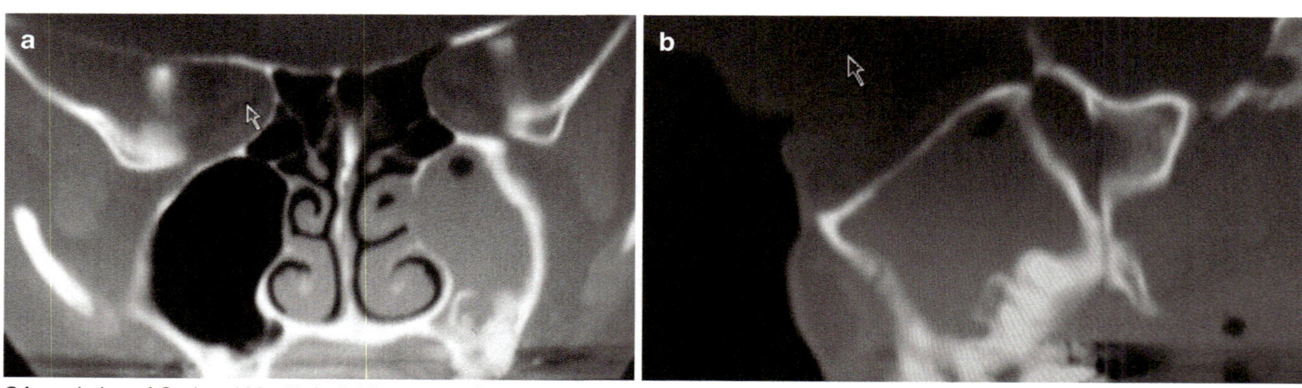




**Fig. 23.5** (**a**) A coronal section of a CT of maxillary sinus showing extensive left-sided maxillary sinusitis. A periapical radiolucency on the upper left first molar with a breach in the cystic area to allow the pus to enter the sinus and causing the sinusitis. (**b**) A sagittal section same image showing the extent of the sinusitis. A periapical radiolucency is noticeable in relation to mesiobuccal root of upper left first molar

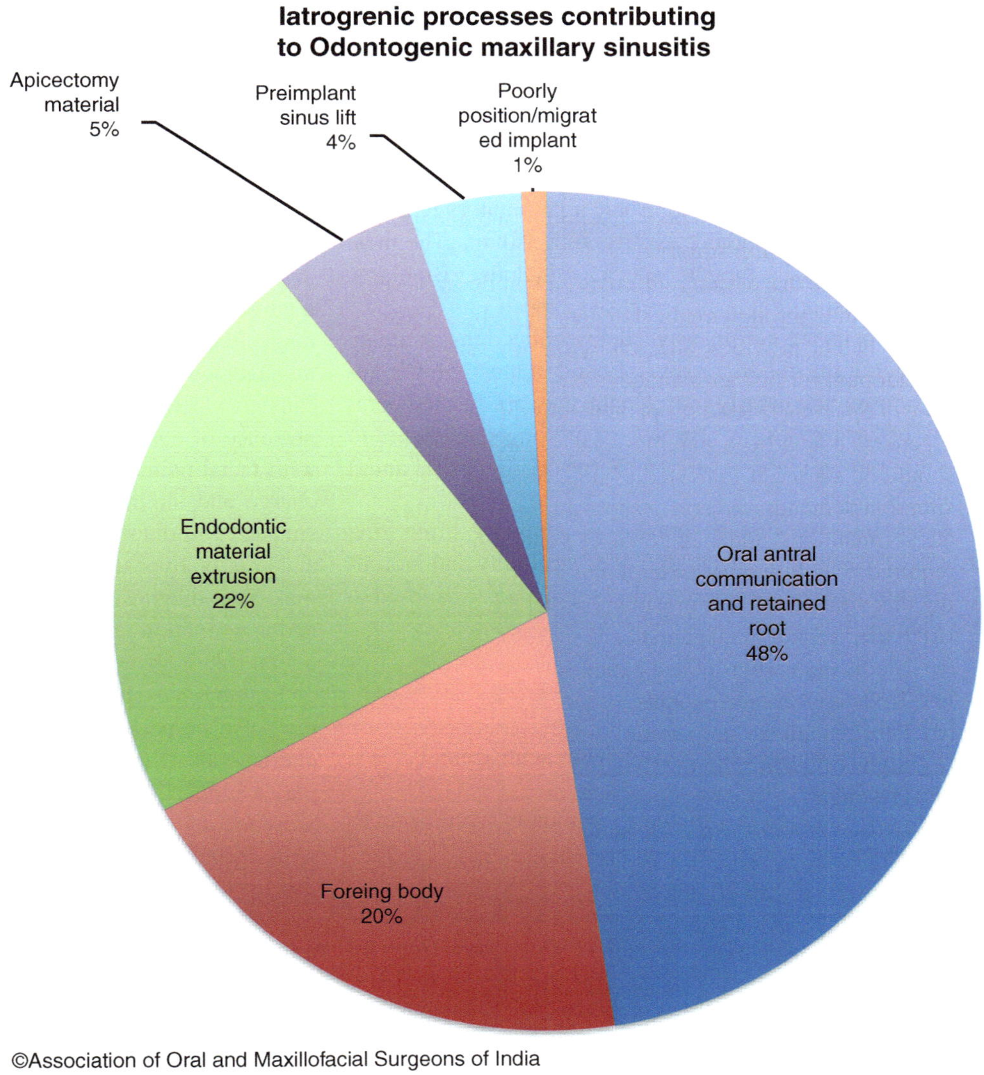


**Fig. 23.6** A pie chart illustrating a distribution of the iatrogenic processes contributing to odontogenic sinusitis [21]

**Table 23.2** Features of rhinosinusitis [14]

| Symptoms | Endoscopic signs of | CT changes |
|---|---|---|
| • Nasal obstruction/ blockage<br>• Nasal congestion<br>• Anterior/ posterior nasal discharge<br>• Anosmia/ Hyposmia<br>• Facial pain/ pressure | • Nasal polyps,<br>• Mucosal oedema/ obstruction of the middle meatus,<br>• Mucopurulent discharge mainly from the middle meatus | • Mucosal change in the sinus Mucosal change in the osteomeatal complex |

### 23.6.3 Fungal Rhinosinusitis

This subtype of chronic rhinosinusitis involves the inflammation of the maxillary sinusitis that is attributed to a fungal pathogen and can be classified into acute fungal rhinosinusitis, fungus balls or fulminant invasive fungal rhinosinusitis.

Acute fungal rhinosinusitis (AFRS), as described by Bent and Kuhn, is characterised by five properties [22]:

1. Nasal polyps.
2. Type I hypersensitivity to fungi (skin test or serum IgE testing).
3. Sample positive for fungal staining.

4. Eosinophilic mucin that does not invade into sinus tissue.
5. Characteristic CT radiopaque sinus findings.

The predicted pathogenesis of AFRS is believed to be an allergic, immediate hypersensitivity reaction to an inhaled fungal organism resulting in a chronic inflammatory response in a predisposed individual, usually with asthma. The most common isolated fungal species include Bipolaris, Curvularia, Aspergillus, and Drechslera species.

Fungal balls are non-invasive, dense collections of fungal debris within the maxillary sinus. Found in mostly immunocompromised and elderly individuals, they are formed commonly of aspergillus, in response to prolonged exposure to the fungi through inhalation of airborne spores or oral antral communication.

Acute invasive fungal sinusitis is a rapidly infiltrating growth of the fungi with a high risk of morbidity and mortality. Immunocompromised individuals that are predisposed to this include those with:

- Diabetes,
- Leukaemia,
- Hard and soft tissue malignancy with neutropenia,
- Steroid therapy,
- Severely impaired cell-mediated immunity (congenital or acquired).

Initial clinical presentation involves an acute onset of facial/head pain, fever, epistaxis and, in severe cases, of bony erosion with extrasinus infiltration and possible mental status change. Urgent surgical management and post-operative antifungal therapy is required.

## 23.7 Clinical Diagnosis

Diagnosis of sinusitis is primarily through clinical history and examination with the possible adjuncts of imaging studies and/or laboratory testing. The signs and symptoms of sinusitis can be categorised in to major and minor. Major features include infraorbital and maxillary facial pain, pressure sensation, congestion/obstruction sensation, purulent rhinorrhoea, hyposmia and fever [23]. Minor features are present in some of the individuals with suspected sinusitis and include headache, fatigue, dental pain, halitosis, cough and ear pain/fullness.

The acute form of rhinosinusitis is indicated usually when a patient has recently suffered with the symptoms of an upper respiratory tract infection that is viral in nature. After an initial 7–10 day phase of viral infection with gradual recovery, patients give history of worsening symptoms. Evaluation of nasal discharges show secretions that were once clear at the initial stages of the viral infection that become yellow, green or grey in nature at the latter aspect of the biphasic disease process. Unilateral disease process provides greater indication towards sinusitis. Palpation over the infraorbital sinus region would elicit tenderness due to the pressure build-up from stasis and inflammation of the sinus cavity.

Patients with suspected chronic rhinosinusitis may present with symptoms of acute rhinosinusitis but to a milder degree, with the absence of a predisposing upper respiratory tract infection including fever. The presenting complaint may often be of the lack of effectiveness in acute medical management techniques [24]. Regardless of whether the causative factor in the chronicity of their sinusitis is from the presence of nasal polyps or not, patients will often present with facial pain or pressure, anterior or posterior nasal discharge and slight fatigue. Those that suffer from chronic sinusitis without the presence of polyps may also experience anosmia or hyposmia. Thus, the ambiguity in presentation makes the diagnosis of chronic sinusitis with clinical history and examination alone challenging, but nonetheless provide a vital role in their diagnosis and long-term management.

Endonasal examination in the form of anterior rhinoscopy may also be performed with headlighting and a speculum; alternatively with the large speculum of an otoscope. It can play a supportive role in visualising inflamed nasal mucosa, presence and quality of nasal discharge and the turbinates with an indication of nasal polyps or anatomical variation that may not have been suspected previously.

Nasal endoscopy provides an enhanced technique for direct visualisation of the nasal passage. Abnormalities in the nasal passage can be seen including the middle, superior turbinates and the osteomeatal mucociliary drainage passage. Where acute rhinosinusitis is diagnosed mainly through clinical history and simple examination, this method is more relevant for incidences of chronic rhinosinusitis. Nasal endoscopy can be used at 3, 6, 9 and 12 monthly intervals in chronic disease process to assess the degree of inflammation, discharge and size of nasal polyps.

Intraoral assessment should include assessment of both soft and hard tissues. The dentition requires close evaluation to rule out primary aetiology which can account for 5–10% of acute rhinosinusitis cases [25]. Detailed assessment for extensive dental caries, periapical and/or periodontal infections for teeth distal to the canine is required. Where multiple teeth are unilaterally tender to percussion with a lack of correlation to dental pathology clinically or radiographically, sinusitis not of dental cause is a probable diagnosis. This sensation may also be elicited with facial or head movements. This is due to the close neural relationship between the maxillary sinus and upper molars. Pain or pressure sensation is also elicited from palpation in the most superior aspect of the maxillary buccal sulcus. In some cases, posterior discharge in to the nasopharynx that is either characteristically

**Table 23.3** Differential diagnosis for maxillary sinusitis, NICE guidelines 2018 [26]

- Upper respiratory tract infection.
- Allergic rhinitis.
- Adenoiditis or tonsillitis.
- Sinonasal tumour.
- Turbinate hypertrophy.
- Migraine.
- Giant cell arteritis.
- Temporomandibular joint dysfunction.
- Neuropathic or atypical facial pain.

clear or coloured in nature can be visualised during intraoral assessment.

Recurring episodes of acute rhinosinusitis (more than three episodes a year) requires wider consideration of the primary causative factor. Peters et al. has attributed recurrent acute rhinosinusitis to various reasons such as immunodeficiency, cystic fibrosis, ciliary dysfunction and anatomic abnormalities [16] (Table 23.3).

Severe episodes of acute rhinosinusitis originating from the maxillary sinuses are a rare presentation. Complications can arise with the involvement of the ethmoidal and frontal sinuses that are in close proximity to vital structures including the anterior cranial cavity and the orbits with associated venous drainage systems [27].

As per Ah- See et al. [28], certain features of sinusitis that require urgent intervention are:

- Bleeding.
- Proptosis/diplopia.
- Maxillary paresthesia.
- Intraorbital/intracranial complications.
- Osteomyelitis.
- Immunocompromised patients.

## 23.8 Clinical Imaging

Clinical imaging is a useful adjunct to the diagnosis of sinusitis. It can provide confirmatory and characteristic information to guide management of the condition.

Plain radiography is an accessible and cost-effective means of visualising the maxillary sinus. An orthopantomogram (OPG), though focusing on the dentition, maxilla and mandible, also includes a significant proportion of the maxillary sinuses and provides an opportunity to identify the presence of pathological features. Indication of sinusitis would be from the presence of unilateral or bilateral generalised diffuse radiopacity within the maxillary sinus. Causative disease process can also be visualised including the proximity of periapical pathology from the maxillary dentition, periodontal disease, cystic lesions of dental origin, foreign body presence, sinonasal mucocele or polyps. The significant level of artefact from overlying structures however limits the usefulness of this imaging modality. Where dental disease is a suspected contributing factor, dental periapical radiographs can be considered for a targeted and enhanced dental evaluation. Consequently, a dental cause for sinusitis can be challenging to diagnose, in particular in cases of chronic sinusitis.

The occipitomental view, also known as the 'Water's view, can additionally offer visualisation of the entire sinus as well as other paranasal sinuses, with fluid collection and mucosal thickening evident at varying angles. Care must be taken to differentiate between a benign mucosal cyst and a fluid level. A diagram showing the difference in the appearances between the two is shown in Fig. 23.7.

Despite the efficiency with which these images can be taken, one should consider whether the overall information gained for sinusitis diagnosis justifies the exposure to radiation. Plain imaging does not offer a comprehensive view of the maxillary sinus ostium, the occlusion of which will often be the causation of subsequent sinusitis. Apart from suggestion in the presence or absence of disease process, it does not offer information on the severity of the condition. With significant overlap, diagnosis of sinus masses can also be difficult.

Computer tomography (CT) (Fig. 23.8) offers the three-dimensional visualisation of the sinuses and can be confirmatory in the presence or absence of sinus disease. These should be considered only where a patient's symptoms are vague or first-line medical management has thus far failed to offer significant relief of symptoms. Contrast medium is not required as they do not offer additional value towards diagnosis or management. It should also be noted that where CT scans of sinuses are taken, maxillary teeth should also be included to assess for their involvement in the disease process.

With appropriate manipulation of imaging sections, the location and severity of sinus disease can be gauged. Mucosal thickening is distinctly evident on CT scans, being more pronounced in cases of sinusitis with polyps. Further diagnostic information is available on the sinus content including air–fluid levels. The patency of the sinus discharge tract can be assessed with detailed view of the osteomeatal complex on coronal sections thus allowing for surgical planning. The presence or absence of nasal masses can be confirmed in CT cases but can be used to differentiate between sinus polyps, cysts or tumours. Generalised thickening or sclerosis of the maxillary sinus walls may be indicative of chronic sinusitis whereby early infective processes cause demineralisation of the sinus wall and prolonged reactive host responses that result in sclerotic bone deposition. Where sclerosis is more localised in the maxillary sinus wall, there may be indication towards enquiry of previous sinus surgery.

Cone beam computer tomography (CBCT) can provide enhanced information on the pathological processes contrib-

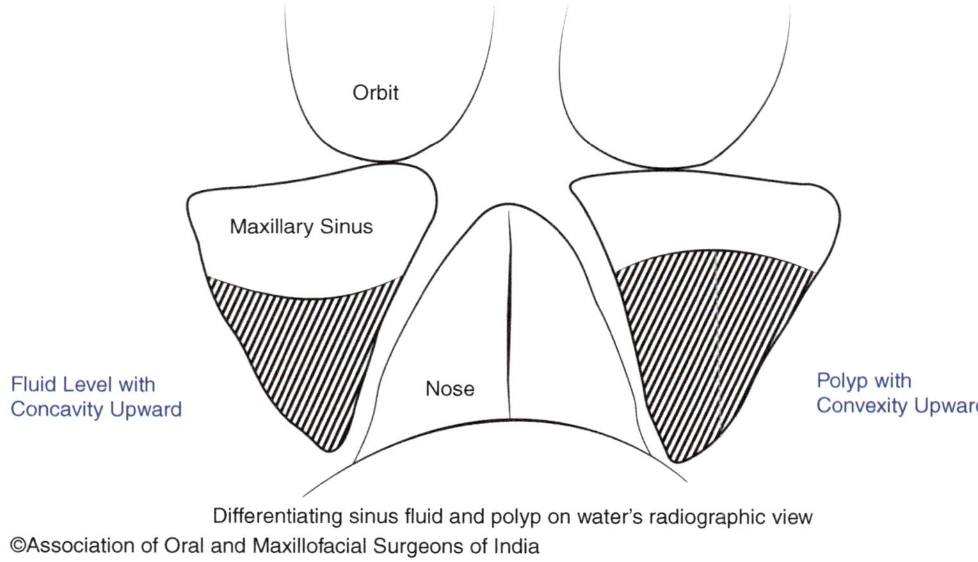


**Fig. 23.7** Diagram showing the difference between the fluid level and the mucosal cyst/polyp

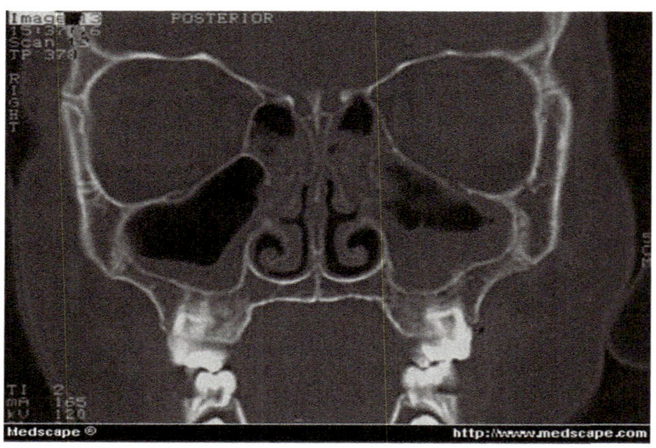


©Association of Oral and Maxillofacial Surgeons of India

**Fig. 23.8** A coronal view of a CT scan showing thickened mucosal lining of the both maxillary sinus with a fluid level on the left maxillary sinus

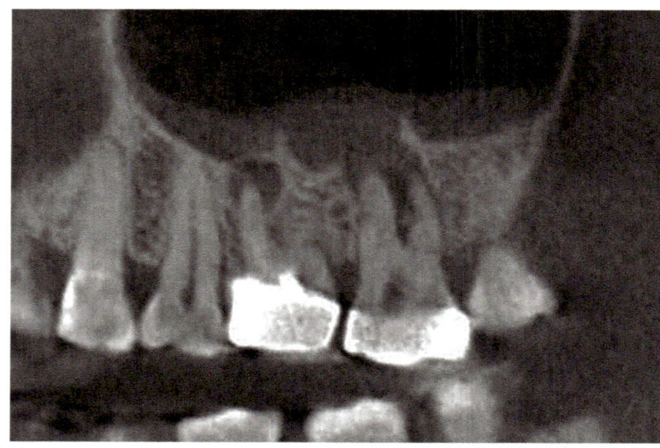

©Association of Oral and Maxillofacial Surgeons of India

**Fig. 23.9** CBCT of the sinuses showing upper second molar with a breach in the periodontal ligament space and periapical area opening into the maxillary sinus causing sinusitis—a classic odontogenic sinusitis

uting towards sinusitis, with slices as fine as 0.4 mm as well as offering a lower radiation dose exposure, in the region of 10%, in comparison to a fine slice CT scan (Fig. 23.9).

This is more relevant for cases of maxillary sinusitis of dental origin in which pathological processes can be tracked from the tooth to the sinus structure.

MRI scans offer an imaging modality that allows some enhanced interpretation in the appearance of the soft tissue within the sinus. This is not relevant in the majority of uncomplicated maxillary sinusitis presentations. The use of MRI is limited to cases where there is opacification of the maxillary sinus with no obvious obstruction, osseous abnormality or odontogenic pathology. It allows the differentiation between mucosal inflammation, complete fluid collection or a tumour within the maxillary sinus as well as its origin.

## 23.9 Treatment

### 23.9.1 Conservative Management

In acute sinusitis cases, with a primary virus and secondary bacterial infection, the aim of treatment focuses around relieving of symptoms including pain, nasal congestion and discharge during the 2–3 week period that it will take to resolve. Antibiotics in the early stages are not recommended. Advice can be offered in the management of systemic virus infection including physical rest, adequate analgesia and increased fluid intake.

The pain sensation from the maxillary sinus region is attributed to pressure changes caused by occlusion of the ostia and thus, treatment to promote unblocking will inherently contribute towards pain reduction. During this process, analgesia in the form of paracetamol and ibuprofen can be utilised for management of pain.

Nasal saline and decongestants have been shown in some literature to be an effective means of opening the ostia and ecouraging ventilation.

Nasal saline mists and irrigations can offer a breakdown of nasal blockages, dilution of irritants and allergens, reduction of postnasal drainage and overall more effective mucociliary clearance [29]. Lavage/irrigation of the nasal passage can be performed using small quantities of salt or bicarbonate dissolved in warm water. These can be administered by inhaling small volumes of the self-made formulation in cupped hands through each nostril until nasal ventilation feels clearer. Alternative over-the-counter devices such as squeeze-bottles and syringes can be used. Humidified air and steam inhalation can also be utilised as a means of nasal secretory blockage breakdown. These irrigative techniques can offer supportive relief to other symptomatic management methods but are not deemed effective as monotherapy [30].

Where there is indication of chronic sinusitis, potential risk factors should be identified and addressed, including avoidance of triggers that may exacerbate allergies and asthmatic flare-ups. Where applicable, patients should be encouraged to stop smoking or being exposed to passive smoke.

## 23.9.2 Medical Management

Where acute sinusitis symptoms last for longer than 10 days, medical treatment modalities can be offered.

### 23.9.2.1 Nasal Decongestants

Topical nasal decongestants can be offered as a means of improving sinonasal ventilation through reducing mucosal secretion, nasal congestion and thus improved patency of the osteomeatal complex. Topical formulations can include phenylephrine (0.25%), oxymetazoline (0.5%) and xylometazoline [31]. These should be limited to use twice a day for up to 3 days. These formulations have a sympathomimetic effect causing vasoconstriction with subsequent reduced fluid secretion and mucosal inflammation. Long-term use of these agents can produce a rebound effect with the absence of sustained vasoconstriction.

### 23.9.2.2 Topical Nasal Glucocorticosteroids

Topical intranasal glucocorticosteroids may be considered in the management of prolonged acute rhinosinusitis or chronic rhinosinusitis as an adjunctive or monotherapy prior to the consideration of antibiotic prescription [32]. These can be utilised for up to 3 months in adult patients depending on the formulation used and especially where allergy is deemed a significant risk factor. Common formulations utilised include budesonide, ciclesonide, fluticasone furoate, fluticasone propionate, mometasone furoate and triamcinolone acetonide. These have been deemed an effective means of clearing nasal and sinus air passages in several studies when used in a retroclined, head tilt action to encourage exposure towards the middle meatus.

### 23.9.2.3 Systemic Glucocorticosteroids

The use of systemic glucocorticosteroids has been reserved for refractory cases of chronic rhinosinusitis, in particular those with allergy [2], as well as initial treatment for patients with suspected allergic fungal rhinosinusitis. It can provide symptomatic relief through improving ventilation through the sinuses, reducing the size of polyps and thus restoring some sense of smell. Current British guidelines suggest prednisolone 0.5 mgk/kg for 5–10 days as well as the adjunct therapy with betamethasone nasal drops [33], taking relevant consideration of those already on steroids for other conditions.

### 23.9.2.4 Antimicrobial Therapy

There is limited evidence to support the use of antibiotics in the short term for acute rhinosinusitis. A Cochrane review of 10 trials based in the primary care environment found that irrespective of treatment modality with or without antibiotics, 71% of patients' symptoms of uncomplicated acute sinusitis had resolved by the 2-week mark [34]. Where symptoms of sinusitis arise, the microbes of dominance usually include aerobic streptococcus pneumonia, haemophilus influenza and Moraxella catarrhalis. Antibiotic therapy should be reserved for cases of acute exacerbations of rhinosinusitis where symptoms haven't resolved after 7–10 days or for severe cases involving signs of systemic spread including fever and severe unilateral facial pain. Though the evidence is limited, some literature supports the use of amoxicillin for 7–14 days. This is mostly effective; however, approximately 20–30% of haemophilus influenza strains have been found to be resistant to amoxicillin due to the production of lactamase [35]. During persistent periods of acute sinusitis or during exacerbations of chronic sinusitis, there is a shift towards a mixture of anaerobic and aerobic pathogenesis. The Infectious Diseases Society of America recommends amoxicillin clavulanate as the first choice of antibiotic for 5–7 days [36], with clindamycin, doxycycline, levofloxacin or moxifloxacin for those with an allergy to penicillin. This can be used in combination with topical glucocorticosteroids to attain more efficient symptom relief [32]. In cases of chronic sinusitis, use of low-dose macrolides has shown some effectiveness [14]. In all cases, where viable, the choice of antibiotic should be guided by microbiological culture growth, attained from discharges from the middle meatus or surgically guided sample collection.

### 23.9.3 Surgery

Surgical intervention is routinely carried out by Ear, Nose and Throat speciality and is usually indicated in the failed medical management of chronic sinusitis or as the first treatment for acute fungal rhinosinusitis. The aim of surgery is to attain normal function through restoration of ventilation and allowing physiological mucociliary drainage of the sinuses. This can be through opening and widening of the osteomeatal complex, removing foreign body and polypoid tissue, clearing the sinus of infected mucin, removal of chronically inflamed mucosal and bony tissue whilst throughout preserving as much of the virgin, healthy mucous membrane in the sinus as possible.

Extra-oral or intra-oral approaches can be taken. The classically used internal access is the Caldwell-Luc approach. George W Caldwell first published this technique in the New York Medical Journal in 1893, where he utilised the canine fossa approach to gain access to the sinus and perform intranasal drainage, significantly improving surgical outcomes. Henry Luc, a french surgeon, further adapted this method in 1897 for surgical treatment of chronic sinusitis where performed antrstomy in the middle meatus whilst Caldwell had performed an inferior meatal antrostomy.

#### 23.9.3.1 Surgical Method: Caldwell-Luc Approach

Advanced imaging like CT or CBCT should be used for the procedure. Particular awareness is required for the presences of any septae that may interfere with the Caldwell-Luc access in to the sinus. In addition, assessment is required of the availability of a window on the anterior wall of maxillary sinus, with short maxillary sinus height creating challenges in this approach.

This procedure can be done either under a general or a local anaesthetic with sedation support; though complete painrelief and anaesthesia with the latter option is difficult to achieve (Fig. 23.10). Once adequate anaesthesia has been achieved, the upper lip is retracted an incision is made 2–3 mm above the mucogingival junction, parallel to the occlusal surface of the teeth. A full-thickness mucoperiosteal flap can be raised with a molt"s periosteal elevator to reveal the underlying bone. Often, bulbosities caused by the root projections of the upper canines and premolars are noticeable and they can be used as anatomical landmarks to avoid damaging the roots of the teeth. The periosteum can be raised elevated all the way to infraorbital foramen and care must be taken not to stretch the infraorbital nerve. Then a bony window can be made with a Rosehead bur 2–3 mm above the root apices of the teeth. On entry in to the sinus, a microbiology swabbing of the sinus content is done for culture and sensitivity. Once the swab has been taken, this is followed by stripping of the sinus lining, especially when treating chronic, persistant sinusitis. The lining can be removed with a microdebrider, Freer's elevator and curettes. Care must be taken not to remove tissue from the roof of the sinus due to the fact infraorbital nerve can be seen through the canal resorbed by maxillary sinusitis.

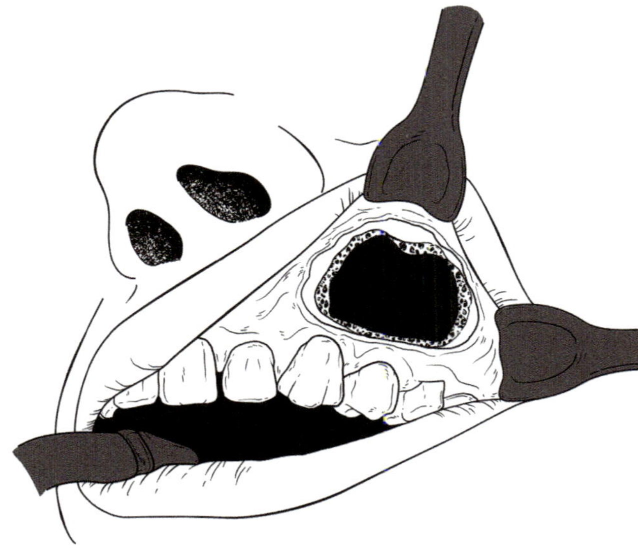



**Fig. 23.10** A diagram showing the intraoral approach for the Caldwell-Luc technique

Any soft tissue curetted from the sinus can be sent for histopathological examination. A 30 or 45 degree endoscope is used to visualise the floor of the sinus which is not feasible with a standard 0 degree FESS. To complete the procedure, an intranasal antrostomy can be done to improve the drainage of the sinus. This procedure can be done by passing a curved haemostat through the nasal aperture to penetrate the lateral nasal wall, 1-1.5cm posterior to the anterior attachment of the inferior nasal turbinate. Care should be taken to avoid injuring the opening of nasolacrimal duct. The projection of the haemostat can be visualised with an endoscope in the sinus simultaneously. Forceps are used to remove the fragments of bone created from the enlargement of the ostium and thus complete the intranasal antrostomy. The intra-oral Caldwell-Luc access is used to provide a final saline-wash within the sinus, prior to achieving haemostasis and would closure, often with resorbable sutures.

#### 23.9.3.2 Complications with Caldwell-Luc approach

Complications associated with this surgical technique include infraorbital nerve parasthesia that is often transient and may last up to 6 months. Similarly there may be numbess of the attached gingivae and associated teeth or even possible devitalisation. If the lacrimal apparatus has been encountered, there may also be the risk of dacryocystitis.

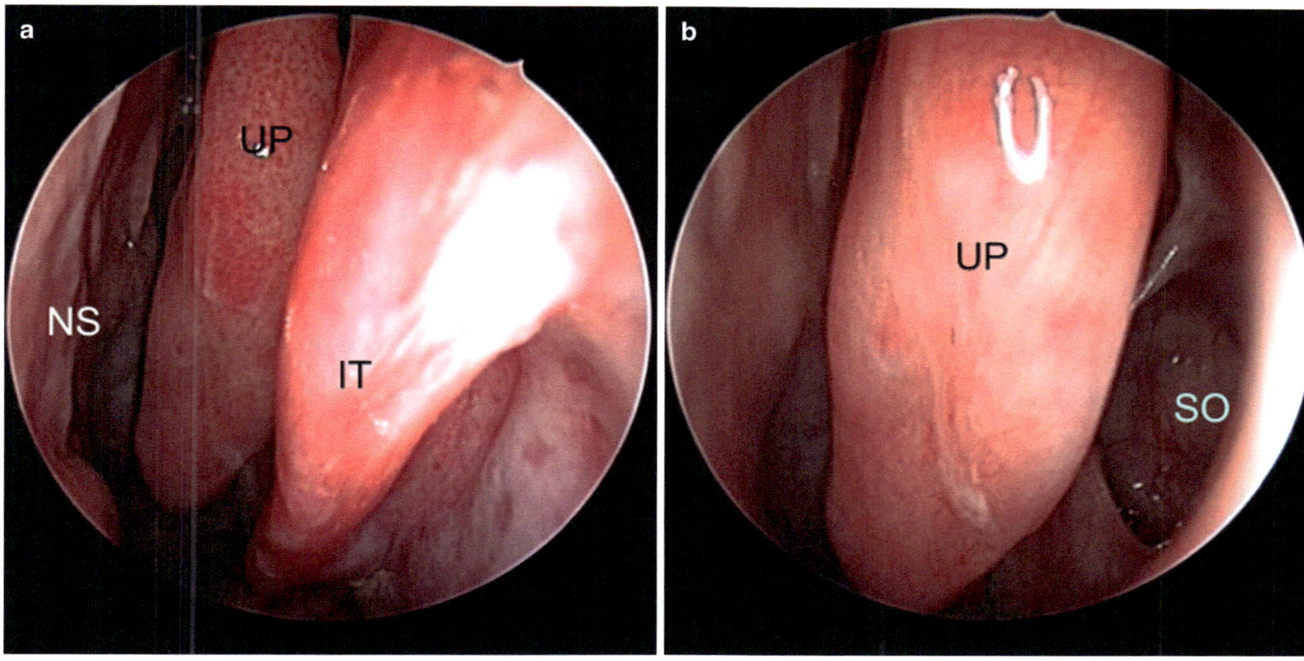




**Fig. 23.11** (**a** and **b**) Naso endoscopic pictures showing as the scope enters the left nostril. Nasal septum (NS) on the left and Inferior turbinate (IT) on the right and the uncinate process (UP). Further up showing maxillary sinus ostium (SO) and Uncinate process (UP)

#### 23.9.3.3 Surgical Method: Functional Endoscopic Sinus Surgery

With technology continually advancing, many prospective studies report functional endoscopic sinus surgery (FESS) (Fig. 23.11) to be a safe and effective means of managing chronic sinusitis. For the FESS approach to be an effective surgical method in the management of chronic sinusitis, appropriate patient and surgical instrumentation related factors require consideration. Standard preparation for FESS involves an oral endotracheal tube which can be positioned based on surgeon's convenience to improve the access. Prior to donning surgical scrubs, the neuro-patties soaked in a vasoconstrictor solution may be placed along the floor and middle portion of the nasal cavity such that it is effective at the start of the operation. In addition, all Encoscopic acumen should be ready for the beginning of the procedure. Endoscopic instrumentation includes a 0, 30, and 70 degree angle scope, a powered debrider with a 4 mm straight and a 60 degree cannula, 4 mm long curved suction, various types of punch forceps, curettes and a monopolar suction cautery.

Before the start of the procedure, neuro-patties are removed and 1% lidocaine and 1:100000 adrenaline injected into the septum, middle turbinate and uncinate process for the maxillary sinus-related issues. To survey the width and depth of the nasal cavity and also to establish the boundaries to avoid any complications, a systematic examination of the nasal cavity carried out with a 30 degree scope attached to an endoscopic tower/viewing screen. All the nasal structures should be visualised including posterior nasal choana and the inferior turbinates.

Systematic intranasal survey with the scope is also carried out as a part of the surgical planning to identify any nasal septal spur, septal deviations and turbinate hypertrophy to improve the access and to prevent any complications. Additionally, any polyps can be removed to improve the access. An angled probe is used to reflect the uncinate process to visualise hiatus semilunaris and infundibulum. Back fracturing the uncinate process finally allows visualisation of the maxillary sinus ostium and medial wall of the orbit. A 4 mm trimmer can be used to remove uncinate and part of the middle turbinate to gain access to maxillary sinus ostium. The superior border of the sinus ostium is an important anatomical landmark as it is the junction of the medial wall of the orbit and the lamina papyracea. At this point of dissection, a decision can be taken to do a minimal or extensive dissection process, and this depends on the extent of the disease process. Mostly, a minimal dissection (expansion of the ostium) is all that is necessary.

#### 23.9.3.4 Complications with the FESS Approach

FESS is an essentially safe procedure in the hands of a trained and experienced surgeon; however there are a wide range of risks associated with this procedure due to the proximity of anatomical structures such as the orbits and their content, major arterial and venous structures and the base of the skull. Severe complications can include orbital content penetration that may lead to fat herniation, enopthalmous and damage to extraocular muscles; penetration in to the skull base can result in cerebrospinal fluid leakage and carotid artery dissection may cause a stroke or even death. Orbital content penetration leading to fat herniation, enophthalmos and damage to extraocular muscles. Crusting, septal perforation, mild bleeding, nasal obstruction, anosmia, minimal fat herniation from orbital wall perforation and crusting of the nasal mucosa are examples of what are believed to be minor complications.

Sinus surgery should be supported with medical management post-operatively to prevent further inflammation developing, particularly in the case of polyp removals that may re-establish without maintenance therapy.

## 23.10 Conclusion

Sinusitis can be a debilitating condition for patients whether acute or chronic. With close proximity to the dentition, symptoms of dental pain can result in presentation to the maxillofacial and dental professional. A succinct clinical history and examination is vital in attaining an accurate diagnosis. Though management is guided by diagnosis, management should commence with symptom relief.

**Acknowledgements** We would like to acknowledge Mr. Martyn Barnes and SurgTec for the endoscopic pictures attached to this chapter. More endoscopic images and videos can be accessed from www.surgtech.net website.

## References

1. Lawson W, Patel ZM, Lin FY. The development and pathologic processes that influence maxillary sinus pneumatization. Anat Rec: Advances in Integrative Anatomy and Evolutionary Biology: Advances in Integrative Anatomy and Evolutionary Biology. 2008 Nov;291(11):1554–63.
2. Ugincius P, Kubilius R, Gervickas A, Vaitkus S. Chronic odontogenic maxillary sinusitis. Stomatologija. 2006;8:44–8.
3. Pommer B, Ulm C, Lorenzoni M, Palmer R, Watzek G, Zechner W. Prevalence, location and morphology of maxillary sinus septa: systematic review and meta-analysis. J Clin Periodontol. 2012 Aug;39(8):769–73.
4. Stallman JS, Lobo JN, Som PM. The incidence of concha bullosa and its relationship to nasal septal deviation and paranasal sinus disease. Am J Neuroradiol. 2004 Oct 1;25(9):1613–8.
5. Benninger MS. Rhinitis, sinusitis and their relationship to allergy. Am J Rhinol. 1992;6:37–43.
6. Aust R, Stierna P, Drettner B. Basic experimental studies of ostial patency and local metabolic environment of the maxillary sinus. Acta Otolaryngol Suppl. 1994;515:7–10. Discussion 1
7. ENT UK and Royal College of Surgeons. Commissioning guide: chronic rhinosinusitis. London: ENT UK and Royal College of Surgeons; 2016.
8. Pawankar R. Nasal polyposis: an update. Curr Opin Allergy Clin Immunol. 2003 Feb 1;3(1):1–6.
9. Norlander T, Fukami M, Westrin KM, Stierna P, Carlsöö B. Formation of mucosal polyps in the nasal and maxillary sinus cavities by infection. Otolaryngol Head Neck Surg. 1993 Sep;109(3):522–9.
10. Drake-Lee AB, McLaughlan P. Clinical symptoms, free histamine and IgE in patients with nasal polyposis. Int Arch Allergy Appl Immunol. 1982;69:268–71.
11. Gwaltney JM Jr, Scheld WM, Sande MA, Sydnor A. The microbial etiology and antimicrobial therapy of adults with acute community-acquired sinusitis: a fifteen-year experience at the University of Virginia and review of other selected studies. J Allergy Clin Immunol. 1992;90:457–61. Discussion 62
12. Finegold SM, Flynn MJ, Rose FV, et al. Bacteriologic findings associated with chronic bacterial maxillary sinusitis in adults. Clin Infect Dis. 2002;35:428–33.
13. Brook I, Foote PA, Hausfeld JN. Increase in the frequency of recovery of methicillin-resistant *Staphylococcus aureus* in acute and chronic maxillary sinusitis. J Med Microbiol. 2008;57:1015–7.
14. Fokkens WJ, Lund VJ, Mullol J, et al. European position paper on rhinosinusitis and nasal polyps 2012. Rhinol Suppl. 2012;(23):3 p preceding table of contents, 1–298.
15. Serrano E, Neukirch F, Pribil C, Jankowski R, Klossek JM, Chanal I, et al. Nasal polyposis in France: impact on sleep and quality of life. J Laryngol Otol. 2005;119(7):543–9.
16. Peters AT, Spector S, Hsu J, Hamilos DL, Baroody FM, Chandra RK, Grammer LC, Kennedy DW, Cohen NA, Kaliner MA, Wald ER. Diagnosis and management of rhinosinusitis: a practice parameter update. Ann Allergy Asthma Immunol. 2014 Oct 1;113(4):347–85.
17. Koskinen OM, Husman TM, Meklin TM, Nevalainen AI. The relationship between moisture or mould observations in houses and the state of health of their occupants. Eur Respir J: Official Journal of the European Society for Clinical Respiratory Physiology. 1999 Dec;14(6):1363–7.
18. Report of the rhinosinusitis task force committee meeting Alexandria, Virginia, August 17, 1996. Otolaryngol Head Neck Surg. 1997;117(3 Pt 2):S1–68.
19. Vestin Fredriksson M, Öhman A, Flygare L, Tano K. When maxillary sinusitis does not heal: findings on CBCT scans of the sinuses with a particular focus on the occurrence of odontogenic causes of maxillary sinusitis. Laryngoscope Investig Otolaryngol. 2017 Dec;2(6):442–6.
20. Patel NA, Ferguson BJ. Odontogenic sinusitis: an ancient but under-appreciated cause of maxillary sinusitis. Curr Opin Otolaryngol Head Neck Surg. 2012 Feb 1;20(1):24–8.
21. Arias-Irimia O, Barona-Dorado C, Santos-Marino JA, Martínez-Rodríguez N, Martínez-González JM. Meta-analysis of the etiology of odontogenic maxillary sinusitis. Med Oral Patol Oral Cir Bucal. 2010 Jan 1;15(1):e70–3.
22. Bent JP III, Kuhn FA. Allergic fungal sinusitis/polyposis. Allergy Asthma Proc. 1996;17:259–68.
23. Rosenfeld RM, Andes D, Bhattacharyya N, et al. Clinical practice guideline: adult sinusitis. Otolaryngol Head Neck Surg. 2007;137(suppl):S1–S31.
24. Tan BK, Chandra RK, Pollak J, et al. Incidence and associated premorbid diagnoses of patients with chronic rhinosinusitis. J Allergy Clin Immunol. 2013;131:1350–60.
25. Williams JW, Simel DL. Does this patient have sinusitis? Diagnosing acute sinusitis by history and physical examination. JAMA. 1993;270:1242–6.
26. National Institute for Health and Care Excellence. Sinusitis. London: NICE; 2018.
27. Cummings CW, Haughey BH, Thomas JR, Harker LA, Flint PW, Haughey BB, et al. Cummings otolaryngology: head & neck surgery. 4th ed. Philadelphia: Mosby; 2005.

28. Ah-See KW, Evans AS. Sinusitis and its management. BMJ: Brit Med J. 2007 Feb 17;334(7589):358.
29. Hauptman G, Ryan MW. The effect of saline solutions on nasal patency and mu- cociliary clearance in rhinosinusitis patients. Otolaryngol Head Neck Surg. 2007;137:815–21.
30. Harvey R, Hannan SA, Badia L, Scadding G. Nasal saline irrigations for the symptoms of chronic rhinosinusitis. Cochrane Database Syst Rev. 2007;3:CD006394.
31. Kretzschmar DP, Kretzschmar CJ. Rhinosinusitis: review from a dental perspective. Oral Surg Oral Med Oral Pathol Oral Radiol Endod. 2003 Aug 1;96(2):128–35.
32. Zalmonovici A, Yaphe J. Steroids for acute sinusitis. Cochrane Database Syst Rev. 2007;(2):CD005149.
33. Scadding GK, Durham SR, Mirakian R, Jones NS, Drake-Lee AB, Ryan D, et al. BSACI guidelines for the management of rhinosinusitis and nasal polyposis. Clin Exp Allergy. 2008;38:260–75.
34. Lemiengre MB, van Driel ML, Merenstein D, Young J, De Sutter AI. Antibiotics for clinically diagnosed acute rhinosinusitis in adults. Cochrane Database Syst Rev. 2012;10:CD006089.
35. Fairbanks DN. Inflammatory diseases of the sinuses: bacteriology and antibiotics. Otolaryngol Clin N Am. 1993;26:549–59.
36. Chow AW, Benninger MS, Brook I, et al. IDSA clinical practice guideline for acute bacterial rhinosinusitis in children and adults. Clin Infect Dis. 2012;54:e72–e112.

# OroAntral Communications and OroAntral Fistula

# 24

Suvy Manuel

*Routine exodontia is a common procedure performed by the general dental practitioner and the oral surgeon alike. Most of the maxillary premolar/molar extractions heal uneventfully but some may cause inadvertent opening into the maxillary sinus, manifesting as immediate oro antral communications (OAC) or delayed oro antral fistulae. The common reasons being difficulty encountered in the extractions intra operatively due to myriad reasons or the OAC may be due to a pre existing pathology in the peri apical region or within the sinus lining. Whatever the reason be , its paramount that the surgeon identifies the problem and approach it in a sequential manner to avoid long term consequences and to attain a perfect closure. The timing of the closure is crucial which is dependent upon the sinus health and the socket condition. This may be complicated by a missing root tip which is lying in the sinus. This chapter aims to walk the reader through these events in a logical fashion, so that they can take appropriate decisions and use the correct surgical technique which will ensure a successful closure of the defect.*

## 24.1 Introduction

Maxillary sinus is an anatomical area, which is intimately associated with the field of oral and maxillofacial surgery. Many of the procedures done violate the integrity of the maxillary sinus, as in orthognathic surgeries, or when the sinus is involved per se as part of midface trauma or in odontogenic pathologies that infringe upon the sinus.

The relevance of the sinus in day-to-day minor dentoalveolar surgical procedures is that the sinus floor is in very close approximation with the roots of the maxillary posterior teeth, especially the molars [1].

Eberhardt, in 1992, did a CT study to evaluate the distance between maxillary sinus floor and the apices of the maxillary pre-molar/molar teeth. The buccal first premolar showed the largest value of 6.18 mm (SD 1.60 mm). It is quite disturbing to know that the mesiobuccal root of maxillary second molar is only 0.83 mm (SD 0.49 mm) away from the maxillary sinus floor, as per this study results. Readers are advised to refer the table in reference [1] to have a better picture of this relevant CT study.

This intimate relation with the root of maxillary molars causes many a time inadvertent communication between the sinus and oral cavity causing acute OroAntral communication (OAC). If the OAC is unrecognized or not dealt with primarily, either it may undergo spontaneous healing if the circumstances are favourable or it may progress into a full-fledged OroAntral fistula (OAF), which will need secondary intervention for closure.

This section of the book deals with OAC and OAF caused during exodontia and minor dentoalveolar surgical procedures, cyst enucleation and small-sized tumour excision.

Communications caused due to excision of moderate to large pathologies, post-oncosurgery defects, major maxillofacial trauma, gunshot/missile injuries, osteoradionecrosis and developmental and congenital deformities usually may require locoregional/free flap transfers and/or prosthetic rehabilitations. Such communications are dealt with elsewhere in this book.

This section is limited to closure of OAF caused after exodontia; however, many surgical techniques used for OAF closure do overlap with surgical closure techniques of oronasal and palatal fistulas. Those techniques are dealt with in relevant sections of the book.

This chapter also deals with managing and retrieving root/root tips, which are inadvertently displaced into the sinus (Root in sinus).

Most of the surgical procedures aimed at correction of OAC/OAF are doomed to fail if the underlying sinus is not

**Electronic Supplementary Material** The online version of this chapter (https://doi.org/10.1007/978-981-15-1346-6_24) contains supplementary material, which is available to authorized users.

S. Manuel (✉)
Department of Oral and Maxillofacial Surgery, Ananthapuri Hospitals and Research Institute, Trivandrum, Kerala, India

Kerala Institute of Medical Sciences, Trivandrum, Kerala, India


K. Bonanthaya et al. (eds.), *Oral and Maxillofacial Surgery for the Clinician*, https://doi.org/10.1007/978-981-15-1346-6_24

healthy before the anticipated closure. The "Antral regime procedures" are aimed at ensuring a disease-free sinus before anticipated elective closure of a post-extraction OAF. When patients are referred to oral surgeons for treatment of OAF, depending upon the duration of complaint, the sinus may be in various stages of the disease. It is difficult to ascertain whether the sinus was diseased primarily at the time of exodontia, accentuating the chance of an OAF formation or whether the sinus had been secondarily infected following the formation of OAF due to direct communication with the oral cavity. Another possibility is that the sinus lining would have been secondarily involved by a periapical pathology and removal of the involved tooth was conducive to the formation of the OAC.

The role of an otorhinolaryngologist cannot be understated, and at times, the closure has to be attempted after consulting with them regarding the sinus health. Their presence may be required during the closure for allied procedures in the sinus like FESS (Functional Endoscopic Sinus Surgery).

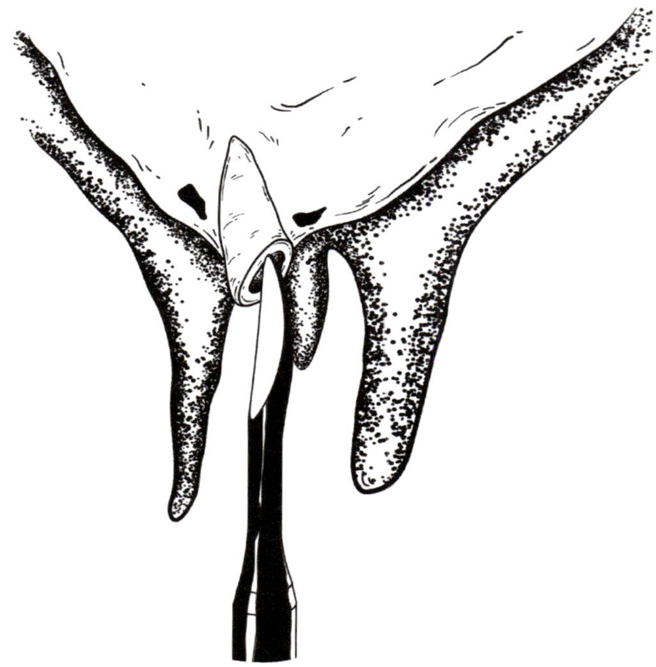



**Fig. 24.1** Improper use of dental elevators causing pushing of root tip into maxillary sinus

## 24.2 Aetiology of OAC

The common causes for OAC during dentoalveolar procedures are

1. Aberrant anatomy causing the sinus floor to dip down between the roots of premolars and molars/decreased thickness of sinus floor.
2. Unusually long roots, which lie in close proximity to the sinus floor/Schneiderian membrane.
3. Dense alveolar bone causing difficult extractions.
4. Removal of root canal-treated maxillary molars is usually difficult due to the brittle nature of the tooth.

   Attempted removal of brittle root tip fractures in such teeth shows an increased chance of getting OAC.
5. Improper use of dental elevators when attempting to remove root tip can cause undue vertical forces, whichmay push the roots into the sinus (Fig. 24.1).
6. Progressive pneumatization of the sinus as age advances, especially around lone standing molars (Fig. 24.2).
7. Progressive pneumatization is also a cause for OAC during removal of maxillary third molars especially when associated with tuberosity fractures.
8. Teeth, which have periapical pathologies, cause bone loss/erosion at the sinus floor and are at a higher chance of causing OAC after extractions. It is imperative that such cases are identified pre-operatively, adequate radiographic examinations are done, the patients are pre-warned and necessary measures are to be taken to close the OAC, if they occur during the procedure (Fig. 24.3a, b and c).
9. Occasionally, odontogenic infections/abscess may spread to the sinus, which may manifest "Fluid levels" in the sinus on paranasal sinus X-rays. Extraction of such teeth involves a greater chance of having OAC.

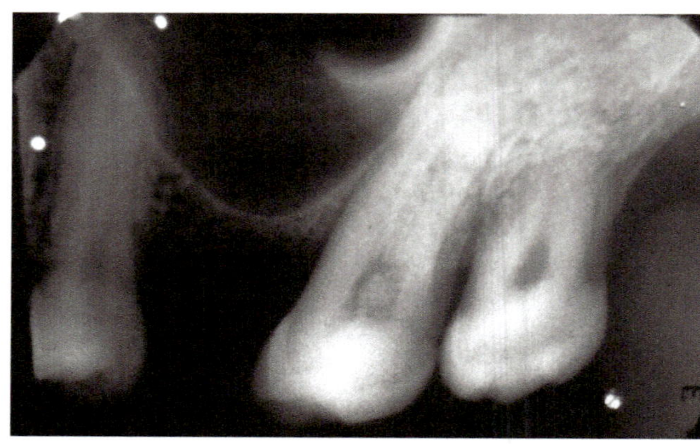



**Fig. 24.2** Sinus dipping down in a long-standing edentulous area of upper left first molar (IOPA)

10. Lack of adherence to basic principles of dentoalveolar surgery or overzealous/aggressive attempts to remove or retrieve fractured root tips of maxillary posterior teeth may cause OAC. It is the judgement of the concerned clinician whether to attempt removal of a fractured root tip; if the clinician can remove the root tip via the socket through closed intra-alveolar technique well and good, if not the clinician should be able to remove the tip via transalveolar technique based on sound dentoalveolar surgical principles and should be able to close the OAC if it occurs. If the clinician feels that he is not able to perform the above-mentioned procedure, it may be wise

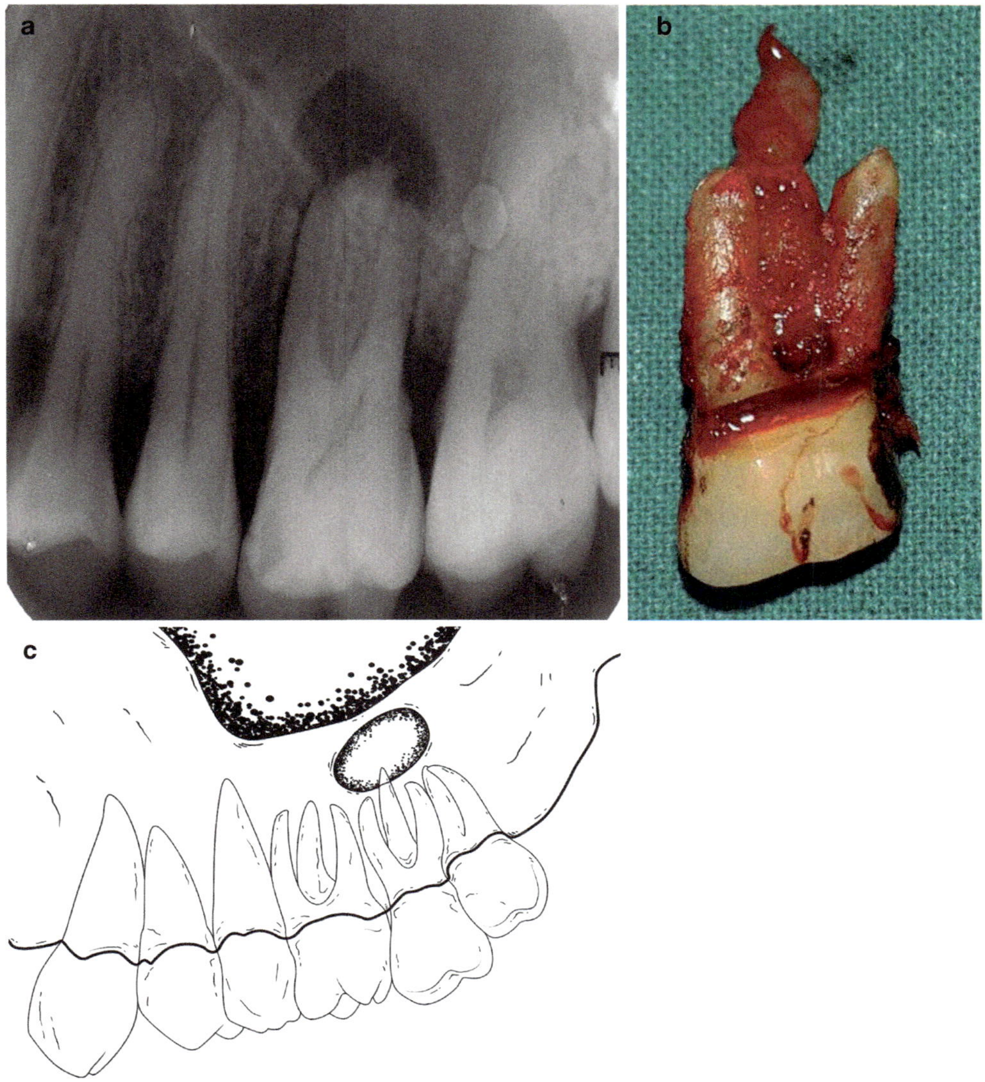



**Fig. 24.3** (**a**) IOPA of a molar showing periapical lesion, (**b**) Extracted molar with the lesion attached to the root tip, (**c**) Diagrammatic representation of periapical lesion close to sinus floor

not to vigorously attempt to remove the root tip. Either he should get expert help or it would be judicious to leave the root tip behind and attempt removal later if required when expert help is available (Fig. 24.4).

11. Teeth, which have aberrant root anatomies, dilacerations, hypercementosis and ankylosis, are all at risk of developing OAC.

## 24.3 Clinical Features of OAC

The basic rule to be followed when we suspect an OAC is never to enlarge or aggravate the existing communication. Most of the time OAC goes unrecognized, and it may heal spontaneously if it is less than 3–5 mm in diameter [2]. If a bigger OAC is not recognized and adequate measures are not taken for closure, it may progress to OAF. Unless it is an evident OAC, confirmatory tests are not done in order to prevent enlarging the OAC. Literature also says that sinusitis will ensue if the OAC is not closed within 24–48 h.

1. Bubbling of mucous or blood may be seen at the socket opening when the patient exerts pressure via a closed nostril (Valsalva manoeuvre).
2. Patient may feel oronasal regurgitation or leaking of oral fluids via nose if they hold water in mouth.
3. There may be unilateral epistaxis on the affected side.
4. Close examination of the socket apex under direct light vision may show the sinus lining or opening into the sinus.
5. There may be changes in the resonance of the voice.
6. An OAC should be suspected if a piece of antral floor is attached to the root end after extraction (Fig. 24.5).

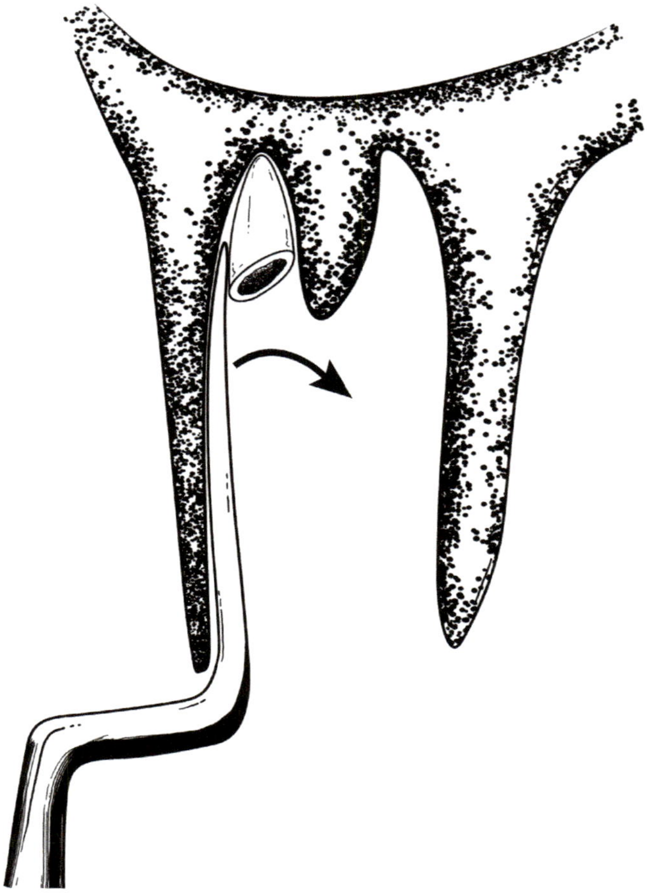

©Association of Oral and Maxillofacial Surgeons of India

**Fig. 24.4** Diagram showing the importance of slow, careful and fine movements to remove root tips with straight probes, fine mosquito forceps or apical fragment ejectors

### 24.3.1 Radiological Features of OAC

There may not be radiological evidence of a small OAC on a routine IOPA, unless there is sizeable loss of antral floor or breach in antral floor, which will manifest as a direct communication between the sinus and socket. It is not advisable to insert a probe or radiopaque marker into the socket and take an x-ray as it may enlarge the OAC.

### 24.3.2 Management of OAC

The OAC may be managed in the following step wise approach:

1. If you suspect an OAC, it is prudent to inform the patient about the anticipated treatment plan and the sequel.

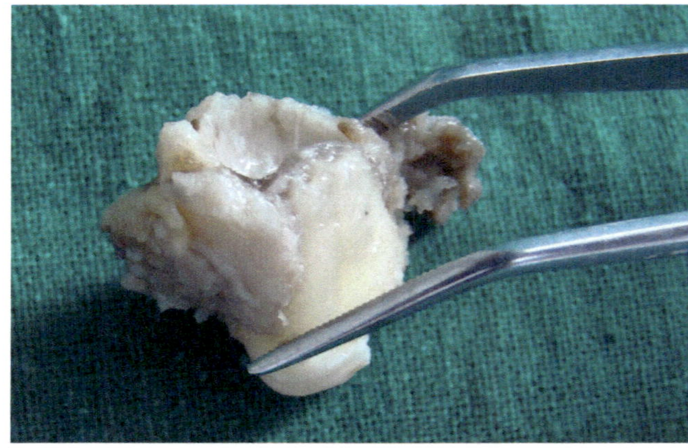

©Association of Oral and Maxillofacial Surgeons of India

**Fig. 24.5** Note the sinus floor attached to the roots of an upper third molar after extraction, with associated tuberosity fracture. It is a definite case of OAC, which warrants primary closure if conditions are favourable

   Patient has to be aware of the condition as post-operative compliance form of the patient is of paramount importance in order to prevent any dehiscence or clot break down at the OAC closure site. *(See antral regime section.)*
2. Openings less than 3–5 mm in size may be left without any intervention hoping for spontaneous healing, or a primary closure may be attempted depending upon individual case scenarios. If left for spontaneous healing, patients are specifically instructed to avoid any manoeuvres, which may increase the intra-sinus pressure.

A routine suturing across the socket in maxillary premolar/molar extraction sites may not suffice in suspected cases of OAC, as the buccal and palatal gingivae may not approximate primarily and healing may be secondary in nature. Suturing in such cases just plays a role in supporting the clot. If aiming at primary closure to treat OAC, the buccal and palatal gingivae may be approximated by the following additional measures:

(a) Reduce the height of the buccal/palatal alveolar bone in order for the sutures to approximate.
(b) As it is the palatal mucoperiosteum that is more adherent, a semilunar relaxing incision may be placed about 5 mm away from the palatal gingival edge and the flap is advanced buccally to meet the buccal gingivae (Fig. 24.6).

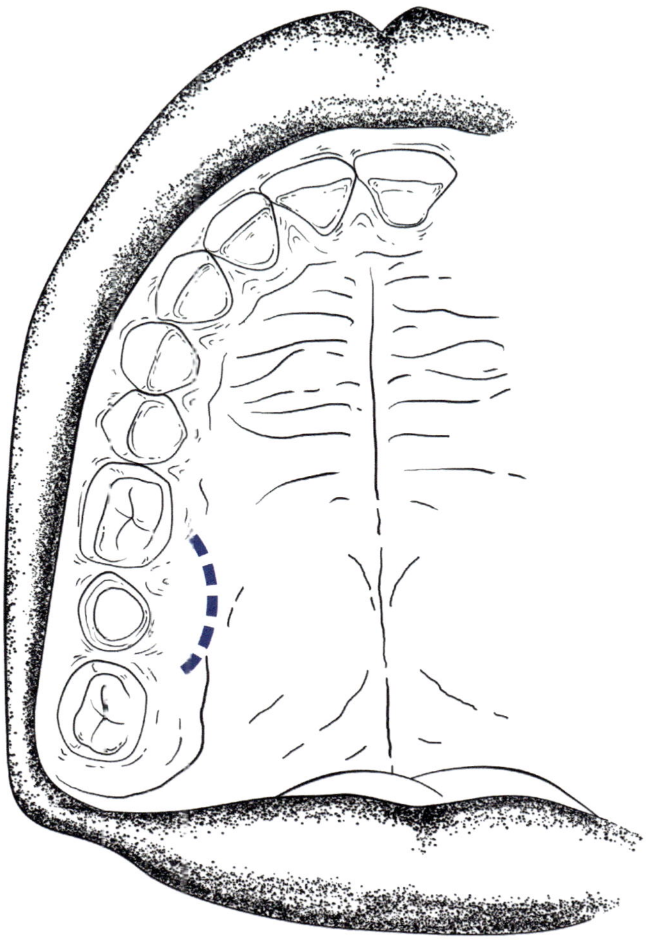
©Association of Oral and Maxillofacial Surgeons of India

**Fig. 24.6** Depicts releasing incision in the palate, to advance the flap in order to achieve primary closure of the socket

Beyond these two steps, any attempt at closing the OAC would mean that the surgeon is using techniques that are common with established techniques of closing an OAF. If primary closure is not obtained by (a) or (b), the next logical step would be to raise a buccal full thickness three-sided (trapezoidal/rectangular/4 cornered) flap and advancing it to the palatal side. At this stage, if adequate relaxation is not present for the flap, the mucoperiosteum may have to be scored and the details of this are given in OAF surgical closure section of this chapter.

If the sinus is healthy, the best chance of closing an OAC is at the time of occurrence and the surgeon may use any of the techniques in his armamentarium, and these decisions are taken on a case-by-case basis.

**Clinical Scenario 1**

A simple clinical scenario is given here as food for thought for the young readers (Fig. 24.7).

I believe that there may be different opinions, with few possible ones being

1. Extract the tooth and allow the lesion to regress/observe periodically.
2. Extract the tooth and curette/attempt enucleation via socket.
3. Extract the tooth via transalveolar technique and enucleate the lesion.
4. Further investigations/imaging before attempting extraction.
5. Assess the sinus condition before performing any extraction.
6. Be aware of the possibility of an OAC after extraction and be prepared for the possible technique of closure.

This case was included just to show how perplexing a routine clinical situation could be and to stress on the importance of a solid pre-operative plan before attempting such cases.

## 24.4 OroAntral Fistula

Intrusion into the maxillary sinus and establishment of direct communication with the oral cavity are referred to as an oroantral fistula (Fig. 24.8a and b). An oroantral fistula is a pathological condition in which the oral and antral cavities have a permanent communication by means of a fibrous connective tissue fistula coated by epithelium. Once an unrecognized OAC does not heal or there is failure of attempted closure, the condition progresses to an OAF, which means that the epithelization of the communicating tract has occurred. Usually, such cases get referred to the oral surgeon from the general dental practice within 2–3 weeks of the occurrence, when patient notices oronasal regurgitation.

### 24.4.1 Aetiology of OAF

The causes for OAF are similar to those of OAC mentioned earlier. Apart from this, if the sinus has pre-existing sinusitis/antral pathology/fungal infections/fungal balls, the

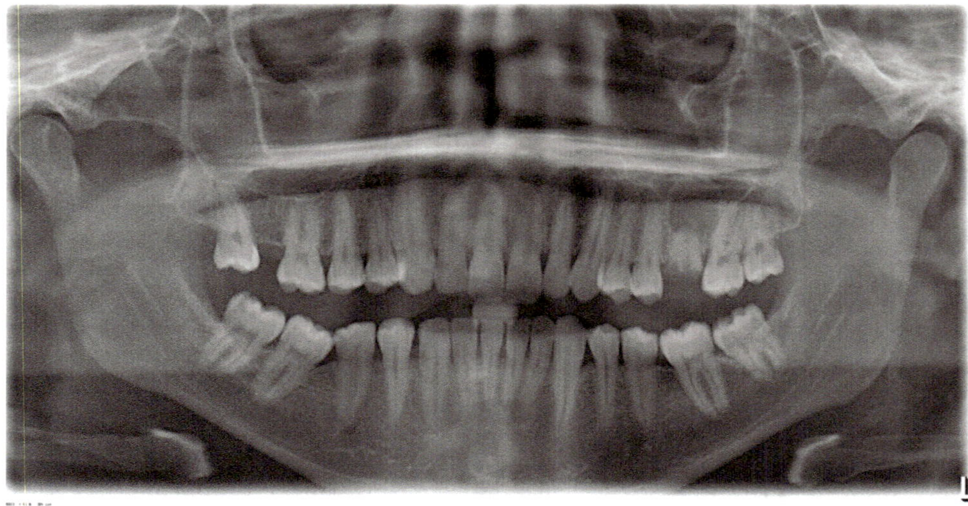



**Fig. 24.7** This is the OPG of a 25-year-old man who reported for routine extraction of root stump of upper left first molar tooth. OPG shows an incidental finding of a periapical lesion (which is probably a periapical cyst that appears to be very close to the sinus floor or probably pushing the sinus lining up). How would you manage this case?

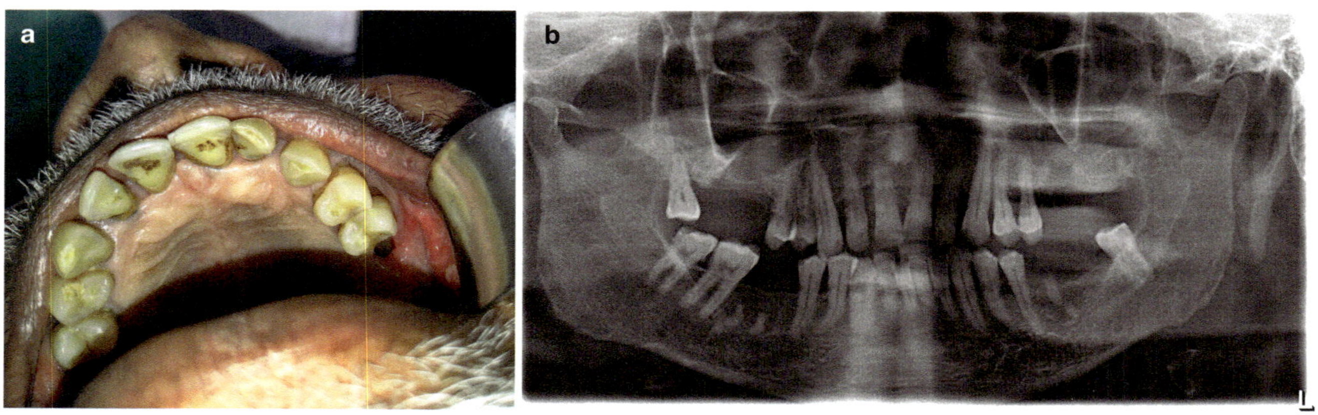



**Fig. 24.8** (**a**) Note the OAF on upper left first molar extraction site. The socket edges are well-healed, epithelized and rounded off. (**b**) OPG of the above case showing a defect in the alveolar ridge in the 26 socket region and direct communication of the sinus with the oral cavity

chance of healing of OAC is decreased and may progress to OAF.

Among patients who do not follow the post-extraction instructions or where the clot is deficient/gets dislodged, chances of OAF are increased in susceptible cases. Failed sinus lift procedures, ailing and failing implants and peri-implantitis are all potential causes for causing OAF.

### 24.4.2 Clinical Features

1. Primary complaints in established OAF cases are mainly oronasal regurgitation and burning sensation in sinus on having food.
2. Patients may visit the ENT surgeon with complaints of acute sinusitis, secondary to infection of sinus via unrecognized OAF.
3. In certain cases, there may localized pain, tenderness, foul smell, unpleasant tasting discharge, persistent nasal discharge and post-nasal drip.
4. In long-standing untreated cases, there will be clinical and radiological features of chronic sinusitis. The antral lining will undergo thickening/hyperplasia, and eventually, sinus gets obliterated or there may be evidence of sinus polyps.

I have seen a case where the patient was referred with a protruding sinus polyp through the socket of an untreated OAF in a maxillary molar site (Fig. 24.9a and b). In this particular case, a root was displaced into the sinus as well. It was not sure whether this polyp ensued secondary to OAF or whether pre-existing sinus polyp leads tothe OAF.

We should also be aware that antral malignancies may protrude through the unhealed socket of maxillary molars. Most of the times, the surgeon being ignorant of the disease would have extracted the tooth due to mobility caused by the erosion due to the malignant lesion, and a few weeks after, the patient may present, with the lesion protruding through the socket (Fig. 24.10).

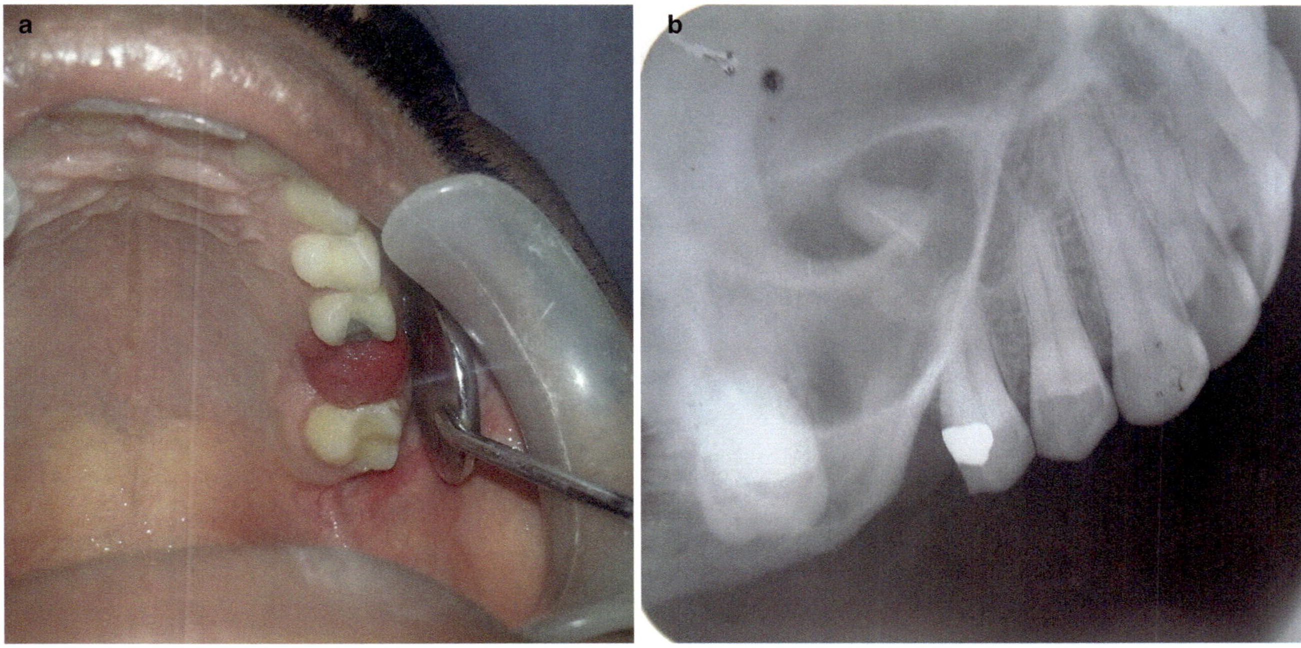




Fig. 24.9 (a) Clinical picture showing an antral polyp protruding through the sinus. Some clinicians may consider this to be a Post-extraction granuloma possibly of a reactive nature due to the root in the sinus. (b) Occlusal X-ray view showing root in the sinus

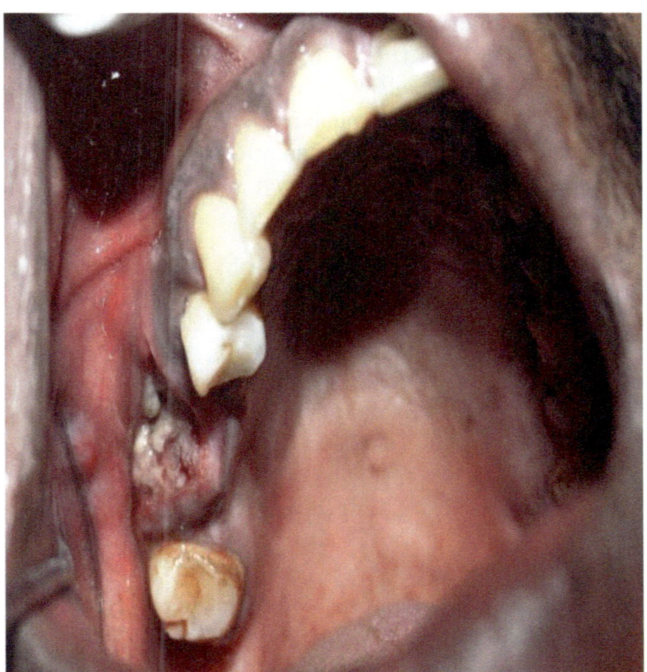



Fig. 24.10 A case of extraction of upper right second molar due to mobility by dental surgeon, who was unaware of the cause of mobility being antral malignancy. Couple of weeks after extraction, the lesion was seen protruding through the socket

5. The mucosal edges of the socket will be rounded off, and an evident opening may be seen via the socket into the sinus.

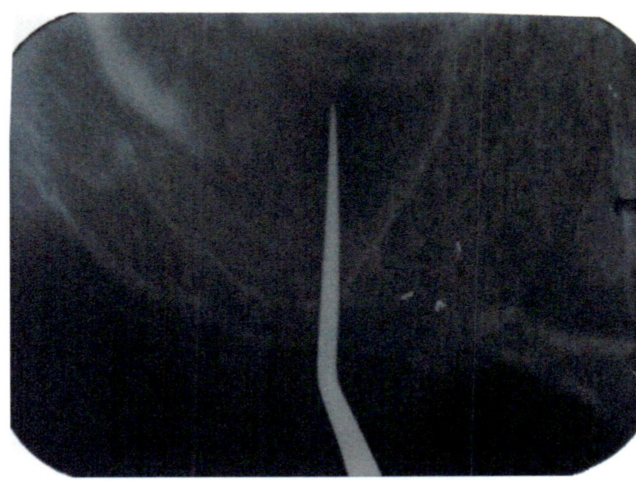



Fig. 24.11 IOPA x-ray showing metal probe entering the sinus via a minute unhealed OAF defect

6. In certain cases, the ridge will clinically look well-healed; however on careful probing, an unhealed tract will be seen, leading to the sinus (Fig. 24.11).

### 24.4.3 Confirmatory Tests of OAF

1. Holding water in the mouth and exerting pressure with mouth closed may elicit oronasal regurgitation.
2. Hold a piece of cotton wisp with tweezers at the OAF opening site, and request the patient to blow through the

nose with the nostril closed. The wisp will vibrate under the flow of air via the OAF (cotton wisp test/butterfly test).
3. The patient may find it difficult to hold pressure within the sinus, and a whistling sound may be appreciated by the examiner during the Valsalva manoeuvre.
4. Holding a mouth mirror near the opening of OAF will cause fogging of the mirror.
5. Place the nozzle of the suction at the opening of the fistulae. A sound similar to blowing through the mouth of an empty bottle may be heard.

### 24.4.4 Treatment Modalities for OAF

Techniques for OAF closure have evolved over a long period of time and have a robust history. Many techniques have been time tested and well-established, form the mainstay of OAF closure and will be discussed in this section. Literature is replete with various technical modifications; it is not possible to discuss all these in detail and will be beyond the purview of this chapter. The reader is advised to look into the references if a thorough review of techniques is required [3, 4]. Figure 24.1, in reference [4] (Visscher et al. JOMS 2010), gives an excellent overview of the various treatment modalities for oroantral communications Awang et al. [5] back in 1988 have published an excellent review of techniques, which were established at that time.

Since a plethora of techniques are available, the surgeon has the freedom to choose the technique, which works well in his hands based on the training received and surgical competence. One cardinal rule, which may be followed in OAF closure, is to start with the simplest technique available and reserve the complex technique in case the first attempt fails. A sequential option may be followed, the patient is to be warned that there are chances of failure and a secondary or tertiary surgery with more complex techniques may be required at times.

At this stage, it is worth remembering a quote which I have come across somewhere: "*Re-operation after past failures at the hands of other surgeons should be approached with due humility*".

The options for treatment can be broadly categorized under the following headings:

- Local flaps.
- Regional flaps.
- Combined with autografts.
- Combined with allografts.
- Prosthetic options.

The most widely used local flaps can be classified as

1. Buccal advancement mucoperiosteal flap (Moczair flap/Rehrmann flap/Berger flap).
2. Buccal advancement flap with buccal fat pad grafting (Two-layer closure).
3. Palatal pedicled flap (Ashley's rotational flap).
4. Tongue flaps: anterior and posterior based.

The multitude of techniques and variations has made the literature on OAF closure a trifle confusing. It is interesting to know that even third molar auto transplantation has been found to be successful in closure of immediate OAC (Kitagawa 2003) [6].

In this chapter, we will only be discussing the time tested and commonly performed buccal/palatal flaps with a reasonable amount of success rate. The tongue flaps are a second option, but the difficulty is caused to the patient in the post-operative period until the pedicle is divided and the need for patient compliance, difficulties in feeding, mastication; speech and maintenance of oral hygiene should be taken into consideration before performing them.

As there are multitude of variations and modifications in OAF closure techniques, the author feels that it is wise to present all the relevant modifications in a sequential order (Box 24.1). If the reader refers to the historical evolution of techniques given in the box format, it is evident that different flap designs have been advised ranging from advancement, sliding, pedicled, rotation, bridge, hinged, transverse buccal, double flaps, island flaps, bipedicled flaps, submucosal connective tissue flap, osteoperiosteal flaps, buccinator myomucosal flaps, etc. Each technique has been presented with its own indications and advantages. The reader is advised to read individual publications to get details of these techniques if required.

Irrespective of the technique used, the success of the closure warrants that the basic sound principles of mucoperiosteal flap design are used. *The flap should have adequate blood supply, should be handled gently, and should lie in the advanced position without tension.*

### 24.4.5 Assessment of OAF

The following factors should be assessed while planning the technique of closure in an OAF.

Size of the communication (Bone defect is always bigger than the visualized soft tissue defect)

- Location of defect.
- Health of the sinus/presence of infection.
- Time of diagnosis of fistula.
- Condition of tissue available.
- Amount of tissue available.

### 24.4.6 Objectives in Treatment of OAF

When treating an OAF, the surgeon should have the following objectives in mind [7]. (This can be called the 4 E's).

1. Elimination of the antral pathology.
2. Elimination of the epithelial lining of the fistulous tract.

3. Establishment of stable closure of fistula.
4. Establishment of satisfactory drainage.

**Box 24.1 Historical Evolution of OAF Closure Techniques**

- Welty CF 1920: buccal mucoperiosteal flap [8].
- Moczair 1930: buccal sliding trapezoidal flap [9].
- von Rehrman 1936: vestibular buccal mucoperiosteal flap [10].
- Berger 1939: Buccal advancement flap [11].
- Ashley 1939: palatal rotation flap [12].
- Kruger GO 1984: V-shaped excision of lesser curvature of palatal rotation flap [13].
- Kazangian 1949: bridge flap [14].
- Mc Clung 1951: tantalum foil [15].
- Schuchardt 1953: transverse buccal flap [16].
- Guerrero- santos 1966: Tongue flaps for OAF [17].
- Rintala 1971: palatal hinged flap (inversion/reverse palatal flap) [18].
- Zeimba 1972: double flaps (reverse palatal & buccal [19]).
- Meyerhoff 1973: gold foil [20].
- Henderson 1974: palatal island flap [21].
- Choukas 1974: Palatal rotational advancement flap [22].
- Gullane P 1975: modified palatal island flap, relieved vessel at greater palatine foramen [23].
- Cockerham 1976: Bone grafting [24].
- Egeydi 1976: bucket handle flap (bipedicled buccal flap) [25].
- Egeydi 1977: Buccal fat pad and split thickness graft [26].
- Sachs 1979: posteriorly based lateral tongue flap [27].
- Ito & Hara 1980: submucosal connective tissue pedicle palatal flap [28].
- Quale 1981: double flap [29].
- Brusati 1982: osteoperiosteal flap + vestibule mucoperiosteal flap [30].
- Al sibahi 1982: used soft polymethacrylate [31].
- Mitchell 1983: used collagen [32].
- Carstens MH 1991: anteriorly based buccinator myomucosal island flap [33].
- Zide 1992: Hydroxyapatite block closure [34].
- Shaker 1995: used Zenoderm [35].
- Hanazawa 1995: pedicled fat pad graft [36].
- Hori M 1995: Deans extended interseptal alveolotomy technique [37].
- Paul salins 1996: anteriorly based palatal flap [38].
- Pandolfi 2000: Three layer closure of oroantral cutaneous defect—palatal flap + buccal fat pad + skin flap [39].
- Lee JJ 2002. Repair of OAC in the third molar region by random palatal flap [40].
- Haas 2003: Monocortical bone grafts [41].
- Kitagawa 2003: third molar transplantation [6].
- Ogunsalu 2005: GTR membrane [42].
- Martin S 2008: metal plates and aluminium foils [43].
- Visscher 2010: biodegradable polyurethane foam [44].
- Sandhya 2016: Resorbable GTR Membrane and FDMB Sandwich Technique [45].
- Ram H 2016: used auricular cartilage [46].

## 24.5 The Buccal Advancement Flaps

The names of Moczair, Berger and von Rehrman have been used interchangeably when speaking of buccal flaps in the literature. The buccal flap designed by Moczair [9] was a sliding trapezoidal flap, while the ones designed by Berger [11] and Von Rehrman [10] were buccal straight advancement mucoperiosteal flaps.

Von Wowern (1982) [47] in a study of 90 patients compared Moczair with Rehrman flaps and advocated the former for treating OAF in edentulous patients. Killey and Kay (1967) [48] proved the efficacy of buccal flap in a large series of 250 cases. The buccal flap technique can be satisfactorily employed in the treatment of small and medium-sized communications where there is clear sinus lavage through OAF, and proper antral regime has been maintained 4–5 days prior to the surgery.

The technique of raising a buccal flap is given along with the 2 layer BFP closure technical note box (Box 24.2) and is essentially the same. A few words are needed to elaborate on the buccal flap and periosteal scoring. The buccal flap raised is a full thickness trapezoidal (rectangular/4 sided) mucoperiosteal flap. There are 2 releasing incisions, one anterior and one posterior. The incisions are put in such a way that the flap looks tongue/funnel-shaped and is feasible for advancement palatally without tension. Great care is given to raise it gently without causing any 'button holing'/fenestrations in the flap. The base should be broad enough to have good random blood supply, and flap margins should be incised sharply in order to avoid ragged edges. It is the periosteum that gives tension and may prevent advancement palatally. In order for the flap to lie passively, the periosteum alone is scored gently with a number 12 or 15 blade, horizontally at the level of the base of the buccal flap. This will release the tension and help in advancement. The scoring is a fine procedure, and the surgeon should be aware that, if the scoring goes deep beyond the level of periosteum, the mucosa may be incised which may even jeopardize the viability of the flap by affecting the blood supply emanating from the base (Fig. 24.12).

**Box 24.2 Technical Notes of a 2 Layer BFP Closure**

- Anaesthesia.
- Fistula tract excision with No 11 BP blade.
- Curette the granulation tissue.
- Buccal and palatal margin freshened with No 15 blade.
- Palatal margin made into a semilunar shape to accept the buccal flap.
- Flap to rest on sound bone on the palatal side.
- Extended trapezoidal flap placed on the buccal side.
- Posterior vertical release of flap slightly curved towards vestibule to facilitate advancement anteriorly.
- Reduction of alveolar bone height if required.
- Periosteal scoring of buccal flap.
- Posterior periosteum teased open to identify the BFP.
- BFP mobilized gently with non-toothed forceps (blunt dissection, avoid tension).
- BFP sutured to palatal margin with 3 'O' non-cutting vicryl rapide.
- Buccal flap advanced palatally to cover the BFP.
- Buccal flap sutured to palatal margin with horizontal mattress vicryl sutures.
- Anterior vertical release sutured.
- Posterior vertical release usually needs no suturing.

One disadvantage of all buccal advancement procedures is the decrease in the vestibular depth, which may be problematic for prosthetic rehabilitation.

### 24.5.1 Step-by-Step Technique of Doing Buccal Advancement Flap + Buccal Fat Pad Grafting (BFP)

The step-by-step procedure for 2 layer closure technique is given in the box format (Box 24.2). The steps of performing a 2 layer closure are similar to the buccal advancement alone, except that the BFP is raised, advanced and sutured primarily to the palatal edge.

The use of the buccal fat pad (BFP) as a grafting source in the closure of intra-oral defects has gained popularity in the last quarter of the twentieth century. Its use as a pedicle graft for oral reconstruction was first reported by Egyedi in 1977 [26]. Studies have proved through a series of cases that the use of buccal pad fat in the closure of oroantral communications has significantly reduced the failure rate of the treatment. The closure of OAF with single-layered buccal mucoperiosteal advancement flaps (Berger/Reherman) has been well documented in the literature. Without much change in the surgical steps, adding a second layer of BFP will enhance the success rate of closure.

The buccal fat pad (BFP) as an anatomic element was first mentioned by Heister in 1732 and was described by Bichat in 1802 [49]. The BFP (Bichat ball) is an anatomically rounded and biconvex structure that is of great importance in the facial contour. It is an adipose tissue surrounded by a thin capsule

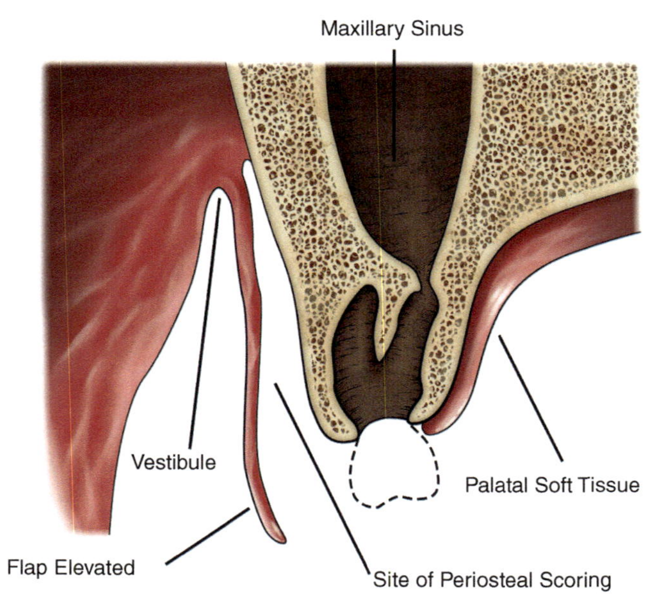




Fig. 24.12 Diagrammatic representation of raising a buccal trapezoidal flap and periosteal scoring

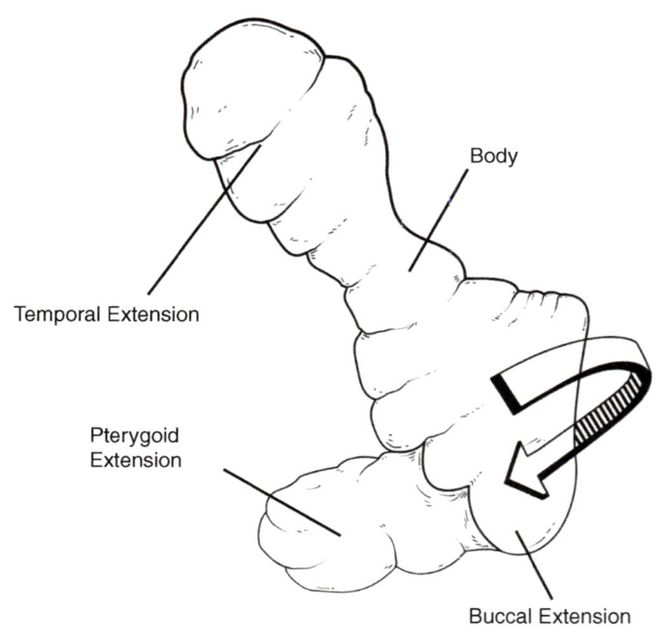




Fig. 24.13 Anatomical representation of the buccal fat pad

and located inside both masticatory spaces in the oro-maxillofacial region (Fig. 24.13). The BFP has a central body with four extensions: pterygopalatine, temporal, pterygoid and buccal. The central body and buccal extension account for approximately 50% of the BFP and are the most clinically significant portions. The BFP has a 10 mL volume, a thickness of 6 mm and an approximate weight of 9.3 g. The BFP is surrounded by a thin fibrous capsule. Blood supply is provided by the vestibular and deep branches of the maxillary artery, the transverse facial branches of the superficial temporal artery and branches of the facial artery. The rich blood supply may explain the high success rate. It also may be one reason for the quick epithelialization of the fat. The buccal fat pad is a mass of specialized fatty tissue called as syssarcosis, a fat that enhances muscular motion. It is distinct from the subcutaneous fat and shows marked similarity to the orbital fat. It can easily cover small to medium sized defects of about 4 cm in diameter. When properly dissected and mobilized, the BFP provides 7 × 4 × 3 cm of a pedicled graft. (Box 24.3).

### 24.5.2 Clinical Pictures Demonstrating 2 Layer Closure Technique with BFP (Fig. 24.14a, b, c, d and e) [50]

Figure 24.14a, b, c, d and e: Reprinted with permission from springer nature customer service centre GmbH: springer publisher: Journal of maxillofacial and oral surgery: The versatility in the use of Buccal Fat Pad in the closure of oro-antral fistulas. Suvy Manuel et al. [COPYRIGHT 4524640093264] (2015).

**Box 24.3 Advantages of Buccal Fat Pad**

- Easy access.
- Relatively easy to perform.
- Minimum dissection.
- Great versatility.
- Good mobility.
- Reliable blood supply.
- Low rate of complication.
- No donor site morbidity.
- Low risk of infection.
- Shortened surgical time.
- No scar.
- Fast cover by epithelium.
- High success rate.

## 24.6 Palatal Rotational Flap (Ashley's Flap)

Among palatal flaps, there are 2 main types: The palatal straight advancement flap (Fig. 24.15) and the palatal rotational flap (Fig. 24.16).

However, the palatal rotational flap proposed by Ashley in 1939 [12] has stood the test of time. It is a pedicled flap, posteriorly based on the greater palatine vessel. A tongue-shaped full thickness mucoperiosteal flap is raised on the side of the OAF. The OAF site is freshened, and the fistula is excised as a preparation to receiving the flap. The flap is rotated and sutured on to the OAF site. In order to avoid kinking at the site of rotation near the palatal margin of the socket, a V-shaped area may be excised (Kruger's [13] modification). The raw site is packed with dressing to allow secondary healing. This is a thick, bulky and vascular flap, which is quite reliable and serves often as a second line of defence when the buccal advancement flap fails. Different authors have given various names for this flap-like rotational, advancement and transposition.

Other types of palatal flaps mentioned or published in the literature are the palatal island flaps (Henderson 1974 [21]), palatal hinged/inverted/reverse flap (Rintala 1971 [18]) and sub-mucous connective tissue flap (Ito & Hara 1980 [28]). Palatal flaps are also used as part of double flap techniques as proposed by Zeimba in 1972 [19] and Quayle in 1981 [29].

## 24.7 Importance of Timing of Closure of OAF

The health and status of the socket edges and margins play an important role in deciding the success of the closure, irrespective of the surgical technique used. An OAF, which is well-rounded margins and does not show any evidence of oedema/inflammation, is a good recipient area for the closure. Oral surgeons may often get referred cases with history of difficult extraction of maxillary molars/attempted removal of fractures root tips/cases with established OAC and/or with missing root tips. Often, the socket may show evidence of traumatic extraction with ragged margins, tissue loss, irregular bony edges, congestion, tenderness and oedema. Such sites are not favoured for an OAC/OAF closure, and surgeons should not be tempted to attempt a closure. The chances of failure of the closure are high due to unhealthy mucosal condition and its prudent to wait for a couple of weeks for good healing of the wound edges and then consider closure. It may be argued that the sinus health may deteriorate during this waiting period, and all these are decisions to be taken by the surgeon on their individual merit (Fig. 24.17a and b).

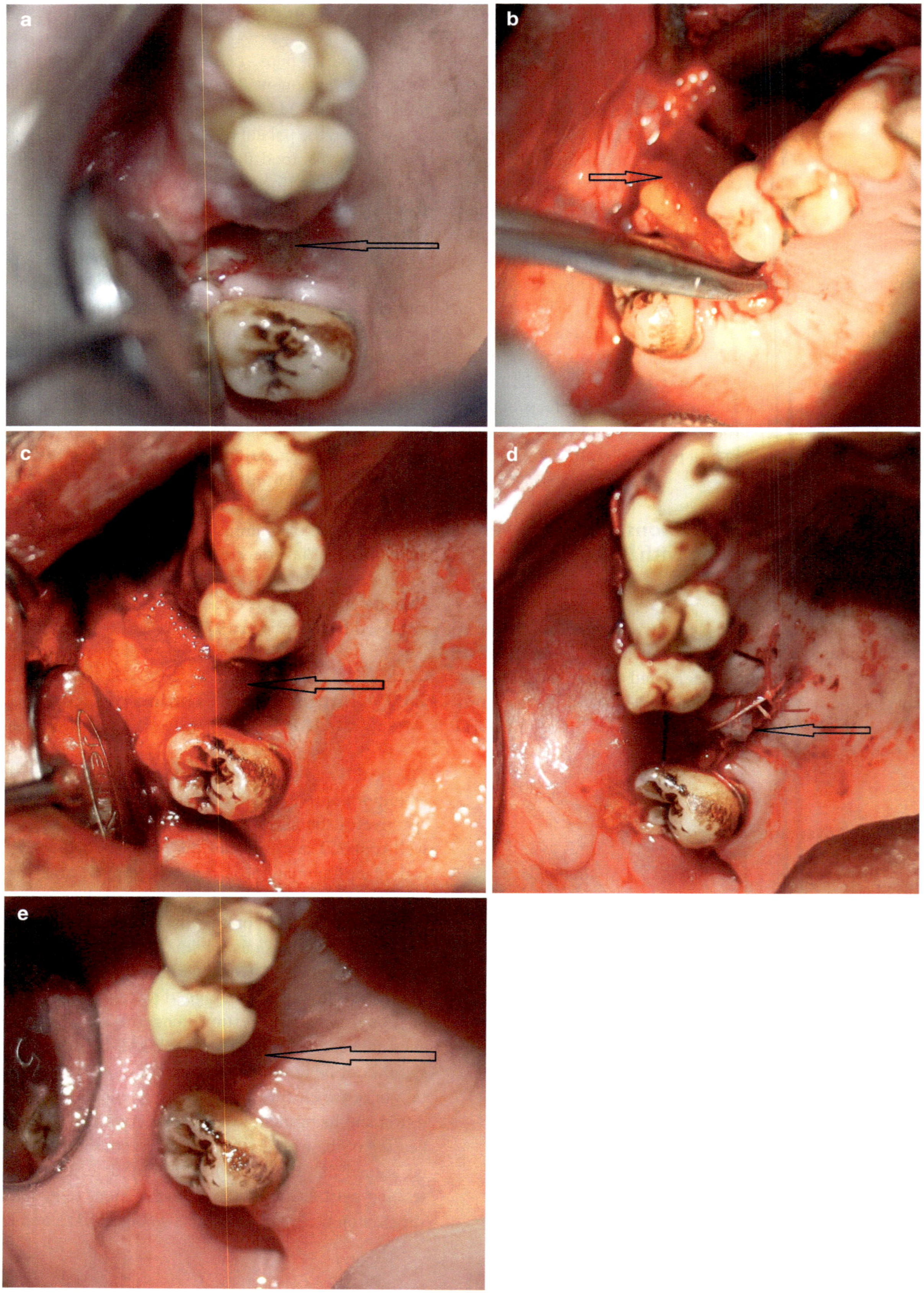
a
b
c
d
e

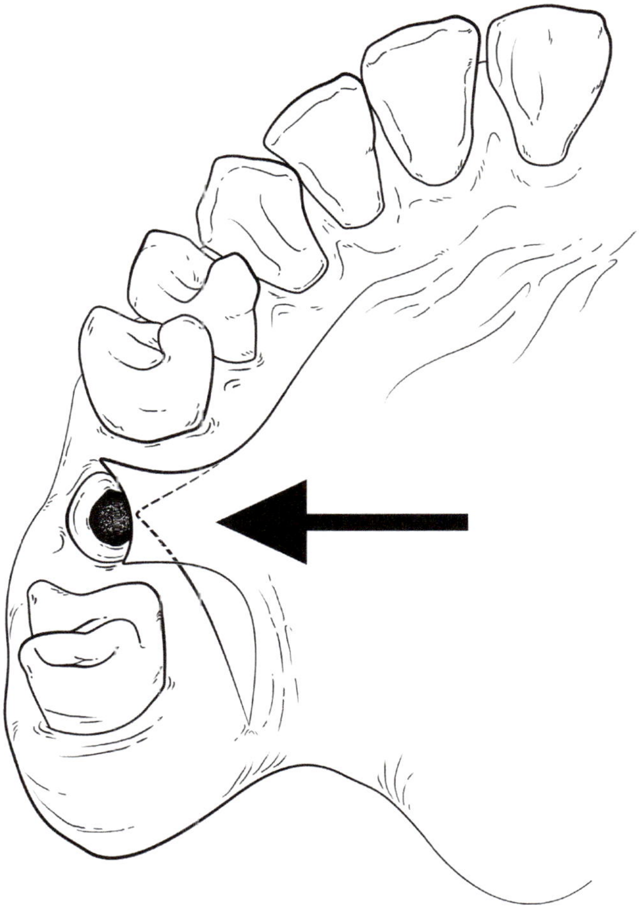


Fig. 24.15 Diagrammatic representation of a palatal straight advancement flap

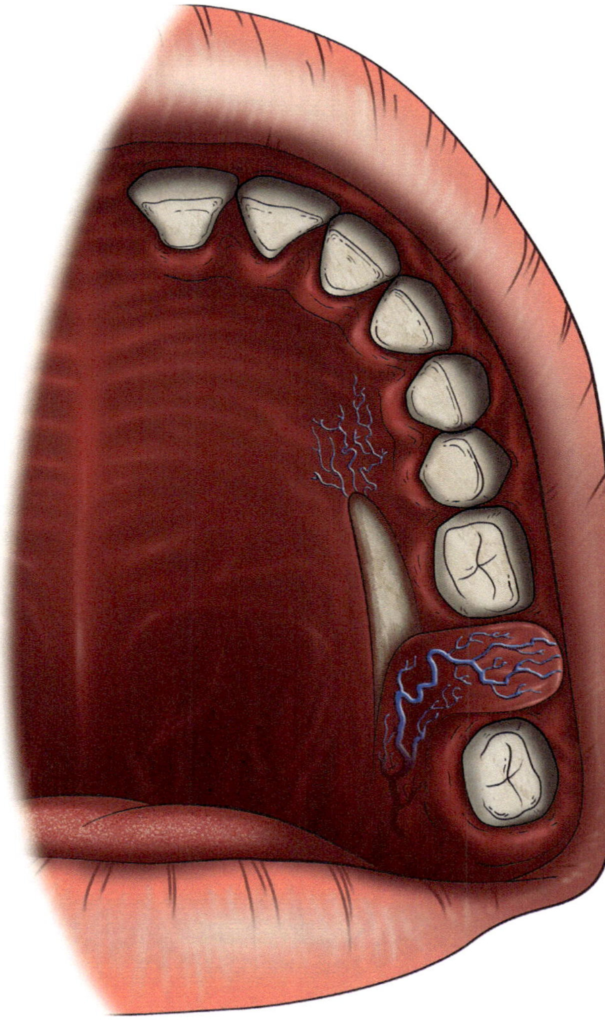


Fig. 24.16 Diagrammatic representation of a palatal rotational flap

### 24.7.1 Role of Health of Sinus and Antral Regime

Depending upon the duration of OAF, the sinus may be in various stages of disease. In acute OAC, unless there is preexisting disease, the closure may be attempted with a fair chance of success. In untreated cases of OAF, patients may have acute episodes of sinusitis or progress into a chronic stage manifesting thickened antral lining and fluid/exudates/pus collection in sinus or antral polyps. In cases of acute nature, the sinusitis has to be under control before closure (Fig. 24.18).

Fig. 24.14 (**a**) Oroantral fistula seen at the maxillary right first molar extraction site (**b**) Buccal fat pad being teased out from the buccal vestibule. (**c**) The buccal fat pad being advanced and sutured to the palatal margin. (**d**) The buccal mucoperiosteal flap sutured to the palatal margin and covering the buccal fat pad. (**e**) Excellent healing of the closure site (2 month post-operative view) [50]

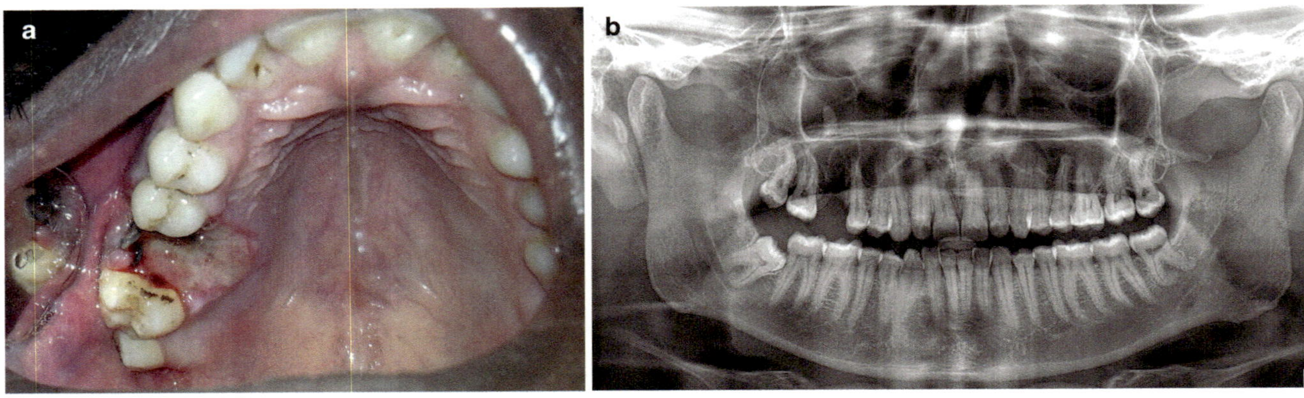


©Association of Oral and Maxillofacial Surgeons of India

**Fig. 24.17** (**a**) Clinical picture of a referred case in a 30-year-old male, who had a traumatic extraction of upper right first molar 1 week back. One complete root has been pushed into the sinus (see OPG, Fig. 24.17b). Note the traumatized, congested, oedematous and ragged sutured wound edges/tissue loss and slough in the palatal tissue. He is not a candidate for closure immediately. It is preferable to wait until complete healing and schedule the procedure electively. (**b**) OPG of the above case showing the root in the sinus cavity

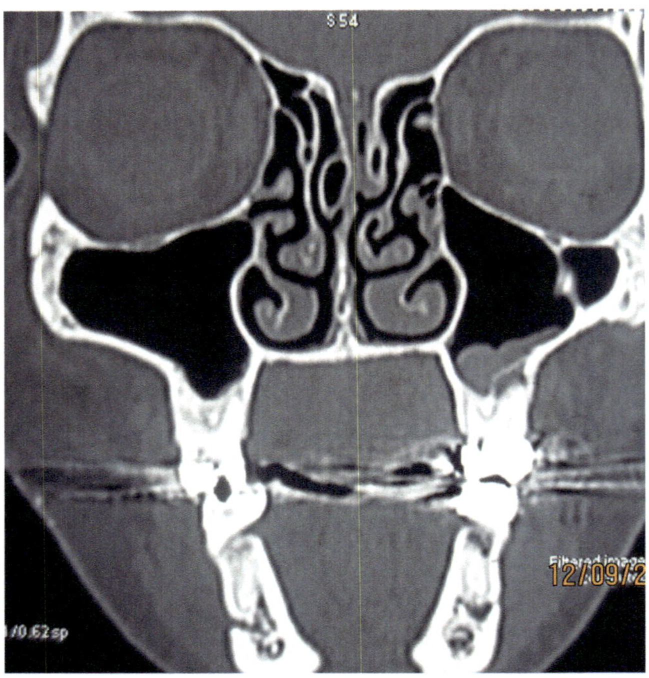

©Association of Oral and Maxillofacial Surgeons of India

**Fig. 24.18** A coronal CT scan, showing periapical widening/lesion in a maxillary left molar, which is close to the sinus floor and reactive sinus lining thickening in that region. Possible OAC resulting from this extraction may have a decreased chance of success after immediate closure

## 24.7.2 The Antral Regime

Antral regime is usually helpful, which is usually started about 5–7 days before the anticipated closure. It includes.

1. Antibiotics to control sinusitis.
2. Anti-inflammatory agents if required.
3. Steam inhalation at prescribed intervals.
4. Nasal decongestant drops to increase the drainage of the sinus and open up closed ostium.
5. Antihistamines to decongest the sinus and also to avoid sneezing, which may increase the sinus pressure and have a deterrent effect on the success of the closure.

The antral regime may be continued for a few days (3–7 days) after the closure as well to ensure a trouble-free healing. After closure, the patient is advised to have certain restrictions in the initial healing phase, in order to avoid break down of the closure, i.e.

1. Avoid vigorous sneezing/coughing/blowing through the nose.
2. If coughing cannot be avoided, do cough with mouth open.
3. Avoid smoking to avoid negative pressure in the oral cavity.
4. Avoid using straws to drink fluids.
5. Avoid vigorous gargling or swishing in the oral cavity.
6. Do not disturb the surgical site with tongue movements.
7. It would be preferable to review the patient at least once in 2–3 days during the initial healing period to assess the healing status. The clinician may irrigate the surgical site with saline removing the collected debris/slough if any.
8. Some author's advice to keep a pre-fabricated custom-made acrylic splint at the site of closure as a support.

However, there are thoughts that the splint may irritate or traumatize the sutured edges on the alveolar ridge and be a deterrent for the healing.

## 24.7.3 Antral Lavage

At times, the antral lavage is done daily or on alternate days along with the antral regime to clear the exudate from the

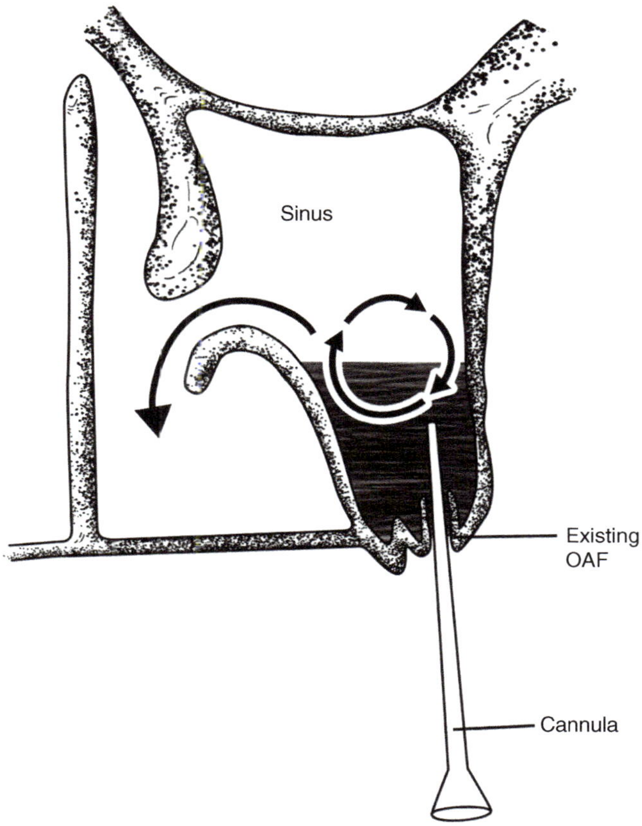


©Association of Oral and Maxillofacial Surgeons of India

**Fig. 24.19** Diagrammatic representation of antral lavage via the existing OAF

sinus. The presence of exudate/pus can be seen as a 'fluid level' in a paranasal sinus X-ray, or there may be generalized opacification of the involved sinus in the X-ray. The closure is attempted, only when the surgeon feels that the antral washouts are clear, and the sinus is reasonably healthy to receive the closure.

ENT books describe different methods of antral lavage, either via a Caldwell Luc opening or via the nasal meatus depending upon the case. However, from an oral surgical perspective for most cases, antral lavage may be done via the existing OAF (Fig. 24.19). 10–20 ml of saline is flushed through the OAF via a syringe, and patient is seated at a forward position with head bent down. The washout will flow out through the nasal cavity or via the OAF, and the washout is collected in a tray positioned before the patient. In the initial days of lavage, the washout will have a cloudy/opaque appearance, and after few days, we should expect the washout to be clear.

## 24.8 Caldwell Luc Procedure

This procedure was developed independently by two surgeons, George Caldwell in New York (1893) and Henry Luc in Paris (1897) (Box 24.4).

**Box 24.4 Technical Note: Caldwell Luc Procedure in Oral Surgery Context**

- Upper lip retracted.
- Horizontal U-shaped incision in the vestibule-few mm above gingival attachment or
- Mucoperiosteal flap-raised upward to the point of emergence of the infra-orbital nerve.
- Do not damage infraorbital nerve
- Chisel or dental bur is used to create a window on anterior wall of sinus above root of teeth of that area.
- Opening enlarged using Rongeur's forceps until it is of the size of an index finger.
- Sinus exposure gained and required procedure performed.
- Soft tissue placed and sutured over bone with resorbable sutures.
- Good closure is important as the dehiscence itself-will cause an OAF.

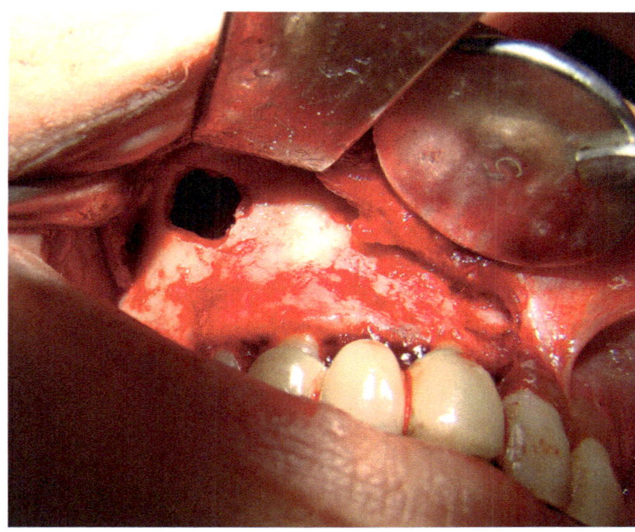

©Association of Oral and Maxillofacial Surgeons of India

**Fig. 24.20** Clinical picture showing a Caldwell Luc procedure via extended crevicular flap for removal of a root in sinus. Note the defect made in the anterior maxilla wall

It involves making an opening in the anterior wall of sinus in the canine fossa region, to get good access to the sinus. The procedure is done either via a sublabial incision or by extended crevicular incisions (Fig. 24.20). In the context of OAF, this approach has relevance when combined along with the closure of OAF. The approach may be used to retrieve root tip or to surgically treat chronic sinusitis as in polyps. In combined cases, the extended crevicular flap with adequate releasing incisions may be used to remove root tip and may be used as a buccal advancement flap with or without buccal fat pad graft for the closure of OAF.

The indications for Caldwell Luc procedure are given below:

1. Recovery of entrapped foreign body from the sinus cavity proper, displaced tooth or root.
2. Excision of sinus polyps, tumours and cysts.
3. Treatment of blowout orbital fracture.
4. Management of haematomas of antrum.
5. Chronic maxillary sinusitis.
6. Neoplasm of maxillary sinus.
7. Removal of impacted canines.

## 24.9 OAF with Chronic Sinusitis

Such cases are more difficult to manage and will need a combined oral surgery/ENT approach. There may be severe antral lining hyperplasia and lack of natural drainage by blockage of the ostium or antral polyps. The line of management has to be decided on an individual basis. Occasionally, the sinus problem may have to be addressed before attempting a closure, which may require two surgeries. Sometimes, the oral surgeon may be in for a surprise during OAF closures to see fungal balls in the sinus. The reasons for c/c sinusitis should be evaluated and addressed accordingly.

The second option is to attempt closure along with the treatment of chronic sinusitis. In such cases, a formal Caldwell Luc opening may be made to remove the unhealthy lining. If that is the case, the buccal flaps are modified as per requirement to get a tension-free closure at the OAF site. In situations where FESS is used, oral surgeon can visualize the sinus and see the OAF from the nasal/antral side. The use of FESS gives a two pronged approach, i.e. the unhealthy lining from the antral side of the OAF can be removed and closure performed. This means that in OAF with c/c sinusitis, a general anaesthesia will be necessary, unlike uncomplicated OAF cases where most of the established techniques may be done under local anaesthesia if required.

Adams (2015) [51] has reported on the success of using combined FESS and BFP closure. The sequence followed by Adams included pre-operative computed tomography, antibiotic therapy, exploration and removal of sinus pathologic tissues, rotation of a pedicled fat pad graft into the oral opening, repair and closure of oral mucosa, exploration of involved sinuses with excision of sinus and nasal tissues necessary for establishment of osteomeatal drainage and follow-up.

Cases of fulminant pansinusitis have been encountered arising from long-standing untreated OAF. This involves the contralateral side, and such cases need a comprehensive joint approach with the allied specialities, before embarking upon closing the OAF.

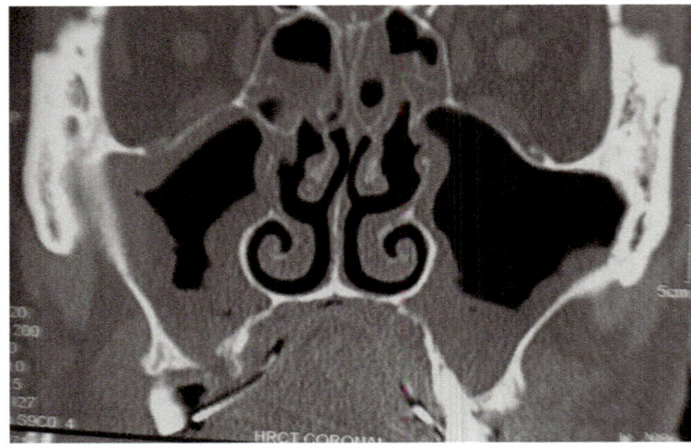


©Association of Oral and Maxillofacial Surgeons of India

**Fig. 24.21** Coronal slice CT scan, showing hyperplasia of sinus lining, especially on the right side, where the OAF can be Appreciated

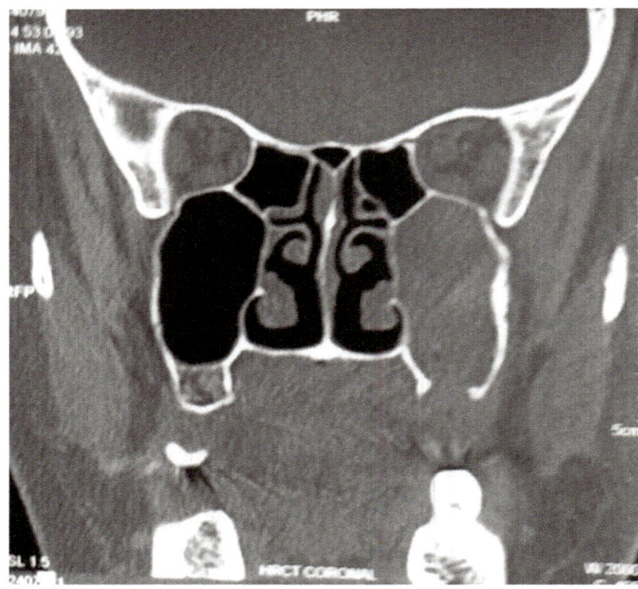


©Association of Oral and Maxillofacial Surgeons of India

**Fig. 24.22** Coronal CT scan of a 50-year-old male, who had normal extraction of upper left second molar, which was followed by break down of clot and resulted in OAF. He later developed infection with pus discharge from socket. CT scan shows the fully opacified left sinus. Under GA (joint case with ENT surgeon), a 2 layer BFP closure was done, accompanied by FESS and Caldwell Luc approach via extended mucoperiosteal flap. Intraoperatively, the sinus was filled with fungal balls, which could have been the cause for the formation of OAF

Figures 24.21, 24.22 and 24.23 show coronal CT slices of different case scenarios where OAF was accompanied by chronic sinusitis.

In Video 24.1, the video contributing Surgeon has managed an OAF associated with chronic sinusitis, by a combination of Caldwell-Luc procedure, Nasal antrostomy, and layered closure by buccal advancement flap. Layered closure has been achieved by suturing of sub mucosa and mucosa of the advanced buccal flap.

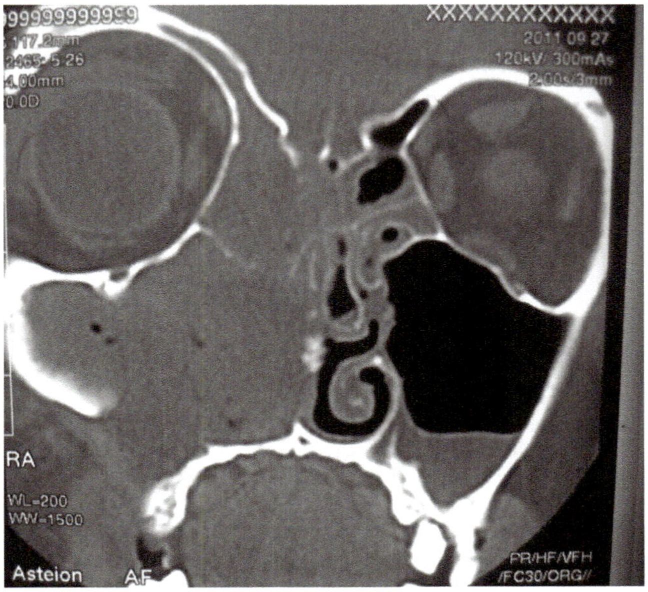




**Fig. 24.23** Coronal CT view showing pan sinusitis in 58-year-old male, who developed an OAF in the anterolateral wall of maxilla from a previous failed surgery, probably for a cyst enucleation in the maxilla (previous records not available)

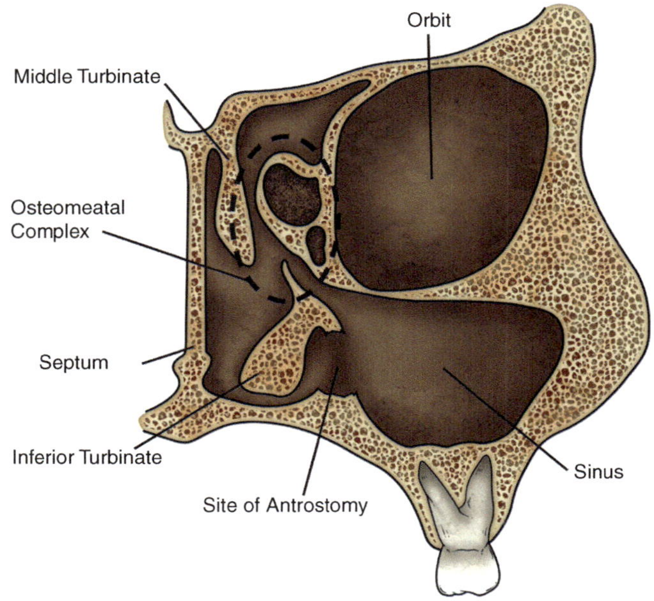




**Fig. 24.24** Diagrammatic coronal section of sinus demonstrating the sinus drainage

## 24.10 Nasal Antrostomy

The ostium of maxillary sinus opens into middle meatus, which is at a higher level than the sinus floor (Fig. 24.24). In normal healthy sinus, this is not a problem as the normal ciliated respiratory epithelium will help in the drainage. Briefly saying, nasal antrostomy is a procedure where an opening is made in the inferior meatus, either from the nasal or sinus side to facilitate drainage of sinus in a dependent manner. Nasal antrostomy is an adjuvant procedure, which can be done along with cyst enucleations of the sinus or in selected cases of OAF closure. The need for nasal antrostomy has decreased now with changing philosophies, the advent of FESS and the importance given to the osteomeatal complex. Recent studies (Huang YC [52] 2012) have also proved the decreased need for inferior meatal antrostomy following sinus surgeries.

For elaborate details of Caldwell Luc and nasal antrostomy procedures, readers are advised to refer the concerned speciality books.

## 24.11 Root in Sinus

In situations where a fragment of a root or a full root or roots is missing during extraction of maxillary premolars or molars, the surgeon will have to take certain decisions and some questions should flash through his or her mind.

(a) Should I locate the root tip and where should I look for it.
(b) If located, should I attempt to retrieve it or decide to leave it.
(c) Will the root retrieval necessitate GA and if so when to schedule the procedure.
(d) Should the root tip left behind be removed later at an elective date or not removed and remove only if any symptoms occur.
(e) If the root has gone into the sinus, an OAC would have been formed. Should I remove the root tip and close the OAC, or should I leave the root tip and close the OAC or plan for a combined removal of root and OAC/OAF closure later on an elective date.

While attempting removal of a root tip, if it suddenly disappears, make sure that the tip is not there in the following places.

(a) Lying freely elsewhere in the oral cavity/vestibules/lingual sulcus.
(b) Tip is not attached with cotton/gauze pieces.
(c) Tip has not stuck to suction drains or bottles.
(d) Tip has not been accidentally swallowed or aspirated.

If the root tip is assumed to be pushed upwards into the sinus cavity, the tip may lodge in the following areas:

(a) A fenestration would have happened in the apical labial/palatal alveolar bone, and the tip would be lodged between the labial/palatal alveolar bone and the mucoperiosteum.

(b) Rarely, the tip would have perforated the buccal mucoperiosteum and get lodged near the buccinator muscle.
(c) Tip would be lying between the sinus lining and the sinus floor. In strict sense, it may be assumed that an OAC is not formed as the integrity of the membrane is not lost.
(d) Tip may have pierced through the sinus membrane and entered the sinus cavity (theoretically causing an OAC).

X-rays in two different planes (IOPA/OPG/Occlusal) will be helpful to give an idea about the root tip position especially when it is inside the sinus. When the root tip is retaining its lamina dura on an IOPA x-ray, it may be assumed that it is still lying within the bone and not have entered the sinus cavity. Paranasal sinus view will confirm that the root is in the sinus and CBCT also may be helpful in localization.

In situation (a), Transalveolar approach will help in removing the root tip.

In situations (c) and (d), the following methods are suggested in the literature and the resulting OAC is closed primarily or at a later stage depending upon the surgeons' choice.

1. If the root tip is visible through the socket, it is gently removed with the help of probes/tweezers/mosquito forceps.
2. If not visible, the sinus is flushed with saline and it is hoped that the root tip will float in the sinus. A metal suction tip is placed at the socket apex, and the clinician may expect the root tip to be lodged at the end of the suction tube.
3. A gauze piece may be inserted into the sinus via the socket and pulled out in a jerky fashion hoping that the-root tip will get entangled in the gauze piece.
4. The tip may be removed through the socket, by enlarging the communication. This may require removal of the inter-radicular bone and visualizing the sinus to get better approach, vision and access. This technique is usually successful, but the flip side is that the chance of failure of closure is increased as the surgeon is dealingwith a communication of considerable size (Fig. 24.25).
5. Another option would be to remove the root via the Caldwell Luc approach or FESS. This is usually done on an elective basis.

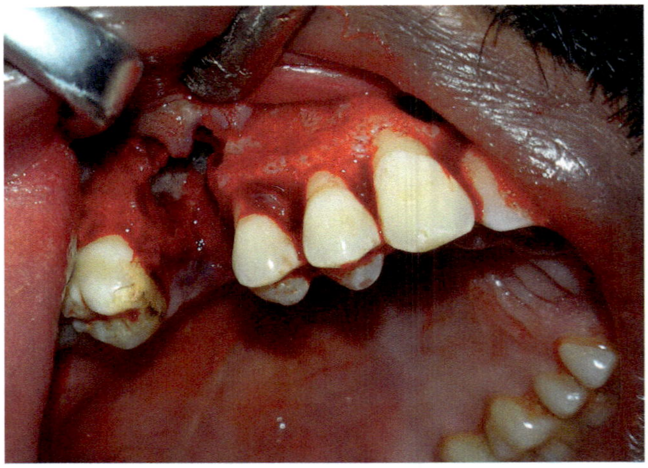



**Fig. 24.25** In this case, the surgeon is attempting to remove the root in sinus, which has been dislodged superiorly during the extraction, by enlarging the socket and an extended mucoperiosteal flap has been raised. The sinus can be visualized via the socket. This technique is usually not recommended as the resulting OAC will be of considerable size; however, in this case, the OAC was closed by a 2 layer BFP technique

## 24.11.1 Policy of Leaving Root Tip In Situ

It is important to say a few words on this topic at this juncture, even though there may be difference of opinion and contentions on the points given below. These can be applied to all root tips being left behind. If the clinician feels that removing a fractured root tip of an upper premolar/molar is beyond his or her level of competence or there is a possibility of causing OAC, which he or she cannot deal primarily, the root tip may be left behind in the following situations;

1. The root tip is less than 2–3 mm in length.
2. It is not associated with any periapical pathology.
3. It may not interfere with any future prosthetic rehabilitation.
4. Aged/patients with considerable medical co-morbidities.
5. Attempts at removal of the tip may cause more damage and surgical procedures when compared to the benefits of removal.

The patient should be well-informed about this situation and should be informed that the tip may be removed later if they wish so. Adequate documentation in the form of x-rays and clinical notes is mandatory, in order to follow up the case and to avoid any future medico-legal issues.

### Clinical Scenario 2

An interesting clinical Scenario for the benefit of young clinicians.

A 40-year-old female had routine extraction of root stumps of upper left first molar. A pre-operative IOPA was not taken. After extraction, to the surprise of the dental surgeon, there was pus discharge through the socket (See Fig. 24.26a and b)

The probabilities are that either there was a pre-existing sinusitis, which was unrecognized, or the root stumps caused the odontogenic infection to spread into the sinus.

### How will you Manage this Case?

There may be different opinions, but the following sequence may be followed in this particular case, which is given as clinical pearl section below.

**Clinical Pearls (Management of Case in Fig. 24.26a and b)**

- Temporary closure of socket and no flap advancement.
- Anti-biotics.
- Discuss with patient.
- Record in case file.
- ENT consultation to assess the sinus health.
- Required radiographs and CT scans.
- Fix elective date for OAC closure.
- Routine work up/lab investigations.
- Decide on type of closure technique/anaesthesia.
- Decide whether there is need for Caldwell luc/FESS/nasal antrostomy after sinus evaluation.
- Start antral regime.
- Start antral lavage until clear washout is achieved.
- Execute the surgery.
- Follow up to assess the status of closure.

### Clinical Scenario 3 (Fig. 24.27a, b, c and d)

Another interesting clinical scenario, which I came across in a maxillofacial trauma case recently, is given as follows:

A 36-year-old male sustained RTA and facial fractures as seen in Fig. 24.27a and b. Tooth numbers 15 and 16 (upper right first pre-molar and molar) were avulsed with comminution of labial cortical plate and the alveolar process creating an oroantral communication (Fig. 24.27c). You can appreciate the bubbling of mucus at the OAC site. CT showed bilateral haemosinus, fracture maxilla and mandible, The right posterior alveolar segment containing 17,18 (upper right second molar and third molar) was mobile and extruded due to a posterior right parasagittal fracture of the maxilla.

It was a challenging case to plan and execute.

The upper sub-labial incision, given for the maxillary fracture exposure, was curved down distal to 14 (upper right first pre-molar) and continued as a full thickness crevicular mucoperiosteal flap. The distal release was not given, for fear of jeopardizing the vascularity of the posterior alveolar segment. The BFP was mobilized in the conventional way (Fig. 24.27d), and a good two-layered primary closure was attained after reduction and fixation of the fractures. The posterior alveolar segment had to be fixed to the main segment via transosseous wiring. This segment was extruded, and to achieve healing and occlusion, post-operative IMF was given. This particular patient was on Ryles Tube feeding for few days, mainly due to other injuries and tracheostomy, which would have helped in the good healing of the OAC closure.

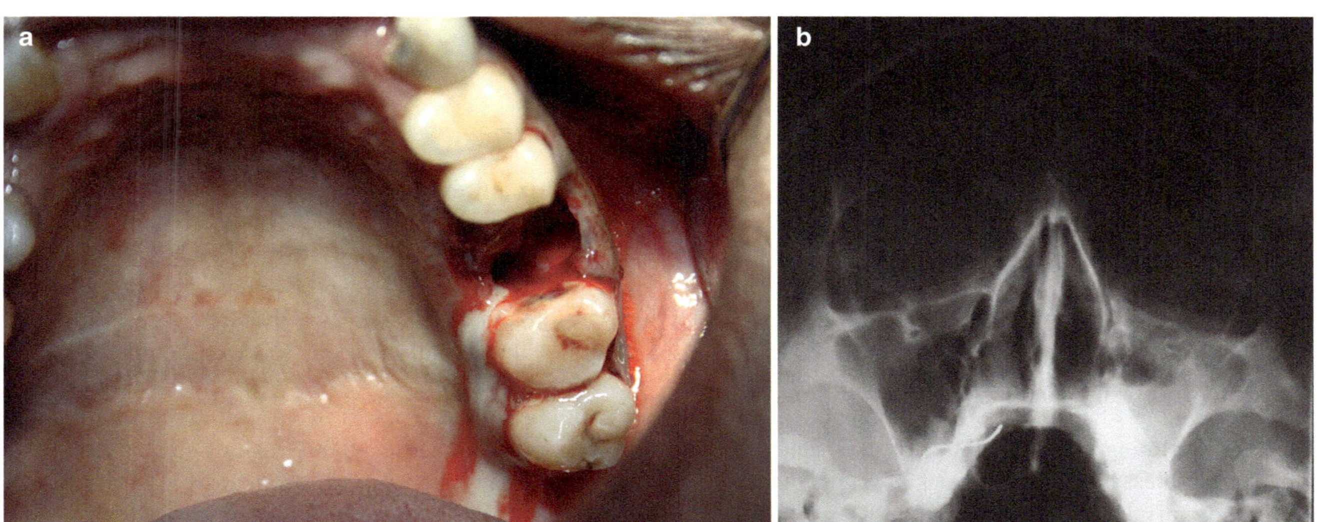




**Fig. 24.26** (**a**) Surprise finding of pus from socket after extraction of upper left first molar root stumps, (**b**) PNS view taken after extraction shows fluid level in the sinus, probably due to pre-existing sinusitis

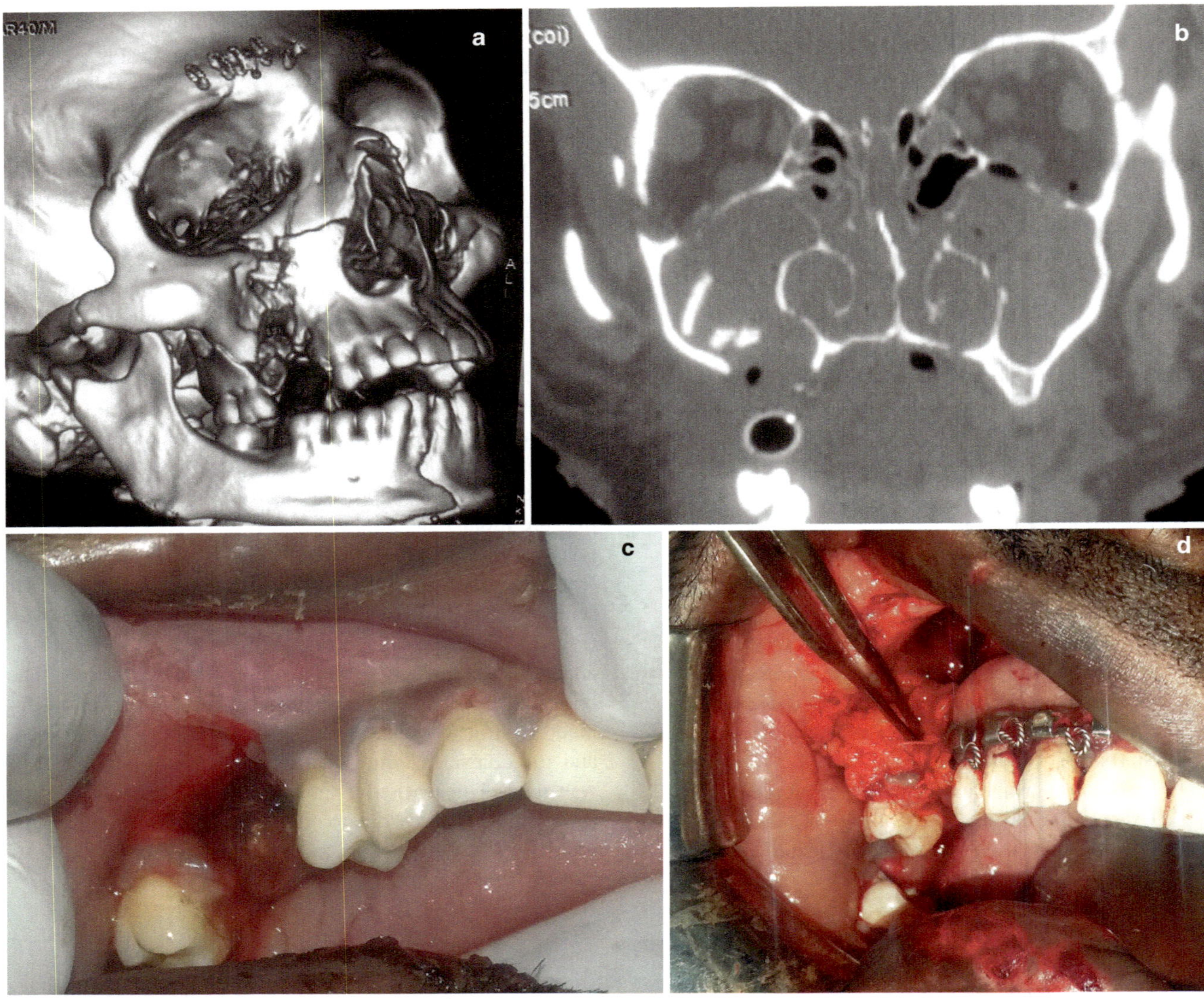




**Fig. 24.27** (**a**, **b**, **c** and **d**) OAC following maxillofacial trauma (see the text for details)

## 24.12 Conclusion

The clinician should be cautious of not deliberately causing an OAC while performing exodontia and dentoalveolar procedures in maxillary posterior region. An OAC should be ruled out in suspected cases, and if it occurred, necessary steps should be taken to ensure a closure primarily if possible. Even as this chapter is going to the publishers, clinicians are exploring the possibilities of new techniques, of which the flapless closure techniques of acute OAC seem to be quite promising. Closing OAC with PRF membrane/collagen composite [53, 54] offers easier, less traumatic methods to close OAC, which may even obviate the need for special surgical expertise. Materials like acellular dermal/bone matrix are also being used recently [55] However, only time will prove the obduracy of these path breaking methods.

Visscher [56] in a retrospective study of 308 oroantral closures found that about 10% needed re-operation, and patients with maxillary sinusitis had 15 times higher risk of developing a recurrence.

Dealing with OAF cases is interesting in the sense that it involves assessing the health of sinus and choosing and performing the most suitable surgical technique, most of which are fine surgeries. It is indeed rewarding to see a symptom-free patient with a well-healed OAF closure site.

## References


1. Eberhardt JA. A computed tomographic study of the distances between the maxillary sinus floor and the apices of the maxillary posterior teeth. Oral Surg Oral Med Oral Pathol. 1992;73(3):345–6.
2. von Wowern N. Correlation between the development of an oro-antral fistula and the size of the corresponding bony defect. J Oral Surg. 1973;31:98.
3. Dym H. Oroantral communication. Oral Maxillofac Surg Clin N Am. 2012 May;24:239–47.
4. Visscher S, et al. Closure of oroantral communications: a review of the literature. JOMS. 2010;68:1384–91.
5. Awang MN. Closure of oroantral fistula. IJOMS. 1988;17:110–5.
6. Kitagawa Y. Use of third molar transplantation for closure of the oroantral communication after tooth extraction: a report of 2 cases. Oral Surg Oral Med Oral Pathol Oral Radiol Endod. 2003;95(4):409–15.
7. Procacci P. Surgical treatment of oroantral communications. J Craniofac Surg. 2016;27(5):1190–6.
8. Welty CF. Closure of fistulous opening through alveolar process in the antrum of Highmore. JAMA. 1920;75:867–9.
9. Moczair L. Nuovo methodo operatiopela chisura delle fistole dei seno mascellase di origina dentale. Stomatol (Roma). 1930;28:1087–8.
10. Rehrmann VA. Eine methods zur Schliessung von Kiejerhohlen perforationen. Deutsche Zahnarztliche Wochenschrift. 1936;39:1136–9.
11. Berger A. Oroantral openings and their surgical corrections. Arch Otolaryngol. 1939;130:400–2.
12. Ashley RE. Method of closing antroalveolar fistula. Ann Otol Rhinol Laryngol. 1939;48:632.
13. Kruger GO. Text book of oral and maxillofacial surgery. 6th ed. St Louis: CV Mosby; 1984. p. 291–3.
14. Kazanjian VZ, Converse JM. The surgical treatment of facial injuries. Baltimore: Williams; 1949.
15. McClung EJ. Tantalum foil used in closing antro-oral fistulas. US Armed Forces Med J. 1951;7:1183.
16. Schuchardt K. Methodik des Verschlus-ses von Defekten im alveolarforsate zahn-lose oberkiefer. Dtsh Zahn Mund Kieferheilk. 1953;17:366–9.
17. Guerrero-Santos J. The use of lingual flaps in repair of fistulas of the hard palate. Plast Reconstr Surg. 1966;38(2):123–8.
18. Rintala A. A double, overlapping hinge flap to close palatal fistula. Scand J Plast Reconstr Surg. 1971;5(2):91–5.
19. Ziemba RB. Combined buccal and reverse palatal flap for closure of oral-antral fistula. J Oral Surg. 1972;30(10):727–9.
20. Meyerhoff W. Gold foil closure of oroantral fistula. Laryngoscope. 1973;83:940.
21. Henderson D. The palatal island flap in the closure of oroantral fistulae. British JOS. 1974;12:141.
22. Choukas NC. Modified palatal flap technique for closure of oroantral fistulas. J Oral Surg. 1974;32(2):112–3.
23. Gullane PJ. Palatal island flap for reconstruction of oral defects. Arch Otolaryngol. 1977;103(10):598–9.
24. Cockerham S. Closure of a large oroantral communication by bone grafting. J Oral Surg. 1976;34(12):1098–100.
25. Egyedi P. The bucket-handle flap for closing fistulae around the premaxilla. J Maxillofac Surg. 1976;4(4):212–4.
26. Egyedi P. Utilization of the buccal fat pad for closure of oro-antral and/or oro-nasal communications. J Maxillofac Surg. 1977;5:241.
27. Sachs SA. Treatment of a persistent oro-antral fistula with a posteriorly based lateral tongue flap. Int J Oral Surg. 1979;8(3):225–8.
28. Ito T, Hara H. A new technique for closure of the oroantral fistula. J Oral Surg. 1980;38(7):509–12.
29. Quayle AA. A double flap technique for the closure of oro-nasal and oro-antral fistulae. Br J Oral Surg. 1981;19(2):132–7.
30. Brusati R. The use of an osteoperiosteal flap to close oroantral fistulas. J Oral Maxillofac Surg. 1982;40(4):250–1.
31. Al-Sibahi A. The use of soft polymethylmethacrylate in the closure of oro antral fistula. J Oral Maxillofac Surg. 1982;40:165–6.
32. Mitchell R. Immediate closure of oro-antral communications with a collagen implant. A preliminary report. Br Dent J. 1983;154(6):171–4.
33. Carstens MH. A new approach for repair of oro-antral-nasal fistulae. The anteriorly based buccinator myomucosal island flap. J Craniomaxillofac Surg. 1991;19(2):64–70.
34. Zide MF. Hydroxylapatite block closure of oroantral fistulas: report of cases. J Oral Maxillofac Surg. 1992;50(1):71–5.
35. Shaker MA. Competent closure of chronic oroantral fistula with Zenoderm. Egypt Dent J. 1995;41(3):1237–42.
36. Hanazawa Y. Closure of oroantral communications using a pedicled buccal fat pad graft. J Oral Maxillofac Surg. 1995;53(7):771–5.
37. Hori M. Application of the interseptal alveolotomy for closing the oroantral fistula. J Oral Maxillofac Surg. 1995;53(12):1392–6.
38. Salins PC, Kishore SK. Anteriorly based palatal flap for closure of large oroantral fistula. Oral Surg Oral Med Oral Pathol Oral Radiol Endod. 1996;82(3):253–6.
39. Pandolfi PJ. Three-layer closure of an oroantral-cutaneous defect. Int J Oral Maxillofac Surg. 2000;29(1):24–6.
40. Lee JJ. Repair of oroantral communications in the third molar region by random palatal flap. Int J Oral Maxillofac Surg. 2002;31(6):677–80.
41. Haas R. A preliminary study of monocortical bone grafts for oroantral fistula closure. Oral Surg Oral Med Oral Pathol Oral Radiol Endod. 2003;96(3):263–6.
42. Ogunsalu C. A new surgical management for oro-antral communication: the resorbable guided tissue regeneration membrane – bone substitute sandwich technique. West Indian Med J. 2005;54(4):261–3.
43. Steiner M. Metal plates and foils for closure of oroantral fistulae. JOMS. 2008;66:1551–5.
44. Visscher SH, van Minnen B, Bos RR. Closure of oroantral communications using biodegradable polyurethane foam: a feasibility study. J Oral Maxillofac Surg. 2010 Feb;68(2):281–6.
45. Sandhya G, et al. Surgical management of oro-antral communications using resorbable GTR membrane and FDMB sandwich technique: a clinical study. J Maxillofac Oral Surg. 2013;12(3):254–9.
46. Ram H. Use of auricular cartilage for closure of oroantral fistula: a prospective clinical study. J Maxillofac Oral Surg. 2016;15(3):293–9.
47. von Wowern N. Closure of oroantral fistula with buccal flap: Rehrmann versus Môczár. Int J Oral Surg. 1982;11(3):156–65.
48. Killey HC, Kay LW. An analysis of 250 cases of oro-antral fistula treated by the buccal flap operation. Oral Surg Oral Med Oral Pathol. 1967;24(6):726–39.
49. Bichat FMX. Anatomie generale: appliquee a la physiologie et la medecine, Paris; 1801. Cited in Stuzin JM, Wagstrom L, Kawamoto HK, Baker TJ, Wolfe A The anatomy and clinical applications of the buccal fat pad. Plast Reconstr Surg 1990;85:29.
50. Manuel S. Surej Kumar LK, Parvathi R Nair: the versatility in the use of Buccal fat pad in the closure of oro-antral fistulas. J Maxillofac Oral Surg. 2015;14(2):374–7.
51. Adams T. Repair of oroantral communications by use of a combined surgical approach: functional endoscopic surgery and buccal advancement flap/buccal fat pad graft. J Oral Maxillofac Surg. 2015;73(8):1452–6.
52. Huang YC. Caldwell-Luc operation without inferior meatal antrostomy: a retrospective study of 50 cases. J Oral Maxillofac Surg. 2012;70(9):2080–4.
53. Gülşen U. Etal. Flap-free treatment of an oroantral communication with platelet-rich fibrin. Br J Oral Maxillofac Surg. 2016;54(6):702–3.

54. Pandikanda R, Singh R, Patil V, Sharma M, Shankar K. Flapless closure of oro-antral communication with PRF membrane and composite of PRF and collagen – a technical note. J Stomatol Oral Maxillofac Surg. 2018 Dec 29;120(5):471–3.
55. Li XY, Wu J, Cao J, Yang W, Wu B, Xie C.Clinical analysis of acellular dermal matrix and acellular bone matrix in oro-antral fistula repair. Hua Xi Kou Qiang Yi Xue Za Zhi 2018 Dec 1;36(6):633–637. https://doi.org/10.7518/hxkq.2018.06.010. Chinese.
56. Visscher SH, van Roon MR, Sluiter WJ, van Minnen B, Bos RR. Retrospective study on the treatment outcome of surgical closure of oroantral communications. J Oral Maxillofac Surg. 2011 Dec;69(12):2956–61.

# Part X

# Nerve Injuries and Neuralgias of Oral and Maxillofacial Region

# Trigeminal Nerve Injuries

# 25

Tara Renton

There are infinite opportunities in dentistry to damage the trigeminal nerve. Nerve damage from surgery can cause chronic post-surgical pain; however, this is limited in dentistry as a result of Local anaesthetic (LA) infiltration injections but more commonly associated with injuries to the nerve trunks of division two and three caused by implants, endodontics and third molar surgery (or other high-risk extractions). Fortunately, painful post-traumatic trigeminal neuropathy (PPTTN) is rare in dentistry compared to other common general surgical procedures where 20–45% of patients experience persistent pain after surgical limb amputation, thoracotomy and breast surgery. This chapter highlights the prevention (using risk assessment, optimal surgical techniques, early post-surgical follow-up protocols and other strategies) and optimal management of trigeminal nerve injuries.

Trigeminal nerve injury (TNI) associated with chronic pain is the most problematic consequence of dental surgical procedures with major medico-legal implications [1]. The incidence of lingual nerve injury has remained static in the UK over the last 30 years, but is increasing in the US, as is the incidence of inferior alveolar nerve injury in the UK, with the latter being due to implant surgery and endodontic therapy [2]. Third molar surgery-related inferior alveolar nerve (IAN) neuropathy or inferior alveolar block injections are usually temporary but can persist and become permanent (by definition at 3 months). There are rare reports of resolution of implant and other cause-related IAN neuropathies at over 4 years, [3] but these are not similar reports of other peripheral sensory nerve injuries [4–7]. In dentistry, frequently, a treat delay is 3–6 months [5], which is inappropriate when compared to other peripheral sensory nerve injuries where immediate repair and exploration are recommended. We now understand that known or suspected, restorative (endo and implant)-induced nerve injuries require intervention ideally immediately, within 30 h or within 3 months, dependent upon the mechanism of injury, to optimize resolution from injury and prevent the permanent central and peripheral changes within the nervous system [6, 7].

Paraesthesia is often inappropriately used in the dental literature to mean neuropathy. However, paraesthesia is only a descriptive term, meaning altered sensation and not a diagnosis. When sensory nerves are injured, a neuropathy (malfunction) may arise, and this may be painful or non-painful.

The trigeminal nerve has the largest representation in the sensory cortex, reflecting the disproportionate sensory input from the orofacial region. It protects vital structures that underpin our very survival, providing sensory supply to the eyes, airway, brain, mouth and ears. It is no 'wonder' that when the threat or actual pain arises in the trigeminal nerve area that the patient is neurophysiologically wired to 'run for the hills' from the dental chair. Latrogenic (caused by surgery or medicine) trigeminal nerve injuries (TNIs) result in 70% pain in patients seen seeking treatment on our clinic [7]. The ongoing or evoked pain results in interference with eating, speaking, sleeping, applying makeup, shaving, kissing, tooth brushing and drinking; just about every social interaction, we take for granted. As a result, these injuries have a significant negative effect on the patient's self-image, quality of life and psychology [7].

With the increasing age of the patient, the time elapsed since the injury and the proximity of the injury to the cell body (the more proximal lesions have a worse prognosis) will dictate the persistence of any peripheral sensory nerve injury.

There are many non-surgical causes for trigeminal neuropathy, and these must be borne in mind if the patient presents with an unclear onset of motor or sensory neuropathy [8].

Sensory nerve injuries caused by implant and endodontic treatments are mainly permanent. Only LA nerve injuries have a 75% likelihood of recovery and lingual access third molar surgery and have 90% potential for recovery [9].

T. Renton (✉)
Oral Surgery, Kings College London, London, UK
e-mail: Tara.renton@kcl.ac.uk


K. Bonanthaya et al. (eds.), *Oral and Maxillofacial Surgery for the Clinician*, https://doi.org/10.1007/978-981-15-1346-6_25

Referral of patients with these nerve injuries before 4 months [2] is too late for optimal resolution or management as inferior alveolar nerve injuries often require an immediate implant or endo-treated tooth removal within 24–30 h. We now understand that after 3 months, permanent central and peripheral changes occur within the nervous system subsequent to injury, which are unlikely to respond to surgical intervention [10].

Nerve damage is likely to result from a combination of poor risk assessment, poor technique, lack of recognition and the acute management of intra-operative and post-operative signs of neuropathy. Risk assessment involves the patient selection, pre-operative planning, both clinical and radiographic, appropriate selection of implant site and type (width and length) and suitable treatment protocol and follow-up.

It is important that the clinician is familiar with the nerve injury risk factors, specific for each of the types of invasive procedures. For example, in the case of protrusion through the IDC and resultant direct IAN mechanical injury by implant drill, a "sudden give" or an "electric shock" type feeling, even with local anaesthesia working, is reported by most of the patients seen in our clinic with post-traumatic neuropathy. This should result in the clinician stopping surgery, not reaching for another LA block injection and reassessing their surgical position with regard to the injured nerve.

The problem with implant-related nerve injuries is that they are entirely avoidable as this is elective surgery, thus negligent, and likely to be permanent and painful for the patient [11]. In addition, persistent nerve injuries cannot be resolved. Surgical intervention for hypoaesthetic nerve injuries does not return the patient to normality [10], and surgery for patients with pain and hyperaesthesia is not appropriate as the pain is not abated and patients are faced with long-term anti-epileptics or anti-depressants for chronic pain [11].

When assessing patients with surgically induced nerve injuries, we recommend a more holistic approach in assessing patients with nerve injury [8]. The definition ICHD 3 (International Craniofacial pain and Headache Disorders) of painful post-traumatic trigeminal neuropathy (PPTTN) includes development of neuropathy within 3 months of injury with sensory neuropathy and pain. The author believes that the neuropathy develops immediately after trauma, unless related to endodontic procedure where there may be a 2–3 days delay in neuropathy development. Features of iatrogenic trigeminal nerve injury worthy of assessment include

- Focal sensory neuropathy (mostly present). There is almost always an area of abnormal sensation (neuropathy with the exception in Trigeminal neuralgia which is NOT post-traumatic), and the maximum reported pain is associated with the area of sensory deficit (i.e. suffering from a mixture of pain, numbness and altered sensation). This is an important diagnostic feature for sensory nerve neuropathy.
- Pain discomfort, altered sensation and numbness (anaesthesia). Neuropathic pain is commonly present with allodynia (pain on non-noxious stimuli), hyperalgesia (increased pain to noxious stimuli) and hyperpathia (continuous altered sensation or pain after stimulation ceases). In 50–70% of patient reports, a combination of numbness, altered sensation and pain is experienced, the pain may be spontaneous ongoing pain, which often had a burning character, spontaneous shooting or electric shock-like sensations (neuralgia) [7]. Evoked pain due to touch or cold often leads patients to have difficulties with daily function, such as eating, socializing, kissing, speech and drinking. As a consequence, patients are often anxious and tearful and had psychological repercussions of surgery. These symptoms were often compounded by the lack of informed consent, which was given by only 30% of patients, most of whom were not specifically warned about potential nerve injury [7].
- Daily function problems (drinking, kissing, eating, sleeping, speaking, tooth brushing and avoidance) [12],
- Psychological (anxiety, stress, post-traumatic stress disorder and anger) [12].

The following sections address the prevention and management of trigeminal nerve injuries related to

- Local anaesthesia.
- Implants.
- Third molar and other high-risk extractions.

## 25.1 Local Anaesthetic-related Nerve Injuries

Local block injection-related nerve injury is an acknowledged complication in relation to surgery [13]. Dentistry is the only speciality that still trains clinicians to aim for nerves rather than avoiding neural contact (often using ultrasound), which likely explains the continued prevalence of LA-related nerve injuries in dentistry. All other block injections are undertaken using ultrasound in order to avoid nerve injury. One report highlights that the prevalence of IDB-related nerve injuries in UK General dental practise is 1:14,000 blocks, or 1:56 K IDB patients experience permanent lingual or inferior alveolar nerve injury of which this 25% of nerve injuries are permanent [9]. It is estimated that every practising dentist will experience causing 4–6 temporary nerve injuries and one permanent nerve injury related to IDBs during their working life based upon current practice.

Nerve injury may be due to many causes including physical (needle, compression due to epineural or perineural haemorrhage), ischaemic or chemical (haemorrhage or LA contents). The site of the injury may also vary and combine peri-, epi- and intra-neural trauma causing subsequent haemorrhage, inflammation and scarring, resulting in demyelination (loss of nerve lining) [14]. Only 1.3–8.6% of patients get an 'electric shock' type sensation on application of an IAN block and 57% of patients suffer from prolonged neuropathy having not experienced the discomfort on injection, and thus, this is not a specific sign [15]. Routine practice in Germany includes warning patients of potential nerve injury in relation to dental block injections. Risk factors for persistent local anaesthesia nerve injuries are summarized in Table 25.1.

The lingual nerve (LN) is at increased risk of permanent injury compared to the IAN during local anaesthesia, possibly related to the reduced number of fascicles in the LN compared to the IAN [16].

Higher concentration agents are more neurotoxic and, therefore, more likely to cause persistent inferior dental block (IDB)-induced nerve injury [17–22]. Irrefutably, Schwann cell death is related to increased concentration and time exposure to LA [22]. Articaine is provided in 4% concentration and Lidocaine in 2% solution in most countries. A recent prospective randomized study reports that there is no benefit or using 4% Articaine IDBs compared to 2% Lidocaine [23], which is substantiated by other evidence [24–27]. Thus, logically why would anyone use a higher concentration agent for an IDB when there is no increased efficacy and higher risk of nerve injury? [28]

Intra-operatively, all clinicians should document unusual patient pain reactions occurring during injections or surgery (such as sharp pain or an electrical shock-like sensation), as neuralgia during injections is associated with increased persistence of nerve injury [15]. Thus, it is important that the clinician uses an appropriate LA method to prevent proximity of the injection/surgical instruments to the IDC, for example, infiltration anaesthesia for implant surgery.

**Table 25.1** Risk factors for persistent neuropathy related to IDBs

In order to minimize complications related to dental LA, you need to consider modifying the following risks:

- **Block anaesthesia:** nerve block injections should be undertaken without intent on direct 'hit' of the nerve. 60% of patients who experience the 'funny bone' neuralgia due to the IDB needle being placed too close to the lingual or inferior alveolar nerves experience persistent neuropathy
- **Lingual nerve > IAN:** is this technique related or anatomically related (less fascicles in LN lower capacity for recovery). Perhaps, the direct IDB approach may place the lingual nerve at increased risk compared to the indirect technique
- **Concentration of LA:** any increased concentration of any agent leads to increased neural neurotoxicity
- **Volume of LA:** there is no evidence to support this suggestion, but all chemicals are neurotoxic, and depending upon the proximity, LA concentration and neural damage, additional volume would add to potential neurotoxicity
- **Multiple injections:** second or subsequent injections that impede directly on or in neural tissue may not be associated with the usual 'funny bone' neuralgic pain. Thus, the patient does not self-protect as effectively possibly rendering the nerves more at risk of direct damage
- **Severe pain on injection:** 60% increased occurrence of persistent neuropathy after IDBs
- **Type of LA:** agent bupivacaine most neurotoxic of all LA agents
- **Type of vasoconstrictor?** The role of vasoconstrictor in nerve damage is unknown
- **Sedated or anaesthetized patients?** There is no evidence to support unresponsive patients, who are less likely to protect themselves when neuralgia (funny bone reaction) occurs as the IDB needle encroaches too close to the nerve
- **Lack of LA aspiration?** There is no evidence to support that aspiration during IDB results in lower persistent neuropathies, but a pragmatic view may infer less chemical injected intraneurally will cause less chemical nerve injury

### 25.1.1 Avoiding Block Anaesthesia by Using Infiltration Dentistry

Daublander et al. reported that in a 2014 [23] survey of German dental LA practise, 74% were using infiltration dentistry routinely and rarely giving IDBs (personal communication). Improved patient comfort is reported by patients with preference for having full lingual sensation and shorter duration LA anaesthesia after dental treatment.

There is further evidence to support the notion of infiltration dentistry can be successful in many aspects of dentistry

- *Maxillary infiltration anaesthesia*
  Studies report that 4% Articaine to be more effective than 2% lidocaine for lateral incisors but not molars [25], differing from other reports [23, 25]. A recent randomized controlled trial reported a statistically significant difference advocating the use of 4% Articaine in place of 2% lidocaine for buccal infiltration in patients experiencing irreversible pulpitis in maxillary posterior teeth [24, 26]. This has been superceded by a metanalysis that reports there is no advantage in using 4% Articaine for maxillary infiltration anaesthesia and that 2% Lidocaine is suffice for dental interventions.
- *Pulpal anaesthesia in the anterior mandible compared to inferior dental block (IDBs) [25].*
  Meechan provides evidence supporting the significantly increased rates of pulpal anaesthesia using infiltration anaesthesia when compared to IDB anaesthesia particularly for premolar and incisor teeth (Fig. 25.1).
- *Pulpitic mandibular molars in adults [23, 25, 29, 30].*
  A recent systematic review reports that Articaine is 3.4 times more effective for pulpitic mandibular molars when compared to lidocaine, but there is no difference between Articaine and Lidocaine maxillary infiltrations or IDBs [31].

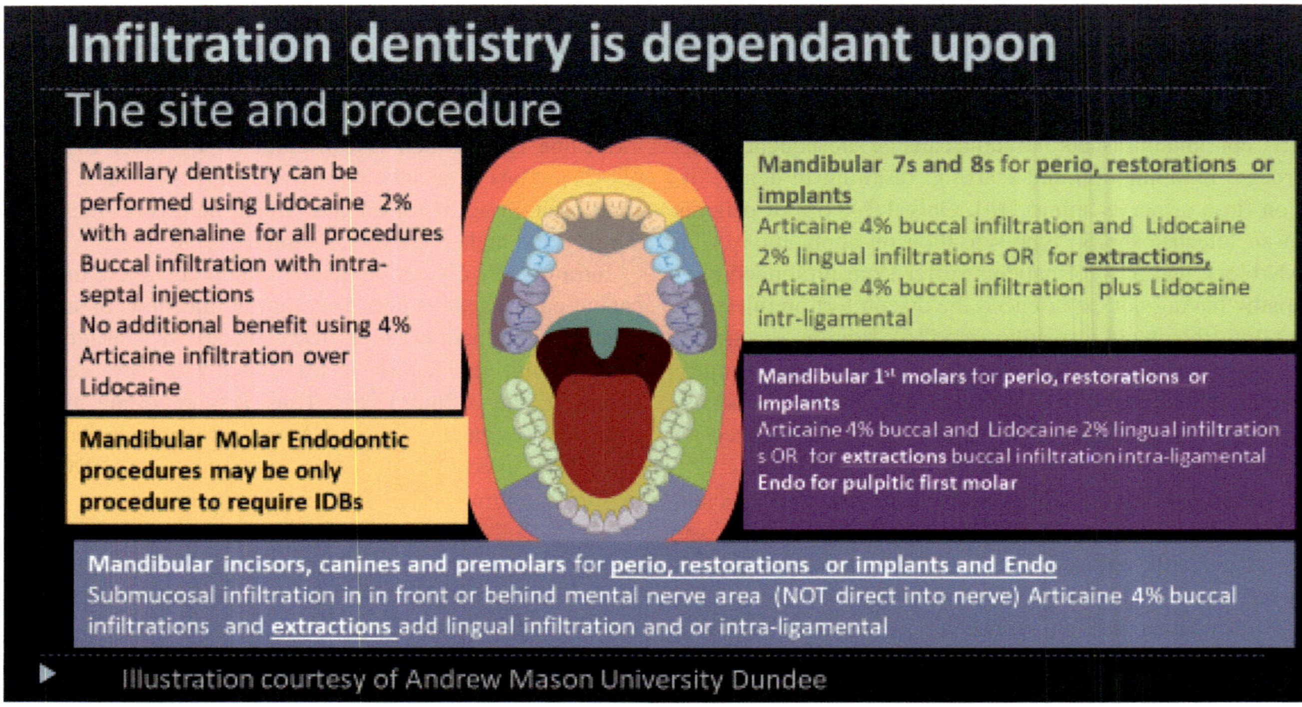



**Fig. 25.1** Summary of infiltration methods to minimize nerve injury

- *for exodontia in adults and children [32].*
  Paedodontic extractions do not require IDBs as the bone is very porous and susceptible to absorption of infiltrative anaesthesia.
- *is ideal for implant surgery,*
  Several reports of supra-periosteal infiltration anaesthesia not only are sufficient for posterior mandible implant surgery but also may be protective of the IAN [33].
- *is suitable for periodontal surgery.*
  The standard care for periodontal and implant surgery is infiltration LA [34].

Intra-ligamental anaesthesia for extractions and avoiding IDBs is also gaining population [34].

**Key Facts for Prevention of local anaesthetic nerve injuries.**

Thus, prevention of LA nerve injuries is possible and some simple steps may minimize LA-related nerve injuries:

- Avoid high concentration LA (Articaine 4%) for block injections and for ID blocks (use 2% Lidocaine as standard) as the efficacy is equal.
- Avoid multiple blocks where possible.
- Avoid nerve contact during block injections.
- Avoid block anaesthesia by using Infiltration dentistry and, thus, prevent LA-related nerve injury, for which there is no cure.

## 25.2 Management of LA Nerve Injuries

Evidence base remains limited for managing dental LA-related nerve injuries; we only know that 25% are permanent and that there is no 'magic bullet' to fix them. A sit and wait approach has to be adopted with reassurance of the patient and therapeutic management of their symptoms

- HOMECHECK—If you cause pain during an IDB injection in your patient, do follow them up the next day and check they are OK. If the patient reports numbness, altered sensation and/or pain, reassure them.
- Continue to support, reassure your patient and advise them to visit to confirm the presence of neuropathy. If the neuropathy affects most of the dermatome ± associated with severe neuropathic pain, nerve injury must be suspected. Reassure your patient that 75% of these injuries resolve.
- Say SORRY as this is NOT an admission of guilt.
- Initiate medical management (recommended for other peripheral sensory nerve injuries).
  – High-dose oral NSAIDs (400–800 mgs Ibuprofen PO QDS) for 2 days only. Bandolier Oxford league table summarizes the optimal analgesia for post-operative pain, and combined Ibuprofen and paracetamol have the smallest number needed to treat.

  - GMP prescription for Prednisolone 5 day step down does 50-40-30-20-10 mg PO (not for patients with contraindications for steroids or NSAIDs).
  - Vitamin B complex (Riboflavin 400 mg once daily for maximum of 3 months plus other Vit B complex).
- Arrange a review of the patient. All advice is summarized on the Trigeminalnerve.org.uk website.
- Long-term management of patients with non-resolving LA nerve injuries. The reality for these patients is that if they have persistent neuropathic pain and have to be treated as such with psychological and medical management. Topical local anaesthetic (Lidocaine 5%) patches may assist the patient in sleeping and playing sports in cold weather [35]. Psychological interventions play a significant role in managing these patients, and recommendations for treatment of trigeminal neuropathic pain are also well described by Renton & Zakzrewska [36].

## 25.3 Implant-related Nerve Injuries

Implant-related IANI's incidence varies from 0–40% [37]. Two recent studies highlight persistent neuropathic pain due to implant IANIs [38, 39]. Prevention of nerve implant IANIs can be attributed to the avoidance of direct damage to the Inferior dental canal (IDC) during preparation [40]. A good clinical and radiographic pre-assessment protocol is required to mitigate damage due to proximity of implant bed preparation to the inferior dental canal (IDC) and are recommended [41, 42]. The risk factors for implant nerve injury are summarized in Table 25.2 [41, 42, 45–52].

A limited window is available to maximize inferior alveolar nerve injury resolution in relation to dental implants, endodontics and mandibular wisdom teeth. A report illustrated that early removal of implants (within 30 h) may maximize neuropathy resolution; however, the evidence remains weak [37]. Prevention of implant-related nerve injuries includes;

- *Pre-operatively*
  - undertake a good risk assessment,
  - ability to read and use CBCT to plan a sufficient safety zone (know difference between drill length and implant length),
  - extra diligence in planning implants in the parasymphyseal region near the mental nerve (loop and incisal branches),
  - Screen out neuropathic pain pre-implant.
- *Operatively:*
  - make sure the implant bed preparation is above the safety zone,
  - stop drilling if patient reports intraoperative pain and reassess depth,
  - use drill guides and stops,
  - intra-operative reassessment of implant bed depth using marker and LCPA films at 60% of planned depth,
  - Record any events that may indicate operative nerve injury,
  - extreme pain during LA IDB, or during implant bed preparation
  - Suddenly give and/or profuse haemorrhage arising from the implant bed (possible breech of IDC).
  - In such situations, stop surgery, do not reach for more LA and reassess your surgical position,

**Table 25.2** Risk factors for implant-related nerve injury

| |
|---|
| *A. Inadequate preoperative assessment and planning due to* |
| • Surgeon lack of knowledge/inexperience/training |
| • Inadequate informed consent-all options provided and related risk benefit for each option of treatment. Implants are elective treatment. Sublingual haematoma that can require the need for tracheostomy post-implant treatment and rare events of death |
| • Lack of identification of existing pre-surgical neuropathy (especially important in edentulous patients) |
| • Poor planning in risk assessment and positioning the implant. A sectional DPT is recommended as a minimum for mandibular implant planning. If there is limited bone depth, a CBCT may be used to quantify and qualify bone density and volume. The clinician must be able to read and analyse the CBCT, depending upon technicians, software or radiologist specialist (who are not present with you intra-operatively) |
| – Bone assessment quality and quantity |
| – Know where the nerve is. Nerve localization, risk factors when assessing IAN position (mental loop, characteristics of IAN position in various sites of mandible) and Parasymphyseal zone that is of high risk. |
| – The accuracy of estimating the position of the IDC based on plain films or CT scans is highlighted in the radiographic assessment section |
| – Safety zone- the recommendation is 2 mm (by ITI and ADI), which may be insufficient considering that most-implant drills are 1.5 mm longer than implants. This increases the risk perforation of a canal surrounding IDC or even direct perforation and damage to the nerve |
| • Selection of implants 10 mm + (short implants <8 mm to simplify procedure and minimize morbidity) |
| *B. Surgical procedure should include the execution of* |
| • Local Anaesthesia (use infiltration LA techniques to allow patients to notify the surgeon or intraoperative neuralgia; if pain is reported, intra-operatively stop surgery and reassess preparation depth and width) |
| • Flap design |
| • Use surgical guides to minimize morbidity |
| • Surgical stents [43] |
| • Using intra-operative radiographs, ITI recommends stopping drilling after 60% of planned depth and reassess with bed marker and Long cone PeriApical radiograph |
| • Drill stops [44] |
| *C. Post-operative care should attend to* |
| • Early post-operative recognition of neuropathy (HOMECHECK). |
| • Prompt management of neuropathy (removal of implant if indicated) [44] |
| – Acute phase |
| – Late phase |
| • Early or late post-operative infection |

- *Post-operatively.*
- take appropriate post-operative periapical radiographs (CBCTs not indicated) to confirm proximity and/or breech of the inferior dental canal or around the mental foramen before patient discharge.
- If nerve injury is suspected or identified, the patient should be informed, Immediate removal of the implant should be arranged and appropriate medical management should be instituted with arranged review with the treating clinician and specialist if required.
- HOMECHECK -Contact must be made by the clinician and the patient between 6 and 24 h after surgery to confirm that the patient is experiencing any persistent neuropathy. This builds on the relationship of the clinician with the patient, which will be premised upon good consent process.
  - Continue to support and reassure your patient and advise them to visit return to your clinic. If the neuropathy affects most of the dermatome ± associated with severe neuropathic pain, nerve injury must be suspected.
  - Say SORRY this is NOT an admission of guilt. When neuropathy is confirmed, check who you must notify as in many countries, IANIs are reportable events. It is essential to be honest with your patient.
  - Additional scanning or radiography may not be essential. Post-traumatic neuropathy is a clinical diagnosis. You will already be aware of the proximity of the implant bed to the IDC, and whether there was likely breach into the IAN canal.
  - If nerve injury is suspected, the implant must be removed within 24–36 hours of placement in order to maximize recovery from nerve injury [37].
  - Arrange a review of the patient to confirm neuropathy.
  - Initiate medical management (recommended for other peripheral sensory nerve injuries).
    High-dose oral NSAIDs (400–800 mgs Ibuprofen PO QDS) for maximum 2 days.
    GMP (General Medical Practitioner) prescription for Prednisolone 5 day step down does 50-40-30-20-10 mg PO (not for patients with contraindications for steroids or NSAIDs).
    Vitamin B complex (Riboflavin 400 mg once daily for a maximum of 3 months plus other Vit B complex).
- Arrange a further review of your patient.
- Long-term management of patients with non-resolving nerve injuries. The reality for these patients is that if they have persistent neuropathic pain and have to be treated as such with psychological and medical management. Psychological interventions play a significant role in managing these patients, and recommendations for treatment of trigeminal neuropathic pain are also well described by Renton & Zakzrewska [36].

## 25.4 Mandibular Third Molar Extraction-related Nerve Injuries

The nerves at risk of damage in mandibular third molar extraction are the terminal nerves of the third branch of the trigeminal nerve [53, 54], i.e. the inferior dental nerve (IDN) and lingual nerve (LN). The reported risk of neurosensory deficit ranges from 0.26 to 8.4% for IDN [55] and from 0.1 to 22% for LN [ 7]. Patients with IDN injury suffer from paresthesia, anaesthesia or dysesthesia in the lip, chin or gingiva on the affected side, while patients with LN injury have a sensitivity deficit at the homolateral half of the tongue, with or without taste alteration [ 7]. Transient and permanent lesions should be differentiated; permanent lesions often remain after 6–12 months, and spontaneous recovery cannot be expected in these cases [ 56].

Damage to the LN or IDN during third molar extraction is among the most frequent causes of litigation in dentistry [57]. Highly varying results have been published by numerous studies on risk factors related to neurosensory deficit in lower third molar surgery. The objective of a recent literature review was to identify and analyse studies on factors related to IDN and/or LN injury in lower third molar extraction, allowing clinicians to take appropriate measures to minimize this risk [58]. Several radiological risk factors have been identified that increases the risk of nerve injury during removal by ten-fold (from 0.2 to 2% permanent injury and 2–20% temporary nerve injury) [59, 60].

**Key Facts**

Factors that may be implicated in nerve injury after lower third molar surgery were classified into four groups:

- Risk assessment—diagnostic radiographic techniques.
- IDN injury risk factors.
- LN injury risk factors.
- Alternative surgical approaches.

### 25.4.1 Risk Assessment

A recent review included three cohort studies and various randomized clinical trials (RCTs) on the influence of diagnostic radiographic techniques. They generally reached similar conclusions, finding that the non-utilization of CBCT was not an additional risk factor for nerve injury in patients examined by conventional panoramic radiography [61–63].

Korkmaz et al. [64] and Lee et al. [65] reported a lower frequency of transient but not permanent IDN damage when

CBCT was also used. This may be because in cases where the relationship between third molar and the IDN is doubtful, there is likely to be no direct contact and the injury would result from pressure due to haemorrhage or haematoma so that the association would be less detectable on panoramic radiology. In contrast, cases of direct contact are readily observed using both radiographic techniques.

### 25.4.2 Patient Factors

Various authors reported a significantly lower frequency of nerve injury with younger age. [66–70] Thus, no cases of nerve injury were observed among patients under 23 years of age in the cohort study of 1050 patients by Zhang et al. [ 71], while Kjølle et al. [66] confirmed a significant association with age ($p = 0.007$), finding a higher frequency of permanent injury in patients over 30 years of age. These findings may be attributable to an increased difficulty of the surgery at older ages due to a greater likelihood of hypercementosis, lower bone elasticity and, above all, completed root formation, in addition to lesser vascularization, reducing the regenerative capacity of the nerve. Nevertheless, other researchers found no significant relationship with age [72] although the sample sizes were smaller than that in the aforementioned studies. All reviewed articles observed a higher frequency of nerve injuries in females [62] although this difference was only statistically significant ($p = 0.005$) in the multiple logistic regression analysis of 320 cases conducted by Selvi et al. [68] Gender differences have been attributed to the generally smaller mandible of females, implying a smaller gap between third molar root and IDN.

### 25.4.3 Anatomical

The mandibular canal is evidently more susceptible to nerve injury with greater depth and, therefore, closer proximity of the impacted third molar, reducing the surgical accessibility and visibility. A statistically significant association was demonstrated by all three articles that studied this risk factor [62]. A higher risk of IDN injury was associated with mesioangular impactions and with horizontal impactions [62], but these associations were not found to be statistically significant.

### 25.4.4 Radiological Factors

In 1990, Rood and Shehab [59] proposed seven radiological signs identifiable by panoramic radiography, which indicate a close relationship between lower third molar and IDN: root narrowing, root darkening, apex darkening and bifid images, changes in root direction, dental canal narrowing, dental canal diversion and interruption of the white line of the dental canal. Only four of these signs were reported to be significant indicators of IDN risk in the reviewed articles: interruption of the radiopaque band of the canal [62, 66, 69, 73–76], canal diversion [59, 74, 76], root darkening [59, 62, 74, 76] and mandibular canal narrowing. [70, 74, 76] In contrast, a retrospective study by Pippi et al. [72] found that none of these signs were significantly associated with nerve injury, even when two or more were observed. CBCT radiological signs have also been associated with IDN damage. Detection of contact between lower third molar and mandibular canal has been found to potentially influence the resulting nerve damage, [62, 68, 69, 72, 77] which is associated by Kim et al. [70] with a 21-fold higher risk of paraesthesia. Various studies [67, 69, 73, 78, 79] have associated nerve injury with the lingual position of the mandibular canal with respect to the third molar root, attributed to the more likely interruption of the mandibular canal cortex due to the direction of extraction manoeuvres. The RCT reported by Ghaeminia et al. [ 62] found the risk of nerve injury to be 16-fold higher when the localization was lingual versus buccal. In addition, some authors have described a higher risk of IDN injury for dumbbell-shaped versus round-, oval- or drop-shaped canals [72, 73, 76, 77].

**Key Facts**

There are seven radiological signs identifiable by panoramic radiography, which indicate a close relationship between lower third molar and IDN: root narrowing, root darkening, apex darkening and bifid images, changes in root direction, dental canal narrowing, dental canal diversion and interruption of the white line of the dental canal.

### 25.4.5 Surgical

Two studies related the type of anaesthesia to IDN injury. Nyugen et al. [67] found a significantly higher ($p = 0.007$) frequency of permanent damage in lower third molar surgery under general versus local anaesthesia, and Costantinides et al. [80] reported a 2–16-fold greater risk of IDN injury under the former. One explanation is that the absence of patient feedback with general anaesthesia means that surgeons are less aware of the force applied. Hasegawa et al. [69] observed a significantly higher ($p < 0.05$) IDN injury rate in patients with versus without nerve exposure during the surgery. However, Pippi et al. [72] reported nerve injuries in only 6.5% of cases in which the nerve was exposed versus

9.3% of cases in which it was not, suggesting that IDN exposure may simply reflect the close proximity of tooth and nerve and cannot per se be considered an indicator of potential nerve damage. Three studies associated haemorrhage during third molar extraction with IDN injury [62, 75, 81], without elucidating whether the bleeding resulted from mandibular canal fracture or a haematoma or other causes of nerve compression.

With respect to the experience of the clinician, Nguyen et al. [67] found a significantly higher frequency of permanent IDN injury ($p = 0.026$) amongst inexperienced dentists in comparison to oral specialists or maxillofacial surgeons, possibly related to inappropriate force and less instrumental control in the hands of those with less experience. The same study also explored the effect of surgery duration, finding a higher nerve injury rate when this was more than 20 min (from incision to completed tooth extraction), mainly because a longer surgical time implies a more challenging extraction. With regard to the surgical approach, Jain et al. [73] reported a significantly ($p = 0.04$) higher nerve injury rate in patients who underwent odontosection versus those who did not. This may be explained by the less extensive ostectomy often associated with this procedure although odontosection can be a direct risk factor for IDN injury in the extraction of horizontal third molars [82].

## 25.5 LN Injury Risk Factors

*Demographics* A prospective study by Charan Babu et al. [83] reported that older age was a significant risk factor for LN injury ($p < 0.05$), but Kjoelle et al. [66] found no differences in permanent nerve damage amongst age groups. No significant gender differences in LN injury rate were found in any study.

*Anatomical* Charan Babu et al. [ 83] observed a significantly ($p < 0.01$) higher risk of LN injury with greater impaction depth, attributed to the more difficult extraction and, therefore, more extensive osteotomy. A higher LN injury rate was observed for distoangular impactions [67, 83] generally due to the more difficult extraction and for horizontal extractions [83], possibly because of the larger amount of bone removed. However, these associations were not statistically significant.

*Surgical* Charan Babu et al. [ 83], Osunde et al. [84] and Yadav et al. [85] reported a significantly higher LN injury rate ($p < 0.01$, $p < 0.001$ and $p < 0.001$, respectively) in patients who had undergone lingual flap retraction before third molar extraction than in those who had not.

This injury was found to be transient in the RCT by Shad et al. [86], who suggested that permanent injury can be produced when the lingual flap is not separated from the bone. Three studies [62, 85, 87] observed a significant association between higher LN injury risk and the requirement for odontosection in third molar surgery.

## 25.6 Role of Alternative Surgical Techniques

Various authors have proposed alternative surgical techniques to avoid nerve damage in lower third molar extraction, but their findings should be considered with caution due to major study limitations (e.g. no control group and small sample size), and there has been little research on this issue. In a study of 53 patients, Bataineh et al. [88] reported a modified flap that appeared to reduce LN lesions caused by flap retraction, considering all known anatomical variations of LN. Ge et al. [89] observed lower nerve injury rates when type III lower third molars in lingual position were extracted by piezosurgery in a lingual split approach in comparison to published rates reported using the conventional lingual split technique. The persistence in defending lingual access third molar surgery is inappropriate, in that it significantly increases the risk of temporary lingual nerve injury and 10–12% of these injuries will be permanent [90]. A recent literature review recommends avoidance of lingual flaps in third molar surgery to minimize lingual nerve injury [91].

A recent surgical technique to mitigate the risk of high risk third molars in close proximity to the IDC is a coronectomy. Coronectomy, in which the dental crown is removed and the root is retained in the jaw, has been recommended to reduce IDN injury risk in cases of close proximity between nerve and third molar, and the majority of the reviewed studies described any IDN injury with the utilization of this approach [60]. Nevertheless, this technique is not free of controversy, even when clearly indicated, given the possibility of infectious complications around the root or its migration [92–95]. Extraction by orthodontic traction may also be useful when there is a high risk of nerve injury, and Wang et al. [96] found no cases of nerve injury in patients undergoing this procedure although account should be taken of study design limitations and the small sample size. There is a strong evidence base to support the prevention of IDN nerve injuries using the coronectomy technique [43, 44, 53, 54, 97].

**Table 25.3** Risk factors for third molar surgery-related nerve injury

| | |
|---|---|
| *Lingual nerve injury* | |
| | Increased patient age |
| | Increased duration surgery |
| | Lingual access surgery |
| | Inexperience of surgeon |
| | Distoangulation of third molar |
| | Depth of impaction |
| *Inferior alveolar nerve injury* | |
| | Proximity of tooth root to inferior dental canal |
| | Increased patient age |
| | Increased duration surgery |
| | Inexperience of surgeon |
| | Distoangulation of third molar |
| | Depth of impaction |

Summary prevention of third molar surgery-related nerve injury (Table 25.3) [98, 99].

- Nerve injury risk does not appear to be influenced by the diagnostic imaging technique used (CBCT or panoramic radiograph) although the utilization of CBCT may possibly reduce the risk of transient injuries. Studies with larger sample sizes are needed to clarify this issue.
- Older age, female sex, mesioangular position, impaction depth, utilization of general versus local anaesthesia, haemorrhage, inexperience of the clinician and certain signs on panoramic radiography and CBCT appear to be associated with a higher risk of IDN injury.
- Lingual flap retraction, older age, horizontal and distoangular positions, impaction depth and odontosection may be possible risk factors for LN injury.
- Coronectomy is evidence based to prevent IDN injuries in selected cases, High-risk third molar, healthy and cooperative patients and vital tooth.
- Definitive conclusions are limited by the variability in study design (with the inclusion of some retrospective studies), reduced sample sizes and differences in the experience of clinicians, amongst other factors. However, buccal approach technique (when undertaken properly) will minimize lingual nerve injury.

## 25.7 Prognosis of Nerve Injuries (Table 25.4) [43]

It is not possible to classify the degree or outcome of a sensory nerve injury based on patients' presentation early post-injury. Just as with phantom limb pain patients, who may express non-existence or existence of a 'normal feeling' limb (after amputation, the most catastrophic nerve injury) with or without pain, numbness or altered sensation, these symptoms do not reflect the degree of injury or prognosis. Thus, in order to assess the end results of nerve injury, the patient must be reassessed and/or treated if indicated. The type and related permanency of trigeminal nerve injuries are summarized in Table 25.4.

**Table 25.4** Resolution rates of inferior alveolar nerve injury (IANI)

| Procedure | Recovery rate |
|---|---|
| Third molar surgery [7] | IANI – 67%; LNI – 72% Buccal access TMS<br>LIN – Lingual access TMS 88% |
| Mandibular fractures [7] | IANI – 91% |
| Orthognathic surgery | IANI – 87%<br>Bilateral sagittal split osteotomy (BSSO) IANI (patients 80–92%) |
| Local anaesthesia inferior dental block (mainly Lidocaine) [14] | 75% |
| Implant-related IANI [87] | Complete recovery – 50%<br>Partial recovery – 44%<br>No change – 6% |

A review of common operations such as groin hernia repair, breast and thoracic surgery, leg amputation and coronary artery bypass surgery found an incidence of chronic post-surgical pain in 10–50% of patients [100].

**Table 25.5** Timing for intervention of Trigeminal nerve injury

| Event | Recovery | |
|---|---|---|
| Endodontic | <24–36 h | Remove tooth and remove over fill or over instrumentation |
| Implant | <24–36 h | Remove implant |
| Wisdom teeth- inferior alveolar nerve injury | <2 weeks | Consider earlier intervention |
| Radiographic evidence of retained tooth fragments or IDC damage | | Access via extraction socket and remove retained roots ± repair nerve |
| Wisdom teeth -lingual nerve injury | >3–6 months | Consider earlier intervention |
| If CBCT confirmation of breech, lingual plate | Consider earlier intervention | Access via extraction socket and remove retained roots ± repair nerve |
| Local anaesthetic nerve injuries (LN or IAN) | | Therapeutic management only |
| Orthognathic nerve injuries | | Therapeutic management only |
| Mandibular fracture nerve injuries | | Therapeutic management only |

A known or suspected sectioned/damaged nerve should undergo immediate exploration repair

*Summary of type and timing of management* (Table 25.5 and Fig. 25.2) Management of third molar-related nerve injuries will depend upon the presentation of the patient (pain, functional and psychological implications) duration and cause of the nerve injury [56, 98]. Figure 25.2 summarizes the management and timing of intervention for trigeminal nerve injuries based upon the current evidence base [56, 98]. It is recognized that neuropathic pain does not respond to surgical intervention, and thus, prevention and early management are paramount in preventing chronic life-long pain after routine surgery in these patients. Advice is summarized on the Trigeminalnerve.org.uk website.

**MANAGEMENT OF TRIGEMINAL NERVE INJURIESRELTED TO DENTAL PROCEDURES**

| Timeline | During surgery | Post surgery 2-6 weeks | 12 weeks | > 12 weeks |
|---|---|---|---|---|

Psychological intervention

Medical intervention

| | | |
|---|---|---|
| High risk nerve injury/ or patient high risk of developing neuropathic pain consider pre-emptive Amitriptyline or Pregabalin | Reported neuropathy immediate post-surgery<br>• NSAIDs Ibuprofen 6—mg TDS 5 days (MH permitting)<br>• step down Prednisolone 50-10mg over 5 days (exclude known risk of DU and or PU)<br>• Vitamin B complex (long term during recovery)<br>• Review | If required: Psychological support (fcr PTSD and sleep disorders) and Therapeutic management of neuropathic pain (NICE Guidance Ne Pain in adults)<br>• Step 1 Amitriptyline or Nortriptyline<br>• Adjunctive topical agents (Lidocaine, Capsaicin)<br>• Step II Gabapentin or Pregabalin |

Surgical intervention

| | | | | | |
|---|---|---|---|---|---|
| Known or suspected nerve Inferior alveolar or lingual injury<br>**Duty of candour inform patient immediately**<br>**Repair nerve immediately Or refer for immediate repair** to a specialist centre | Post Local anaesthesia or orthognathic surgery or trauma<br>**Duty of candour inform patient immediately**<br>**Surgery not indicated**<br>**Medical and psychological therapies** | Post Implant or endodontic surgery<br>Patient presents with nerve injury early postoperatively<br>Confirm extensive dermatome affected, anaesthesia, +/- paraesthesia, +/- neuropathic pain<br>**Within 30 hours**<br>**Remove implant or endodontically treated tooth** and reassess patient combined with medical intervention above | Post M3M surgery<br>Patient presents with nerve injury early postoperatively<br>Confirm extensive dermatome affected, anaesthesia, +/- paraesthesia, +/- neuropathic pain<br>**Inferior alveolar nerve** DPT confirms retained roots or bony defect of IDC<br>**Lingual nerve (buccal approach)** DPT confirms retained roots CBCT confirms lingual plate defect due to M3M surgery<br>**Consider early exploration (IAN via M3M socket) +/- nerve repair dependent upon surgical findings** | Patient presents with persistent non-resolving **LINGUAL nerve injury** after lingual access(lingual retraction +/- lingual split) surgery<br>Confirm extensive dermatome affected, anaesthesia, +/- paraesthesia, +/- neuropathic pain<br>**Consider exploration @ 12 weeks +/- nerve repair dependent upon surgical findings** | Patient presents with persistent non-resolving **Inferior alveolar nerve injury** OR **LINGUAL nerve injury** after M3M surgery<br>Confirm extensive dermatome affected, anaesthesia, +/- paraesthesia, +/- neuropathic pain<br>Consider medical and psychological therapeutic measures<br>**N.B Surgical repair DOES NOT IMPROVE neuropathic pain** |

- *New developments*
- *MRI micro neurography may assist in confirmation of damage to IAN and LN (currently available in US under development London)*
- *Larger IAN defects can be optimally repaired using Axogen cadaveric nerve graft (currently NICE approved for hand surgery in UK)*



**Fig. 25.2** suggested management of nerve injuries related to mandibular third molar surgery

The patient with the nerve injury must be treated, NOT the nerve injury in isolation. The neuropathy, pain, numbness or paraesthesia, with associated functional and psychological impact, will be the driving force behind the patient seeking treatment [98]. These factors must be assessed, and the potential outcomes, good or bad, should be discussed and agreed with the patient [99].

Patients sustaining LA, orthognathic, oncology and trauma-related nerve injuries will mainly be managed therapeutically [101–104].

Overall, there is poor evidence to support late surgical intervention for Trigeminal nerve injuries [6, 105]. Most studies report on repair procedures undertaken too late, and early repair is imperative to minimize central irreversible changes and possibly chronic pain. Generally, surgical repair of the trigeminal nerves never returns the patient to peroperative neural function; in addition, there is a risk of making a numb patient into one with chronic post-surgical pain [100, 106]. As with other post-trauma sensory neuropathies, it is recognized that immediate repair is optimal; [107, 108] however, this is rarely applied to dental nerve injuries with the misconception that we should sit and wait for resolution (only for 3 months for lingual nerve injuries related to lingual access third molar surgery), resulting in long delays before surgical intervention [109–111].

Some recent studies have highlighted immediate repair with cadaveric-treated human nerve graft successful in managing various sized defects in planned resection of nerves related to benign tumour resection or trauma [112, 113].

Recent reports have also concluded that, similar to other surgical sites, neuropathic pain does not resolve with surgery, with this being the main driver for surgical repair [114, 115].

Many reports have recommended the use of conduits (venous, prosthetic), sural nerve grafts and other techniques without sufficient evidence and many with poor outcomes including neuropathy and pain from the donor sites! The future may prove that nerve growth factors, other growth-promoting chemical and anti-neuropathic pain agents and specialized conduits may play a role in improving repair of trigeminal nerve injuries, and the overall conclusion from reviews in this area is that we have a lot of evidence base to harness [105, 106, 116]. The singular consensus is that prevention of these nerve injuries is possible and optimal.

The timing of intervention and mechanism of injury are paramount in decision making in the treatment of trigeminal nerve injuries (summarized in Table 25.5).

1. Counselling is the most useful effective tool for managing patients with problematic permanent sensory nerve injuries.
2. Medical intervention is indicated for patients with pain or discomfort or with anxiety and/or depression in relation to chronic pain. However, due to the multiple noxious side effects of chronic pain medication, less than 18% of patients remain adherent with medication.
   - acute (medical),
   - late (chronic pain management with psychological interventions).
3. Surgical intervention is indicated for:
   - Immediate surgical repair for suspected or known nerve injury or intended surgical defect after removal of benign tumour or recent trauma [98].
     - Removal of implant.
     - or overfill or RCT-treated tooth with 36 h if related to the development of neuropathy [99].
   - Within 2–4 week, exploration if clinical presentation of persistent neuropathy is paramount and radiographic follow-up is not necessary; however, if there is CBCT evidence of breech of lingual plate or IDC, consider immediate action-nerve exploration ± repair;
     - Lingual nerve neuropathy patients with CBCT evidence of damage to lingual plate adjacent to third molar surgical site.
     - Inferior alveolar nerve with retained roots or evidence of bone inclusions or compression of IDC.
   - Within 3 months of injury;
     - Non-resolving lingual or inferior dental nerve injuries: Exploratory surgery for lingual or inferior alveolar nerve injuries within 3 months post-injury. Surgical intervention is not effective for neuropathic pain, and if this is the driving force behind seeking surgery, it should be reconsidered.
     - There are reported exciting results of allografting lingual and inferior alveolar nerve injuries. Using a pre-prepared human-treated cadaveric allograft, the IDN and LN can be repaired with minimal tension. This is undertaken using microscopy and described in several publications by John Zuniga and Michael Miloro [109]. This is likely to be the treatment of choice if repair is indicated and direct re-anastomosis cannot be undertaken most commonly for the IDN. One of the main issues regarding nerve repair is the early identification of the neuroma related to the patients 'symptoms and the connectivity of the nerve itself, i.e. is the nerve actually functioning. Recent developments with Magnetic Resonance Neurography (MRN) have availed the surgeon to identify the nerve lesion and neural functionality to facilitate appropriate and earlier nerve repair intervention [117, 118].

## 25.8 Conclusions

Unfortunately, none of these interventions 'fix' the patient, but the aim is to manage their symptoms as best as possible, improve function and allow them time to accommodate to these unfortunate events, which is often not very satisfactory.

This chapter was intended to acknowledge and share some key issues around iatrogenic trigeminal nerve injuries and to provide some key take home messages including:

- Neuropathic pain as well as altered sensation and numbness is what most patients experience with iatrogenic sensory nerve injury. This has a significant and unpleasant effect on the patient (improve your consent!)
- The majority of iatrogenic nerve injuries are avoidable.
- Inferior alveolar nerve injuries in relation to implant and endodontic dentistry are permanent and 'unfixable' unless treated quickly within 30 h.
- Owing to the significant problems following nerve injury, pre-operative strategies for minimizing this risk of nerve damage need to be considered carefully. Peri-operative planning, operative execution and post-operative care need improving to minimize and hopefully abolish these injuries.
- Several strategies are presented to assist in preventing nerve injuries.
- There is a need for a consensus and standardization of risk assessment and management, a holistic approach in managing the pain, related effect on functionality and psychological implications caused to the patients affected by iatrogenic nerve injury.

## References


1. Caissie R, Goulet J, Fortin M, Morielle D. Iatrogenic paresthesia in the third division of the trigeminal nerve: 12 years of clinical experience. J Can Dent Assoc. 2005;71(3):188–92.
2. Hillerup S. Iatrogenic injury to oral branches of the trigeminal nerve: records of 449 cases. Clin Oral Investig. 2007 Jun;11(2):133–42. Epub 2006 Dec 22.

3. Elian N, Mitsias M, Eskow R, Jalbout ZN, Cho SC, Froum S, Tarnow DP. Unexpected return of sensation following 4.5 years of paresthesia: case report. Implant Dent. 2005 Dec;14(4):364–7.
4. Loescher AR, Robinson PP. The effect of surgical medicaments on peripheral nerve function. Br J Oral Maxillofac Surg. 1998 Oct;36(5):327–32.
5. Hegedus F, Diecidue RJ. Trigeminal nerve injuries after mandibular implant placement--practical knowledge for clinicians. Int J Oral Maxillofac Implants. 2006;21(1):111–6.
6. Ziccardi VB, Assael LA. Mechanisms of trigeminal nerve injuries. Atlas Oral Maxillofac Surg Clin North Am. 2001;9(2):1–11.
7. Renton T, Yilmaz Z. Profiling of patients presenting with posttraumatic neuropathy of the trigeminal nerve. J Orofac Pain. 2011 Fall;25(4):333–44.
8. Carter E, Yilmaz Z, Devine M, Renton T. An update on the causes, assessment and management of third division sensory trigeminal neuropathies. Br Dent J. 2016 Jun;220(12):627–35.
9. Renton T, Adey-Viscuso D, Meechan JG, Yilmaz Z. Trigeminal nerve injuries in relation to the local anaesthesia in mandibular injections. Br Dent J. 2010;209(9):E15. https://doi.org/10.1038/sj.bdj.2010.978.
10. Zuniga JR, Yates DM, Phillips CL. The presence of neuropathic pain predicts postoperative neuropathic pain following trigeminal nerve repair. J Oral Maxillofac Surg. 2014 Dec;72(12):2422–7.
11. Leung YY, Cheung LK. Longitudinal treatment outcomes of microsurgical treatment of neurosensory deficit after lower third molar surgery: a prospective case series. PLoS One. 2016 Mar 4;11(3):e0150149.
12. Smith JG, Elias LA, Yilmaz Z, Barker S, Shah K, Shah S, et al. The psychosocial and affective burden of posttraumatic neuropathy following injuries to the trigeminal nerve. J Orofac Pain. 2013;27(4):293–303.
13. Renton T, Janjua H, Gallagher JE, Dalgleish M, Yilmaz Z. Uk dentists' experience of iatrogenic trigeminal nerve injuries in relation to routine dental procedures: why, when and how often? Br Dent J. 2013;214(12):633–42. https://doi.org/10.1038/sj.bdj.2013.583.
14. Pogrel MA, Schmidt BL, Sambajon V, Jordan RC. Lingual nerve damage due to inferior alveolar nerve blocks: a possible explanation. J Am Dent Assoc. 2003;134(2):195–9.
15. Smith MH, Lung KE. Nerve injuries after dental injection: a review of the literature J Can Dent Assoc 2006 Jul–Aug;72(6):559–564. Review.
16. Pogrel MA, Thamby S. Permanent nerve involvement resulting from inferior alveolar nerve blocks. J Am Dent Assoc. 2000;131(7):901–7.
17. Haas DA, Lennon D. A 21 year retrospective study of reports of paresthesia following local anesthetic administration. J Can Dent Assoc. 1995;61(4):319–20, 323–316, 329–330
18. Hillerup S. Iatrogenic injury to oral branches of the trigeminal nerve: records of 449 cases. Clin Oral Investig. 2007;11(2):133–42.
19. Hillerup S, Jensen R. Nerve injury caused by mandibular block analgesia. Int J Oral Maxillofac Surg. 2006;35(5):437–43. https://doi.org/10.1016/j.ijom.2005.10.004.
20. Pedlar J. Prolonged paraesthesia. Br Dent J. 2003;195(3):119. https://doi.org/10.1038/sj.bdj.4810421.
21. Perez-Castro R, Patel S, Garavito-Aguilar ZV, Rosenberg A, Recio-Pinto E, Zhang J, Blanck TJ, Xu F. Cytotoxicity of local anesthetics in human neuronal cells. Anesth Analg. 2009 Mar;108(3):997–1007.
22. Kämmerer PW, Schneider D, Palarie V, Schiegnitz E, Daubländer M. Comparison of anesthetic efficacy of 2 and 4% articaine in inferior alveolar nerve block for tooth extraction-a double-blinded randomized clinical trial. Clin Oral Investig. 2017 Jan;21(1):397–403.
23. Daubländer M, Kämmerer PW, Willershausen B, Leckel M, Lauer HC, Buff S, Rösl B. Clinical use of an epinephrine-reduced (1/400,000) articaine solution in short-time dental routine treatments--a multicenter study. Clin Oral Investig. 2012 Aug;16(4):1289–95.
24. Evans G, Nusstein J, Drum M, Reader A, Beck M. A prospective, randomized, double-blind comparison of articaine and lidocaine for maxillary infiltrations. J Endod. 2008 Apr;34(4):389–93.
25. Oliveira PC, Volpato MC, Ramacciato JC, Ranali J. Articaine and lignocaine efficiency in infiltration anaesthesia: a pilot study. Br Dent J. 2004 Jul 10;197(1):45–6.
26. Vähätalo K, Antila H, Lehtinen R. Articaine and lidocaine for maxillary infiltration anesthesia. Anesth Prog. 1993;40(4):114–6.
27. Srinivasan N, Kavitha M, Loganathan CS, Padmini G. Comparison of anesthetic efficacy of 4% articaine and 2% lidocaine for maxillary buccal infiltration in patients with irreversible pulpitis. Oral Surg Oral Med Oral Pathol Oral Radiol Endod. 2009 Jan;107(1):133–6.
28. Meechan JG The use of the mandibular infiltration anesthetic technique in adults. J Am Dent Assoc. 2011 Sep;142 Suppl 3:19S–24S. Review.
29. Zain M, et al. Comparison of Anaesthetic efficacy of 4% Articaine primary Buccal infiltration versus 2% Lidocaine inferior alveolar nerve block in symptomatic mandibular first molar teeth. J Coll Physicians Surg Pak. 2016 Jan;26(1):4–8.
30. Poorni S, et al. Anesthetic efficacy of four percent articaine for pulpal anesthesia by using inferior alveolar nerve block and buccal infiltration techniques in patients with irreversible pulpitis: a prospective randomized double-blind clinical trial. J Endod. 2011 Dec;37(12):1603–7.
31. Kung J, McDonagh M, Sedgley CM. Does articaine provide an advantage over lidocaine in patients with symptomatic irreversible pulpitis? A systematic review and meta-analysis. J Endod. 2015;41(11):1784–94.
32. Thakare A, Bhate K, Kathariya R. Comparison of 4% articaine and 0.5% bupivacaine anesthetic efficacy in orthodontic extractions: prospective, randomized crossover study. Acta Anaesthesiol Taiwanica. 2014 Jun;52(2):59–63.
33. Etoz OA, Er N, Demirbas AE. Is supraperiosteal infiltration anesthesia safe enough to prevent inferior alveolar nerve during posterior mandibular implant surgery? Med Oral Patol Oral Cir Bucal. 2011 May 1;16(3):e386–9.
34. Dumbrigue HB, Lim MV, Rudman RA, Serraon A. A comparative study of anesthetic techniques for mandibular dental extraction. Am J Dent. 1997 Dec;10(6):275–8.
35. Khawaja N, Yilmaz Z, Renton T. Case studies illustrating the management of trigeminal neuropathic pain using topical 5% lidocaine plasters. Br J Pain. 2013;7(2):107–13.
36. Renton T, Zakrzewska JM Chapter 22 Orofacial pain. In: Shaw I, Kumar C, Dodds C, editors. Oxford textbook of anaesthesia for oral and maxillofacial surgery. Oxford: Oxford University Press; 2010. p. 283–298 isbn:978-0-19-956421-7.
37. Khawaja N, Renton T. Case studies on implant removal influencing the resolution of inferior alveolar nerve injury. Br Dent J. 2009;206(7):365–70. https://doi.org/10.1038/sj.bdj.2009.258.
38. Alhassani AA, AlGhamdi AS. Inferior alveolar nerve injury in implant dentistry: diagnosis, causes, prevention, and management. J Oral Implantol. 2010;36(5):401–7.
39. Fukuda K, Ichinohe T, Kaneko Y. Pain management for nerve injury following dental implant surgery at Tokyo dental college hospital. Int J Dent. 2012;2012:209474. https://doi.org/10.1155/2012/209474.
40. Renton T, Dawood A, Shah A, Searson L, Yilmaz Z, Renton T, Yilmaz Z. Post-implant neuropathy of the trigeminal nerve. A case series. Br Dent J. 2012;212(11):E17. https://doi.org/10.1038/sj.bdj.2012.497.
41. Juodzbalys G, Kubilius M. Clinical and radiological classification of the jawbone anatomy in endosseous dental implant treatment. J

Oral Maxillofac Res. 2013 Jul 1;4(2):e2. https://doi.org/10.5037/jomr.2013.4202.N.
42. Harris D, Horner K, Gröndahl K, Jacobs R, Helmrot E, Benic GI, Bornstein MM, Dawood A, Quirynen M. EAO guidelines for the use of diagnostic imaging in implant dentistry 2011. A consensus workshop organized by the European Association for Osseointegration at the Medical University of Warsaw. Clin Oral Implants Res. 2012 Nov;23(11):1243–53.
43. Leung YY, Cheung LK. Coronectomy of the lower third molar is safe within the first 3 years. J Oral Maxillofac Surg: Official Journal of the American Association of Oral and Maxillofacial Surgeons. 2012;70(7):1515–22.
44. Cervera-Espert J, Pérez-Martínez S, Cervera-Ballester J, Peñarrocha-Oltra D, Peñarrocha-Diago M. Coronectomy of impacted mandibular third molars: a meta-analysis and systematic review of the literature. Med Oral Patol Oral Cir Bucal. 2016 Jul 1;21(4):e505–13.
45. Greenstein G, Tarnow D. The mental foramen and nerve: clinical and anatomical factors related to dental implant placement: a literature review. J Periodontol. 2006 Dec;77(12):1933–43.
46. Thoma DS, Cha JK, Jung UW. Treatment concepts for the posterior maxilla and mandible: short implants versus long implants in augmented bone. J Periodontal Implant Sci. 2017 Feb;47(1):2–12.
47. Bartlett G, Mansoor J. Articaine buccal infiltration vs lidocaine inferior dental block – a review of the literature. Br Dent J. 2016 Feb 12;220(3):117–20.
48. Al-Ani O, Nambiar P, Ha KO, Ngeow WC. Safe zone for bone harvesting from the interforaminal region of the mandible. Clin Oral Implants Res. 2013 Aug;24(Suppl A100):115–21.
49. Van Assche N, van Steenberghe D, Guerrero ME, Hirsch E, Schutyser F, Quirynen M, Jacobs R. Accuracy of implant placement based on pre-surgical planning of three-dimensional cone-beam images: a pilot study. J Clin Periodontol. 2007;34(9):816–21.
50. De Kok IJ, Thalji G, Bryington M, Cooper LF. Radiographic stents: integrating treatment planning and implant placement Dent Clin N Am. 2014 Jan;58(1):181–192. https://doi.org/10.1016/j.cden.2013.09.008. Review.
51. Burstein J, Mastin C, Le B. Avoiding injury to the inferior alveolar nerve by routine use of intraoperative radiographs during implant placement. J Oral Implantol. 2008;34(1):34–8.
52. Greenstein G, Greenstein B, Desai RN. Using drill stops on twist drills to promote safety and efficiency when creating osteotomies for dental implants. J Am Dent Assoc. 2014 Apr;145(4):371–5.
53. Szalma J, Lempel E. Protecting the inferior alveolar nerve: coronectomy of lower third molars. Rev Orv Hetil. 2017 Nov;158(45):1787–93.
54. Ali AS, Benton JA, Yates JM. Risk of inferior alveolar nerve injury with coronectomy vs surgical extraction of mandibular third molars-a comparison of two techniques and review of the literature. J Oral Rehabil. 2018 Mar;45(3):250–7.
55. Cheung LK, Leung YY, Chow LK, Wong MC, Chan EK, Fok YH. Incidence of neurosensory deficits and recovery after lower third molar surgery: a prospective clinical study of 4338 cases. Int J Oral Maxillofac Surg. 2010;39(4):320–6.
56. Renton T, Yilmaz Z. Managing iatrogenic trigeminal nerve injury: a case series and review of the literature. Int J Oral Maxillofac Surg. 2012;41(5):629–37. https://doi.org/10.1016/j.ijom.2011.11.002.
57. Koskela S, Suomalainen A, Apajalahti S, Venta I. Malpractice claims related to tooth extractions. Clin Oral Investig. 2017 Mar;21(2):519–22.
58. Leung YY, Cheung LK. Risk factors of neurosensory deficits in lower third molar surgery: a literature review of prospective studies. Int J Oral Maxillofac Surg. 2011;40(1):1–10.
59. Rood JP, Shehab BA. The radiological prediction of inferior alveolar nerve injury during third molar surgery. Br J Oral Maxillofac Surg. 1990;28(1):20–5.
60. Renton T. Notes on coronectomy. Br Dent J. 2012;212:323–6.
61. Petersen LB, Vaeth M, Wenzel A. Neurosensory disturbances after surgical removal of the mandibular third molar based on either panoramic imaging or cone beam CT scanning: a randomized controlled trial (RCT). Dentomaxillofac Radiol. 2016;45(2):20150224.
62. Ghaeminia H, Gerlach NL, Hoppenreijs TJ, Kicken M, Dings JP, Borstlap WA, et al. Clinical relevance of cone beam computed tomography in mandibular third molar removal: a multicentre, randomised, controlled trial. J Cranio-Maxillo-Fac Surg: Official Publication of the European Association for Cranio-Maxillo-Fac Surgery. 2015;43(10):2158–67.
63. Matzen LH, Schou S, Christensen J, Hintze H, Wenzel A. Audit of a 5-year radiographic protocol for assessment of mandibular third molars before surgical intervention. Dentomaxillofac Radiol. 2014;43(8):20140172.
64. Korkmaz YT, Kayipmaz S, Senel FC, Atasoy KT, Gumrukcu Z. Does additional cone beam computed tomography decrease the risk of inferior alveolar nerve injury in high-risk cases undergoing third molar surgery? Does CBCT decrease the risk of IAN injury? Int J Oral Maxillofac Surg. 2017;46(5):628–35.
65. Lee B, Park Y, Ahn J, Chun J, Park S, Kim M, et al. Assessment of the proximity between the mandibular third molar and inferior alveolar canal using preoperative 3D-CT to prevent inferior alveolar nerve damage. Maxillofac Plast Reconstr Surg. 2015;37(1):30.
66. Kjolle GK, Bjornland T. Low risk of neurosensory dysfunction after mandibular third molar surgery in patients less than 30 years of age. A prospective study following removal of 1220 mandibular third molars. Oral Surg Oral Med Oral Pathol Oral Radiol. 2013;116(4):411–7.
67. Nguyen E, Grubor D, Chandu A. Risk factors for permanent injury of inferior alveolar and lingual nerves during third molar surgery. J Oral Maxillofac Surg: Official Journal of the American Association of Oral and Maxillofacial Surgeons. 2014;72(12):2394–401.
68. Selvi F, Dodson TB, Nattestad A, Robertson K, Tolstunov L. Factors that are associated with injury to the inferior alveolar nerve in high-risk patients after removal of third molars. Br J Oral Maxillofac Surg. 2013;51(8):868–73.
69. Hasegawa T, Ri S, Shigeta T, Akashi M, Imai Y, Kakei Y, et al. Risk factors associated with inferior alveolar nerve injury after extraction of the mandibular third molar--a comparative study of preoperative images by panoramic radiography and computed tomography. Int J Oral Maxillofac Surg. 2013;42(7):843–51.
70. Kim JW, Cha IH, Kim SJ, Kim MR. Which risk factors are associated with neurosensory deficits of inferior alveolar nerve after mandibular third molar extraction? J Oral Maxillofac Surg: Official Journal of the American Association of Oral and Maxillofacial Surgeons. 2012;70(11):2508–14.
71. Zhang QB, Zhang ZQ. Early extraction: a silver bullet to avoid nerve injury in lower third molar removal? Int J Oral Maxillofac Surg. 2012;41(10):1280–3.
72. Pippi R, Santoro M. A multivariate statistical analysis on variables affecting inferior alveolar nerve damage during third molar surgery. Br Dent J. 2015;219(4):E3.
73. Jain N, Thomas S, Prabhu S, Jain S, Pathak AD, Pillai A, et al. Influence of tooth sectioning technique and various risk factors in reducing the IAN injury following surgical removal of an impacted mandibular third molar. Oral Maxillofac Surg. 2016;20(2):149–56.
74. Huang CK, Lui MT, Cheng DH. Use of panoramic radiography to predict postsurgical sensory impairment following extraction of impacted mandibular third molars. J Chin Med Assoc. 2015;78(10):617–22.
75. Pathak S, Mishra N, Rastogi MK, Sharma S. Significance of radiological variables studied on orthopantomogram to predict

post-operative inferior alveolar nerve paresthesia after third molar extraction. J Clin Diagn Res. 2014;8(5):ZC624.
76. Ueda M, Nakamori K, Shiratori K, Igarashi T, Sasaki T, Anbo N, et al. Clinical significance of computed tomographic assessment and anatomic features of the inferior alveolar canal as risk factors for injury of the inferior alveolar nerve at third molar surgery. J Oral Maxillofac Surg: Official Journal of the American Association of Oral and Maxillofacial Surgeons. 2012;70(3):514–20.
77. Shiratori K, Nakamori K, Ueda M, Sonoda T, Dehari H. Assessment of the shape of the inferior alveolar canal as a marker for increased risk of injury to the inferior alveolar nerve at third molar surgery: a prospective study. J Oral Maxillofac Surg: Official Journal of the American Association of Oral and Maxillofacial Surgeons. 2013;71(12):2012–9.
78. Ye Z, Yang C, Abdelrehem A. Prediction of inferior alveolar nerve injury in complicated mandibular wisdom teeth extractions: a new classification system. Int J Clin Exp Med. 2016;9(2):3729–34.
79. Kim HG, Lee JH. Analysis and evaluation of relative positions of mandibular third molar and mandibular canal impacts. J Korean Assoc Oral Maxillofac Surg. 2014;40(6):278–84.
80. Costantinides F, Biasotto M, Maglione M, Di Lenarda R. Local vs general anaesthesia in the development of neurosensory disturbances after mandibular third molars extraction: a retrospective study of 534 cases. Med Oral Patol Oral Cir Bucal. 2016;21(6):e724–30.
81. Xu GZ, Yang C, Fan XD, Yu CQ, Cai XY, Wang Y, et al. Anatomic relationship between impacted third mandibular molar and the mandibular canal as the risk factor of inferior alveolar nerve injury. Br J Oral Maxillofac Surg. 2013;51(8):e215–9.
82. Mavrodi A, Ohanyan A, Kechagias N, Tsekos A, Vahtsevanos K. Influence of two different surgical techniques on the difficulty of impacted lower third molar extraction and their post-operative complications. Med Oral Patol Oral Cir Bucal. 2015;20(5):e640–4.
83. Charan Babu HS, Reddy PB, Pattathan RK, Desai R, Shubha AB. Factors influencing lingual nerve paraesthesia following third molar surgery: a prospective clinical study. J Maxillofac Oral Surg. 2013;12(2):168–72.
84. Osunde O, Saheeb B, Bassey G. Indications and risk factors for complications of lower third molar surgery in a Nigerian teaching hospital. Ann Med Health Sci Res. 2014;4(6):938–42.
85. Yadav S, Verma A, Sachdeva A. Assessment of lingual nerve injury using different surgical variables for mandibular third molar surgery: a clinical study. Int J Oral Maxillofac Surg. 2014;43(7):889–93.
86. Shad S, Shah SM, Alamgir AMM. Frequency of lingual nerve injury in mandibular third molar extraction: a comparison of two surgical techniques. J Ayub Med Coll Abbottabad. 2015;27(3):580–3.
87. Agrawal A, Yadav A, Chandel S, Singh N, Singhal A. Wisdom tooth complications in extraction. J Contemp Dent Pract. 2014;15(1):34–6.
88. Bataineh AB, Batarseh RA. The effect of modified surgical flap design for removal of lower third molars on lingual nerve injury. Clin Oral Investig. 2016;21(6):2091–9.
89. Ge J, Yang C, Zheng J, Qian W. Piezosurgery for the lingual split technique in lingual positioned impacted mandibular third molar removal: A retros pective study. Medicine. 2016;95(12):e3192.
90. Blackburn CW, Bramley PA. Lingual nerve damage associated with the removal of lower third molars. Br Dent J. 1989 Aug 5;167(3):103–7.
91. Pippi R, Spota A, Santoro M. Prevention of lingual nerve injury in third molar surgery: literature review. J Oral Maxillofac Surg. 2017 May;75(5):890–900.
92. Leung YY, Cheung LK. Long-term morbidities of coronectomy on lower third molar. Oral Surg Oral Med Oral Pathol Oral Radiol. 2016;121(1):5–11.
93. Agbaje JO, Heijsters G, Salem AS, Van Slycke S, Schepers S, Politis C, et al. Coronectomy of deeply impacted lower third molar: incidence of outcomes and complications after one year follow-up. J Oral Maxillofac Res. 2015;6(2):e1.
94. Monaco G, De Santis G, Pulpito G, Gatto MR, Vignudelli E, Marchetti C. What are the types and frequencies of complications associated with mandibular third molar coronectomy? A follow-up study. J Oral Maxillofac Surg: Official Journal of the American Association of Oral and Maxillofacial Surgeons. 2015;73(7):1246–53.
95. Frenkel B, Givol N, Shoshani Y. Coronectomy of the mandibular third molar: a retrospective study of 185 procedures and the decision to repeat the coronectomy in cases of failure. J Oral Maxillofac Surg: Official Journal of the American Association of Oral and Maxillofacial Surgeons. 2015;73(4):587594.
96. Wang Y, He D, Yang C, Wang B, Qian W. An easy way to apply orthodontic extraction for impacted lower third molar compressing to the inferior alveolar nerve. J Cranio-Maxillo-Fac Surg: Official Publication of the European Association for Cranio-Maxillo-Facial Surgery. 2012;40(3):234–7.
97. Long H, Zhou Y, Liao L, Pyakurel U, Wang Y, Lai W. Coronectomy vs. Total removal for third molar extraction: a systematic review. J Dent Res. 2012;91(7):659–65.
98. Renton T. Oral surgery: part 4. Minimising and managing nerve injuries and other complications. Br Dent J. 2013 Oct;215(8):393–9.
99. Ziccardi VB, Zuniga JR. Nerve injuries after third molar removal. Oral Maxillofac Surg Clin North Am. 2007 Feb;19(1):105–15, vii. Review.
100. Kehlet H, Jensen TS, Woolf CJ. Persistent postsurgical pain: risk factors and prevention. Lancet. 2006;367(9522):1618–25. https://doi.org/10.1016/s0140-6736(06)68700-x.
101. Greenstein G, Carpentieri JR, Cavallaro J. Nerve damage related to implant dentistry: incidence, diagnosis, and management. Compend Contin Educ Dent 2015 Oct;36(9):652–659. quiz 660.
102. Juodzbalys G, Wang HL, Sabalys G, Sidlauskas A, Galindo-Moreno P. Inferior alveolar nerve injury associated with implant surgery. Clin Oral Implants Res. 2013;24(2):183–90. https://doi.org/10.1111/j.1600-0501.2011.02314.x.
103. Bede SY, Ismael WK, Al-Assaf DA, Omer SS. Inferior alveolar nerve injuries associated with mandibular fractures. J Craniofac Surg. 2012;23(6):1776–8. https://doi.org/10.1097/SCS.0b013e318266fda3.
104. Iannetti G, Fadda TM, Riccardi E, Mitro V, Filiaci F. Our experience in complications of orthognathic surgery: a retrospective study on 3236 patients. Eur Rev Med Pharmacol Sci. 2013;17(3):379–84.
105. Kushnerev E, Yates JM. Evidence-based outcomes following inferior alveolar and lingual nerve injury and repair: a systematic review. J Oral Rehabil 2015 Oct;42(10):786–802. https://doi.org/10.1111/joor.12313. Epub 2015 Jun 7.
106. Coulthard P, Kushnerev E, Yates JM, Walsh T, Patel N, Bailey E, Renton TF. Interventions for iatrogenic inferior alveolar and lingual nerve injury. Cochrane Database Syst Rev. 2014 Apr 16;4:CD005293.
107. Susarla SM, Kaban LB, Donoff RB, Dodson TB. Does early repair of lingual nerve injuries improve functional sensory recovery? J Oral Maxillofac Surg. 2007;65(6):1070–6. https://doi.org/10.1016/j.joms.2006.10.010.
108. Ziccardi VB, Steinberg MJ. Timing of trigeminal nerve microsurgery: a review of the literature. J Oral Maxillofac Surg. 2007 Jul;65(7):1341–5.
109. Zuniga JR. Sensory outcomes after reconstruction of lingual and inferior alveolar nerve discontinuities using processed nerve allograft--a case series. J Oral Maxillofac Surg 2015

Apr;73(4):734–744. https://doi.org/10.1016/j.joms.2014.10.030. Epub 2014 Nov 13.
110. Bagheri SC, Meyer RA, Khan HA, Kubmichel A, Steed MB. Retrospective review of microsurgical repair of 222 lingual nerve injuries. J Oral Maxillofac Surg. 2010;68:715–23.
111. Strauss ER, Ziccardi VB, Janal MN. Outcome assessment of inferior alveolar nerve microsurgery: a retrospective review. J Oral Maxillofac Surg. 2006;64(12):1767–70. https://doi.org/10.1016/j.joms.2005.11.111.
112. Salomon D, Miloro M, Kolokythas A. Outcomes of immediate allograft reconstruction of Long-span defects of the inferior alveolar nerve. J Oral Maxillofac Surg 2016 Dec;74(12):2507–2514. https://doi.org/10.1016/j.joms.2016.05.029. Epub 2016 Jun 14.
113. Yampolsky A, Ziccardi V, Chuang SK. Efficacy of Acellular nerve allografts in trigeminal nerve reconstruction. J Oral Maxillofac Surg. 2017 Oct;75(10):2230–4.
114. Zuniga JR, Yates DM, Phillips CL. The presence of neuropathic pain predicts postoperative neuropathic pain following trigeminal nerve repair. J Oral Maxillofac Surg 2014 Dec;72(12):2422–2427. https://doi.org/10.1016/j.joms.2014.08.003. Epub 2014 Aug 11. PMID:25308410.
115. Zuniga JR, Renton T. Managing post-traumatic trigeminal neuropathic pain: is surgery enough? J Neurol Neuromed. 2016;1(7):10–4.
116. Rosén A, Tardast A, Shi TJ. How far have we come in the field of nerve regeneration after trigeminal nerve injury? Curr Oral Health Rep. 2016;3(4):309–13.
117. Zuniga JR, Mistry C, Tikhonov I, Dessouky R, Chhabra A. Magnetic resonance Neurography of traumatic and nontraumatic peripheral TrigeminalNeuropathies. J Oral Maxillofac Surg 2018 Apr;76(4):725–736. https://doi.org/10.1016/j.joms.2017.11.007. Epub 2017 Nov 16.
118. Chhabra A, Madhuranthakam AJ, Andreisek G. Magnetic resonance neurography: current perspectives and literature review. Eur Radiol 2018 Feb;28(2):698–707. https://doi.org/10.1007/s00330-017-4976-8. Epub 2017 Jul 14.

# Trigeminal Neuralgia

# 26

Kandasamy Ganesan and Asha Thomson

## 26.1 Introduction

Neuralgia can be defined as paroxysmal, intense intermittent pain that is usually confined to specific nerve branches of the head and neck. The trigeminal nerve is responsible for sensory innervation of the scalp, face and mouth, and damage or disease to this nerve may result in sensory loss and/or pain. Trigeminal Neuralgia (TN), also referred to as 'Tic Douloureux,' is sought to be the most intense and well-known neuralgias, which displays classical features of intense sharp, stabbing sensations with or without burning pain throughout the face. It is considered as one of the most chronic painful conditions known within the body. The pain, which is often initiated by just a light touch to an area of skin, can occur at any time without warning and depending on the severity of the condition, the frequency of the attacks can vary.

This severe medical condition affects one or more branches of the fifth cranial nerve known as the trigeminal nerve, which is the largest cranial nerve and has both sensory and motor functions. >85% of cases of trigeminal neuralgia are of the classic type known as classical trigeminal neuralgia (CTN), while the remaining cases can be separated to secondary trigeminal neuralgia (STN). STN is thought to be initiated by multiple sclerosis or a space-occupying lesion affecting the trigeminal nerve, whereas the leading cause of CTN is known to be compression of the trigeminal nerve in the region of the dorsal root entry zone by a blood vessel.

Investigation of the cause of the neuralgia present and treatment planning of these symptoms can pose a challenge for any clinician and the importance of detailed assessment and history taking of orofacial pain should be highlighted. Extreme care must be taken to identify the underlying cause of the symptoms experienced by the patient, who may often present in distress, as suffering from head and neck neuralgia can severely affect a patient's quality of life.

There is no guaranteed cure for the condition of trigeminal neuralgia, but there are several treatment options that may give symptomatic relief. In this chapter, we will review the common neuralgias occurring within the oral and maxillofacial region with specific emphasis on trigeminal neuralgia. We will discuss the historical evolution of treatment including the medical and surgical modalities with the use of current literature and newer developments. This highlights the need for further studies and investigation into the phenomenon of neuralgia to improve patient management and treatment outcomes.

This chapter will also cover surgical interventions such as, peripheral neurectomies, which can be done by an Oral and Maxillofacial Surgeon.

## 26.2 Anatomy of the Trigeminal Nerve

This is the largest cranial nerve with both sensory and motor components. It provides sensory nerve supply to the face, the scalp, the nasal cavity and the oral cavity including the teeth. It carries proprioception from the periodontal ligaments of the teeth and masticatory muscles. The trigeminal nerve provides motor supply to the muscles of mastication, tensor tympani, tensor veli palatini, mylohyoid and anterior belly of digastric. Its name is derived from its three main

**Electronic Supplementary Material** The online version of this chapter (https://doi.org/10.1007/978-981-15-1346-6_26) contains supplementary material, which is available to authorized users.

K. Ganesan (✉)
Department of Oral and Maxillofacial Surgery, Southend University Hospitals NHS Trust, Southend-on-Sea, UK

University of Leeds, Leeds, UK
e-mail: mailme@kandyganesan.com

A. Thomson (✉)
Norfolk and Norwich University Hospitals, Norfolk, UK
e-mail: ashathomson1@nhs.net


K. Bonanthaya et al. (eds.), *Oral and Maxillofacial Surgery for the Clinician*, https://doi.org/10.1007/978-981-15-1346-6_26

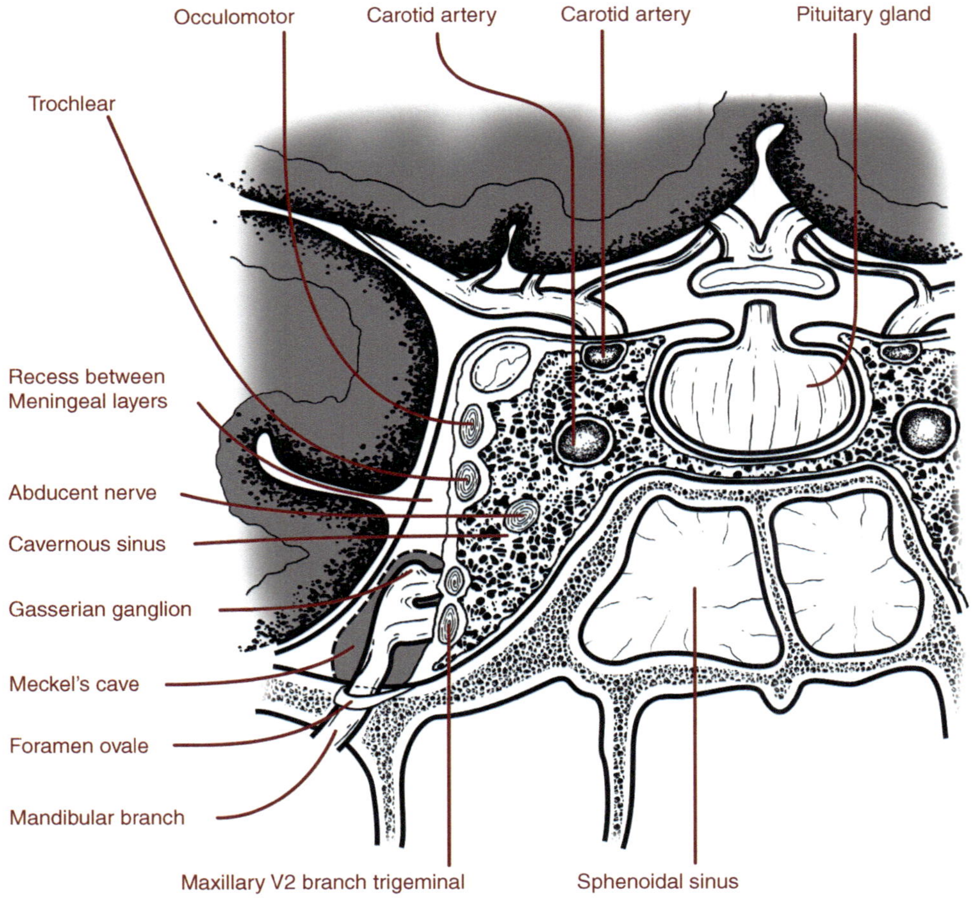


**Fig. 26.1** Schematic diagram showing the Meckel's cave within the dura layer lateral to cavernous sinus

branches ophthalmic, maxillary and mandibular. This nerve can be divided into various anatomical segments by its course from the brain stem, cisternal, Meckel's cave, ganglionic and finally to peripheral divisions (Ophthalmic, maxillary and mandibular). For trigeminal neuralgia, understanding of the anatomy of cisternal and Meckel's cave segments is important.

The trigeminal ganglion is located in the Meckel's cave, which is a recess between the two layers of the dura in the posteromedial portion of the middle cranial fossa. Any disease process in and around the Meckel's cave can develop the symptoms of trigeminal neuralgia. The anatomy of the Meckel's cave is detailed through the use of Fig. 26.1.

Arachnoid membrane from the posterior cranial fossa extends into the Meckel's cave and continues along the rootlets of the trigeminal nerve to as far as the trigeminal ganglion [1].

### 26.2.1 Peripheral Distribution of Trigeminal Nerve (Fig. 26.2 and Table 26.1)

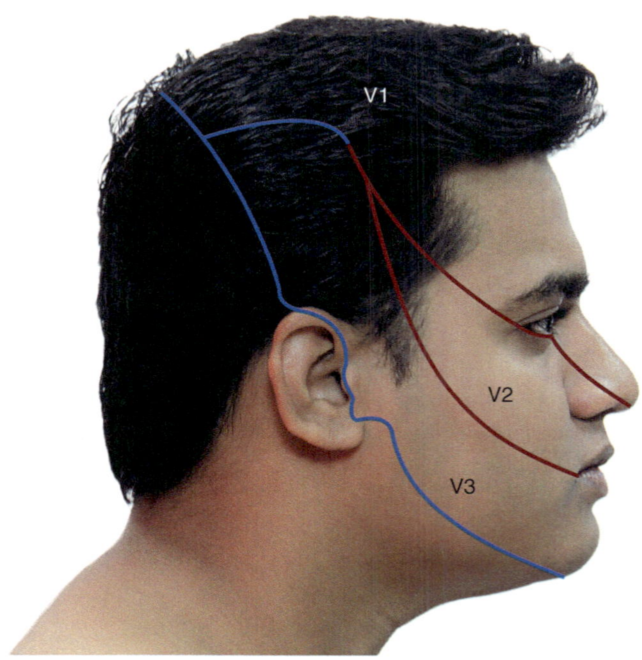


**Fig. 26.2** Diagram showing peripheral distribution of trigeminal nerve

Table 26.1 Branches of the 3 divisions of the trigeminal nerve

| Nerve | Branches |
|---|---|
| *V1—Opthalmic* | |
| 1. Frontal nerve | a. Supraorbital nerve<br>b. Supratrochlear nerve |
| 2. Lacrimal nerve | |
| 3. Nasociliary nerve | a. Long Ciliary nerve<br>b. Anterior and Posterior Ethmoidal nerves<br>c. Infratrochlear nerve |
| *V2—Maxillary* | |
| 1. Meningeal Branches | |
| 2. Ganglionic Branches | a. Greater Palatine nerve<br>b. Lesser Palatine nerve<br>c. Nasopalatine nerve<br>d. Nasal Branches |
| 3. Posterior Superioer Alveolar nerve | |
| 4. Infraorbital nerve | a. Anterior Superior Alveolar nerve<br>b. Middle Superior Alveolar nerve |
| 5. Zygomatic nerve | a. Zygomaticofacial nerve<br>b. Zygomaticotemporal nerve |
| *V3—Mandibular* | |
| 1. Nervous Spinosus | |
| 2. Motor Branches | |
| 3. Anterior Division | a. Nerve to Lateral Pterygoid<br>b. Masseteric nerve<br>c. Deep Temporal nerve<br>d. Buccal nerve |
| 4. Posterior Division | a. Auriculotemporal nerve<br>b. Lingual nerve<br>c. Inferior Alveolar nerve<br>i. Nerve to Mylohyoid<br>ii. Mental nerve |

## 26.3 Aetiology of Trigeminal Neuralgia

### 26.3.1 Neurovascular Compression

Myelin sheath surrounds the cranial nerves formed by oligodendrocytes in the central nervous system and Schwann cells in the peripheral nervous system. The main function of the myelin sheath is to provide mechanical insulation and metabolic support for the axons. This myelin sheath at the transition zone (TZ), between the central and peripheral nervous systems is a vulnerable area in the context of neurovascular compressions. The TZ is more relevant and not always located in the same position as root entry zone (REZ) [2].

Neurovascular compression at the REZ is found to be a reason for 80% of the TN but not a consistent finding in all the TN patients. This neurovascular contact at the REZ is also found in non-TN patients. A superior cerebellar artery alone or in association with another vessel is found in 88% as a source for vascular compression. Other vessels such as anterior cerebellar artery, the basilar artery and vertebral artery are also found to be in contact with RTZ [3].

### 26.3.2 Multiple Sclerosis (MS)

In 1950, the first finding of a connection with multiple sclerosis is reported [4]. A comprehensive review of pain in MS patients identified the prevalence to be TN to be 3.8%, which is lower than headaches (43%) and neuropathic extremity pain (26%) [5].

From this review, TN was the first symptom of MS in 9–14% of patients and the mean age of onset ranged from 33 to 51, highlighting younger patients than patients with TN alone. In addition to this, TN due to MS is often associated with numbness and paraesthesia [6]. Neuralgic pain, over a period of time, evolves with atypical features and involves an increase in the number of divisions of trigeminal distribution. Additionally, 6% became bilateral and literature shows MS precedes TN, however several studies showed TN as a first symptom before any other MS symptom [7, 8].

Electrophysiologic testing of MS-related TN patients showed up to 89% abnormal trigeminal reflexes such as the blink reflex compared to 3% in idiopathic TN patients. In MS, plaques result in neural damage causing TN but not as a result of neurovascular compression however, both can play a role in the aetiology of TN [9].

In MS, ephaptic nerve conduction is effected due to an increase in inflammatory activity in the plaques with a high T-cell activity [10].

### 26.3.3 Tumour and Cyst

Tumours alone are shown to be aetiology in TN from 0.8 to 11.6%, but this increased to 5.7 to 13.4% when aneurysms, angiomas or vascular malformations are present. Tumours may cause TN by compression, wrapping around the nerve root, neurovascular compression and/or neoplastic factor-related chemical irritation [6].

### 26.3.4 Diabetes Mellitus

The involvement of diabetic neuropathy is more common in the 3rd, 4th and 6th cranial nerves than in the trigeminal nerve. Diabetic patients tend to have more of a neuropathic pain than neuralgic pain, which may present as hot, burning, electric with a pins and needles sensation, especially in the peripheral areas such as the hands and legs. Often, this tends to be bilateral, and may present worse at night [11].

Hyperglycaemia is known to cause aggravated nerve damage, and this also applies for the increased risk of developing TN however, more studies need to be done in order to validate the underlying pathophysiology between the association of diabetes and TN [12].

### 26.3.5 Herpes Simplex

Post-herpetic TN after herpes zoster-shingles has been documented [13] and can present as a burning persistent severe pain for the patients. The reactivation of the latent herpes zoster virus from the dorsal root ganglion results in TN affecting the ophthalmic branch in over 80% of cases. When antivirals are administered within 72 h from the onset of the rash, they are known to reduce the duration of the rash, pain and also the incidence of post-herpetic neuralgia [14–17].

## 26.4 Pathophysiology of TN

The exact aetiopathogenesis of TN remains unclear. The most common hypothesis is the "ignition theory," which is a result of abnormalities in the afferent neurones of the trigeminal root or ganglion. Injury to the axons can make them hyperexcitable and also cause central sensitisation, leading to TN [18].

Demyelination at the trigeminal REZ where central and peripheral myelin meets results in generation of ectopic impulses. This in turn can cause cross-talk between touch and pain sensations which is thought to decrease the central pain gating mechanisms. Which, can conversely result in trigeminal nerve remyelination. This may explain the spontaneous remission in some patients; however, the same cannot be applied for rapid electrophysiologic recovery and pain relief after microvascular decompression treatment [6].

The affected (demyelinated) nerves can spontaneously discharge electric impulses. Touch sensation carrying A-β fibres aligned near the pain carrying (nociceptive pathway) A-δ and C fibres in the REZ, leading to ephaptic cross-talk between the two pathways. This may explain how trivial touch sensation triggers pain in TN [18].

The trigeminal ganglion itself can show pathological changes such as hypermyelination [19, 20]. Demyelination is common in many patients with TN and is caused by a compression by vascular structures, MS, tumours and vascular malformations.

Compression on the REZ should cause a continuous pain, but TN patients suffer paroxysmal attacks, which are most likely to be caused by spontaneous discharges where the threshold for the repetitive firing has been altered. It is also notable in TN that such firing occurs not only spontaneously but also by trivial tactile stimuli. This type of firing behaviour is also observed within in dorsal root ganglions [20].

Rappaport and Devor [21] explained that the development of atypical features of the TN may be due to central sensitization following a prolonged barrage of nerve impulses and also from progressive damage to trigeminal afferents, which become the source of continuous ectopic discharges [20].

Interestingly, literature shows that different treatments of TN yield similar results in pain control however, the long-term results show that decompression provides prolonged pain relief compared to destructive peripheral procedures [20]. In addition, destructive procedures may cause some degree of sensory loss along with the same duration of pain relief [22].

## 26.5 Historical Perspective

Historically, reviews dating back to 2 AD demonstrates the existence of TN or a similar condition described by Aretaeus of Cappadocia, a contemporary of Galen. The same author is known for the description of migraine, and in the 11th century [23], an Arab physician Jujani describes a unilateral facial pain causing spasms and anxiety. He explains that the cause of the pain is 'proximity of the artery to the nerve' [24].

Wells Cathedral, an Anglican cathedral in Wells, Somerset, England, dedicated to St Andrew the Apostle, contains the tomb of Bishop Button, who died in 1274. He was canonized, and many pilgrims and toothache sufferers left offerings at the tomb, in commemoration of which the capitals of the pillars bear carvings of people depicted with facial neuralgia. One is famed as the toothache figure and because of the surprising rarity of dental caries at that time (confirmed when the sarcophagus was opened in 1848), Wilfred Harris pointed out the probable relevance to trigeminal neuralgia [25].

A first Royal account in relation to TN is by John Locke, the famous philosopher and physician who wrote a series of letters to Dr John Mapletoft in 1677 [26] describing TN suffered by Countess of Northumberland, wife of Ambassador to France.

Nicolas Andre invented the term *tic douloureux* in 1756 in a book, Observations pratiques sur les maladies de l'urethre et surplusiers faits convulsifs [27].

*John Fothergill* publishes the first account of TN to the Medical Society in London in 1773 and described TN as a 'paroxysmal unilateral facial pain, evoked by eating, speaking or touching, starting and ending abruptly, and associated the condition with anxiety [23].

Between the eighteenth and nineteenth centuries, Pujol, Chapman and Tiffany completed the clinical picture and differentiated TN from other facial pain conditions. Later, Oppenheim highlighted the association between TN and MS [28].

Treatment of TN including microvascular decompression has been available since 1925 [29]; however, it took another 50 years to become an accepted neurosurgical intervention. During 1950 to 60, Gardner and Miklos [30] promoted neurovascular decompression theory and continued to modify the technique, but a major shift in this practice happened after a large clinical series published by Jannetta [31]. Throughout the last century, ablative neurosurgical procedures continued to evolve to balance the best possible outcome between pain control and adverse effects. The latest in this process is radiosurgery. And even although surgical practice was continuing to evolve, medical therapy had little success in the same period. In 1942, Bergouignan's discovery of phenytoin was the first medical intervention in effective control of pain paroxysms [32]. In 1953, Walter Schindler discovered Carbamazepine and marketing was started in 1962. Although it was originally used for epilepsy, trials showed their effectiveness in TN pain control.

## 26.6 Clinical Presentation

Within the maxillofacial region, neuralgias can present in different severities and can affect patients from any race, gender and age. Certain conditions may be distinctive to certain groups of people, but there is no current classification followed for the diagnosis and management of neuralgic pain; however, groups do exist in order to distinguish the categories that they may be separated into.

These pain episodes experienced may last from seconds up to several minutes and can be described by the patient as an 'electric shock' feeling. This sensation may occur frequently per day (up to hundreds of times) over weeks and months and then suddenly stop with pain-free periods in between. It may also present infrequently with periods of remission, which may possibly last for years [13]. The pain often occurs unilaterally, does not usually cross the midline of the face and is often unbearable for the patient. It has been shown that only 3% of cases are known to be bilateral in nature [13].

### 26.6.1 Risk Factors

**Sex**
It has been highlighted that TN affects females more than males [13].

**Age**
In patients over 80 years old, males tend to have a higher incidence (45/100,000) [13, 33–36].

It can be prominent within all age ranges, but most frequently, TN affects individuals over the age of 50. Approximately 70% of the patients develop TN after they reach 60 years of age and it is known that the incidence of TN increases with age, and has been emphasised that this condition is rare to affect people younger than 40 years old [36, 37]. This is therefore highly important in suggesting that multiple sclerosis may be present in younger patients who suffer from TN [38].

#### 26.6.1.1 Initiating Factors

The pain felt can be precipitated by trigger areas or factors of light touch on specific areas of the face, and patients often avoid these actions, which they may feel causes the attacks.

These activities may include:

Shaving
Applying make-up or face cream
Brushing the teeth
Speaking
Smiling
Yawning
Face washing
Swallowing
Vibration
Exposure to cold such as cold wind, breeze on the face or air conditioning
Eating, chewing or biting into something
Touching or washing certain areas of the face

### 26.6.2 Prevalence

A systematic review highlighted that the range of TN prevalence was 0.03–0.3%, mostly women were affected, and the affected age range was 37–67 years old. The affliction was marked by unilateral symptoms, most commonly in the maxillary and mandibular branches [39].

NICE guideline data and studies [13] indicate that a survey carried out within general practice in the United Kingdom, which highlighted that the annual incidence of trigeminal neuralgia was 8 per 10,000.

The true prevalence of this condition remains unclear as there is little data to support the evidence of how common this condition is [13]. It is evident that even with studies carried out, further research is required to validate the prevalence of trigeminal neuralgia due to the complexity of the condition including diagnosis difficulties and heterogeneity of the disease characteristics [39].

### 26.6.3 Clinical Diagnosis

#### 26.6.3.1 Pain History

Accurate diagnosis relies greatly on a detailed history of symptoms from the patient, with pattern and nature of the pain highlighting the condition as there is no definitive diagnostic test yet available. SOCRATES is a useful assessment tool (Table 26.2), which is often used to help clinicians in achieving an accurate pain history.

**Table 26.2** SOCRATES assessment tool

| | |
|---|---|
| Site/localization | Can the pain be localized to a specific area? |
| Onset | Sudden or gradual? when—day/night/ spontaneous? |
| Characteristic of pain | Sharp, stabbing and dull ache |
| Radiation | Does the pain radiate elsewhere? |
| Associated signs and symptoms | Any associated signs or symptoms? |
| Timing/duration | Seconds/minutes/hours? (constant, paroxysmal-recurrent and slowly/rapidly progressive) |
| Exacerbating or relieving factors | Does anything make it better/worse? |
| Severity | How intense is the pain? Scale 1–10 |

Trigeminal neuralgia may be misdiagnosed for dental pathology, and so it is important that unnecessary dental treatment is not carried out without full investigation of the source of the pain. When patients suffer from the condition, it often becomes apparent that their quality of life decreases as they may be unable to carry out their normal daily activities and suffer from weight loss due to problems in eating, and as a result the condition may lead to depression and/or isolation.

On clinical examination, trigeminal reflex testing may be used to test all three divisions of the nerve and may reveal loss of sensitivity in the cutaneous region, which may be related to the affected nerve. This may present as partial numbness (hypoesthesia) or complete numbness (anaesthesia) and occasionally may present as hyperaesthesia causing considerable discomfort.

*The classical symptoms of trigeminal neuralgia are as follows:*

- Severe shooting or stabbing pain, which may feel like an 'electric shock' on a focussed part or wider area of the face.
- Pain usually only affects one side of the face at one time.
- Bouts of pain may last from a few seconds to several minutes.
- Spontaneous attacks of pain may occur with or without triggers.
- As time progresses, the painful attacks may increase in frequency and intensity.

#### 26.6.3.2 Other Causes

Trigeminal neuralgia can occur as a result of several causes such as trauma, tumours, infectious or demyelinating diseases, connective tissue diseases and can also be idiopathic in nature. This poses a challenge to the clinician when trying to investigate the cause of the pain. The importance of the causative factors may highlight the possibility that trigeminal neuralgia can present as the first manifestation of an underlying systemic disease. This emphasises that careful and in-depth investigations with detailed history taking are required in order to appropriately treat this life-affecting condition. A referral to a specialist in pain management or neurologist should be considered in severe cases [13, 38].

As trigeminal neuralgia is uspected when a patient has severe and intense pain in the orofacial region, other reasons may need to be explored for patients who have physical signs of motor or sensory problems. Neoplasms, infective conditions such as HIV, multiple sclerosis and even cerebrovascular disease may cause neuralgic pain, and so it is important to be aware of the differential diagnosis that could be derived from neuralgia within the head and neck.

TN is restricted to one or more branches of the trigeminal nerve distribution with an exception of TN in MS patients, where one side of the face may be affected. It is sudden in onset and typically lasts for a few seconds to a maximum of 2 min. Pain can be spontaneous but can also be triggered by innocuous mechanical stimuli or facial movements. In between the episodes, patients can remain pain-free and very rarely, patients suffer continuous pain in TN.

### 26.6.4 Glossopharyngeal Neuralgia

Glossopharyngeal neuralgia (GPN) is a rare uncommon painful neuralgic condition involving pharyngeal/orofacial region including the ear, base of the tongue, tonsillar fossa and submandibular region. It has similar etiopathogenesis to TN with neurovascular compression and demyelination of the 9th or the 10th cranial nerves. The prevalence rate is 0.2–0.7 per 100,000 and accounts for 0.2–1.3% of the orofacial neuralgias [40].

Clinical history taking is important to differentiate different types of neuralgias. GPN clinically presents as a unilateral, severe and paroxysmal pain involving the ear, base of the tongue, tonsillar fossa and submandibular region. Painful symptoms are described very similar to TN symptoms such as, sharp, stabbing or electric shock like pain. Similar to TN, GPN is triggered by innocuous stimuli/function like swallowing, chewing, talking, coughing and yawning.

According to the criteria put forward by the International Classification of headache disorders (ICHD) [41]:

- TN pain should be unilateral with at least three attacks
- Occurring in one or more divisions of the trigeminal nerve, with no radiation beyond the trigeminal distribution.
- Pain should have at least three of the following characteristics
  - recurring in paroxysmal attacks lasting from a fraction of a second to 2 min
  - severe intensity
  - electric shock-like, shooting, stabbing or sharp in quality
  - precipitated by innocuous stimuli to the affected side of the face
- There should be no clinically evident neurological deficit

The International Association for the Study of Pain (IASP) current classification

| | |
|---|---|
| Classical TN | Caused by vascular compression of the trigeminal nerve root, resulting in morphological changes of the root |
| Secondary TN | Caused by major neurological disease, e.g. a tumour of the cerebellopontine angle (TN attributed to space-occupying lesions) or MS |
| Idiopathic TN | No apparent cause |

The readers may access the detailed classification at the following open access publication [42]. https://doi.org/10.1007/s40265-018-0964-9.

## 26.7 Investigations

A thorough pain history and a clinical examination including cranial nerve examinations are important for the diagnosis of TN due to the fact that MS and tumours may be found in this cohort. Any deficiency in the cranial nerve examination, especially a sensory loss, should prompt further imaging.

In order to rule out possible diseases, specific tests may be carried out in adjunct by radiographic examinations such as plain radiographs including intra-oral (periapicals) and orthopantograms. These may be carried out in the first instance to rule out dental pathology, and orthopantograms may also be able to detect temporomandibular joint pathology. Cranial computed tomography scan (CT) may also be used in order to identify any changes of the maxillary sinus.

Magnetic resonance imaging (MRI) is an important investigation to investigate and to differentiate between patients suffering from trigeminal neuralgia due to tumours and MS [18]. It may demonstrate the close and potentially causative relationship between the trigeminal root and adjacent blood vessel and can be of specific value to exclude posterior cranial fossa lesions [38]. TN caused by MS should be ruled out, specifically in the younger patient, and this may be aided by MRI. Clinical Knowledge Summaries (CKS). NICE [13] guidelines recommend MRI assessment specifically for younger people, patients presenting atypical symptoms, non-responders to initial therapy or anyone for whom neurosurgery is being considered. Even though MRI is commonly used, from previous studies carried out, the suggestion of its sensitivity and specificity seems to be variable [43–50]. As a result, emphasis is placed on the challenge in identifying the cause of trigeminal neuralgia as a relationship between the clinical symptoms and radiological findings as this may not be clear.

In idiopathic forms of trigeminal neuralgia, it is typical for no cause to be detected with the patient having both normal neurological and MRI examinations, which can cause difficulty with treatment planning. MRI finding of an aberrant loop of a blood vessel at RTZ is the most common cause, and this is reported in about 60–90% of the cases described in neurosurgical/neuroradiological series [51–54].

Meaney et al. have designed a set of specific parameters to visualise the blood vessels using thin slices to create the reconstruction of nerve and vessel in any orientation. This is called magnetic resonance tomographic angiography (MRTA) [55]. This reconstruction between the vessels and the nerves allowed us to identify the neurovascular compression. In comparison to MRTA, MR angiography only provides image of the blood vessels. Meaney et al. then validated their findings by comparing the MRTA findings with surgical findings. In a series of 52 consecutive cases, MRTA findings were comparable to surgical finding in 50 out of 52 cases. In four cases, MRTA misclassified veins as arteries; otherwise, MRTA is a sensitive and specific method in demonstrating neurovascular compression [44].

## 26.8 Management

### 26.8.1 Medical Management

It has been highlighted that first line of treatment for trigeminal neuralgia is still pharmacological treatment. The desired outcome of these patients is to treat the pain experienced, manage the symptoms and with time preferably, eradicate these symptoms in order to improve the patient's quality of life. Where appropriate, referral to a specialist pain service and/or neurologist may be necessary with clear information and given to the patient.

There are several drugs that have been delivered systemically or topically in the use of treating trigeminal neuralgia, which include:

Baclofen
Dextromethorphan
Lamotrigine
Gabapentin
Pregabalin
Sumatriptan
Levetiracetam
Eslicarbazepine
Pimozide
Proparacaine
Tizanidine
Tocainide
Topiramate

The most common therapy of choice is Carbamazepine for pain control [56] and after carrying out a systematic review of the literature, The American Academy of Neurology and the European Federation of Neurological Societies support Carbamazepine (200–1200 mg/day) [57] as the first-line treatment to be offered due to strong evidence supporting this pharmacological treatment. In addition to this, another drug of preferred choice is Oxcarbazepine (600–1800 mg/day) [57], which is known to have better tolerability and is also supported by existing guidelines [13, 58].

All the above drugs have been evaluated using RCTs, whereas other drugs such as capsaicin cream, phenytoin, clonazepam, gabapentin, oxcarbazepine, mexiletine and tramadol have been assessed from case reports and case series. Studies involving many of these drugs regarding the full benefit and effect on the treatment of trigeminal neuralgia are limited, and so further evaluation is required [59, 60]. The response to the drugs mentioned is unique to each patient, and it is evident that the doses also vary between patients in order to achieve a beneficial effect to counteract the symptoms experienced. It has been highlighted that it may be helpful for the patient to keep a pain diary in order to record episodes and help the patient and clinician identify possible trigger factors and timing of the pain. This may aid treatment planning and may give patients back a sense of control, which has been lost due to their condition.

#### 26.8.1.1 Carbamazepine and Oxcarbazepine

Based on existing evidence, carbamazepine also known with the trade name 'Tegretol' is an anti-convulsant drug used primarily in the treatment of epilepsy [61] and remains the drug of choice for standard first-line treatment of trigeminal neuralgia in patients over 18 years of age [13, 57, 58]. It is considered to be of diagnostic help if complete resolution or reduction of symptoms occurs after its use [38]; however, carbamazepine must be used prophylactically and continuously for long periods, with tiered dosages prescribed to suit individual patients in regard to their response. Carbamazepine should be used with caution, and as it not an analgesic, it is not appropriate to use this medication during a pain episode for relief as it will not have an analgesic effect on symptoms. Patients can often misinterpret what the purpose of the medication is, and so this in turn highlights the importance of patient communication. The mechanism of the medication, the instructions in terms of dosage titration, timing of effects and the possible adverse side effects associated with its use should be highlighted. From current guidelines such as—NICE [13], it has been advised that if no sinister or red flag symptoms are evident and carbamazepine is not contraindicated for the patient, then, the following dosage guideline can be offered:

- 100 mg up to twice daily, titrated in increments of 100–200 mg every 2 weeks until pain has been relieved
- 200 mg three of four times daily (600–800 mg daily) is seen in the majority of people to be the dosage of choice sufficient to manage pain
- 1600 mg maximum dose daily
- Once pain is in remission, the dosage should be gradually reduced to the lowest possible maintenance level or even discontinued until a further episode occurs.

Frequent side effects have been reported with the use of carbamazepine drug therapy with specific emphasis on elderly patients [61–63]. When patients are treated with carbamazepine, it is strongly advised that a full blood count and liver function tests are carried out prior to starting treatment and then reviewed periodically in order to monitor the possible effects of the drug. Hyponatraemia, which refers to low sodium levels, is thought to occur in 20% of patients, and NICE guidelines [13] suggests that carbamazepine in concurrent use with sertraline can also increase this risk. Serum levels of the drug are not routinely monitored unless carbamazepine toxicity is suspected but within the \ British National Formulary (BNF), all information is available in regard to drug interactions, adverse effects and contraindications and cautions. Within primary care settings, this is the standard first choice of treatment if the physician is confident with the diagnosis; otherwise, it is advised to refer the patient to a secondary care specialist for further investigations and treatment.

In several studies, the effectiveness of carbamazepine was demonstrated with specific outcomes found in the reduction of both intensity and frequency of the painful paroxysms [36, 57, 64–68]. In addition to this, the pharmacological drug of choice was found to be equally effective on the reduction of both trigger touch and spontaneous attacks [59, 66]. Due to the possible side effects from carbamazepine, oxcarbazepine may often be used as initial treatment due to the decreased potential drug interactions and possible greater tolerability acceptance [57, 63, 68].

#### 26.8.1.2 Gabapentin

It is known for its effective role in the management of neuropathic pain especially post-herpetic neuralgia, but there is a lack of evidence on its role in the management of TN. There is one randomized-controlled trial showing improvement in pain control with fewer side effects. This study compared the use of combination of both gabapentin and ropivacaine injected to trigger points and gabapentin alone [18].

#### 26.8.1.3 Baclofen

Baclofen is used to control the symptoms in MS, and therefore, it is generally accepted to use in TN patients with MS [59]. It may well control the symptoms without adding carbamazepine. Its side effects including sedation and loss of muscle tone and abrupt discontinuation may cause seizures and hallucinations.

#### 26.8.1.4 Lamotrigine

Lamotrigine is used when Carbamazepine is not tolerated well, or it is used in addition to carbamazepine when it is not effective on its own. There is not enough evidence to support the use of lamotrigine from studies carried out with relation to patients with TN [18].

#### 26.8.1.5 Evolving Medical Therapy

Due to the known difficulty in treating trigeminal neuralgia, new therapeutic modalities are being investigated and have been tried [57]. It has been evident from recent reviews [18] that the combination of the pharmacological drug gabapentin with the addition of regular ropivacaine injections into specific sites, which may be 'trigger sites,' has had a positive outcome on pain control with an improvement in quality of life.

Botulinum Toxin A (BTX-A) has also been suggested as an effective treatment of trigeminal neuralgia from a systematic review [69] carried out on patients suffering from this condition No major adverse events were reported, and it was concluded that with an approximate 60–80% reduction in mean pain intensity and frequency, this medical treatment may be a future recommendation. Cruccu and Truini [42] were in agreement with these findings who have also reviewed the literature on possible medical treatments for Trigeminal Neuralgia. It was highlighted that there is possible increasing evidence for BTX-A injections as a treatment option, specifically prior to considering surgical options or for patients who do not want surgery. In relation to this, it is emphasised that further evidence is needed with regard to this treatment option with more investigation and well-designed studies to take place.

Finally, it has been highlighted that local anaesthesia injected into the specific trigger area, 8% lidocaine spray and the use of intravenous infusion of fosphenytoin may be an option to provide temporary relief for patients suffering from severe pain [18].

### 26.8.2 Surgical Management

A successful surgical intervention of TN is determined by elimination of pain. Currently available surgical options are

1. Invasive technique:
   (a) Open:
      (i) Microvascular decompression
   (b) Percutaneous:
      (i) Radiofrequency rhizotomy
      (ii) Retrogasserian glycerol rhizotomy
      (iii) Balloon compression of trigeminal nerve
      (iv) Stereotactic radiosurgery—Gamma knife
2. Non-invasive technique:
   (i) Peripheral neurectomy
   (ii) Alcohol injections
   (iii) Cryotherapy
   (iv) Selective radiofrequency thermocoagulation

#### 26.8.2.1 Microvascular Decompression (MVD)

The original theory was outlined by Dandy in 1925, and vascular decompression of the trigeminal nerve was first described by Gardner and Miklos in 1959 [70] and was further refined by Jannetta et al. in 1967 [71]. Advances in anaesthesiology, use of operating microscopes and evolving surgical techniques allowed the MVD as a safer and effective procedure. MVD further evolved in the next 50 years to become accepted as one of the best surgical options.

Surgical target is the trigeminal nerve-pons junction. To reach this target, the posterior cranial fossa needs to be accessed via suboccipital craniotomy. On entering via craniotomy site, cerebrospinal fluid will be aspirated. Further advancing is done towards the nerve by gently retracting part of the cerebellum (Fig. 26.3). It is common to find a segment of superior cerebellar artery compressing on the REZ. Less

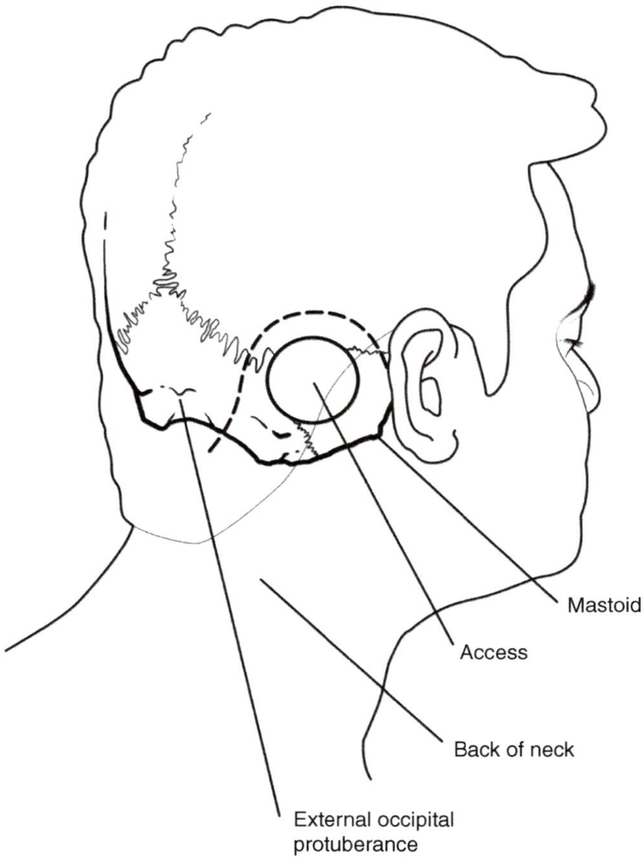




**Fig. 26.3** Diagram showing suboccipital access

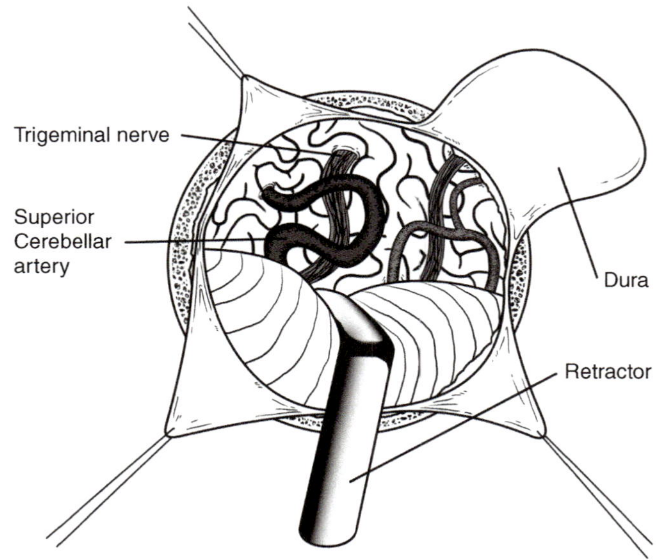




**Fig. 26.4** Craniotomy access showing a retracted and a cerebellar artery resting on the nerve. A piece of Teflon to be placed between the vessel and the nerve

commonly, a variation with an anterior inferior cerebellar artery or the superior petrosal vein can be found as a cause of the neurovascular compression [72]. Once the vessel is freed of the REZ, a piece of Teflon is placed to keep the nerve and the vessel apart (Fig. 26.4).

Utmost care should be taken to avoid any post-operative hearing loss. This is usually done by monitoring the brainstem evoked potential as hearing loss is due to the pressure on the eight cranial nerve due to retraction. A timely release of retraction improves this and literature recommends the removal of a section of the root when there is no vascular compression or there may be difficulties in mobilizing the artery. Deliberate Bruising of the nerve in addition to decompression is also recommended [73].

Literature shows that MVD can be done in any age group. Both Resnick et al. and Roski et al. concluded that MVD can be done with good outcomes in the paediatric population [74, 75]. It is also unique that in the paediatric population, venous compression is more common than arterial.

The long-term outcome of MVD for TN suggests 87–98% have immediate pain relief but this is reduced slightly to 75–80% in a 1–2 year review [76–82]. This proportion of patients with pain relief further reduced to 58–64% this is also associated with 4–12% of recurrence.

Several studies showed that the outcome of MVD is better with an arterial compression compared to venous [77, 79, 83]. Lee et al. showed a recurrence rate of 31% when there is TN due to venous compression and mostly recurred within the first 12 months [83]. Literature shows that there are poor outcomes on patients who have had previous neurosablative surgery, but this is not substantiated by other studies [76, 84, 85]. Review of literature in the management of recurrence following MVD in TN did not provide a general consensus but suggested re-exploration and neuroablative procedures [86–88]. A good quality imaging system may enable the surgeon to pinpoint the reason for the recurrence and choose an appropriate remedial surgical intervention.

In terms of the outcomes, complication rates seem to be minimal with an experienced neurosurgical team with innovations. Although a rate of 0.2–1% mortality is shown in the earlier literature, two large studies with a patient population of 444 [79] and 1995 [52] showed 0% mortality. A recent retrospective study listed other complications such as cerebellar injury (0.45%) 8th cranial nerve injury (0.8%) and CSF leak (1.85%) [52].

Although this study showed low complication rates, other centres reported higher complication rates [80, 81]. This wide range in the outcomes is likely due to the experience of the surgical team and their advanced perioperative monitoring systems.

Despite the increasing popularity of MVD, its advantage over the neuroablative procedures continues to be debated at various levels [22, 89]. In the absence of well-structured clinical studies, varying interventions will be preferred based on the individual centre experience.

#### 26.8.2.2 Gamma Knife Radiosurgery (GKRS)

In the 1950s, the term and the concept of radiosurgery and Gamma Knife were introduced by Lars Leksell. GKRS is used to treat various benign and malignant brain tumours and also various non-neoplastic conditions such as vascular malformations without an open intracranial surgical access. For the next few decades, GKRS is evolved with technology as the precision targeting has improved [90]. The 'Gamma Knife' technique was based on the fact that radiation may block the conduction of excessive sensory information responsible for triggering the pain episodes [91]. This would affect the radiosurgery targets with no significant change outside the target nerve, with the myelin sheath being primarily affected by radiosurgery [92]. It is indicated in typical or atypical TN, with or without vascular compression, failed MVD, TN patients in MS and patients with significant medical comorbidities.

This procedure [90–92] is done under local anaesthetic with or without sedation. Once the patient is supine under the collimator head, local anaesthetic is used to secure the stereotactic frame to the patient's head. MRI is then performed to locate the trigeminal nerve. Gamma knife is made up of 201 intercepting beams of gamma radiation with a dose of 70–100 Gy, and it is targeted at REZ of trigeminal nerve. Radiosurgery can be done with or without frame-based method, with MRI or computerized tomography (CT) planning when there is contraindication to MRI.

GKRS can also be given using one or two isocenters/target areas and targeting radiosurgery posteriorly at dorsal REZ or anteriorly in retrogasserian zone. Lower dosages to the root can be associated with fewer side effects, whereas higher dosages provide better pain control with less risk of recurrence but more side effects such as facial numbness. The benefits and risks of a higher dose must be carefully discussed with patients since bothersome facial numbness may be an acceptable option for patients with severe pain.

Two studies showed that approximately it takes a month for pain relief [91]. One of them is a multicentre study of 50 patients with a median follow-up of 18 months, which showed the results of 58% pain free and 36% had significant pain relief with a 6% failure rate.

However, when recurrence is evident after GKRS, repeat GKRS provides a similar rate of pain relief as the first procedure. The best responses are observed when there is good pain control after first procedure, with new sensory dysfunction and in single division nerve distribution typical TN.

#### 26.8.2.3 Percutaneous Balloon Compression (PBC)

PBC was described by Mullen in 1980 [93]. It relieves TN pain by injuring the large myelinated fibres involved in the sensory trigger. It is especially useful in managing TN with first division involvement as it selectively spares small myelinated fibres, which mediate the corneal/blink reflex. It gained its role in management of TN due to its low cost and simplicity.

The procedure is performed under a short general anaesthetic, with a fluoroscopic control. A 14-gauge cannula is inserted into foramen ovale but does not pass beyond. A negative cerebrospinal fluid confirms it further. A catheter advanced through the needle, and balloon inflated slowly up to a pressure of 1.3–1.6 atm. Balloon can also be inflated with 0.5–1.0 ml of contrast dye until it occupies Meckel's cave, and radiographic confirmation of its position is achieved. Up to 6 min of duration of compression is achieved. Typically, patients awaken with a mild subjective sensory loss with immediate pain relief up to 80–90% [94, 95]. This subjective numbness resolves in few weeks.

PBC is most helpful when pain involves multiple divisions including the first division, patients with MS, significant comorbidities and failed MVD.

#### 26.8.2.4 Radiofrequency Thermocoagulation (RFTC)

Failures and complications in failing to control the spread of alcohol in ganglionolysis led to thermocoagulation of the Gasserian ganglion. This procedure thermocoagulates the ganglion at temperatures above 65 °C, which selectively ablates the Aδ and C pain fibres [96, 97].

The procedure is carried out under a short-intermittent general anaesthesia either under fluoroscopic control or radiologically guided. Patients are awake for the part of the procedure to ensure correct positioning of the needle. The radiofrequency needle with a stylet is introduced through the foramen ovale into Meckel's cave using bony landmarks. Transient bradycardia may occur at this juncture. Once the needle position at the trigeminal rootlet is confirmed by fluoroscopy and radiographs, the stylet can be removed to introduce the electrocoagulation needle. The patient is awakened, and the stimulation of the nerve root can be tested. A mapping of the paraesthesia is carried out to the trigger zones of the neuralgia. Then, the patient is anaesthetized again for thermocoagulation, which is achieved with 0.2–1 V. The same procedure is repeated for 45–90s cycles at temperatures of 60–90 °C. After each episode of thermocoagulation, the patient is awakened and the sensory mapping is repeated again [19].

#### 26.8.2.5 Glycerol Rhizotomy

This procedure was a chance finding by Håkansson and colleagues whilst working on stereotactic gamma radiation for TN. They used glycerol mixed with tantalum dust as a radio-opaque marker to visualize the trigeminal cistern and discovered that it also abolished pain. They published the first series of 75 patients with a mean follow-up of 18 months [98].

This procedure is done under local anaesthesia with sedation. Similar to other percutaneous in the treatment of TN, the aim is to safely place the needle at the gasserian ganglion [99]. The advantage of being done awake allows the patient to sit up, and a small dose of sterile glycerol is injected in small increments. Up to a total of 0.1–0.4 ml can be used based on the number of divisions involved. Patients remain seated for up to 2 h to allow glycerol to reach the intended root.

This method is well tolerated with negligible mortality. Commonly reported complications are meningitis, cranial nerve palsies, local haematomas, reactivation of herpes labialis and permanent masseter weakness [100].

## 26.9 Peripheral Nerve Procedures

### 26.9.1 Infraorbital Neurectomy

Peripheral neurectomies are a safe and cost-effective option for patients with medical co-morbidities, elderly and for population where there is lack of highly skilled neurosurgical centres. Pain relief can be lasting from 15 to 24 months. Loss of sensation and recurrences are associated with peripheral neurectomy. These are carried out by oral and maxillofacial surgeons, and it is under reported to evaluate its benefits over central neurosurgical interventions.

Access to infraorbital nerve is gained through a maxillary vestibular approach. The infraorbital foramen is identified as it is exiting foramen and the nerve is released from the foramen by raising the periosteum around it. Care should be taken as to ensure that there is no 'pull' to trunk of the nerve from the infraorbital canal. Reeling of the nerve is also a common practice, but sectioning of the nerve is done to eliminate the touch sensation, and there is no need to remove the infraorbital canal portion of the nerve.

The nerve is then sectioned using diathermy to have a bloodless field and nerve branches on the soft tissue side may be closed over by releasing the surrounding periosteum to avoid regeneration. Similarly, infraorbital canal can be obturated with bone wax or chips of the bone carved around the canal.

Khanna and Galinde [101] published their successful experience of 118 patients with 75% pain relief at a 1–5 year follow-up.

Oturi et al. published their 7 years follow-up series comparing alcohol block, neurectomy and thermocoagulation. They have found that up to 78% had recurrence with the neurectomy cohort, and sadly, one of half of it recurred within a month. They reported the complications rate under 10% (dysesthesia and eye problems) on thermocoagulation and alcohol ganglionolysis patients [102].

### 26.9.2 Inferior Alveolar Nerve or Mental Nerve Neurectomy

Ali FM et al. [103] suggest peripheral neurectomy in a rural set-up where there is a lack of highly trained and equipped neurosurgical facilities. It is an effective option for elderly patients and who are reluctant for opting for neurosurgical intervention.

#### 26.9.2.1 Inferior Alveolar Neurectomy via Ginwala's Access [103] (Video 26.1)

This procedure is done under local anaesthesia, with access gained to the medial aspect of the ramus using an inverted Y-shaped incision. Once the incision is made, the mucoperiosteal flap is raised along the anterior aspect of the ramus. The tendon of the temporalis and the medial pterygoid muscle is raised off the bone for access to the lingula and once the inferior alveolar nerve is dissected free off the surrounding tissues, the neurovascular bundle is clamped and cut below the clamp by electrocoagulation to achieve haemostasis. Following this, a separate buccal sulcus incision is made to identify the mental foramen and the end of inferior vascular bundle is identified and dissected off the surrounding tissues. The bundle is then clamped and sectioned to avulse the neurovascular bundle from the canal.

Based on the available literature, there is a role for peripheral neurectomy in selective cases where other treatments have failed, and in patients with comorbidities and where there is reluctancy of either clinician or the patient to opt for neurosurgical procedures. However, it is difficult to conclude its role as a primary interventional procedure.

### 26.9.3 Cryotherapy

Peripheral procedures in the management of TN result in permanent sensory loss with the aim of achieving pain free results, and therefore, alternative forms were sought. Cryofreezing is performed on the surgically exposed nerve endings with temperatures of −50 to −70 °C [104]. Literature shows that this procedure is well tolerated by the patients; however, the results are sub-optimal. In a study published in 1988, 145 patients underwent 348 sessions of which 56%

had more than one session. The pain-free effect lasted less than 6 months in one half of patients, and at 12 months, only 27% were pain-free [105]. It is also important to note that 61% of the patients remained on their previous medications. The treatment it is well tolerated by the patients and were willing to undergo repeated cryofreezing and the distinct advantage is that the nerve damage is reversible. It is likely that adjacent nerve branch reconnecting is the reason for the recurrence of the pain. Although the sensation is preserved and nerve injury is reversible, its outcomes fall short of other peripheral procedures. It is reported that 4% of the patients developed post-operative infections warranting antibiotic therapy and about 40% had suffered, some from pain ranging from burning sensation, pins and needles to symptoms such as a dull ache [105].

In summary, despite patient outcomes with this procedure and preserved sensation, there is little evidence to support this procedure in the role of management of TN where other surgical procedures are available.

### 26.9.4 Alcohol Block

Percutaneous ganglionic ganglionic blocks and peripheral blocks have been used since the 1930s. Direct deposition of alcohol into the affected nerve peripheral branch causes chemical ablation of the nerve. Essentially, alcohol causes destruction of nerve fibres. It can seep into the adjacent tissues and cause necrosis, resulting in pain and local oedema. With a high-risk recurrence of pain and with a moderate risk of developing dysesthesia, its use is restricted only in the elderly or patients with comorbidities or those who are reluctant to undergo extensive neurosurgical procedures.

An injection of 0.5–1.0 ml of absolute alcohol is injected directly into the affected nerve bundle under local anaesthesia and injections have to be placed accurately to avoid dissipation, which may result in local damage. Utmost care must be taken to avoid intravascular injections and not to inject into the subcutaneous tissues [106].

The duration of pain relief varies from 6 to 24 months, and there is variation with different peripheral branches. Only a short pain relief with third division is observed compared to the second with a longer duration of pain relief with in the first division [106].

### 26.9.5 Other Peripheral Procedures

Other peripheral neurolysis procedures seen in the literature are radiofrequency coagulation and chemical neurolysis with glycerol. phenol, mixture of lignocaine with streptomycin and high concentration of tetracaine. Evidence in the literature fails to support their true efficacy and long-term benefits.

## 26.10 Conclusion

TN is the most severe type of pain humans ever face for an innocuous touch without any force, and it is debilitating to an extent that it was described historically as "suicide disease" until the development of the medications and various surgical procedures in the 1950s.

As an OMF surgeon, obtaining a good clinical history is to rule out other potential pathologys including dental focus. Patients may be initially present to a primary care dentist or a physician with facial pain, and they should be aware of the medical management and the secondary care team (oral medicine specialists, OMFS and neurologists) involved to deliver the appropriate course of action. Usually, only those who are refractory to the drug therapy or unacceptable drug-related side effects will be escalated further to tertiary care for the consideration of complex central surgical procedure.

Peripheral surgical procedures are suitable for those who are unable or unwilling to undergo complex and expensive neurosurgical procedures. Peripheral procedures are safe with minimal morbidity and almost no mortality; however, there is a lack of evidence to show the recurrence rate and associated long-term complications.

The management of TN patients should be carried out in a multidisciplinary setting to allow the patients to choose the best-suited option for them. It is also important to set up self-help groups to enable them to share knowledge and information for themselves and their family members for the best possible outcomes.

## References


1. Joo W, Yoshioka F, Funaki T, Mizokami K, Rhoton AL Jr. Microsurgical anatomy of the trigeminal nerve. Clin Anat. 2014;27:61–88.
2. Haller S, Etienne L, Kovari E, Varoquax AD, Urbach H, Becker M. Imaging of neurovascular compression syndromes: trigeminal neuralgia, hemifacial spasm, vestibular paroxysmia, and glossopharyngeal neuralgia. AJNR Am J Neuroradiol. 2016;37:1384–92.
3. Sindou M, Howeidy T, Acevedo G. Anatomical observations during microvascular decompression for idiopathic trigeminal neuralgia (with correlations between topography of pain and site of the neurovascular conflict): prospective study in a series of 579 patients. Acta Neurochir. 2002;144:1–12.
4. Harris W. Rare forms of paroxysmal trigeminal neuralgia, and their relation to disseminated sclerosis. Br Med J. 1950;2:1015–9.
5. Foley PL, Vesterinen HM, Laird BJ, Sena ES, Colvin LA, Chandran S, et al. Prevalence and natural history of pain in adults with multiple sclerosis: systematic review and meta-analysis. Pain. 2013;154:632–42.

6. Toda K. Aetiology of trigeminal neuralgia. Oral Sci Int. 2007;4:10–8.
7. Mohammad-Mohammadi A, Recinos PF, Lee JH, Elson P, Barnett GH. Surgical outcomes of trigeminal neuralgia in patients with multiple sclerosis. Neurosurgery. 2013;73:941–50.
8. Zakrzewska J, Jianhua WU, Tricia S, Brathwaite L-A. Systematic review of the management of trigeminal neuralgia in patients with multiple sclerosis. World Neurosurg. 2018;111:291–306.
9. Cruccu G, Biasiotta A, Di RS, Fiorelli M, Galeotti F, Innocenti P, et al. Trigeminal neuralgia and pain related to multiple sclerosis. Pain. 2009;143:186–91.
10. Reder AT, Arnason BG. Trigeminal neuralgia in multiple sclerosis relieved by a prostaglandin E analogue. Neurology. 1995;45:1097–100.
11. Tesfaye S, Selvarajah D. Advances in the epidemiology, pathogenesis and management of diabetic peripheral neuropathy. Diabetes Metab Res Rev. 2012;38:8–14.
12. Xu Z, Zhang P, Long L, He H, Zhang J, Sun S. Diabetes mellitus in classical trigeminal neuralgia: a predisposing factor for its development. Clin Neurol Neurosurg. 2016;151:70–2.
13. NICE. NICE Guidance (online). 2017. Available at http://guidance.nice.org.uk/CG173
14. Dworkin RH, Nagasako EM, Johnson RW, Griffin DR. Acute pain in herpes zoster: the famciclovir database project. Pain. 2001;94:113–9.
15. Beutner KR, Friedman DJ, Forszpaniak C, Andersen PL, Wood MJ. Valaciclovir compared with aciclovir for improved therapy for herpes zoster in immunocompetent adults. Antimicrob Agents Chemother. 1995;39:1546–53.
16. Davis LE, King MK. Shingles (herpes zoster) and post-herpetic neuralgia. Curr Treat Options Neurol. 2001;3:401–11.
17. Schmader K. Herpes zoster in older adults. Clin Infect Dis. 2001;32:1481–6.
18. Zakrzewska JM, Linskey ME. Trigeminal neuralgia. BMJ Clin Evid. 2014;10:1207.
19. Nurmikko TJ, Eldridge PR. Trigeminal neuralgia—pathophysiology, diagnosis and current treatment. Br J Anaesth. 2001;87:117–32.
20. Amir R, Michaelis M, Devor M. Membrane potential oscillations in dorsal root ganglion neurons: role in normal electrogenesis and neuropathic pain. J Neurosci. 1999;19:89–96.
21. Rappaport ZH, Devor M. Trigeminal neuralgia: the role of self-sustaining discharge in the trigeminal ganglion. Pain. 1994;56:127–38.
22. Taha JM, Tew JM, Buncher CR. A prospective 15-year follow up of 154 consecutive patients with trigeminal neuralgia treated by percutaneous stereotactic radiofrequency thermal rhizotomy. J Neurosurg. 1995;83:989–93.
23. Rose FC. Trigeminal neuralgia. Arch Neurol. 1999;56:1163–4.
24. Amir R, Devor M. Functional cross-excitation between afferent A- and C-neurons in dorsal root ganglia. Neuroscience. 2000;95:189–95.
25. Harris W. The facial neuralgias. London: Oxford University Press; 1937. p. 13–4.
26. Pearce JMS. HISTORICAL NOTE—Trigeminal neuralgia (Fothergill's disease) in the 17th and 18th centuries. J Neurol Neurosurg Psychiatry. 2003;74:1688.
27. André N. Traité sur les maladies de l'urèthre. Paris: Delaguette; 1756.
28. Fromm GH, Sessle BJ. Introduction and historical review. In: Fromm GH, Sessle B, editors. Trigeminal neuralgia: Current concepts regarding pathogenesis and treatment. Boston: Butterworth-Heinemann; 1991. p. 1–26.
29. Dandy WE. Section of sensory root of the trigeminal nerve at the pons. Bull Johns Hopkins Hosp. 1925;36:105.
30. Gardner WJ, Miklos MV. Response of trigeminal neuralgia to 'decompression' of sensory root: discussion of cause of trigeminal neuralgia. JAMA. 1959;170:1773–6.
31. Jannetta PJ. Treatment of trigeminal neuralgia by suboccipital and transtentorial cranial operation. Clin Neurosurg. 1977;24:538–49.
32. Bergouignan M. Cures heureuses de neÂvralgies faciales essentielles par le diphennyl-hydantoinate de soude. Rev Laryngol Otol Rhinol (Bord). 1942;63:34–41.
33. MacDonald BK, Cockerell OC, Sander JW, Shorvon SD. The incidence and lifetime prevalence of neurological disorders in a prospective community-based study in the UK. Brain. 2000;123(Pt 4):665–76.
34. Katusic S, Beard CM, Bergstralh E, Kurland LT. Incidence and clinical features of trigeminal neuralgia, Rochester, Minnesota, 1945–1984. Ann Neurol. 1990;27:89–95.
35. Katusic S, Williams DB, Beard CM, Bergstralh EJ, Kurland LT. Epidemiology and clinical features of idiopathic trigeminal neuralgia and glossopharyngeal neuralgia: similarities and differences, Rochester, Minnesota, 1945–1984. Neuroepidemiology. 1991;10:276–81.
36. Zakrzewska JM. Trigeminal neuralgia. Clin Evid. 2003;9:1490–8.
37. White JC, Sweet WH. Pain and the neurosurgeon: a 40-year experience. Springfield, IL: Charles C Thomas; 1969. p. 123–5.
38. Coulthard P, Horner K, Sloan P, Theaker E. Facial pain, oral and maxillofacial surgery, radiology, pathology and oral medicine, Second Edition Master Dentistry Volume One, Edinburgh: Churchill Livingstone Elsevier, Chapter 14. pp. 228–9; 2008.
39. De Toledo I, Conti Réus J, Fernandes M, Porporatti A, Peres M, Takaschima A, Linhares M, Guerra E, De Luca Canto G. Prevalence of trigeminal neuralgia-A systematic review. J Am Dent Assoc. 2016;147(7):570–6.
40. Lu VM, Goyal A, Graffeo CS, Perry A, Jonker BP, Link MJ. Glossopharyngeal neuralgia treatment outcomes after nerve section, microvascular decompression, or stereotactic radiosurgery: a systematic review and meta-analysis. World Neurosurg. 2018;120:572–82.
41. Headache Classification Committee of the International Headache Society (IHS). The International Classification of Headache Disorders, 3rd edition. Cephalalgia. 2018;38:1–211.
42. Di Stefano G, Truini A, G. Cruccu current and innovative pharmacological options to treat typical and atypical trigeminal neuralgia. Drugs. 2018;78:1433–42.
43. Meaney JF, Miles JB, Nixon TE, Whitehouse GH, Ballantyne ES, Eldridge PR. Vascular contact with the fifth cranial nerve at the pons in patients with trigeminal neuralgia: detection with 3D FISP imaging. Am J Roentgenol. 1994;163:1447–52.
44. Meaney JF, Eldridge PR, Dunn LT, Nixon TE, Whitehouse GH, Miles JB. Demonstration of neurovascular compression in trigeminal neuralgia with magnetic resonance imaging: comparison with surgical findings in 52 consecutive operative cases. J Neurosurg. 1995;83:799–805.
45. Masur H, Papke K, Bongartz G, Vollbrecht K. The significance of three-dimensional MR-defined neurovascular compression for the pathogenesis of trigeminal neuralgia. J Neurol. 1995;242:93–8.
46. Korogi Y, Nagahiro S, Du C, et al. Evaluation of vascular compression in trigeminal neuralgia by 3D time-of-flight MRA. J Comput Assist Tomogr. 1995;19:879–84.
47. Majoie CB, Hulsmans FJ, Castelijns JA, et al. Symptoms and signs related to the trigeminal nerve: diagnostic yield of MR imaging. Radiology. 1998;209:557–62.
48. Boecher-Schwarz HG, Bruehl K, Kessel G, Guenthner M, Perneczky A, Stoeter P. Sensitivity and specificity of MRA in the diagnosis of neurovascular compression in patients with trigeminal neuralgia: a correlation of MRA and surgical findings. Neuroradiology. 1998;40:88–95.

49. Jawahar A, Kondziolka D, Kanal E, Bissonette DJ, Lunsford LD. Imaging the trigeminal nerve and pons before and after surgical intervention for trigeminal neuralgia. Neurosurgery. 2001;48:101–6.
50. Patel NK, Aquilina K, Clarke Y, Renowden SA, Coakham HB. How accurate is magnetic resonance angiography in predicting neurovascular compression in patients with trigeminal neuralgia? A prospective, single-blinded comparative study. Br J Neurosurg. 2003;17:60–4.
51. Jannetta PJ. Neurovascular compression in cranial nerve and systemic disease. Ann Surg. 1980;192:518–25.
52. McLaughlin MR, Jannetta PJ, Clyde BL, Subach BR, Comey CH, Resnick DK. Microvascular decompression of cranial nerves: lessons learned after 4400 operations. J Neurosurg. 1999;90:1–8.
53. Love S, Coakham HB. Trigeminal neuralgia: pathology and pathogenesis. Brain. 2001;124:2347–60.
54. Zakrzewska JM. Diagnosis and differential diagnosis of trigeminal neuralgia. Clin J Pain. 2002;18:14–21.
55. Meaney JF, Watt JW, Eldridge PR, Whitehouse GH, Wells JC, Miles JB. Association between trigeminal neuralgia and multiple sclerosis: role of magnetic resonance imaging. J Neurol Neurosurg Psychiatry. 1995;59:253–9.
56. Montano N, Conforti G, Di Bonaventura R, Meglio M, Fernandez E, Papacci F. Advances in diagnosis and treatment of trigeminal neuralgia. Ther Clin Risk Manag. 2015;11:289–99.
57. Cruccu G, Gronseth G, Alksne J, Argoff C, Brainin M, Burchiel K, Nurmikko T, Zakrzewska J. AAN-EFNS guidelines on trigeminal neuralgia management. Eur J Neurol. 2008;15(10):1013–28.
58. Zakrzewska JM. Trigeminal neuralgia. In: Clinical evidence. Issue 7. London: BMJ Publishing; 2002. p. 1221–31.
59. Fromm GH. Baclofen as an adjuvant analgesic. J Pain Symptom Manag. 1994;9:500–9.
60. Wiffen P, Collins S, McQuay H, Carroll D, Jadad A, Moore A. Anticonvulsant drugs for acute and chronic pain. Cochrane Database Syst Rev. 2000;3:CD001133.
61. Wiffen P, McQuay H, Moore R. Carbamazepine for acute and chronic pain. Cochrane Database Syst Rev. 2005;3:CD005451.
62. Jensen TS. Anticonvulsants in neuropathic pain: rationale and clinical evidence. Eur J Pain. 2002;6(Suppl A):61–8.
63. Killian JM, Fromm GH. Carbamazepine in the treatment of neuralgia. Use of side effects. Arch Neurol. 1968;19(2):129–36.
64. Nicol CF. A four-year double-blind study of tegretol in facial pain. Headache. 1969;9(1):54–7.
65. Rockliff BW, Davis EH. Controlled sequential trials of carbamazepine in trigeminal neuralgia. Arch Neurol. 1996;15(2):129–36.
66. Wiffen PJ, Derry S, Moore RA, Kalso EA. Carbamazepine for chronic neuropathic pain and fibromyalgia in adults. Cochrane Database Syst Rev. 2014;4:CD005451.
67. McQuay H, Carroll D, Jadad AR, Wiffen P, Moore A. Anticonvulsant drugs for management of pain: a systematic review. BMJ. 1995;311(7012):1047–52.
68. Kutluay E, McCague K, D'Souza J, Beydoun A. Safety and tolerability of oxcarbazepine in elderly patients with epilepsy. Epilepsy Behav. 2003;4(2):175–80.
69. Hu Y, Guan X, Fan L, et al. Therapeutic efficacy and safety of botulinum toxin type A in trigeminal neuralgia: a systematic review. J Headache Pain. 2013;14:72.
70. Gardner WJ, Miklos MV. Response of trigeminal neuralgia to decompression of sensory root: discussion of cause of trigeminal neuralgia. J Am Med Assoc. 1959;170:1773–6.
71. Jannetta PJ. Arterial compression of the trigeminal nerve at the pons in patients with trigeminal neuralgia. J Neurosurg. 1967;26:159–62.
72. Rhoton AL. The cerebellopontine angle and posterior fossa cranial nerves by the retrosigmoid approach. Neurosurgery. 2000;47(Suppl):S93–129.
73. Adams CBT. Trigeminal neuralgia: pathogenesis and treatment. Br J Neurosurg. 1997;11:493–5.
74. Resnick DK, Levu EI, Jannetta PJ. Microvascular decompression for paediatric onset trigeminal neuralgia. Neurosurgery. 1998;43:804–8.
75. Roski RA, Horwitz SJ, Spetzler RF. Atypical trigeminal neuralgia in a 6-year-old boy. J Neurosurg. 1982;5:424–5.
76. Barker FG, Jannette PJ, Bissonette DJ, Larkins MV, Jho HD. The long-term outcome of microvascular decompression for trigeminal neuralgia. N Engl J Med. 1996;334:1077–83.
77. Burchiel KJ, Clarke H, Haglund M, Loeser JD. Long-term efficacy of microvascular decompression in trigeminal neuralgia. J Neurosurg. 1988;69:35–8.
78. Kolluri S, Heros RC. Microvascular decompression for trigeminal neuralgia. A five-year follow-up study. Surg Neurol. 1984;22:235–40.
79. Kondo A. Follow-up results of microvascular decompression in trigeminal neuralgia and hemifacial spasm. Neurosurgery. 1997;40:46–52.
80. Lee KH, Chang JW, Park YG, Chung SS. Microvascular decompression and percutaneous rhizotomy in trigeminal neuralgia. Stereotact Funct Neurosurg. 1997;68:196–9.
81. Platt JH, Wilkins RH. Treatment of tic douloureux and hemifacial spasm by posterior fossa exploration: therapeutic implications of various neurovascular relationships. Neurosurgery. 1984;14:462–71.
82. Slettebø HJ, Eide PK. A prospective study of microvascular decompression for trigeminal neuralgia. Acta Neurochir. 1997;139:421–5.
83. Lee SH, Levy EI, Scarrow AM, Kassam A, Jannetta PJ. Recurrent trigeminal neuralgia attributable to veins after microvascular decompression. Neurosurgery. 2000;46:352–6.
84. Barba D, Alksne JF. Success of microvascular decompression with and without prior surgical therapy for trigeminal neuralgia. J Neurosurg. 1984;60:104–7.
85. Hunn MK, Eldridge PR, Miles JB, West B. Persistent facial pain following microvascular decompression of the trigeminal nerve. Br J Neurosurg. 1998;12:23–8.
86. Kureshi SA, Wilkins RH. Posterior fossa exploration for persistent or recurrent trigeminal neuralgia or hemifacial spasm: surgical findings and therapeutic implications. Neurosurgery. 1998;43:1111–7.
87. Liao J-J, Cheng W-C, Chang C-N, Wei K-C, Hsu Y-H, Lin T-K. Reoperation for recurrent trigeminal neuralgia after microvascular decompression. Surg Neurol. 1997;47:562–70.
88. Rath SA, Klein HJ, Richter H-P. Findings and long-term results of subsequent operations after failed microvascular decompression for trigeminal neuralgia. Neurosurgery. 1996;39:933–40.
89. Kitt CA, Gruber K, Davis M, Woolf CJ, Levine JD. Trigeminal neuralgia: opportunities for research and treatment. Pain. 2000;85:3–7.
90. Kondziolka D. Functional neurosurgery. Neurosurgery. 1999;44:12–20.
91. Kondziolka D, Lunsford LD, Flickinger JC, Young R, Vermeulen S, Duma C, Jacques D, Rand RW, Regis J, Peragut JC, Manera L, Epstein M, Lindquist C. Steretotactic radiosurgery for trigeminal neuralgia: a multi-institution study using the gamma unit. J Neurosurg. 1996;84:940–5.
92. Kondziolka D, Perez P, Flickinger JC, Habeck M, Lunsford LD. Gamma knife radiosurgery for trigeminal neuralgia. Arch Neurol. 1998;55:1524–9.

93. Mullan S, Duda EE, Patronas NJ. Some examples of balloon technology in neurosurgery. J Neurosurg. 1980;52(3):321–9.
94. Tatli M, Satici O, Kanpolat Y, Sindou M. Various surgical modalities for trigeminal neuralgia: literature study of respective long-term outcomes. Acta Neurochir. 2008;150(3):243–55.
95. Bergenheim AT, Asplund P. Linderoth B percutaneous retrogasserian balloon compression for trigeminal neuralgia: review of critical technical details and outcomes. World Neurosurg. 2013;79(2):359–68.
96. Sweet WG. Proceedings: analgesia dolorosa after differential retrogasserian thermal or mechanical rhizotomy: tactics employed to decrease its influence. J Neurol Neurosurg Psychiatry. 1975;38(4):407.
97. Liu JK, Apfelbaum RI. Treatment of trigeminal neuralgia. Neurosurg Clin N Am. 2004;15(3):319–34.
98. Håkansson S. Trigeminal neuralgia treated by the injection into the trigeminal cistern. Neurosurgery. 1981;9:638–46.
99. Young RF. Glycerol rhizolysis in the treatment of trigeminal neuralgia. J Neurosurg. 1988;69:39–45.
100. North RB, Kidd DH, Piantadosi S, Carson BS. Percutaneous retrogasserian glycerol rhizotomy. Predictors of success and failure in treatment of trigeminal neuralgia. J Neurosurg. 1990;72:851–6.
101. Khanna JN, Galinde JS. Trigeminal neuralgia. Report of 140 cases. Int J Oral Surg. 1985;14(4):325–32.
102. Oturai AB, Jensen K, Erikson J, Marsden F. Neurosurgery for trigeminal neuralgia: comparison of alcohol block, neurectomy and radiofrequency coagulation. Clin J Pain. 1996;12:311–5.
103. Ali FM, Prasant MC, Pai D, Aher VA, Kar S, Safiya T. Peripheral neurectomies: a treatment option for trigeminal neuralgia in rural practice. J Neurosci Rural Pract. 2012;3:152–7.
104. Nally FF. A 22-year study of paroxysmal trigeminal neuralgia in 211 patients with a 3-year appraisal of the role of cryotherapy. Oral Surg. 1984;58:17–23.
105. Zakrzewska JM, Nally FF. The role of cryotherapy (cryoanalgesia) in the management of paroxysmal trigeminal neuralgia: a six-year experience. Br J Oral Maxillofac Surg. 1988;26:18–25.
106. McLeod NMH, Patton DW. Peripheral alcohol injections in the management of trigeminal neuralgia. Oral Surg Oral Med Oral Pathol Oral Radiol Endod. 2007;104(1):12–7.

# Part XI

# Benign Pathologies of the Oral and Maxillofacial Region

# Cysts of the "Oro-Maxillofacial Region"

# 27

Neelima Malik

**Learning Targets**

1. Definition and classification of the Cysts of the Oro-maxillofacial region.
2. Etiopathogenesis, general features, and management of cysts in general
3. Pathogenesis, clinical features, radiological picture, histopathology, and surgical management of common cystic lesions.

## 27.1 Introduction

A cyst is essentially an enclosed sac formed by the cluster of cells, which group together. The unique characteristic of a cyst is that the cells that form the outer covering of the sac are abnormal from the surrounding normal cells of that specific region. There are various categories of cysts, which can occur almost anywhere within the human body's hard and soft tissues, and their occurrences are very common. They vary in size from tiny microscopic to huge macroscopic varieties, and the large cysts can displace the adjoining normal anatomical structures.

Once formed, sometimes, a cyst may resolve on its own, but in most cases, it keeps growing and needs surgical intervention depending on its type and location. Cysts are usually nonaggressive, but certain groups of cysts show aggressive behavior. The cysts of the oral and maxillofacial region are the commonest pathological entities. Historically, mummified specimens in Egypt (400 BC to 2800 BC) showed the presence of cysts [1].

**Electronic Supplementary Material** The online version of this chapter (https://doi.org/10.1007/978-981-15-1346-6_27) contains supplementary material, which is available to authorized users.

N. Malik (✉)
Department of Oral and Maxillofacial Surgery, Krishna Institute of Medical Sciences "Deemed to be University", Karad, Maharashtra, India

## 27.2 Definition

A cyst is explicitly defined as "A pathological (uni- or multilocular) sac that may or may not be lined by an epithelium and filled with a fluid, semifluid, or gaseous contents and not created by the accumulation of pus" [1, 2].

## 27.3 General Histopathological Common Components of a Cyst

Cysts can be found in the facial bones as well as in the soft tissues of the orofacial region.

Cysts lined by an epithelium are more common in both jawbones than any other regions of the body because of great many epithelial cell rests present in close proximity to the developing jaw bones, and they are called True Cysts, e.g., radicular cyst, dentigerous cysts, etc.

Pseudocysts do not have an epithelial lining, e.g., solitary bone cysts, Cysts of maxillary antrum, etc. [1] (Fig. 27.1).

A cyst is a tissue-space occupying lesion/sac with a cavity in the center known as a Lumen. There is an outer fibrous connective tissue wall that separates the cyst from surrounding normal tissues. On the inner aspect of this wall, there is a cystic lining of epithelium, mostly made up of stratified squamous epithelium (Fig. 27.2). In some cases, there can be lining other than squamous epithelium.

## 27.4 Etiopathogenesis

The etiopathogenesis of orofacial cysts basically originates from the remnants of the complex processes of embryonic tissue responsible for jaw and dental development. Such a conversion does not occur in any other part of the body.

All True Cysts have their genesis from the epithelial remnants along with strong proliferative impetus and capability for bone remodeling. Odontogenic cysts are derived from


K. Bonanthaya et al. (eds.), *Oral and Maxillofacial Surgery for the Clinician*, https://doi.org/10.1007/978-981-15-1346-6_27

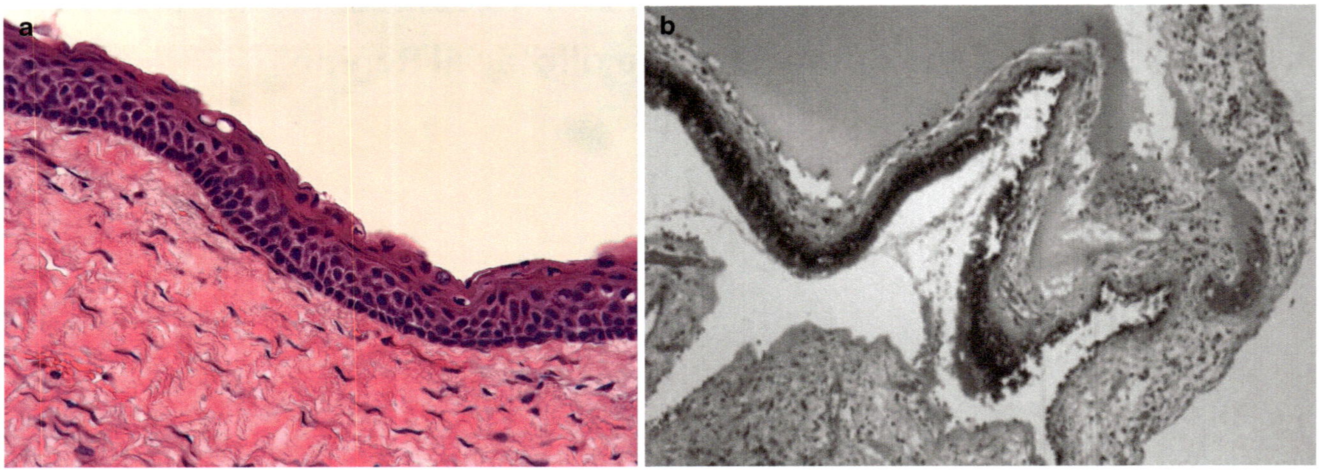




**Fig. 27.1** Histological picture of a true (**a**) and pseudocyst (**b**)

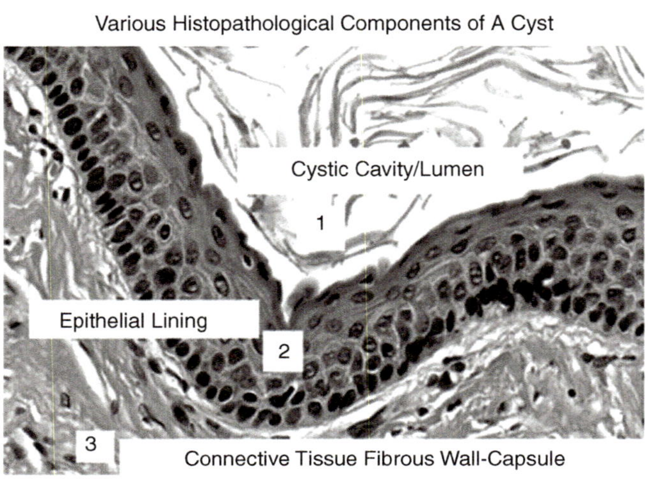




**Fig. 27.2** General broad histopathological characteristic components of a Cyst; Epithelial lining-various types of epithelium can line a cyst

**Table 27.1** Classification of cysts based on the embryological derivation sources (modified from Regezi et al. [3])

| Type | Source | Origin of cell rest | Cyst variety |
|---|---|---|---|
| Odontogenic rests | Cell rests of malassez | Epithelial hertwig's root sheath | Periapical (radicular) cyst |
| | Reduced enamel epithelium | Enamel organ | Dentigerous cyst |
| | Rests of dental lamina (rest of Serres) | Epithelial connection between mucosa and enamel organ | Glandular odontogenic cyst, Lateral periodontal cyst, Odontogenic keratocyst, and Gingival cyst of newborn & adult |
| Nonodontogenic Rests | Remnants of nasopalatine duct | Paired nasopalatine duct-vestigial | Nasopalatine canal cyst and Fissural cysts |
| | Remnants of maxillary sinus epithelium | | Cysts of the maxillary sinus |

remnants of odontogenic epithelium of stomodeum, and inflammatory cysts are derived from infective process (Table 27.1).

Pathogenesis of a cyst is mainly divided into three stages:

(1) Cyst Initiation, (2) Cyst Formation, and (3) Cyst enlargement or expansion

1. *Cyst Initiation*—unknown stimulus promotes the rapid increase of epithelial rest cells via cytokine synthesis. The factors, which are suggested to be responsible for cyst initiation phase, are mainly genetics, loss of immunological surveillance, inflammatory mediators, or some local factors like decreased oxygen tension along with increased CO2 tension.

   The residual epithelial cells (Table 27.1) are implicated to initiate the process of cyst formation. Initiation is followed by the rapid growth of the epithelial cells and the development of a cystic lesion.
2. *Cyst Formation*—Nutritional deficiency theory
   After initiation, proliferating epithelial cells form a mass inside the sac and the innermost central cells become deprived of nutrients/blood supply, as they are far from the source of nutrients. The innermost cells do not get adequate blood supply, and so there is an ischemic liquefactive necrosis in the center, leading to a cavity for-

mation, which is surrounded by growing epithelial cells. Enhancement in intercellular edema and acid phosphatase activity leads to the formation of microcysts, which slowly start to form a larger cyst [4].

3. *Cyst enlargement or expansion*
   Once formed, the cyst continues to enlarge slowly, over the months.
   The process is similar for all epithelial lined cysts with some variations. Many debatable hypotheses have been put forward regarding the definitive mechanism of cyst enlargement.

## 27.4.1 Theories of Cyst Enlargement/ Expansion

### 27.4.1.1 Mural Growth & Peripheral Cell Division

(a) Epithelial proliferation-peripheral cell division, (b) Accumulation of the contents within the lumen.

Due to Proliferation or rapid increase in the number of cells and by the active division of peripheral lining epithelial cells, surface area of cystic sac increases and the enlargement of a cyst at the circumference is noted along with the accumulation of cellular contents [4, 5].

### 27.4.1.2 Hydrostatic Enlargement

**Biomechanical Theory**

Intraluminal concentration and pressure differences between the cystic cavity and the peripheral growth surroundings influence fluid movement into the cyst, bringing about an increase in size.

Cyst starts expanding and growing in size, with the increase in intracystic pressure due to the intake of fluids inside the cyst from the surrounding area. (The center of the cyst has higher concentration of sodium than the surrounding serum, and so it tends to absorb water.)

This increase in cyst size process is different from the true autonomous growth, which is found in tumor cells [5, 6].

Secondary proliferation of epithelial cells is, thus, a result of increased volume pressure within the cystic cavity, as a result of osmosis. An osmotic concentration gradient is created as a result of degradation and metabolic by-products, which are taken up inside the cyst.

Due to the rapid increase in the osmotic gradient, the fluid from the surrounding region diffuses in the cystic cavity, increasing internal hydrostatic pressure and thereby resulting in the expansion of the cyst (Fig. 27.3).

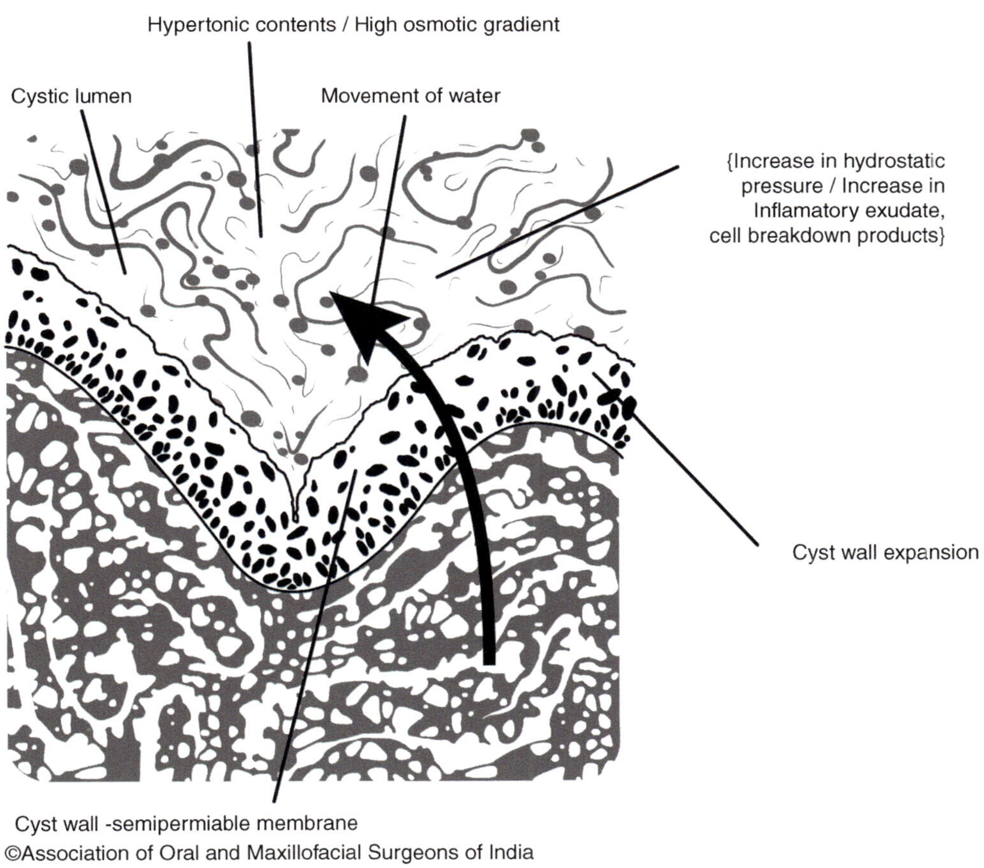


**Fig. 27.3** The phase of enlargement of a cyst

#### 27.4.1.3 Bone Resorbing Factor

In intraosseous cysts, resorption of the surrounding bone also increases the size of bony cavity.

**Biochemical and Cellular Aspects of the Cyst Proliferation**

Newer research points to the role of molecular biology in cyst proliferation, over older theories of bone loss resulting from osmotic gradient. The cystic capsule produces bone resorbing factors like prostaglandins, leukotrienes, and osteoclasts.

(A) Bone degeneration in the jaw bone is brought by Collagenase (breakdown of collagen), providing room for cysts to develop. Body's immune mechanism releases cytokines and growth factors due to the connective tissue breakdown, which contributes to the mobilization and proliferation of epithelial cells in the area.

Evidence-based studies showed that collagenase activities in cystic capsule result in bone degeneration by destruction of the collagen [6, 7].

(B) Prostaglandin theory—Bone resorption caused by metabolism of acidic matter produced in the cysts lends to the cystic growth. These are the substances produced by the cyst itself, which include Prostaglandin-2 and Interleukin-1. Along with the epithelial cell division, the cyst enlarges within the jaw bone due to bone resorption caused by Prostaglandin-induced osteoclastic activity. Bone resorption is mediated as a result of production of PGE-2 and PGE-3 by dental cysts. Prostaglandin-2 and other by-products are part of arachidonic acid metabolism [8].

The production of prostaglandin-2 can be triggered by Interleukin-1. Meghji et al. [9] summarized that odontogenic cysts produce interleukin-1, which in turn triggers the production of Prostaglandin-2, resulting in osteoclastic bone resorption and cyst enlargement. Most dental cysts demonstrate a common growth mechanism though radicular and developmental cysts may be initiated by different factors (Flow Chart 27.1).

## 27.5 Historical Evolution of the WHO Classification Systems

Many researchers including WHO have tried to put forward a uniform, globally accepted nomenclatures and classifications for the cysts of orofacial region. But still there is a continuous debate going on, and therefore, various classifications are cited in the literature. WHO in 1992 [2] had classified cysts into two main categories as odontogenic and nonodontogenic, with further subsets as developmental and inflammatory (Flow Charts 27.2 and 27.3).

**Flow Chart 27.1** Potential mechanism of bone resorption in a radicular cyst

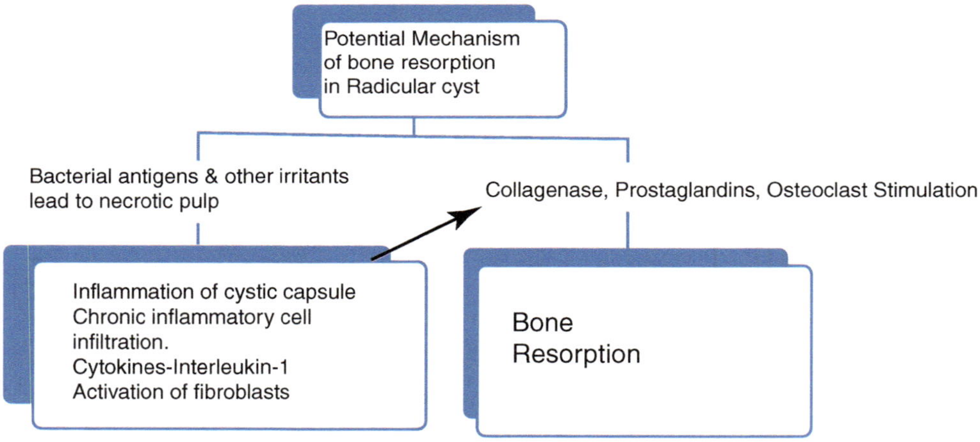


**Flow Chart 27.2** Basic classification of cysts of jaws

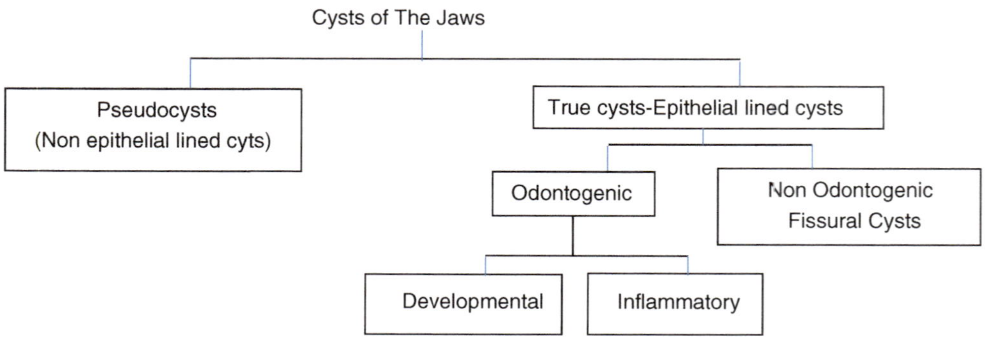

**Flow Chart 27.3** Classification of pseudocysts

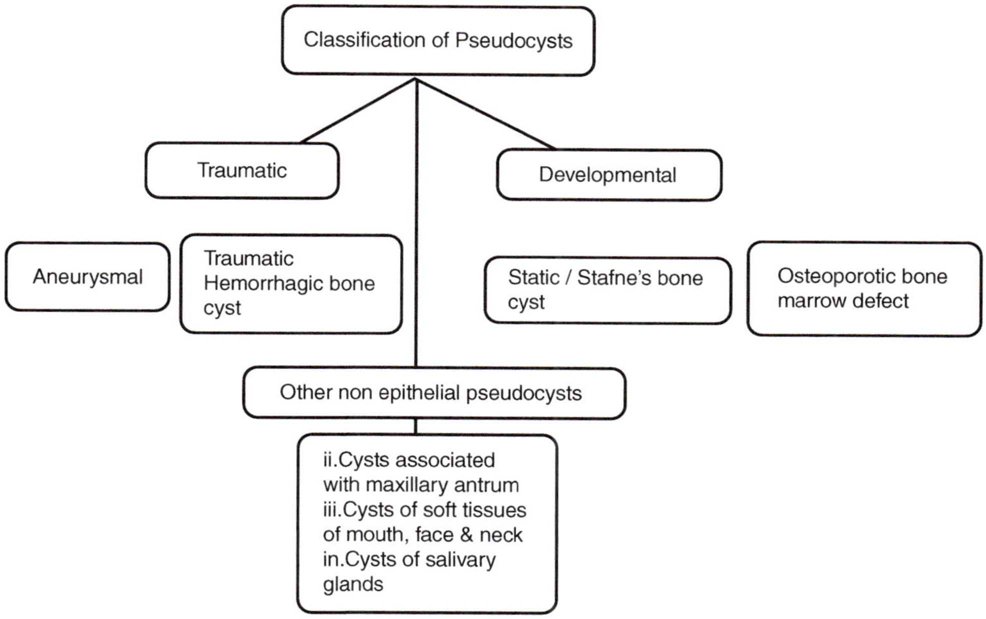


**Table 27.2** According to Shear [1], cysts of orofacial region are categorized under three major groups:

| | |
|---|---|
| I. | Cysts of the jaws |
| II. | Cysts associated with the maxillary antrum |
| III. | Cysts of the soft tissues of the mouth, face, and neck. |

This simple classification did not include Calcifying odontogenic cyst (COC), cysts involving maxillary sinus and nonodontogenic soft tissue cysts. WHO in 2005 [10] reclassified the cysts into epithelial and nonepithelial varieties, which were further divided into odontogenic and nonodontogenic types. At this time, COC—calcifying odontogenic cyst—and Odontogenic Keratocysts (OKCs) were not considered as cystic entities, but they were listed as keratocystic odontogenic tumors—KCOT—and calcifying cystic odontogenic tumors—CCOT—respectively. The justification for this new OKC designation was the high recurrence rate and aggressive behavior along with association with mutations in PTCH gene. This reclassification led to a lot of confusion, and it was not accepted by many. But in 2017, the peer group of WHO did not think that there was sufficient affirmation for classifying both OKC and COC as neoplasms. Therefore, in 2017 again, both these lesions were put back in the cyst category [11].

Among so many classifications, Shear (2007) has suggested a comprehensive classification of cysts with good understanding of cystic lesions of mouth, face, and neck region [1] (Table 27.2).

The cysts of the jaws are divided into those that are:

I. Cysts of the jaws
  A. Epithelial-lined cysts
    1. Developmental origin
      (a) Odontogenic Developmental cysts
        (i) Odontogenic keratocyst
        (ii) Dentigerous cyst
        (iii) Developmental lateral periodontal cyst
        (iv) Gingival cyst of infants
        (v) Eruption cyst
        (vi) Gingival cyst of adults
        (vii) Glandular odontogenic cyst
        (viii) Calcifying odontogenic cyst
        (ix) Botryoid odontogenic cyst
      (b) Nonodontogenic Developmental cysts
        (i) Midpalatalraphé cyst of infants
        (ii) Nasolabial cyst
        (iii) Nasopalatine duct cyst
    2. Odontogenic Inflammatory origin
      (i) Radicular cyst, apical, and lateral
      (ii) Paradental cyst and juvenile paradental cyst
      (iii) Residual cyst
      (iv) Inflammatory collateral cyst
  B. Nonepithelial-lined pseudocysts
    (i) Solitary bone cyst
    (ii) Aneurysmal bone cyst
II. Cysts associated with the maxillary antrum
  (i) Retention cyst
  (ii) Mucocele

III. Cysts of the soft tissues of the mouth, face, and neck
 (i) Dermoid and epidermoid cysts
 (ii) Thyroglossal duct cyst
 (iii) Lymphoepithelial (branchial) cyst
 (iv) Anterior median lingual cyst (intralingual cyst of foregut origin)
 (v) Nasopharyngeal cyst
 (vi) Oral cysts with gastric or intestinal epithelium (oral alimentary tract cyst)
 (vii) Cystic hygroma
 (viii) Thymic cyst

## 27.6 Prevalence of Cysts

Quite a large number of studies are conducted on jaw cysts, but detailed information on demographic profiles in different populations is limited and most have focused on odontogenic cysts [12, 13] (Box 27.1 and Fig. 27.4).

**Box 27.1 Prevalence of Dento-orofacial Cysts**

*Incidence*:

- The jaw cysts are more common than cysts of other bones in the body [12].
- Prevalence of odontogenic cysts is higher (90%) than nonodontogenic cysts in the jaws [12, 13]
- The commonest varieties are periapical cyst (65%), dentigerous cyst (24%), and OKC (5–8%) [12, 13]
- Inflammatory cysts account for 36%, whereas developmental cysts represent 27% of all cysts. 4% cysts are either unclassifiable or nonepithelial (Lucas and WHO classification) [12, 13]

*Age*: Range from the 1st to 9th decades. Peak incidence is seen between 21 and 30 years of age.

*Sex*: More prevalent in males, with a male to female ratio of 1.4:1 [12, 13]

*Site*: Review of literature suggests mandibular preponderance and may imply a higher tendency for activation of cell rests to cystic degeneration in the mandible.

**Box 27.2 Diagnosis of the Cystic Lesion Can Be Arrived by the Following Steps**

A. History
B. Clinical Examination (signs and symptoms, site, inspection, palpation, percussion, teeth vitality check, and aspiration of the cystic content)
C. Radiographic examination
D. Biopsy (to ascertain histopathological features leading to final diagnosis)

**Box 27.3 History**

History: Duration of the complaints/progress is also important. History of pain, loose teeth, occlusion change, intraoral/extraoral swelling/discharge, or sinus track, missing teeth, and delayed eruption of teeth should be noted.

## 27.7 General Key Attributes Regarding an Oro-maxillo-Facial Cyst-Signs & Symptoms (Boxes 27.2 and 27.3)

Signs and symptoms of a cyst depend on its size and site. Small cysts are detected as an incidental finding during routine radiographic examination. Large cyst after enlargement can be noticed first by the patient himself, or there can be facial disfigurement noticed by others. Generally, cysts are symptoms free, unless they get infected secondarily.

If the cyst has not enlarged beyond its normal anatomical boundaries of the jaw bone, then its lump cannot be palpated intraorally or extraorally. The majority of cysts expand very slowly, and the surrounding bone gets time to form fresh subperiosteal new bony layer around the lesion, which isolates the lesion.

**On Palpation**

1. During early stage, smooth, bony hard, and painless prominence can be felt.

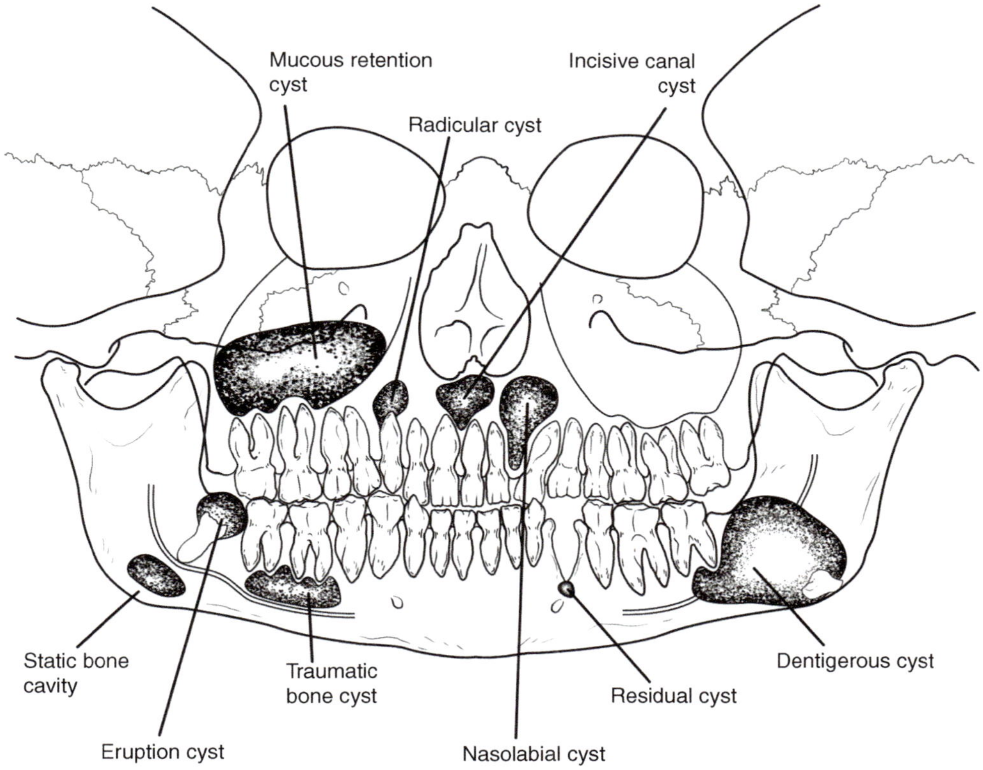


**Fig. 27.4** Typical locations of odontogenic and nonodontogenic cysts

2. Later on "eggshell crackling" can be felt at the thinned out less mineralised *cortex*.
3. When the cyst grows in volume, the outer cortex is thinned out, due to the loss of bone mineral content and may show "Ping Pong/Table Tennis Ball" springy consistency, or
4. Fluctuation can be felt in its center, where the cyst has eroded the bone and the cystic sac fuses with oral mucosa. Cysts, which show buccal cortical expansion, are still mostly covered with a thin layer of the new bone. Cysts are typically slow growing and tissue space occupying lesions and have the capacity to displace or replace normal tissues. They form compressible, fluctuant swelling, if encroached into the soft tissues, and if they are very close to the mucosal surface, then bluish tinge is seen. A majority of cysts show buccal cortical expansion as the cyst grows in size, but in some aggressive cases, lingual or both buccal and lingual expansion can be seen, which produces facial disfigurement.

A cyst may become secondarily infected, and pus discharge may be seen into the oral cavity via a sinus tract. Examination of the sinus track and discharge from sinus track should be checked for cholesterol crystals or pus. Salty, sweet, or unpleasant taste of the discharge is noted.

At this stage, patient may complain of pain. Loosening of adjacent teeth or displacement of the teeth out of their normal arch alignment can happen. Very rarely, depending on the variety of cyst, as it enlarges to an enormous size, it may resorb adjoining teeth/roots, as well as bone, and may end up in pathological fracture of the jaw bone. As most cysts enlarge at a slow pace, and even in the large lesions, the inferior alveolar canal usually gets displaced and there will be no altered sensation (anesthesia or paraesthesia). Paraesthesia and/or anesthesia of the lower lip can exist in aggressive or acutely infected cysts. Percussion of involved teeth will produce a dull or hollow sound. Usually, high-pitched sound is obtained on the uninvolved teeth. Edentulous patient will complain of ill-fitting denture due to the bulge. Periapical cysts are always seen in relation to one or more nonvital teeth. A large maxillary anterior region cyst may cause distortion of nostril shape and show nasal congestion. Diagnosis can vary as per the site of the lesion,

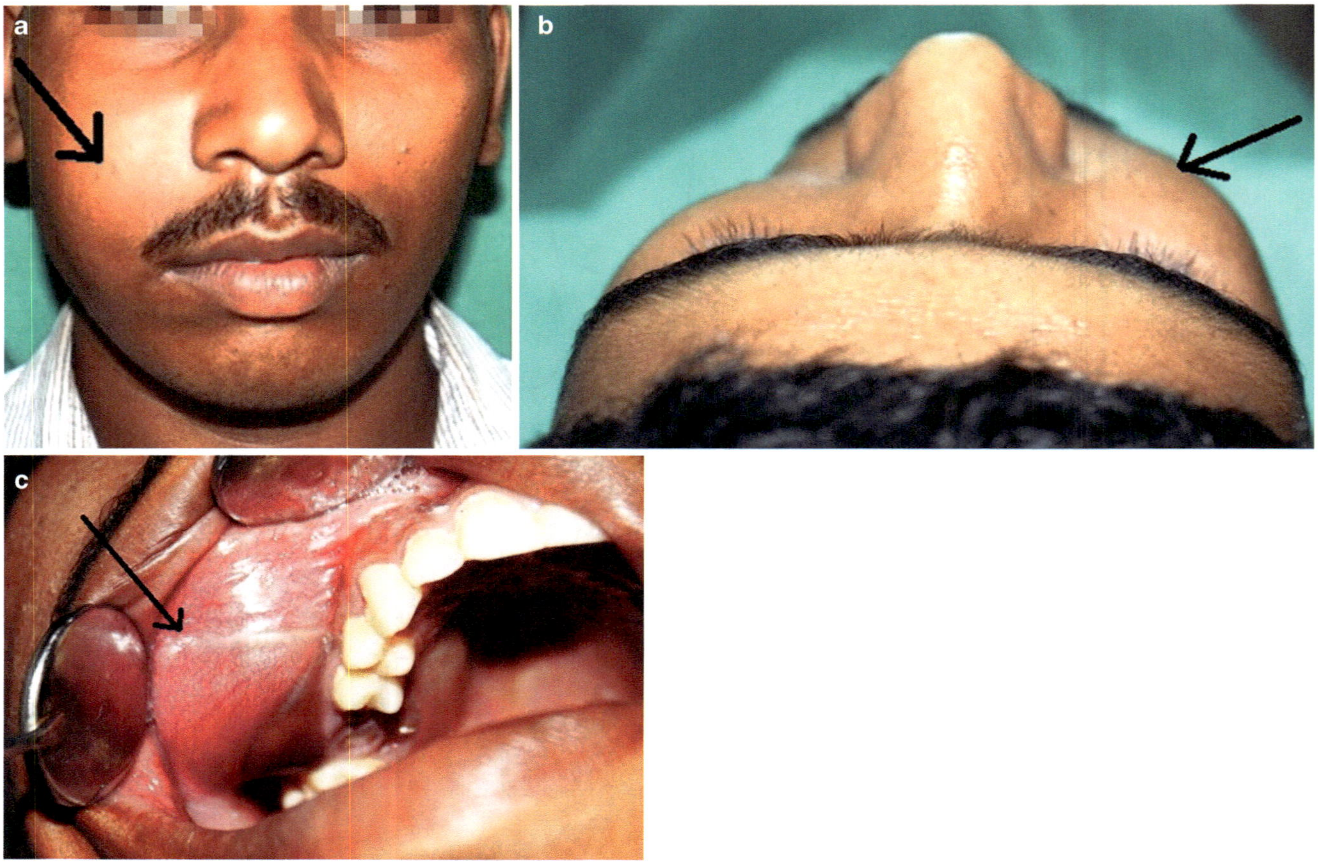



**Fig. 27.5** Clinical examination: extraoral inspection; (**a**) extraoral swelling on the right cheek area, (**b**) head position for inspection of swelling and comparison with normal side, and (**c**) intraoral examination showing obvious bulge in right buccal vestibule. *(Courtesy Dr, Kumar Nilesh, SDS, Karad)*

age of the patient, clinical, radiological, and histopathological examination (Fig. 27.5).

### 27.7.1 Vitality Test of the Involved Teeth in the Lesion

In cysts other than radicular cysts or inflammatory periodontal cyst, there is no compromise in blood supply of the teeth, and so teeth vitality is preserved. Vital teeth are associated with odontogenic keratocyst, solitary bone cyst, lateral periodontal cyst, etc. In inflammatory cysts, the vitality of all involved and adjoining teeth should be checked.

### 27.7.2 Radiographic Examination

Radiographic picture of a cyst is not always pathognomonic. It will depend not only on cyst category, but also the variants related to its duration, location, and degree of expansion and the presence or absence of infection. When the patient is referred for X-rays, the type of film used will depend on the size of a lesion. Dental panoramic or maxillofacial Cone Beam CT provides good imaging for most of these cystic lesions. They help to define site, size, extent, and marginal outline of the lesion.

Intraoral film: For smaller lesions, minimum of two films are taken at right angles to one another. Periapical and occlusal views may be taken.

Extraoral film-used for larger lesions. Panoramic/ Orthopantograms, Lateral oblique views, and Water's view may be taken.

Patient may be referred for CT scan or MRI in cases of extensive aggressive lesion or recurrent lesions to know the exact expanse, proximity to the important vital structures/ adjacent anatomical structures, perforations, and multilobulated/multicystic character. If there is suspicious extraosseous lesion with soft tissue extension or malignancy, then it is also indicated. Postoperative imaging helps to assess the rate of regression and bone regeneration.

#### 27.7.2.1 General Radiographic Picture

1. Radiographically, intrabony cysts, small or large, form sharply defined unilocular or multilocular radiolucency with or without cortication.

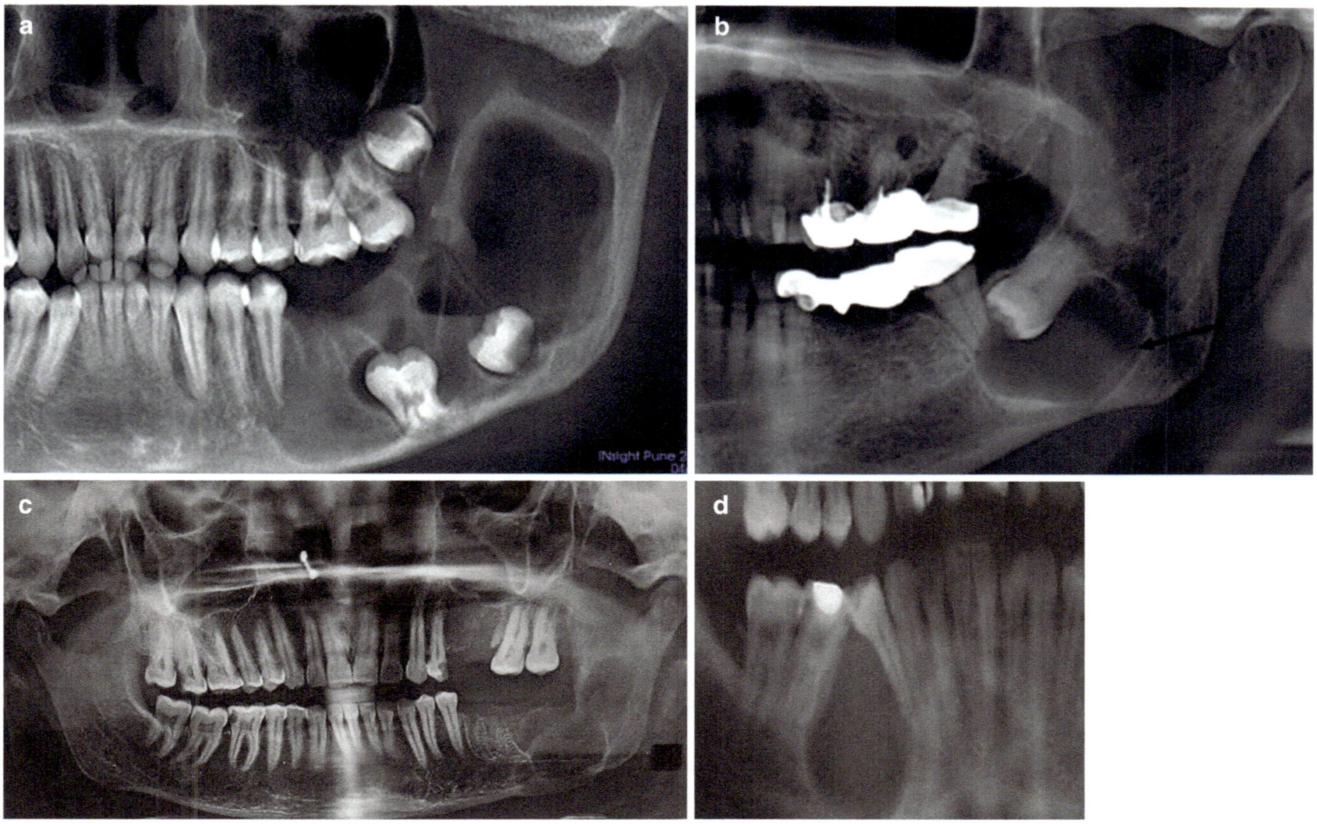




**Fig. 27.6** Different radiological picture of the cystic lesions as per the types: (**a**) replacement type (cyst in place of third molar), (**b**) envelopmental type (cyst enveloping lower third molar), (**c**) extraneous type (ascending ramus cyst away from teeth), and (**d**) collateral type (adjacent to the roots of the teeth)

2. The presence of septae can be seen.
3. The shape of a cyst will vary, depending on the type; round or oval in radicular or dentigerous cysts, scalloped margins in odontogenic keratocyst, traumatic bone cyst, pear-shaped, heart-shaped in nasopalatine or incisive canal cyst.
4. Cortical expansion, perforations, or pathological fractures may be seen.
5. Displacement or compression may be noticed on the adjacent dentition, maxillary sinus, or neurovascular bundle.

#### 27.7.2.2 Radiological Classification of Jaw Cysts (Shear) [1]

- Replacement type: cyst that forms in place of normal tooth
- Envelopmental type: cyst that embraces an adjacent unerupted tooth
- Extraneous type: cyst that occurs in ascending ramus away from the teeth
- Collateral type: cyst that occurs near the roots of the teeth (Fig. 27.6)

### 27.7.3 Aspiration

The orofacial cyst contains fluid in its cystic cavity, which varies in consistency, color, and protein content, and helps in differentiating and arriving at a provisional diagnosis based on these observations. These findings should be remembered to be able to diagnose any cyst, which may be encountered in the clinical practice. An aspiration biopsy of a cyst is the norm for initial diagnosis of all cysts.

- Aspiration with syringe is always positive for most of the odontogenic cysts. Aspiration can be carried out after the clinical examination is over or at the time of planned incisional biopsy. Aspiration and excision biopsy can be done in the same sitting for small lesions.
- Aspiration of Intralesional fluid is done using a wide bore needle of 18 gauge and 5 ml syringe under local anesthesia. It is a very valuable provisional diagnostic aid with simple procedure with least discomfort. Inability to retract the plunger may be due to a solid mass. Introduce a needle occlusally, as this area is usually thinner than buccal or lingual side (Fig. 27.7).

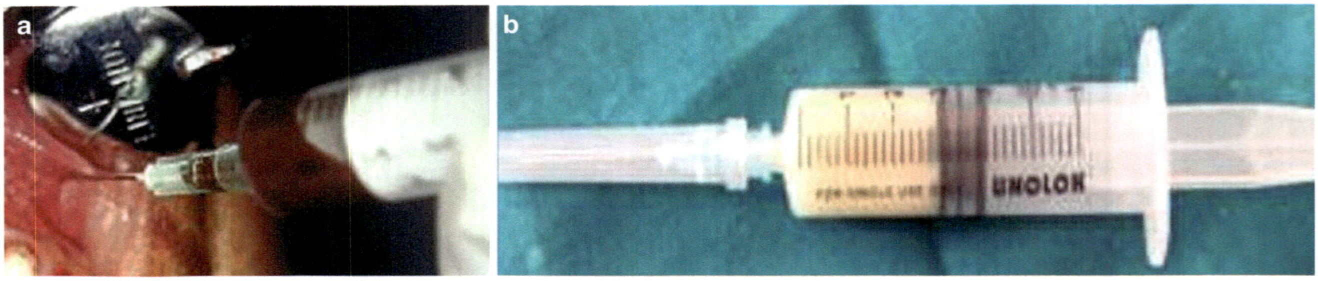




**Fig. 27.7** Aspirated cystic fluid; (**a**) aspiration from infected radicular cyst, (**b**) aspiration from infected keratocyst

### 27.7.4 Cystic Fluids

Cystic contents are different ranging from clear yellow fluid to a creamy or cheese like semisolid liquid. The content can be examined for its color, consistency and for the existence shimmering cholesterol clefts or crystals (microscopic examination of cholesterol crystal shows an envelope with cut-corner appearance). Electron microscopic examination reveals the presence of various protein fractions like alpha and beta globulin , albumin, flecks of keratin, as well as total protein content along with inorganic phosphates [14] (Table 27.3).

#### 27.7.4.1 Biochemical Analysis of the Cystic Fluid

Toller has opined that by an active cellular transport mechanism, the proteins are drawn into the cystic fluid by immunoglobulin (Ig) producing cells. Estimation of IgA, IgG, and IgM levels in cystic fluid can be done quantitatively [15]. Smith et al. [16] concluded in their study that the most of the cystic fluids show the presence of proteins with higher molecular weight. This is due to the fact that the semipermeable intraepithelial channels facilitate the passage of lactoferrin into the cystic lumen.

The cystic fluid, which is collected via aspiration biopsy, can be biochemically analyzed for their protein content estimation by Cellulose acetate membrane (CAM) electrophoresis. First, the cystic fluid is transferred to the centrifuge machine for the removal cell debris and deposits at 2000 rev/min for 5 min.

Since electrophoresis studies the movement of charged particles through an electrolyte, which is subjected to an electric field, and it separates different proteins as per their physical properties, the fluid free of debris is then studied qualitatively and quantitatively. The protein mixture is applied to the end of the CAM strip. Scanning of these impregnated CAM strips can be carried out using a densitometer for the quantitative estimation of protein fractions.

**Table 27.3** Various cystic lesions and their aspirates

| Types of cysts | Aspirate color | Aspirates' other findings |
|---|---|---|
| Dentigerous Cyst Inflammatory Cyst | Absolutely Clear and faint straw/golden color liquid | Shimmering Cholesterol crystals. Resembles serum. Aggregate Total protein >4 gm/100 ml. |
| Odontogenic Keratocyst | Dirty, creamy white, and viscoid/thick suspension | Floating of desquamated keratin flakes, Less than 4 gm/100 ml of Aggregate Total protein. The predominant presence of Albumin is seen, which is less soluble. |
| Periodontal Cyst | Absolutely Clear and faint straw/golden color liquid | Cholesterol clefts/crystals. Aggregate Total protein 5–11 gm per 100 ml. |
| Infected radicular Cyst | Presence of Pus or brown color fluid | Polymorphonuclear leukocytes and cholesterol crystals |
| Mucocele and Ranula | Sticky, viscous, and thick Mucus | Secreted by salivary glands |
| Gingival Cysts | Clear fluid | |
| Solitary Bone Cyst | Serous type of fluid; sometimes, blood is aspirated, or empty cavity is found | Necrotic material in blood clot |
| Stafne's Bone Cyst Idiopathic bone cavity | On aspiration air is drawn—Empty cavity | |
| Dermoid Cyst | Sebaceous thick material | |
| Fissural Cysts | Mucoid liquid | |
| Unicystic ameloblastoma | chocolate brown fluid | |
| Hemangioma-intramedullary cavernous | Syringe full of fresh venous blood | |
| A-V malformation Arterial or arteriovenous malformation | Bright red blood, pulsatile, pushes plunger | |

### 27.7.5 Biopsy

Incisional (for large lesions) or excisional (for small lesions) biopsy and histopathological examination of the specimen is the gold standard to arrive at final diagnosis.

## 27.8 Various Surgical Treatment Modalities for Cystic Lesion

With all the investigation results in hand, the surgeon will have a clear idea of the type, the location, extent, and behavior of the lesion. A final diagnosis is then obtained, and a suitable surgical line of treatment is decided upon (Boxes 27.4, 27.5, 27.6, 27.7, 27.8, 27.9, and 27.10).

**Box 27.4 Clinical Tips**

Incisional Biopsy: For large lesions, a "representative" section of the lesion is incised with the help of a scalpel along with the normal tissue and sent for histopathological evaluation. An elliptical, wedge-shaped tissue is obtained with the "V" of the wedge converging into the deeper tissues. The depth of the biopsy should be enough to obtain a representative area of the lesion.

Excisional Biopsy: It is a combination of diagnostic and curative procedure and is suitably smaller for lesions <1 cm. In these cases, the entire lesion is excised in toto at the same sitting and sent for histopathological examination.

**Box 27.5 Reasons for the Definitive Treatment**

- Cysts continue to grow and show a tendency to increase slowly in size
- They can get secondarily infected
- Cyst can make the jaw bone weak, leading to pathological fracture
- Few cysts can undergo transformation to aggressive pathological lesions like ameloblastoma or squamous cell carcinoma
- Cysts prevent eruption of teeth (as in the case of a dentigerous cyst)
- Cysts can involve neighbouring structures like teeth, maxillary sinus, nasal cavity, inferior alveolar nerve, etc.

**Box 27.6 Goals of Surgery**

- Complete elimination of the pathology, minimizing the recurrence rate & morbidity for the patient, and improving the quality of life postsurgically
- Minimum trauma to the adjacent important structures like dentition and nerves
- Restore/Preserve/Maintain function & esthetics

**Box 27.7 Factors for the Choice of Optimum Surgical Strategy/Treatment**

*Patient factors & lesion characteristics*

- Patient's age & general health and coexistence of NBCCS-Nevoid Basal Cell Carcinoma Syndrome/ any other syndrome
- Patient's reliability to follow up
- Size of the lesion & whether solitary/multiple
- Uni/multilocular
- Location of the lesion-surgical access
- Cortical perforation/Soft tissue/adjacent structure involvement
- Presence or absence of infection
- History of recurrence/previous surgery
- Histological variant

**Box 27.8 Conservative Surgical Treatment**

- Decompression alone-placement of a drainage tube-palliative (decrease in lesion size)
- Decompression followed by Enucleation along with adjuvant therapy (two-staged procedure)
- Marsupialization Alone (creating a pouch)
- Marsupialization followed by Enucleation (Waldron's method) [17] (two-staged procedure)
- Enucleation Alone with packing, with primary closure, or with primary closure with bone grafting/ reconstruction
- Enucleation along with excision of overlying oral mucosa (Stoelinga protocol [18])
- Enucleation followed by various Adjuvant Therapies

**Box 27.9 Enucleation with Adjunctive Modalities to Eliminate the Microscopic Pathologies**

- Peripheral ostectomy (Mechanical/physical methods, Hand instruments like curettes, & use of rotary bur for removal of perimeter of investing bone)
- Chemical cauterization treatment with Carnoy solution (1.5 mm depth of bone penetration/5 min)
- Electrocauterization is used for buccal and lingual perforation area.
- Cryotherapy (use of liquid nitrogen after enucleation)
- Multidisciplinary Sequential treatment (MST) Approach (decompression, enucleation, peripheral ostectomy, and cauterizing bone cavity by carbolic acid) (Sun et al. [19])

**Box 27.10 Aggressive Surgical Treatment**

- Resection without causing a continuity defect-peripheral ostectomy
- Resection with a continuity defect–segmental resection
- Resection along with disarticulation of condyle

### 27.8.1 Conventional Surgical Options

The objective of the choosing any particular surgical method is to minimize patient morbidity and reduce the recurrence rate. Surgical procedures for treating cystic lesions are often put into two categories; conservative or aggressive (Boxes 27.8, 27.9, and 27.10).

***Decompression and marsupialisation (cystotomy)***: Partsch I operation of the cysts is presumably the earliest treatment. Enucleation or cystectomy with primary closure is also known as Partsch II procedure (Partsch 1892, 1910) [17].

***Decompression, marsupialisation***: both methods achieve evacuation of the cystic contents by creating a surgical opening in the cystic wall. These procedures preserve the continuity of the cystic lesion with the oral/nasal cavity or maxillary sinus.

#### 27.8.1.1 Decompression

Decompression of a cyst is achieved by a minor surgical procedure, which decreases the intracystic hydrostatic pressure, which is responsible for cyst expansion. Subsequently, decompression allows for the bone remodeling and bone fill.

Decompression can be achieved under L.A. by creating a small opening in the cystic wall and keeping it patent with a surgical drain. Acrylic tubes, Luer syringes, polyethylene tubes, nasopharyngeal airways, or nasal cannula or intravenous tubes have been used by fixing them with sutures or wires to keep the opening in the cyst patent, through which the cystic lumen is flushed twice/thrice everyday with saline/antiseptic wash.

Cysts of the lower jaw are normally evacuated through opening into the oral cavity, and maxillary cysts can be drained either into the oral cavity, the maxillary sinus or nasal cavity [17] (Fig. 27.8).

#### 27.8.1.2 Marsupialization

It is a surgical procedure, whereby a cystic sac is modified or deroofed to convert it into a pouch. This results in a self-sustaining stoma/opening or outlet, which in turn reduces intracystic hydrostatic pressure. It is basically a surgical externalization of the cystic cavity by creating an opening in the superficial aspect of the cyst. The resected portion is sent for histopatholgical study. The remainder borders of the cystic wall are then sutured to the surrounding edges of the oral mucosa, thus converting an enclosed sac, into an open pouch, exposing the cystic lining or epithelium to the oral environment. This procedure decreases the volume and size of the lesion and promotes the speedy healing and new bone formation. This option is more precise compared to the decompression method. Marsupialization may be used as a solo treatment regime for a cyst or as a prior step to final second stage enucleation [17].

*Surgical Procedure* In Marsupialization, after locally anesthetizing the buccal/labial area, an oval/elliptical incision is taken to make a surgical window spanning 1 cm into a cyst; the window cover consisting of oral mucosa, thinned out bony cortex and cystic lining, is removed, and the boundaries of the cystic lining around the surgical opening are sutured to the surrounding oral mucosa. In the case of a thick bony cover over a cyst, an inverted U-shaped incision is planned with a wider base in the buccal sulcus, mucoperiosteal flap is reflected, and bony window is removed cautiously with burs or rongeurs. The excised tissue of the window created must be subjected to histopathological study. The contents of the cyst are sucked out, and the residual lining of the cyst is inspected. The remainder cystic cavity is irrigated thoroughly to lavage any residual debris. The residual cystic cavity is inspected carefully for any abnormal findings like ulcerative lesions or possible dysplastic/neoplastic areas.The cystic cavity is then packed with ribbon gauze strip soaked with tincture of benzoin or iodoform/white head's varnish or paraffin, or an antibiotic ointment, or bismuth iodine paraffin paste-BIPP, with its end protruding through the opening.

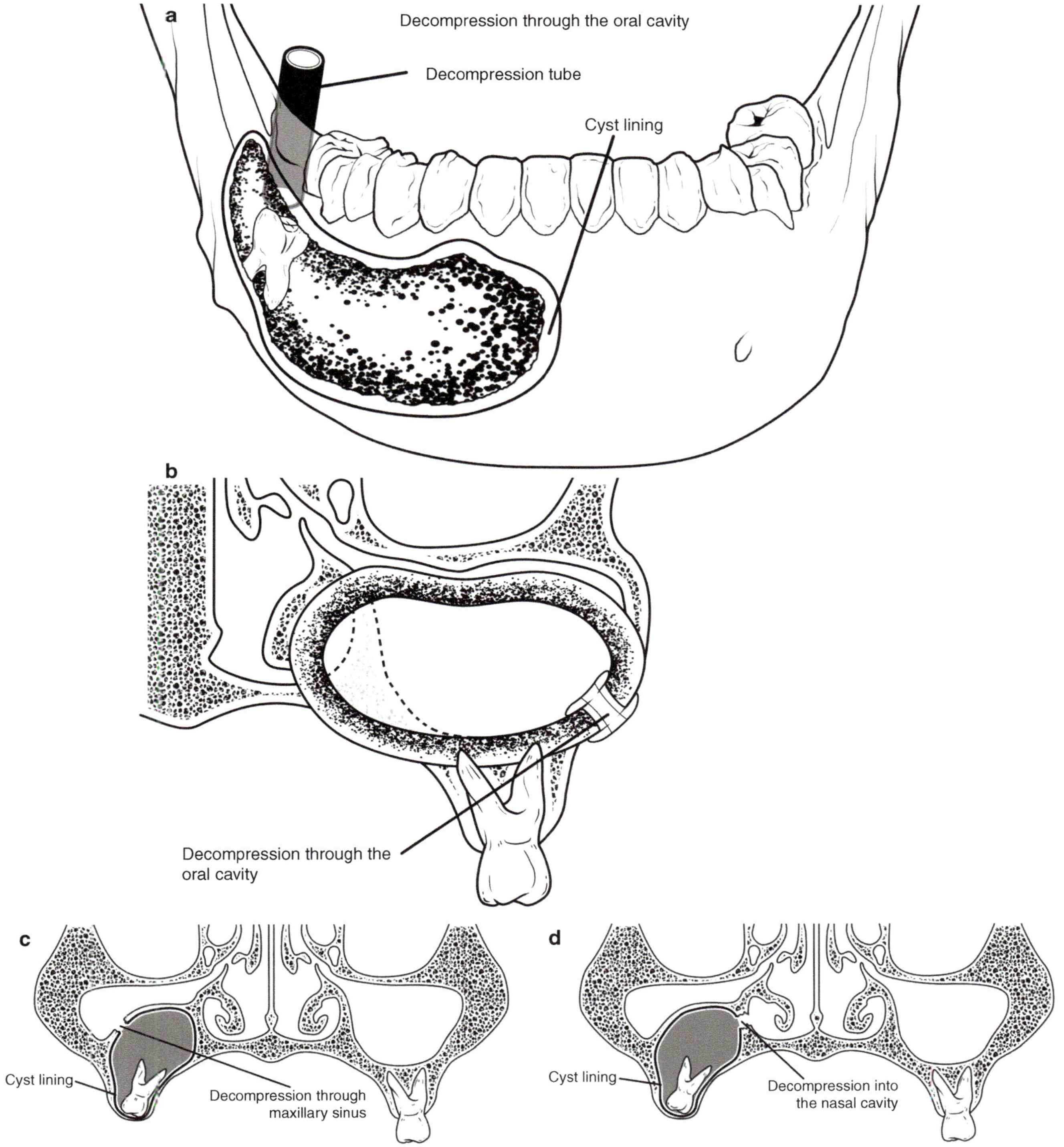




**Fig. 27.8** Decompression of a cystic lesion by creating a small opening and keeping it patent by inserting a drain. (**a**, **b**) Decompression through oral cavity, (**c**) maxillary sinus, (**d**) nasal cavity

This packed gauze strip is left in situ for 2 weeks, until the line of junction between the cystic lining and oral mucosa is healed. After it is removed from the cystic cavity, the patient needs to irrigate/gargle with antiseptic mouthwash frequently in a day to prevent food accumulation. The flushing has to be continued for many following months, until the bone fill and complete healing is noticed.

Later on, acrylic plate or plug/obturator can be prepared to protect the healing cavity and used until it gets obliterated over a period of time, but as the healing progresses, the plug needs periodic adjustments (Table 27.4).

**Table 27.4** Indications, advantages & disadvantages of decompression & marsupialization

| Indications | Advantages | Disadvantages |
|---|---|---|
| • Very large cyst in proximity to vital structures<br>• When apices of many adjacent teeth are involved in large cyst<br>• Guided Assistance for eruption of developing teeth- young children with developing teeth buds or unerupted teeth<br>• Possibility of creating a pathological fracture of a jaw bone<br>• Difficult Surgical access for large multilocular cyst<br>• Medically compromised or debilitated patients<br>• To detect any occult Pathology by visual inspection | • Very simple procedures, not much skill needed, and done under L.A.<br>• Prevents iatrogenic injury to vital structures<br>• Avoids pathological fracture<br>• Gradually decreases the cystic cavity, preserving adjacent oral tissues<br>• Maintains the pulp vitality, avoiding dental extractions<br>• There is a change in the nature of the fragile cystic lining, which becomes thick or converts to normal mucosa, and thereby, secondary enucleation becomes easy.<br>• Reduce the intracystic pressure and induce endosteal bone formation | • Leaves pathological tissue behind<br>• It takes longer healing time<br>• Needs patient commitments to maintain hygiene with repeated irrigations and for long follow-up<br>• Second surgical intervention may be needed.<br>• Not recommended for mentally challenged patients with multiple cystic lesions.<br>• Inability to examine the whole cystic lining histopathologically is also a matter of concern sometimes and may miss out mural pathologic changes |

### 27.8.2 Modification of Marsupialization-Waldron's Method—Two-Staged Procedure [17]

Usually, once the cystic lesion regresses in size after initial marsupialization procedure, enucleation is carried out as a second stage surgery.

The larger or inaccessible cyst is initially marsupialized, and bony healing in progress is observed. As the cystic cavity decreases to a relatively small size, then complete surgical removal is possible by enucleation. The proper time for secondary enucleation is when bone covers adjoining vital structures. This protective shield of new bone prevents their injury during secondary enucleation, also provides adequate strength to the basal jaw bone, and prevents pathological fracture.

In a cyst associated with developing tooth bud, as soon as the tooth erupts into the dental arch alignment, there may not be any residual cystic lining left to enucleate. Decompression and/or marsupialization with less morbidity and preservation of adjoining vital structures has a good rate of success over many other aggressive treatments (Figs. 27.9 and 27.10).

### 27.8.3 Enucleation or Cystectomy or Partsch II (Videos 27.1 and 27.2)

*Enucleation or Cystectomy or Partsch II* with and without adjunct procedures has been validated as the most appropriate surgical modality for almost all cysts of the orofacial region, with various adjunct procedures as deemed fit for individual case.

To enucleate is "complete removal or excision in toto from its envelope without rupture." With this, no bone, other than required for surgically accessing the lesion, is removed.

It is the most versatile treatment modality, and many researchers have said that the surgical enucleation of a cyst in one piece has been known to reduce the rate of recurrence.

An enucleation procedure is possible because of the presence of a fibrous connective tissue layer in between the epithelial lining of a cyst and cystic cavity bony wall. This layer acts as a cleavage point for separating the cystic lining from the jaw bone and makes surgical procedure of enucleation easy, as we carry out stripping of periosteal layer from the jaw bone. The surgical cavity gets filled with the blood clot and eventually gets organized into bone formation.

#### 27.8.3.1 Surgical Procedure

The small cysts can be treated with local anesthesia, but larger cysts need to be treated under general anesthesia. As per the size and site of the lesion, the mucoperiosteal flap is designed, following the right surgical principles. If the bone over the lesion is thinned out, access can be gained by removal of the cortical bone by rongeurs. But if the bony cortex overlying the access area is hard and thick, then the osseous window is created by using rotary burs.

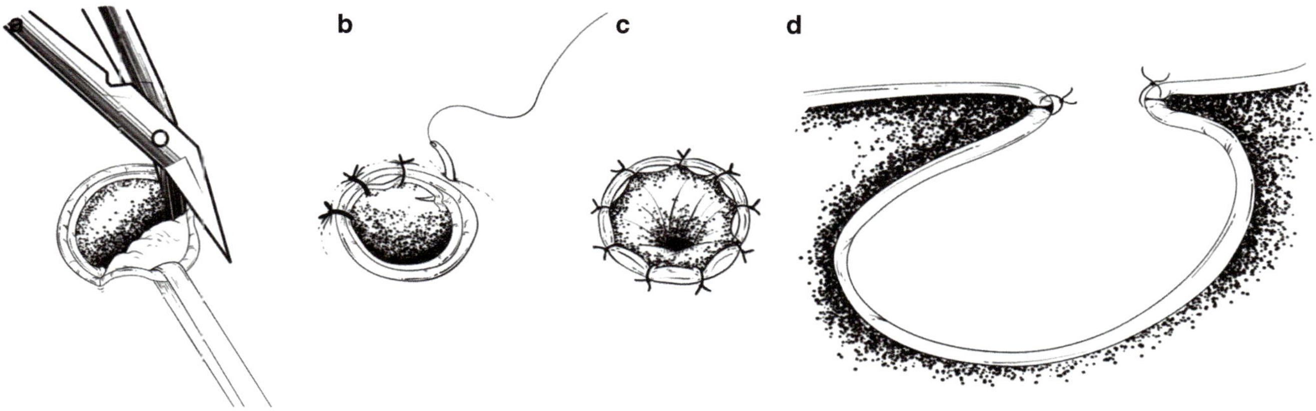




**Fig. 27.9** Diagrammatic representation of Marsupialization procedure; (**a**) creation of opening on the buccal side of a cyst, (**b**) suturing remaining cystic lining to oral mucosa, (**c**) final suturing to keep the cystic cavity open into oral cavity, and (**d**) diagrammatic representation of Marsupialization procedure

After complete enucleation procedure is over, the entire cavity is inspected for proximity of the adjoining vital structures and for the remnants of the pathological tissues.. In large extensive cysts, usually the neurovascular bundle is pushed to one side by the slowly growing lesion, and in these cases, atraumatic enucleation should be carried out. Irrigation and cleaning of the entire bony cavity with saline will assist in visualising/inspecting it. The roughened bony edges of the cavity are then smoothened with a file or rotary bur before final suturing.

Cysts that include tooth roots or certain areas of the jaws, which are surgically inaccessible, require thorough curettage, in order to remove fragile cystic lining fragments. If devitalization of the teeth is brought about during enucleation, then the affected teeth should be treated with root canal fillings.

*Clinical Tips*: If the patient is young and the lesion is involving multiple anterior teeth, the teeth can be retained after root canal treatment and apicectomy, provided thorough inter-radicular curettage by using small periodontal instruments.

If the teeth show a great degree of mobility and in the case of recurrent lesion, they should be extracted.

Enucleation of a cyst is followed by watertight suturing over the sound bone. To achieve this, sometimes, mobilization of the soft tissue flaps with advancement is required. If complete surgical suturing is not possible, then the defect should be packed with stripped ribbon gauze soaked with an antibiotic ointment or BIPP/White head's varnish. Frequent change of this packing is advocated after irrigating the cavity, until new granulation tissue has filled up the cavity and complete epithelisation of the wound has taken place (Fig. 27.11).

#### 27.8.3.2 Enucleation Along with the Adjunct Procedures

Enucleation with different adjuncts has been carried out since many years.

A. *Enucleation with Peripheral Ostectomy*

It is basically used as an additional adjunctive step for peripheral bone trimming for avoiding resection, as almost all hypotheses for recurrence point out toward the possibility of leaving residual pathological fragments behind, especially, in the large cyst with scalloped borders or cysts with difficult access. Here, a greater risk of incomplete excision may exist. Adjunct procedure of peripheral ostectomy may be carried out in cases of cysts, which have high recurrence rate, e.g., Odontogenic Keratocyst. A peripheral ostectomy with rotary bur with sterile irrigation helps to remove all the microscopic residual pathological tissue. The procedure is followed to remove the lesion in one piece along with an enveloping border of bone, and hence, the possibility of iatrogenic rupture of the cystic capsule or leaving its fragments behind is greatly reduced. A minimum 2–5 mm bony margin inclusion for peripheral ostectomy is supposed to be adequate. In the case of thin inferior border of mandible, reinforcement with reconstruction plate is advocated. This can also be accomplished by means of mechanical hand instruments like a sharp curette. The recurrence of the cyst can be prevented by this procedure.

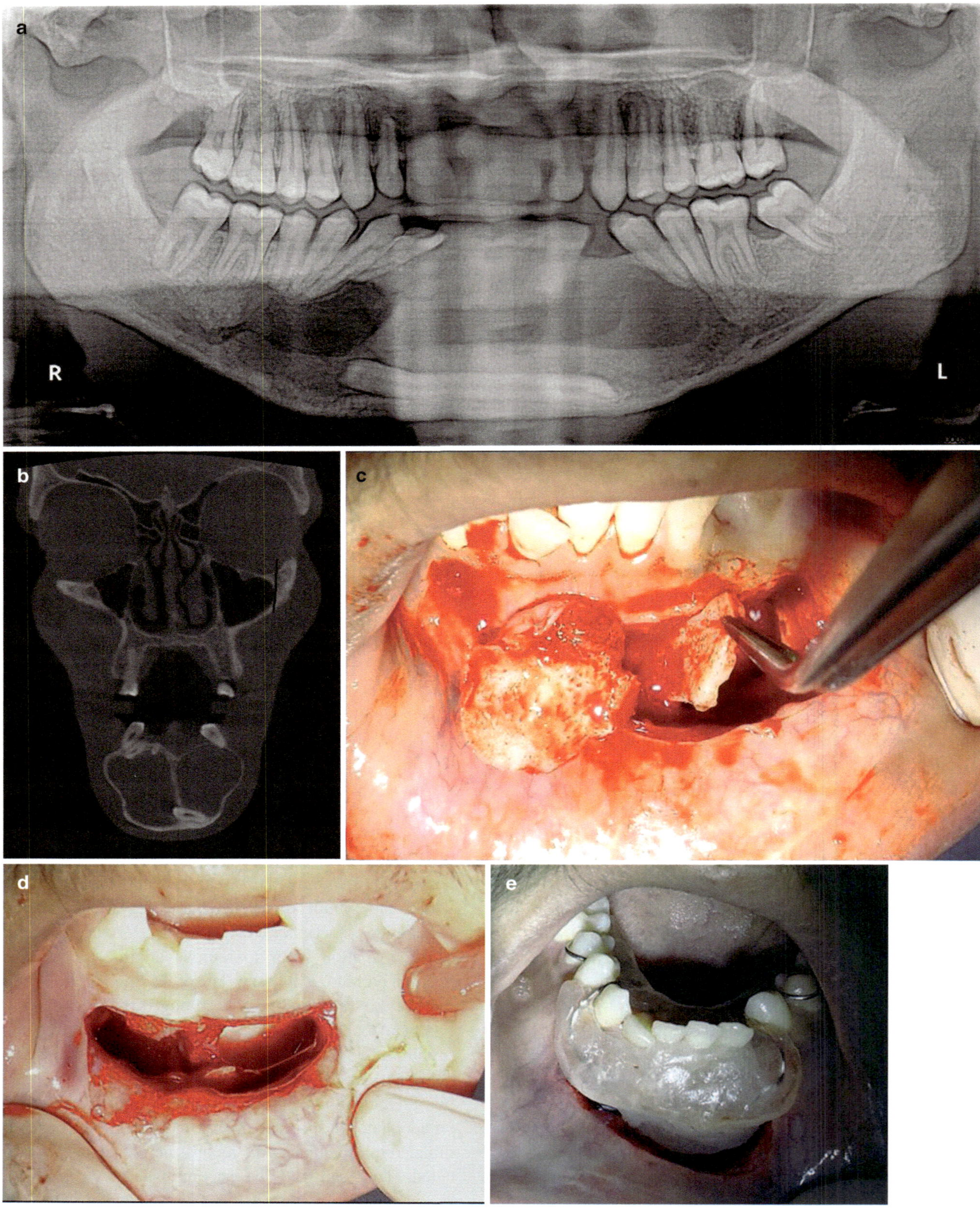


Fig. 27.10 *(CLINICAL CASE SCENARIO)*: (**a**) OPG showing the large radiolucent lesion extending in the mandibular body with impacted canine at the inferior border, (**b**) CT scan of the same patient showing multilocular radiolucent lesion with embedded canine, (**c**) a large opening was created in the anterior body mandible region, and roof of the cyst along with oral mucosa was removed along with the evacuation of the cystic content, (**d**) healing of the wound after marsupialisation, (**e**) acrylic plate was constructed to cover the wound, (**f**) 6 months follow-up, lesion reducing in size, and (**g**) OPG after six months showing the reduction in size of the cyst. The patient is advised to undergo second stage surgery for enucleation and extraction of impacted canine. *Courtesy-Prof. Vidya Rattan, PGI, Chandigarh*

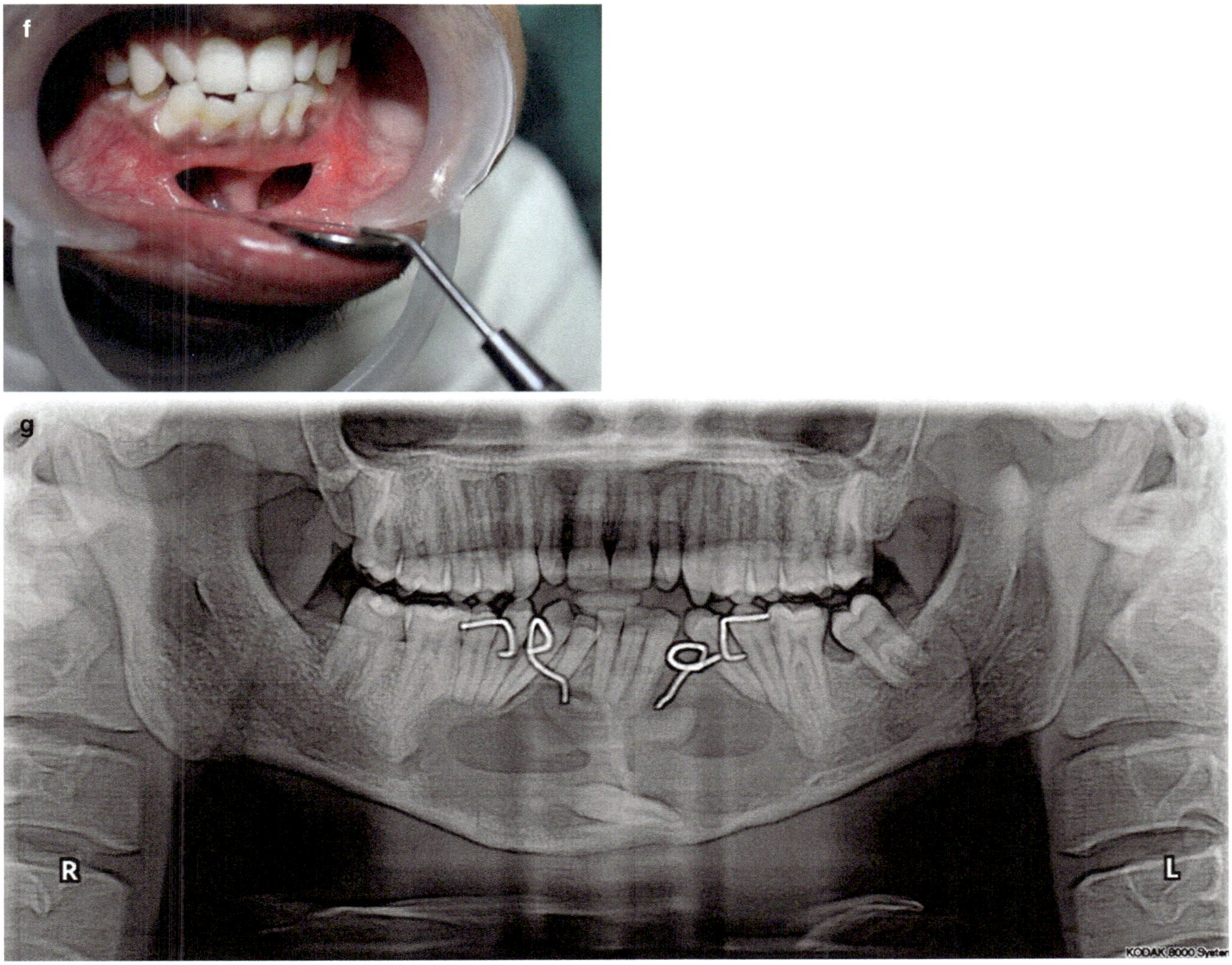




**Fig. 27.10** (continued)

B. *Enucleation and application of Carnoy solution to the bony defect*

Many a times, due to the thin, friable wall and the presence of many small satellite cysts, there is a difficulty of enucleating it in one piece. Hence, the surgical treatment is focused on eliminating all residual epithelial fragments. In order to achieve this, a mild, judiciously penetrating, and cauterizing agent like Carnoy's solution is utilized. It has a mean bone penetration depth of 1.54 mm, with an application time of 5 minutes. (Carnoy's solution's composition is 3 ml of chloroform, 6 ml of absolute ethanol, 1 ml of glacial acetic acid, and 1 g of ferric chloride) [18, 20–22]. This is adequate to bring about chemical cauterization of the residual pathologic fragments. Literature shows the use of modified Carnoy's solution without chloroform, as it is currently listed as a carcinogenic agent.

The protocol of carrying out enucleation followed by the application of Carnoy's solution in the treatment of locally aggressive cysts, like OKCs, lowers the recurrence rate and morbidity. During the application of Carnoy's solution, the neurovascular bundle can be protected by using bone wax cover or wooden spatula or paraffin gauze.

Dashow et al. studied and compared the use of Carnoy's solution versus modified carnoy's solution in cases of OKCs and stated that the recurrence is almost eliminated, and the results are comparable to those of the resection without carrying out the morbid surgery [22].

C. *Enucleation followed by liquid nitrogen cryotherapy*

The aggressive cysts are best treated by enucleation followed by cryotherapy, using liquid nitrogen. This therapy is commonly used for the treatment of many locally aggressive jaw lesions, such as ameloblastoma, OKC, or ossifying fibroma [23]. Cryotherapy destroys the residual

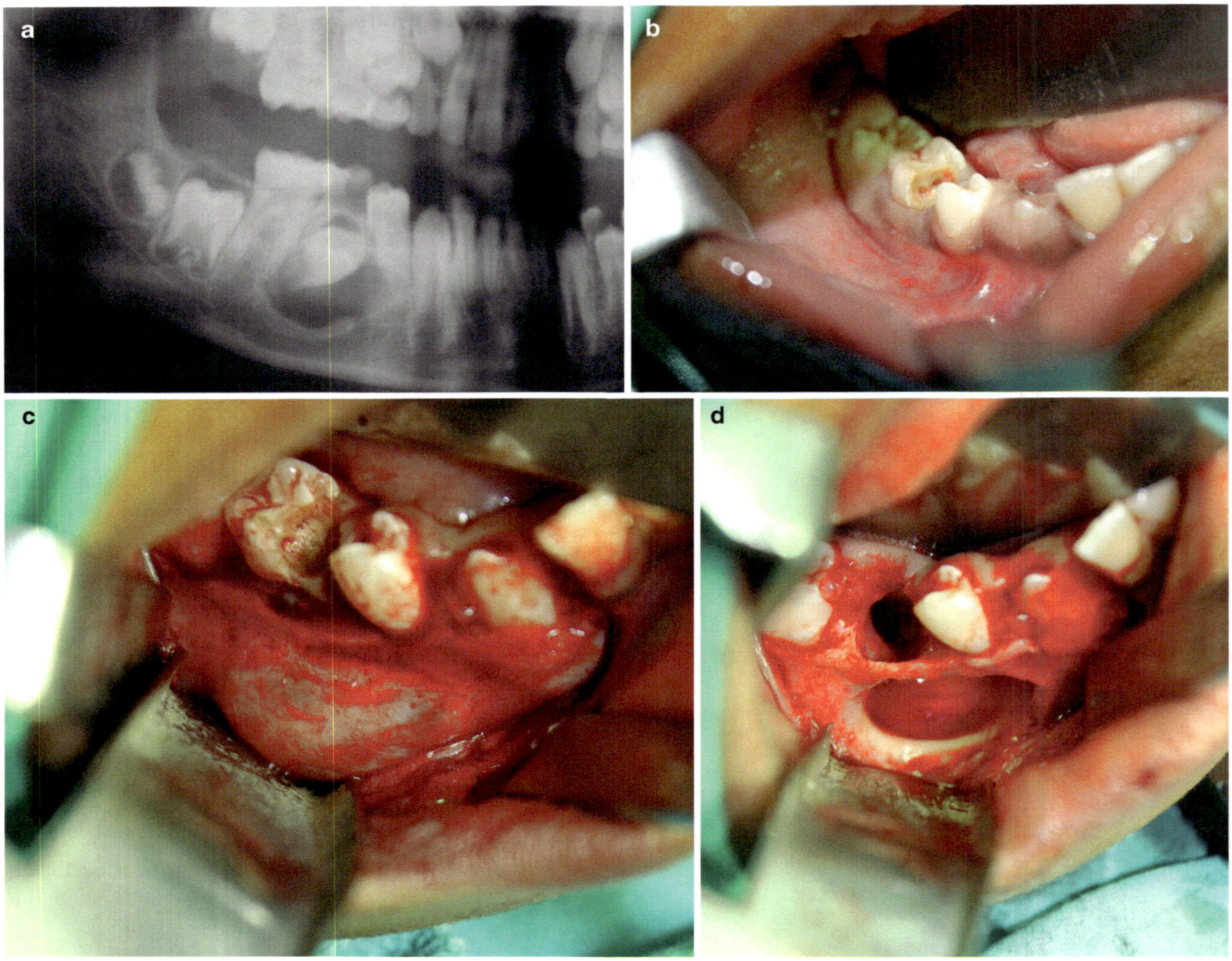

©Association of Oral and Maxillofacial Surgeons of India

**Fig. 27.11** *(CLINICAL CASE SCENARIO)* (**a**) OPG showing the presence of a dentigerous cyst in a 7 years old child, (**b**) clinical intraoral picture of the same, (**c**) reflected flap to expose the underlying expanded buccal cortex, and (**d**) enucleation of the lesion in toto. *Courtesy Dr, Kumar Nilesh, SDS, Karad*

epithelial lining cells or satellite cysts and leaves behind the inorganic bony matrix intact, which is helpful for osteoconduction. Liquid nitrogen causes bone devitalization due to direct effect/damage from ice crystal formation, which takes place in the cellular and extracellular compartments and due to the subsequent osmotic and electrolyte disturbances [23]. The routine first step in surgery of the lesion is enucleation of a cyst, followed by cryotherapy. The adjoining tissues are then shielded by sterile wooden spatula and gauze strip, and the residual cavity is treated with liquid nitrogen spray—two swipes for 1 min each, with a 5 min thaw break between two spray freezes. After cryotherapy, it is possible to place the bone graft in the cystic cavity to strengthen the jaw bone. Finally, the wound is sutured in a watertight manner [23] (Box 27.11 and Table 27.5).

**Box 27.11 The Advantages and Disadvantages of Liquid Nitrogen Cryotherapy After Enucleation**

*Advantages*:

1. The matrix shell of basal bone is left behind, which acts as a scaffold and induces new bone formation.
2. In order to accelerate the bony healing and strengthening the jaw bone, immediate bone grafting can be done. This avoids pathological fracture.
3. It decreases bleeding and scarring.

*Disadvantages*:

1. Unpredictable results are usually due to utilization of uncontrolled spray of liquid nitrogen to the area. This may lead to bone necrosis and postoperative swelling.
2. If liquid nitrogen comes into contact with unprotected inferior alveolar nerve, there will be altered sensation/paraesthesia or total anaesthesia. In most of the cases,partial or total recovery of sensation is expected within 3 months [23].

#### 27.8.3.3 Enucleation Followed by Bone Grafting

*Indications*

1. To avoid pathological fracture,
2. To avoid long-term esthetics and functional problems in larger cystic cavity, more than 4 cm.

Autogenous bone grafts possess characteristic osteoconductive and osteoinductive qualities due to the presence of abundant osteoprogenitor cells. The use of Autogenous cancellous bone grafts for large defects to obliterate the cavity and stimulate osteogenesis is the gold standard, but the issue of donor site morbidity is always there. The dead space elimination after enucleation of a large defect is recommended by packing the defect with autogenous bone graft or its synthetic substitute. Calcium phosphates, α- and β-tricalcium phosphate (TCP), bioactive glasses, calcium sulfate, glass ionomers, hydroxyapatite (HA), etc. are some of the synthetic graft materials available in the market, which can be used instead of autogenous bone grafts, for filling up the defect after enucleation. The blood clot in the cystic cavity is stabilized by these synthetic grafts, thereby minimizing the postoperative infection. These synthetic grafts are also osteoconductive in nature and promote new bone formation by facilitating the migration of osteoprogenitor cells [24, 25].

**Table 27.5** Indications, advantages, & disadvantages of enucleation along with adjunct procedures

| Indications | Advantages | Disadvantages |
|---|---|---|
| 1. For smaller and accessible lesions.<br>2. Medically fit patients with larger lesions.<br>3. If it is possible to enucleate without jeopardizing the vitality & integrity of teeth & adjacent vital structures.<br>4. Enucleation as a second stage procedure after decompression or marsupialization.<br>5. Enucleation along with adjunct procedures. | 1. Better alternative than radical treatment.<br>2. Cyst-oriented treatment<br>3. Entire pathological tissue is removed, which is available for histopathological examination.<br>4. Chances of recurrence are reduced with adjunct procedures. (Elimination of satellite cysts & epithelial remnants)<br>5. Healing period is reduced.<br>6. Maintainance of oral hygiene is easy.<br>7. Enucleation with water tight suturing eliminates the need for long postoperative treatment.<br>8. Good patient compliance.<br>9. Comfortable for patient. | 1. After primary closure, it is not possible to observe the healing cavity.<br>2. In younger patients, erupting teeth have to be extracted.<br>3. Large cyst enucleation may end up in fracture or perforation/damage to adjoining soft tissues.<br>4. Possibility of damaging adjacent vital structures.<br>5. May lead to pulpal necrosis/ devitalization of adjacent teeth.<br>6. Enucleation with fragmentation in inaccessible areas may end up in recurrence. |

### 27.8.4 Block Resection, With or Without Preservation of the Continuity of the Jaw

Resection of a jaw bone can be done either as (1) marginal resection procedure or (2) segmental resection procedure. In marginal resection procedure, the lesion is smaller, which is excised in toto, and hence, it is possible to maintain the continuity of the jaw bone by preserving the portion of the uninvolved bone. In segmental resection procedure, since the lesion is extensive, the complete segment/portion of maxilla or mandible is sacrificed, and hence, continuity of the jaw bone is lost after this radical treatment. Since this procedure ends up in considerable morbidity, there is always a need for rehabilitating the patient functionally and esthetically by various reconstructive measures [26]. Many researchers felt that there is no need for aggressive therapy in the case of cystic lesions, as their management can be done by using relatively noninvasive means [26].

Blanas et al. [21] carried out a systematic review and found that following resection, there was 0% recurrence rate, but it is always associated with the high morbidity rate. Their study suggested that enucleation followed by the use of Carnoy's solution gives similar low recurrence rates, as resection, without unwarranted radical surgery. Complete resection of the mandibular/maxillary bone is considered as morbid overtreatment for large locally aggressive cysts. The only main disadvantage of a conservative treatment is prolonged therapeutic time [27].

In this chapter, we will be discussing only briefly Dentigerous and Keratocyst varieties prototypes.

## 27.9 Dentigerous Cysts or Follicular Cysts

*Dentigerous Cysts or Follicular Cysts*, The term dentigerous is a Latin word, literally means "tooth bearing/producing". Paget in 1853 first coined the term "Dentigerous cyst", in this entity, there is an enclosure of the crown of a tooth, which is unerupted, and cyst is attached to the CE junction and is formed by the enlargement of its follicle [1]. There is always an association of this cyst with the crown of fully or partially impacted or submerged tooth (Fig. 27.12).

Depending on the location and extent of the cystic degeneration in relation to the crown of an unerupted tooth, the cyst can have central, lateral, or circumferential variety [28]. In central type, initially, the crown may be enclosed by a cyst symmetrically, but as it expands, crown of the mandibular third molar may be shifted to the inferior border of the mandible or migrated high up in the ascending ramus and similarly, maxillary canine or third molar may be seen at the orbital floor or high in maxillary sinus. The lateral type will be because of expansion of cyst only on one particular side of the crown, and it will be seen in cases of partially erupted mandibular third molars. In circumferential type, the radiograph will show a radiolucency enveloping the entire tooth (Fig. 27.13).

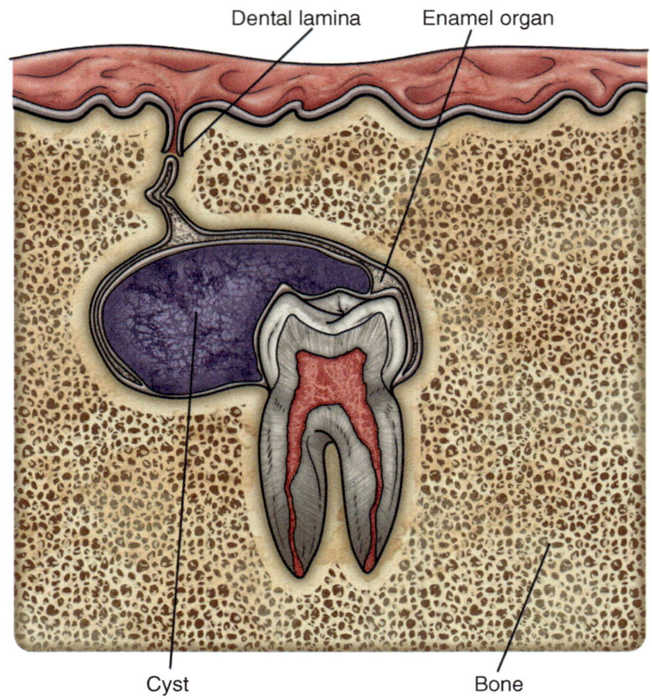



**Fig. 27.12** Formation of a dentigerous cyst

### 27.9.1 Differential Diagnosis

Hyperplastic follicle-Normal follicular space size is 2–3 mm; if it exceeds 5 mm, then dentigerous cyst should be suspected.

Differential diagnosis of unicystic ameloblastoma, an odontogenic keratocyst, Calcified odontogenic cyst, Ameloblastic fibroma, Adenomatoid odontogenic tumor, or radicular cyst must be considered in such cases comparable to the radiographic details, but the incidence of all the above lesions is rare in the first decade of life. Since radiographs alone cannot differentiate the above-mentioned lesions, a histopathological examination should be performed.

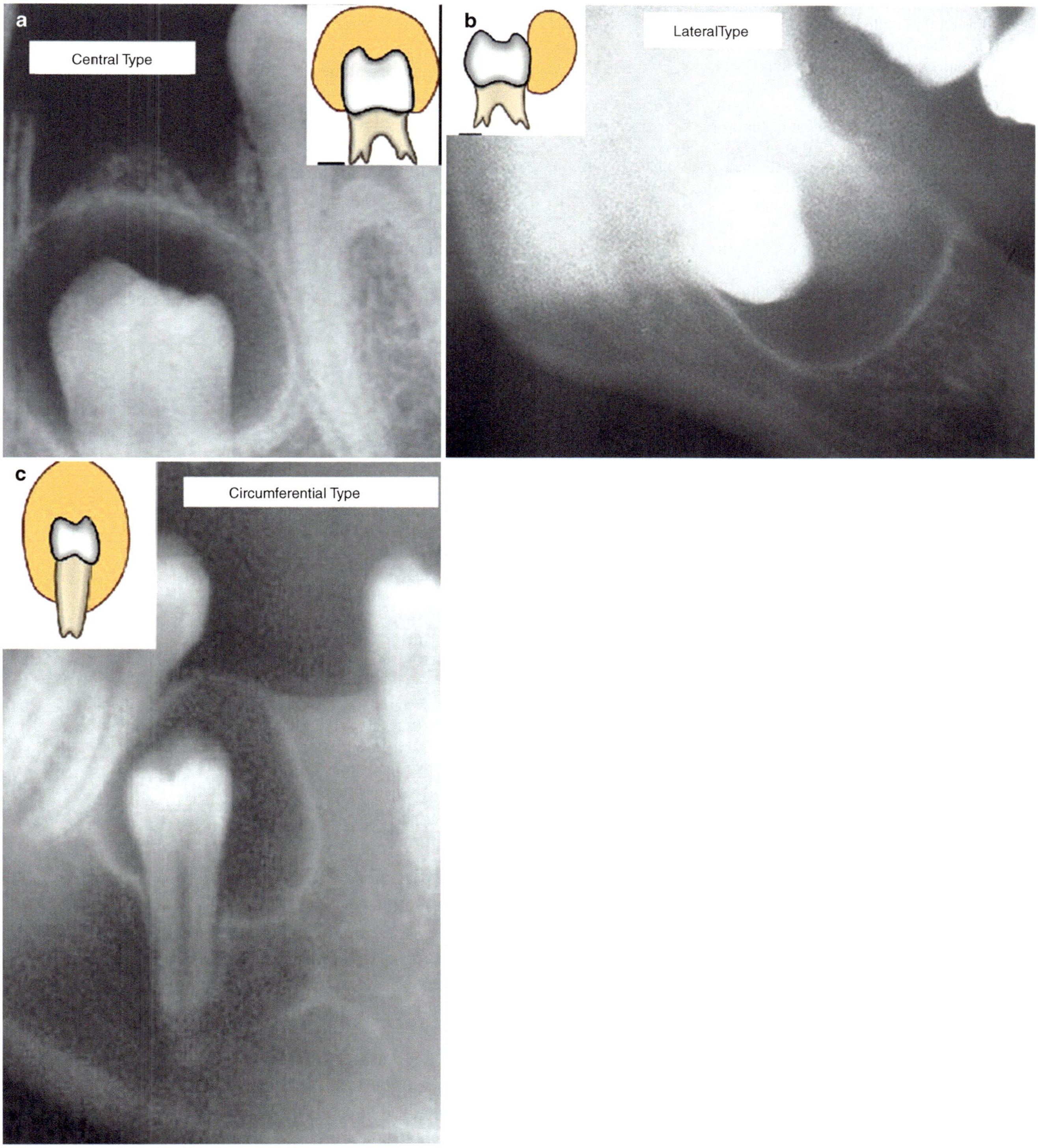




**Fig. 27.13** Types of dentigerous cysts and their radiological picture of central, lateral, and circumferential type (**a**–**c**)

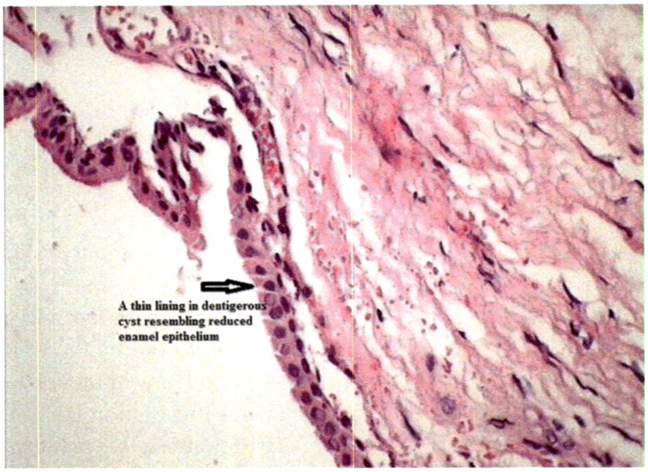




**Fig. 27.14** Arrow pointing to a thin lining in dentigerous cyst resembling reduced enamel epithelium histologically

### 27.9.2 Histology

Thin layer of nonkeratinizing stratified squamous epithelium lining the lumen is seen, and no rete ridges are seen. Connective tissue wall shows bundles of collagen fibers; sometimes, many odontogenic epithelial islands are seen. The cystic lumen contains thin, watery, and yellowish fluid (Fig. 27.14).

### 27.9.3 Potential Complications of Dentigerous Cyst

1. As it is known that dentigerous cysts have potential for neoplastic proliferation in the form of cystic or mural ameloblastoma, in these cases, there is a nodular thickening at some places in the cystic wall, which cannot be discerned clinically, but is a tumor manifestation itself, and therefore, histopathologist is requested to carry out thorough gross and microscopic examination of the whole specimen for nodular thickening, etc. in the cystic wall.
2. Epidermoid carcinoma—cyst lining, which shows longstanding keratin metaplasia, should be considered as a marker for the initiation of carcinomatous changes.
3. Mucoepidermoid carcinoma—dentigerous cyst may contain cells with the potential of mucus secreting ability, which may transform into mucoepidermoid carcinoma [28].

## 27.10 Odontogenic Keratocyst

OKC has got its name because it exhibited keratinization of cystic lining. Its lumen contains a cheesy material resembling keratin debris and clear fluid. It is a Dilemmatic, Distinctive, Odontogenic Developmental, and Intraosseous cyst of epithelial origin of Oral & maxillofacial region, with specific characteristics, such as rapid Infiltrative growth, aggressive nature, high recurrence rate and defined histopathological features [26, 27]. Since 1956, for the last six decades, many researchers started focusing on this entity. Journey of this changing nomenclature is pretty interesting (Box 27.12).

**Box 27.12 History of OKC**

| | |
|---|---|
| 1774 | Dental cyst (John Hunter) |
| 1876 | Dermoid cyst (Mikulicz) identified & described as a part of familial jaw condition |
| 1926 | Cholesteatoma (Hauer) |
| 1945 | Primordial cyst as per origin |
| 1956 | Odontogenic Keratocyst (OKC) (Philipsen first coined the word) |
| 1963 | Aggressive growth/high tendency for recurrence rate (described by Pindborg & Hansen) |
| 1967 | Regarded OKC as a benign tumor (Toller) |
| 1992 | OKC as preferred term for keratinized cysts (WHO) |
| 2004 | Keratinizing Cystic Odontogenic Tumor( KCOT) (Reichart & Philipsen) |
| 2005 | Keratocystic Odontogenic Tumor (KOT) (WHO working group) |
| 2017 | Odontogenic Keratocyst (WHO) |

In 2004, Reichart and Philipsen suggested a new classification for the odontogenic tumors, redesignated OKC as Keratinizing cystic Odontogenic Tumor (KCOT), and put it under the subcategory of "benign neoplasm of odontogenic epithelium with mature, fibrous stroma "due to its propensity for local destruction, aggressive biological behavior, and high recurrence rate and mitotic figures seen in the suprabasal layers [29]. Shear had re-emphasized that OKC shows increased proliferative activity & high recurrence tendency and stressed on association of OKC with the Gorlin-Goltz syndrome/Nevoid Basal Cell Carcinoma syndrome (NBCCS). Some of these OKCs had association with the PTCH 1 gene mutation and increased immunohistochemical expression of proliferation markers Ki 67 and presence of PCNA (Proliferating cell nuclear antigen marker of cell replication) and p53 in KCOT. All this evidence led to change in nomenclature by WHO in 2005 [10].

This shift in tumor category suggested change in management protocol for OKC, which created a lot of skepticism, and the concept was not widely accepted, with the reason being not all OKCs possess identifiable PTCH mutation. There were no clear-cut suggestions such as neoplastic title was to be applied to all OKC or to just a small subset. All relevant sequencing data on the odontogenic keratocysts has not yet been presented and still under research.

Researchers have suggested that marsupialization can revert the fragile cystic lining epithelium to normal oral mucosa or from parakeratin to orthokeratin type [30, 31].

Extensive debate (for 12 years) over putative neoplastic nature of the lesion took place. So, in 2017, a WHO expert panel declared that there is no strong affirmation to rationalize to label OKC as a neoplasm, and therefore, Odontogenic Keratocyst-OKC should be put back in cyst category and the term keratocystic odontogenic tumor (KCOT) was eliminated from the new classification (Boxes 27.13, 27.14, 27.15, 27.16, 27.17 and 27.18).

**Box 27.13 Epidemiology of OKC**

*Incidence*: Second most prevalent cysts of odontogenic origin (10–12% of all odontogenic cysts) [32].

*Age*: Wide age range. Range of occurrence between the 1st and 9th decades of life. Bimodal age distribution (first peak at 20–30 & second at 50–60 years of age) and Predominantly in younger patients in syndromic cases.

*Sex*: Male predilection (1.6:1 ratio), More Female predilection in syndromic cases.

*Race*: predominantly in white population.

**Box 27.14 Site Predilection of OKC**

*Central intraosseous Lesion*—Thrice more prevalent in mandible. Seen more at various sites in following order-angle-ascending ramus, maxillary third molar region (*may involve sinus, nasal floor premaxilla, presence of impacted third molar seen, and occasionally floor of orbit involvement*), mandibular, premolar area, and maxillary canine.

*Peripheral OKC in buccal gingiva* (female predominance 2.2:1 ratio [33])

**Box 27.15 Number of Cysts in OKC**

- Usually solitary/sporadic/nonsyndromic lesions
- *Syndromic*: Multiple OKCs are often one of the manifestations of genetically inherited Nevoid Basal cell Carcinoma Syndrome (NBCCS), Gorlin-Goltz syndrome, etc. [In syndromic cases, multiple cysts can be seen in one patient at a time or during lifetime occurrence, many cysts can happen at different times [34].
- *Nonsyndromic multiple cysts* [34]

**Box 27.16 Syndromic Associations of OKC**

- Basal cell nevus syndrome, Nevoid Basal cell Carcinoma Syndrome (NBCCS), or Gorlin-Goltz syndrome
- Marfan syndrome
- Noonan syndrome
- Orofacial Digital Syndrome
- Simpson–Golabi-Behmel syndrome

**Box 27.17 Latest Histopathological Groups of OKC**

As per the occurrence of satellite/daughter cysts & squamous islands found in the cystic wall (Kahraman et al. [35]) (Fig. 27.17)

*Group I*: Unicystic, without any satellites (63%)

*Group II*: With few satellite/microcysts & squamous islands in the cystic lining less than (10–27%)

*Group III*: Abundant presence of satellite/daughter cysts and squamous islands (6–10%)

### 27.10.1 Etiology and Pathogenesis

Various origins—Two sources are implicated.

1. Remnants of dental lamina and
2. It can originate from downgrowth or implantation following trauma of the offshoots of epithelial basal layer of the oral gingiva and mucosa [27]. Islands of Epithelium and/or daughter cysts are seen in 50% of the cases, in overly-

**Box 27.18 Reasons for Recurrence of OKC (13–62%; Nakamura et al. [36])**

1. Thin walls and fragile epithelial lining
2. Epithelial lining is weakly attached to capsule
3. Extension of the cyst into cancellous bone
4. Dental lamina remnants in bone/overlying mucosa
5. In the case of perforation of the cortex, cyst lining adheres to adjoining bone or buccal or lingual mucosa (especially, lingual perforation is difficult to access during enucleation)
6. In dentate area (residual remnants in intraradicular areas)
7. Scalloped margins in multilocular variety
8. Desire to preserve adjacent vital structures
9. Location with difficult access
10. Extensive lesion involving coronoid/ascending ramus (difficult access)

ing mucosa. (In the past designated as basal cell hamartias). Genetic factors are also always key players, especially PTCH gene aberration.

### 27.10.2 Unique Growth Pattern—Peculiar Behavior—Pattern of Bone Involvement in OKC

Unlike other cysts, lesion grows by extension in medullary space in anteroposterior direction, compared to osmotic expansion.

Finger-like projections are seen in marrow spaces, and enlargement goes on relentlessly along the path of least resistance. When it reaches a considerable size, it expands buccolingually also (Figs. 27.15 and 27.16).

### 27.10.3 Radiographic Differential Diagnosis

OKC is a great mimic; many times, the radiographic picture is nonpathognomonic. Radiographically, the following differential diagnosis for Odontogenic Keratocyst has been suggested:

Dentigerous cyst, residual cyst, radicular cyst, lateral periodontal cyst, Nasopalatine cyst, Unicystic/multicystic ameloblastoma, A-V malformation, fibro-osseous lesion at initial stages, Benign intraosseous neoplasms, traumatic cyst. Patients with multiple jaw cysts should always be evaluated for basal cell nevus syndrome.

### 27.10.4 Aspiration

- Cheesy, straw color, caseous, dirty milky white semifluid, and viscoid content-Keratin-varying consistencies reflect various densities of keratinous debris.
- Protein content less than 3.5/4 g per 100 ml by electrophoresis, mostly albumin is present.
- Protein-53 is positive in NBCC Syndrome, indicating active proliferation of cells.
- Exfoliative cytology/smear is stained & examined for keratin cells, and Estimation of Keratocyst Antigen (KCA) and Lactoferrin levels is helpful.
- Immunohistochemistry for cytokeratin is also a useful diagnostic tool

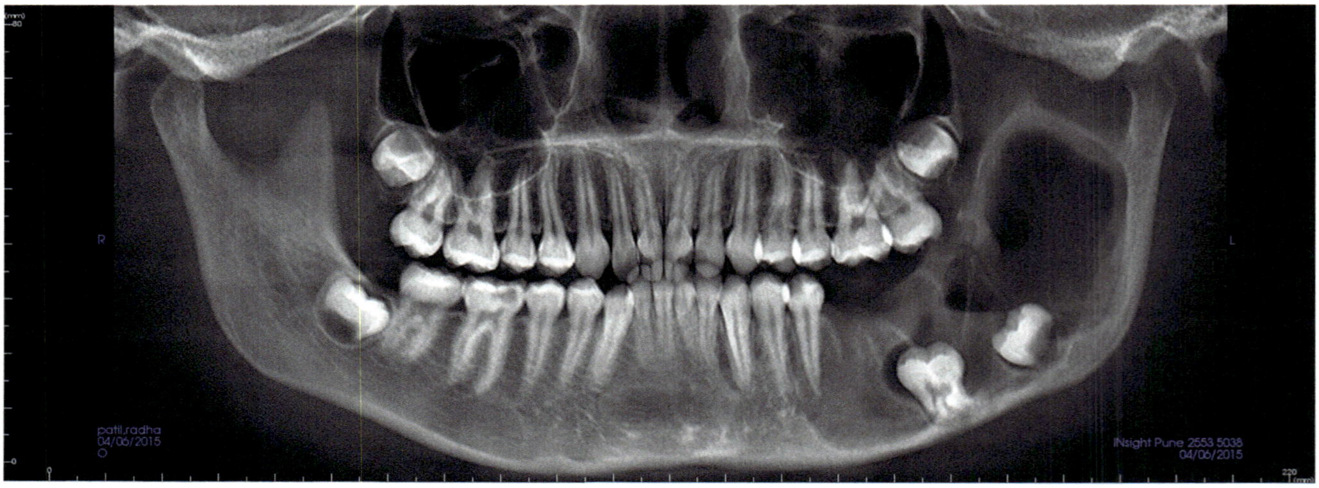




**Fig. 27.15** OPG showing how lesion grows in medullary space (in anteroposterior direction), multiloculated radiolucency in left angle, and ascending ramus with impacted teeth diagnosed as OKC

### 27.10.5 Surgical Treatment

Incidence of these lesions is seen more in younger age group and the supportive evidence of success of conservative treatment options like marsupialisation for large expanding OKCs or two-staged surgical procedures, plus the fact of alteration of the remaining epithelium, i.e., return to more normal oral epithelium after decompression/marsupialisation has prompted many to opt for these procedures. The lesions, which are easily accessible, can be enucleated by adjunctive methods.

#### 27.10.5.1 Resection

- It should be used as a last alternative method
- Resection of the jaw bone results in morbidity and requires extensive reconstruction/rehabilitation, which is unwarranted in the treatment of benign lesions, and hence, most of the times, more conservative approaches are sought.

*Absolute indications*

- Multiple recurrences

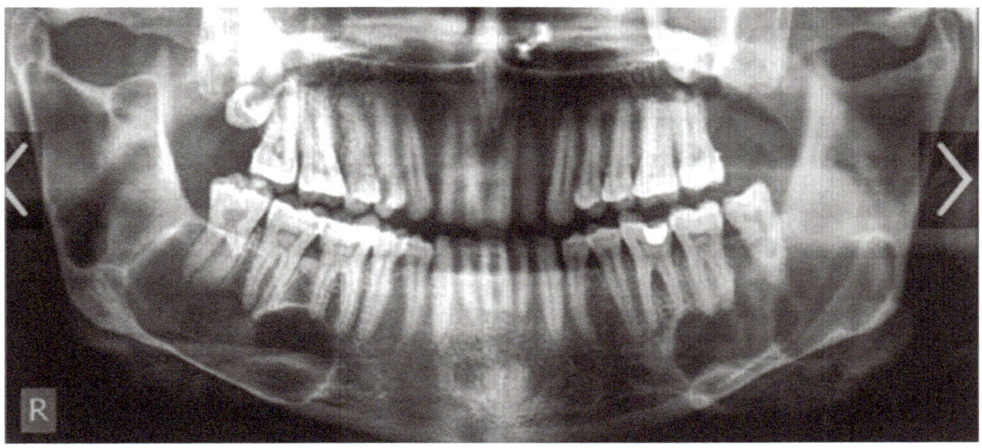




**Fig. 27.16** Multiple cysts in the same individual, involving both maxilla and mandible

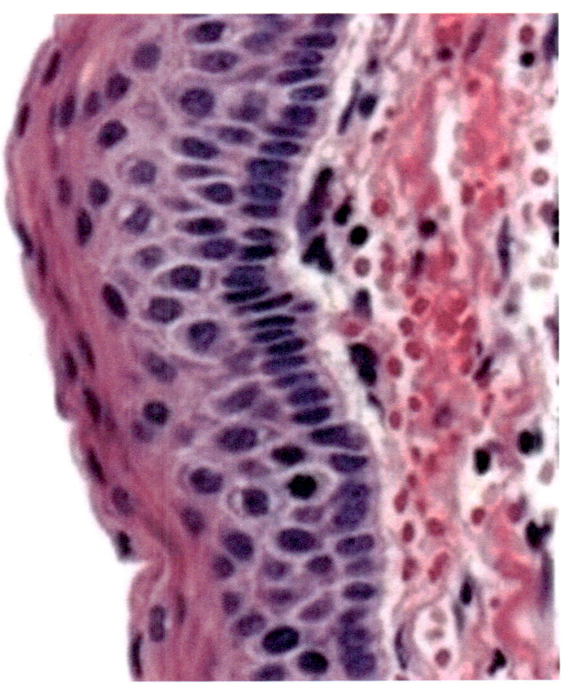

**HISTOPATHOLOGIC CRITERIA OF OKC-SHEAR & PINDBORG (1960–62)**

- Thin, collapsed and folded, corrugated lining
- Zone of uniform parakeratinized stratified squamous epithelium 5–8 cell layers with no rete pegs
- Picket fence / tombstone appearance of hyperchromatic palisaded basal cells with reversed polarity
- Weak epithelial connective tissue interface
- Presence of daughter satellite cyst



**Fig. 27.17** Typical histopathological picture of OKC showing all the features

- Extensive soft tissue invasion and multiple large perforations
- Resection is used only in aggressive extensive cases or under extraordinary situations
- Condylar involvement or lesions that have undergone ameloblastomatous/malignant transformation

*Follow-up*

- After surgery, yearly follow-up till 5 years postoperatively
- After 5 years of follow-up, once in 2 years as long as patient cooperates
- Lifelong follow-up is a must-more than 10–20 years

### 27.10.6 Basal Cell Nevus Syndrome/Nevoid Basal Cell Carcinoma Syndrome

It is also known as bifid rib syndrome or Gorlin and Goltz syndrome or multiple jaw cyst syndrome. This is a genetically inherited uncommon affliction with autosomal dominant trait/inheritance and high penetration.

This syndrome's complex manifestations include relative frontal bossing, Ocular hypertelorism, brain tumors, midface hypoplasia, mandibular prognathism, mental retardation, schizophrenia, multiple basal cell nevi/epitheliomas on the skin, calcification of the falx cerebri, bifid ribs and vertebral anomalies, palmar pitting (the pits later develop into basal cell carcinoma), ovarian tumors, CNS disturbances, hypogonadism in males,cleft lip and palate, etc., and 50% of cases show multiple KCOT-now OKCs. Multiple KCOTs (OKCs) are indicative of basal cell nevus syndrome until diagnosed otherwise. 5% of the patients with KCOT/OKC are diagnosed having basal cell nevus syndrome. Early identification of these patients with their associated manifestations along with proper treatment planning and long-term follow-up will improve the long-term survival rate and quality of life.

## 27.11 Conclusion

Cysts of the jaw bones are considered as one of the most common pathologies in the oral and maxillofacial region. Various tumors mimic the clinical features of cysts and, thus, can be confused with the same. Radiography alone cannot be the diagnostic tool to distinguish various jaw cysts. Cysts are benign lesions, but few will show locally aggressive and destructive behavior. The detailed present and past history of the patient accompanied by a thorough clinical examination along with aspiration biopsy will lead to probable differential diagnosis. Both conservative and aggressive surgical treatment modalities have been used in the past to treat orofacial cysts with variable results, depending on the type of cyst. Correct final diagnosis, thorough planning, meticulous surgery with stringent protocols, and watchful long-term postoperative follow-up will ensure high success rate.

## References

1. Shear M, Speight PM, editors. Cysts of the oral and maxillofacial regions. 4th ed. Oxford: Blackwell Munksgaard; 2007.
2. Kramer IRH, Pidborg JJ, Shear M. Histological typing of odontogenic tumors. Berlin: Springer-Verlag; 1992.
3. Regezi J, Sciubba J, Jordan R. Oral pathology: clinical pathological correlations. 4th ed. St. Louis: Elsevier Health Sciences; 2016. p. 244–54.
4. Browne RM. The pathogenesis of odontogenic cysts: a review. J Oral Pathol. 1975;4(Suppl 1):31–46.
5. Harris M, Toller P. The pathogenesis of dental cyst. Br Med Bull. 1975;31(Suppl 2):159–63.
6. Shrestha P, Yamada K, Higashiyama H, Takagi H, Mori M. Epidermal growth factor receptor in odontogenic cysts and tumors. J Oral Pathol Med. 1992;21(Suppl 7):314–7.
7. Sakamoto S, Sakamoto M, Goldhaber P, Glimcher M. Collagenase and bone resorption: isolation of collagenase from culture medium containing serum after stimulation of bone resorption by addition of parathyroid hormone extract. Biochem Biophys Res Commun. 1975;63(Suppl 1):172–8.
8. Harvey W, Guat-Chen F, Gordon D, Meghji S, Evans A, Harris M. Evidence for fibroblasts as the major source of prostacyclin and prostaglandin synthesis in dental cyst in man. Arch Oral Biol. 1984;29(Suppl 3):223–9.
9. Meghji S, Harvey W, Harris M. Interleukin 1-like activity in cystic lesions of the jaw. Br J Oral Maxillofac Surg. 1989;27(Suppl 1):1–11.
10. Barnes L, Eveson JW, Reichart P, Sidransky D. Pathology and genetics of head and neck tumours: WHO classification of tumours. 3rd ed. Lyon: IARC Press; 2005. p. 107–62.
11. Wright JM, Vered M. Update from the 4th edition of the World Health Organization; classification of head and neck tumours: odontogenic and maxillofacial bone tumors. Head Neck Pathol. 2017;11(Suppl 1):68–77.
12. Martin L, Speight PM. Mini-symposium: pathology of the jaws. Odontogenic cysts. Diagn Histopathol. 2015;21:359–69.
13. Olojede O, Adisa AO, Effiom O, Warith AA. Cysts of the orofacial region: a clinicopathologic review of 403 Nigerian cases. East Afr Med J. 2017;94(Suppl 2):116–24.
14. Das AK, Prajapati VK. Concentration of proteins in intra osseous jaw cysts as an adjunct to diagnosis. Int J Sci Stud. 2015;2:150–5.
15. Toller PA, Holborow EJ. Immunoglobulins and immunoglobulin containing cells in cysts of the jaws. Lancet. 1969;2(Suppl 7613):178–81.
16. Smith AJ, Matthews JB, Mason GI, Browne RM. Lactoferrin in aspirates of odontogenic cyst fluid. J Clin Pathol. 1988;41(Suppl 10):1117–9.
17. Pogrel MA. Treatment of keratocysts: the case for decompression and marsupialization. J Oral Maxillofac Surg. 2005;63(Suppl 11):1667–73.
18. Voorsmit RA, Stoelinga PJ, van Haelst UJ. The management of keratocysts. J Maxillofac Surg. 1981;9:228–36.
19. Sun J, Wu J, Zhou N, Meng N, Lin Y. A prospective study of jaw odontogenic keratocyst treated by multidisciplinary sequential treatment. Int J Oral Maxillofac Surg. 2009;38(Suppl 5):537.

20. Morgan TA, Burton CC, Qian F. A retrospective review of treatment of odontogenic keratocyst. J Oral Maxillofac Surg. 2005;63(Suppl 5):635–9.
21. Blanas N, Freund B, Schwartz M, Furst IM. Systematic review of the treatment and prognosis of the odontogenic keratocyst. Oral Surg Oral Med Oral Pathol Oral Radiol Endod. 2000;90(Suppl 5):553–8.
22. Dashow JE, McHugh JB, Braun TM, Edwards SP, Helman JI, Ward BB. Significant decreased recurrence rates in keratocystic odontogenic tumour with simple enucleation and curettage using carnoy's versus modified carnoy's solution. J Oral Maxillofac Surg. 2015;73(Suppl 11):2132–5.
23. Schmidt BL, Pogrel MA. The use of enucleation and liquid nitrogen cryotherapy in the management of odontogenic keratocysts. J Oral Maxillofac Surg. 2001;59(Suppl 7):720-5–6-7.
24. Ochandiano CS. Bone cavity filling with alloplastic material in maxillofacial surgery. Rev Esp Cir Oral Maxillofac. 2007;29(Suppl 1):21–32.
25. Ettl T, Gosau M, Sader R, Reichert TE. Jaw cysts—filling or no filling after enucleation? A review. J Craniomaxillofac Surg. 2012;40(Suppl 6):485–93.
26. Stolinga PJ. Long term follow-up on keratocysts treated according to a defined protocol. Int J Oral Maxillofac Surg. 2001;30(Suppl 1):14–25.
27. Giuliani M, Grossi GB, Lajolo C, Bisceglia M, Herb KE. Conservative management of large odontogenic keratocyst: report of a case and review of the literature. J Oral Maxillofac Surg. 2006;64(Suppl 2):308–16.
28. Neville BW, Damn DD, Allen CM, Bouquot JE. Oral and maxillofacial pathology. 3rd ed. Philadelphia: WB Saunders; 2004.
29. Reichart P, Philipsen H. Odontogenic tumours and allied lesions. 3rd ed. New Malden: Quintessence Publishing; 2004.
30. Wushou A, Zhao YJ, Shao ZM. Marsupialization is the optimal treatment approach for keratocystic odontogenic tumour. J Craniomaxillofac Surg. 2014;42(Suppl 7):1540–4.
31. Maurette PE, Jorge J, de Moraes M. Conservative treatment protocol of odontogenic keratocyst: a preliminary study. J Oral Maxillofac Surg. 2006;64(Suppl 3):379–83.
32. Chirapathomsakul D, Sastravaha P, Jansisyanont P. A review of odontogenic keratocysts and the behaviour of recurrences. Oral Surg Oral Med Oral Pathol Oral Radiol Endod. 2006;101(Suppl 1):5–9.
33. Chuong R, et al. The odontogenic keratocyst. J Oral Maxilllofac Surg. 1982;40:797–802.
34. Auluck A, Suhas S, Pai KM. Multiple odontogenic keratocysts: report of a case. J Can Dent Assoc. 2006;72(7):651–6.
35. Kahraman D, Gunhan O, Celasun B. A series of 240 odontogenic keratocysts: should we continue to use the terminology of "keratocystic odontogenic tumour" for the solid variant of odontogenic keratocyst? J Craniomaxillofac Surg. 2018;46(6):942–6.
36. Nakamura N, et al. Marsupialization for odontogenic keratocyst: long term follow up analysis of the effects and changes in growth characteristics. Oral Surg Oral Med Oral Pathol Oral Radiol Endod. 2002;94(Suppl 5):543–53.

# Benign Odontogenic Tumours

# 28

Anjan Kumar Shah

## 28.1 Introduction

The region of Head and Neck has a wide range of pathological disorders due to the complex nature of the tissues in this region. The tooth-forming tissues can give rise to a wide array of tumours, both benign and malignant. They vary in size from tiny swelling to a large variety, causing cortical bone perforation with the displacement of the adjoining normal anatomic structures. Odontogenic tumours are slow growing and generally non-aggressive, with aggressive behaviour shown by certain tumours.

It is important for the clinician to have a thorough knowledge of the pathology, clinical as well as radiological presentation in order to manage these conditions.

**According to W.H.O** [1]
'Odontogenic tumours and tumour-like lesions constitute a group of heterogeneous diseases that range from hamartomatous or non-neoplastic tissue proliferations to benign neoplasms and finally malignant tumours with metastatic potential. They are derived from epithelial, ectomesenchymal and/or mesenchymal elements of the tooth-forming apparatus. Odontogenic tumours are rare, some being extremely rare, but can pose a significant diagnostic and therapeutic challenge.'

The WHO first classified benign odontogenic tumours in 1971 followed by in 1992, 2005 and the recent classification was in 2017. The origin-based sub-classification was first defined in 1992, which is still in use, i.e. the tumours are sub-classified into Epithelial origin, Mixed origin and Mesenchymal origin. The metastasising (malignant) ameloblastoma is included in epithelial origin tumour in 2017 WHO classification and desmoplastic ameloblastoma was excluded from the classification of benign odontogenic tumour. In 1992 classification, adenomatoid odontogenic tumour (AOT) was considered under mixed origin but in 2005 and 2017 classification, it is included in the epithelial origin tumour [2].

The dentinogenic ghost cell tumour (DGCT) comes under the spectrum of ghost cell lesions. Gorlin et al. in 1962 first described calcifying odontogenic cyst (COC) as the earliest ghost cell lesions. In 2005 WHO classification, COC is renamed as calcifying cystic odontogenic tumour (CCOT). Fejerskov and Krogh used the term calcifying ghost cell odontogenic tumour for DGCT in 1972. Dentigerous ghost cell tumour term was given by Praetorious et al. in 1981, which is still retained in 2005 and 2017 WHO classification. In between, Shear in 1983 used the term dentinoameloblastoma, whereas Ellis and Shmookler proposed epithelial odontogenic ghost cell tumour. Hong et al. in 1991 suggests the term epithelial odontogenic ghost cell tumour [3, 4].

## 28.2 WHO (2017) Classification of Odontogenic Tumours [5]

### 28.2.1 Benign Odontogenic Tumours

#### 28.2.1.1 Epithelial Origin

- Ameloblastoma, conventional
  Ameloblastoma, unicystic type
  Ameloblastoma, extraosseous/peripheral type
  Metastasising (Malignant) ameloblastoma
- Squamous odontogenic tumour
- Calcifying epithelial odontogenic tumour
- Adenomatoid odontogenic tumour

**Electronic Supplementary Material** The online version of this chapter (https://doi.org/10.1007/978-981-15-1346-6_28) contains supplementary material, which is available to authorized users.

A. K. Shah (✉)
Department of OMFS, Rajarajeswari Dental College, Bangalore, India

Bhagwan Mahaveer Jain Hospital, Bangalore, India


K. Bonanthaya et al. (eds.), *Oral and Maxillofacial Surgery for the Clinician*, https://doi.org/10.1007/978-981-15-1346-6_28

#### 28.2.1.2 Mixed (Epithelial-Mesenchymal) Origin

- Ameloblastic Fibroma
- Primordial odontogenic tumour
- Odontoma, complex type
- Odontoma compound type
- Dentinogenic ghost cell tumour

#### 28.2.1.3 Mesenchymal Origin

- Odontogenic Fibroma
- Odontogenic myxoma/myxofibroma
- Cementoblastoma

### 28.2.2 Malignant Odontogenic Tumours

- Ameloblastic carcinoma
- Primary intra-osseous carcinoma, NOS
- Sclerosing odontogenic carcinoma
- Clear cell odontogenic carcinoma
- Ghost cell odontogenic carcinoma
- Odontogenic carcinosarcoma
- Odontogenic sarcomas

## 28.3 Ameloblastoma

### 28.3.1 Introduction

It is the most common odontogenic tumour arising from odontogenic epithelium.

Ameloblastoma originates from sources, which include [6]

- Epithelial cell rests of Malessez, which are the residual epithelium of the tooth-forming apparatus.
- Epithelium of the enamel origin and of odontogenic cysts
- Surface epithelium of the basal cells
- Heterotopic epithelium from the extra-oral sites such as pituitary gland

Edited 2017 WHO classification of odontogenic tumours has simplified the classification of Ameloblastomas. It has removed the various pathologically descriptive classification terminologies such as follicular, plexiform, basaloid, granular or desmoplastic as these terminologies do not have any relevance to clinical behaviour. Conventional-type Ameloblastomas are characterised by multilocular, expanding behaviour. The histological margin is characterised by the infiltrating margin, requires wide excision with a margin of 0.5–1 cm of normal bone, or one anatomical layer if grown out of the confines of the bone. That is if bony cortex invaded, then take muscle or subcutaneous tissue to maintain periosteum as anatomical barrier.

### 28.3.2 Definition

'It is a true neoplasm of enamel organ-type tissue, which does not undergo differentiation to the point of enamel formation" proposed by WHO. Robinson [7] defined it as a "Non-functional, unicentric, intermittent in growth, anatomically benign and clinically persistent type of tumour'

### 28.3.3 Incidence

It represents 19.3–41.5 % of all odontogenic tumours [8, 9]. Posterior Mandible is the commonest site of occurrence in almost 80% of ameloblastomas [10]. It occurs over a broad range; cases ranging from adults older than 90 to the children younger than 10 years. Most frequently, they occur in the second and fourth decade of life. Some authors found no gender predilection [11] while many studies showed female predilection [12] between the first and the third decade of life [13].

### 28.3.4 Clinical Features

1. Swelling of maxilla or mandible
2. Facial disfigurement
3. Tooth displacement and mobility
4. Paraesthesia
5. Ulceration or Nasal obstruction

### 28.3.5 Radiological Features

- Ameloblastomas commonly originate within the bone, thus often they are detected on routine dental x-rays or on orthopantomogram (OPG).
- Root resorption of the involved teeth
- The solid/multilocular-type ameloblastomas, which is most common, classically shows "soap bubble appearance" [14]
- Computed tomography (CT) is very helpful in surgical planning by giving exact cortical destruction and soft tissue extension, it typically demonstrates well-defined radiolucent uni/multilocular lesions [15]
- Magnetic resonance imaging (MRI) is very helpful in maxillary lesions for defining the extension of ameloblastomas into paranasal sinuses, orbit and skull base [16]
- PET–CT generally indicated in patients with metastatic ameloblastomas.

## 28.4 Solid/Multicystic Ameloblastoma

In 2005 WHO classification, the Ameloblastoma, solid/multicystic type, was mentioned, which is replaced by Ameloblastoma alone in 2017 classification again. Historically, the Ameloblastoma is classified into Unicystic and Multilocular or Solid.

The solid/multicystic or intra-osseous ameloblastoma is locally invasive, slow-growing and odontogenic tumour of epithelial origin with a high rate of recurrence if not removed or treated properly. It has no tendency to metastasise. It invades the bone marrow spaces.

It has no gender predilection and occurs equally in both sexes. Most commonly diagnosed between 30 and 60 years of age. The posterior mandible region affected in more than eighty percent of the tumour cases. It may present as variably sized swelling of jaws. Pain and paraesthesia are rare. It usually appears multilocular (soap bubble appearance) in radiographs.

It occasionally is associated with an impacted tooth and causes expansion of the bony cortex, with the possibility of resorption of roots of the involved teeth [17, 18]. The most common histological patterns found are plexiform and follicular types. The others are desmoplastic, acanthomatous, granular and basal [2]. To confirm the diagnosis, the combination of imaging (plain as well as computed tomography) and biopsy can be performed.

The tumour infiltrates through the medullary spaces and might erode the cortical bone. After resorbing the cortical bone, it may extend into the adjacent tissues. The maxillary tumours of the posterior region tend to obliterate the maxillary sinus and may extend to infiltrate the skull base.

### 28.4.1 The Treatment Goals

- Complete removal of tumour
- Aesthetic reconstruction with minimal disfigurement
- Good prognosis
- Long-term follow-up

The treatment depends on the best judgement of the surgeons and individual status of the patient. The surgical planning should be based on the lesions present in the mandible or maxilla. The maxilla has got higher percentage of cancellous bone, which facilitates the spread of tumour in comparison to the mandible having thick and dense cortical plates, which limit the spread of neoplasm.

The treatment of the conventional/multicystic variant is classified into radical and conservative. The conservative methods include

- Curettage
- Enucleation
- Peripheral ostectomy with surgical excision
- Surgical excision with other adjuvant therapy such as cryotherapy or use of carnoy's solution
- Liquid nitrogen therapy [19]
- Marsupialisation

Radical treatment includes resection of bone. At least 1 cm of the surrounding healthy tissues should be removed along with the tumour in cases of cortical bone perforation because if tumour cells are left behind, they may give rise to locoregional recurrence even several years after resection [20]. There is a 1.26-fold increase in the chance of the recurrence rate with the increase in the size of every 10 mm of tumour [21].

In mandible, resection can be carried out on the basis of the extension of the lesion in the form of alveolectomy, marginal mandibulectomy, segmental resection, hemimandibulectomy or hemimandibulectomy with disarticulation depending on the extension of the tumour. Based on the extension of tumour, maxillectomy (partial, total or subtotal) has been performed in radical treatment of maxillary lesions [22].

Enucleation and curettage are inadequate because the tumour invades the adjoining cancellous bone. However, some conditions in which it is carried out are given below:

#### 28.4.1.1 Indications of Enucleation and Curettage

1. In medically compromised patient or conditions in which patient is unfit for general anaesthesia.
2. Very young or old patient who is not willing for segmental resection.

If enucleation and curettage has to be done, it is preferable to be carried out in association with chemical cauterisation with the help of modified carnoy' solution and peripheral ostectomy.

The surgical treatment of solid/multicystic variant is controversial. A high rate of recurrence is reported if it is not adequately excised or resected. According to some authors, the initial treatment should be conservative as the tumour has low metastatic potential and the radical treatment should be done in cases of recurrence. While others believe that whenever possible complete removal of the tumour with preservation of lower border of the mandible will be the treatment of choice [23].

Conservative treatment has a recurrence rate ranging from 33 to 90%, as compared to the rate of recurrence by radical treatment, i.e. 7–25% in the literature. However, the patients experience serious functional and aesthetic impairments with radical treatment [24, 25]. Hasegawa et al. [26] also reported the recurrence rate of 43.5% following conservative management.

Enucleation alone showed the highest rate of recurrence amongst all the modalities of conservative management [27]. According to Esquillo ME [28], small multicystic and solid lesions can be treated by marsupialisation with good results. This will maintain good facial aesthetics of the patient, lessening the treatment cost but patients have to keep on long-term follow-up.

About 40% of intra-osseous Ameloblastomas did not recur after conservative management, which led to the conclusion that the small intra-osseous ameloblastomas can be treated with conservative management initially, leading to fewer post-operative complications and if the lesion recurs, the radical treatment can be carried out in the second-stage surgery aggressively [29].

Almeida AC et al. [30] in the systematic review and meta-analysis concluded that the bone resection should be the treatment of choice for primary multicystic ameloblastoma, also the chances of recurrence were 3.15 fold more when the conservative treatment was performed in comparison to radical treatment. Hendra FN et al. also suggest that the rate of recurrence was less when radical treatment was opted for the treatment of intra-osseous ameloblastoma in their systematic review and meta-analysis [31].

Antonoglou GN and Sandor GK [32] in the systematic review and meta-analysis concluded that no strong recommendations have been made regarding the treatment options regarding the intra-osseous ameloblastoma. However, radical treatment in the form of resection is the treatment of choice for solid/multicystic ameloblastoma.

Pogrel MA and Montes DM [33] concluded that Enucleation alone should not be the choice of treatment for multicystic or solid lesions. In the case of maxilla, partial maxillectomy and in mandibular lesions, segmental resection with 1 cm margin will be preferred to avoid recurrence.

Sampson DE and Pogrel MA [34] suggested the management algorithm for management of mandibular ameloblastoma, which is, in the case of mandibular ameloblastoma, if lesion is less than 1 cm, in plain radiograph, then curettage and cryotherapy is the treatment of choice and patient is to be kept on long-term clinical and radiological follow-up. If the lesion is more than 1 cm, CT scan is to be done. If findings are positive, then segmental resection with involved soft tissue is carried out with suitable reconstruction and patient is to be kept on long-term clinical and radiological follow-up.

Sammartino et al. advocated the following treatment plan in Mandibular tumour management [24]. In the cases of small lesions, box resection has to be done and the patient has to keep for long-term follow-up to 10 years. For large lesions if cortical perforation is there on CT examination. Then segmental or marginal resection has been carried out along with excision of overlying soft tissues, if cortical perforation is absent then curettage is the choice of treatment with 0.5–1 cm of clinically uninvolved surrounding bone. In both cases, 10-year followup of patients is mandatory. If no recurrence occurs, orthopantomogram has to be done in every 2–3 years on the other hand if recurrence occurs, then the first or second small recurrence can be treated with marginal resection while for the third recurrence, the segmental resection is the choice of treatment.

### 28.4.2 Surgical Management of Ameloblastoma According to the Anatomic Locations

#### 28.4.2.1 Mandibular Anterior Region (Canine to Canine)

According to Gardner, anterior mandible should be approached conservatively because no important major anatomic structures are present in the anterior mandible. However, if curettage is used as a choice of treatment, recurrence is anticipated and it is preferred in smaller lesions. Always an attempt should be made to preserve the inferior border of mandibular in the anterior region because the tumour infiltration is less, due to the thick cortical bone of the symphyseal region. In large lesions with cortical perforation, marginal mandibulectomy will be the choice of treatment followed by long-term follow-up (Fig. 28.1). After marginal mandibulectomy, the lower border of mandible is reinforced with a reconstruction plate, to avoid pathological fracture in future (Videos 28.1 and 28.2).

#### 28.4.2.2 Posterior Mandible (Bicuspid to Condyle)

Marginal mandibulectomy should be the choice of surgical treatment for the posterior mandible and body region while maintaining the inferior and posterior border whenever possible for solid/multilocular variant. Maxillomandibular fixation might be required after marginal resection without

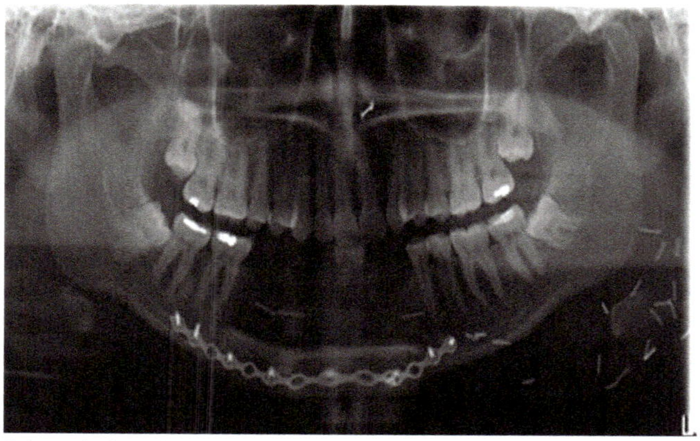



**Fig. 28.1** Orthopantomogram representing marginal mandibulectomy, lower border protected with reconstruction plate

continuity defects to avoid the chances of pathological fracture. A reconstruction plate may be contoured before resection, in order to maintain the normal anatomic relationship between proximal and distal segments by marking the points of screw fixation on the normal bone. In recent years, mandibular reconstruction using intra-oral microvascular anastomosis following segmental resection in cases of ameloblastomas has been carried out with great success. Most commonly, free fibular graft has been used for the same, followed by dental rehabilitation with the help of dental implants [35, 36].

#### 28.4.2.3 Anterior Maxilla (Canine to Canine)

Goodcell JF reported 2% ameloblastomas in anterior maxilla [37]. However, Sehdev MK et al. show 9% of ameloblastomas occurs in the canine and incisor region [38]. Less-aggressive treatment has been advocated in anterior maxilla when compared to posterior, because a sufficient distance from the vital structures allows being less radical. Radical treatment in the form of partial or total maxillectomy may result in significant deformity.

#### 28.4.2.4 Posterior Maxilla (Bicuspid to Pterygoid Plates)

Ameloblastoma occurs 47% in the molar region, 15% in the maxillary antrum and floor of the nose, while 9% in the premolar region.

Lack of cortical bone in maxilla makes it much more dangerous than mandibular ameloblastomas. The definitive treatment becomes difficult in the posterior maxillary region because tumours are not well confined by the thin maxillary cortical bone and easily spread beyond the maxillary bone boundaries. Early detection is also very difficult. Posterior maxillary tumours are rarely treated by conservative management. Extra-oral or intra-oral resection of the tumour is carried out, sometimes Le fort I down fracture is required to access the tumours of maxillary sinus or the tumour invades the posterolateral wall of the maxillary sinus.

Weber Fergusson incision and mandibulotomy can be used for accessing the tumors of maxilla, pterygoid and infra temporal fossa. When reconstruction of the defect after maxillectomy has been planned by temporalis muscle, Rai A et al. [39] advocated use of Borle's extension weber fergusson incision.

**Various surgical options in management of maxilla/ mandible tumours.**

**Benign Mandible Tumours**

Type or surgery depends on number of factors

1. Type of pathology—Benign/Benign aggressive
2. Extent of involvement—e.g. Sufficient lower border of mandible present or not
3. Site of tumour—Anterior mandible/Posterior mandible

Based on this options starting from the most conservative to most radical are:

1. Marsupialisation
2. Enucleation or curettage
3. Peripheral ostectomy or En bloc resection
4. Segmental resection

**Access incisions:**

1. Intraoral transmucosal access
2. Combined Intraoral and extraoral submandibular access
3. Combined Intraoral and Visor incision

**Repair:**

1. Primary mucosal closure
2. Packing cavity and healing by secondary intention
3. Reconstruction plate with primary mucosal closure
4. Reconstruction plate with free bone graft
5. Vascularised Bone free flap

**Benign Maxillary Tumours**

Type or surgery depends on number of factors

1. Type of pathology—Benign/Benign aggressive
2. Extent of involvement—e.g. Involvement of sinus/pterygoids/infratemporal fossa
3. Site of tumour—Anterior maxilla/Posterior maxilla

Based on this the following excision options are possible:

1. Marsupialization into Oral cavity/Maxillary Sinus
2. Enucleation/Curretage
3. Enbloc resection—Low level/High level maxillectomy

**Access incisions:**

1. Transoral accesss
2. Weber Ferguson incision—Good for anterior tumours
3. Mandibulotomy access approach—This provides excellent access for posterior tumours especially when access to the pterygoids/intratemporal region is required

**Repair:**

1. Primary closure
2. Packing cavity to allow healing by secondary intention with a Healing plate
3. Obturator
4. Local flap—e.g. Temporalis
5. Free flap reconstruction

## 28.5 Reconstructive Modalities After Surgical Resection of Ameloblastoma

*Need for Reconstruction:*

1. For restoration of movements and equilibrium of mandible
2. For maintenance of normal occlusal plane, floor of the mouth and tongue's anatomical position
3. For restoration of near normal feeding
4. For acceptable aesthetics and function.
5. For more favorable social acceptance
6. To establish the arch form, width and alveolar height.
7. To establish the bone continuity and maintain facial contours

### 28.5.1 Timing of Reconstruction

Immediate reconstruction is usually performed with the help of microvascular-free flaps, harvested from fibula, scapula, iliac crest and ribs. For the reconstruction of the mandible, free fibula flap is the treatment of choice. It is superior to iliac crest graft. Scapula flap for maxillary reconstruction may be a good alternative because of its long pedicle and good bone quality. For soft tissue reconstruction, the radial forearm-free flap is the choice of treatment. Most of the surgeons still prefer to use Titanium reconstruction plate for reconstruction when free flaps are not possible as an immediate reconstruction modality. Delayed reconstruction (second stage) can be performed for reconstruction with the help of a titanium reconstruction plate. The immediate reconstruction significantly improves the patients' health-related quality of life, many patients prefer immediate reconstruction [40].

Lawson et al. [41] reported 90% success rate with delayed reconstruction in comparison to immediate, which is 46% using non-vascularised bone grafts.

Autogenous bone graft selection (Vascularised free flaps vs non-vascularised bone graft) depends on following factors

1. Experience of the surgeon
2. Contour and size of the defect
3. Size and quality of the soft tissue available

The HCL classification [42, 43] is used as an aid in classifying mandibular defects. The defect from canine to canine, i.e. the central defect is designated as 'C'. The lateral segment defect excluding condyle designated as 'L' and when condyle is included in resection with lateral mandible the defect is designated 'H' (Fig. 28.2). The importance of this classification indicates that reconstruction of lateral defect can be done by straight bone segment while defect located centrally required osteotomies.

#### 28.5.1.1 Case Scenario 1 (Fig. 28.3a–g)

A 38 year old male patient reported to our outpatient department with the chief complaint of painless swelling of lower jaw since last 6 months (Fig. 28.3a). History of present illness represents swelling initially was of lemon size and increasing gradually to reach the present size, extending from right side of the body region of the mandible to the ramus region of the opposite side. On intra-oral examination, a diffuse swelling was present from one side of the molar region extending to the other side of the molar region of the mandible (Fig. 28.3b).

The orthopantomogram (Fig. 28.3c) and the CT scan (Fig. 28.3d) showing the multilocular lesion extending from the right side of the first molar to the ramus region of the contralateral side. The incisional biopsy of the lesion confirmed the diagnosis of solid/multicystic ameloblastoma. Under general anaesthesia, the resection of the lesion was done, the complete resection of lesion was confirmed in the specimen radiography (Fig. 28.3e). The reconstruction of the

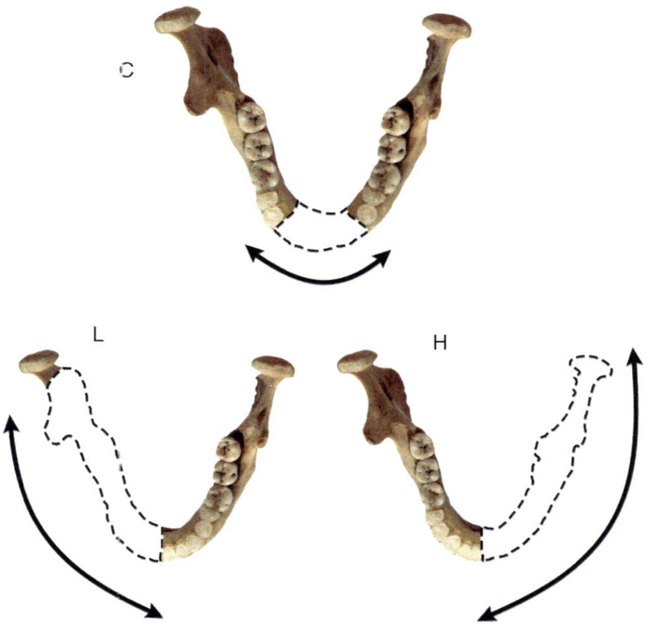


**Fig. 28.2** The HCL Classification

defect was done with the help of microvascular free fibula flap and with the titanium reconstruction plate (Fig. 28.3f), post-operative OPG representing reconstruction (Fig. 28.3g).

### 28.5.2 Bone Graft Substitutes

The calcium phosphate cement (Hydro set) is the commonly used material, which converts in situ to hydroxyapatite, serving as an effective osteoontegrative and osteoconductive material [44]. The other implantable material options include high-density porous polyethylene implants [45]. Using rapid prototype models, the custom-made implants are commonly used for the reconstruction of maxillofacial defects with good results [46].

The titanium mesh tray filled with autologous cancellous bone blocks fixed with the residual segment of bone and also titanium mesh cage filled with fresh bone marrow, recombinant human bone morphogenic protein (BMP) and xenogenic bone mineral are used for reconstruction of mandibular defect. The BMP is the key activator of bone induction [42].

Recent advances in mandibular reconstruction include transport disc distraction osteogenesis, modular endoprosthesis and tissue engineering. Dental implants are commonly used in autogenous bone grafts for the rehabilitation of masticatory functions [42].

## 28.6 Unicystic-Type Ameloblastoma

Robinson and Martinez [47] first described Unicystic Ameloblastoma (UA) in 1977.

In 1988, Ackermann GL et al. [48] reclassified UA with prognostic and therapeutic implications into three types

Type 1: Unilocular cystic lesions lined by epithelium exhibiting features of ameloblastoma.
Type 2: Epithelial nodules arising from cystic lining and projecting into the cyst lumen.
Type 3: The presence of invasive islands of ameloblastomatous epithelium in the connective tissue wall of the cyst and these islands may or may not be connected to the cyst lining.

### 28.6.1 Clinical and Radiographic Features

Most of the UA clinically and radiographically resemble denigerous cysts in behaviour. Embedded teeth are associated with some UA and hence resembles residual or primordial cysts.

UA most commonly occurs in the second and third decade of life and have predilection to mandible [48]. UA many times are associated with mandibular third molars. There will be well-corticated unilocular and often pericoronal radiolucency

In some cases, root resorption can occur.

#### 28.6.1.1 Case Scenario 2 (Fig. 28.4a, b)

A 14 year old female reported with swelling on the left side of the ramus region for the past 3 weeks. OPG (Fig. 28.4a) and PA view (Fig. 28.4b) showed a large unilocular radiolucent lesion involving the whole of the ramus of the left mandible. Tooth bud of lower left third molar was absent. The lesion seemed to arise from the impacted tooth bud of lower left second molar and the lesion was also involving the roots of lower left first molar. Under the provisional diagnosis of a dentigerous cyst, the lesion was enucleated under anaesthesia and primary closure was done and the impacted tooth bud was removed in this case. The histopathology report was that of an unicystic ameloblastoma with mural changes. The child was on follow-up with no evidence of recurrence.

On histological examination, various situations may be found such as shown in Fig. 28.5

1. The ameloblastomatous epithelial lining
2. An ameloblastoma nodule projects into the lumen (Luminal Ameloblastoma)
3a. Ameloblastoma islands present in the connective tissue wall of an apparently non-neoplastic cyst.
3b. Proliferation of ameloblastoma into the connective tissue wall from cystic lining. (One of the Mural variant)

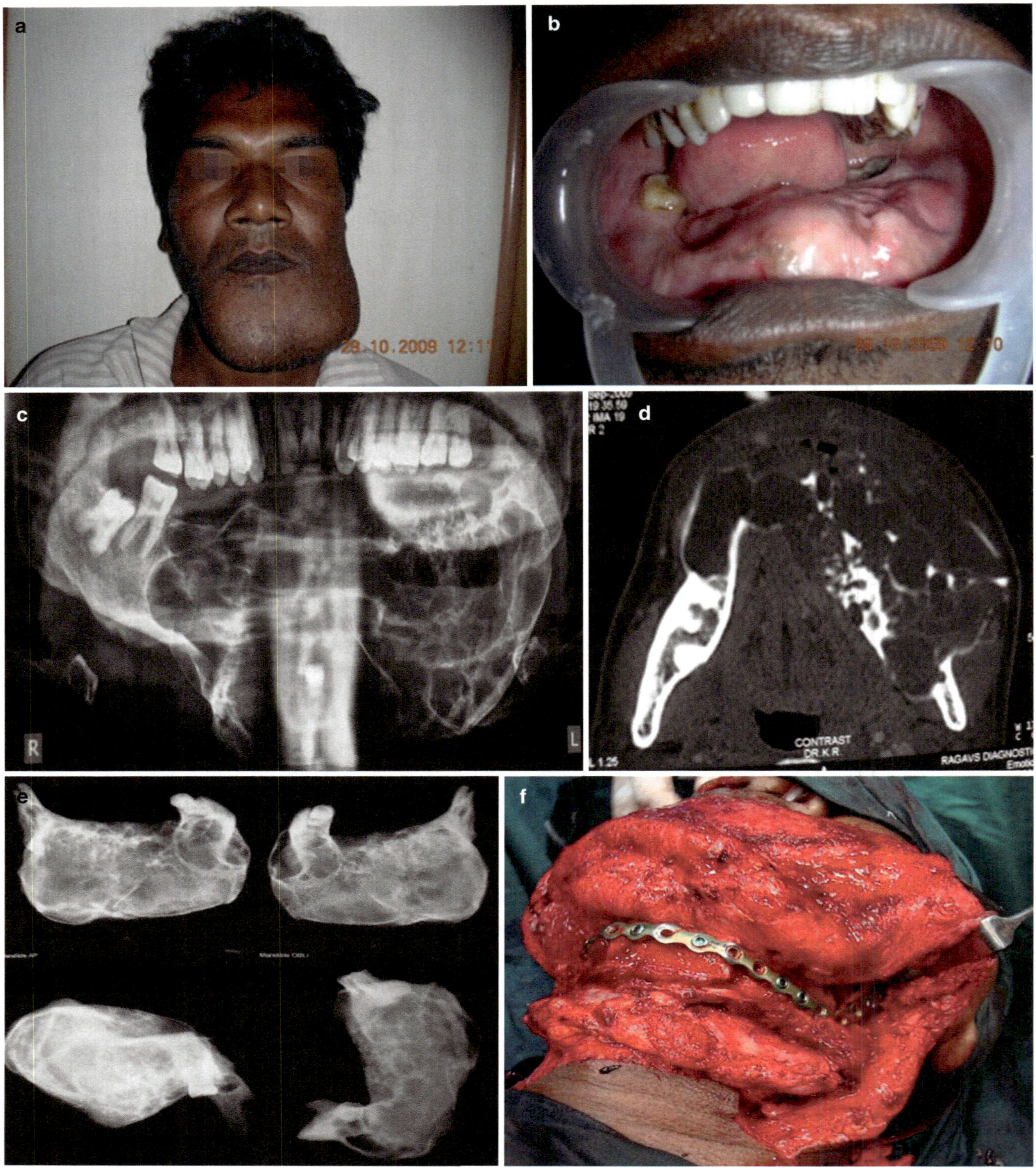


**Fig. 28.3** (**a**) Pre-operative extra-oral view. (**b**) Pre-operative intra-oral view. (**c**) Pre-operative OPG. (**d**) Pre-operative CT Scan of the patient. (**e**) Specimen Radiography. (**f**) Clinical picture showing reconstruction with the reconstruction plate. (**g**) Post-operative OPG

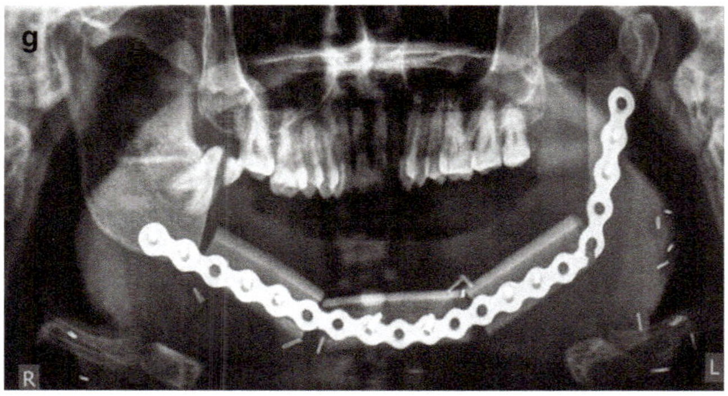


©Association of Oral and Maxillofacial Surgeons of India

**Fig. 28.3** (continued)

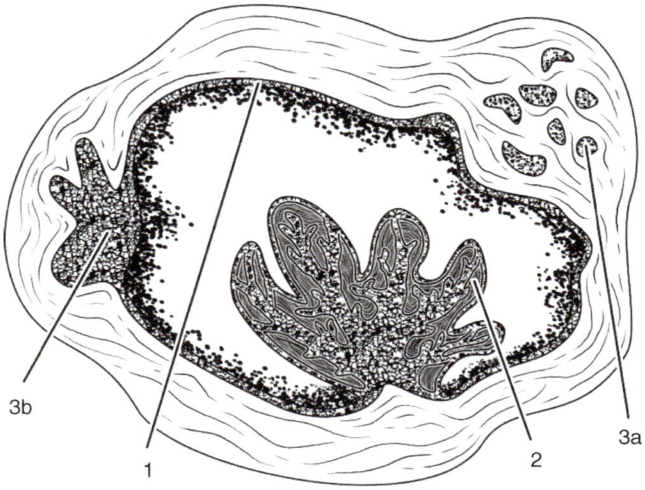


©Association of Oral and Maxillofacial Surgeons of India

**Fig. 28.5** Various situations of Unicystic Ameloblastoma found on Histological examination. 1. The ameloblastomatous epithelial lining. 2. An ameloblastoma nodule projects into the lumen (Luminal Ameloblastoma). 3a. Ameloblastoma islands present in the connective tissue wall of an apparently non-neoplastic cyst. 3b. Proliferation of ameloblastoma into the connective tissue wall from cystic lining. (One of the Mural variant)

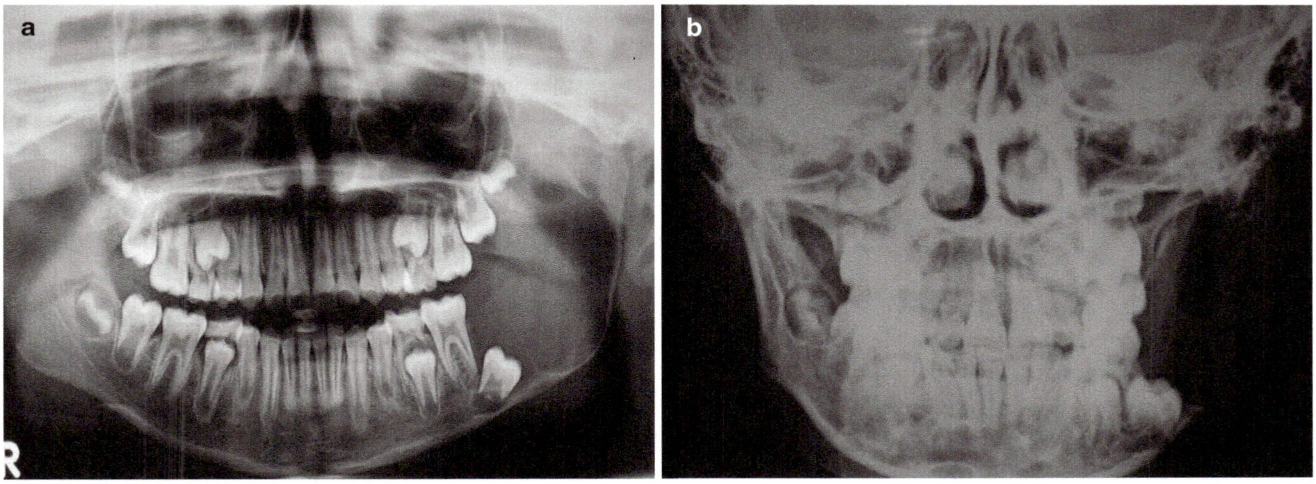


©Association of Oral and Maxillofacial Surgeons of India

**Fig. 28.4** (**a**, **b**) OPG and PA view showing Unicystic Ameloblastoma

## 28.6.2 Management

UA treatment is controversial and can be grouped into

- Enucleation
- Marsupialisation or decompression
- Radical resection

Conservative management has been advocated by cakarer et al. in their study on large benign aggressive lesions of the jaws, where they performed decompression followed by curettage if required [49].

Zheng et al. in 2019 published a long-term follow-up study on 116 cases of UA and have concluded that marsupialisation as an effective treatment option for UA. They found the recurrence rate more for the mural sub-types and the predictors for outcomes were resorption of the root, perforation of the cortical bone and histopathological sub-types [50].

Usually, initial treatment for UA is enucleation because they appear clinically as cysts, and the histopathology type is known only in the excision biopsy report as mural changes can be picked by the pathologist only when the full specimen is available. For histologic type showing luminal changes, the treatment of choice is Enucleation, but has to be followed up for 5–10 years. In types where the ameloblastoma infiltrates the adjacent cancellous bone, marginal resection is the treatment of choice after initial Enucleation and curettage [51]. This means that patient has to undergo two surgeries based on the histopathological examination.

There is some controversy on its management, with some authors advocating aggressive management, especially for the mural variant, while others advocating conservative management such as curettage, peripheral ostectomy and various adjuvant materials such as Carnoy's solution and Liquid Nitrogen [33, 52, 53]. If adequate follow-up is possible, the UA of posterior mandible can be treated conservatively with curettage or peripheral ostectomy.

According to LAU and Samman [54], 30.5% recurrence rate reported with enucleation alone. Application of carnoy's solution along with Enucleation decrease the recurrence rate to 16% and the least percentage of recurrence was seen with resection of tumour, i.e. only 3.6%

## 28.7 Use of Carnoy's Solution in Ameloblastomas

- Stoelinga and Bronkhorst [55] in 1987 suggested the use of carnoy's solution for UA as a chemical cauterisation. The carnoy's solution consists of chloroform 3 ml, absolute Alcohol 6 ml, 1 ml glacial acetic acid, sclerosing agent ferric chloride 1 gm for the management of fistulae and cysts as a fixative.
- The modified carnoy's solution avoids the use of chloroform due to concerns about its carcinogenicity [56]. However, the recurrence rate is lower with application of conventional carnoy's solution after enucleation and curettage in comparison to modified carnoy's solution [57].
- The use of carnoy's solution reduces the risk of recurrence by fixing the residual tumour tissues after enucleation of UA with mural invasion, but conventional multicystic ameloblastoma and some UA are unlikely to be effective by carnoy's solution. The recurrence experienced more in patients treated with Enucleation alone without the application of carnoy's solution.
- The solution is applied for 5 min with the help of cotton applicator or gauze soaked in carnoy's solution in the bony cavity. Irrigation with normal saline is done after that. The nerve and vessels should be avoided by contact of the carnoy's solution as much as possible. The method and duration of application of carnoy also is contentious where different regimes have been proposed by various authors.

### 28.7.1 Case Scenario 3 (Fig. 28.6a–i)

Case scenario 3 is provided to show that conservative management with adjunctive procedures will give reasonably good results thereby avoiding major resective and reconstructive surgeries. A 21-year male reported with gradually growing swelling right side body mandible (Fig. 28.6a). OPG (Fig. 28.6b) showed an unilocular expansile lesion in right side body mandible with resoprtion of the associated roots. There was intra-oral vestibular swelling and it was fluctuant on palpation due to thinning of the labial cortex. CT views (Fig. 28.6c–e) show the lesion to be unilocular, expansile with loss of both labial and lingual cortices. An incisional biopsy was performed, which gave the report as Unicystic ameloblastoma. This could be considered as an aggressive form as there was root resorption. Considering the age of the patient, a less-radical approach was taken, which involved excision of the lesion by raising an intra-oral crevicular mucoperiosteal flap (Fig. 28.6f), extraction of all the involved teeth (Fig. 28.6i), performing a peripheral ostectomy and applying carnoy's solution (Fig. 28.6g) and also excising the overlying mucosa, which was in direct contact with the lesion. The excised cystic lesion was quite thick walled and an in toto enucleation was possible (Fig. 28.6h). A reasonable thickness of the lower border of mandible was left behind and as the alveolar part of labial and lingual cortices was removed, excess tissue was available for achieving a tension-free primary closure. The postoperative OPG at one and half years (Fig. 28.6j) shows no evidence of recurrence and prosthetic rehabilitation performed. The patient is recurrence free for past 7 years.

### 28.7.2 Case Scenario 4 (Fig. 28.7a–f)

This case scenario is given to show that at times complex resection and reconstructive procedures may be avoided in amelobalstomas considering, the patients age and general health and other social background. In such cases where a conservative approach is used, the adjunct measures of peripheral ostectomy and carnoys solution will serve as adjunct methods to give an overall good prognosis (readers are also advised to refer chapter 27 on odontogenic cysts for use of these adjunct measures in odontogenic keratocyst).

A 67 year old male patient presented with loosening of teeth and swelling of gums in the anterior mandible

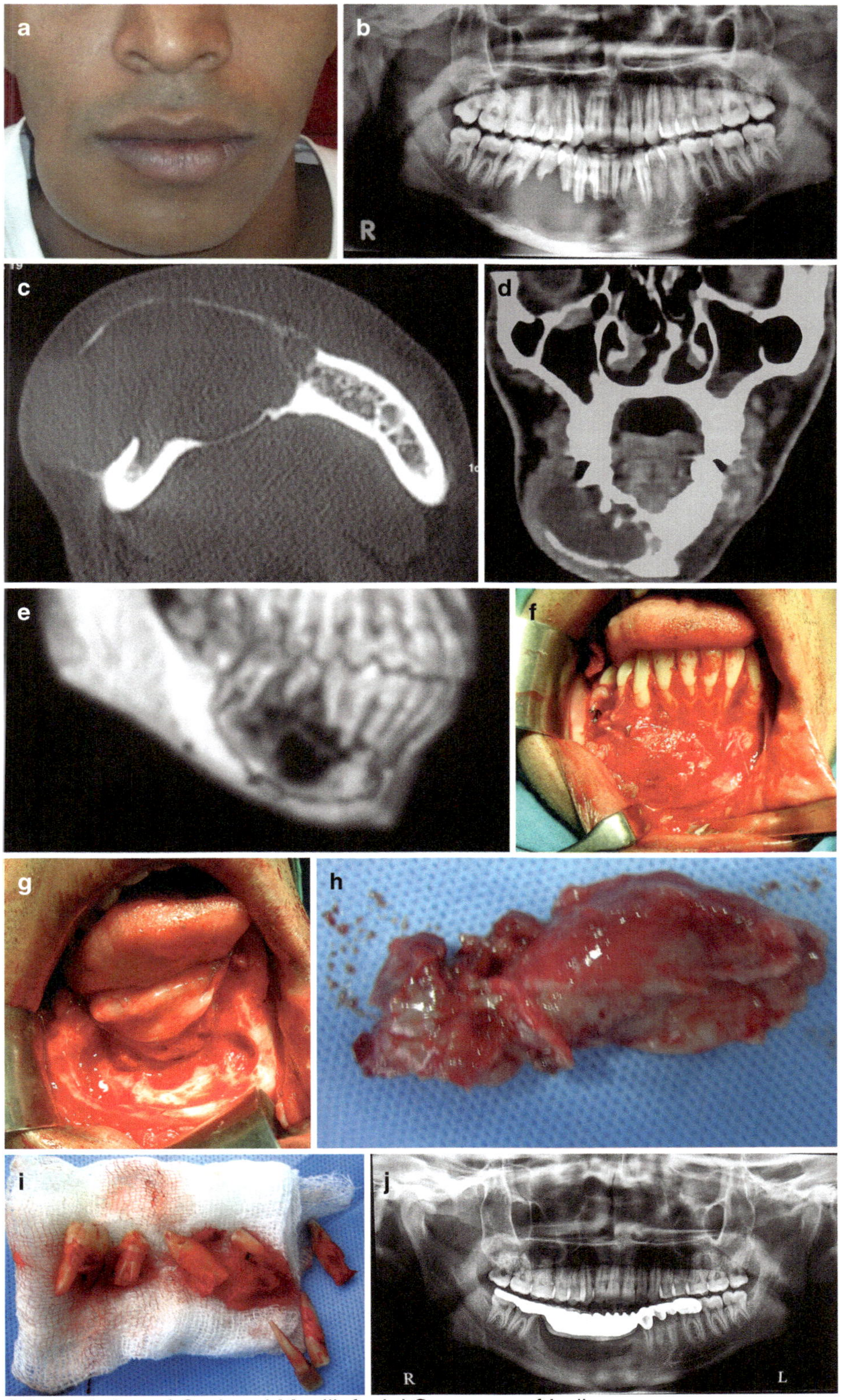



**Fig. 28.6** (**a**) Clinical image showing swelling right body mandible. (**b**) opg showing the radiolucent lesion right body mandible with root resorption (**c**) Axial CT image showing the expansile lesion with thinning of the labial cortex. (**d**) Coronal CT image showing the expansile nature of the lesion. (**e**) 3D CT showing the erosion of both labial and lingual cortical walls. (**f**) Intra-oral intra-operative view showing the lesion exposed by crevicular flap. (**g**) Intra-oral view of the surgical bed after extraction of teeth, excision of lesion and peripheral ostectomy. (**h**) Image of the excised cystic lining, with thick walls. (**i**) Images of the extracted teeth showing the root resorption, (**j**) post operative radiograph after prosthetic rehabilitation

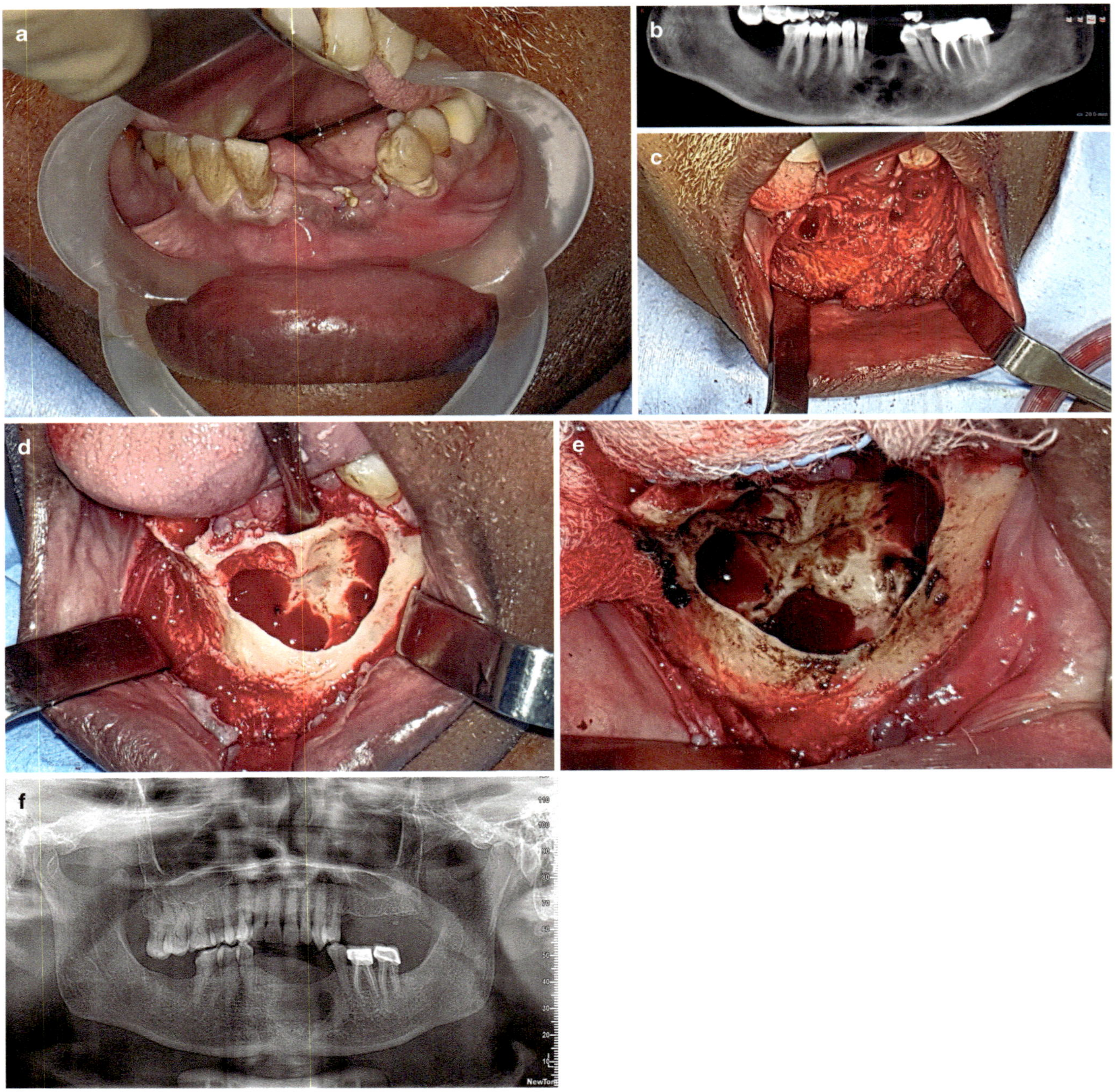

**Fig. 28.7** (**a**) loosening of teeth and expansion of the gums in the anterior lower mandible. (**b**) A OPG and CBCT showing multilocular radiolucency in the anterior mandible. (**c**) Lesion exposed (**d**) lesion excised and peripheral ostectomy done (**e**) carnoys solution applied to surgical bed (**f**) sixteen month post operative OPG

(Fig 28.7a). A CBCT scan (Fig 28.7b) confirmed the presence of a multilocular radiolucency in between right lateral incisor and left first premolar region. An incisional biopsy confirmed a diagnosis of a plexiform ameloblastoma.

Considering the patient's age and general health, it was decided to follow a conservative line of treatment to avoid the need for complex reconstruction.

The lesion was exposed under general anesthesia (Fig 28.7c) and the involved teeth and tumour lining was removed. A Large round bur was then used to remove 3mm of bony walls around the locules left by the lesion (Fig 28.7d). The lesion was treated with modified carnoy's solution for 3 minutes (Fig 28.7e) followed by irrigation with normal saline and primary closure achieved.

Excision pathology confirmed the diagnosis of a Plexiform ameloblastoma. The healing was uneventful. A 16 month post operative radiograph showed good bony healing (Fig 28.7f) without any recurrence and the patient is on long term follow-up.

## 28.8 Extraosseous/Peripheral Ameloblastoma (PA)

The tumour was first described by Kuru [58] 1911. The PA is defined as the tumour having intra-osseous ameloblastoma characteristics histologically but occurs in the soft tissues overlying the tooth-bearing areas of mandible and maxilla. In comparison to the intra-osseous solid/multicystic ameloblastoma, it is the extraosseous counterpart [59].

PA representing only 1–5% of all ameloblastomas considering it as a very rare odontogenic tumour. It is also called ameloblastoma of soft tissue, mucosal origin ameloblastoma and gingival ameloblastoma. It arises from the remnants of the odontogenic epithelium with in the lamina propria gingival or from the gingival epithelium of the basal cell layer.

It is painless, firm and exophytic growth with a smooth, granular and warty surface. Most commonly located in the oral mucosa or the gingiva. It occurs in wide age range groups, i.e. from 1 to 92 years with more than 64% of cases occurring in the fifth to seventh decade of life. In edentulous areas, it affects the alveolar mucosa. The ratio of 2.4:1 is noted in mandible: maxilla. Intra-osseous ameloblastoma rarely extends to the gingival tissues and merge with gingival epithelium creating PA of the exophytic type [60]. Histopathologically same histomorphic cell types of odontogenic epithelium seen in solid/multicystic variant as consist in PA.

### 28.8.1 Differential Diagnosis

1. Peripheral odontogenic fibroma
2. Peripheral variant squamous odontogenic tumour

It does not show invasive behaviour and the treatment of choice will be conservative excision with adequate disease-free margins. The recurrence is low, but patients are to be kept on long-term follow-up.

## 28.9 Metastasising (Malignant) Ameloblastoma

'Malignant Ameloblastoma (MA)' term was proposed by Slootweg and Muller [61] in 1984. According to them, it is well-differentiated ameloblastoma that metastasises but which maintains the characteristic cytologic features of original tumour [62]. The ameloblastic tumour that undergoes malignant cytologic transformation; the term 'Ameloblastic carcinoma' is used.

Metastasis is the only factor that distinguishes ameloblastoma from MA. Its clinical behaviour is helpful in diagnosing the tumour.

Lung shows maximum 75% metastatic deposits, 15% each by spine and cervical lymph nodes followed by cervical lymph nodes and spine (15% each) [63]. Small bowel, liver, skull, brain and kidneys were the other locations, which show metastases but with lower incidence [64].

MA is very rare with an occurrence rate of 2% of all benign ameloblastomas [65]. The age ranges from 5 years to 74 with 34.4 years mean age. 1:1.2 is the male to female ratio. The majority cases were localised in the mandible. The survival time ranges from 3 months to 5 years after the appearance of metastases. Most MA are histologically plexifom type but not significantly different from the metastatic type in their histologic and cytologic features [66].

The initial tumours were treated with Enucleation and curettage while advanced with resection (block or segmental). Open thoracotomy is indicated in discrete and isolated lung metastases and wedge resection. Occasionally, chemotherapy gives successful results. Inoperable metastatic deposits can be treated with radiation therapy but having an unpredictable response [67, 68].

## 28.10 Squamous Odontogenic Tumours

### 28.10.1 Introduction

Squamous odontogenic tumour (SOT) was first described by Pullon et al. [69] as a rare benign odontogenic tumour in 1975. It affects all the age group and equally occurs in both the jaws. SOT histologically characterised by squamous epithelial islands, which are surrounded by mature connective tissue stroma. The SOT is occasionally misdiagnosed as squamous cell carcinoma, keratocanthoma, ameloblastoma and verrucous carcinoma. It is hamartomatous epithelial proliferation, arising probably from cell rests of Malessez [70]. The differential diagnosis of SOT may be acanthomatous and desmoplastic ameloblastoma variants, squamous cell carcinoma (well differentiated).

### 28.10.2 Definition

"SOT is a locally infiltrative, benign neoplasm consisting of islands of well-differentiated squamous epithelium in a fibrous stroma. The epithelial islands shows foci of central cystic degeneration occasionally" (WHO).

### 28.10.3 Clinical Features [71]

1. Swelling, which is painless
2. Mildly painful gingival swelling
3. Loosening of involved teeth
4. Occurs in the mean age of 38 years with age ranges from 8 to 74 years.

5. Multiple SOT, which involves several quadrant of mouth in few patients have been reported, a family of 3 siblings having multiple lesions has been reported.
6. Absence of periodontal ligament between the lesion & the root of the tooth, suggesting that lesion arises from Malassez rests cell in the periodontal ligament or closely adjacent mucous membrane.
7. Equally affects maxilla and mandible, but most commonly involves incisor-cuspid area in maxilla and bicuspid-molar area in mandible

### 28.10.4 Radiographic Features [72]

1. Unilocular radiolucency of the triangular or semicircular type located in alveolar bone along the roots' lateral surface.
2. In some cases, vertical bone loss appears
3. The radiolucent area may show ill-defined or well-defined margins
4. Sometimes, tumour appears as an intra-bony pocket between the teeth
5. Peripheral lesions may cause saucerisation of underlying bone, which is likely because of the pressure phenomenon rather than infiltration of the tumour.
6. Few extensive lesions show multilocular radiolucency, pushing the maxillary sinus and involving the mandibular body region.

### 28.10.5 Treatment and Prognosis

Conservative treatment in the form of local excision, enucleation and curettage may be done for the successful management of SOT. Recurrent and clinically aggressive lesions have been treated with en bloc excision. Extraction of the associated teeth along with the conservative treatment is mandatory. It has a very low recurrence rate [73].

Cortical bone erosion of maxilla and mandible exhibits aggressive biological behaviour. Aggressive treatment should be followed for the lesions, which show early recurrence [74].

## 28.11 Calcifying Epithelial Odontogenic Tumour

Pindborg in 1955 first introduced the calcifying epithelial odontogenic tumour (CEOT) in the scientific literature [75]. It is well known as 'Pindborg Tumor' since then. CEOT is slow growing, benign and occasional locally invasive odontogenic neoplasm, which is epithelial in its origin.

WHO accepted and adopted the term calcifying epithelial odontogenic tumour (CEOT) in its first edition of 'Histological typing odontogenic tumours, jaw cysts and allied lesions', and recognised it as a distinct entity [76]. It may be extra-osseous or intra-osseous.

### 28.11.1 Definition

CEOT is a epithelial odontogenic neoplasm, which is locally invasive and is characterised by the presence of amyloid material that may become calcified (WHO)

### 28.11.2 Epidemiology

It accounts for less than 1% of all odontogenic tumours, hence considered uncommon. It commonly occurs between the age of 8 and 92 years with the mean age of 36.9 years.

The intra-osseous variant occurs in the third, fourth and fifth decade of life in 64% of patients [77]. CEOT has no gender predilection, and occurs equally in both the sexes. Premolar and molar regions are the commonest site of occurrence, although can occur at any site. Anterior gingiva is most commonly affected by the peripheral lesions. Maximum cases reported are of intra-osseous lesions, only 6% arise in extra-osseous locations. Mandible is affected by intra-osseous lesions more frequently than maxilla, with a ratio of 2:1.

### 28.11.3 Clinical Features

CEOT is slowly growing, painless, expansile and hard bony swelling, which can cause thinning of the cortical bone and infiltration of soft tissue subsequently. It can cause rotation, tipping, migration or mobility of tooth secondary to resorption of roots. In the anterior region, there is also a distinctly uncommon peripheral variant of CEOT, limited to soft tissue only, presenting as a nodular mass on the gingiva.

### 28.11.4 Radiographic Features

The larger or the mature tumour will be mixed radiolucent—radiopaque, although the early tumour may be completely radiolucent. CEOT is often associated with unerupted teeth. It may be unilocular and cystic in appearance. It can demonstrate a mixture of large and small multilocular spaces described as 'soap bubble' and 'honey comb' in appearance. The radiographic borders in almost all cases between surrounding tissues and tumour appear to be circumscribed and well defined [78].

CEOT on CT examination demonstrating thinning and expansion of lingual and buccal cortical plates with well-defined mass containing scattered radiopaque areas of different size and signal intensity in mandible. Pindborg tumour on MRI reveals predominantly a hypointense lesion on T1-weighted images and mixed hyperintense lesion on T2-weighted images [79].

### 28.11.5 Treatment

Surgical management is the treatment of choice for CEOT. Conservative treatment in the form of Enucleation or curettage followed by judicious removal of the thin layer of bone adjacent to the tumour is the choice of treatment in small, intra-bony lesions with well-defined borders. However, the tumours treated with curettage and enucleation show a recurrence rate ranging from 15 to 30% after 2–4 years with the overall recurrence rate of 14% [77].

According to Melrose RJ [80], even the small CEOTs are infiltrating in nature. A margin of about 1 cm normal bone should be removed along with the tumour excision. Peripheral tumours are treated with smaller margins 0.5 cm because they are less aggressive. Few recurrences have been reported with the tumours treated with jaw resection. However, the patient should be kept for follow-up upto 5–10 years.

The recurrent lesions and the tumours, which are diagnosed late in their clinical course, which over an extended time becomes larger and extensive (more than 4 cm in size) may not respond well to conservative management-like surgical excision only. Segmental resection such as partial or hemimandibulectomy or hemimaxillectomy will be the treatment of choice. However, it may leave a significant bony discontinuity requiring grafting or extensive soft tissue reconstruction.

The incidence of malignant transformation is very low; however, Veness et al. [81] reported a case of metastatic spread and malignant transformation with CEOT.

## 28.12 Adenomatoid Odontogenic Tumour

Stafne in 1948, first described the adenomatoid odontogenic tumour (AOT) as an odontogenic neoplasm [82]. It was referred as ameloblastic adenomatoid tumour or adenoameloblastoma initially, because it was considered as a variant of ameloblastoma [83]. The term AOT, which is generally accepted today suggested by Philipsen and Birn [84].

### 28.12.1 Definition [85]

A neoplasm of locally invasive nature was characterised by ameloblastoma-like islands of epithelial cells in a mature connective tissue stroma. Aberrant keratinisation may be found in the form of ghost cells in association with varying amounts of dysplastic dentin (WHO).

Three variants of AOT are recognised, i.e. Follicular, Extra follicular and peripheral.

The peripheral type arises from the gingival tissues and is very rare. The follicular type is commonly associated with impacted tooth and found in 75% of cases; on the other hand, the extrafollicular type is located between the roots of adjacent teeth and is not related to an unerupted teeth [86].

### 28.12.2 Clinical Features

- AOT commonly occurs in the anterior region of jaws, particularly the maxilla.
- It occurs commonly in young patients, two-thirds of the cases occurring between 10 and 19 years of age. However, the age ranges from 3 to 82 years [87].
- Females are affected more than males with a ratio of 5.6:1.
- Size of AOT ranges from 2 to 7 cm with more than 60% involving the entire quadrant [88].
- The most common tooth associated with AOT is impacted canine followed by premolars and lateral incisors [89].

Radiographically, the most common appearance will be a well-demarcated unilocular radiolucency associated with unerupted tooth. Sometimes, intra-bony cases show scattered radiopacities within the radiolucency. Intra-oral periapical radiographs found to be better than OPG are best suited for showing discrete calcified deposits [90].

The AOT is usually well-encapsulated tumour so the treatment of choice will be Enucleation and Curettage. The recurrence is extremely rare [91].

## 28.13 Mixed (Epithelial-Mesenchymal) Origin

### 28.13.1 Ameoblastic Fibroma

Ameloblastic Fibroma (AF) was first reported by Kruse in 1891 [92]. AF consists of odontogenic ecto-mesenchyme resembling the dental papilla, epithelial strands and nests resembling dental lamina and enamel organ. Dental hard tissues are absent in it. The lesion is referred to as ameloblastic fibro-dentinoma if there is dentin formation. It is a rare odontogenic mixed tumour in which ectomesenchymal and epithelial elements are neoplastic. It accounts only 2% of all odontogenic tumours [93].

#### 28.13.1.1 Clinical Features

AF occurs in young adults and children with an age range from 1.5 to 42 years, with the average age ranging from 14.5 to 15.5 years [94]. It was occasionally reported in middle-aged individuals. There is no gender predilection. More than 50% of patients present with a sign of swelling. Failure of tooth eruption, pain, tenderness and discharge are the other common findings [95]. Posterior mandible is the commonest site of occurrence and first permanent molar and second primary molar areas were involved in more than 70% of cases.

#### 28.13.1.2 Radiographic Features

Multilocular radiolucency with sclerotic margins is the most common radiographic appearance. Unilocular radilolucency is the feature of small tumours, while large tumours extend through the bony cortices. The size typically ranges from 1 to 8 cm [96]. Ameloblastic fibrosarcoma is the differential diagnosis of AF.

Enucleation and curettage of the adjacent bone along with the extraction of affected teeth is the treatment of choice for AF. They occur rarely but required a long-term followup. In order to preserve the teeth involved in the tumour, the chances of recurrence increase after conservative management [97, 98].

The ameloblastic fibro-odontoma is composed of connective tissue characteristic of an ameloblastic fibroma and calcified tissue identifying the tumour as a complex odontoma. The ameloblastic fibro-odontoma diagnosis is based on the histologic evidence of ameloblastic fibroma with active odontogenic epithelium embedded in an embryonal connective tissue. The differential diagnosis of ameloblastic fibroma and ameloblastic fibro-odontoma is based on the absence (ameloblastic fibroma) and presence (ameloblastic fibro-odontoma) of enamel and dentin. A tumour is called ameloblastic fibro-dentinoma when exclusive dentin formation is observed. A tumour is called an ameloblastic fibro-odontoma in the presence of both enamel and dentin. In ameloblastic fibroma, no dental hard tissues are present [99]. AFO is similar to AF described by the WHO, and [they also show inductive changes that lead to both enamel and dentin formations]. Moreover, AFO and AF are defined as hamartomatous lesions and they are believed to be stages of formation of odontoma. That means the above-mentioned lesions should not be considered as distinct entities [100].

### 28.13.2 Odontoma (Compound, Complex Types)

In 1866, Broca coined the term 'Odontome' [101]. The term 'Odontoma' was given by Thoma and Goldman, to include tumours that were composed of well-differentiated tooth structure [102]. Odontoma defined as a tumour that differentiated and developed enough to produce dentin, enamel and cementum in varying proportions [103].

Compound odontoma is defined by the WHO as a malformation in which all the dental tissues represented in a more orderly pattern than complex odontoma, so that lesions consist of many tooth-like structures.

Complex odontoma is a type of malformation in which all dental tissues are represented and individual tissues are well formed, but occur in a disorderly pattern [104].

Compound-type odontomas are more common than complex odontomas [105]. According to Regezi, the compound odontomas are 37% and complex odontomas were 30% of all the reported odontogenic tumours [106]. Odontomas occur equally in both sexes. They are rarely associated with deciduous teeth but more frequently associated with permanent teeth. Anterior maxilla is the most common site for the occurrence of compound-type odontome while posterior mandible (Fig. 28.8) is affected more commonly in complex odontomes followed by anterior maxilla [107].

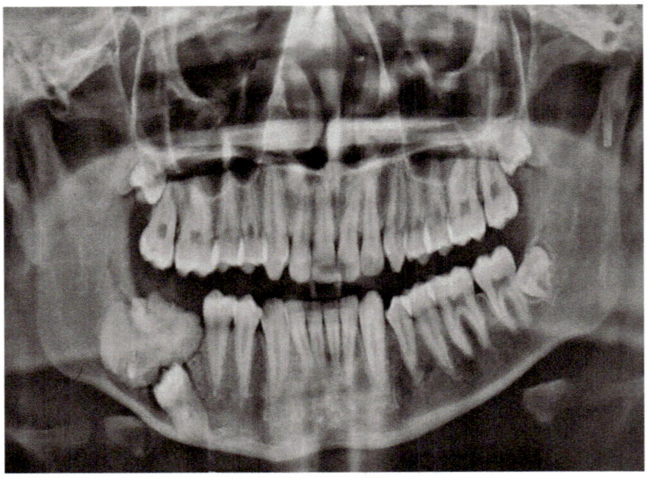



**Fig. 28.8** OPG showing complex odontome in mandible right molar region

They are small, painless and hard mass. Permanent impacted or retained deciduous teeth are present as a common symptom. The second most common complaint is swelling. Complex odontoma may become large and produce asymmetry with bone expansion [108, 109].

On radiological examination, the lesion consists of densely opaque masses of varying size, usually associated with unerupted or impacted teeth. The radiolucent line surrounds the opaque masses. The collections of tooth-like structures of different shapes and sizes are the features of compound odontomes, the teeth are of diminutive sizes. The complex-type odontomes appear as calcified masses that have consistency the same as the tooth structure.

The treatment of choice for odontomes is surgical excision and recurrence is very rare.

## 28.14 Mesenchymal Origin Tumours

### 28.14.1 Odontogenic Myxoma

Myxoma is very uncommon. It accounts for 0.5 to 20% of all odontogenic tumours and has a incidence of 0.07/million [110]. It arises from mesenchymal stroma and is a benign, locally aggressive tumour. Bone, soft tissues and most frequently the myocardium are favourite sites for myxomas. Jaws myxomas are both odontogenic and osseous in the origin . Myxoma according to WHO is defined as a locally invasive neoplasm, consisting of angular and rounded cells that lie in an abundant mucoid stroma [111].

#### 28.14.1.1 Clinical Features

The myxomas have a predilection for molar and premolar regions of mandible and maxilla, however they can occur anywhere in the jaws. One third of myxomas located in the maxilla while two third in mandible. In maxillary myxomas, the cortical expansion and perforation of bone are common and often extend into the sinus [112].

It is reported to have a slight female predilection (1.5:1) while other authors reported equal gender predilection between females and males. Odontogenic myxomas most commonly occur in the second and third decade of life with the average age ranging from 25 to 30 years [113].

The periapical radiographs and OPGs are the first indicators of myxomas of jaws. Odontogenic myxomas radiographically present as unilocular lesions to large multilocular neoplasms, which often cause displacement of teeth but resorb the roots less frequently. The unilocular lesions are small in size on the other hand multilocular myxomas are greater than 4 cm in size. 5% Myxomas have association with unerupted tooth [114].

#### 28.14.1.2 Treatment and Prognosis

Surgical excision is the treatment of choice of odontogenic myxomas. The rate of recurrence is quite high, i.e. nearly 25% during first two years after removal. Atleast 1 cm of medullary bone should be resected along with tumour and always try to involve one tumour-free anatomic barrier at its periphery [78]. Subramaniam S [115] used endoscopes in the resection of pterygoid plates for the complete treatment of odontogenic myxoma. Use of endoscopes eliminates the use of extra-oral incisions.

### 28.14.2 Cementoblastoma

Dewy in 1927 first described Benign cementoblastoma [116]. It is a rare tumour of mesenchymal origin. Cementum-like tissue formation around the roots of the teeth is its important characteristic.

Cementoblastoma has predilection of mandible with 79.5% and most commonly in the premolar and molar region. They rarely occur in maxilla.

The roots of vital erupted permanent tooth are affected by the cementoblastoma. The most common tooth involved is the mandibular first molar. It has slight male predilection and occurs most commonly in the second and third decade of life. Cementoblastoma can cause teeth displacement, expansion of bone and maxillary sinus invasiveness, and aggressive tumours usually present with the symptoms of swelling and pain [117].

The diagnosis of cementoblastoma is very challenging as hypercementosis is also associated with roots of the teeth, that is the reason why hypercementosis is always included in the differential diagnosis. Cementoblastoma is slow growing, but can cause perforation and expansion of the cortices. The most common symptom is pain [118]. Radiographically the lesion will appear as a radiopaque mass fused with roots of the teeth , surrounded and limited peripherally by a radiolucent halo.

Complete excision of cementoblastoma is the gold standard treatment with extraction of the involved teeth [119]. It must be removed early, otherwise it may continue to grow. Maxillary lesions at times can involve the entire maxillary sinus making the prognosis poor. Recurrence is very rare, however incomplete removal may result in recurrence.

The tooth associated with cementoblastoma may be preserved under the following conditions [120]

1. In slow-growing tumour
2. In asymptomatic patients, with no pain
3. Perforation of cortical plates is absent
4. Patient refusal for teeth extraction

## 28.15 Recent Advances

Genetic marking has helped identify gene mutations, which may in the future help with histological and clinical management of these lesions. The most promising of these is the BRAF V600E mutation that is present in 90% of ameloblastomas and in the unicystic mural variant, suggesting predisposition to infiltrative behaviour. In the future, gene therapy may be possible using this gene marker [121].

The sonic hedgehog (SHH) and PI3K/Akt/Mtor signaling pathways may soon provide non-surgical options for treatment of ameloblastoma. The tumours that depend on active SHH signalling for growth/survival and maintenance may be susceptible targets for combined chemotherapy with SHH-specific inhibitors together with PI3K, Akt or mTOR blocking agents [122]. Jhamb T and Kramer JM advise to check molecular markers and accordingly decide the treatment plan [123]. Effiom OA et al. reported that explanation of molecular factors that arrange pathogenesis and recurrence of ameloblastoma will lead to new targeted drug therapies and diagnostic markers for ameloblastoma [124].

## 28.16 Case Scenario 5 (Fig. 28.9a–j)

A 25 year old male patient presented with an expanding lesion around the left upper posterior teeth (Fig. 28.9a). Radiographs suggested a cystic lesion and a CT scan confirmed bony destruction by a multilocular lesion extending from the first molar to the tuberosity (Fig. 29.8b). An incisional biopsy of the lesion confirmed a diagnosis of follicular ameloblastoma.

The patient had excision of the lesion with a posterior partial maxillectomy, with a mandibular split [125] for access (Fig. 28.9c, d). The defect was reconstructed with a temporalis muscle flap (Fig. 28.9e, f, g). The mandibulotomy site was fixed with titanium plates (Fig. 28.9h).

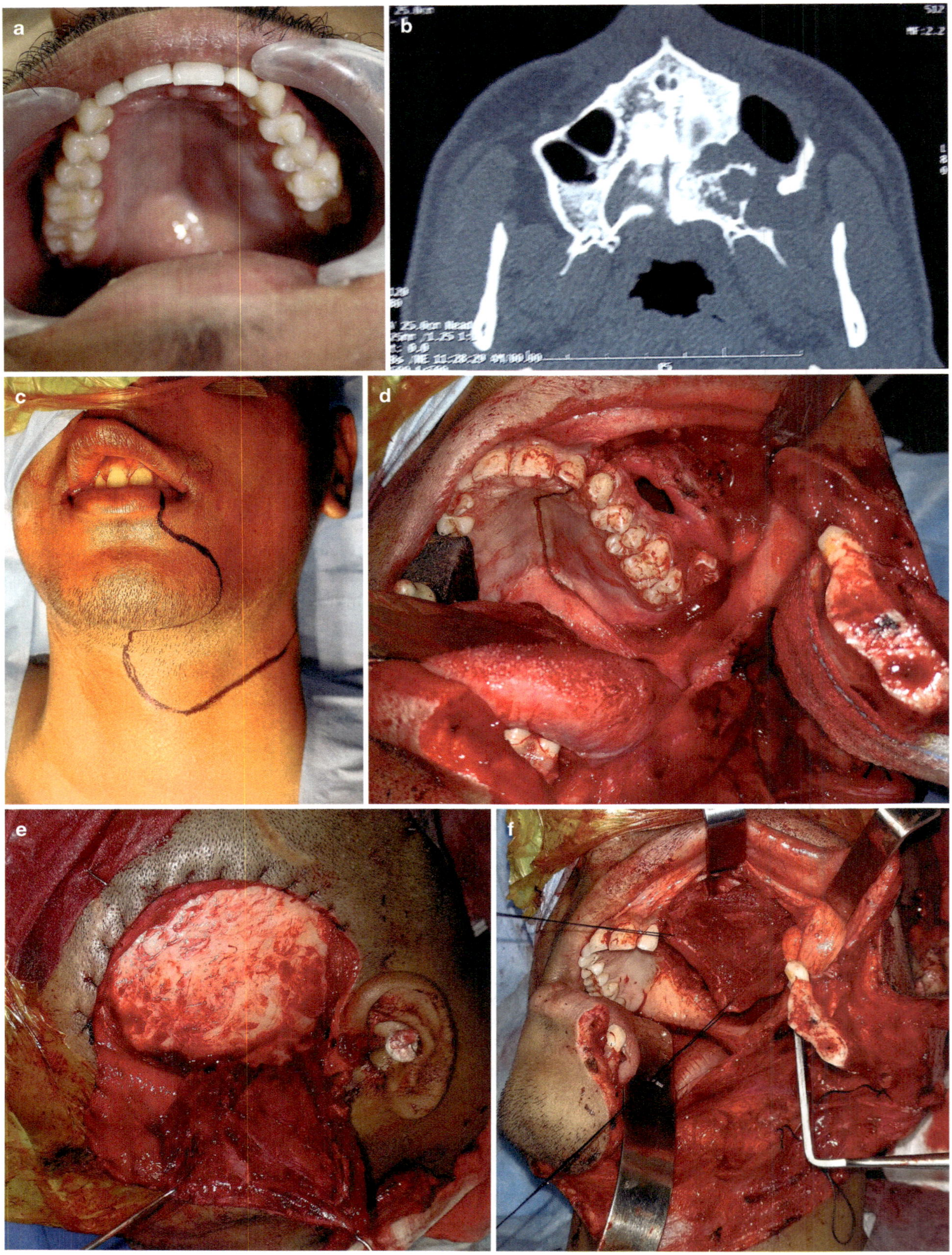

**Fig. 28.9** (**a**) expanding lesion around the left upper posterior teeth. (**b**) CT scan confirmed bony destruction by a multilocular lesion extending from the first molar to the tuberosity. (**c**) Incision marked for partial maxillectomy via mandibular split access (**d**) left posterior partial maxillectomy being performed (**e**) temporalis muscle flap being harvested (**f**) temporalis flap being advanced to the partial maxillectomy defect (**g**) Introperative view after suturing of the temporalis flap to cover the defect. (**h**) Fixation done at the mandible split region (**i**) post-operative intra oral view showing good healing (**j**) extra oral view showing good cosmetic and functional result

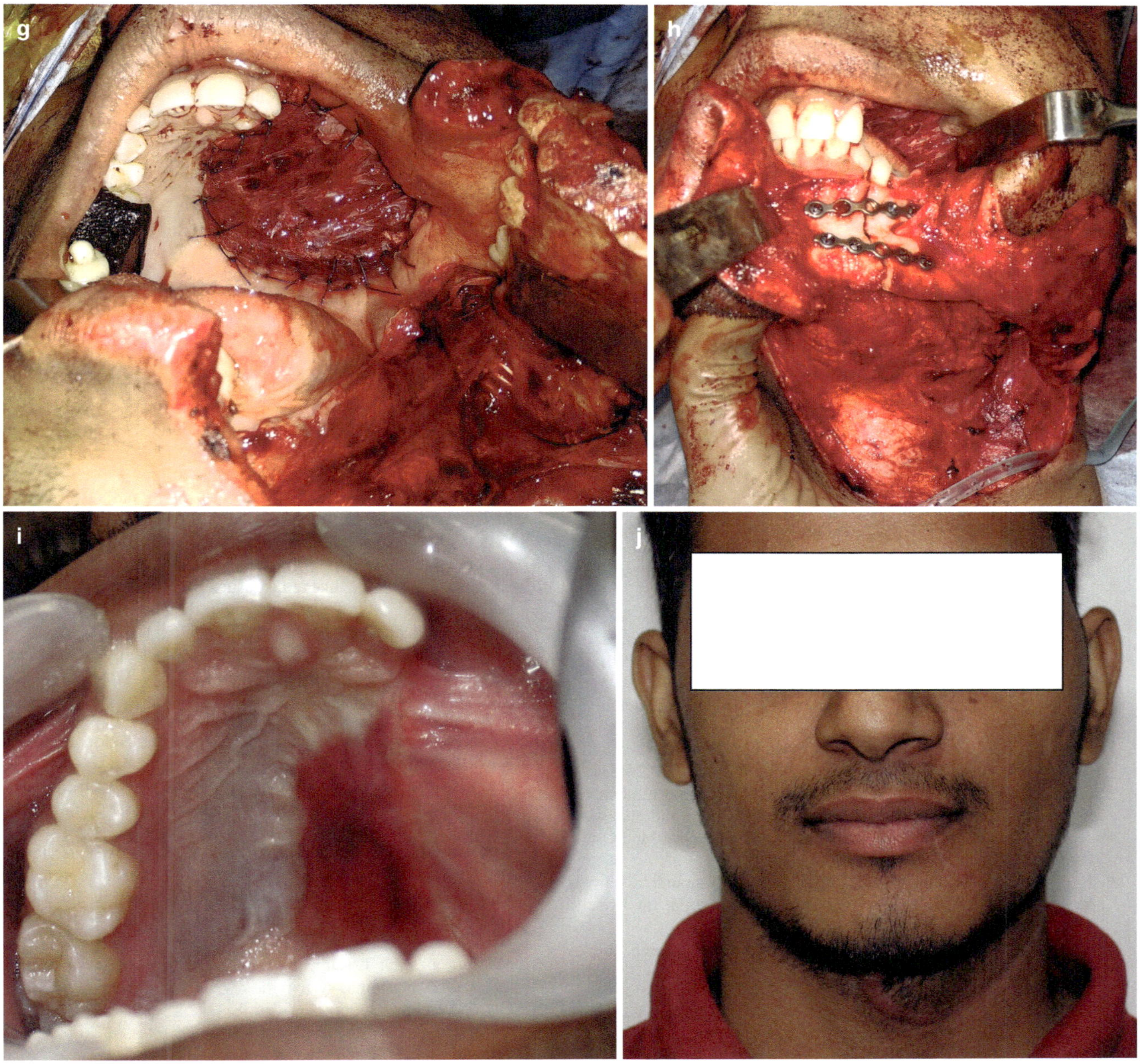


Fig. 28.9 (continued)

The healing was uneventful. Pathology reports confirmed the diagnosis of Follicular Ameloblastoma with clear excision margins. He had an excellent intra oral and cosmetic (extra oral) post-operative result (Fig. 28.9i, j).

Maxillectomy through mandibulotomy approach has been followed by author in a series of cases [125].

The readers are advised to refer chapter 85 of this book for detailed reading on access surgeries and osteotomies for the maxillofacial region.

## 28.17 Conclusion

Posterior mandible and cuspid areas of maxilla are the most common sites for the odontogenic tumours to occur. However, they can occur anywhere in the tooth-forming apparatus. The detailed history, thorough radiological and clinical evaluation is important in making the probable diagnosis. Conservative and aggressive surgical management has been used according to the size and extent of the tumour.

Proper aesthetic reconstruction should be carried out to avoid facial disfigurement. To check for recurrence, patients should be kept on regular follow-up and ensure long-term successful results.

**Acknowledgements** for Figs. 28.4 and 28.6 (case scenarios 2 and 3) to suvy manuel

## References


1. Barnes L, Eveson JW, Reichart PA, Sidransky D. WHO Classification. Head and neck tumors. In: Odontogenic tumors. Lycon: IRAC Press; 2005. p. 283–318.
2. Wright JM, Soluk TM. Odontogenic tumors: where are we in 2017? J Istanb Univ Fac Dent. 2017;51(3 Suppl 1):S10–30.
3. Gorlin RJ, Pindborg JJ, Clausen FP, et al. The calcifying odontogenic cyst: a possible analogue of the cutaneous calcifying epithelioma of Malherbe. Oral Surg Oral Med Oral Pathol Oral Radiol Endod. 1962;15:1235–43.
4. Ledesma-Montes C, Gorlin RJ, Shear M, Praetorius F, Mosqueda-Taylor A, Altini M, et al. International collaborative study on ghost cell odontogenic tumours: calcifying cysticodontogenic tumour, dentinogenic ghost cell tumour and ghost cell odontogenic carcinoma. J Oral Pathol Med. 2008;37:302–8.
5. Wright JM, Vered M. Update from the 4th Edition of the World Health Organization Classification of head and neck tumours: odontogenic and maxillofacial bone tumors. Head Neck Pathol. 2017;11:68–77.
6. Ritchie A. Boyd's text book of pathology. 9th ed. Philadelphia: Lea and Febiger; 1990.
7. Robinson HBG. Ameloblastoma: a survey of three hundred and seventy-nine cases from the literature. Arch Pathol. 1937;23:831.
8. Osterne RL, Brito RG, Alves AP, et al. Odontogenic tumors: a 5-year retrospective study in a Brazilian population and analysis of 3406 cases reported in the literature. Oral Surg Oral Med Oral Pathol Oral Radiol Endod. 2011;111:474.
9. Jing W, Xuan M, Lin Y, et al. Odontogenic tumours: a retrospective study of 1642 cases in a Chinese population. Int J Oral Maxillofac Surg. 2007;36:20.
10. Reichart PA, Philipsen HP, Sonner S. Ameloblastoma: biological profile of 3677 cases. Eur J Cancer B Oral Oncol. 1995;31B(2):86–99.
11. Avelar RL, Antunes AA, Santos T, et al. Odontogenic tumors: clinical pathology study of 238 cases. Braz J Otorhinolaryngol. 2008;74:668.
12. Fernandes AM, Duarte EC, Pimenta FJ, et al. Odontogenic tumors: a study of 340 cases in a Brazilian population. J Oral Pathol Med. 2005;34:583.
13. LFA A, et al. Clinical, radiographic, histological characteristics and ameloblastoma treatment: retrospective study. Int J Oral Maxillofac Surg. 2019;48:279–80.
14. Underhill TE, Katz JO, Pope TL Jr, Dunlap CL. Radiologic findings of diseases involving the maxilla and mandible. AJR Am J Roentgenol. 1992;159(2):345–50.
15. Cohen MA, Hertzanu Y, Mendelsohn DB. Computed tomography in the diagnosis and treatment of mandibular ameloblastoma: report of cases. J Oral Maxillofac Surg. 1985;43(10):796–800.
16. Kawai T, Kishino M, Hiranuma H, Sasai T, Ishida T. A unique case of desmoplastic ameloblastoma of the mandible: report of a case and brief review of the English language literature. Oral Surg Oral Med Oral Pathol Oral Radiol Endod. 1999;87(2):258–63.
17. Hertog D, Bloemena E, Aartman IHA, van-der-Waal I. Histopathology of ameloblastoma of the jaws: some critical observations based on a 40 years single institution experience. Med Oral Patol Oral Cir Bucal. 2012;17:76–82.
18. Bataineh AB. Effect of preservation of the inferior and posterior borders on recurrence of ameloblastomas of the mandible. Oral Surg Oral Med Oral Pathol Oral Radiol Endod. 2000;90:155–63.
19. Pogrel MA. The use of liquid nitrogen cryotherapy in the management of locally aggressive bone lesions. J Oral Maxillofac Surg. 1993;51(3):269–73.
20. Lello GE, Smith I. Ameloblastoma with multiple delayed recurrences: a case report. Head Neck Surg. 1987;9:295–8.
21. Au SW, et al. Risk factors fo rrecurrence of ameloblastoma: a long-term follow-up retrospectivestudy. Int J Oral Maxillofac Surg. 2019;48:1300–6.
22. Rastogi V, Pandilwar PK, Maitra S. Ameloblastoma: an evidence based study. J Maxillofac Oral Surg. 2010;9:173–7.
23. Carlson ER, Marx RE. The ameloblastoma: primary, curative surgical management. J Oral Maxillofac Surg. 2006;64:484–94.
24. Sammartino G, et al. Effectiveness of a new decisional algorithm in managing mandibular ameloblastomas: a 10-years experience. Br J Oral Maxillofac Surg. 2007;45:306–10.
25. Nakamura N, Higuchi Y, Mitsuyasu T, Sandra F, Ohishi M. Comparison of long-term results between different approaches to ameloblastoma. Oral Surg Oral Med Oral Pathol Oral Radiol Endod. 2002;93:13–20.
26. Hasegawa T, Imai Y, Takeda D, Yasuoka D, Ri S, Shigeta T, et al. Retrospective study of ameloblastoma: the possibility of conservative treatment. Kobe J Med Sci. 2013;59:E112–21.
27. Fregnani ER, et al. Clinicopathological study and treatment outcomes of 121 cases of ameloblastomas. Int J Oral Maxillofac Surg. 2010;39:145–9.
28. Esquillo ME. Conservative management of ameloblastoma using modified marsupialization and radical marsupialization. Int J Oral Maxillofac Surg. 2019;48:91–2.
29. Hammarfjord O, et al. Surgical treatment of recurring ameloblastoma, are there options? Br J Oral Maxillofac Surg. 2013;51(8):762–6.
30. Almeida Rde A, Andrade ES, Barbalho JC, Vajgel A, Vasconcelos BC. Recurrence rate following treatment for primary multicystic ameloblastoma: systematic reviewand meta-analysis. Int J Oral Maxillofac Surg. 2016;45(3):359–67.
31. Hendra FN, Natsir Kalla DS, Van Cann EM, de Vet HCW, Helder MN, Forouzanfar T. Radical vs conservative treatment of intraosseous ameloblastoma: systematic review and meta-analysis. Oral Dis. 2019;12:1683–96.
32. Antonoglou GN, Sándor GK. Recurrence rates of intraosseous ameloblastomas of the jaws: a systematic review of conservative versus aggressive treatment approaches and meta-analysis of non-randomized studies. J Craniomaxillofac Surg. 2015;43(1):149–57.
33. Pogrel MA, Montes DM. Is there a role for enucleation in the management of ameloblastoma? Int J Oral Maxillofac Surg. 2009;38(8):807–12.
34. Sampson DE, Pogrel MA. Management of mandibular ameloblastoma: the clinicalbasis for a treatment algorithm. J Oral Maxillofac Surg. 1999;57(9):1074–7.
35. Nkenke E, et al. Mandibular reconstruction using intraoral microvascular anastomosis following removal of an ameloblastoma. J Oral Maxillofac Surg. 1983;72:1992.
36. Vayvada H, Mola F, Menderes A, et al. Surgical management of ameloblastoma in the mandible: segmental mandibulectomy and immediate reconstruction with free fibula or deep circumflex iliac artery flap (evaluation of the long-term esthetic and functional results). J Oral Maxillofac Surg. 2006;64:1532.
37. Goodsell JF, Yamashita DD, Moody R. Ameloblastoma of the anterior maxillae. J Surg Oncol. 1977;9:407.

38. Sehdev MK, Huvos AG, Strong EW. Ameloblastoma of maxilla and mandible. Cancer. 1974;33:324.
39. Rai A, et al. Modified Weber-Fergusson incision with Borle's extension. Br J Oral Maxillofac Surg. 2010;48(5):e23–4.
40. Li X, Zhu K, Liu F, Li H. Assessment of quality of life in giant ameloblastoma adolescent patients who have had mandible defects reconstructed with a free fibula flap. World J Surg Oncol. 2014;12:201.
41. Lawson W, Loscalzo LJ, Baek SM, et al. Experience with immediate and delayed mandibular reconstruction. Laryngoscope. 1982;92:5.
42. Kumar BP, Venkatesh V, Kumar KA, Yadav BY, Mohan SR. Mandibular reconstruction: overview. J Maxillofac Oral Surg. 2016;15(4):425–41.
43. Jewer DD, Boyd JB, Manktelow RT, Zuker RM, Rosen IB, Gullane PJ, Rotstein LE, Freeman JE. Orofacial and mandibular reconstruction with the iliac crest free flap: a review of 60 cases and a new method of classification. Plast Reconstr Surg. 1989;84(3):391–403.
44. Takagi S, Chow LC, Markovic M, Friedman CD, Costantino PD. Morphological and phase characterizations of retrieved calcium phosphate cement implants. J Biomed Mater Res. 2001;58(1):36–41.
45. Rai A, et al. Utility of high density porous polyethylene implants in maxillofacial surgery. J Maxillofac Oral Surg. 2014;13(1):42–6.
46. Arora A, et al. Custom-made implant for maxillofacial defects using rapid prototype models. J Oral Maxillofac Surg. 2013:71:e104–10.
47. Robinson L, Martinez MG. Unicystic ameloblastoma: a prognostically distinct entity. Cancer. 1977;40:2278.
48. Ackermann GL, et al. The unicystic ameloblastoma: a clincopathological study of 57 cases. J Oral Pathol. 1988;17:541–6.
49. Cakarer S, Isler SC, Keskin B, et al. Treatment for the large aggressive benign lesions of the jaws. J Maxillofac Oral Surg. 2018;17:372–3.
50. Zheng CY, et al. Marsupialisation for the treatment of unicystic ameloblastoma of the mandible: a long-term follow up of 116 cases. Br J Oral Maxillofac Surg. 2019;57(7):655–62.
51. Gardner DG. A pathologist's approach to the treatment of ameloblastoma. J Oral Maxillofac Surg. 1984;42:161–6.
52. Haq J, Siddiqui S, McGurk M. Argument for the conservative management of mandibular ameloblastomas. Br J Oral Maxillofac Surg. 2016;54:1001–5.
53. Rosenstein T, Pogrel MA, Smith RA, Regezi JA. Cystic ameloblastoma—behaviorand treatment of 21 cases. J Oral Maxillofac Surg. 2001;59(11):1311–6.
54. Lau SL, Samman N. Recurrence related to treatment modalities of unicystic ameloblastoma: a systemic review. Int J Oral Maxillofac Surg. 2006:35:681–90.
55. Stoelinga PJW, Bronkhorst FB. The incidence: multiple presentation and recurrence of aggressive cysts of jaws. J Craniomaxillofac Surg. 1987;15:184–95.
56. Ecker J, et al. Current role of Carnoy's solution in treating keratocystic odontogenic tumors. J Oral Maxillofac Surg. 2016;74:278–82.
57. Dashow JE, et al. Significantly decreased recurrence rates in keratocystic odontogenic tumor with simple enucleation and curettage using Carnoy's versus modified Carnoy's solution. J Oral Maxillofac Surg. 2015;73:2132–5.
58. Kuru H. Ueber das adamantinoma. Zentralbl Allg Pathol. 1911;22:291.
59. Buchner A, Sciubba JJ. Peripheral epitherial odontogenic tumors: a review. Oral Surg. 1987;63:688.
60. Philipsen HP, Reichart PA, Nikai H, et al. Peripheral ameloblastoma: biological profile based on 160 cases from the literature. Oral Oncol. 2001;37:17.
61. Slootweg PJ, Muller H. Malignant ameloblastoma or ameloblastic carcinoma. Oral Surg Oral Med Oral Pathol. 1984;57:168.
62. Lee FE, White WL, Totten RS. Ameloblastoma with distant metastasis AMA Arch Pathol. 1959;68:23.
63. Laughlin EH. Metastasizing ameloblastoma. Cancer. 1989;64:776–80.
64. Reichart PA, Philipsen HP. Metastasizing, malignant ameloblastoma. Odontogenic tumours and allied lesions. London: Quintessence Publishing; 2004. p. 207–13.
65. Houston G, Davenport W, Keaton W, Harris S. Malignant (metastatic) ameloblastoma: report of a case. J Oral Maxillofac Surg. 1993;51:1152–5.
66. Kunze E, Donath K, Luhr HG, Engelhardt W, De Vivie R. Biology of metastasizing ameloblastoma. Pathol Res Pract. 1985;180:526–35.
67. Lanham RJ. Chemotherapy of metastatic ameloblastoma. A case report and review of the literature. Oncology. 1987;44:133–4.
68. Miyamoto CT, Brady LW, Markoe A, Salinger D. Ameloblastoma of the jaw. Treatment with radiation therapy and a case report. Am J Clin Oncoll. 1991;14:225–30.
69. Pullon PA, et al. Squamous odontogenic tumor. Report of six cases of a previously undescribed lesion. Oral Surg. 1975;40:616–30.
70. Baden E, Doyle J, Mesa M, et al. Squamous odontogenic tumor. Oral Surg Oral Med Oral Pathol. 1993;75:733.
71. El-Naggar AK, JKC C, Grandis JR, et al., editors. World Health Organization classification of head and neck tumours. 4th ed. Geneva: World Health Organization Press; 2017.
72. Philipsen HP, et al. Squamous odontogenic tumour: a benign neoplasm of the periodontium. A review of 36 reported cases. J Clin Periodontol. 1996;23:922–6.
73. Lin Y-L, White DK. Squamous odontogenic tumor. Oral Maxillofac Surg Clin North Am. 2004;16:355.
74. Moussa M, ElShafei MM. Squamous odontogenic tumor: a case report. Int J Case Rep Images. 2013;4:607.
75. Pindborg JJ. Calcifying epithelial odontogenic tumour. Acta Pathol Microbiol Scand. 1955;111:71.
76. Philipsen HP, Reichart PA. Calcifying epithelial odontogenic tumor: biological profile based on 181 cases from the literature. Oral Oncol. 2000;36:17–26.
77. Franklin CD, Pindborg JJ. The calcifying epithelial odontogenic tumor: a review and analysis of 113 cases. Oral Surg Oral Med Oral Pathol. 1976;42:753.
78. Marx RE, Stern D. Oral and maxillofacial pathology. Chicago, IL: Quintessence Publishing; 2003. p. 635–703.
79. Cross JJ, Pilkington RJ, Antoun NM, et al. Value of computed tomography and magnetic resonance imaging in the treatment of a calcifying epithelial odontogenic (Pindborg) tumour. Br J Oral Maxillofac Surg. 2000;38:154.
80. Melrose RJ. Benign epithelial odontogenic tumors. Semin Diagn Pathol. 1999;16:271.
81. Veness MJ, Morgan G, Collins AP, et al. Calcifying epithelial odontogénico (Pindborg) tumor with malignant transformation and metastatic spread. Head Neck. 2001;23:692.
82. Stafne EC. Epithelial tumors associated with developmental cysts of the maxilla: report of 3 cases. Oral Surg. 1948;1:887.
83. Neville BW, Damm DD, Allen CM, et al. Oral & maxillofacial pathology. Philadelphia, PA: Saunders; 1995. p. 529.
84. Philipsen HP, Birn H. The adenomatoid odontogenic tumor; ameloblastic adenomatoid tumor; or adenoameloblastoma. Acta Pathol Microbiol Scand. 1969;75:375.
85. Barnes L, Eveson JW, Reichart P, et al., editors. World Health Organization classification of tumors. Pathology and genetics of head and neck tumors. Lyon: IARC Press; 2005. p. 304–5.
86. Bedrick AE, Solomon MP, Ferber I. The adenomatoid odontogenic tumor: an unusual clinical presentation. Oral Surg. 1979;48:143.
87. Rick GM. Adenomatoid odontogenic tumour. Oral Maxillofac Surg Clin North Am. 2004;16:333–54.
88. Mohamed A, et al. Adenomatoid odontogenic tumour: review of the literature and an analysis of 33 cases from South Africa. Int J Oral Maxillofac Surg. 2010;39:843–6.
89. Jeong KL. Adenomatoid odontogenic tumor: a case report. J Oral Maxillofac Surg. 2000;58:1161–4.

90. Philipsen HP, Reichart PA, Siar CH, et al. An updated clinical and epidemiological profile of the adenomatoid odontogenic tumour: a collaborative retrospective study. J Oral Pathol Med. 2007;36:383–93.
91. Chuan-Xiang Z, Yan G. Adenomatoid odontogenic tumor: a report of a rare case with recurrence. J Oral Pathol Med. 2007;36: 440–3.
92. Neville BW, et al. Odontogenic cysts and tumors. In: Oral maxillofacial pathology. 2nd ed. Philadelphia: W B Saunders; 2002. p. 626–32.
93. Blankestijn J, Panders AK, Wymenga JP. Ameloblastic fibroma of the mandible. Br J Oral Maxillofac Surg. 1986;24:417.
94. Gorlin RJ, Chaudhry AP, Pindborg JJ. Odontogenic tumors. Classification, histopathology, and clinical behavior in man and domesticated animals. Cancer. 1961;14:73.
95. Trodahl JN. Ameloblastic fibroma. Oral Surg. 1972;33:547.
96. Cawson RA, Binnie WH, Speight PM, et al. Lucas's pathology of tumors of the oral tissues. 5th ed. Hong Kong: Churchill Livingstone; 1998. p. 65–9.
97. Leider AS, Nelson JF, Trodahl JN. Ameloblastic fibrosarcoma of the jaws. Oral Surg Oral Med Oral Pathol. 1972;33:559.
98. Dallera P, Bertoni F, Marchetti C, et al. Ameloblastic fibroma: a follow-up of six cases. Int J Oral Maxillofac Surg. 1996;25: 199.
99. Friedrich RE. Recurrent ameloblastic fibro-odontoma in a 10-year-old boy. J Oral Maxillofac Surg. 2001;59:1362–6.
100. Surej Kumar LK, Manuel S, Khalam SA, Venugopal K, Sivakumar TT, Issac J. Ameloblastic fibro-odontoma. Int J Surg Case Rep. 2014;5(12):1142–4.
101. Broca P. TraiteV des tumeurs, vol. 1. France: P. Asselin; 1866. p. 350.
102. Thoma KH, Goldman HM. A classification based on observations of the epithelial, mesenchymal, and mixed varieties. Am J Pathol. 1946;12:433–71.
103. Gorlin RJ, Goldman HM. Thoma's oral pathology, vol. 1. 6th ed. St, Louis: The C. V. Mosby; 1970. p. 481–507.
104. Kramer IRH, Pindborg JJ, Shear M. The WHO histological typing of odontogenic tumours. Cancer. 1992;70:2988–94.
105. Miki Y, Oda Y, Iwaya N, Hirota M, Yamada N, Aisaki K, et al. Clinicopathological studies of odontoma in 47 patients. J Oral Sci. 1999;41:173–6.
106. Regezi JA, Kerr DA, Courtney RM. Odontogenic tumors: analyses of 706 cases. J Oral Surg. 1978;36:771–8.
107. Philipsen HP, Reichart RP, Pratorius F. Mixed odontogenic tumors and odontomas: considerations on interrelationship. Review of the literature and presentation of 134 new cases of odontomas. Oral Oncol. 1997;33:86–99.
108. Shafer WG, Hine MK, Levy BM. Cysts and tumors of odontogenic origin. In: A textbook of oral pathology. 4th ed. Philadelphia: WB Saunders; 1983. p. 258–317.
109. Blinder D, Peleg M, Taicher S. Surgical considerations in cases of large mandibular odontomas located in the mandibular angle. Int J Oral Maxillofac Surg. 1993;22:163–5.
110. Gomes CC, Diniz MG, Duarte AP, et al. Molecular review of odontogenic myxoma. Oral Oncol. 2011;47:325–8.
111. Kramer IRH, Pindborg JJ, Shear M. Histological typing of odontogenic tumors. 2nd ed. New York: Springer-Verlag; 1992.
112. Kaffe I, Naor H, Buchner A. Clinical and radiological features of odontogenic myxomas of jaws. Dentomaxillofac Radiol. 1997;26:299–303.
113. King TJ, et al. Pediatric maxillary odontogenic myxoma: a report of 2 cases and review of management. J Oral Maxillofac Surg. 2008;66:1057–62.
114. Williams T. Aggressive odontogenic cysts and tumors. In: Oral and maxillofacial surgery clinics of North America, vol. 9. Philadelphia, PA: WB Saunders; 1997.
115. Subramaniam S. Endoscopic resection of the pterygoid plates following incomplete transoral resection of an odontogenic myxoma. Br J Oral Maxillofac Surg. 2017;55:e19–20.
116. Dewey KW. Osteoma of a molar. Dentisuto Cosmos. 1927;69:1143.
117. Ulmansky M, Hjorting-Hansen E, Praetorius F, Haque MF. Benign cementoblastoma. A review and five new cases. Oral Surg Oral Med Oral Pathol. 1994;77:48.
118. Ohki K, Kumamoto H, Nitta Y, et al. Benign cementoblastoma involving multiple maxillary teeth: report of a case with a review of the literature. Oral Surg Oral Med Oral Pathol Oral Radiol Endod. 2004;97:53.
119. Iannaci G, Luise R, Iezzi G, et al. Multiple cementoblastoma: a rare case report. Case Rep Dent. 2013;2013:828373.
120. Borges DC. Conservative treatment of a periapical cementoblastoma: a case report. J Oral Maxillofac Surg. 2019;77:272.e1–7.
121. Brown NA. Rolland D, McHughJb, Weigelin HC, Zhao l, limMs, Elenitoba-Johnson ks, Betz Bl. Activating FGFr2-ras-braF mutations in ameloblastoma. Clin Cancer Res. 2014;20:5517–26.
122. Sauk JJ, Nikitakis NG, Scheper MA. Are we on the brink of nonsurgical treatment for ameloblastoma? Oral Surg Oral Med Oral Pathol Oral Radiol Endod. 2010;110(1):68–78.
123. Jhamb T, Kramer JM. Molecular concepts in the pathogenesis of ameloblastoma: implications for therapeutics. Exp Mol Pathol. 2014;97(3):345–53.
124. Effiom OA, Ogundana OM, Akinshipo AO, Akintoye SO. Ameloblastoma: current etiopathological concepts and management. Oral Dis. 2018;24(3):307–16.
125. Nair S et al . Maxillectomy through mandibulotomy–a retrospective clinical review. J Oral Maxillofac Surg 2011;69(7):2040–7.


## Additional Reading


Haq J, Siddiqui S, McGurk M. Argument for the conservative management of mandibular ameloblastomas. Br J Oral Maxillofac Surg. 2016;54(9):1001–5.

Soluk-Tekkeşin M, Wright JM. The World Health organization classification of odontogenic lesions: a summary of the changes of the 2017 (4th) edition. Turk Patoloji Derg. 2018;34(1):1–18.

Troiano G, et al. Conservative vs radical approach for the treatment of solid/multicystic ameloblastoma: a systematic review and meta-analysis of the last decade. Oral Health Prev Dent. 2017;15(5):421–6.

# 29 Reactive Lesions of Oro-Maxillofacial Region

Raja Sekhar Gali

## 29.1 Introduction

The tissues of the oral and maxillofacial region are constantly exposed to a plethora of inflammatory stimuli that can be of bacterial, physical, chemical or immunologic in the origin. Chronic/long-standing, low-grade inflammatory stimuli can induce a heightened/escalated reparative response in the oral tissues resulting in the occurrence of non-neoplastic, hyperplastic lesions that are collectively referred to as reactive lesions [1].

Though the occurrence of exophytic reactive proliferation in the oral cavity is relatively common, certain malignant (metastatic/primary) and benign tumours, vascular lesions can closely mimic these lesions leading the clinician to misdiagnosis and sub-optimal treatment. A thorough understanding of the clinical presentation, differential diagnosis and the required diagnostic workup is the key to appropriate treatment.

**Additional features of the chapter:**

- Pearls, Perils & Pitfalls
- Case Scenarios
- Recent Advances

## 29.2 Classification

These lesions can be peripheral/extra-osseous (Soft tissues-Gingiva, oral mucosa etc.) or Central (intra-osseous) in occurrence.

***Peripheral reactive lesions:***

Eversole classified the common peripheral hyperplastic lesions of gingiva and other oral mucosal sites into the following categories [2, 3].

1. Pyogenic Granuloma
2. Peripheral Giant Cell Granuloma
3. Peripheral Ossifying Fibroma
4. Peripheral fibroma (Focal Fibrous hyperplasia/ Fibrous Epulis) [2].

***Central reactive lesions:***

The intra-osseous reactive lesions include the following categories [4, 5].

1. Central giant cell Granuloma
2. Aneurysmal Bone Cyst
3. Brown's Tumour of hyperparathyroidism
4. Chronic Sclerosing Osteomyelitis and Garre's osteomyelitis/Proliferative Periosteitis [4, 5].

## 29.3 Pyogenic Granuloma

### 29.3.1 Clinical Features and Aetiopathogenesis

Pyogenic Granuloma presents as a painless pedunculated or sessile, soft fleshy mass that bleeds easily with a normal or occasionally ulcerated overlying surface (Fig. 29.1). Gingiva is the most common intra-oral site, although it can affect lips, mucosa and tongue [3].

It is a localised proliferative mass occurring as a result of an exuberant reparative response to various stimuli such as chronic local irritation (calculus, overhanging restoration, a sharp margin of crown etc.), trauma, hormonal changes (Pregnancy), bone marrow transplants and reac-

R. S. Gali (✉)
Department of Oral and Maxillofacial Surgery, Narayana Dental College and Hospital, Nellore, Andhra Pradesh, India

Medicover Hospital, Nellore, Andhra Pradesh, India


K. Bonanthaya et al. (eds.), *Oral and Maxillofacial Surgery for the Clinician*, https://doi.org/10.1007/978-981-15-1346-6_29

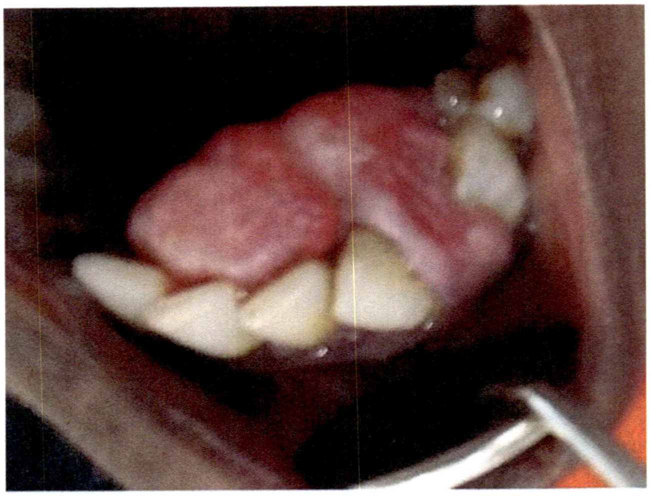



**Fig. 29.1** Exophytic gingival growth associated with chronic gingivitis with heavy bands of calculus. The lesion easily bleeds on palpation and can occasionally cause displacement of teeth

tion to grafts. Pulp polyp or hyperplastic pulpitis is also a type of pyogenic granuloma arising in response to low-grade chronic infection [1]. The term pyogenic granuloma is a misnomer as it does not contain pus and it is not a true granuloma [1, 3].

It can occur across all the age groups and both genders, but with a distinct predominance in females in the 2nd decade of life due to the increased levels of circulating hormones like oestrogen and progesterone [6]. Equal incidence has been reported in both the jaws with a slight predilection to anterior maxilla [1].

### 29.3.2 Differential Diagnosis

Other peripheral reactive lesions that resemble pyogenic granuloma are peripheral giant cell granuloma and peripheral ossifying fibroma [3]. Peripheral ossifying fibroma has a firm consistency and a lesser tendency to bleed. Specific proliferative malignant lesions can closely mimic pyogenic granuloma misguiding the clinician leading to sub-optimal treatment. These can be primary or metastatic squamous cell carcinomas, fibrosarcoma, Kaposi's sarcoma, oral metastatic deposits from distant primary foci like thyroid, lung kidneys etc [1].

### 29.3.3 Diagnostic Workup

*Radiological Features* Appreciable radiological changes are generally not seen in pyogenic granuloma, but occasionally cup-like resorption of underlying alveolar bone can be seen in a peri-apical view or an orthopantomogram. Ruling out the presence of large osteolytic lesions is required to exclude malignant lesions.

*Histopathological Features* Histologically pyogenic granulomas are classified into two distinct sub-types- the non-lobular capillary haemangioma type (non-LCH type) and Lobular capillary haemangioma (LCH) type [6]. The non-LCH type comprises of highly vascular proliferation that is similar to granulation tissue with foci of fibrous tissue whereas the LCH type shows proliferation of blood vessels that are aggregated in a lobular fashion without any signs of inflammation and or reparative response.

### 29.3.4 Recent Concepts

Epivatianos A et al. had demonstrated that these two subtypes have a different origin, clinical behaviour and immunohistochemical properties [7]. Their study had shown that non-LCH pyogenic granuloma presented clinically as a pedunculated mass and was mostly associated with identifiable aetiologic factors and showed a histological picture of a reparative response. However, LCH pyogenic granuloma presented as a non-ulcerated sessile mass without any identifiable aetiology and histological evidence of lobulated vessel pattern and the absence of inflammatory reaction. This has led to the concept that LCH pyogenic granuloma represents a benign tumour of the vascular origin that develops due to unknown factors just like other benign tumours.

### 29.3.5 Treatment

Surgical excision of the lesion followed by removal of local irritants such as calculus, foreign body etc. is the standard treatment. Excision up to the periosteum is required in gingival lesions followed by either primary closure by mobilisation of adjacent mucoperiosteum, or surgical defect is left to heal by secondary intention by the placement of Coe pack. Brisk bleeding is often encountered during excision that would require electrocoagulation. Other treatment options include electrocautery, cryosurgery, sclerotherapy and laser-assisted excision.

### 29.3.6 Prognosis

Complete excision of the lesion till the periosteum and removal of local aetiological factors will eliminate the chances of recurrence.

## 29.4 Peripheral Giant Cell Granuloma

Peripheral giant cell granuloma is the most commonly encountered giant cell containing lesion of the oral cavity that closely resembles pyogenic granuloma.

### 29.4.1 Clinical Features and Aetiopathogenesis

It is thought to originate mainly from the connective tissue of the gingiva or the periosteum of the alveolar ridge. It has been reported in all age groups but with a peak incidence in the 3rd and 4th decades of life with a female predominance [8]. The lesion presents as a soft proliferative mass occurring at gingiva or even at edentulous alveolar ridge. It has a tendency to bleed and may or may not be pedunculated [9].

The term 'reparative' was dropped from its nomenclature as the reparative nature could not be demonstrated histopathologically. The aetiology of this lesion remains unclear, but irritating local factors such as poor restorations, prostheses calculus etc. are thought to contribute to its origin (Fig. 29.2).

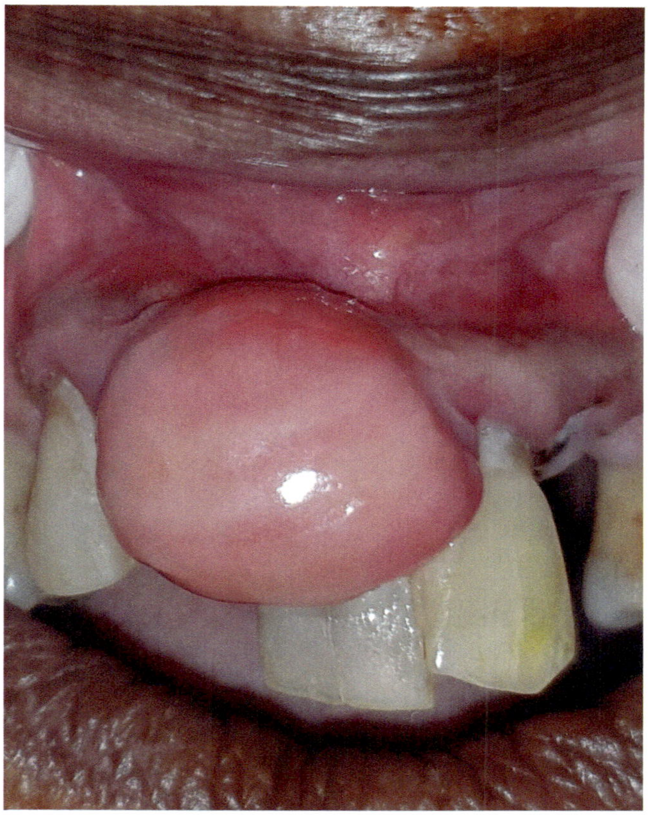



Fig. 29.2 Peripheral giant cell granuloma, presenting as an exophytic gingival growth firm to hard in consistency causing displacement of adjacent teeth

### 29.4.2 Differential Diagnosis

Clinically pyogenic granuloma and peripheral giant cell granuloma are indistinguishable. Erosion of cortical bone is more commonly seen with peripheral giant cell granuloma than with pyogenic granuloma.

Histopathologically, the lesion is very similar to central giant cell granuloma, its intra-osseous counterpart [9].

### 29.4.3 Radiologic Features

Since the lesion is peripheral in the origin and location, radiologic changes are rarely seen. Longstanding, larger lesions can exhibit superficial cortical erosion and may also show widening of adjacent periodontal ligament space.

### 29.4.4 Histopathological Features

Hyperplasia of fibroblasts with abundant multi-nucleated giant cells, with scattered areas of chronic inflammatory cells and neutrophils are seen [9]. Controversy exists about the origin of the giant cells; some believe that they are of the osteoclast origin while others state that they are formed by the fusion of mono-nuclear cells. Irrespective of their origin, they are non-functional in these lesions as they are not involved either in phagocytosis or bone resorption [9].

### 29.4.5 Treatment

Complete surgical excision including the periosteum or periodontal ligament as applicable followed by the removal of local factors is the optimum treatment for peripheral giant cell granuloma. Recurrences are rare, but have been reported and are believed to be due to non-inclusion of periosteum or periodontal ligament during excision.

### 29.4.6 Prognosis and Complications

Recurrence of PGCG is infrequent, ranges as little as 5–11% have been reported. Extensive clearing of the base of the lesion, eradication of the source of irritation prevents recurrence [9].

### 29.4.7 Recent Advances

Increasing incidence of peripheral giant cell granulomas occurring in association with dental implants has been reported [10, 11]. Local irritant factors, inflammation of peri-implant tissues are the causative factors. Clinically, these proliferations are similar to the classic peripheral giant cell granulomas and usually develop within months to years following placement of dental implants. If early detection and complete surgical excision are not performed, such lesions can lead to peri-implantitis, ultimately leading to failure of the implant necessitating its removal.

## 29.5 Peripheral Ossifying Fibroma

The peripheral ossifying fibroma is a reactive gingival proliferation presenting as nodular mass firm in consistency with or without ulceration. It contains fibroblastic cellular tissue with varying amounts of mineralised content that can be either bone, cementum or dystrophic calcification.

The term 'peripheral ossifying fibroma' literally means a benign tumour of fibrous connective tissue origin. However, this lesion is a non-neoplastic reactive proliferative lesion, so this term is a misnomer for this pathology [12].

### 29.5.1 Clinical Features and Aetiopathogenesis

The lesion presents as a slow-growing solitary gingival growth commonly seen during the second decade of life, predominantly in women in the anterior region of either of the jaws. The lesion is believed to originate from periodontal ligament in response to local irritation or inflammation, commonly seen at the inter-dental region as a pedunculated or sessile mass (Fig. 29.3). The exact pathogenesis of peripheral ossifying fibroma is controversial. Some authors believe that it initially develops as a pyogenic granuloma that subsequently undergoes fibrous maturation and calcification. It is thought that these two lesions represent progressive stages of the same reactive pathology [13].

### 29.5.2 Differential Diagnosis

Histopathology is the only method by which one can distinguish a peripheral ossifying fibroma from a pyogenic granuloma or peripheral giant cell granuloma [14].

### 29.5.3 Radiologic Features

Radiographs may occasionally demonstrate specks of calcifications in these lesions (Fig. 29.4a–c).

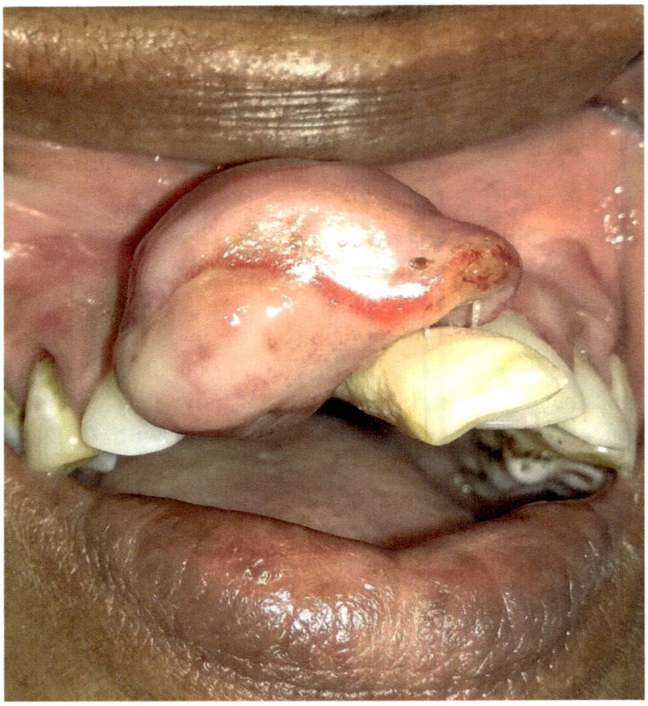



**Fig. 29.3** Exophytic sessile mass over gingiva at anterior maxilla associated with heavy bands of calculus and is seen to be causing displacement of teeth

### 29.5.4 Histopathologic Features (Fig. 29.4c)

The peripheral ossifying fibroma consists of rich fibro-cellular tissue with focal areas of mineralised deposits containing bone, cementum or dystrophic calcification. A chronic inflammatory cell infiltrate is observed at the periphery of the lesion.

### 29.5.5 Treatment

Complete surgical excision of the lesion with circumferential margins of 3mm of healthy gingival tissue and deep margins down to the bone, including the adjacent periosteum and periodontal ligament has to be performed to reduce the chances of recurrence [1]. Extraction of the involved teeth is to be considered in the cases of recurrent or multi-focal lesions of peripheral ossifying fibromas.

### 29.5.6 Prognosis and Complications

The reported reccurrence rate for peripheral ossifying fibroma is surprisingly high for a reactive proliferation. The recurrence rate has varied from 4 to 75% [15, 16].

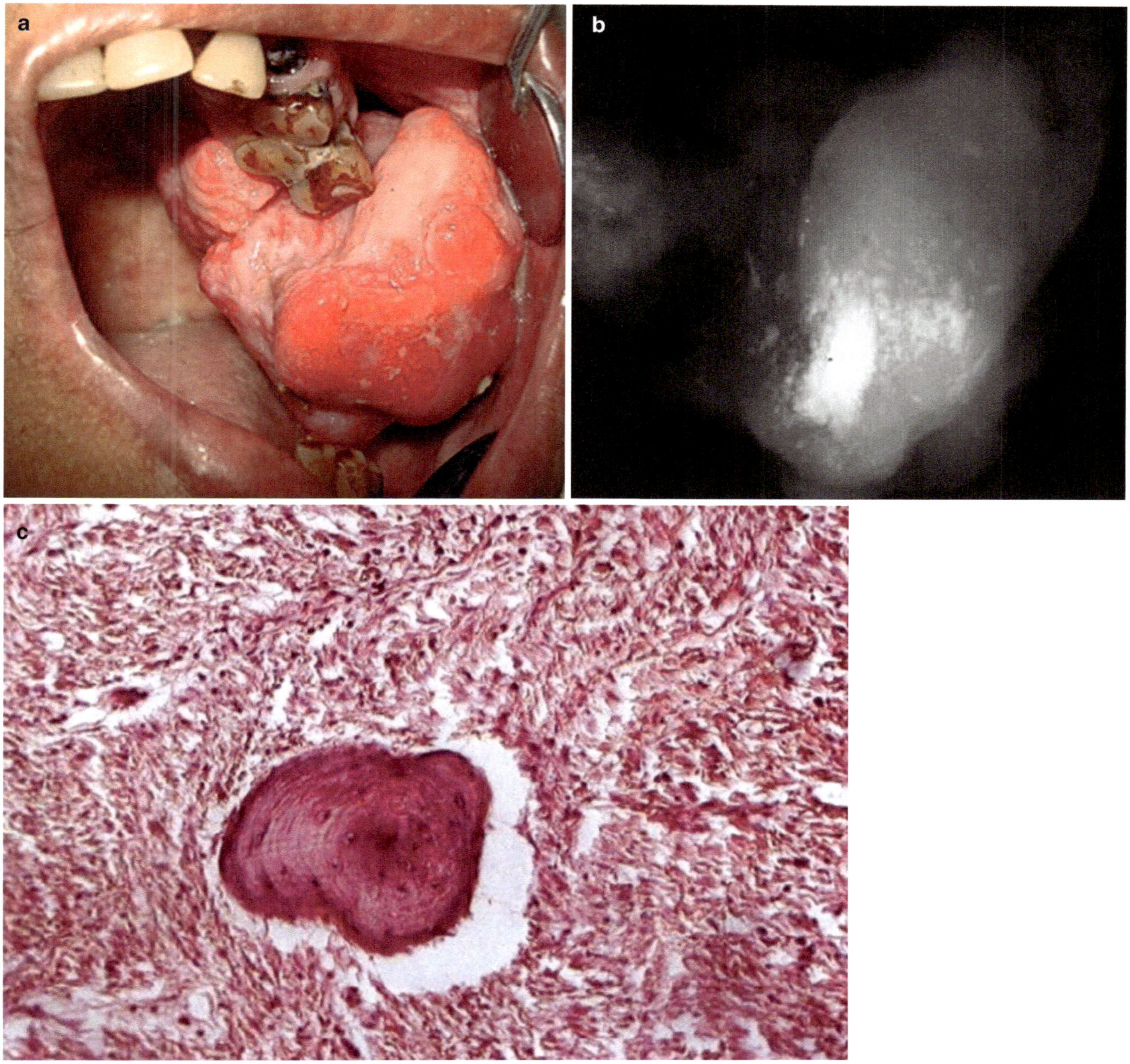




**Fig. 29.4** (**a**) Large peripheral ossifying fibroma of 6 × 7 cm in size, in a 64-year-old female, 5 years duration presenting as firm mass. (**b**) Radio-opacities on the radiograph observed in the excised lesion. (**c**) Histopathological view showing the woven bone (H&E stain, original magnification 400×). (Adapted from A rare massive exophytic gingival growth: Suvy Manuel et al.; Clinics and Practice. 2012 Mar 30; 2(2): e38. Open Access DOI https://doi.org/10.4081/cp.2012.e38 , copy right S. Manuel et al, CC BY-NC 3.0, Licensee PAGEPress Italy)

*Pearls, Perils and Pitfalls: Peripheral Reactive Lesions:*

1. The most common proliferative masses of Gingiva are a Triad of reactive lesions—The 3 P's—Pyogenic Granuloma, Peripheral giant Cell granuloma & Peripheral Ossifying fibroma.
2. Pyogenic granulomas and peripheral giant cell granulomas are more vascular, which is reflected by their tendency to bleed and their red or reddish-blue colour.
3. Unlike pyogenic granuloma, peripheral giant cell granuloma can occur on edentulous alveolar ridges arising from the periosteum
4. POF is firm to hard in consistency due to the mineralised content like cementum/bone/dystrophic calcification
5. Complete Surgical excision of these lesions with circumferential margins of 3 mm of healthy gingival tissue and deep margins down to the bone, including the adjacent periosteum & periodontal ligament has to be performed to reduce the chances of recurrence. This should be followed by removal of putative local factors like calculus, plaque faulty restoration/prosthesis etc.
6. Extraction of the involved but firm teeth should be considered in the cases of recurrent/multi focal lesions.

## 29.6 Central Giant Cell Granuloma (Figs. 29.5 and 29.6)

*Synonyms* Central giant cell Lesion, Central reparative giant cell granuloma and Giant cell tumour of jaw bones.

### 29.6.1 Introduction

The central giant cell granuloma is one of the few maxillofacial pathologies that have generated a significant amount of discussion and controversy. The true biological nature of the lesion remains to be understood and the debate about labelling it as a tumour still exists [12].

Initially, it was described as Giant cell 'reparative' granuloma by Jaffe in 1953 [17] suggesting that it was a reactive response to intra-bony haemorrhage and inflammation. Later, the term 'reparative' was dropped, as prior traumatic/inflammatory episodes could not be elicited in most cases and clinical progression of disease was inconsistent with the repair process of bone.

The aggressive clinical behaviour of specific lesions demonstrated by osteolysis, cortical expansion, perforation and extension into soft tissue has led to the view that it is a benign tumour similar to the giant cell tumour of long bones [18]. The exact relationship between these two pathologies remains to be understood. The concept that these lesions represent two points in the spectrum of a single-disease process has been putforth [19, 20]. Considering the variability in clinical presentation, individual authors have classified it as a rapidly growing & destructive—aggressive form and a slow-growing, incidentally picked up lesion—the non-aggressive form [19, 20].

Since the true neoplastic nature is yet to be established and the histologic features do not represent a true granulomatous lesion, the term central giant cell 'lesion' had been proposed by Whitaker & Waldron [20].

### 29.6.2 Clinical Features and Aetiopathogenesis

The lesion can occur in any age group but, children and young adults are more commonly affected and with a female predominance [19]. The anterior mandibular region is the most frequent site of occurrence almost twice as compared to the maxilla. The most common presentation is that of an asymptomatic, slow-growing, bony hard and expansile swelling of the involved jaw [19, 20]. This can be accompanied by progressive displacement/loosening of teeth, paresthesia, nasal obstruction and secondary infection leading to pain (Fig. 29.5a, b).

### 29.6.3 Differential Diagnosis

Histopathologically, central giant cell granulomas and brown tumour of hyperparathyroidism are indistinguishable from each other, and this can be very misguiding to the clinician and the pathologist. Hence, biochemical tests like serum calcium, phosphate and parathormone levels are to be evaluated to rule out brown's tumour. In all cases of multi-focal and or recurrent central giant cell granulomas of jaws, the possibility of primary or secondary hyperparathyroidism is to be ruled out, so that unnecessary surgical procedures and their added morbidity can be avoided.

### 29.6.4 Radiological Features

The central giant cell granuloma presents as multi-locular radiolucency with scalloped margins that are usually non-corticated [19]. The cortical expansion, thinning followed by perforation, root resorption and displacement of adjacent teeth can be seen in aggressive variants [20] (Fig. 29.5c, d).

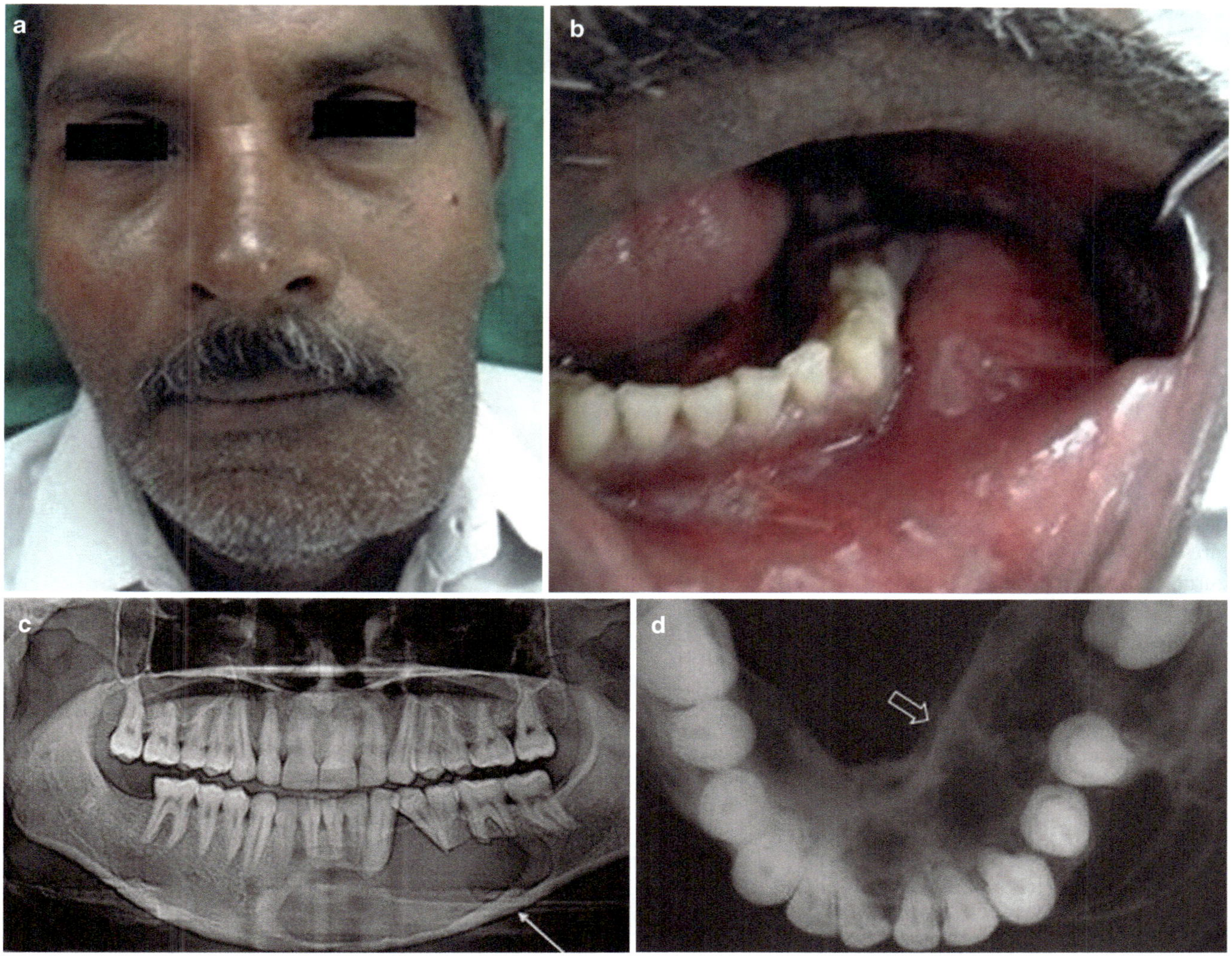




**Fig. 29.5** (**a**, **b**) Central Giant cell granuloma presenting as hard bony mass over the left body of the mandible with bi-cortical expansion. (**c**) Central Giant cell granuloma presenting as a unilocular osteolytic lesion with sclerotic border and thinning of lower border. (**d**) Occlusal radiograph demonstrating bi-cortical expansile lytic lesion with incomplete septae

### 29.6.5 Histopathologic Features

The lesion consists of a proliferation of spindle-shaped fibroblasts in fibrous and fibromyxoid/vascular stroma [20]. Clusters of multi-nucleated giant cells are scattered throughout connective tissue stroma especially around vascular channels. These cells are believed to originate from osteoclasts or by the fusion of mono-nuclear cells [9]. Focal deposits of metaplastic bone are seen. The histological picture is precisely identical to brown's tumour of hyperparathyroidism [1].

### 29.6.6 Treatment

The most commonly practised and favoured treatment for central giant cell granuloma has been aggressive surgical curettage. Recurrence rates ranging from 20 to 50% have been reported following curettage [21]. Adjuvant treatments to curettage-like peripheral ostectomy or marginal resection have been advocated to reduce the chances of recurrence [22]. Aggressive surgical treatment options such as en bloc resection/segmental mandibulectomy/maxillectomy are presently reserved for locally advanced lesions & recurrent lesions [22, 23]. Significant vascularity and intra-operative bleeding are frequently associated with these lesions. Aggressive surgical resection with 0.5 cm margins of healthy tissue is advocated to reduce the chances of recurrence [24]. However, the morbidity associated with surgical resection such as functional, cosmetic impairment, loss of teeth, teeth buds and neurosensory disturbances questions the need for such aggressive treatments in a benign reactive lesion-like central giant cell granuloma [24].

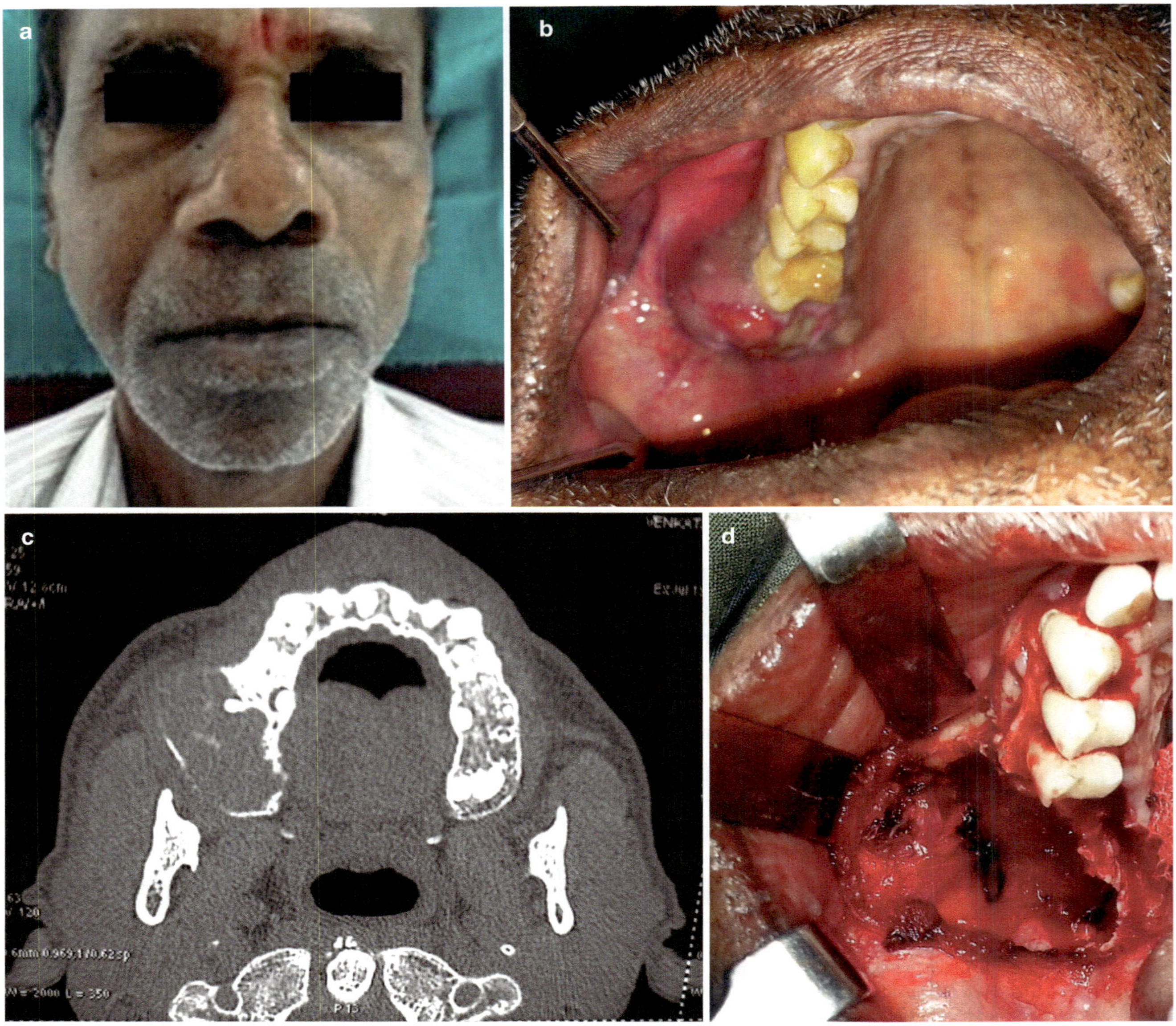




**Fig. 29.6** (**a**) Swelling right side face. (**b**) Intra oral view of lesion right posterior maxilla. (**c**) CT axial cut showing changes in posterior right maxilla. (**d**) Intra operative view

*Medical Methods of Treatment* Based on the premise that osteoclastic activity steers the progression of the disease process, medical treatments aimed at antagonising the activity and proliferation of osteoclasts have been used with varying rates of success [25–27].

*Intra-lesional Steroids* Steroids have demonstrated the ability to inhibit bone resorption and induce apoptosis of osteoclasts. Weekly intra-lesional injections of triamcinolone acetonide for six weeks have shown highly variable results from partial shrinkage, in complete remission, to complete resolution leading to hypercalcification of the area [28, 29]. The protocol described involves the use of a 50% mixture of local anaesthetic and 10 mg/ml triamcinolone acetonide. Two ml of this solution has to be used for every 1cc of the lesion visible on orthopantomogram [29, 30].

*Systemic Calcitonin Therapy* Based on the observations that calcitonin receptors were found in the multi-nucleated giant cells of central giant cell granuloma and the role of calcitonin in inhibiting osteoclast function, systemic administration of calcitonin has been practised to treat central giant cell granuloma [31]. Calcitonin is administered through a sub-cutaneous or intra-nasal route. Subcutaneous administration involves 100 units per day for a period of 18–21 months during which sequential radiographs are obtained to monitor the remission of the lesion.

Unlike sub-cutaneous administration, the intra-nasal route has better patient compliance but unpredictable absorption rates [31].

Results with calcitonin therapy have been highly variable. In some instances, they have been used to shrink the lesions first, later to be followed by curettage.

*Interferon Therapy* Owing to the prominent vascular component in central giant cell granuloma, the anti-angiogenic properties of interferon alpha have been used as adjuvant therapy following enucleation/curettage of the lesion. Isolated interferon therapy without prior surgical procedure led to partial resolution of lesions and is of limited value. Kaban et al. had proposed a protocol that involved treatment of aggressive central giant cell granulomas of the mandible by a staged treatment of conservative surgical enucleation (sparing the inferior alveolar nerve and teeth). This is followed by administration of interferon Alpha 2 or beta (3,000,000 units/m$^2$) 48–72 h after surgery, given once daily by a sub-cutaneous route for a period of 6 months or till a period when CT scan showed complete regeneration of bony defect [32]. Their study was based on the hypothesis that these lesions are vascular proliferations, thus explaining the high success rate in response to anti-angiogenic therapy in their experience [32].

*Bisphosphonates* Bisphosphonates that have an antagonising effect on the osteoclastic activity. Owing to the virtue of this property, bisphosphonates have been used in conjunction with intra-lesional steroids in central giant cell granuloma with promising results [33].

*Denosumab* Denosumab is a human monoclonal antibody that binds to the RANK ligand located on the surface of osteoclasts and deactivates them. The stromal cells of giant cell tumour have been shown to secrete RANKL and upregulate osteoclast activity and development. Recent Phase-II clinical trials on the use of denosumab in giant cell tumours of long bones showed that it reduces the need for morbid surgeries [34, 35]. A single report on the use of denosumab in central giant cell granulomas of jaws in two patients was recently published and had claimed very promising results involving complete remission of jaw lesions. However, studies involving a larger sample with longer follow-up periods are awaited to know the exact risk-benefit status of this novel treatment option [36].

## 29.7 Aneurysmal Bone Cyst (Fig. 29.7a–f)

The aneurysmal bone cyst is a controversial lesion believed to be a non-neoplastic and exaggerated reactive response of vascular tissues of bone. It is a pseudocyst that presents as expansile, osteolytic lesion often characterised by ballooning distension of the cortex, that consists of blood-filled cavernous spaces showing occasional osteoid material and multi-nucleated giant cells [37].

### 29.7.1 Clinical Features

The aneurysmal bone cyst generally occurs in patients less than 30 years of age with a reported higher incidence during the second decade of life with almost equal gender predilection. Aneurysmal bone cysts of the jaws are relatively rare comprising of only 1–3% of all aneurysmal bone cysts occurring in the skeleton. The posterior region of the mandible is the preferred site compared to maxilla (6:1).

Most of these lesions present as expansile swellings with or without perforation of the involved jaw bone, causing facial asymmetry or displacement of adjacent teeth and malocclusion. Pain, paresthesia and rapid progression of swelling can be seen occasionally. Dark venous blood is generally obtained on aspiration (Fig. 29.7a–c).

Pulsatile nature, thrill and bruit are generally not seen in these lesions despite the prominent vascular component associated with aneurysmal bone cysts. The presence of these signs in an expansile, osteolytic jaw lesion would rather indicate a high flow vascular malformation. The clinician should recognise this and not mistake it for an aneurysmal bone cyst, because doing an aspiration or incisional biopsy of such high flow vascular malformations can lead to disastrous bleeding and potentially fatal outcomes.

### 29.7.2 Aetiopathogenesis

The exact mechanism regarding the origin of aneurysmal bone cysts remains controversial. The reported hypotheses include post-traumatic, reactive malformation, genetic predisposition causing chromosomal translocation and minor vascular injury in a pre-existing bone lesion leading to pooling of blood in the stromal spaces creating bone destruction [38].

This lesion can occur de novo as a primary aneurysmal bone cyst or as a secondary phenomenon arising in pre-existing lesions like central giant cell granuloma, ossifying fibroma, fibrous dysplasia, osteosarcoma, fibrosarcoma and other lesions [38]. It has been postulated that injury to the capillary network in these lesions leads to extravasation of blood. The associated capillary blood pressure readily destroys unsupported stroma resulting in a blow out reaction thereby producing the expansile and destructive aneurysmal bone cyst.

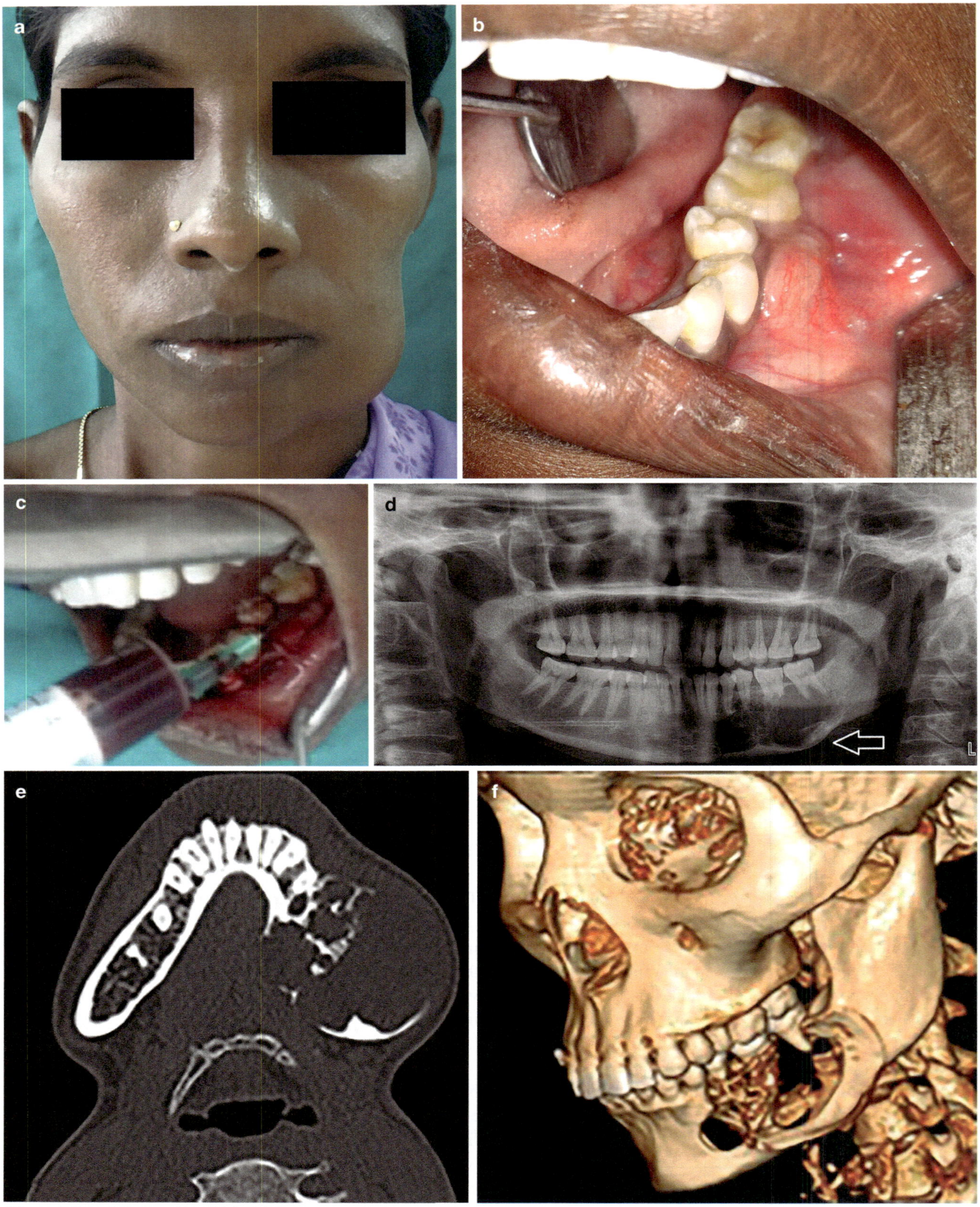




**Fig. 29.7** (**a**) Swelling left side body mandible. (**b**) Intra oral view of swelling left lower posterior buccal cortex. (**c**) Aspirate showing blood tinged fluid. (**d**) OPG showing lesion left body mandible. (**e**) Axial CT scan showing the expansile lesion. (**f**) 3D CT showing the destruction of bone

### 29.7.3 Radiologic Features

Owing to its osteolytic nature, aneurysmal bone cyst presents as unilocular or multi-locular radiolucency often associated with cortical thinning and perforation with resorption of roots seen occasionally. A classic sign commonly seen is the 'ballooning' distension of the thinned out cortex occurring as a result of a thin outline of reactive sub-periosteal bone formation. CT and MRI scans of such lesions often demonstrate blood and free fluid in these cavities (Fig. 29.7d, e, f).

These typical features can sometimes be masked in those aneurysmal bone cysts occurring as secondary phenomena in pre-existing bone lesions. Such aneurysmal bone cysts present as mixed radiolucent-radiopaque lesions.

### 29.7.4 Histopathological Features

Histopathologically, it consists of variable amounts of fibrous connective tissue stroma with blood-filled sinusoidal spaces, multi-nucleated giant cells and reactive woven bone/osteoid. Correlating the histopathological and clinical features, three variants of aneurysmal bone cysts were proposed namely, the solid type, vascular type and mixed type [39]. The solid type is associated with a dense stroma, few sinusoidal spaces and blood vessels that correlates with the absence of cortical perforation clinically and minimal bleeding observed intra-operatively. The vascular variant falls into the other end of the spectrum that shows loose fibrous tissue stroma with large blood-filled cavernous spaces causing extensive osteolysis and cortical perforation that is frequently associated with brisk intra-operative bleed. The mixed variant shows characteristics of both these sub-types.

### 29.7.5 Treatment

Complete Surgical curettage of the lesion is the most commonly followed treatment modality. Adjuvant therapies like cryosurgery and electrocauterisation have been used to reduce the chances of recurrence. Due to its vascular nature, brisk bleeding is often encountered during surgery that generally ceases after complete removal of the lesion. Pre-operative embolisation had been advocated in extensive, vascular variants of aneurysmal bone cysts to reduce intra-operative blood loss.

Resection is generally reserved for aggressive aneurysmal bone cysts that have extensively resorbed the lower border of the mandible or have caused a pathological fracture and lesions that have recurred following conservative therapy. The decision to perform segmental resection is also influenced by the nature and extent of primary jaw pathology in which the aneurysmal bone cyst has arisen. Segmental resection has been recommended as the treatment option for secondary aneurysmal bone cysts occurring in ossifying fibromas, giant cell granulomas and osteoblastomas [40].

### 29.7.6 Prognosis and Complications

Aneurysmal bone cysts have relatively higher recurrence rates compared to central giant cell granuloma [38]. This has been attributed to incomplete removal of the lesion during curettage/marginal mandibulectomy. The multi-locular nature of the lesion can sometimes limit the access leading to residual pathological tissue that causes increased intra-operative bleeding and also gives rise to recurrences usually in the first year following surgery.

## 29.8 Brown Tumour of Hyperparathyroidism (Fig. 29.8)

Brown tumour is a misnomer as it is not a true neoplasm, but a localised area of osteolytic defect caused by increased osteoclastic activity and demineralisation of bone that is induced by excessive secretion of parathyroid hormone. It is considered to be an intra-osseous reactive lesion [4].

### 29.8.1 Etiopathogenesis

Hypersecretion of parathyroid hormone can occur due to Primary (benign/malignant adenoma of parathyroid gland), secondary (pre-existing kidney disease leads to compensatory overactivity of parathyroid) or tertiary causes (parathyroid tumours arising due to prolonged hyperactivity induced by secondary causes). Irrespective of the origin, the resultant effect is hypercalcaemia (caused by mobilisation of calcium from bone to bloodstream) and altered phosphate levels that give rise to the entire spectrum of signs and symptoms of this disease. These include disturbances in ion metabolism, demineralisation of bone, kidney stones, gastrointestinal disorders and muscle weakness. Hence, hyperparathyroidism is also referred to as the 'disease of bones, stones, abdominal groans and psychic moans' [41].

### 29.8.2 Clinical Features

Brown tumour is a localised, lytic bone defect characterised by a mass of reactive fibrous tissue that presents as swelling with cortical expansion, perforation occasionally associated with pain and pathological fracture. The lesion occurs in adults above 50 years of age and has a female to the male pre-dilection of 5:2 and can occur in any bone but more common sites are long bones, pelvis, ribs, maxilla and mandible [42]. Co-existing multiple synchronous lesions in the jaws and at other skeletal sites can also occur

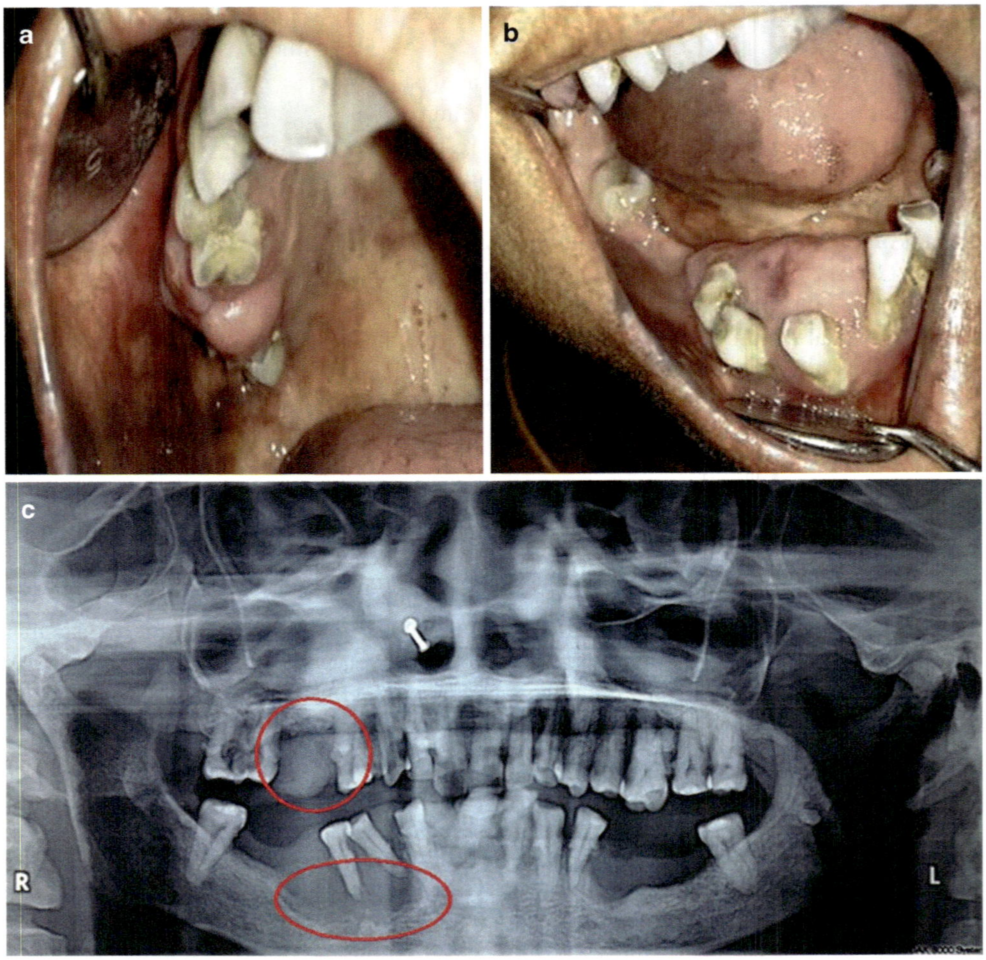


**Fig. 29.8** (**a**) Lesion right posterior maxilla. (**b**) Lesion anterior mandible. (**c**) OPG showing the changes (red circles)



[43] (Fig. 29.8a–c). Bone manifestations usually occur in the late stages of hyperparathyroidism, and brown tumours are picked up during the diagnostic work-up for the same. Rarely, brown tumour of the jaw may be the first manifestation of primary hyper parathyroidism [44, 45]. They can cause significant bone destruction leading to facial asymmetry, displacement of teeth, malocclusion pathological fracture etc.

### 29.8.3 Diagnostic Workup

Since it is not possible to histopathologically distinguish brown tumour from central giant cell granuloma, biochemical tests are mandatory to confirm its diagnosis. Elevated serum calcium (>10.4 mg/dl), decreased serum phosphate level, elevated parathormone levels, ultrasonography to identify parathyroid adenomas (primary hyperparathyroidism), and renal function tests to rule out renal disease (secondary hyperparathyroidism) constitute the sequence of diagnostic work up to diagnose hyperparathyroidism [45].

### 29.8.4 Differential Diagnosis

- Giant cell granuloma
- Giant cell tumour
- Aneurysmal bone cyst

### 29.8.5 Radiographic Features

It shows a well-defined mono-locular or multi-locular well-demarcated lesion that is purely lytic. There are significant root resorption and loss of lamina dura.

### 29.8.6 Histopathology

Brown tumour very closely resembles central giant cell granuloma, and these two lesions are indistinguishable on histopathology. Features such as the proliferation of multi-nucleated giant cells, osteoclasts present in a rich fibro-cellular and vascular connective tissue stroma with scattered areas of haemorrhagic foci and haemosiderin pigmentation are seen. The presence of haemosiderin renders this lesion its characteristic brown/brownish yellow colour and hence the name brown tumour.

### 29.8.7 Treatment

Spontaneous resolution/remission of brown tumour generally occurs after treatment of the underlying cause of hyperparathyroidism. Primary hyperparathyroidism is treated by excision of parathyroid adenoma/gland. Treatment of renal disease, vitamin D deficiency is done in the cases of secondary hyperparathyroidism. Refractory lesions that fail to resolve or incomplete remissions after treatment of underlying cause would require surgical curettage [44, 45].

### 29.8.8 Prognosis

Brown tumours are generally slow-growing lesions that can be locally destructive. Invasion into surrounding structures may cause a variety of symptoms. Small lesions usually resolve spontaneously once the underlying condition (hyperparathyroidism) is treated whereas large lesions take about 6–12 months to subside.

*Pearls, perils and pitfalls:*

1. Central Giant cell granuloma (CGCG) and brown tumour are indistinguishable histologically. An incisional biopsy report of CGCG should prompt the clinician to ask for biochemical investigations to rule out the brown tumour, that is characterised by increased serum levels of calcium, phosphate, alkaline phosphatase and parathyroid hormone.
2. It is crucial to diagnose brown tumours that are invariably reported as CGCG on incisional biopsy because treatment of hyperparathyroidism will generally lead to spontaneous resolution of brown jaw tumours, thereby avoiding unnecessary surgical procedures of jaw lesions.
3. Aneurysmal bone cysts have varied clinical, radiological and histological presentations.
4. Secondary aneurysmal bone cysts that arise in pre-existing pathologies have a higher tendency to recur if treated by conservative surgical methods like curettage.

## 29.9 Chronic Sclerosing Osteomyelitis and Garre's Osteomyelitis

Chronic sclerosing type of osteomyelitis occurs as a result of low-grade and long-standing infection of the marrow spaces that is characterised by areas of reactive bone sclerosis extending over a larger area (diffuse sclerosing) or localised to one or two teeth (focal sclerosing) [4].

Garre's osteomyelitis also known as proliferative periostitis is a sub-type of osteomyelitis that occurs in children. It is characterised by reactive sub-periosteal bone formation in response to chronic low-grade infection. Predominantly occurring in the posterior region of the mandible, it is best seen on an occlusal radiograph or an axial section CT scan as onion skin-layered appearance of the expanded bony cortex.

Rarely, malignancies like osteosarcoma (juxtacortical and parosteal), chondrosarcoma, fibrosarcoma and others can closely mimic Garre's osteomyelitis leading to a diagnostic dilemma and sub-optimal treatment.

These lesions are discussed in detail in other chapters of the book.

## 29.10 Conclusion

A variety of reactive soft tissue and bony pathologies occur in the oro-facial region that arises in response to chronic low-grade inflammation, trauma, metabolic and hormonal influences. These lesions very closely mimic benign and malignant neoplasms in their clinical, radiological and histological presentations. Knowledge about their etiopathogenesis, clinical behaviour patterns is of paramount importance for providing appropriate treatment.

## Case Scenario 1 (Fig. 29.5)

A 53-year-old male patient reported with a chief complaint of bony hard swelling over the left side lower jaw of 8 month duration.

**Clinical Examination**

Bony hard swelling over the left body of the mandible was noted with the expansion of buccal and lingual cortical plates (Fig. 29.5a, b).

**Pre-operative Diagnostic Work-up**

*Imaging*: Orthopantomogram revealed unilocular radiolucency with a sclerotic border and x-ray occlusal view showed a bicortical expansile, osteolytic lesion at the left body of mandible, with areas of osteosclerosis (Fig. 29.5c, d).

*Incisional Biopsy*: Incisional biopsy done under local anaesthesia proved it to be central giant cell granuloma. Biochemical tests for assessment of serum parathormone, calcium, phosphate levels were performed, and the possibility of brown tumour of hyperparathyroidism was ruled out.

*Diagnosis*: Central Giant cell granuloma of mandibular body.

*Surgical Plan*: Considering bi cortical perforation and thinning of lower border caused by the lesion, segmental mandibulectomy through submandibular approach + mandibular reconstruction plate fixation was performed.

*Postoperative Period*: Post-operative period was uneventful. The patient was last seen three years after surgery and was found to be recurrence-free.

## **Case Scenario 2** (Fig. 29.6a–d)

A 60-Year-old male with a complaint of an asymptomatic slow-growing swelling in the upper jaw of 10 months duration.

### Clinical Examination

A single firm to hard swelling measuring approximately 4 × 3 cm located over the right maxillary posterior alveolus causing buccolingual expansion, vestibular obliteration was found. It was extending from the mesial aspect of right maxillary 1st molar to the maxillary tuberosity area. The swelling was non-tender, firm to hard in consistency, with normal overlying mucosa. There was associated odontogenic focus of sepsis, but there was grade-II mobility of right maxillary 1st molar.

### Pre-operative Diagnostic Work-up

*Imaging*: A pre-operative CT scan revealed a unilocular radiolucency with scattered areas of radio-opacity located at right maxillary posterior alveolus that was causing buccal cortical expansion, thinning and even perforation with denuding of the roots of the 1st molar. Superiorly the lesion was found to be extending till the body of the zygoma and just abutting the floor of the maxillary sinus.

*Histopathological and Biochemical Evaluation*: An incisional biopsy of the lesion was performed under local anaesthesia, that was reported as a central giant cell granuloma of the maxilla. A thorough biochemical evaluation was done to rule out brown tumour of hyperparathyroidism as both the lesions are indistinguishable histopathologically. Serum calcium, parathormone, and phosphate were within the normal limits.

*Diagnosis*: *Central Giant cell granuloma*—Right maxillary posterior alveolus.

*Surgical Plan*: Extended alveolectomy of the right posterior maxillary alveolus + nasal antrostomy + two-layered closure of the resultant defect with oroantral communication by mobilisation of the buccal fat pad and adjacent Bucco-palatal mucoperiosteum. Following excision of the lesion, since maxillary sinus was breached, the resultant defect was packed with ribbon gauzed soaked in whitehead's varnish, and a trans nasal inferior meatal antrostomy was done, through which the tip of the pack was brought outside and knotted for removal on the 12th day. A two-layered watertight closure of the wound was achieved.

*Post-operative Period*: The wound healed uneventfully. The patient was last seen 4 years post-operatively and was free of disease.

## **Case Scenario 3** (Fig. 29.7)

A 38-year-old female with a complaint of swelling at the left side lower jaw of 1-year duration.

### Clinical Examination

Figure 29.7a A single firm to hard swelling was located over the left body of mandible, non-tender with normal overlying skin & mucosa. On palpation, buccal and lingual cortical plate expansion (Fig. 29.7b) with eggshell crackling sign-positive suggestive of expanded and thinned out cortical plates causing microfractures on digital pressure.

### Pre-operative Diagnostic Work-up

*Imaging*: Orthopantomogram revealed a radiolucent lesion in the left body of the mandible with focal radio-opacities located in the anterior aspect of the lesion. The lesion was causing root resorption, thinning of mandibular lower border and was extending from lower left 2nd molar to lower left lateral incisor (Fig. 29.7d).

CT scan confirmed the presence of an expansile, lytic lesion with a characteristic 'ballooning distension of the buccal and lingual cortical plates'. It also showed scattered areas of radio-opacities & multilocularity in the anterior region of the lesion and bi-cortical perforation along its posterior aspect.

'Ballooning distension' of the cortex with scattered areas of radio-opacities within a radiolucency was suggestive of secondary aneurysmal bone cyst arising in a pre-existing lesion (Fig. 29.7e).

Reconstructed CT scan showing bi-cortical perforation and lower border thinning at the mandibular body (Fig. 29.7f).

*Aspiration*: Figure 29.7c Dark venous blood of about 8–10 ml could readily be aspirated from the lesion.

*Incisional Biopsy*: Correlating the bloody venous aspirate, clinical & radiological findings, a clinical diagnosis of the aneurysmal bone cyst was made. However, owing to the change in radiodensity in the anterior aspect of the lesion (as evident on CT scan), an incisional biopsy was performed to rule out the presence of a hybrid lesion or co-existing pathology.

*Diagnosis*: A histopathological diagnosis of *secondary aneurysmal bone cyst arising in ossifying fibroma* of the mandible has been made.

*Surgical Plan*: Considering the hybrid nature of the lesion, bi-cortical perforation, thinning of lower border, the proposed surgical plan was segmental mandibulectomy and reconstruction.

## Case Scenario 4 (Fig. 29.8)

A 40-year-old female patient reported with a complaint of swelling over the lower jaw of 18 months duration and swelling over the right side of the upper jaw of 6 months duration.

### Clinical Examination

A firm to hard swelling was noted in the mandibular anterior dentoalveolar region extending from right lower 2nd premolar to lower left lateral incisor (Fig. 29.8a). There was a displacement of lower anterior teeth. Another similar firm swelling was noted in the right maxillary posterior dentoalveolar region in the region of missing right 1st maxillary molar (Fig. 29.8b). Overlying mucosa appeared normal in both the swellings.

### Pre-operative Diagnostic Work-up

*Imaging*: Figure 29.8c Orthopantomogram revealed a unilocular radiolucency with a sclerotic border located in relation to the periapical region of right lower premolars. A poorly defined mixed lesion (radiolucent lesion with foci of radio opacities) was noted in the right maxillary posterior region.

*Incisional Biopsy*: An incisional biopsy of both the lesions was performed under local anaesthesia. Both the lesions were reported as central giant cell granulomas.

*Biochemical Evaluation*: Since synchronous giant cell granulomas are generally rare and as these lesions are histopathologically similar to browns tumour, biochemical evaluation was performed. Serum parathormone was remarkably elevated along with raised serum calcium levels, while renal function parameters were well within normal limits.

*Ultrasound Evaluation of Neck*: An ultrasound evaluation of neck revealed parathyroid adenoma on the left side.

*Diagnosis*: After correlating the biochemical and sonographic examination, a diagnosis of primary hyperparathyroidism is made. The osteolytic lesions of mandible and maxilla were diagnosed as *Synchronous brown tumours of maxilla and mandible*.

*Surgical Plan*: The patient was advised parathyroidectomy for primary hyperparathyroidism followed by the wait and watch policy for synchronous brown jaw tumours to undergo self-resolution. But spontaneous resolution the jaw lesions was very slow following eight months after parathyroidectomy and the patient wanted surgical removal of the brown jaw tumours. They were treated by marginal mandibulectomy and alveolectomy of posterior maxilla.

## References

### Reactive Lesions of Oro-facial Soft Tissues


1. Marx RE, Stern D. Oral and maxillofacial pathology: a rationale for diagnosis and treatment. Hanover Park, IL: Quintessence Publishing; 2012.
2. Eversole LR, Rovin S. Reactive lesions of the gingiva. J Oral Pathol Med. 1972;1(1):30–8.
3. Neville BW. Soft tissue tumours. In: Oral and maxillofacial pathology. London: Elsevier; 2009. p. 507–70.
4. Wick MR, McDermott MB, Swanson PE. Proliferative, reparative, and reactive benign bone lesions that may be confused diagnostically with true osseous neoplasms. Semin Diagn Pathol. 2014;31(1):66–88. WB Saunders
5. Hoch B, Montag A. Reactive bone lesions mimicking neoplasms. Semin Diagn Pathol. 2011;28(1):102–12. WB Saunders
6. Sternberg SS, Antonioli DA, Carter D, Mills SE, Oberman H. Diagnostic surgical pathology. 3rd ed. Philadelphia, PA: Lippincott Williams & Wilkins; 1999.
7. Epivatianos A, Antoniades D, Zaraboukas T, Zairi E, Poulopoulos A, Kiziridou A, et al. Pyogenic granuloma of the oral cavity: comparative study of its clinicopathological and immunohistochemical features. Pathol Int. 2005;55:391–7.
8. Motamedi MH, Eshghyar N, Jafari SM, Lassemi E, Navi F, Abbas FM, Khalifeh S, Eshkevari PS. Peripheral and central giant cell granulomas of the jaws: a demographic study. Oral Surg Oral Med Oral Pathol Oral Radiol Endod. 2007;103:39–43.
9. Katsikeris N, Kakarantza-Angelopoulou E, Angelopoulos AP. Peripheral giant cell granuloma. Clinicopathologic study of 224 new cases and review of 956 reported cases. Int J Oral Maxillofac Surg. 1988;17(2):94–9.
10. Hernandez G, Lopez-Pintor RM, Torres J, de Vicente JC. Clinical outcomes of peri-implant peripheral giant cell granuloma: a report of three cases. J Periodontol. 2009;80:1184–91.
11. Hirshberg A, Kozlovsky A, Schwartz-Arad D, Mardinger O, Kaplan I. Peripheral giant cell granuloma associated with dental implants. J Periodontol. 2003;74(9):1380–4.
12. Subramanyam RV. Misnomers in oral pathology. Oral Dis. 2010;16(8):740–6.
13. Prasad S, Reddy S, Patil SR, Kalaburgi NB, Puranik RS. Peripheral ossifying fibroma and pyogenic granuloma. Are they interrelated? N Y State Dent J. 2008;74:50–2.
14. Buchner A, Hansen LS. The histomorphologic spectrum of peripheral ossifying fibroma. Oral Surg Oral Med Oral Pathol Oral Radiol. 1987;63(4):452–61.

15. Mergoni G, Meleti M, Magnolo S, Giovannacci I, Corcione L, Vescovi P. Peripheral ossifying fibroma: a clinicopathologic study of 27 cases and review of the literature with emphasis on histomorphologic features. J Indian Soc Periodontol. 2015;19(1):83–7.
16. Cuisia ES, Brannon RB. Peripheral ossifying fibroma-a clinical evaluation of 134 pediatric cases. Pediatr Dent. 2001;23(3):245–8.

## Central Giant Cell Granuloma

17. Yamaguchi T, Dorfman HD. Giant cell reparative granuloma: a comparative clinicopathologic study of lesions in gnathic and extragnathic sites. Int J Surg Pathol. 2001;9(3):189–200.
18. Schlorf RA, Koop SH. Maxillary giant cell reparative granuloma. Laryngoscope. 1977;87(1):10–7.
19. Chuong R, Kaban LB, Kozakewich H, Perez-Atayde A. Central giant cell lesions of the jaws: a clinicopathologic study. J Oral Maxillofac Surg. 1986;44(9):708–13.
20. Whitaker SB, Waldron CA. Central giant cell lesions of the jaws: a clinical, radiologic, and histopathologic study. Oral Surg Oral Med Oral Pathol Oral Radiol. 1993;75(2):199–208.
21. Eisenbud L, Stern M, Rothberg M, Sachs SA. Central giant cell granuloma of the jaws: experiences in the management of thirty-seven cases. J Oral Maxillofac Surg. 1988;46(5):376–84.
22. Tosco P, Tanteri G, Iaquinta C, Fasolis M, Roccia F, Berrone S, Garzino-Demo P. Surgical treatment and reconstruction for central giant cell granuloma of the jaws: a review of 18 cases. J Cranio-Maxillofac Surg. 2009;37(7):380–7.
23. Bataineh AB, Al-Khateeb T, Ma'amon AR. The surgical treatment of central giant cell granuloma of the mandible. J Oral Maxillofac Surg. 2002;60(7):756–61.
24. de Lange J, van den Akker HP, van den Berg H. Central giant cell granuloma of the jaw: a review of the literature with emphasis on therapy options. Oral Surg Oral Med Oral Pathol Oral Radiol Endod. 2007;104:603–15.
25. Pogrel AM. The diagnosis and management of giant cell lesions of the jaws. Ann Maxillofac Surg. 2012;2(2):102–6.
26. Suárez-Roa LM, Reveiz L, Ruíz-Godoy LR, Asbun-Bojalil J, Dávila-Serapio JE, Menjívar-Rubio AH, Meneses-García A. Interventions for central giant cell granuloma (CGCG) of the jaws. Cochrane Database Syst Rev. 2009;4:CD007404.
27. Vered M, Buchner A, Dayan D. Immunohistochemical expression of glucocorticoid and calcitonin receptors as a tool for selecting therapeutic approach in central giant cell granuloma of the jawbones. Int J Oral Maxillofac Surg. 2006;35(8):756–60.
28. Jacoway JH, Howell FV, Terry BC. Central giant cell granuloma: an alternative to surgical therapy. Oral Surg Oral Med Oral Pathol. 1988;66:572.
29. Terry BC, Jacoway JR. Management of central giant cell lesions: an alternative to surgical therapy. Oral Maxillofac Surg Clin North Am. 1994;6(3):579–600.
30. Abdo EN, Alves LC, Rodrigues AS, Mesquita RA, Gomez RS. Treatment of a central giant cell granuloma with intralesional corticosteroid. Br J Oral Maxillofac Surg. 2005;43(1):74–6.
31. Pogrel MA. Calcitonin therapy for central giant cell granuloma. J Oral Maxillofac Surg. 2003;61(6):649–53.
32. Kaban LB, Troulis MJ, Ebb D, August M, Hornicek FJ, Dodson TB. Antiangiogenic therapy with interferon alpha for giant cell lesions of the jaws. J Oral Maxillofac Surg. 2002;60(10):1103–11.
33. Da Silva NG, Carreira AS, Pedreira EN, Tuji FM, Ortega KL, Pinheiro JD. Treatment of central giant cell lesions using bisphosphonates with intralesional corticosteroid injections. Head Face Med. 2012;8(1):23.
34. Thomas D, Henshaw R, Skubitz K, Chawla S, Staddon A, Blay JY, Roudier M, Smith J, Ye Z, Sohn W, Dansey R. Denosumab in patients with giant-cell tumour of bone: an open-label, phase 2 study. Lancet Oncol. 2010;11(3):275–80.
35. Chawla S, Henshaw R, Seeger L, Choy E, Blay JY, Ferrari S, Kroep J, Grimer R, Reichardt P, Rutkowski P, Schuetze S. Safety and efficacy of denosumab for adults and skeletally mature adolescents with giant cell tumour of bone: interim analysis of an open-label, parallel-group, phase 2 study. Lancet Oncol. 2013;14(9):901–8.
36. Naidu A, Malmquist MP, Denham CA, Schow SR. Management of central giant cell granuloma with subcutaneous denosumab therapy. J Oral Maxillofac Surg. 2014;72(12):2469–84.

## Aneurysmal Bone Cyst

37. Rosenberg AE, Nielson GP, Fletcher JA. Aneurysmal bone cyst. In: CDM F, Unni KK, Mertens F, et al., editors. WHO classification of tumours: pathology and genetics of head and neck tumours, vol. 9. 3rd ed. Lyon: IARC; 2005.
38. Struthers PJ, Shear M. Aneurysmal bone cyst of the jaws:(II). Pathogenesis. Int J Oral Maxillofac Surg. 1984;13(2):92–100.
39. Motamedi MH, Navi F, Eshkevari PS, Jafari SM, Shams MG, Taheri M, Abbas FM, Motahhari P. Variable presentations of aneurysmal bone cysts of the jaws: 51 cases treated during a 30-year period. J Oral Maxillofac Surg. 2008;66(10):2098–103.
40. Sun ZJ, Zhao YF, Yang RL, Zwahlen RA. Aneurysmal bone cysts of the jaws: analysis of 17 cases. J Oral Maxillofac Surg. 2010;68(9):2122–8.

## Brown Tumor

41. Abdelrahman TE. Brown jaw tumors: challenges and outcomes. Int Surg J. 2017;4(11):3586–9.
42. Ullah E, Ahmad M, Ali SA, Redhu N. Primary hyperparathyroidism having multiple Brown tumors mimicking malignancy. Indian J Endocrinol Metab. 2012;16(6):1040.
43. Chami B, Benrachadi L, El Omri N, El Qatni M, El Wady W, El Mohtarim B. Brown tumor of the palate as first manifestation of primary hyperparathyroidism: a case report. Méd Buccale Chir Buccale. 2011;17(4):287–91.
44. Arunkumar KV, Kumar S, Deepa D. Brown tumor in mandible as a first sign of vitamin D deficiency: a rare case report and review. Indian J Endocrinol Metabo. 2012;16(2):310.
45. Scott SN, Graham SM, Sato Y, Robinson RA. Brown tumor of the palate in a patient with primary hyperparathyroidism. Ann Otol Rhinol Laryngol. 1999;108:91–4.

# Fibro-osseous Lesions in the Maxillofacial Region

30

Taranjit Kaur

Fibro-ossoeus lesions have posed a diagnostic dilemma since the beginning, when first case was reported in late 19th century. Since then various lesions are included in this group, yet the understanding of the lesions remains obscure for the clinican/surgeon. The main reason for this, is their histological resemblance with one another, where they all show varying degrees of healthy bone replaced by fibrous tissue and some amount of bone/cementum like tissue intermingled in between. This chapter is written with the aim of simplifying these group of bony lesions for its readers and highlighting the key idea of interdisciplinary approach in the management of these lesions where the oral pathologist along with radiologist and clinician play a pivotal role in differentially diagnosing these lesions, for the maxillofacial surgeon to chose and perform her/his duty of managing them, rightfully, for their patients. The spectrum of these lesions have seen several changes during the course of history yet there is still ample scope for ambiguity in identification and classification of the lesions, hence the authors have chosen few most commonly encountered lesions in Indian subcontinent, for the description and discussion.

## 30.1 Introduction

Fibro-osseous lesions (FOLs) are miscellaneous and challenging group of intra-osseous lesions posing a diagnostic dilemma for the clinician as well as the pathologist and this makes them interesting to treat and manage for the surgeon [1]. It was Boyko who first reported a case of craniofacial fibrous dysplasia, diagnosed at that time as osteofibroma, in 1936, which was called leontiasis ossea, the term first described by Virchow in 1862, for bony lesions involving upper facial bones resulting in lion-like faces. Clinicians and pathologists have gone through a drastic change in their understanding of these lesions since then yet pathogenesis and progression still needs further investigation [2].

One thing that is common in all these lesions is that normal bone is replaced by connective tissue and fibroblasts; occasional foci of mineralisation is seen, with varying degrees of bone- or cementum-like tissue. The biological behaviour of these lesions ranges from benign and indolent to aggressive, inflammatory and neoplastic [1].

The diagnosis is difficult to obtain on the basis of histopathology alone, clinical history and radiographic details have an important role to play in the decision-making of the management. Most often than not, pathologists may not be able to comment more than just benign fibro-osseous lesion in the absence of additional clinical and radiographic information [1].

Though considered as one of the most confusing and challenging pathological processes, it was the meticulous hard work of Charles A Waldron, an American Oral Pathologist, who was first to describe these lesions in a systematic way and propose the classification, in the year 1985, which was later revised by himself in the year 1993 [3, 4].

With the evolution of technology and a better clinical understanding of the lesions as well as the availability of ample literature, various other classifications have emerged from time to time [5, 6].

## 30.2 Classifications

Fibro-osseous lesions have undergone a turbulent phase with regard to its classification and categorisation and in this chapter, it may not be possible to include all the available classifications, but the major ones have been referred to. The major changes in classifications are seen in the publications by Waldron [5], Waldron [6], Slootweg [7], WHO [8], Speight

**Electronic Supplementary Material** The online version of this chapter (https://doi.org/10.1007/978-981-15-1346-6_30) contains supplementary material, which is available to authorized users.

T. Kaur (✉)
Department of Oral and Maxillofacial Surgery, Government Dental College and Hospital, Jamnagar, Gujarat, India



K. Bonanthaya et al. (eds.), *Oral and Maxillofacial Surgery for the Clinician*, https://doi.org/10.1007/978-981-15-1346-6_30

and Carlos [9] and Eversole et al. [1]. As all the changes in classifications have not been included in the chapter, readers are encouraged to refer the concerned publications. Some of the commonly used classifications are as follows.

### 30.2.1 Waldron's Classification, 1985 [5, 10]

1. Fibrous dysplasia (FD)
   (a) Monostotic
   (b) Polyostotic
2. Fibro-osseous (cemental) lesions' plausible origin in the periodontal ligament
   (a) Periapical cemental dysplasia
   (b) Localised fibro-osseous-cemental lesions (presumably reactive in nature)
   (c) Florid cemento-osseous dysplasia (gigantiform cementoma)
   (d) Ossifying and cementifying fibroma
3. Fibro-osseous neoplasms of uncertain or detectable relationship to those arising in the periodontal ligament
   (a) Cementoblastoma, osteoblastoma and osteoid osteoma.
   (b) Juvenile active-ossifying fibroma and other so called aggressive-ossifying/cementifying fibromas.

### 30.2.2 WHO Classification of FOLs, 2005 [8]

At the core of these classifications is the spectrum of clinicopathological entities in which the diagnosis can only be made by the correlation of clinical, radiological and histological features.

1. Ossifying fibroma (OF)
2. Fibrous dysplasia
3. Osseous dysplasia
   (a) Periapical osseous dysplasia
   (b) Focal osseous dysplasia
   (c) Florid osseous dysplasia
   (d) Familial gigantiform cementoma
4. Central giant cell granuloma
5. Cherubism
6. Aneurysmal bone cyst
7. Solitary bone cyst

### 30.2.3 Speight and Carlos Classification (2006) [9]

1. Fibrous Dysplasia
   (a) Monostotic FD
   (b) Polyostotic FD
   (c) Craniofacial FD
2. Osseous Dysplasia
   (a) Periapical Osseous Dysplasia
   (b) Focal Osseous Dysplasia
   (c) Florid Osseous Dysplasia
   (d) Familial Gigantiform Cementoma
3. Ossifying Fibroma
   (a) Conventional Ossifying Fibroma
   (b) Juvenile Trabecular-Ossifying Fibroma
   (c) Juvenile Psammomatoid-Ossifying Fibroma

### 30.2.4 Eversole Classification, 2008 [1]

In 2008, Eversole et al. gave a comprehensive classification by including developmental lesions, neoplastic lesions and inflammatory/reactive processes. This classification emphasised that final diagnosis can be attained by the correlation of microscopy, imaging and clinical features together and not on the basis of histopathological features alone.

1. Bone dysplasias
   (a) Fibrous dysplasia
      (i) Monostotic
      (ii) Polyostotic
      (iii) Polyostotic with endocrinopathy (McCune-Albright)
      (iv) Osteofibrous dysplasia
   (b) Osteitis deformans or Pagets disease
   (c) Pagetoid heritable bone dysplasias of childhood
   (d) Segmental odontomaxillary dysplasia
2. Cemento-osseous dysplasias
   (a) Focal cemento-osseous dysplasia
   (b) Florid cemento-osseous dysplasia
3. Inflammatory/reactive processes
   (a) Focal sclerosing osteomyelitis
   (b) Diffuse sclerosing osteomyelitis
   (c) Proliferative periostitis
4. Metabolic disease
   (a) Hyperparathyroidism
5. Neoplastic lesions (ossifying fibromas)
   (a) Ossifying fibroma
   (b) Hyperparathyroidism jaw lesion syndrome
   (c) Juvenile-ossifying fibroma
      (i) Trabecular type
      (ii) Psammomatoid type
   (d) Gigantiform cementomas

Based on the above-mentioned classification systems, author have selected few most commonly occurring BFOLs (Benign fibro-osseous lesions), which will allow a better understanding of these lesions, from a maxillofacial surgeon's point of view.

It is apparent from this wide spectrum of FOL that a diagnosis cannot be made from pathology reports alone and it has to be correlated with the clinical and radiological findings [11]. BFOL form a wide spectrum of diseases, which occur intra-osseously and is characterised by similar microscopic pictures with hypercellular fibroblastic stroma and varying amounts of bone, cementum and other calcified structures. El Mofty stated that reactive, dysplastic, developmental and neoplastic processes are included under the broad umbrella of BFOLs and the treatment given varies from case to case [12].

## 30.3 Fibrous Dysplasia (FD)

Fibrous Dysplasia is a benign dysplastic disease with a well-approved genetic cause in GNAS 1 (Guanine nucleotide-binding protein alpha-stimulating activity polypeptide 1) gene. The clinical severity of the disease depends on the stage of foetal life (prenatal/postnatal) at which gene mutation occurs. So far, the identification of *GNAS1* mutations are the most useful molecular tool to differentiate fibrous dysplasia from other fibro-osseous lesions [13].

### 30.3.1 Clinical Features

There are four main clinical subtypes of FD depending on the time of mutation in GNAS 1

(a) Monostotic FD, which affects single bone: Post-natal life mutation.
(b) Polyostotic FD affecting multiple bones at the same time: Mutation in the late embryonic stages of life.
(c) McCune—Albright syndrome in which multiple bony lesions are seen along with skin pigmentations and endocrinopathies presenting itself as precocious puberty and hyperthyroidism: Due to mutation in early embryonic stages of life.
(d) Craniofacial FD confined to bones of craniofacial complex.

Craniofacial variant will be discussed in detail, as it is the most common FD encountered in the maxillofacial region.

FD is the disease of growing bones and the majority of lesions are diagnosed in first two decades of life, without any predilection for gender or race. Though mandibular lesions are purely monostotic, but the lesions involving maxilla, which invariably involve zygoma, sphenoid and other adjoining bones of the craniofacial skeleton, are not truly monostotic and hence may be suitably referred to as Craniofacial FD. Since multiple adjoining bones are involved of the same anatomic region, term polyostotic is avoided. Craniofacial FD appears in few commonly seen patterns,

One, involving maxilla-zygoma-sphenoid-frontal-nasal bones. Another, involving frontal-temporal-sphenoid-zygoma bones

Clinically, painless expansion of the affected area with facial asymmetry is the common presentation of FD. Rarely does a lesion expand the bone to cause structural weakening. Thickening of the skull bones and obliteration of the foramina of the base of the skull occasionally can present variously as headache, proptosis, visual loss, anosmia and hearing loss.

### 30.3.2 Radiographic Features

Radiographic features vary depending on the stage at which the lesion is diagnosed. Early onset lesions appear radiolucent and later as they age, the classical 'ground glass appearance' (Fig. 30.1) is the identifying feature.

The lesion is ill defined and is radiologically imperceptible from the adjoining normal bone. Ground glass appearance is due to radiodensity caused by abundance of woven bone, which also leads to fuzziness of the boundaries, and strict delineation of lesion from the normal bone is difficult on the radiograph. Poorly defined borders are the diagnostic clue for FD and also differentiate it from Ossifying fibroma, which has well-defined appearance on the radiograph. Publications have stressed on the importance of CT and CBCT as investigative modalities of FOLs [14].

The clinical case scenarios 1 and 2 are provided for the readers to appreciate the difference in the CT images between early and long-standing lesions

***Clinical case scenario 1*** (Fig. 30.2a–e)

A 17-year-old male with noted swelling in the upper right maxilla posterior vestibule region and he was aware of the swelling for about 1 month.

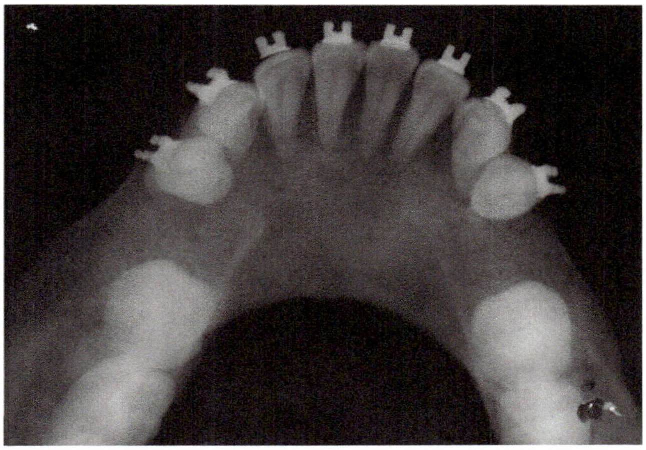



**Fig. 30.1** Occlusal image showing ground glass appearance in a 36-year-old female, who had aymptomatic bilateral body region mandible swelling

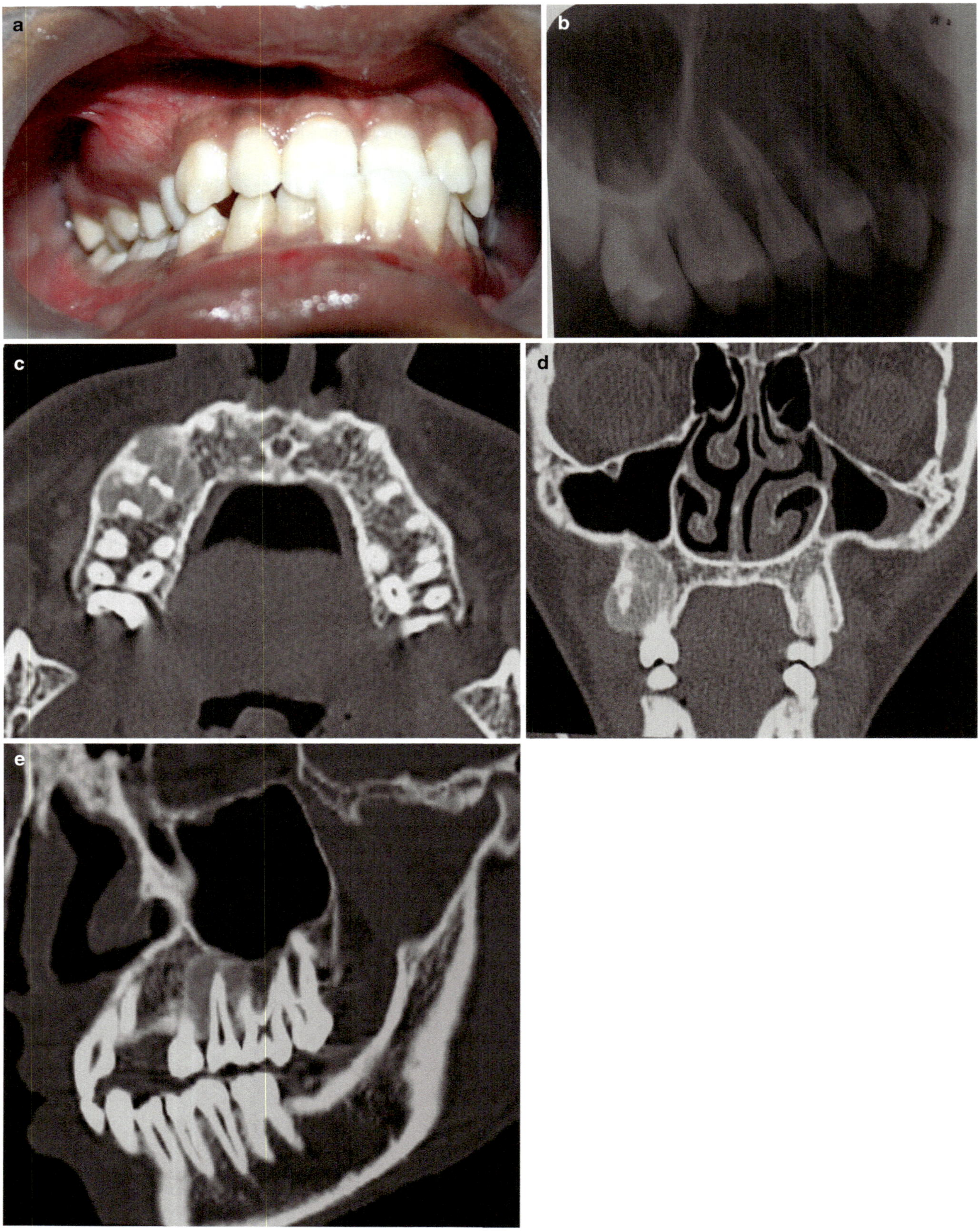




**Fig. 30.2** (**a**) Clinical picture of FD right upper posterior buccal sulcus. (**b**) Occlusal view showing ground glass appearance, no root resoprtion, no root displacement, hazy margins, lamina dura appeared to be lost in IOPA. (**c**) Axial view CT. (**d**) Coronal view CT. (**e**) Sagittal view CT

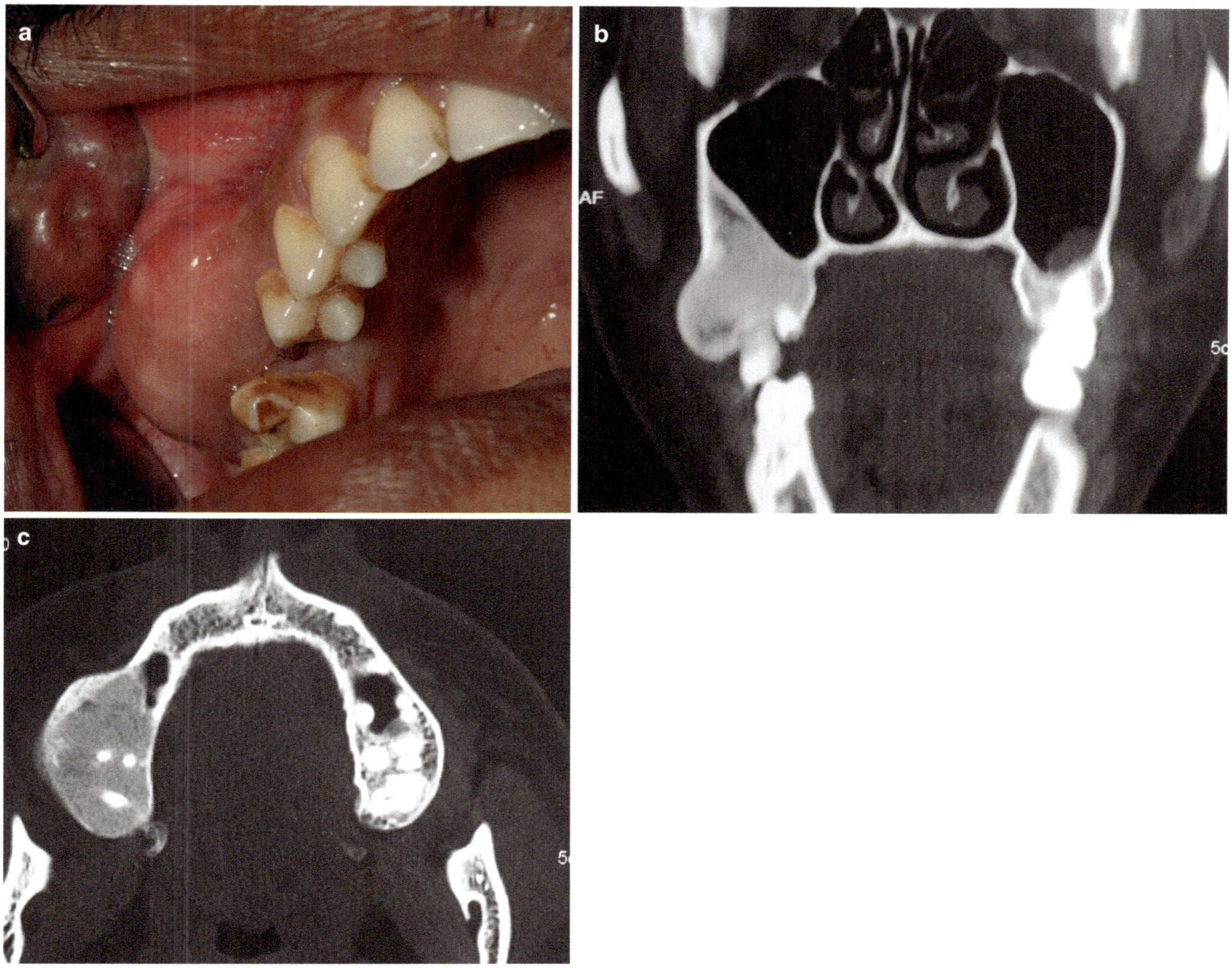




**Fig. 30.3** (**a**) Clinical image. (**b**) Coronal CT showing more dense/opaque appearance of the lesion. (**c**) Axial image

Clinically, the lesion was Ovoid, well defined, non-tender and firm with no palatal expansion, involving the buccal sulcus of tooth 13–16 (Fig. 30.2a).

Occlusal X-ray showed ground glass appearance (Fig. 30.2b), There was no root resorption, no root tilting, margins were hazy and lamina dura lost.

CT scan shows well-defined lesion (Fig. 30.3c–e—axial, coronal and sagittal views, respectively).

The Calcium and Phosphorous values were normal.

A bone incision biopsy was done and the final diagnosis was that FD. It was decided to observe the lesion till growth is completed; however, the patient was lost for follow up

***Clinical case scenario 2*** (Fig. 30.3a–c)

This patient in his late thirties was aware of the swelling on the right posterior upper jaw for past 5-6 years. After an initial biopsy proved it to be FD, the lesion was excised completely under GA.

### 30.3.3 Histological Features

Histologically, FD shows irregularly shaped trabeculae of immature woven bone dispersed in cellular fibroblastic stroma. The bone trabeculae evolve directly from stroma and assume delicate curvilinear patterns, which appear like 'Chinese letters' [15]. The osteoid is generally not rimmed with osteoblasts and develops into lamellar bone as the lesion matures. Such may not be the case with extra gnathic lesions.

### 30.3.4 Treatment and Prognosis

In a large majority of cases, lesions show the tendency of slow growth and eventually stabilise with the cessation of the growth phase. Indications for surgical treatment include functional deficits or significant cosmetic deformity. The aim of treatment is to restore function and cosmetic symmetry.

The involvement of the bone may range from minimal to functional and/or esthetic deformity being present. Based on patient's age, the presence/absence of cosmetic and functional deficits and the growth rate, the treatment is currently designed in the following way [16] (Video 30.1).

1. Observation
2. Conservative approach in the form of surgical recontouring and reshaping.
3. Radical surgical approach involving resection and reconstruction.

In the case of minimal involvement, no surgical intervention may be needed but when involvement is more significant, surface shaving of excess bone, for cosmetic reasons may be done. Radical surgical approach is preferred in the case of significant functional and aesthetic deficit.

A treatment scheme offered by Chen in 1990 [17] is helpful in determining the approach depending on the extent of conditions. The lesions are defined as per the regions, in Zone 1, i.e. frontomaxillofacial are, it is advised that they are completely excised and reconstructed henceforth. In Zone 2, i.e. hair-bearing cranium, observation and conservative or radical approach as and when needed. Whereas in Zone 3, which is central cranial base, more conservative or observational approach is required due to the difficult location of neurovascular bundle, lastly Zone 4 lesions involving dentate maxilla and mandible are advised conservative treatment in the form of surgical recontouring and shaping. Optic canal decompression was advised on patients with orbital dysplasia and decreasing visual acuity.

Riclade in 2001 in his review article stated that in craniofacial dysplasia, early treatment is advised in progressive sensory disturbances, in order to reduce the problems caused by decompression at a later stage [18].

Non-surgical treatment has a limited role, radiotherapy is contraindicated. Steroids show some effectiveness in reducing bone pain and temporary relief from symptoms due to nerve compression. Calcitonin and pamidronate have shown some promise in recent studies but the results of long term trials are awaited [16].

Monostotic lesions of the craniofacial complex need to be differentiated from other FOLs like cemento-ossifying fibroma (COF) and diffuse-sclerosing osteomyelitis of the mandible [15] while COF most commonly appears in young adults in tooth bearing areas of mandible and maxilla, it is well defined and can be separated or scooped out from the adjoining healthy bone easily.

***Clinical case scenario 3*** is a 14-year-old boy who reported with a recurrent lesion on upper left buccal posterior alveolus. The clinical, radiological and surgical findings were suggestive of a COF; however, the pathology report was that of FD. This case is shown to highlight the varied pathology reports, which can be expected in dealing with lesions under the BFOL spectrum (Fig. 30.4a–d).

***Clinical case scenario 4*** (Fig. 30.5a–c) is given to show lesion, which had initial differential diagnosis of FD, but pathology report showed it to be sclerosing osteomyelitis

In 2008, eversole classification inflammatory reactive process containing focal sclerosing osteomyeliotis/diffuse sclerosing osteomyelitis (DSOM) and proliferative periostitis were categorised under BFOL.

Figure 30.6 is an OPG of a 11-year-old child who presented with recurrent pain and swelling left side body mandible. OPG shows a diffuse ground glass appearance, with changes in the trabecular pattern on the whole of the left ramus and body mandible. A provisional diagnosis of DSOM can be made. Unfortunately, the patient didn't report for further investigations. OPG is included to demonstrate the alteration of the trabecular pattern.

## 30.4 Ossifying Fibroma/Cementifying Fibroma/Cemento-Ossifying Fibroma (COF) and Juvenile (Aggressive)-Ossifying Fibroma

### 30.4.1 Clinical Features

These were traditionally a group of Fibro-osseous lesions with neoplastic tendencies. COF has had its own share of controversies, being included previously under BFOLs. The recent update in 2018; however, accepts COF as odontogenic in origin and had been placed under mesenchymal odontogenic tumours [19]. Another entity with a similar clinical picture is central odontogenic fibroma, which is also under benign mesenchymal tumours. Lesion that produces cementum including COF and cementoblastoma, thus, currently has found a new place.

In 2017, the consensus group felt that the term cemento-ossifying fibroma is suitably descriptive and indicates that these lesions are specific to the tooth-bearing areas of the jaws and can be distinguished from the two juvenile variants of ossifying fibroma. This clearly distinguishes it from ossifying fibromas that are non-odontogenic and are classified under benign fibro- and chondro-osseous lesions. The three variants are, therefore, defined as cemento-ossifying fibroma, juvenile trabecular-ossifying fibroma and juvenile psammomatoid-ossifying fibroma [20–22].

COF progressive painless buccal and lingual plate expansion. COF affects dentate segment of mandible and maxilla.

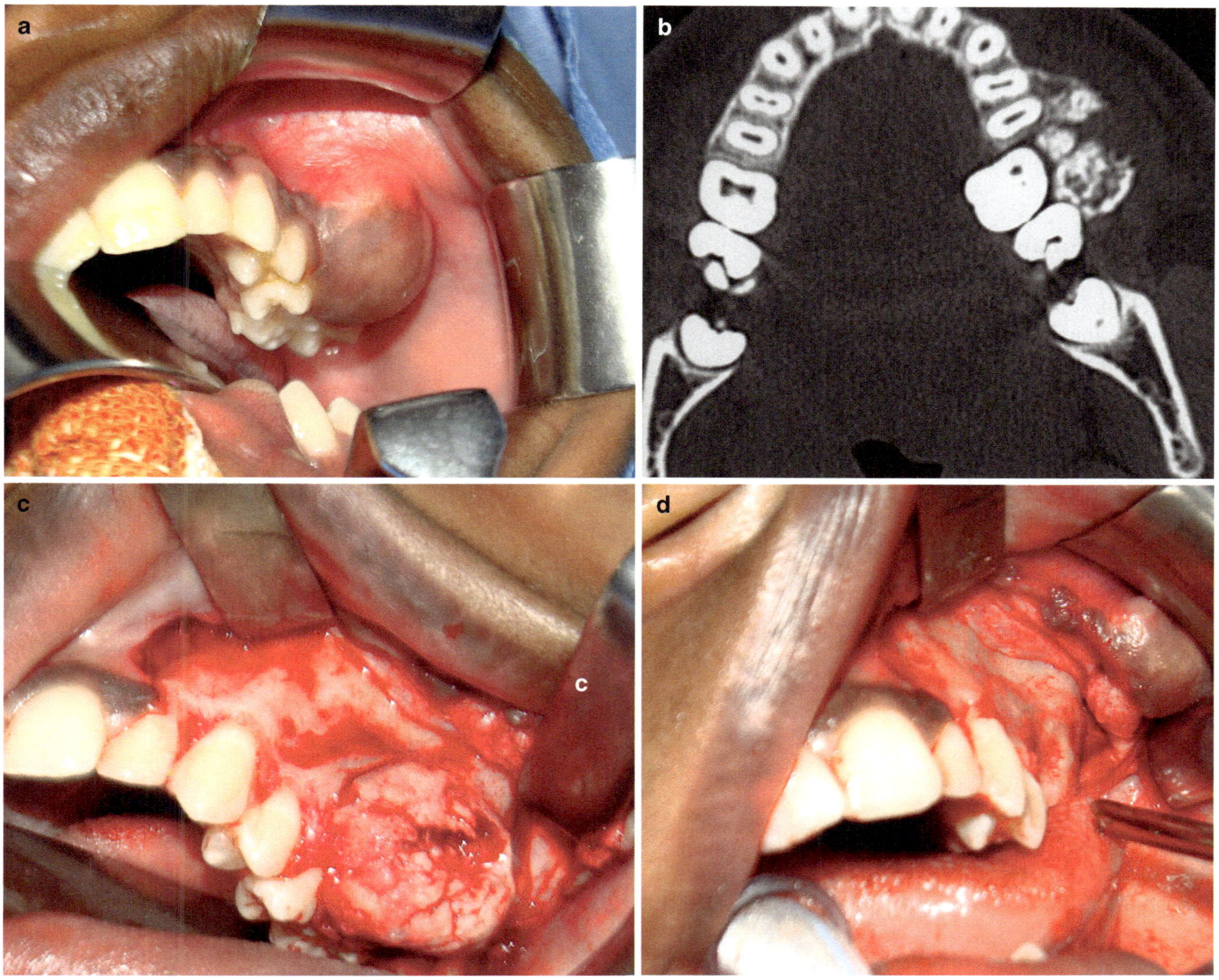




**Fig. 30.4** (**a**) Clinical image of swelling left upper buccal alveolus in a 14-year-old boy. (**b**) Axial CT image showing flecks of radiopacities. (**c**) Shows the lesion exposed, note the gritty nature, which could be easily shelled out with relative ease, in this case. (**d**) Intra-operative image where the lesion was shaved out from the alveolar bone via a mucoperiosteal flap approach

They are slow growing in nature in adults, but show aggressiveness in the younger age group. The teeth are generally displaced. Ossifying Fibromas demonstrate a well delineated or encapsulated cellular fibrous connective tissue with varying amounts of osseous products like bone and cementum (spherical calcification).

Lesions are more commonly seen in mandible (77%) especially the molar region and are found exclusively in jaws. The peak age is 3rd and 4th decades of life and very strong female pre-dilection (almost 5:1). The juvenile variant (Juvenile-Ossifying Fibroma), which is also more aggressive, is seen in the younger age group [23].

### 30.4.2 Radiological Features

It is a well-demarcated radiolucent lesion, in the initial stages, separated from the surrounding healthy bone. Usually, a solitary lesion and is unilocular. The well-demarcated radiolucent/radiopaque appearance is the main differentiating consideration with Fibrous Dysplasia. Appearance is dependent on the maturity of the lesion, i.e. purely radiolucent (initial stages); mixed with radiopaque foci or radiopaque. The radiographic presentation of bowing of mandible with thinning and weakening of the lower border, particularly in large expansive lesions, is seen. Resorption or divergence of roots may result due to continued growth.

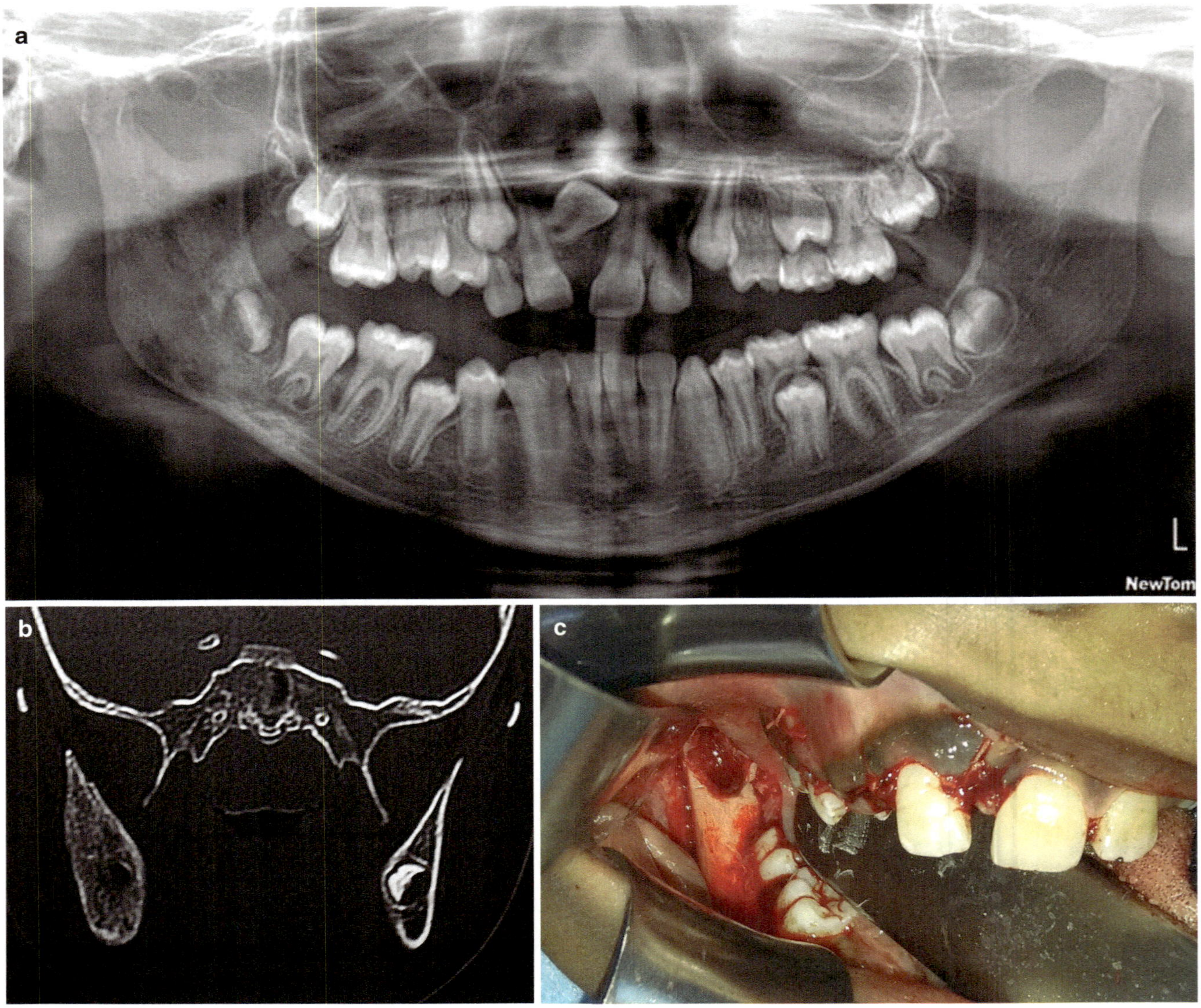




**Fig. 30.5** (**a**, **b**) OPG ant coronal CT cuts show evident changes in the right ramus of a 10-year-old girl, who presented with progressing facial asymmetry on the right side ramus region. The provisional diagnosis was of FD, but the bone biopsy (**c**) report was suggestive of sclerosing osteomyelitis

### 30.4.3 Histologic Features

Ossifying fibromas of craniofacial skeleton are divided into two categories depending on the cell of origin.

(A) Cemento-ossifying Fibroma (COF): OF with odontogenic origin.
(B) Juvenile (aggressive)-Ossifying Fibroma [9, 24–26]: subcategorised as (Table 30.1) (Fig 30.7)
   1. Juvenile trabecular-Ossifying Fibroma (JTOF)
   2. Juvenile Psammomatoid-ossifying fibroma (JPOF)

### 30.4.4 Treatment and Prognosis

COF is a slowly growing benign neoplasm commonly seen in the 3rd to 4th decades of life, if left untreated can enlarge to a significant size. Since it is radiographically as well as microscopically well circumscribed and shells out from the surrounding bone with little effort, it is curettage or enucleation a preferred initial treatment option. An important feature is, it is well defined and can be easily shelled out from the adjoining normal bone, grossly the lesion can be separated out in one piece or a few large chunks. The recurrence rate is variable and unpredictable. Surgical curettage is an

**Fig. 30.6** OPG in a 11-year-old child showing the diffuse change in the trabecular pattern at the left body/ramus region of mandible

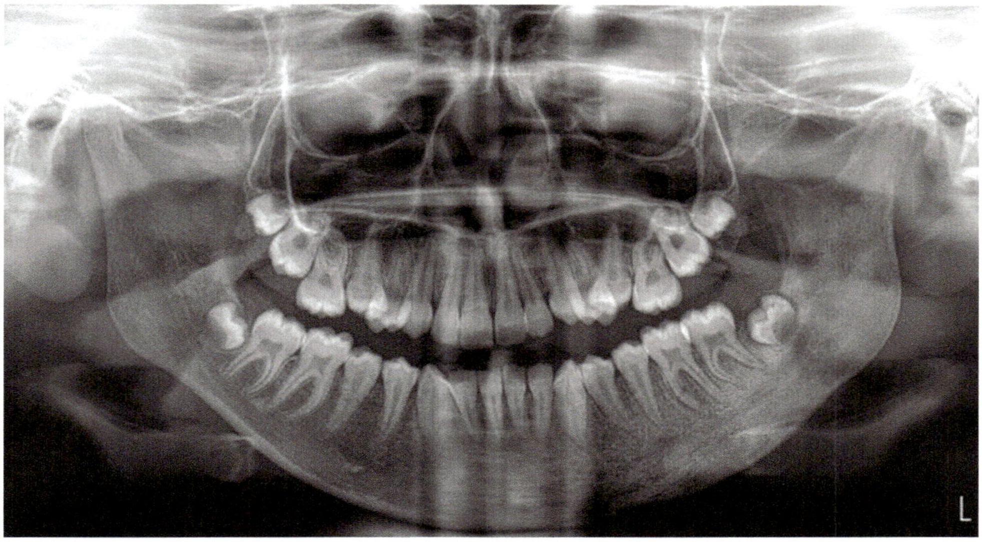




**Table 30.1** Comparing the main features of JTOF and JPOF (adapted from Speight and Carlos [9])

| | JTOF | JPOF |
|---|---|---|
| Age ( mean) | 2–30 years (10) | 3 months–72 years (20) |
| Female: male | 1.2:1 | 1.3:1 |
| site | Maxilla 50%<br>Mandible 44%<br>Sino-nasal 6% | Sino-nasal 62%<br>Maxilla 20%<br>Mandible ramus 10%<br>Cranium 8% |
| Radiology | Well circumscribed<br>Speckled calcifications | Well circumscribed, aggressive, expands and occupies the paranasal sinuses |
| Histopathology | Densely cellular, immature bone and osteoid in a trabecular pattern, osteoblast rimming seen | Densely cellular, spherical cementum-like psammomatoid calcifications |
| Clinical features | Progressive and rapid expansion of lesion, pain may not be present, in maxilla can produce nasal obstruction and epistaxis | Affects predominantly extragnathic bones of craniofacial skeleton, particularly the paranasal, orbital, frontal and ethmoid bones.<br>Orbital extension of sino-nasal tumors may present as proptosis, visual complaints nasal stuffiness etc |

acceptable trteatment [27]. Lesions exhibiting more aggressive behaviour and recurrence may need to undergo resection. The anatomical location and age of the patient and aggressiveness of the lesion have a role in deciding the treatment modality of the lesion.

***Clinical case scenario 5*** (a case of COF affecting the right side body of the mandible) (Fig. 30.8a–e).

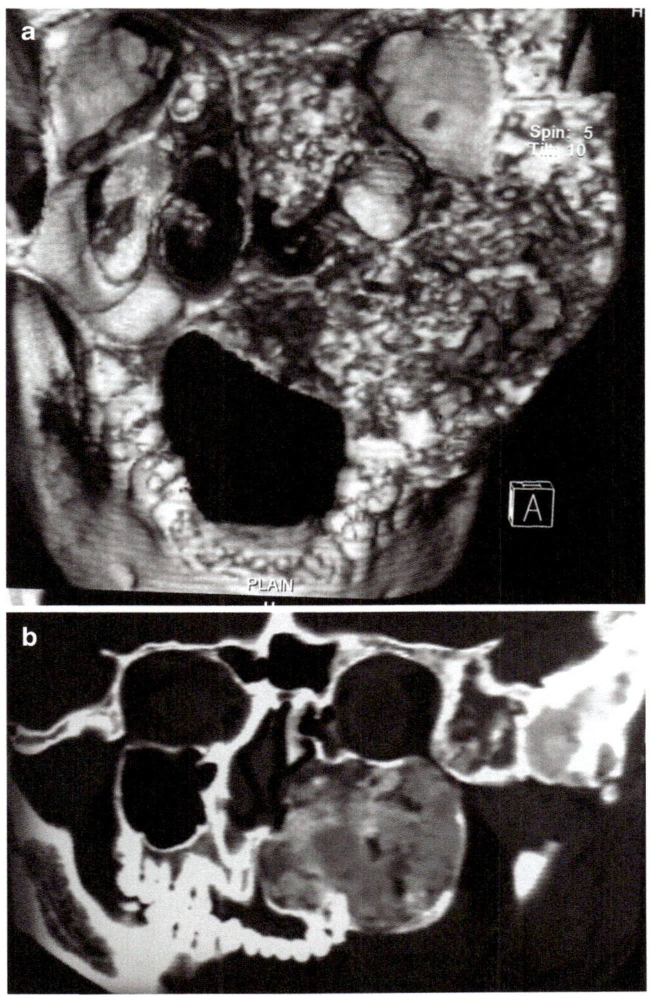




**Fig. 30.7** (**a**, **b**) Coronal and panoramic CT views in a 26-year-old man with long-standing swelling of the left side maxilla and cheek bone—the case of JOF—lesion fills the left hand side of the nose and paranasal sinuses

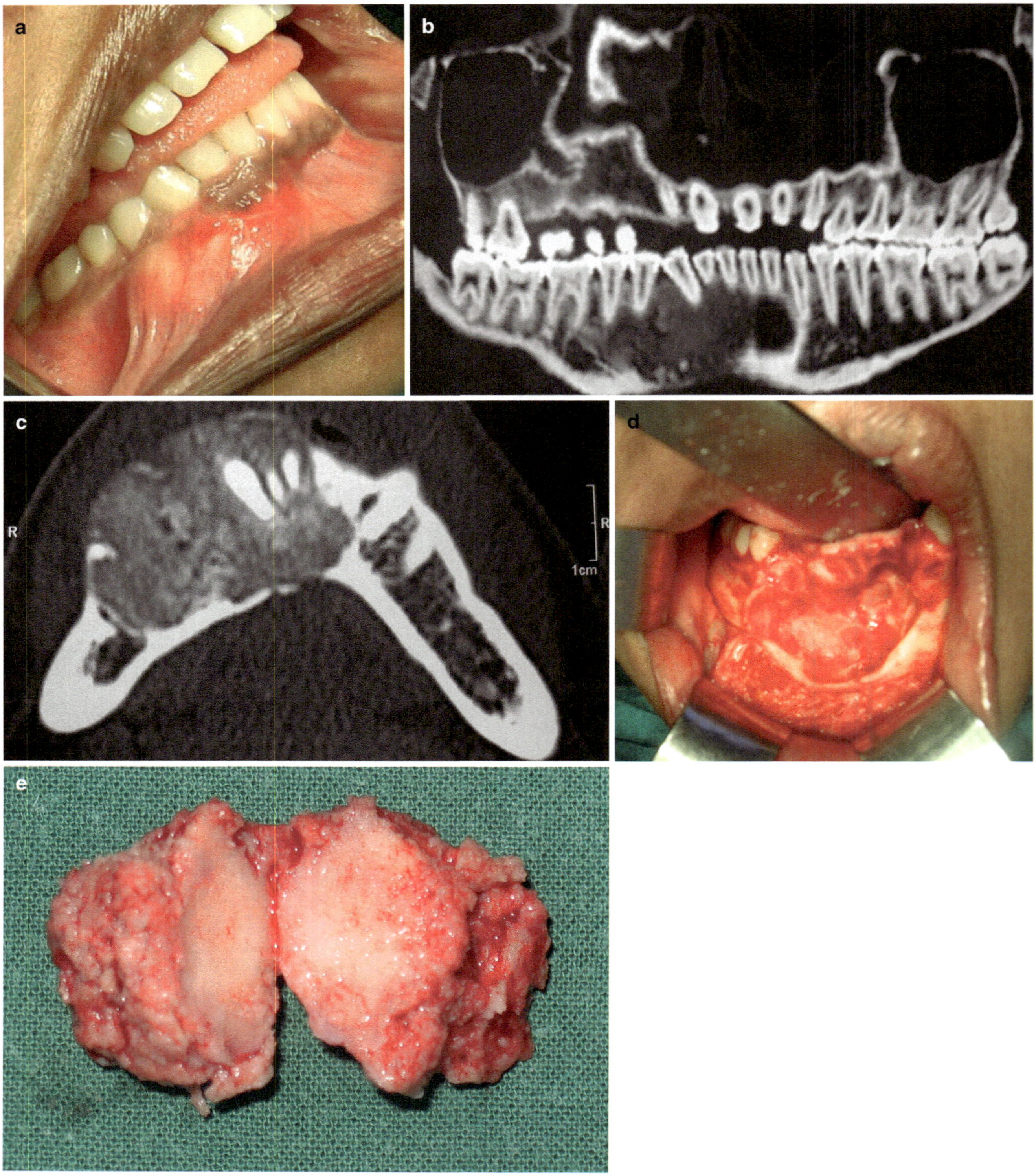




**Fig. 30.8** (**a**) Swelling rt body mandible in 29-year-old female, clinical picture. (**b**) Panoramic image of the CT scan. (**c**) Axial CT image showing the bone destruction. (**d**) Surgical bed after excision of the lesion. (**e**) Cut section of the fibrous lesion

## 30.5 Cemento-Osseous Dysplasia (Osseous Dysplasia)

Osseous dysplasia is a non-neoplastic, commonest, least understood fibro-osseous lesion occurring in tooth-bearing areas of the jaws. The cause of misunderstanding lies at the similarities shared at the clinical and histological levels with other fibro-osseous lesions like fibrous dysplasia and ossifying fibroma and even few neoplasias [28].

Since these lesions lie in close association with the periodontal ligaments of the tooth-bearing segment of the jaws, and histopathologically as well, they bear close similarity with PDL, the strong suspicion of the origin in PDL cannot be ruled out.

Two main types are recognised, based on the clinical and radiological features.

1. Localised and
2. Generalised.

Localised variety includes

(a) Periapical cemento osseous dysplasia (PCOD)
(b) Focal cemento osseous dysplasia (FCOD)

Generalised variety includes
Florid cemento osseous dysplasia

Ideally, these lesions can be identified clinically and radiographically without the need for the biopsy, as the presentation is pathognomonic

Su et al. in 1997 have published a series of 316 cases to distinguish the clinical, radiological and pathological features of the cement osseous dyplasias [29, 30].

## 30.6 Periapical Cemento-Osseous Dysplasia

### 30.6.1 Clinical, Radiological and Histological Presentation

The clinical and radiographic presentation of PCOD is well established. There is a marked predilection for females (14:1) and Afro-Caribbean women [2], and commonly seen in and around the third decade of life, rarely before the age of 20.

Predominantly involves periapical region of anterior mandible, frequently involving more than one tooth at a time though solitary lesions may be occasionally seen.

These are non-expansile asymptomatic lesions and teeth in association are invariably vital and are discovered accidently when radiographs are taken for other purposes.

Radiographically, maturation of the lesion can be appreciated, when examined at various stages.

Initially, they appear as periapical radiolucencies, which can be easily mistaken for a periapical cyst or a granuloma.

Over a period of time, the mixed radiolucent radiopaque picture may emerge and as the lesion matures further, eventually show dense periapical calcifications at the end stage, which is surrounded by a narrow radiolucent rim. The lesions seldom reach beyond 1–1.5 cm diameter and growth is self-limiting. The lesions remain separated from the periodontal ligament of the tooth throughout their growth phase.

The histological features are coincidental with radiographic findings and categorised as three stages.

Stage 1: Osteolytic stage/Radiolucent phase
Which shows ample fibrous connective tissue, highly cellular and with numerous small vessels.
Stage 2: Cementoblastic stage/radiolucent radiopaque phase
Various trabecular-woven bone and cementum-like tissues seen.
Stage 3: Mature stage/radiopaque phase
Consolidation of bone- or cementum-like tissue.

## 30.7 Focal Cemento Osseous Dysplasia

For several years, pathologists were aware of the lesions occurring in the mandibular posterior region, often occurring in the tooth-bearing areas and in relation with recently extracted teeth sockets. Waldron recognised them to be, localised fibro-osseous cemental lesions, supposedly reactive in nature. The present understanding of these lesions is hard work of Summerlin and Tomich, besides naming them as Focal cemento osseous dysplasia, they clinically defined them for a better understanding and differentiation from other lesions especially Ossifying Fibroma [31].

### 30.7.1 Clinical, Radiological and Histopathological Features

Focal osseous dysplasia is more commonly seen in Afro-Caribbean females. Male to female preponderance is 1:8. Mainly occurs in the 4th to 5th decades of life with 38 years being an average age of occurrence.

The lesion appears as painless, non-expansile, localised condition especially in posterior mandible, both tooth-bearing areas as well as edentulous mandible where tooth was extracted in the recent past. A clinical, radiographic and histopathological differential diagnosis of Focal osseous dysplasia is Ossifying fibroma. Since both are more common in posterior mandible and may appear as radiolucent, mixed or radiopaque, well-circumscribed lesions, the clinical and radiological differentiation can be confusing provided one notices the centrifugal growth pattern of and focal osseous dysplasias barely grow beyond 1.5 cm. Radiographically, focal osseous dysplasias tend to be well defined with slightly irregular borders.

On histological examination, one finds connective tissue stroma comprising of loose collagen fibers, interspersed with irregular shaped cementoid calcifications. Free haemorrhage is noticed throughout, intermixed with collagen background.

## 30.8 Florid Cemento-Osseous Dysplasia

When the lesions, similar in microscopic and radiographic appearance to Focal cemento osseous dysplasia, are found in more than one location in a mandible or in both the quadrants simultaneously, they are identified as Florid cement osseous dysplasia. Radiographs displayed a spectrum of sclerotic and ground-glass opacities limited to alveolar processes but not to root apices [32]. Chronic osteomyelitis may infrequently complicate the disease. These cases appear to represent the most exuberant manifestation of reactive fibro-osseous jaw disease. Many times, these diseases are an incidental finding and patient may be asymptomatic (Figs. 30.9 and 30.10)

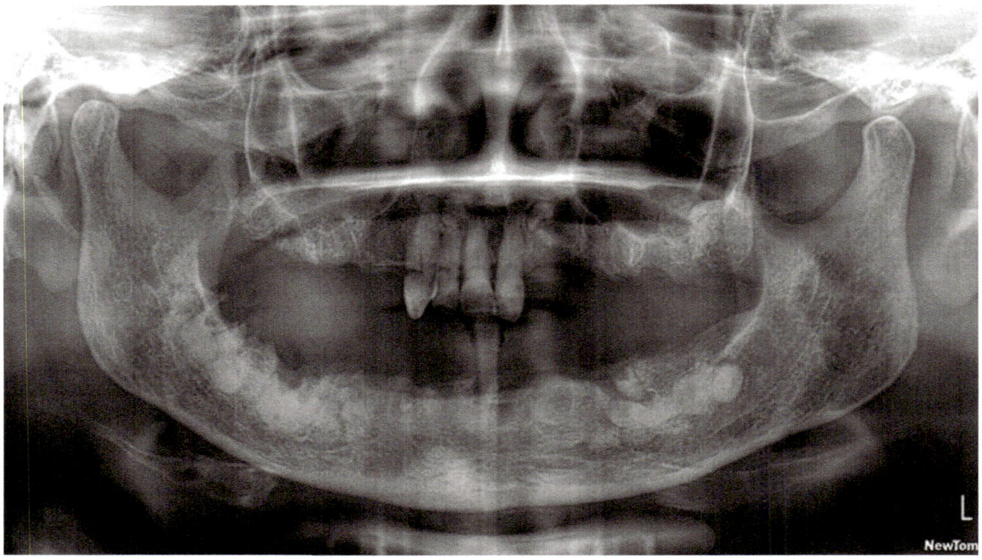




**Fig. 30.9** OPG of a 73-year-old Asian female, who had x-ray taken for removal of lower right third molar. X-ray shows diffuse florid COD-like lesions

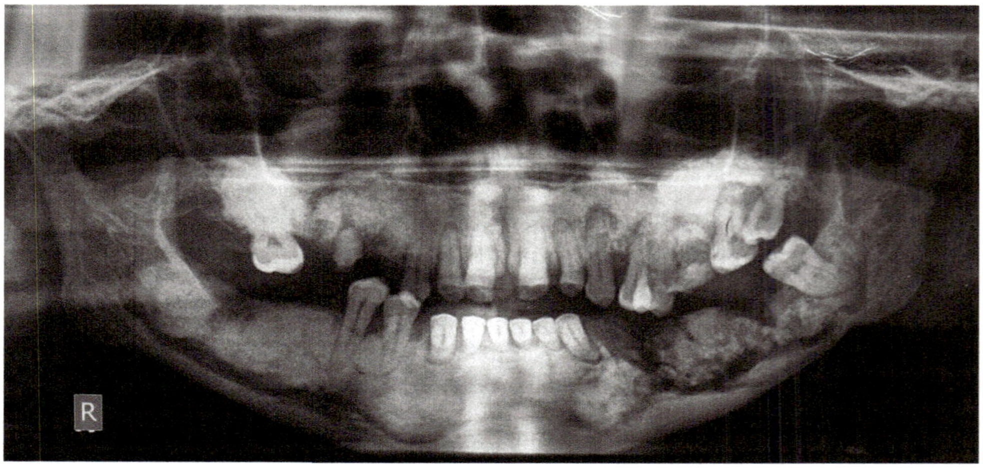




**Fig. 30.10** OPG of a 55-year-old Asian female who reported for dental extractions due to pain. Xray reveals florid COD-like lesions in both jaws

### 30.8.1 Clinical, Radiological and Histological Features

Florid cemento osseous dysplasia shows predilection for Afro-Caribbean women in the fourth to fifth decades of life, with a mean age of 42 years. The lesion has a propensity for bilateral symmetrical involvement of mandible. Occasional maxillary involvement is not rare.

The patients are usually edentulous and lesions are usually non-expansible, if cortical expansion is present then it is limited in nature.

The diagnosis of Florid OD is mainly clinical and radiographic, Melrose [32] suggests the involvement of two jaw quadrant is imperative for the diagnosis of Florid COD. Radiographically, the lesion undergoes stages of maturation as seen in the other types of OD, initially, the lesions are mainly radiolucent and with time progressively become first mixed radiolucent radiopaque and then in later stages turn into radiopaque sclerotic masses. Simple bone cyst that appears as sharply defined radiolucent areas may be intermixed with the lesional tissue, is a frequent finding in Florid OD. The most commonest radiographic presentation is of multiple sclerotic lobular opacities mixed ill defined with radiopaque radiolucent masses involving the alveolar process of mandible and maxilla sparing the lower border of the mandible and vertical rami.

Histologically, the lesion has similar features like other two forms of OD. The lesion specimen consists of cellular mesenchymal connective tissue, with numerous spindle-shaped fibroblasts and blood vessels. Multiple haemorrhagic sites are a common finding in the connective tissue background along with lamellar-, woven- and cementum-like particles. Depending on the extent of maturation of the lesion, they become more sclerotic and the ratio of fibrous connective tissue to mineralised material decreases.

### 30.8.2 Treatment/Management

The modified osseous tissue is prone to infection, hence any local causes of infection-like periapical pathosis, periodontal disease, ill-fitting dentures can lead to osteomyelitis of the underlying altered bone and fistula and sequestra formation. It is recommended to avoid any surgical intervention for diagnostic purposes, as the diagnosis is generally made on clinical and radiographic presentation. As for the treatment of symptomatic lesions like the presence of underlying osteomyelitis, conservative care in the form of removal of sequestra and prolonged antibiotic therapy is recommended. Extractions are not recommended for the same reason, as the socket heals by replacement with cementum-like tissue, which is mainly avascular.

Surgical intervention in terms of the debulking procedures is only recommended where there is obvious facial deformity resulting in reduced quality of life [33].

## 30.9 Conclusion

FOLs form a diverse wide spectrum of lesions, which are still evolving; in their classifications. Maxillofacial surgeons usually come across intra-oral lesions at various stages and many of them can be managed easily by routine surgical modalities. Certain lesions show aggressive nature and involve mid-face and sino-nasal areas. Such cases will need a multi-disciplinary approach for optimal treatment outcomes. Close interaction with the pathologist and adequate radiological investigations are needed to ascertain the diagnosis in many cases. The lack of clarity in classification and the similar radiological and histological picture of various lesions add to the difficulty in reaching a diagnosis.

**Acknowledgments** Suvy Manuel for Figures 30.1, 30.2, 30.3, 30.4, 30.5, 30.6, and 30.9
Oommen A Jacob-Figures 30.7, 30.8
Sooraj S- Figure 30.10

## References

1. Eversole R, Su L, ElMofty S. Benign fibro-osseous lesions of the craniofacial complex a review. Head Neck Pathol. 2008;2:177–202.
2. Brannon RB, Fowler CB. Benign fibro-osseous lesions: a review of current concepts. Adv Anat Pathol. 2001;8:126–43.
3. Waldron CA. Fibro osseous lesions of the jaws. J Oral Maxillofac Surg. 1985;43:249–62.
4. Waldron CA. Fibro-osseous lesions of the jaws. J Oral Maxillofac Surg. 1993;51:828–35.
5. Rajpal K, Agarwal R, Chhabra R, Bhattacharya M. Updated classification schemes for fibro-osseous lesions of the oral & maxillofacial region: a review. IOSR J Dent Med Sci Ver.
6. Srichinthu KK, Yoithapprabhunath TR, Chitturi RT, Yamunadevi A, Potsangbam AD, Singh DN. Fibro osseous lesions—classifications, pathophysiology and importance of radiology: a short review. Int Biol Biomed J. 2016;2:11–20.
7. Slootweg PJ. Maxillofacial fibro-osseous lesions: classification and differential diagnosis. Semin Diagn Pathol. 1996;13:104–12.
8. Barnes L, Eveson JW, Reichart P, Sidransky D. World Health Organization classification of tumours. Pathology and genetics—head and neck tumours. Lyon: IARC; 2005. p. 319–23.
9. Speight P, Carlos R. Maxillofacial fibro-osseous lesions. Curr Diagn Pathol. 2006;12(1):1–10.
10. Waldron CA, Giansanti JS. Benign fibro-osseous lesions of the jaws: a clinical-radiologic-histologic review of sixty-five cases. II. Benign fibro-osseous lesions of periodontal ligament origin. Oral Surg Oral Med Oral Pathol. 1973;35(3):340–50.
11. Hall G. Fibro-osseous lesions of the head and neck. Diagn Histopathol. 2012;18(4):149–58.
12. El-Mofty SK. Fibro-osseous lesions of the craniofacial skeleton: an update. Head Neck Pathol. 2014;8:432–44.

13. Pereira TDSF, Gomes CC, Brennan PA, Fonseca FP, Gomez RS. Fibrous dysplasia of the jaws: integrating molecular pathogenesis with clinical, radiological, and histopathological features. J Oral Pathol Med. 2019;48:3–9.
14. MacDonald DS. Maxillofacial fibro-osseous lesions. Clin Radiol. 2015;70(1):25–36.
15. Slootweg PJ, Müller H. Differential diagnosis of fibro-osseous jaw lesions. A histological investigation on 30 cases. J Craniomaxillofac Surg. 1990;18(5):210–4.
16. Orten SS, Hanna E. Fibrous dysplasia: biology and indications for surgery. Oper Tech Otolaryngol Head Neck Surg. 1999;10(2):109–12.
17. Chen YR, Noordhoff MS. Treatment of craniomaxillofacial fibrous dysplasia: howearly and how extensive? Plast Reconstr Surg. 1990;86(5):835–42; discussion 843–4.
18. Ricalde P, Horswell BB. Craniofacial fibrous dysplasia of the fronto-orbitalregion: a case series and literature review. J Oral Maxillofac Surg. 2001;59(2):157–67; discussion 167–8.
19. Speight PM, Takata T. New tumour entities in the 4th edition of the World Health Organization classification of head and neck tumours: odontogenic andmaxillofacial bone tumours. Virchows Arch. 2018;472(3):331–9.
20. Zegalie N, Martin L, Speight PM. Ossifying fibromas of thejaws and craniofacial bones. Diagn Histopathol. 2015;2015(21):370–8.
21. Wright JM, Odell EW, Speight PM, Takata T. Odontogenictumors, WHO 2005: where do we go from here? Head Neck Pathol. 2014;8(4):373–82.
22. El-Mofty SK, Nelson B, Toyosawa S. Ossifying fibroma. In: El-Naggar AK, JKC C, Grandis JR, Takata T, Slootweg PJ, editors. WHO classification of head and neck tumours. 4th ed. Lyon: IARC; 2017. p. 251–2.
23. Eversole LR, Leider AS, Nelson K. Ossifying fibroma: a clinicopathologic studyof sixty-four cases. Oral Surg Oral Med Oral Pathol. 1985;60(5):505–11.
24. El-Mofty S. Psammomatoid and trabecular juvenile ossifying fibroma of thecraniofacial skeleton: two distinct clinicopathologic entities. Oral Surg Oral Med Oral Pathol Oral Radiol Endod. 2002;93(3):296–304.
25. Slootweg PJ, Panders AK, Koopmans R, Nikkels PG. Juvenile ossifying fibroma. An analysis of 33 cases with emphasis on histopathological aspects. J Oral Pathol Med. 1994;23(9):385–8.
26. Slootweg PJ, Panders AK, Nikkels PG. Psammomatoid ossifying fibroma of theparanasal sinuses. An extragnathic variant of cemento-ossifying fibroma. Reportof three cases. J Craniomaxillofac Surg. 1993;21(7):294–7.
27. Titinchi F, Morkel J. Ossifying fibroma: analysis of treatment methods and recurrence patterns. J Oral Maxillofac Surg. 2016;74(12):2409–19.
28. Neville BW, Damm DD, Allen CM, Chi AC. Oral and maxillofacial pathology. 4th ed. St Louis: Saunders; 2016.
29. Su L, Weathers DR, Waldron CA. Distinguishing features of focalcemento-osseous dysplasias and cemento-ossifying fibromas: I. A pathologic spectrum of 316 cases. Oral Surg Oral Med Oral Pathol Oral Radiol Endod. 1997;84(3):301–9.
30. Su L, Weathers DR, Waldron CA. Distinguishing features of focalcemento-osseous dysplasia and cemento-ossifying fibromas. II. A clinical and radiologic spectrum of 316 cases. Oral Surg Oral Med Oral Pathol Oral Radiol Endod. 1997;84(5):540–9.
31. Summerlin DJ, Tomich CE. Focal cemento-osseous dysplasia: a clinicopathologic study of 221 cases. Oral Surg Oral Med Oral Pathol. 1994;78(5):611–20.
32. Melrose RJ, Abrams AM, Mills BG. Florid osseous dysplasia. A clinical-pathologic study of thirty-four cases. Oral Surg Oral Med Oral Pathol. 1976;41(1):62–82.
33. Shah A, Modgill O, et al. Cemento-osseous dysplasia: to treat or not to treat? J Oral Maxillofac Surg. 2016;74(9):e60.

# Vascular Anomalies of the Oro-Maxillofacial Region

# 31

Sanjiv Nair and Sunil S. Shroff

## 31.1 Introduction

Vascular anomalies are lesions arising from the arterial and/or venous and/or lymphatic circulation. These have a wide array of histological and clinical features and constitute one of the commonest congenital anomalies in infants and children [1].

In the context of iatrogenic creation of arteriovenous fistulas by phlebotomists, William Hunter in the mid-eighteenth century first described vascular anomalies. Haemangiomas and vascular malformations are different entities of vascular anomalies and this was first recognised by James Wardrop in 1818 [2]. In spite of Dr. Wardrop's work, subjective words like 'strawberry hemangioma' and 'salmon patch' were used for a long time. These terms only reflected the appearance and did not correlate clinically or histologically [2].

Anomalies presenting in different age groups with varying clinical behaviours needing different treatments were often given the same or overlapping names by clinicians. Commonly used terms are: haemangioma, arterial malformation, venous malformation, capillary malformation and lymphatic malformation.

Haemangioma (Figs. 31.1 and 31.20): Is a benign tumour of blood vessels comprising arterioles with endothelial cells, which are proliferative and hyperplastic in nature.

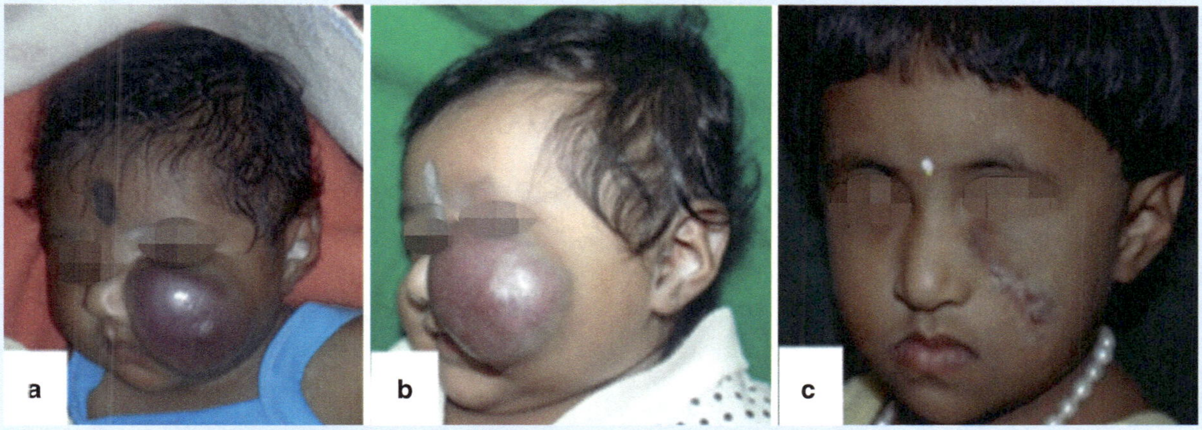




**Fig. 31.1** Non-involuting congenital Haemangioma (NICH) of left cheek ((**a**) initial therapy with propanolol 10 days post-birth, (**b**) 6 months following propanolol therapy, (**c**) excision of lesion at 2 years age)

S. Nair (✉) · S. S. Shroff (✉)
Department of Oral and Maxillofacial Surgery, Bhagwan Mahaveer Jain Hospital, Bengaluru, Karnataka, India


K. Bonanthaya et al. (eds.), *Oral and Maxillofacial Surgery for the Clinician*, https://doi.org/10.1007/978-981-15-1346-6_31

This terminology has been used by many as a common term for any vascular anomaly especially in childhood. These develop within the initial few weeks of life but often resolve with time. It is necessary for one to be able to differentiate between haemangioma and other vascular anomalies.

Arterial malformation (Fig. 31.2): These are dilated, overlapping and tortuous arteries having a coil-like appearance and/or a collection of arterial loops without any venous component. They are also described as 'high flow lesions'.

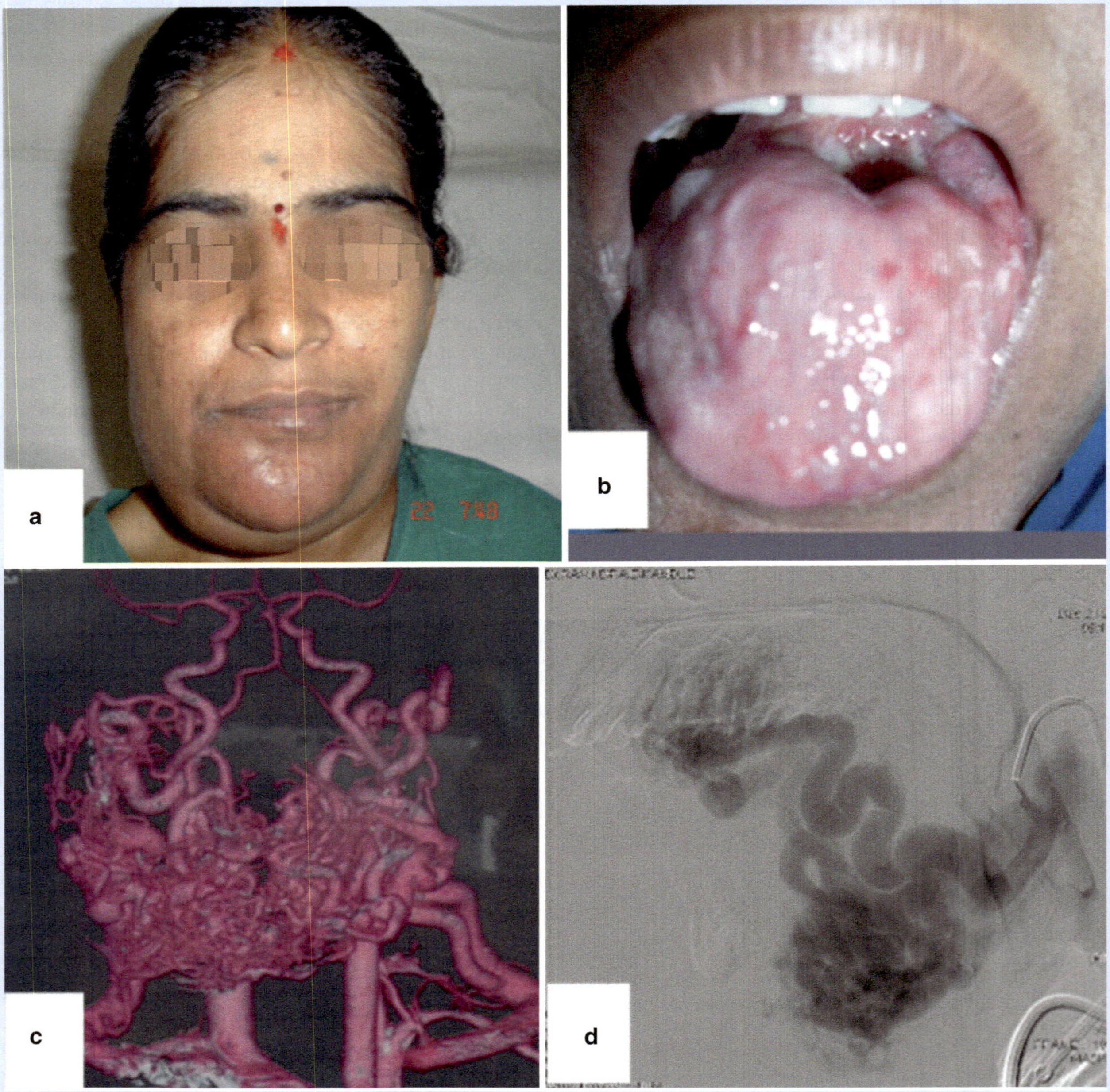




Fig. 31.2 Arterial malformation ((**a**, **b**) tongue high flow lesion, (**c**) DSA, (**d**) embolisation)

Venous malformation (Fig. 31.3): These are commonest type of vascular malformations caused by ectatic venous channels, also called 'low flow lesions'.

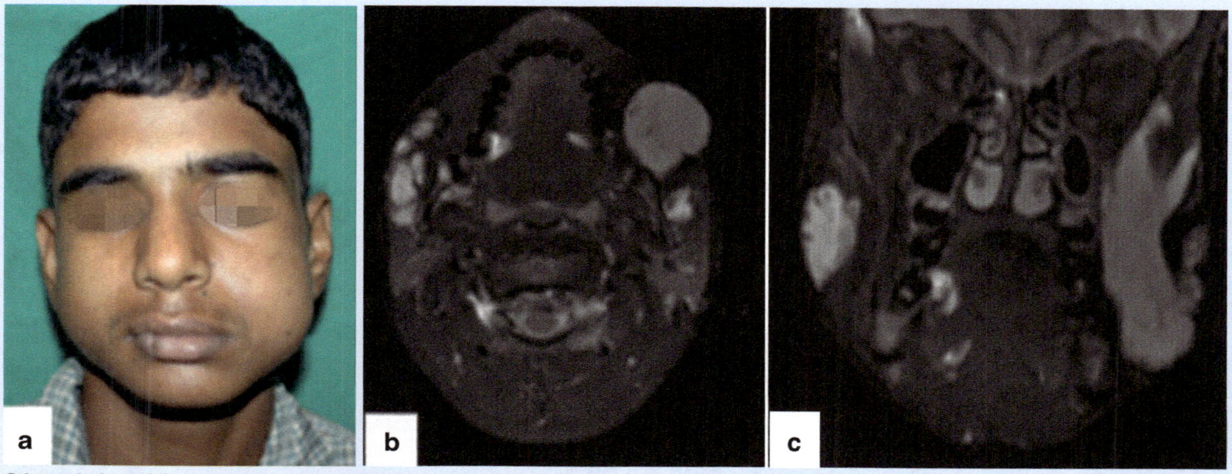


©Association of Oral and Maxillofacial Surgeons of India

**Fig. 31.3** Left cheek venous malformation ((**a**) pre-operative Left cheek VM, (**b**) axial and (**c**) coronal STIR sequence MRI)

Capillary malformations (Fig. 31.4): These are commonly known as, *'port wine stain'*. It is a flat, well-defined vascular stain of skin seen early in development when vessels of skin form abnormally which can increase in size and give a nodular appearance as a late presentation.

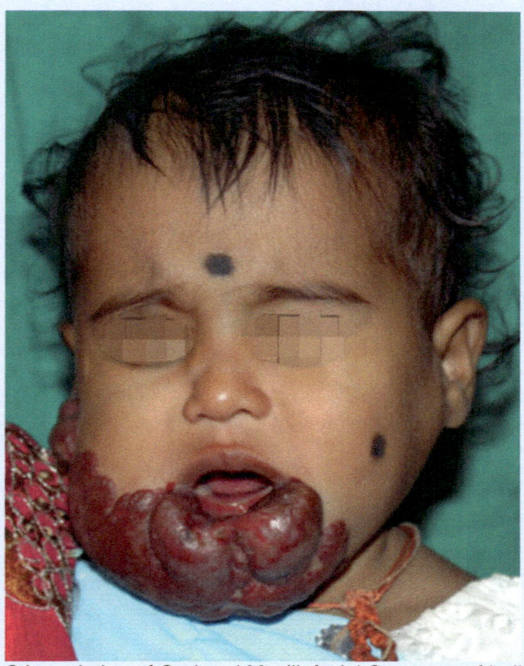

©Association of Oral and Maxillofacial Surgeons of India

**Fig. 31.4** Capillary malformation of lower lip, chin and right cheek

Lymphatic malformation (Fig. 31.5a, b): These are lesions containing fluid-filled spaces or channels, thought to be caused by abnormal development of the lymphatic system.

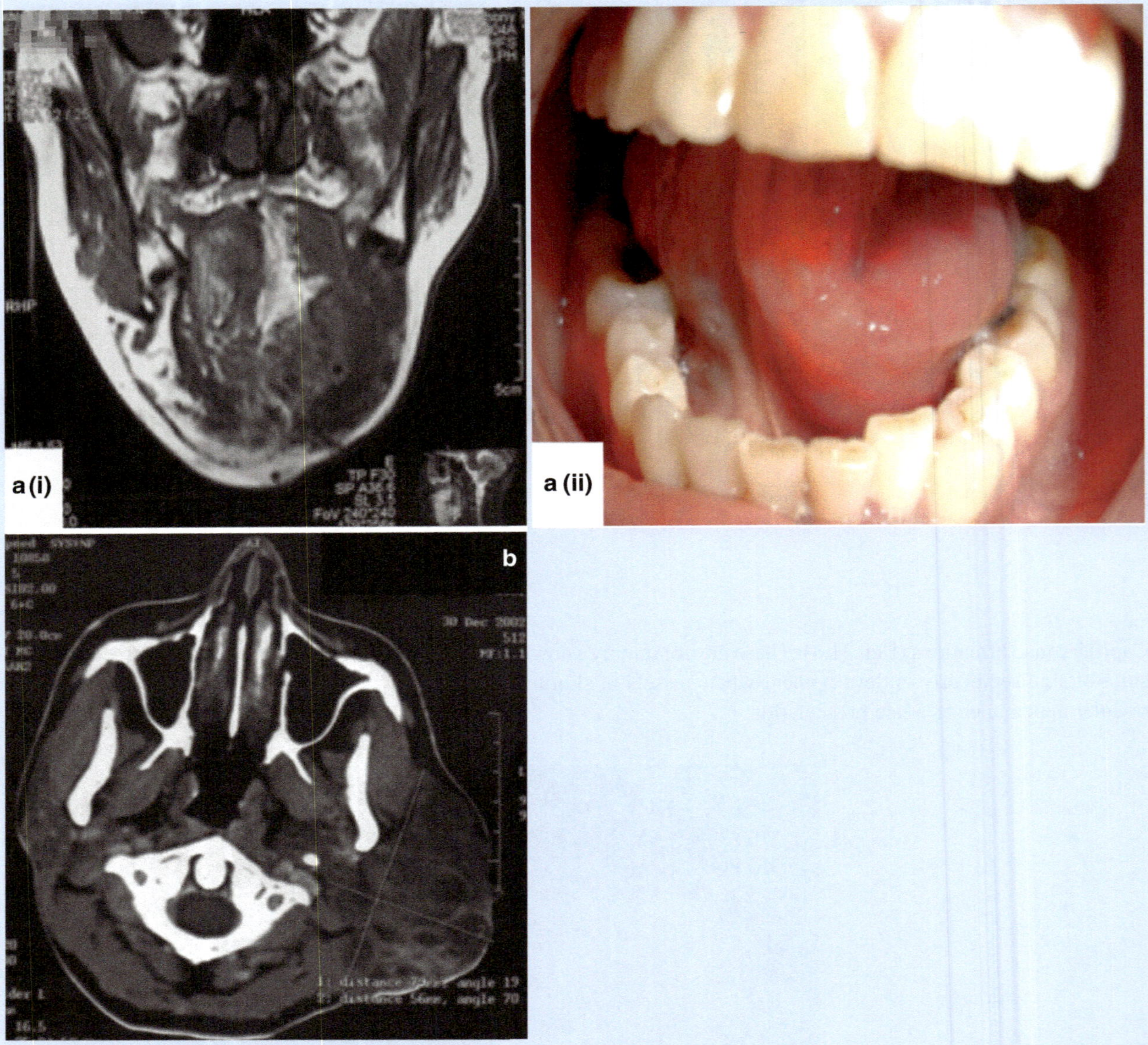




**Fig. 31.5** (**a**) Micro-cystic lymphatic malformation of tongue ((i) coronal T2 weighted MRI image, (ii) pre-operative clinical). (**b**) Axial post-contrast image of macro-cystic lymphatic malformation of left Parotid. Copyright: Authors own publication from IJOMS 2018

The above lesions in different combinations make up for 'arteriovenous' (Fig. 31.6) and 'lymphovenous' malformations.

## 31.2 Pathogenesis

Histologically, vascular anomalies are seen as a localised increase in vasculature with abnormal tortuosity and enlargement. This is known to be caused by defects in the formation of these vessels during vasculogenesis [3].

'Vasculogenesis' is defined as growth of vessels from precursor cells like, haemangioblasts that further give rise to angioblasts and haemocytoblasts.

Fusion takes place in islands of vasculature leading to the formation of primary capillary plexus, which then extends and matures during angiogenesis. This involves the proliferation of endothelial cells and the recruitment of mural cells to form fully developed and functional lymphatic and vascular trees [4].

Angiogenesis is regulated by factors like VEGFs (vascular endothelial growth factors), FGFs (fibroblast growth factors), PDGF-beta (platelet derived growth factor beta) and ANGPT-1 and ANGPT-2 (angiopoietins). These factors cause activation of precursor cells, leading to migration, proliferation and differentiation of the primary capillary plexus [5].

VEGFs, angiopoietins, and their endothelial tyrosine kinase receptors are known to be the central regulators of vasculogenesis, angiogenesis and lymphangiogenesis [4].

**Haemangiomas** have currently 2 dominant theories [6], although unclear. These are:

1. Endothelial cells are formed from deranged placental tissue present in foetal soft tissues during gestation.
2. Stem cells and endothelial progenitor cells which give rise to haemangiomas, are found in circulation of patients with haemangiomas.

Abnormal levels of matrix metalloproteinases (MMP9) and proangiogenic factors (VEGF, b-FGF and TGF-beta 1) are involved in the pathogenesis of haemangioma. Genetic errors involving growth factor receptors are also known to influence the development of these lesions [6].

There are 3 stages in the life cycle of haemangiomas [7], each characterised by biological markers and processes. These stages are clinically seen and distinguished microscopically and immunohistochemically [8] as,

1. *Proliferative phase—0–1 year of age*
2. *Involuting phase—1–5 years of age*
3. *Involuted phase—more than 5 years of age*

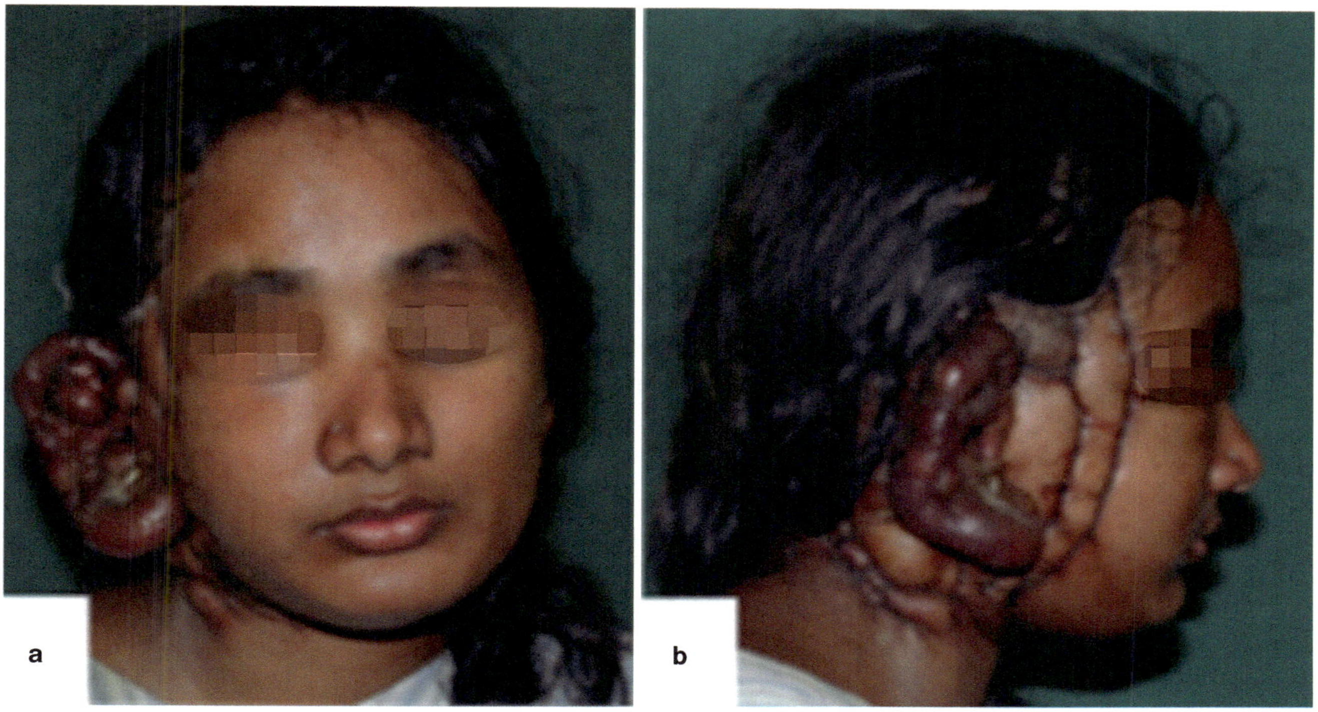


**Fig. 31.6** Arteriovenous malformation of pinna of right ear ((**a**, **b**) previous Popescu suturing as reported, (**c**) coronal CT angiography image, (**d**) contrast MR angiography image). Copyright: Authors own publication from IJOMS 2018

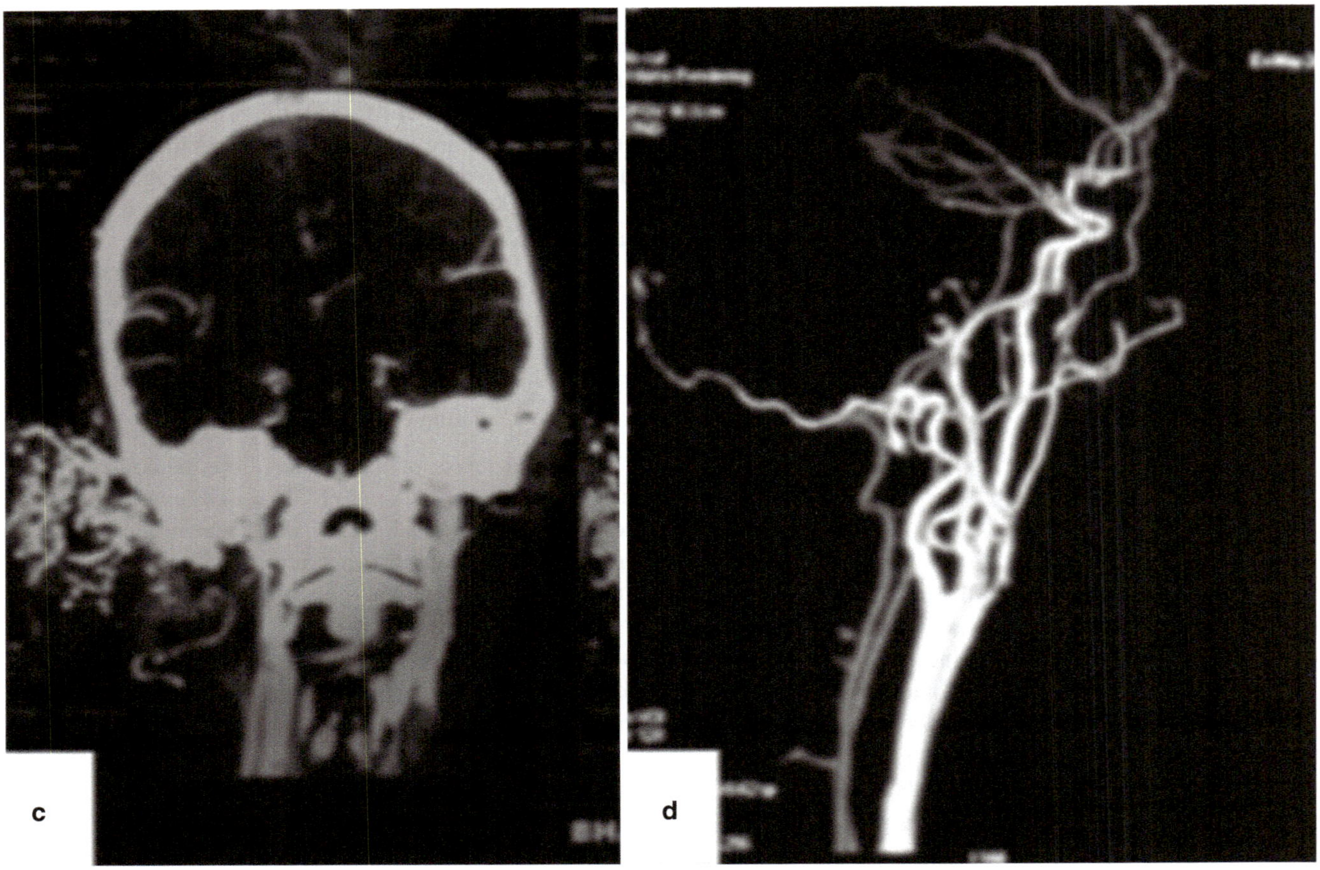

©Association of Oral and Maxillofacial Surgeons of India

**Fig. 31.6** (continued)

**Venous malformations (VMs)** are known to be autosomally dominant showing high penetrance. Abnormal venous connections cause venous congestion, thrombosis and slow expansion of these lesions. VMs commonly have a sporadic occurrence, but research has suspected a genetic locus to be involved in their development [6]. Chromosome 9p has been localised to cause inherited forms of VMs. The loss of functional mutation on the angioprotein-receptor gene TIE2/TEK and upregulation of many factors like tissue growth factor beta (TGF-beta) and basic fibroblast growth factor (beta-FGF) is seen [6]. Progesterone receptors are also found in VMs, which explains their propensity to enlarge rapidly during hormonal changes.

The pathogenesis of *capillary malformations (CMs)* is not clearly understood. These can be seen anywhere on the body, localised to a dermatome or extensive in nature. A familial pattern has been identified with a locus on chromosome 5q in a genome-wide linkage analysis [9].

**Lymphatic malformations (LMs)** show a focal pattern of occurrence. The aetiology is not clearly understood. Although most cases are congenital, there is no evidence of associated familial pattern. There have been cases of LMs following trauma or infection. Receptors like VEGFR3 and Prox-1, likely play a role in their development [10].

The pathogenesis of *arterio-venous malformations (AVMs)* is also not clearly understood. A defect in vascular stabilisation is known to potentially cause AVMs. Intracranial AVM is seen most commonly, followed by AVMs involving extracranial head and neck, extremities, trunk and viscera. These are seen at birth and are frequently misdiagnosed as a CM or haemangioma. These lesions have been seen following trauma in adults. Defects in signalling of TGF-Beta and genetic two-hit hypothesis are the existing theories [11, 12].

## 31.3 Classifications

Mulliken and Glowacki [13] in 1982 introduced a biological classification, which classified vascular lesions into two distinct entities: haemangiomas and vascular malformations.

Haemangiomas demonstrate endothelial hyperplasia unlike vascular malformations, which show progressive dilatation of abnormal vessels lined by flat endothelium on a thin basal lamina. A more practical classification amalgamating their biological behaviour and flow dynamics was later introduced [14] (Table 31.1).

**Table 31.1** Modified Mulliken and Glowacki classification [14]

| |
|---|
| **A. Haemangioma** |
| Superficial (Capillary haemangioma) |
| Deep (Cavernous haemangioma) |
| Compound (capillary cavernous haemangioma) |
| **B. Vascular Malformations** |
| *Simple lesions* |
| Low-flow lesions |
| Capillary malformations (capillary haemangioma, port-wine stain) |
| Venous malformation (cavernous haemangioma) |
| Lymphatic malformation (lymphangioma, cystic hygroma) |
| *High-flow lesions* |
| Arterial malformation |
| *Combined lesions* |
| Arteriovenous malformations |
| Lymphovenous malformations |
| Other combinations |

**Table 31.2** International Society for the study of Vascular Anomalies classification system (ISSVA) [15]

| |
|---|
| **Vascular tumors** |
| Benign |
| Locally aggressive or borderline |
| Malignant |
| **Vascular malformations** |
| *Slow-flow* |
| Capillary malformations |
| Lymphatic malformations |
| Venous malformations |
| Arteriovenous malformations |
| Arteriovenous fistula |
| *Combined (2 or more VMs in one lesion)* |
| CVM, CLM, LVM, CLVM, CAVM, CLAVM, others (C-capillary, V-venous, L-lymphatic, AV-arteriovenous) |
| *Anomalies of major named vessels* |
| *Vascular malformations associated with other anomalies* |

This system was later revised and adopted by the ISSVA [15] (*International Society for the study of Vascular anomalies*). This is currently the most widely accepted and divides vascular anomalies into: vascular tumors and vascular malformations (Table 31.2). The online version of the classification, is available on the ISSVA website (www.issva.org), contains hypertext links that facilitate the navigation in the classification and its appendices. These vascular neoplasms show an increased turnover of endothelial cells, which undergo division by mitosis, unlike vascular malformations. Vascular malformations can be capillary, venous, lymphatic and arterial, which progress in proportion to the child.

We proposed a practical classification of vascular lesions based on anatomy and depth of location in the head and neck region [1] (Table 31.3), which helped not only in understanding the extent of lesion but also in determining the surgical approach and reconstruction necessary. This classification is found to be most useful for the surgical management of these complex lesions.

**Table 31.3** Anatomical classification of Vascular malformations [1] (IJOMS 2011: 40)

| | |
|---|---|
| Type-I | Mucosal/cutaneous |
| Type-II | Sub-mucosal/sub-cutaneous |
| Type-III | Glandular |
| Type-IV | Intra-osseous |
| Type-V | Deep visceral |

Type-I lesions (Fig. 31.7) are superficial involving the epidermis and dermis. These can be excised in toto and reconstructed with local flaps where necessary. Lasers have some use in such surface lesions.

Type-II lesions (Fig. 31.8) involve sub-cutaneous tissue and facial planes. These can be widespread sometimes and approached by meticulously raising a superficial skin flap. The lesion is either debulked, excised or corseted as necessary (discussed in surgical management).

Type-III lesions (Fig. 31.9) are deeper involving salivary glands, usually parotid and sub-mandibular, demand-raising flaps in sub-cutaneous and sub-dermal planes. The lesion is either debulked, excised or corseted as necessary (discussed in surgical management).

Type-IV lesions (Fig. 31.10) involve bone and are either curetted or excised followed by reconstruction. These are usually high-flow lesions and require ECA control or endovascular embolisation to achieve adequate haemostasis (intra-operative dye administration in Fig. 31.10 demonstrates the efficacy of intra-operative ECA control in treating such high-flow vascular lesions).

Type-V lesions (Fig. 31.11) involve deeper visceral spaces like parapharyngeal, retropharyngeal, glottis and laryngeal. These can be rarely excised intoto and require access osteotomies of maxilla, mandible or zygoma (see Chap. 85 on access osteotomies).

## 31.4 Clinical Findings (Table 31.4)

A comprehensive and holistic understanding of the true nature of lesion is important to adequately manage these patients. The different types will be discussed according to the ISSVA classification for simplicity here, while the surgical management will be discussed according to the anatomical classification, as it was found to be more helpful than other available classifications.

Superficial *haemangiomas* (Fig. 31.20) can appear as raspberry-coloured birthmarks or reddish discolouration of the skin. The bright red strawberry-like classic appearance may not be seen in deeper lesions involving sub-cutaneous tissues. These deep lesions are wrongly diagnosed as vascular malformation, with normal appearing overlying skin. Superficial lesions were previously called ‘capillary hemangiomas’, and deeper lesions ‘cavernous hemangiomas’. These terms do not reflect the clinical nature or influence the

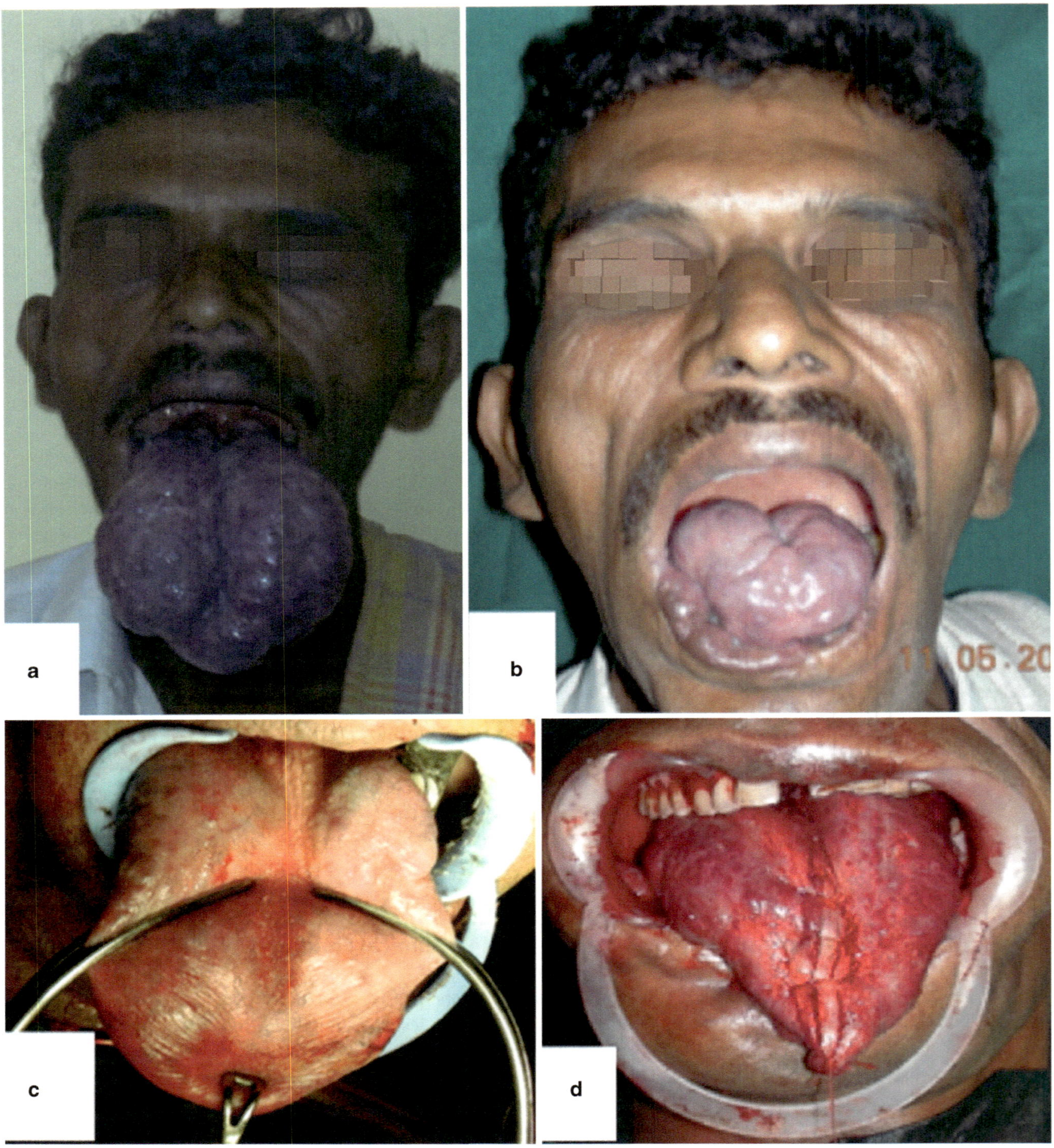




**Fig. 31.7** Type-I vascular lesion ((**a**) pre-operative tongue VM, (**b**) debulking, (**c**) closure and (**d**) post-operative). Copyright: Authors own publications from IJOMS 2011

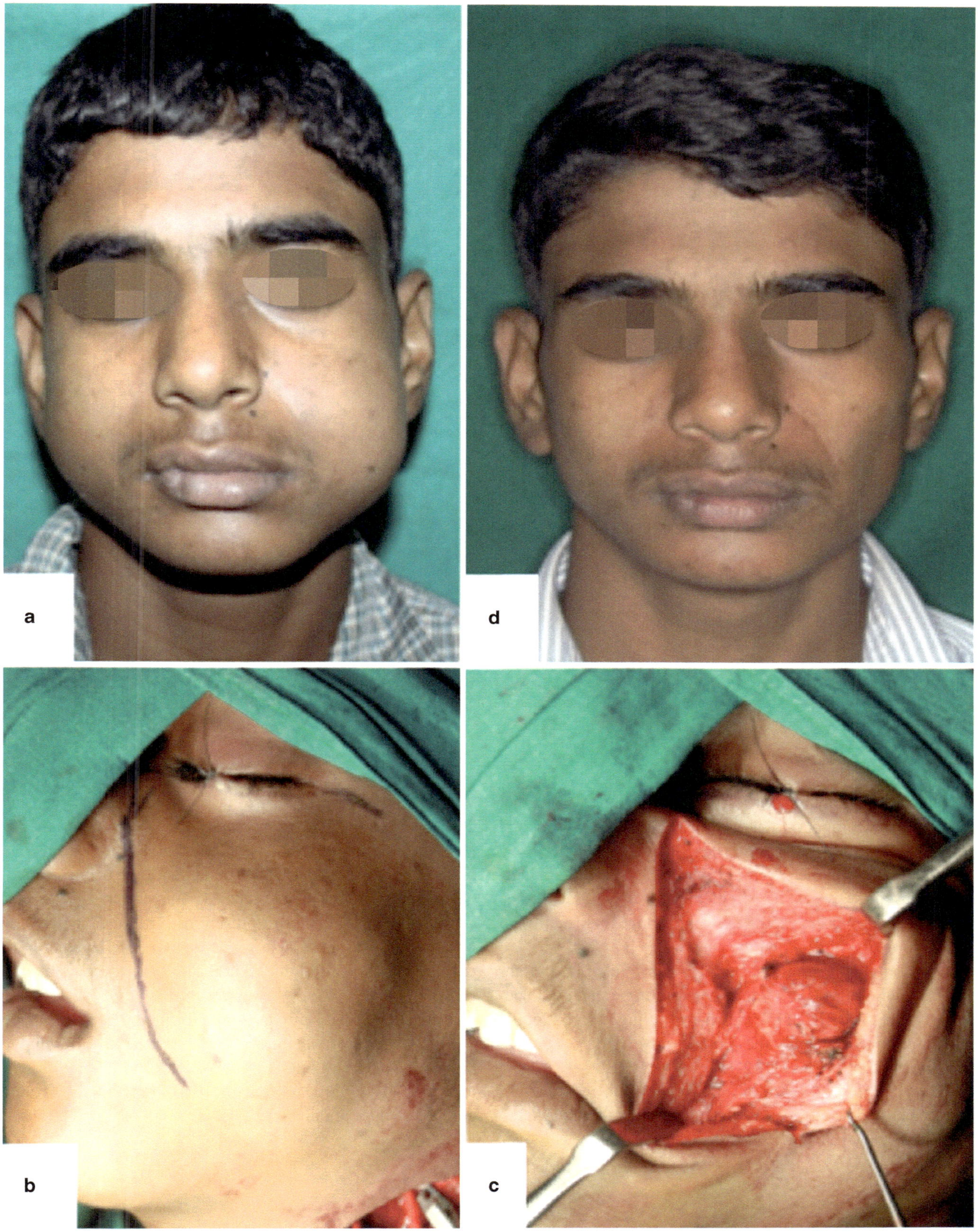




**Fig. 31.8** Type-II vascular lesion ((**a**) pre-operative Left cheek VM, (**b**) incision, (**c**) exposure and excision and (**d**) Post-operative)

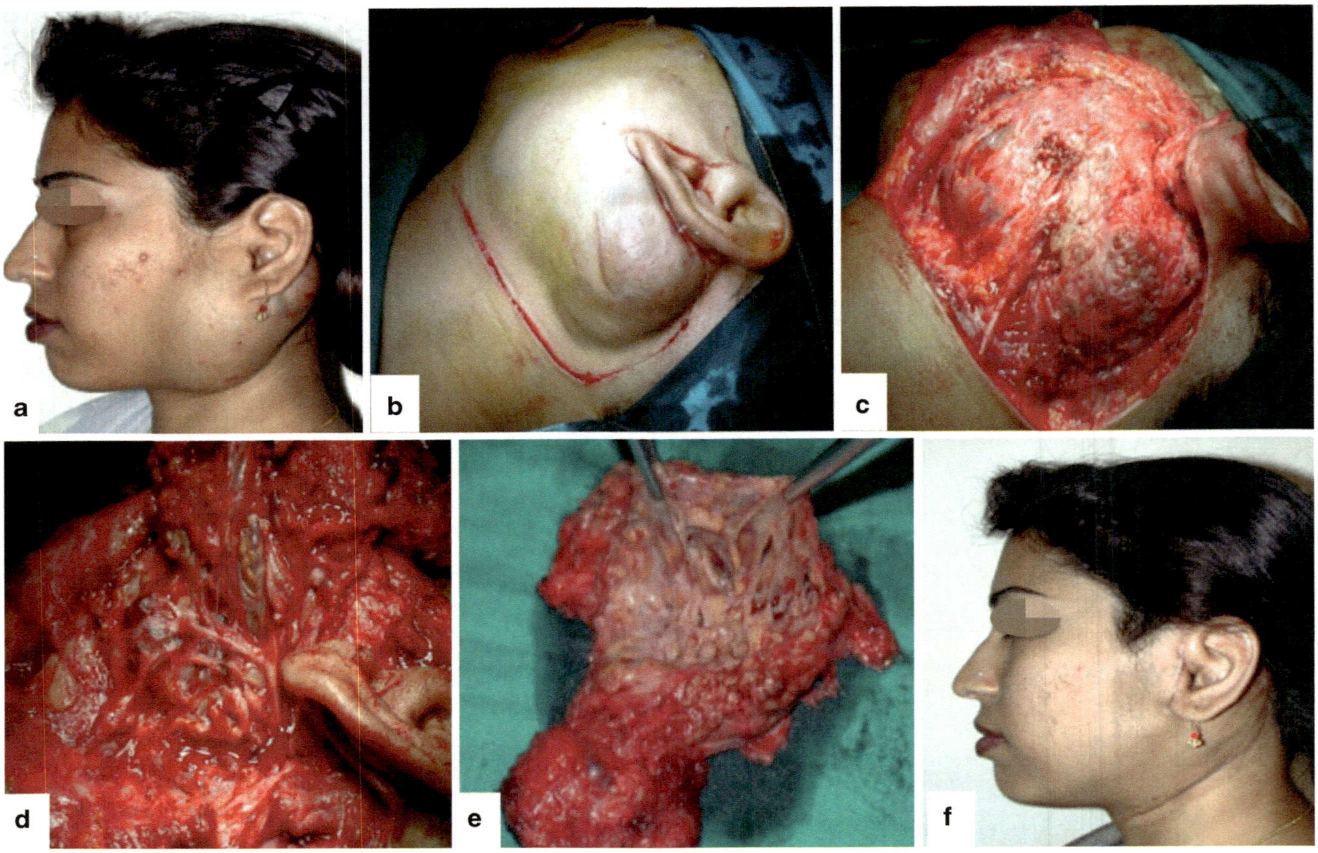


©Association of Oral and Maxillofacial Surgeons of India

**Fig. 31.9** Type-III vascular lesion ((**a**) pre-operative Left parotid AVM, (**b**) incision, (**c**) exposure, (**d**) facial nerve dissection, (**e**) excision specimen and (**f**) post-operative). Copyright: Authors own publications from IJOMS 2011

treatment and should be reserved only for histological description. Compound lesions involving superficial and deeper tissues are also seen. The clinical appearance may vary depending on the depth of tumour. Growing haemangiomas can show organ involvement and cause ulcerations, bleeding, hearing problems, vision changes, difficulty in mastication, dysphagia and dyspnea.

Congenital haemangiomas are further divided into infantile haemangiomas (IHs), rapidly involuting congenital haemangiomas (RICHs), non-involuting congenital haemangiomas (NICHs) and partially involuting congenital haemangiomas (PICHs) [15, 16].

IHs are commonly seen in infants and occur in 5–10% of children [17]. They appear anywhere between a few days to 3 weeks after birth. 80% of these cutaneous lesions are single and 20% are multiple. They grow rapidly and then enter an inactive phase at about 6 months of age. They then begin to shrink and involute after 1 year of age and sometimes leave behind a residual lesion. These residual lesions take longer to resolve.

RICHs (Fig. 31.20) are present at birth and involute by 6–14 months of age. Occasionally, they cause haematological irregularities like the Kasabach-Merritt phenomenon (KMP).

NICHs (Fig. 31.1) are present at birth and get larger with age. It is best to wait until 1 year of age to differentiate between RICH and NICH by looking at the involution pattern. PICHs initially present as RICH but fail to involute completely and remain as NICH.

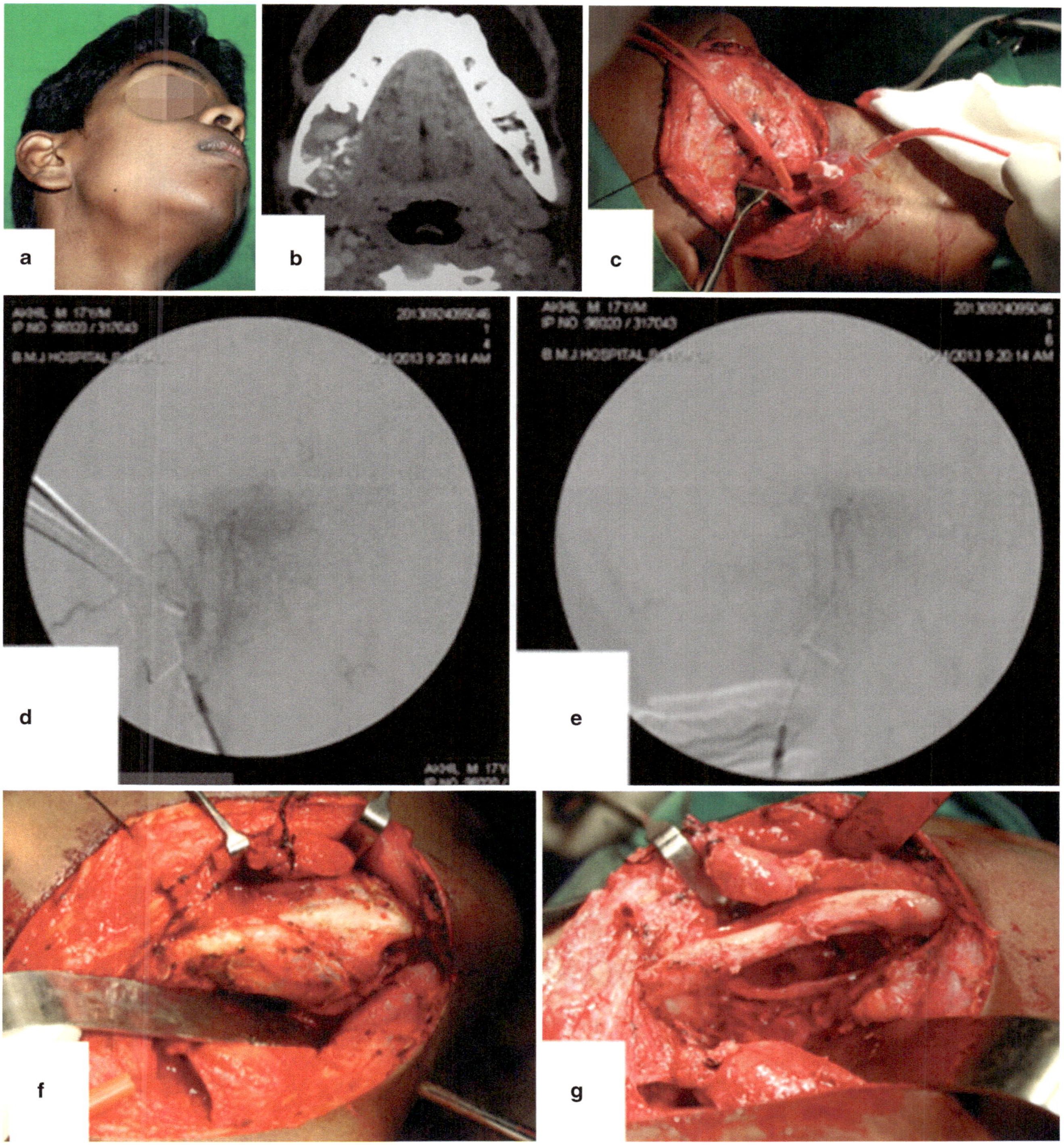




**Fig. 31.10** Type-IV vascular lesion ((**a**) pre-operative AVM right mandible, (**b**) axial post-contrast CT image, (**c**) ECA control and injection of radiopaque dye, (**d**) intra-operative C-arm picture following dye injection before occluding of ECA, (**e**) intra-operative C-arm picture following dye injection and occlusion of ECA, (**f**) lesion exposure and (**g**) currettage of lesion)

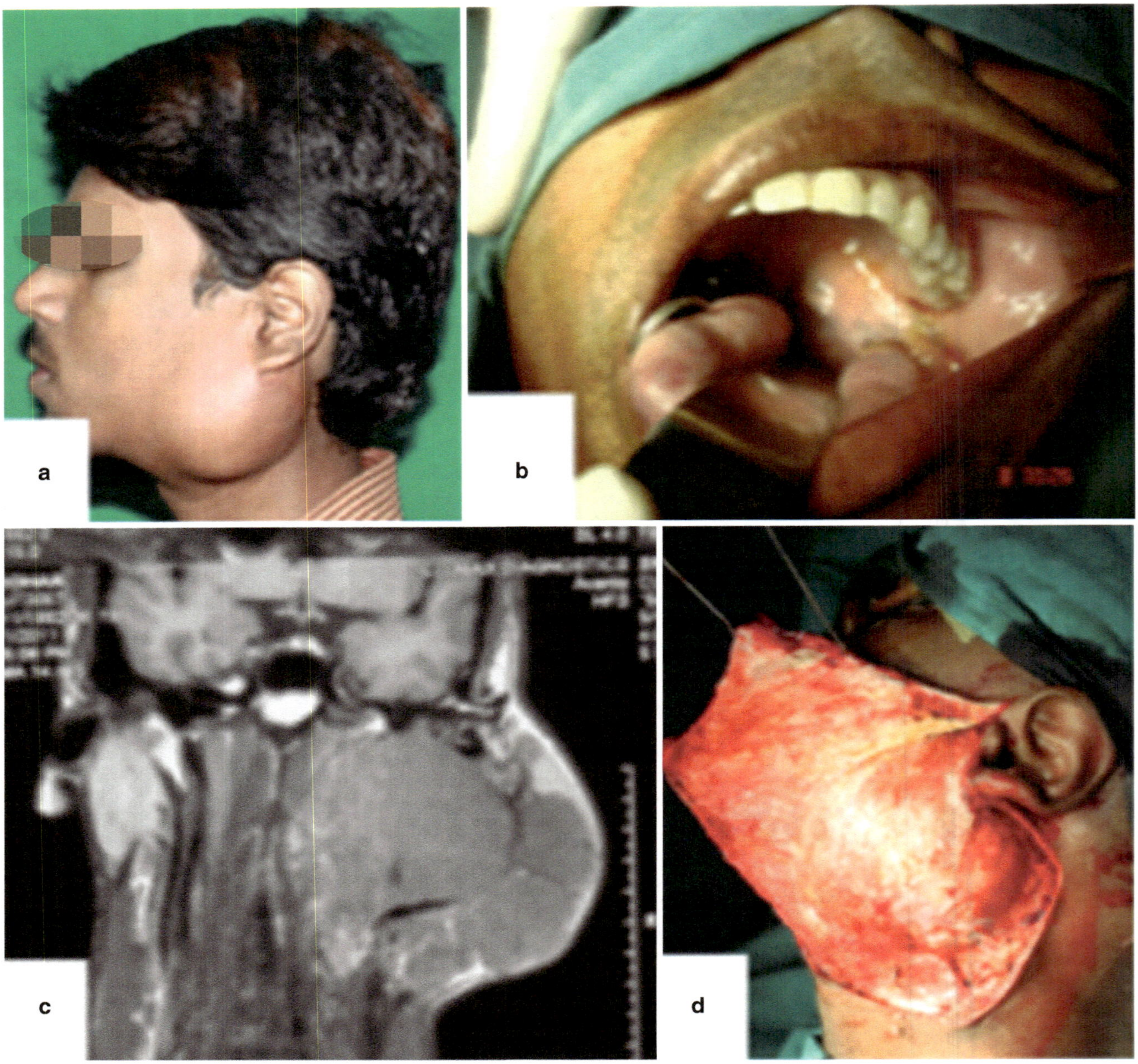

**Fig. 31.11** Type-V vascular lesion ((**a**) pre-operative VM left parotid, (**b**) parapharyngeal extension, (**c**) coronal T1 weighted MRI image, (**d**) exposure, (**e**) lesion exposure with mandibulotomy and ECA control, (**f**) lesion complete currettage, (**g**) mandibulotomy closure and (**h**) post-operative). © Association of Oral and Maxillofacial Surgeons of India

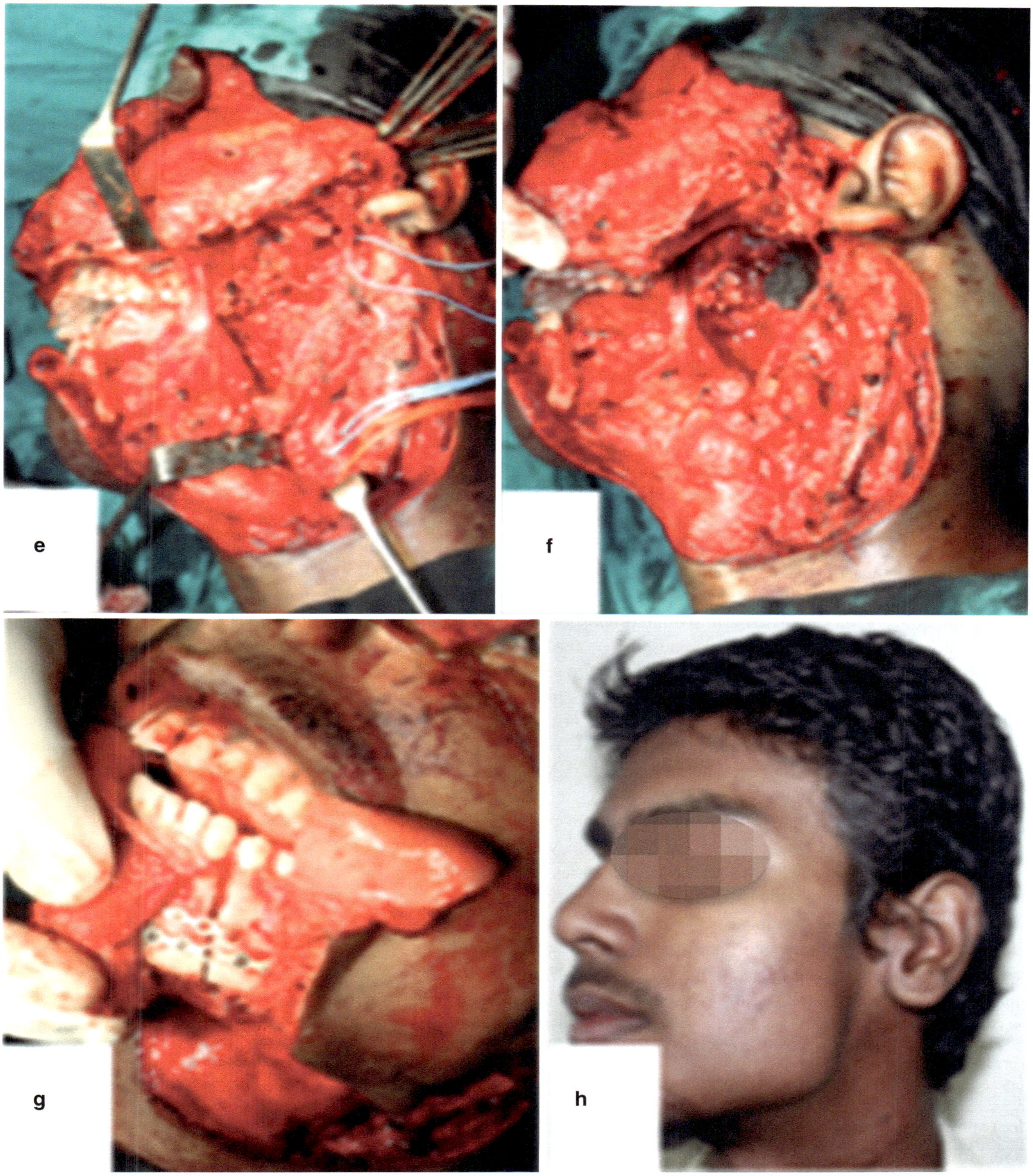




**Fig. 31.11** (continued)

**Table 31.4** Clinical findings of Vascular anomalies of Head and Neck

| | Haemangioma | VM's | CM's | LM's | AVM's | KHE's |
|---|---|---|---|---|---|---|
| Age | Birth, few days to 3 weeks after birth | Birth | Birth | Birth, later in life | Later in life | Neonate |
| Appearance | Reddish discolouration of skin | Bluish | Red or purple patch | Diffuse swelling | Pink to bluish | – |
| Depth | Skin, subcutaneous tissues | Superficial, deep | Cutaneous only | Deep tissues | Superficial, deep | – |
| Types | IH, RICH, NICH | – | Medial, lateral | Macrocystic, microcystic | – | – |
| Behaviour | Slow growing, involute in 12–14 months | Slow growing, low flow, local blood stasis | Painless, can involve deeper structures | Expansile, infiltrative | Pulsatory, thrill | Large, more than 5 cm in size |
| Functional problems | Ulceration, vision/hearing/swallowing/airway issues | Painful thrombophlebitis, phlebolith formation | Cosmetic disfigurement, involve other areas like in Sturge Weber syndrome, Klippel Trenaunay syndrome | Airway problems, pain, dysphagia, difficulty in mastication | Coagulopathy LIC/DIC, throbbing pain, ulceration | Thrombocyte penia, Kasabach-Merritt phenomenon |

**Venous malformations (VMs)** (Fig. 31.3) are most commonly seen vascular malformations, which are slow-growing, low-flow lesions present at birth and demonstrate a network of serpiginous inter-woven veins. These can grow extensively, become palpable, discoloured or bluish in colour with local blood stasis, which sometimes lead to painful thrombophlebitis. VMs can increase in size, in proportion to the increase in pressure within vessels caused by valsalva manoeuvre, dependency, exercise or agitation. VMs are usually compressible on palpation. They can demonstrate 'pheboliths', which are nothing but small calcifications formed due to, prolonged intra-vascular coagulation (Fig. 31.12).

Phleboliths are the commonest cause of pain in VMs. There is progressive lamellar fibrosis following intra-vascular thrombus formation. Calcium phosphate and carbonate are deposited in the core of the thrombus with peripheral mineralisation [18], which slowly increases in size. They are clinically palpable intra-orally, bi-manually in the cheek and over bony prominences. These are present as multiple oval or round laminated bodies (Fig. 31.12) with radiolucent or radiopaque corners, radiologically. Phleboliths can be areas of resistance to injecting sclerosants and should be excised separately.

**Capillary malformations (CMs)** (Fig. 31.4), can be seen in the neonatal period and should not be mistaken with infantile haemangiomas (IHs). They occur in around 0.3% of children presenting with vascular anomalies. CMs usually present congenitally as a flat, red or purple cutaneous patch with asymmetric borders. They are painless and do not bleed spontaneously. They are categorised as 'medial' or 'lateral' lesions, based on their location in head and neck. Lateral lesions involve areas of face along the distribution of trigeminal nerve. They present as portwine stains, usually increase in size to involve deeper sub-cutaneous tissues causing the lesions to become darker, more raised and nodular. CMs may be part of a syndrome, commonly the Sturge-Weber syndrome, which is characterised by CM involving the ophthalmic branch of trigeminal nerve, leptomeningeal angiomatosis and choroid angioma. CMs may also be seen in the Klippel-Trenaunay syndrome with multiple vascular (lymphatic, venous and capillary) abnormalities.

**Lymphatic malformations (LMs)** (Fig. 31.5) are usually congenital and not always detected until later in life. LMs are slow-flow lesions and can be *macro-cystic* (>2 cm) (Fig. 31.5b), *micro-cystic* (<2 cm) (Fig. 31.5a) or *mixed*, depending on the size of predominant cysts within them. Macro-cystic LMs can show expansion and compression of adjacent anatomical structures in the head and neck causing dysphagia, dyspnea and masticatory problems. Micro-cystic LMs were previously called lymphangiomas and demonstrate an infiltrative nature. LMs with local haemorrhage and infection can cause significant pain. LMs of the head and neck are further described by the *de Serres classification scheme* [19], which classifies disease severity based on the location and prognosis.

Fast-flow *arterio-venous malformations* (AVMs) (Fig. 31.6), usually present with a pulsatile local swelling. These AVMs along with some slow-flow lesions are at an increased risk of haematological complications like coagulopathies due to disturbances in haemostasis and thrombosis. Blood pools in abnormal slow-flow vessels, resulting in activation of the coagulation system, resulting in a process known as 'localized intravascular coagulopathy' (LIC), which shows low fibrinogen, elevated D-dimer levels and mild thrombocytopaenia. This can further cause, 'disseminated intravascular coagulopathy' (DIC) and consumption of various coagulation factors.

AVMs are known to behave aggressively in later life, which can be stimulated by pubertal changes, pregnancy or trauma. They may present with throbbing pain, ulceration

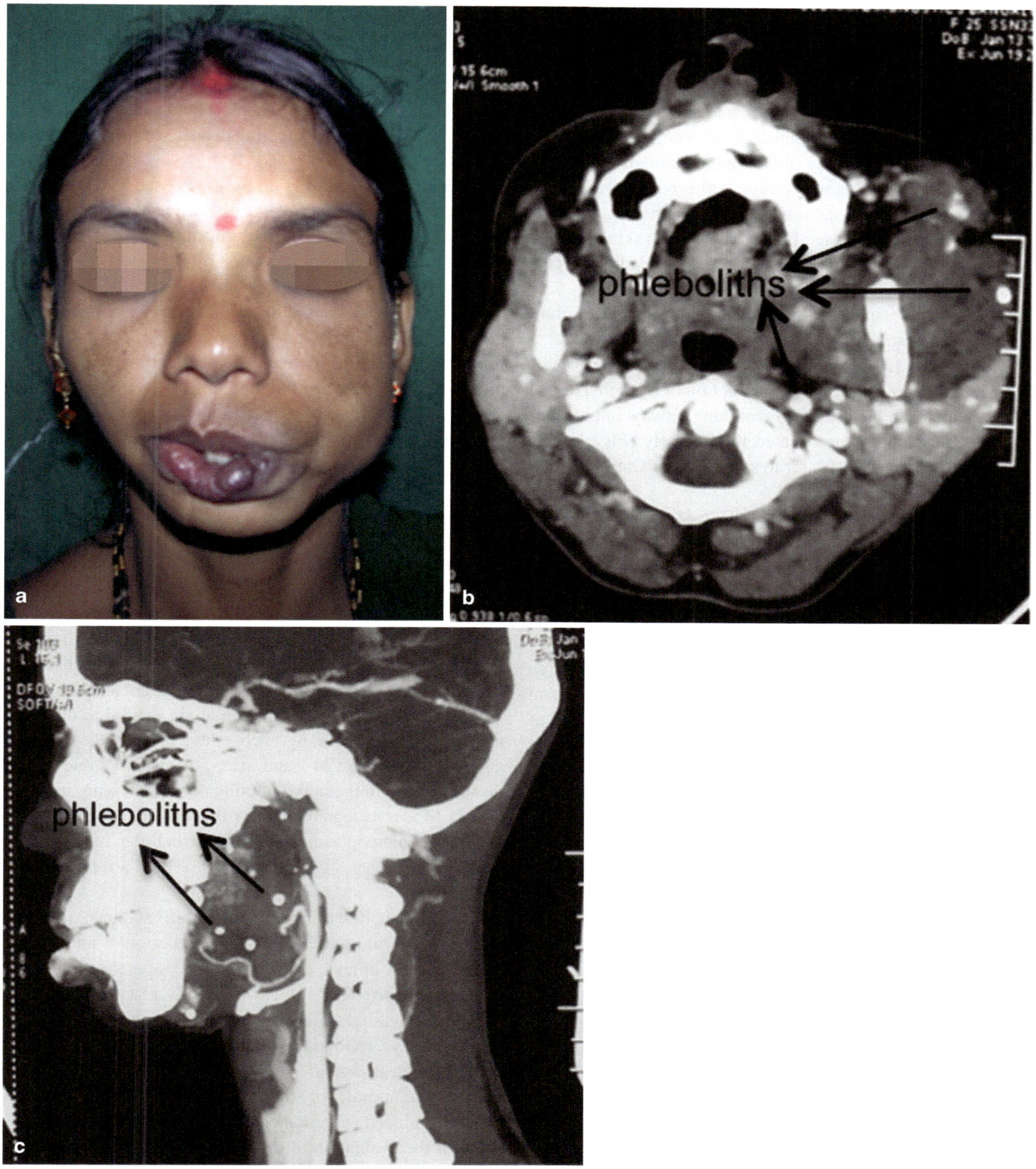




**Fig. 31.12** Left cheek and lower lip VM ((**a**) clinical picture, (**b**, **c**) post-contrast axial and sagittal CT images showing multiple phleboliths)

and bleeding. Significant bleeding can sometimes be a cause of cardiac failure, in affected individuals.

A useful clinical staging system was introduced by Schobinger [20] in 1990. This system is widely used for describing the clinical presentation and evolution of AVMs:

*Stage I* (quiescence): pink-bluish stain, warmth and arterio-venous shunting by way of Doppler examination

*Stage II* (expansion): same as stage I, plus enlargement, pulsations, thrill, bruit and tense/tortuous veins

*Stage III*: the same as stage II, plus dystrophic skin changes, ulceration, (destruction) tissue necrosis, bleeding or persistent pain

*Stage IV*: the same as stage III, plus cardiac failure (decompensation)

Undiagnosed AVMs of bone are occasionally the cause of increased bleeding during/after extraction of teeth in a dental office, which can lead to life-threatening airway and haematological problems if not treated immediately (Fig. 31.13). These warrant urgent transfer to a hospital and embolisation or ECA control.

Hereditary haemorrhagic telangiectasia (HHT) is autosomally dominant and presents with the formation of expanding arterio-venous fistulas. These patients usually present with superficial (skin, mucosal) or deep (visceral) telangiectatic lesions. They may sometimes present with aneurysms causing epistaxis or intra-cranial haemorrhage.

Kaposiform haemangioendotheliomas (KHEs) are large lesions (greater than 5 cm), which are present in the neonatal period. They are extremely rare and have a low incidence of occurrence. Hence, there are no clear guidelines on their management. These are aggressive vascular tumours, which can be complex in their management due to thrombocytopaenia secondary to platelet trapping. This phenomenon is known as KMP (Kasabach-Merritt phenomenon). 70% of patients with KHEs demonstrate this phenomenon [21].

## 31.5 Radiological Assessment

Clinical and radiological assessment go hand in hand to accurately diagnose and manage these diverse groups of head and neck vascular anomalies. Selection of the imaging should be tailored according to the indication, advantages, disadvantages and availability of resources. Good knowledge of all the available radiological modalities is essential to treat these lesions.

*Commonly used imaging modalities are*
Ultrasound (US)
Coloured Doppler ultrasound
Computed tomography (CT) with contrast
Digital subtraction angiography (DSA)
Magnetic resonance imaging (MRI)
MRI angiogram
Multi-planar dynamic contrast enhanced MRI

**US** (Fig. 31.14) is the least invasive modality of imaging available for assessment of vascular anomalies. It is used as a baseline investigation for superficial head and neck vascular lesions. In addition to the above, the US has a high sensitivity in diagnosing these lesions. The disadvantages of the US are its limitation in detecting deeper soft tissue and bony lesions.

**Doppler ultrasound** (Fig. 31.15) is used to demonstrate high-flow lesions. Flow towards the ultrasound transducer is seen in red and away from the transducer seen in blue. The arterial feeder is usually identified by increased colour flow, high doppler shift and low resistance.

**CT** (Fig. 31.16) is used to diagnose bony lesions, provide cross-sectional details and detect the presence of calcifications like phleboliths in venous malformations and haemangiomas. Most scans can be done in less than a minute with quick acquisition time. Reduced imaging time and low cost compared to MRI make contrast CT widely used for diagnosing soft tissue vascular lesions. Surveillance imaging with CT is not recommended due to increased exposure to ionising radiation.

**MRI** (Fig. 31.17) is the most preferred and accepted imaging for diagnosing and monitoring soft-tissue vascular lesions of head and neck. Its superior contrast resolution, in-depth soft-tissue assessment and non-exposure to ionising radiation, makes it the investigation of choice for these lesions. Haemangiomas and VMs show intense enhancement with MRI. AVMs and LMs show minimal enhancement.

Fat-suppressed T2-weighted imaging is used to discriminate these lesions among each other. Intense T2-weighted signal is seen with VM's and macro-cystic LM's due to cystic spaces within them and pooling of slow-flowing blood or lymph. Moderate signal intensity is seen with haemangiomas and vascular neoplasms due to their cellular composition. Mild T2-weighted signal is seen with AVM's reflecting tissue oedema.

Long acquisition time (at least 30 min) and increased cost of imaging limit its use [22]. Use of sedation or anaesthesia is required for infants, children and uncooperative adults.

**Angiography** (Fig. 31.18) is usually reserved for therapeutic endovascular interventions. Angiography includes arteriography, venography and injection of direct intra-lesional contrast agent. This provides good resolution (spatial and temporal) of the vascularity and also permits catheter-induced percutaneous therapy. Arteriography is used for the evaluation of high-flow vascular lesions. Its use is limited due to the invasive nature and use of ionising radiation.

**DSA** (Fig. 31.19) should be reserved for patients undergoing endovascular treatment. DSA is used for diagnosis of AVM's where the feeding artery, draining vein, nidus connecting artery and vein can be clearly imaged [23] and simultaneous embolisation can be performed, by an interventional radiologist.

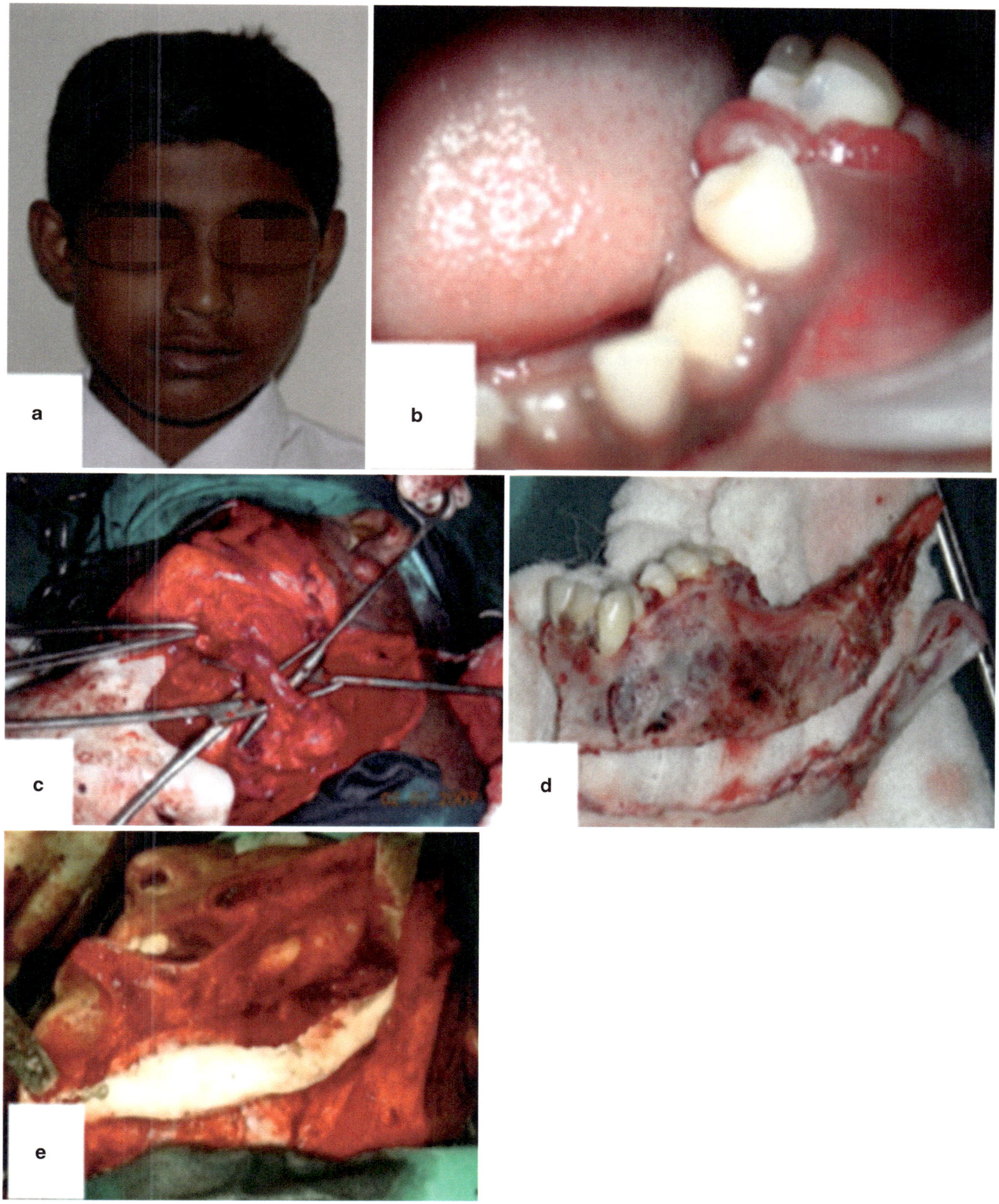




**Fig. 31.13** Bleeding following dental extraction—Extracorporeal currettage of high-flow bony vascular lesion and fixation of mandible ((**a**) pre-operative, (**b**) intra-oral, (**c**) ligation of main feeder, (**d**) extra-corporeal currettage and excision of diseased bone and (**e**) fixation of mandible as the free graft)

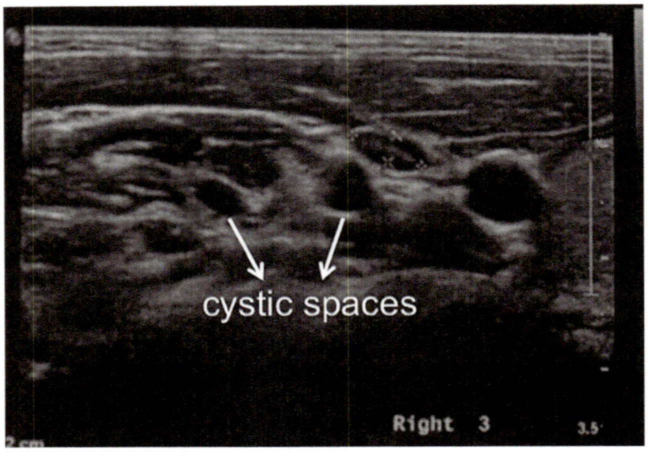




**Fig. 31.14** Ultrasound image-Venous malformation of submandibular region showing multiple cystic spaces

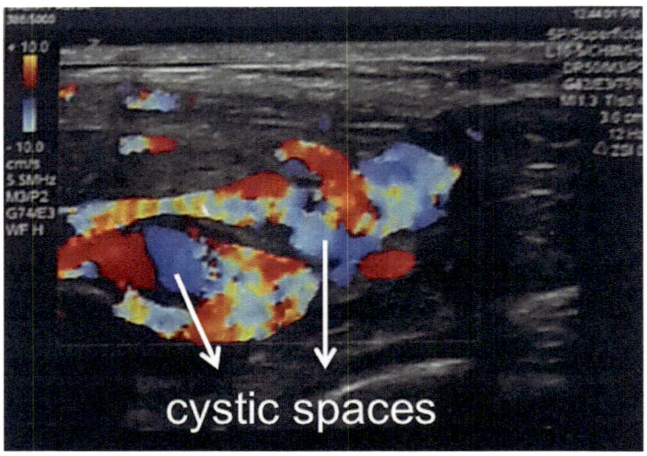




**Fig. 31.15** Coloured Doppler Ultrasound image of AVM of neck showing multiple cystic spaces filled with colour (flow towards the transducer seen in 'red' and away in 'blue', lighter shades of colour depict higher velocity)

Multi-planar dynamic contrast-enhanced MRI is preferred for extensive vascular malformations of the head and neck, especially in lesions involving aerodigestive tract, neural and vascular structures.

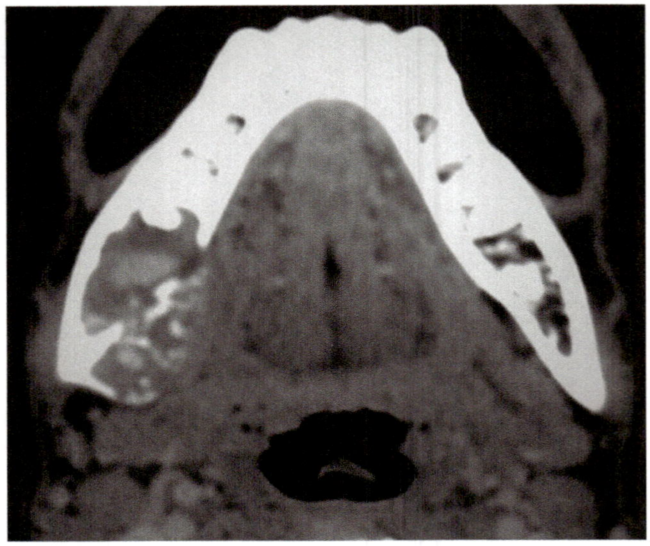



**Fig. 31.16** CT with contrast, Right mandible Type-IV lesion

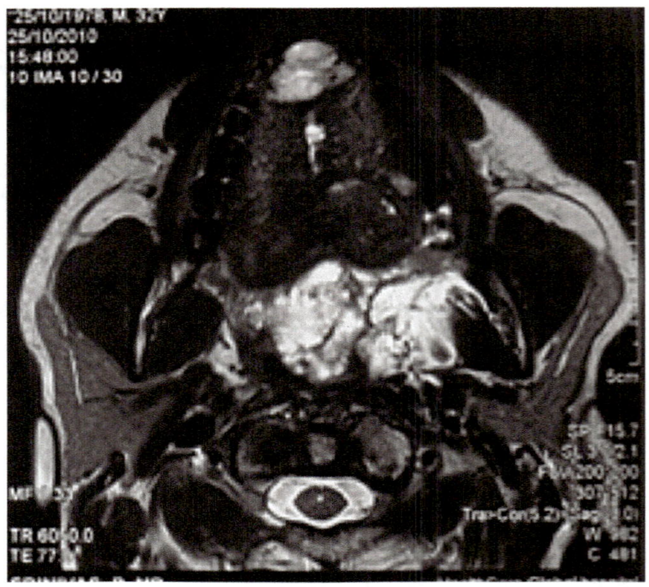




**Fig. 31.17** T2-weighted MRI, left parapharyngeal venous malformation

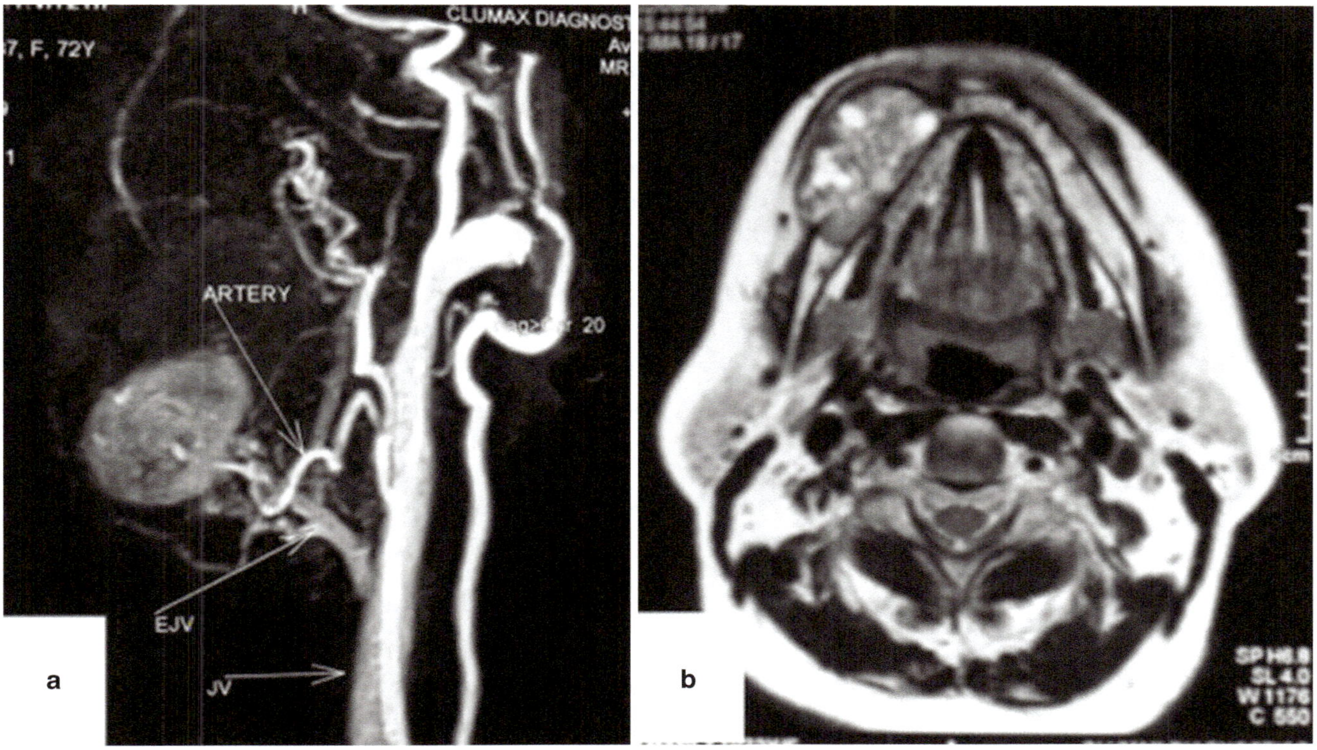




**Fig. 31.18** AVM of right mandible ((**a**) Contrast MR angiography image, (**b**) T2-weighted MRI image). Copyright: Authors own publications from IJOMS 2011

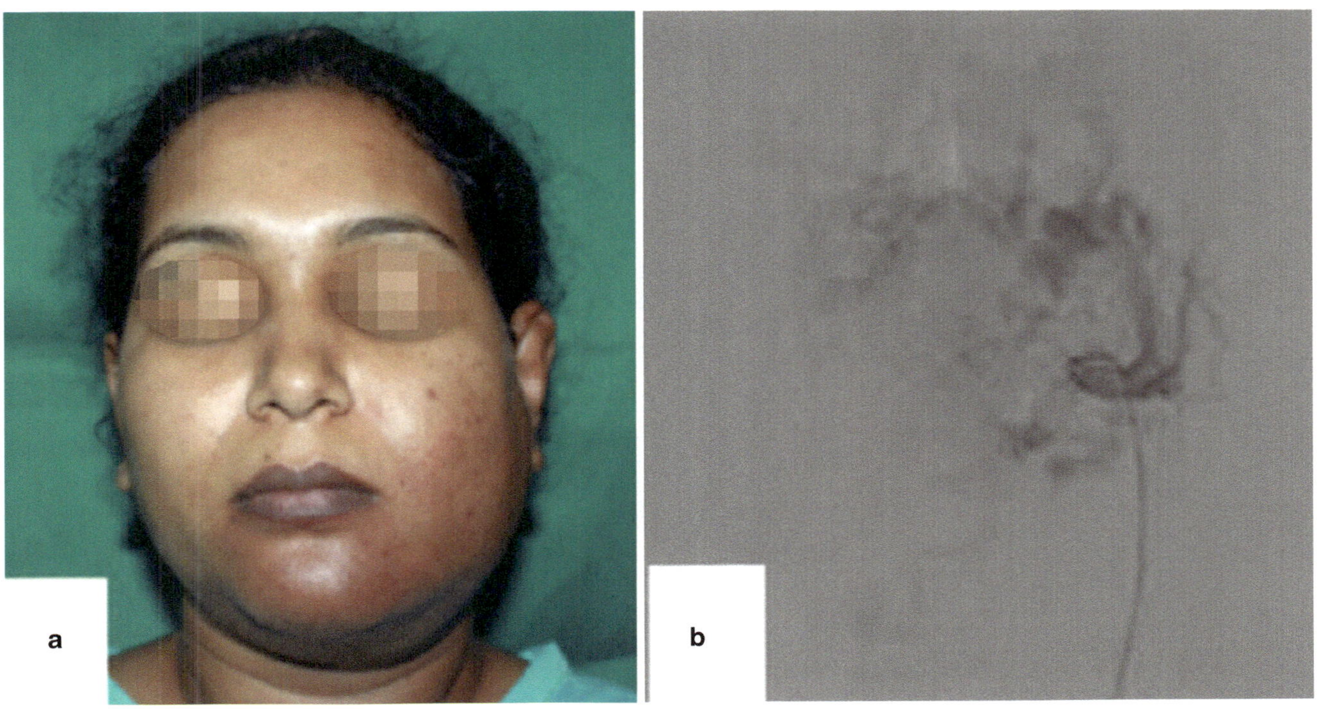




**Fig. 31.19** AVM left cheek ((**a**) clinical image, (**b**) DSA image during embolization)

## 31.6 Medical and Interventional Management

Correct diagnosis is important for selecting the appropriate therapy for vascular anomalies.

> The aim of managing complex vascular lesions should be to relieve acute symptoms like pain, swallowing and airway problems, prevent and treat thromboembolic events and correct the cosmetic impairment caused by them.

> The type of vascular anomaly and its flow characteristics, determine the mode of management.

> These mostly fall into:
> - Medical line of management,
> - Interventional therapy and
> - Surgical management.

Congenital haemangiomas, low flow venous malformations and lymphangiomas can be considered for treatment with systemic and sclerotherapy. Residual and large lesions are usually treated with surgery. AVM's and high-flow malformations have been mostly treated using embolisation with or without surgical excision/debulking successfully.

The author's wide experience in the surgical management of most low- and high-flow lesions has provided acceptable and predictable results.

In *haemangiomas*, a '*wait and observe*' strategy is preferred. Involution is seen in more than 85% of patients. If a malignant lesion is suspected, a biopsy with a request for GLUT-1 immunostaining is required to confirm its true nature [24]. Active intervention is considered if the lesion is

- Large in size causing obvious facial asymmetry
- Multiple with systemic changes like high-output cardiac failure.
- Adjoining or involving important structures like airway, eye and ear causing—vision, hearing, airway or swallowing problems.
- Recurrent and persisting ulcerations

**Propranolol** (Fig. 31.20) is the first line of treatment and is best to involve a paediatrician to monitor the dosage and systemic complications associated with it. Propranolol causes vasoconstriction and possibly reduced expression of pro-angiogenic factors of the haemangioma growth phase, leading to apoptosis of capillary endothelial cells.

Treatment during the proliferating phase is given to prevent impending functional or aesthetic complications especially

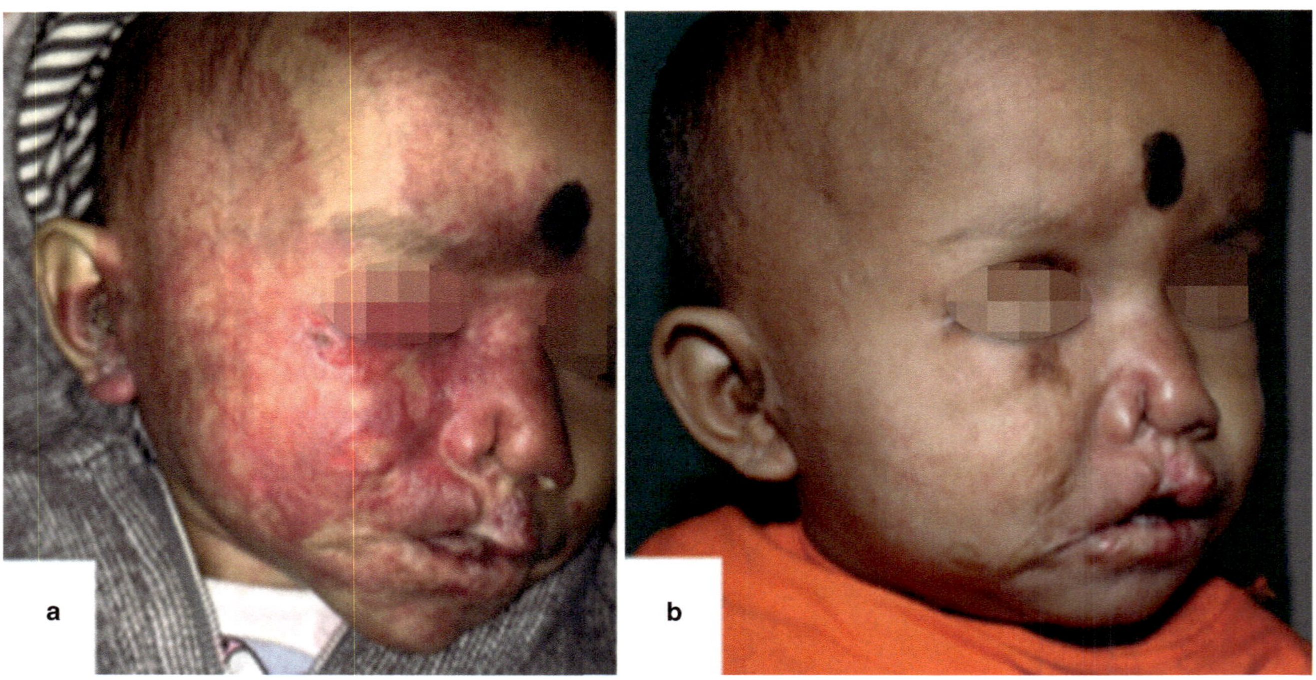




**Fig. 31.20** Rapidly involuting congenital Haemangioma (RICH) of right face treated with propanolol therapy ((**a**) pre-treatment, (**b**) post-treatment)

near vital areas like eyes and ear. In the absence of contra-indications to propranolol like sensitivity to beta-blockers, bronchospasm, hypotension or bradycardia and after having a routine haematological and biochemical assessment by the paediatrician, a dose of 1 mg/kg/day in three divided doses may be initiated and titrated up to 2 mg/kg/day. This is given for 12 months or longer according to the response. Meticulous dose adaptation is important to prevent adverse effects. These could be bradycardia, increased airway resistance, bronchial obstruction and hypotension.Long-term effects of propranolol are still not known and other drugs like timolol have been tried for superficial and peri-ocular lesions. Invasive therapies are almost never required to treat these lesions.

Although propranolol has replaced the use of *systemic steroids* as the first line therapy for haemangiomas, intra-lesional therapy for localised lesions with, Triamcinolone may be used with a dose of 2 mg/kg every 4–6 weeks depending on the response. It is known that one-third of patients do not respond to treatment with steroids. Systemic steroids are sometimes given in conjunction with propranolol after consulting with the paediatrician.

Rebound growth being a problem with systemic therapy using propranolol and/or steroids, the dose is always preferred to be tapered-off before discontinuing following resolution of the lesion.

Embolisation is considered in patients with high-output cardiac failure and large-aggressive lesions causing problems with haemostasis.

Surgery is considered between 2 and 4 years of age after having attempted medical treatment to minimise deformity involving eyes, nose and lips and other areas of face.

Pulsed dye laser was used in past for coagulating the surface of ulcerated lesions. This is now used for the treatment of surface residual telangiectasia, usually after 10 years of age (Algorithm 31.1).

**Minimally invasive percutaneous sclerotherapy** is used widely for the treatment of venous malformations. A wide range of agents are known to be used in the literature. There is no consensus on choice of sclerosant to be used. Commonly used sclerosants [25] are pingyangmycin (PYM), absolute ethanol, OK-432 (picibanil), ethanolamine oleate, bleomycin, polidocanol, doxycycline and STS (Sodium tetradecyl sulphate).

**PYM** [25], also known as Bleomycin A5, is the most commonly used single-drug therapy for the treatment of cervicofacial malformations. Transient fever and swelling are commonly seen side effects. Skin ulceration and subcutaneous tissue atrophy are scarcely seen complications.

**Absolute ethanol** [25] causes alteration in cellular proteins and hence damages the endothelium of the vascular wall leading to obliteration of its lumen. Common complications include, nerve injury, necrosis and ulceration of skin.

**OK-432** [25] is a lyophilised preparation of low-virulence bacteria, group A Streptococcus pyogenes, incubated with benzyl- penicillin. It causes, induction of various cytokines. The inflammatory response caused by this remains localised and causes endothelial damage. The complications include local swelling and transient facial nerve palsy.

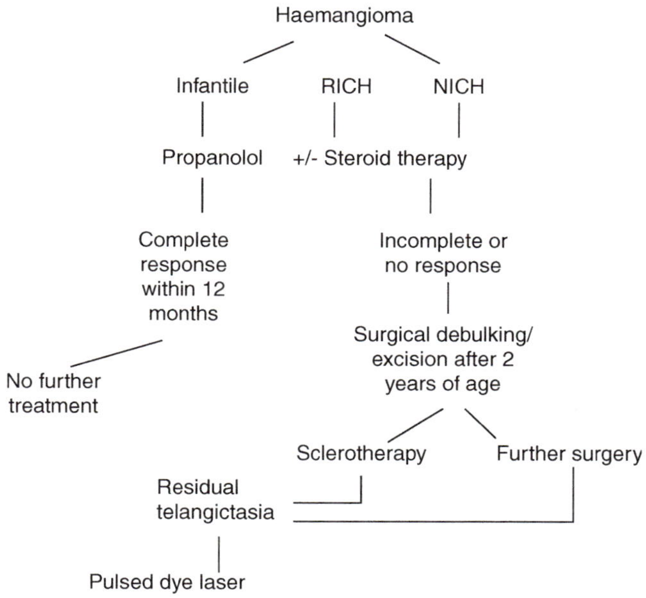


**Algorithm 31.1** Management of Haemangioma

**Ethanolamine oleate** [25] is an emulsion of fatty acids, which induces thrombosis and damages the endothelium. Complications like ulceration and necrosis of skin are known but infrequently observed.

**Bleomycin** [25] was first used in the treatment of cystic hygromas (now lymphatic malformation). It is now used widely for management of lymphatic and venous malformations. It inhibits DNA synthesis and has a non-specific inflammatory reaction on the endothelial cells. Adverse effects of bleomycin are minimal and transient, mostly being localised pain and swelling. Skin infections in the area of injection are seen less commonly. Some people report with occasionally severe nausea.

**Polidocanol** [25] is a non-ionic detergent, causes absorption at the cell membrane and leads to lysis of endothelial lining. Superficial necrosis of skin or mucosa is a known complication with Polidocanol.

**Doxycycline** [25] belongs to the tetracycline group of antibiotics. Its mode of action is not yet clear, but its effects are known to be due to inhibition of matrix metalloproteinases and cell proliferation. It also causes suppression of vascular endothelial growth factor during angiogenesis and lymphangiogenesis. This further leads to dense adhesions and fibrosis due to collagen and fibrin deposition. Macro-cystic LM's show a better response to treatment with doxycycline in comparison to micro-cystic LM's. Haemorrhage, cellulitis, pain and transient oedema are commonly seen complications. Scarring, skin excoriation and horner syndrome are seen less commonly. These adverse effects are self-limiting and likely to be related to the sclerosing effect rather than a side effect of the medication itself.

**STS** [25], also known as *sotradecol*, causes denaturation of proteins like clotting factors due to disruption of the normal architecture of the lipid bilayer in cell membranes of endothelial cells. This causes fibrosis and occlusion of vessels. It is not known to have any major complications so far.

*Lymphatic malformations* are treated depending on the type and location in head and neck. As mentioned previously, these lesions can cause pressure on the airway, aerodigestive tract and enlarge due to repeated infection or haemorrhage into the lesion. In the majority of patients with macro-cystic LMs, sclerotherapy with *Picibanil (OK-432)* has shown good results. Patients may develop inflammation at the site of injection and fever, which is managed symptomatically. Micro-cystic LMs may require systemic therapy with *Sirolimus* or surgery as they do not always respond to Picibanil. Sirolimus is a natural macrolide secluded from Streptomyces genus (Streptomyces hygroscopicus). It causes a decrease in the vascular endothelial growth factor (VEGF) and is a key regulator in lymphangiogenesis and angiogenesis.

**Bleomycin** is used widely for the treatment of VMs and microcystic LMs. The mechanism of action on micro-cystic disease is not completely understood and may involve derangement of tight junctions between endothelial cells or induction of endothelial mesenchymal transition. The overall response is favourable but complete response is seen in only about 20–57% [25]. The author follows a protocol of intralesional injection of 15 IU Bleomycin in 5 ml of fresh normal saline, administered every 15 days. Most patients show a response in 3–4 sittings (Fig. 31.21). Lymphatic malformations are known to cause sec-

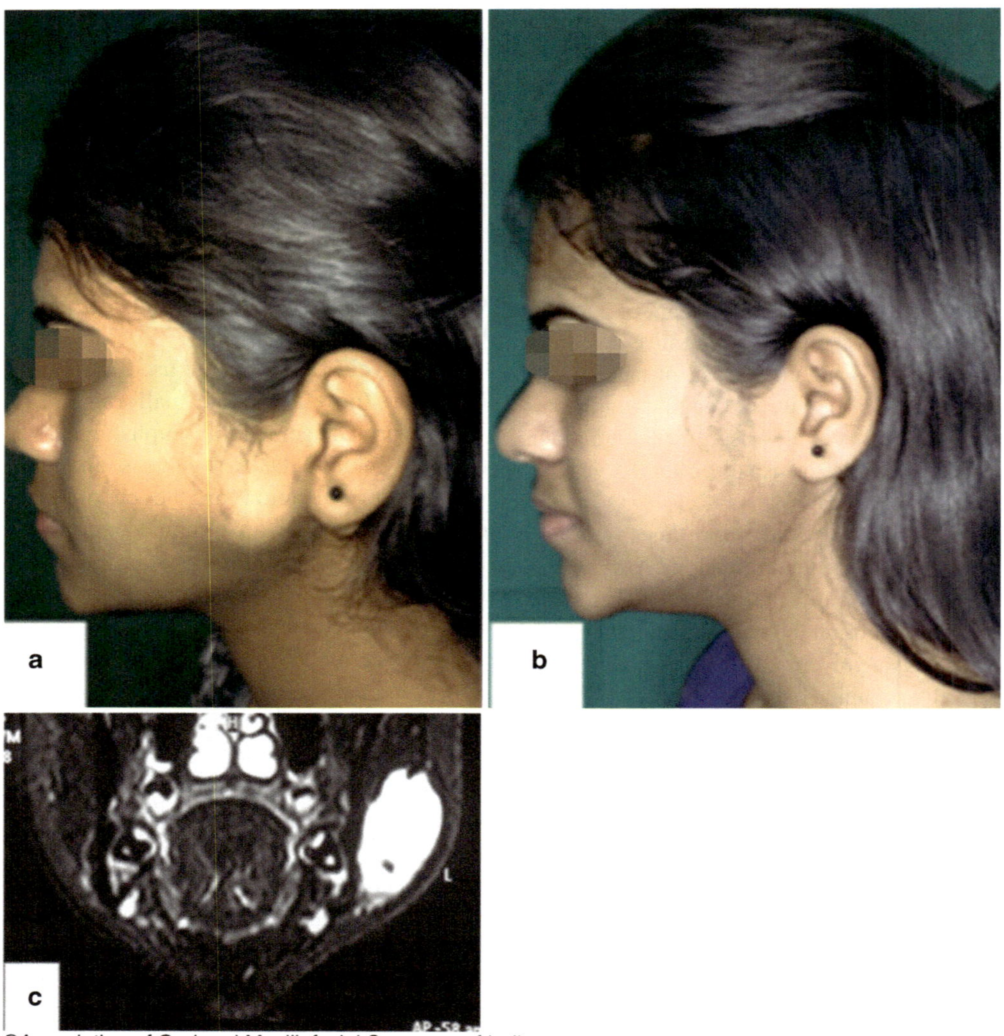




**Fig. 31.21** Venous malformation-Left cheek ((**a**) before sclerotherapy, (**b**) after sclerotherapy, (**c**) pre-treatment T2-weighted MRI image)

ondary skeletal deformities, which are addressed due to functional or cosmetic reasons as necessary.

**AVMs** are the most challenging type of vascular malformations to manage due to their aggressive nature. They tend to cause progressive facial deformity and pose a significant systemic risk. They are high-flow lesions that typically demonstrate a nidus with arterial feeders, arteriovenous connections and enlarged veins. Schobinger's class III and IV demand aggressive management with combined embolisation, surgical excision and reconstructing the residual defect. Trans-arterial and trans-venous catheter angiography are commonly used for assessment, examination of the nidus and location of arterio-venous shunting. A few lesions can be controlled with frequent embolisation. The nidus must be treated to get control over the lesion. *Catheter embolisation causes* obliteration of the nidus in order to prevent a further increase in size and haemorrhagic complications. This can be either *endovascular* (Fig. 31.22) as used for large AVM's with aberrant feeders or *percutaneous* (Fig. 31.23) used for more superficial lesions. The feeders are sequentially embolised from distant to proximal feeders. Embolisation can be used for pre-surgical occlusion of feeder vessel on the same day of planned surgery to minimise intra-operative blood loss.

Commonly used embolic agents are:

Ethanol,
Cyanoacrylate (glue),
Coils, polyvinyl particles,
Onyx—a liquid ethylene vinyl alcohol copolymer.

Kaposiform Haemangioendotheliomas (KHEs) are treated with hematological agents such as *vincristine, steroids or sirolimus*. These systemic medications help in the resolution of KHE and associated KMP (Kasabach Merritt phenomenon). Surgical management of these lesions is usually not required but small lesions can be removed in toto with early intervention.

## 31.7 Surgical Management

Unlike in the past, most low- and high-flow vascular anomalies are amenable to surgical management by either excision or debulking. Smaller-sized lesions are almost always excised completely. In contrast, larger-sized lesions are mostly debulked and need multiple procedures. External carotid artery (ECA) control is used to have reasonable control before and during procedures involving high-flow lesions. This is partly because of collateral blood supply from the opposite side.

For simplicity, the author's own anatomical classification is followed as it makes the understanding of the surgical approaches and the rationale behind them more lucid and comprehensible. Also, the concept of 'Corset suturing' will be explained, which has been proved to be an asset in management of large low-flow vascular anomalies.

### 31.7.1 Surgical Anatomy

An understanding of the different layers and planes of dissection in the head and neck is important to approach and treat these vascular anomalies. The commonest areas involved in the head and neck are cheek, lower and upper lips, eyelids, pre-auricular, mandible, submandibular, submental, upper neck, posterior and lateral oropharynx. The glottis, sub-glottis and lower neck are less commonly involved. Lymphovascular malformations are seen occupying scalp and orbit commonly.

Layers of face from superficial to deep are—skin, subcutaneous tissue, SMAS layer, parotid fascia (pre-auricular)/deep cervical fascia (sub-mandibular), salivary gland (parotid and sub-mandibular regions), muscle, periosteum and bone. The scalp has a loose areolar plane and all other tissues attached. The neck has vital structures like the carotid artery, jugular vein, spinal accessory nerve, cervical plexus and other muscles superficial and deep to them.

### 31.7.2 Case Selection

According to the author's classification, vascular malformations were categorised into five types based on their anatomy and depth of location in the head and neck. This is a good guide for selecting the type of surgical management and reconstruction.

- In type-I, superficial lesions require excision of skin or mucosa. Local or regional flaps have been used in reconstruction of the residual defect.
- Type-II, sub-mucosal lesions require complete excision after elevation of skin flaps.
- Type-III, lymphovenous malformations or venous malformations involve salivary glands and are excised along with the affected gland.
- Type-IV, intra-osseous lesions require excision with removal of involved bone and reconstruction of the residual defect as necessary.

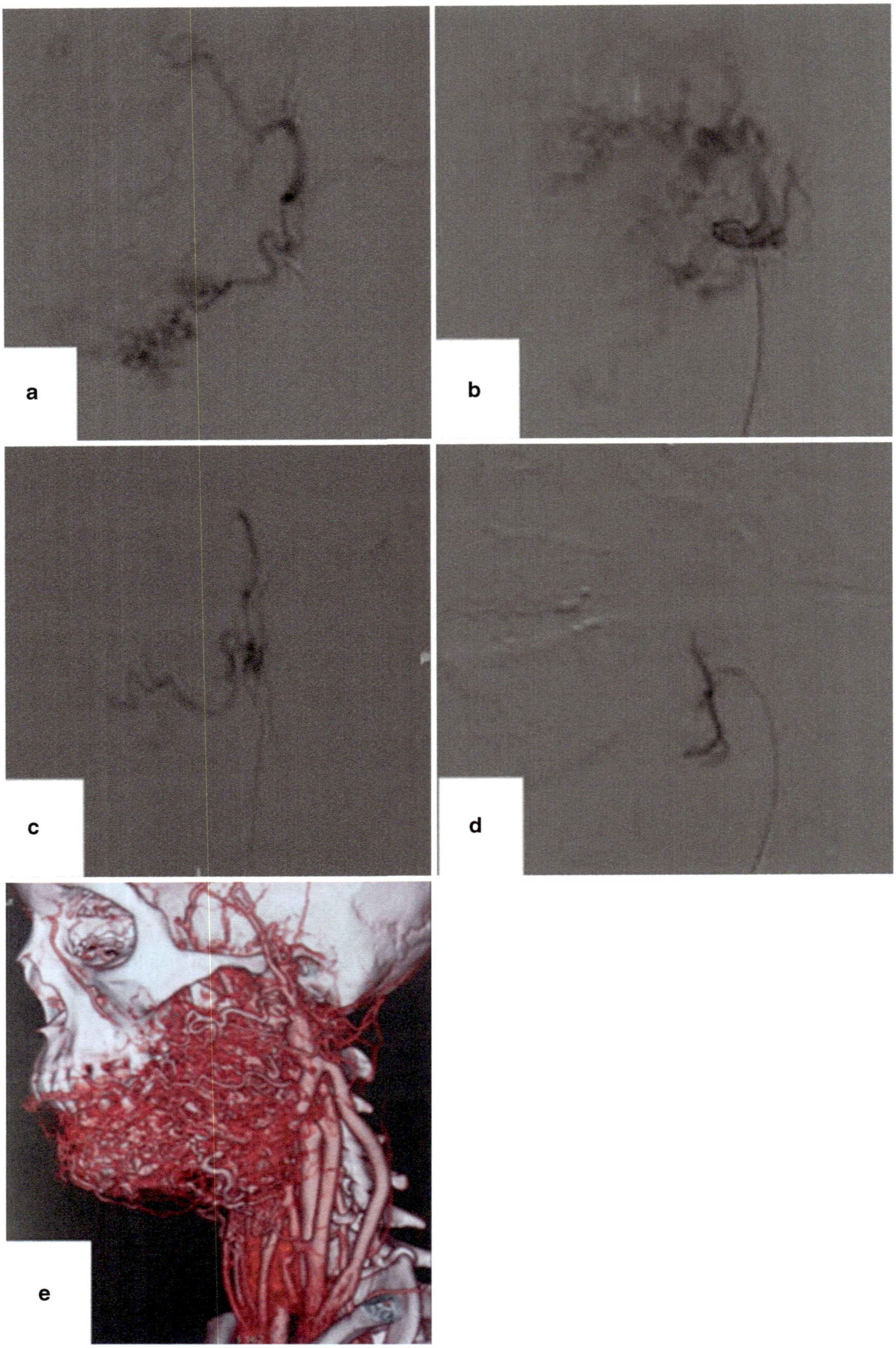




Fig. 31.22 Sequential endovascular embolisation of left cheek AVM ((**a**–**d**) progressing blockage of blood supply to AVM, (**e**) 3D reconstructed view of the vascular network)

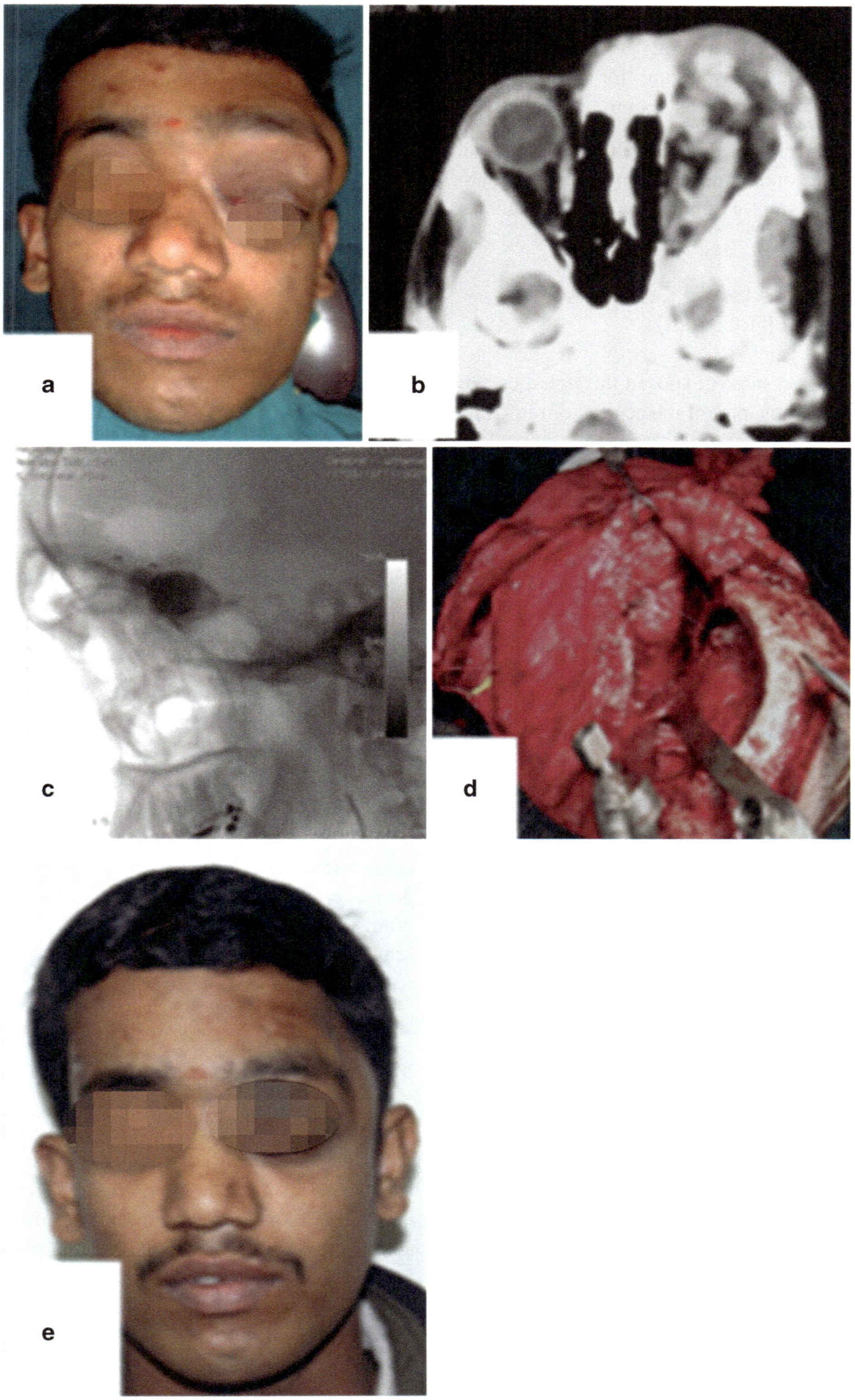




Fig. 31.23 AVM of left supra-orbit ((**a**) pre-operative, (**b**) CT with contrast, (**c**) percutaneous embolisation, (**d**) Surgical excision via haemicoronal approach, (**e**) post-operative)

- Type-V lesions involve deep visceral spaces, such as the parapharyngeal or infra-temporal fossa and usually require mandibular access osteotomy for complete exposure and complete removal of the lesion.

The above procedures can demand either endovascular embolisation, intra-lesional embolisation or ECA control prior to attempting excision or debulking of these lesions.

### 31.7.3 Technique of External Carotid Artery (ECA) Control (Fig. 31.24)

The ECA of the involved side is exposed through a cervical incision, which often forms, part of the access for removal of the malformation. The sternocleidomastoid muscle is retracted posteriorly at the level of the greater cornu of the hyoid bone, exposing the carotid sheath. The external carotid distal to the carotid bifurcation is identified. The vessel is snared with a vascular sling passed through a rubber catheter. Gentle strangulation of the vessel can be accomplished by advancing the catheter. This additional compression of the vessel serves to reduce blood flow to the lesion. In demanding situations, the ECA can be ligated. Many times due to risk of collateral blood supply to these lesions, ECA control is an adjunct to achieving haemostasis along with aggressive local control.

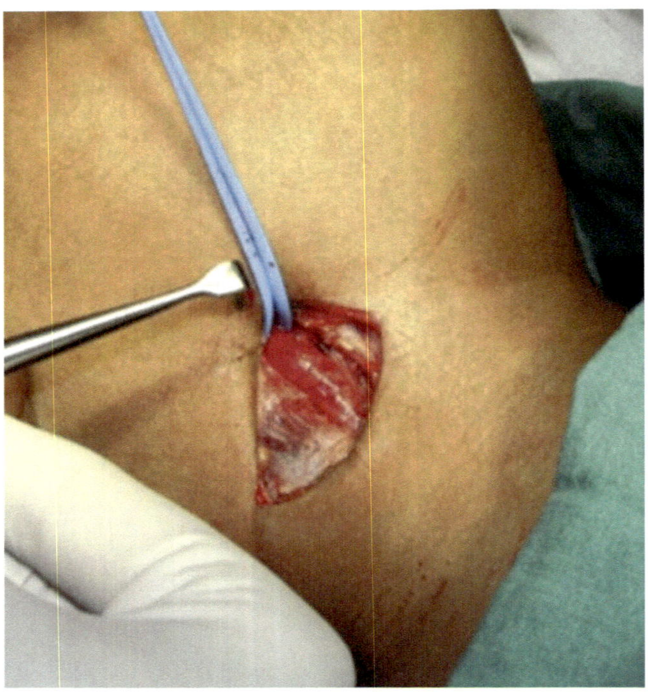



**Fig. 31.24** ECA control. Copyright: Authors own publications from IJOMS 2011

### 31.7.4 Corset-Suturing Technique (Fig. 31.25)

Corset suturing [26] is a proven technique in management of large low-flow venous malformations of head and neck, especially in lesions where complete excision is not practically possible and also those in close proximity to important structures like airway, facial nerve, spinal accessory nerve, internal jugular vein and in medically compromised individuals.

'Corset', is a garment worn to hold and train the torsoin to a desired shape for aesthetic or orthopaedic purposes. The procedure employed is raising a flap in the sub-SMAS or sub-cutaneous plane depending upon the type of lesion followed by placement of a bioresorbable suture (polydiaxanone) that runs in a continuous vertical looping fashion from sub-cutaneous to deep layer and from one end to another, incorporating the lesion within the suture. The suturing is advanced at regular and equidistant intervals to involve the bulk of lesion resulting in compression of the vascular spaces and causing obstruction of the afferent and efferent vessels. This reduces the risk of bleeding, swelling and size of lesion. The blood supply gets interrupted due to obstruction of afferent vessels. In large lesions, this suturing should be done parallel to each other covering the whole lesion from superior to inferior and medial to lateral, which would occlude the regional vascular channels, interrupting and obstructing the blood circulation in the tumour. These sutures must be tightened cautiously, slowly and progressively to achieve gradual and complete strangulation of vascular channels until complete closure of their lumen is assured. This procedure decompresses the lesion completely and reduces the risk of post-operative haemorrhage. The excess skin flap is excised, drains are secured followed by primary closure. The final scar is fairly acceptable, as all incisions are originally placed within the skin tension lines.

### 31.7.5 Approaches and Excision/Debulking

Superficial Type-I (Fig. 31.7) lesions mostly derive from the reticular dermis and is treated with direct excision and closure or local-flap reconstruction. Care is taken to place incisions along the skin tension lines of the face and neck to avoid unaesthetic results. It is challenging to select these lines in young individuals and every attempt is made to lay these incisions on prominent skin creases like nasolabial, mentolabial, pre-auricular and lower skin crease of neck.

Type-II (Fig. 31.8) lesions are approached by raising skin flaps using the following incisions, commonly—pre-auricular with either neck skin crease extension or temporal extension, neck crease incision alone, nasolabial skin crease incision, mid-face Weber-fergusson incision and coronal approach. Every attempt is made to maintain a sub-SMAS

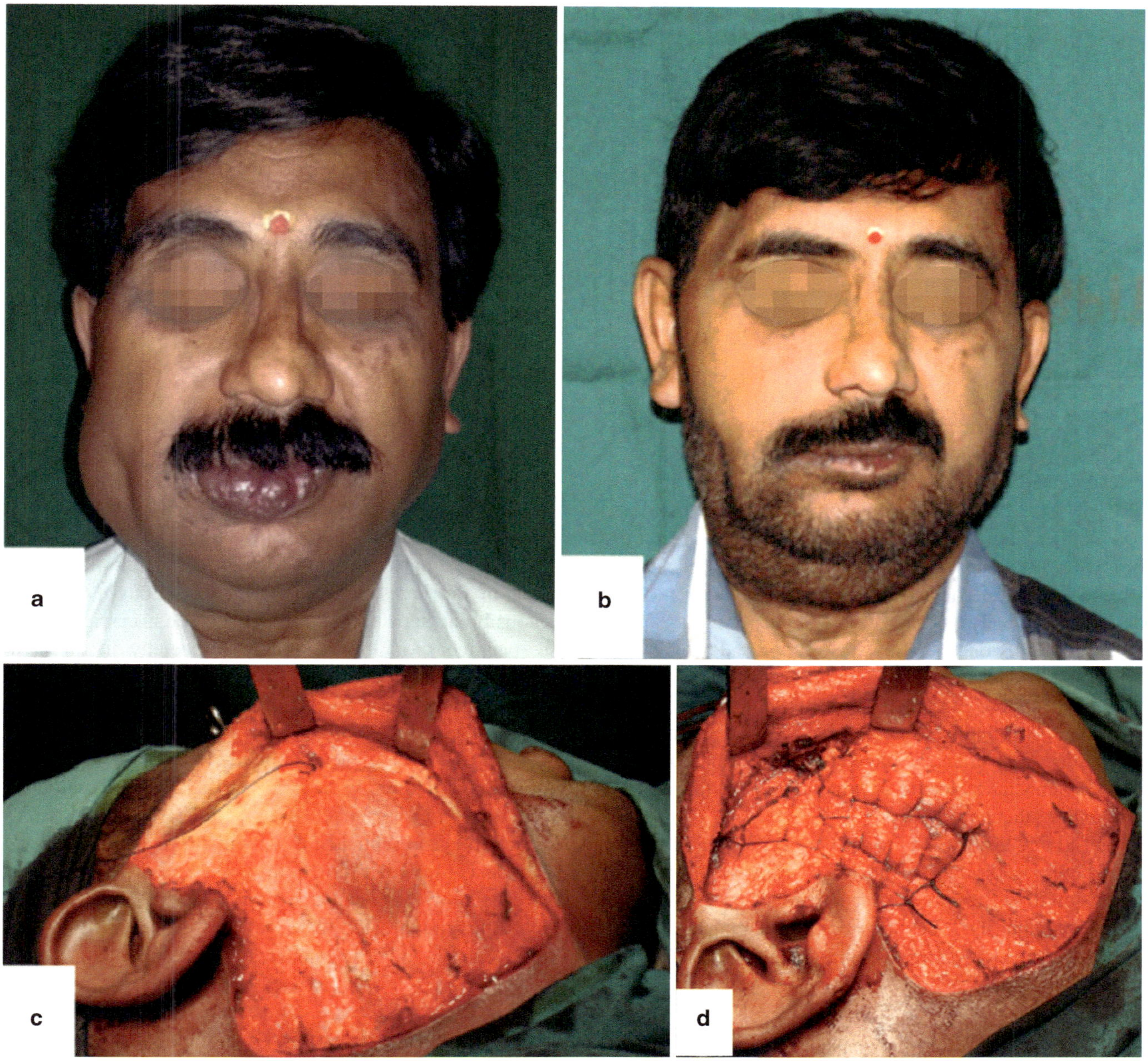




**Fig. 31.25** Venous malformation right face, lower lip ((**a**) pre-operative, (**b**) post-operative, (**c**) lesion exposure and (**d**) corset suturing of lesion). (Fig. 31.25 a,b,d - copyright authors own publication IJOMS 2018)

plane but vascular anomalies being composite in nature can demand modifications. There is always a risk of thinning the skin flap excessively and care should be taken to avoid button-holing and avoiding avascular necrosis. The lesion is excised completely or debulked depending on the size. Corseting is used for large low-flow malformations as described above.

Tongue lesions are mostly excised in toto or debulked in a V shaped fashion to achieve primary closure.

Type-III (Fig. 31.9) lesions are approached the same way as Type-II. Being deeper in nature, the gland is sacrificed with some risk of permanent facial nerve damage. Use of 'corseting' in these cases has shown good results with complete recovery of facial nerve weakness over a period of 1 year.

Type-IV (Fig. 31.10) lesions like other types are rarely seen on their own and are usually in combination with Type I, II or V. These lesions are treated with curettage or segmen-

**Algorithm 31.2**
Management of Vascular malformations

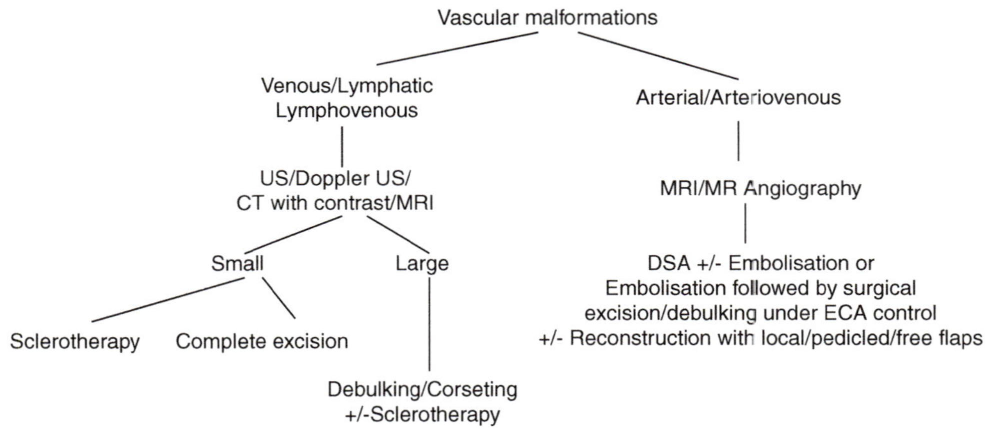


tal resection of bone followed by reconstruction (Fig. 31.13). There are reports of extra-corporeal curettage of segmentally resected lesions and re-fixation to maintain bone continuity.

Type-V (Fig. 31.11) lesions commonly require access to osteotomies like mandibulotomy, segmental or complete Lefort-I, rhinotomy or zygomatic swing osteotomies to gain adequate access. The lesions are uncapsulated and rarely excised completely but improve the quality of life and reduce risk of mortality due to airway obstruction and haemorrhage. In the authors' experience, use of corseting has proven to be beneficial in these cases.

Excess skin flap is always excised to give a near normal appearance. Use of an adequate number of drains and meticulous haemostatic closure is imperative to achieve acceptable and aesthetic results.

Most large lesions require further excision and debulking procedures as the age advances until growth is achieved. Large low-flow lesions have potential to be excised completely secondarily, following prior corset suturing.

Algorithm 31.2 summarises the management of vascular malformations.

## 31.8 Complications

Vascular lesions can have complications ranging from none (like in haemangiomas) to bleeding, ulcerations and infection. Superficial lesions and ulcerations benefit with the use of pulsed-dye laser. Bleeding can usually be managed with compression dressings.

Large venous and lymphatic malformations can cause local swelling, pressure effects on trachea and oesophagus, pain and infection, demanding immediate treatment like embolisation or surgical debulking along with control of airway and infection.

The two common complications of LMs are bleeding within the lesion and infection. Bleeding can be seen spontaneously or as a result of trauma. This further causes immediate and painful enlargement of the lesion with associated ecchymosis. Analgesia and observation usually suffice for symptomatic management. Prophylactic antibiotics can be given in the case of profuse bleeding. Long-term intravenous broad spectrum antibiotics may be necessary covering pathogens of head and neck, especially in high-risk patients. Haemorrhage and infection can sometimes transform a macro-cystic lesion into a micro-cystic type with associated scarring. LMs are known to increase in size in the presence of a viral or bacterial infection. This is usually self-limiting and thought to be due to changes in the lymphatic flow. Bacterial superinfections can be fatal causing ascending cellulitis and septicaemia. Any infection in cervicofacial LMs can cause obstruction of the upper airway and oesophagus causing dyspnea and dysphagia.

Incompletely treated AVMs tend to recur and continue to grow. They should not be underestimated.

## 31.9 Recent Advances

Micro-cystic lymphatic malformations have always been challenging cases to be treat, especially involving extra- and intracranial areas of head and neck. Currently available treatments have limited effectiveness and high risk of complications. Techniques using lymphography and idiocyanine green have been used to locate the exact location of afferent and efferent lymphatic flow and performing a lymphatic-venous anastomosis has been described in treating these lesions [27].

Vascular-disrupting agents (VDA's) [28] are a group of 'vascular targeting' agents that show selective activity against tumour vascular networks, causing severe obstruction in their blood flow and subsequent necrosis. These have been investigated for a long time but haven't yet actively been used in the treatment of vascular lesions of the head and neck. Micro-tubule-depolymerising agents are the largest group of small molecular weight VDAs, which include lead compound disodium combretastatin A-4 3-O-phosphate (CA-4-P) [28], and are under clinical development for cancer. VDAs can also interfere with angiogenesis and can be potentially used as novel drugs for the treatment of conditions with excessive angiogenesis, in addition to cancer.

3D remodelling and bioprinting of areas affected by vascular anomalies with their feeder vessels are under study, for training and familiarising one with possible complications during procedures like embolisation and surgery.

## 31.10 Conclusion

Vascular anomalies are a diverse group of lesions requiring knowledge and skill to identify, accurately diagnose and treat adequately. Most of these lesions present as a complex problem with a combination of different types and other systemic complicating features. This demands a multi-disciplinary team comprising maxillofacial surgeon, vascular surgeon, pediatrician, reconstructive surgeon, anaesthetist and speech and language therapist with extensive training, understanding and experience to tailor an appropriate treatment plan. Selection of sclerosants should be with caution to minimise their side effects. Surgery has an important role in achieving quicker and long-term stable results in most cases.

## References


1. Nair SC, Spencer NJ, Nayak KP, Balasubramaniam K. Surgical management of vascular lesions of the head and neck: a review of 115 cases. Int J Oral Maxillofac Surg. 2011;40:577–83.
2. Mulliken JB, Young AE. Vascular birthmarks. Hemangiomas and malformations. Philadelphia: Saunders; 1988.
3. Brouillard P, Vikkula M. Vascular malformations: localized defects in vascular morphogenesis. Clin Genet. 2003;63:340.
4. Lohela M, Bry M, Tammela T, et al. VEGFs and receptors involved in angiogenesis versus lymphangiogenesis. Curr Opin Cell Biol. 2009;21 154.
5. Boon LM, Ballieux F, Vikkula M. Pathogenesis of vascular anomalies. Clin Plast Surg. 2011;38:7–19.
6. Richter GT, Friedman AB. Hemangiomas and vascular malformations: current theory and management. Int J Pediatr. 2012;2012:645678.
7. Marler JJ, John B. Mulliken current management of hemangiomas and vascular malformations. Clinic Plast Surg. 2005;32:99–116.
8. Takahashi K, Mulliken JB, Kozakewich HP, Rogers RA, Folkman J, Ezekowitz RA. Cellular markers that distinguish the phases of hemangioma during infancy and childhood. J Clin Invest. 1994;93:2357–64.
9. Eerola LMB, Watanabe S, Grynberg H, Mulliken JB, Vikkula M. Locus for susceptibility for familial capillary malformation ("port-wine stain") maps to 5q. Eur J Hum Genet. 2002;10(6):375–80.
10. Pavlov KA, Dubova EA, Shchyogolev AI, Mishnyov OD. Expression of growth factors in endotheliocytes in vascular malformations. Bull Exp Biol Med. 2009;147(3):366–70.
11. Corti P, Young S, Chen CY, et al. Interaction between alk1 and blood flow in the development of arteriovenous malfor- mations. Development. 2011;138(8):1573–82.
12. Kim H, Su H, Weinsheimer S, Pawlikowska L, Young WL. Brain arteriovenous malformation pathogenesis: a response-to-injury paradigm. Acta Neurochir Suppl. 2011;111:83–92.
13. Mulliken J, Glowacki J. Hemangiomas and vascular malformations in infants and children: a classification based on endothelial charecteristics. Plast Reconstr Surg. 1982;69(3):412–20.
14. Ethunandan M, Mellor TK. Hemangiomas and vascular malformations of the maxillofacial region—review. Br J Oral Maxillofac Surg. 2006;44:263–72.
15. ISSVA Classification of Vascular Anomalies ©2018 International Society for the Study of Vascular Anomalies Available at "issva.org/classification".
16. Johnson AB, Richter GT. Vascular anomalies. Clin Perinatol. 2018;45(4):737–49.
17. Kilcline C, Frieden IJ. Infantile hemangiomas: how common are they? A systematic review of the medical literature. Pediatr Dermatol. 2008;25(2):168–73.
18. Mohan RPS, Dhillon M, Gill N. Intraoral venous malformation with phleboliths. Saudi Dent J. 2011;23:161–163).
19. de Serres LM, Sie KC, Richardson MA. Lymphatic malformations of the head and neck. A proposal for staging. Arch Otolaryngol Head Neck Surg. 1995;121(5):577–82.
20. Kohout MP, Hansen M, Pribaz JJ, Mulliken JB. Arteriovenous malformations of the head and neck: natural history and management. Plast Reconstr Surg. 1998;102(3):643–54.
21. Croteau SE, Liang MG, Kozakewich HP, et al. Kaposiform hemangioendothelioma: atypical features and risks of Kasabach-Merritt phenomenon in 107 referrals. J Pediatr. 2013;162(1):142–7.
22. Steinklein JM, Shatzkes DR. Imaging of vascular lesions of head and neck. Otolaryngol Clin N Am. 2018;51:55–76.
23. Baek HJ, Hong JP, Choi JW, Suh DC. Direct percutaneous alcohol sclerotherapy for venous malformations of head and neck region without fluoroscopic guidance: technical consideration and outcome. Neurointervention. 2011;6:84–8.
24. Hoff SR, Rastatter JC, Richter GT. Head and neck vascular lesions. Otolaryngol Clin N Am. 2015;48:29–45.
25. Horbach SER, Lokhorst MM, Saeed P, de Goüyon Matignon de Pontouraude CMF, Rothová A, van der Horst CMAM. Sclerotherapy for low-flow vascular malformations of the head and neck: A systematic review of sclerosing agents. J Plast Reconstr Aesthet Surg. 2016;69:295–304.
26. Nair SC, Chawla JP, Shroff SS, Kumar B, Shah A. Corseting: a new technique for the management of diffuse venous malforma-

tions in the head and neck region. Int J Oral Maxillofac Surg. 2018;47(12):1534–40.
27. Kato M, Watanabe S, Iida T, Watanabe A, Megumi F. Peri-orbital lymphangioma treated by lymphatic-venous anastomosis with indocyanine green lymphography analysis. J Pediatr Surg Case Rep. 2017;23:9e14.
28. Kanthou C, Tozer GM. Microtubule depolymerizing vascular disrupting agents: novel therapeutic agents for oncology and other pathologies. Int J Exp Pathol. 2009;90:284–94.

# Part XII

# Aesthetic Procedures in Oral and Maxillofacial Region

# Non-surgical Modalities of Facial Rejuvenation and Aesthetics

32

Arun Kumar Panda and Aarti Chowdhary

## 32.1 Introduction to Ageing Face

### 32.1.1 Facial Changes Due to Ageing

The Face is a mirror of what we are from inside. It is like an opera that reveals a person's inner self, nature, personality and health. The signs and symptoms of age, illness, deficiencies and personality traits show on our faces. A lot can be postulated by just observing the different facial expressions of a person. A minuscule defect on the face engraves an exaggerated long-lasting impression on a person's mind and soul.

Ageing is a process which cannot be defied. With the passage of time, every individual goes through a phenomenon of complex transformations which takes away the youthfulness. The various signs of ageing seen on the face include recession of hairline, wrinkles on the forehead, drooping of the upper eyelid, hollowness in the under-eye area, deepening of nasolabial fold, folds on the face, sagginess of skin at the border of mandible, etc. (Fig. 32.1). Today, with the changing cultures and requirements in the profession, every individual wants to look better than what he or she is.

As the saying goes "Beauty has no age", more and more elderly people also want to have their face rejuvenated. So, today we have a range of patients of vast age variations who want to have a more rejuvenated look. The various modalities for rejuvenating the ageing face require fine skill and artwork combined with scientific knowledge and understanding of the whole face including scalp, forehead, periorbital area, perioral area, neck, etc., so as to achieve a more youthful appearance.

Time and technology has evolved. For many years the standard had been chemical peels as the non-invasive procedure to facelift as the invasive modality for face rejuvenation. Today, we have a vast range of procedures and technologies to counter ageing phenomenon and provide a rejuvenated appearance. We shall discuss the various non-surgical modalities in this section which physicians are adopting to treat patients with a wide range of Facial Aesthetic concerns.

The ageing of human face is a highly complex, irreversible and progressive biologic phenomenon that occurs with the ticking of time. The main factors leading to facial ageing include gravity, bone remodelling, subcutaneous fat redistribution and loss, hormonal imbalance, chronic sunlight, pollution and smoking. Other environmental factors that allegedly affect facial appearance include mental stress, nutritional deficiencies, work habits, drug abuse and disease. This dynamic process is a synergistic effect of various factors and actually takes place at 4 distinct levels (the 4 S levels): Skin, Subcutaneous tissue, SMAS and facial Skeleton.

### 32.1.2 Ageing of Skin

The epidermis contains keratinocytes and dead corneocytes. The basal cells at the stratum basal divide to form keratinocytes, produce keratins and drift upwards as they mature. By the time keratinocytes reach the most superficial layer, they lose their nucleus and cytoplasmic organelles and are known as corneocytes. In a total period of 40–50 days, the keratinocytes come to the surface and corneocytes exfoliate. This time taken for the process of keratinisation, that is maturation of keratinocytes along with shedding of corneocytes, is known as the turnover time.

The natural process of desquamation sheds off the dry, old, hardened skin cells and gives way to the new cells to

**Electronic Supplementary Material** The online version of this chapter (https://doi.org/10.1007/978-981-15-1346-6_32) contains supplementary material, which is available to authorized users.

A. K. Panda (✉)
Department of Oral & Maxillofacial Surgery,
SD Dental College and Hospital, Parbhani, Maharashtra, India

A. Chowdhary
Department of Periodontology, SD Dental College and Hospital,
Parbhani, Maharashtra, India



K. Bonanthaya et al. (eds.), *Oral and Maxillofacial Surgery for the Clinician*, https://doi.org/10.1007/978-981-15-1346-6_32

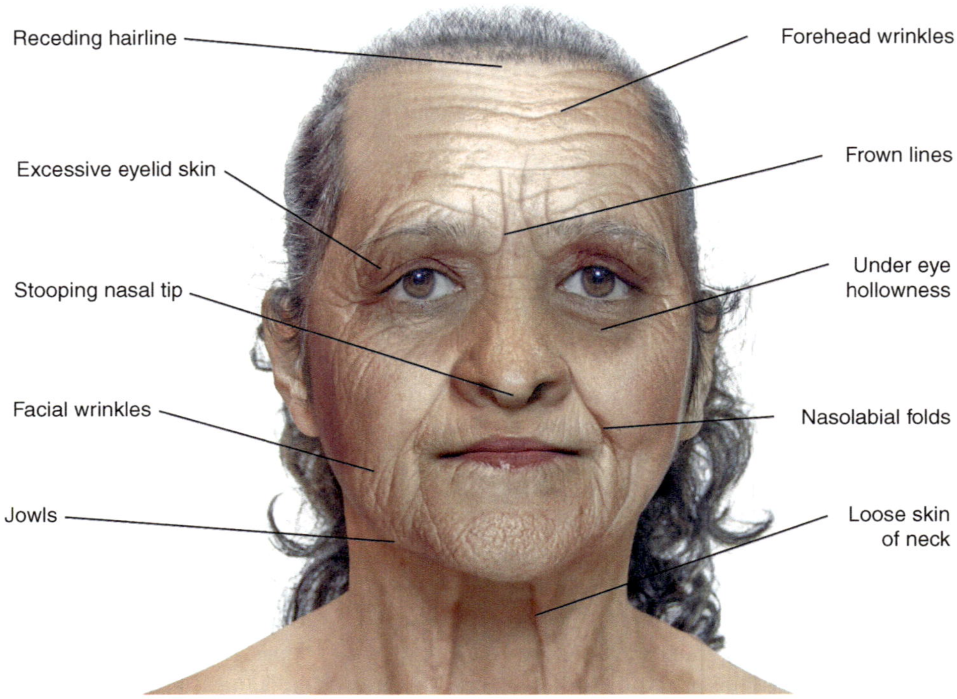


©Association of Oral and Maxillofacial Surgeons of India

**Fig. 32.1** Various signs of an ageing face include but not limited to forehead wrinkles, droopy eyelids, under-eye hollowness, deep nasolabial folds, jowl formation, loose neck skin and thin lips

come to the surface. This process also eliminates damaged and contaminated cells that carry pollutants and microorganisms from the environment.

The specialised fibroblasts in the dermal layer produce two key proteins-collagen and elastin. Collagen constitutes 80% of the dermis and provides strength and firmness to the skin. While elastin, as the name implies, provides elasticity to the skin and enables the skin to bounce back to its original shape after it is stretched, thus preventing wrinkles.

Skin ageing is a dynamic mechanism that transpires due to two basic factors:

- Intrinsic or Innate factors are insidious deteriorating elements that are influenced by internal metabolic processes, genetic programming, cellular metabolism and hormones;
- Extrinsic or Exogenous factors include Ultraviolet rays in the sunlight, cigarette smoking, environmental pollution, etc.

Intrinsic ageing is an inevitable natural ageing process which commences as early as mid-20s. It consists of internal physiological factors that cause inherent degenerative process in the body. Dead corneocytes do not desquamate as swiftly as expected and the turnover of new epidermal cells decreases somewhat. In the dermis, the production of collagen and elastin slows down. The cumulative effect which is seen in case of the inherent ageing includes fine wrinkling, parched, thin and transparent skin and depleted elastic nature of the skin.

Extrinsic ageing is because of the aggregated damage caused by environmental factors such as sun's UV radiation, gravity, sleeping posture, pollution, smoking, exposure to chemicals, etc. These exogenous factors along with the innate factors cause premature ageing of our facial skin. The face, which is most commonly exposed part of the human body to the UV radiations of the sun, undergoes ageing prematurely than any other part. Photoageing with recurrent sun exposure causes the skin to lose its capability to renovate and thereby accumulating damage. Recurrent and continual UV exposure disintegrates collagen and impedes the synthesis of new collagen. Alongside, there is a breakdown of elastin. This causes the facial skin to become slack, wrinkled and leathery much earlier than a sun-protected skin.

Gravity constantly works on different parts of our facial skin. As the skin elasticity reduces with age, the effects become evident. It precipitates jowls, nasolabial fold, drooping of eyelids, elongation of ears, etc. (Fig. 32.2).

Sleep lines are wrinkles that are etched on the facial skin of the people who sleep with the face pressed on the cushion or sleep on the sides.

Cigarette smoking over a period of time causes many biochemical alterations in our body. It has deleterious effects on skin and expedites the ageing process. The nicotine causes vasoconstriction thereby impairing the supply of oxygen and

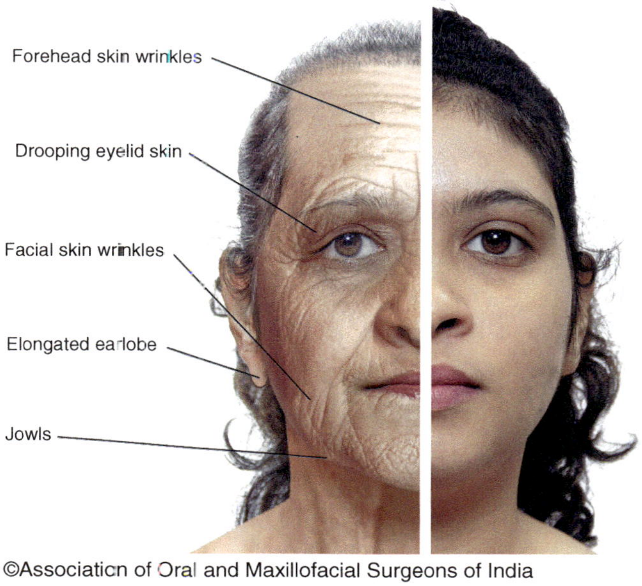


Fig. 32.2 Influence of ageing on skin. Facial wrinkling, jowls and droopy eyelids clearly demonstrate the ageing process

important nutrients, such as vitamin A to the skin. Many of the over 7000 chemicals released from the burning cigarettes cause increased production of matrix metalloproteinases (MMP) that causes degradation of collagen and causes abnormal creation of elastosis materials. These cause premature facial skin wrinkling.

### 32.1.3 Ageing of Subcutaneous Tissue

The subcutaneous fat gives the volume and shape to the face. As explained by Rohrich and Pessa [1], the subcutaneous fat is distributed throughout the face in a multidimensional fashion and is highly compartmentalised. A youthful face is characterised by a smooth transition between these subcutaneous compartments. The superficial musculoaponeurotic system (SMAS) divides this fat into superficial and deep layers. As explained anatomically by Rohrich and Pessa [1], the external recess is in between the skin and SMAS while the internal recess lies under the SMAS and is adherent to the periosteum. The superficial and deep fat recesses are as explained in Fig. 32.3.

Furnas in 1989 first described the osteocutaneous ligaments within the cheek that anchor the dermis to the underlying fibro-osseous structures [2]. He outlined the zygomatic ligaments (McGregor's patch), the mandibular ligament, the platysma auricular ligament and the anterior platysma-cutaneous ligament that anchor the dermis and also support the midface soft tissue. Two theories explain the characteristic soft tissue changes that are distinguished during the mid-face ageing. The gravitational theory advocates that with the attenuation of the osteocutaneous ligaments, there is vertical descent of facial soft tissue which contributes to the deep creases of the ageing face [3]. The diminished strength of the ligaments is because the age-related elastosis and also because of the repeated animation of the muscles of facial expression.

Donofrio explained the volumetric theory in 2000. He suggested that it's the corresponding volume loss or gain in the adjoining areas of the face is what creates the deep creases of age [4]. This theory was later in 2007 reinforced by Lambros who stated that the ageing process was due to the relative deflation of certain fat pads, especially the deep fat pads [5].

### 32.1.4 Ageing of SMAS

The superficial musculoaponeurotic system is a multidimensional scaffold of organised fibrous tissue that connects the facial muscles with the dermis [6]. This fibromuscular layer also segregates the superficial and deep facial fat pads. Anatomically, the SMAS lies in the midface, inferior to the zygomatic arch and superior to the muscular belly of the platysma. It blends with the superficial temporal fascia and frontalis muscle superiorly, and with the platysma muscle inferiorly. Since it connects the facial muscles to the dermis, its purpose is to transmit, distribute and amplify the activity of all facial muscles [7].

As we age, and with the continuous use of the muscles of facial expression, the SMAS weakens and the strength diminishes. So, the ability to hold up the muscles, fat and the skin gets impaired. Combined with the effect of gravitational forces, the weakening causes the structures of the face to slump. The youthful appearance of the face changes as jowls are formed, the nasolabial fold deepens and the mandibular line angle becomes ill defined.

### 32.1.5 Ageing of Facial Skeleton

The bony skeleton serves as a framework for the soft tissues of the face including the skin, muscles and subcutaneous fat. The facial skeleton keeps changing anatomically throughout life with only degenerative and catabolic changes occurring after adolescence.

With ageing, the facial skeleton keeps resorbing in a very predictable manner and that contributes to the appearance of an aged face. Areas with strong tendency to resorb include the periorbital area, the midface, the perinasal area and the mandible (Fig. 32.4).

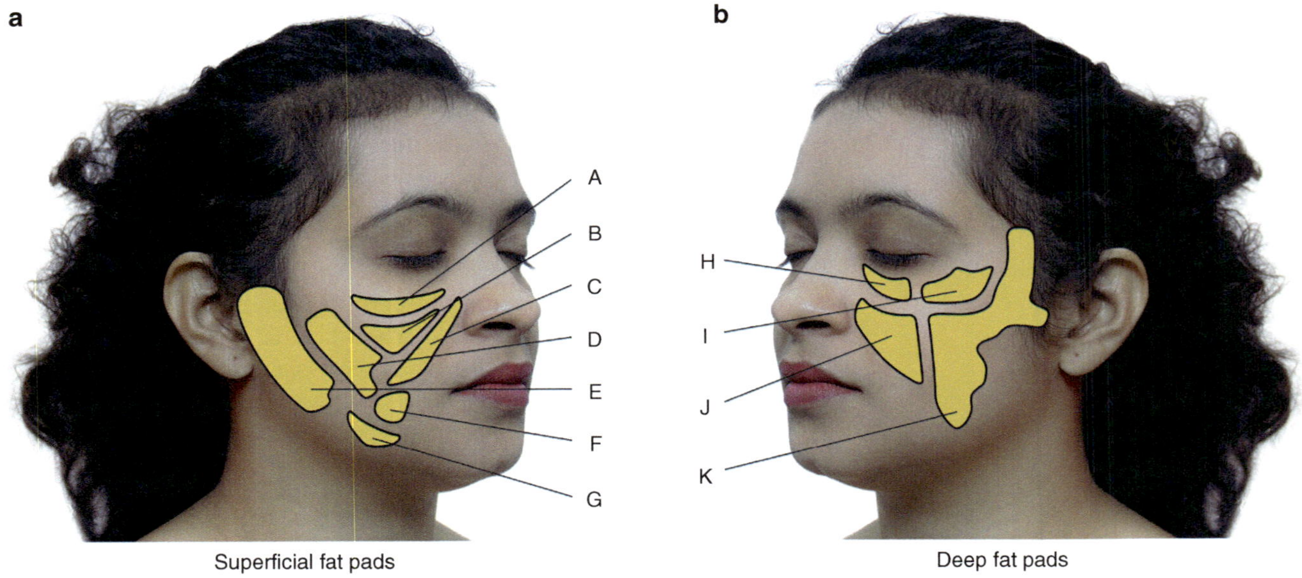




**Fig. 32.3** (a, b) (**A**) Infraorbital fat, (**B**) Medial cheek fat, (**C**) Nasolabial fat, (**D**) Medial cheek fat, (**E**) Lateral cheek fat, (**F**) Superior jowl fat, (**G**) Inferior jowl fat, (**H**) Medial sub-orbicularis fat, (**I**) Lateral sub-orbicularis fat, (**J**) Deep medial cheek fat, (**K**) Buccal fat

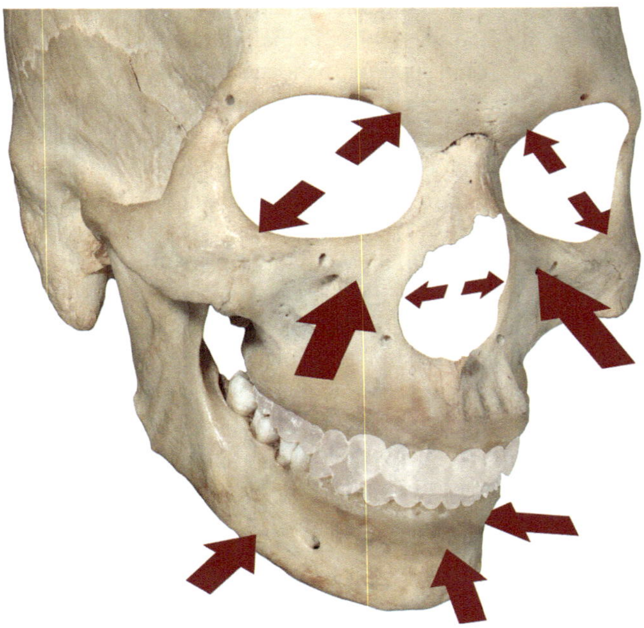



**Fig. 32.4** Various areas of facial skeleton as marked are predominantly destined to resorb contributing to the appearance of aged face

The orbital aperture enlarges with age in all dimensions. The superomedial and inferolateral aspects tend to recede more which imparts the stigmata of periorbital ageing such as increased prominence of the medial fat pad, elevation of the medial brow and lengthening of the lid cheek junction [8].

The midface skeleton is formed by the maxilla medially and the zygoma laterally. With age, the maxilla recedes and the maxillary angle decreases by about 10° between the age of 30 and 60 years [9]. The piriform aperture enlarges with age, as the edges of the nasal bones recede [10]. The anterior nasal spine also retreats which reduces the skeletal support and thereby contributing to retraction of the columella, with a downward rotation of nasal tip and apparent lengthening of the nose [11]. In regards to the mandible, it is well established that the mandibular angle increases, the ramus height and mandibular body height and length decreases with age [12]. The above-mentioned skeletal resorption patterns contribute significantly to the appearance of an ageing face.

In the recent years, the demand for facial rejuvenation has increased exponentially. Individuals from every socioeconomic strata and from all age groups today desire a younger and rejuvenated look. Evolution of numerous surgical and non-surgical procedures has led to an increase in patient demands and expectations. Every aesthetic physician should understand the facial anatomy and the facial ageing process well so as to perform the procedures that would best suit the requirement of the individual to deliver the best of the results. The various non-surgical modalities of facial rejuvenation include the use of Botulinum toxin, dermal fillers, thread lifts, platelet concentrates and radiofrequency waves. Botulinum toxin and fillers are elaborated in the subsequent chapter. The following is a detailed description of the role of thread lifts, platelet concentrates and radiofrequency waves in achieving facial rejuvenation.

## 32.2 Non-surgical Facelift with Threads

Age-related changes on the face include remodelling in the facial skeleton and reorganisation of musculature, connective tissues, fat and skin. The dynamic process of ageing is unstoppable and it induces an ever-progressing slackness in the soft tissues that leads to a ptotic brow, jowl formation, ill-defined mandibular margin and deep nasolabial folds.

Gravity is an important factor that causes drooping of the upper, mid- and lower-facial soft tissue, which adds to the effect of an aged appearance. The hollowness of the midfacial and infra-orbital area is because of the downward shift of the malar fat pad. To manage this ptotic situation, surgical facelift procedures have been the most effective treatment as they not only excise the redundant tissues but also haul the soft tissue in the opposite vector of ageing process. The other non-invasive procedures cannot be as effective as the facelift procedure. But because of the significant downtime, cost and risks involved, facelift is not accepted by patients very readily. To have a way in between the surgical and non-invasive modalities, thread lift has become a popular procedure to manage drooping tissue of the face because of ageing.

### 32.2.1 Introduction to Thread Lift

Thread lifting modality is a minimally invasive cosmetic procedure that utilises a biocompatible implant placed into the deeper layers of face to predictably shift and realign tissues in a predetermined direction or vector. When compared to a surgical facelift procedure, this elevates the drooping tissues with least amount of risks and complications, immediate results and rapid recovery.

Historically, Ruff in Durham, North Carolina, in 1992 and Sulamanidze et al. in Moscow, Russia, in 1996 independently developed barbed sutures for correcting facial ptosis. FDA in 2004 approved Ruff's clear, barbed, unidirectional, polypropylene sutures for treating ptotic skin of face and neck [13].

### 32.2.2 Classification

(A) Depending on the modality of their action (Fig. 32.5):
- Redefinition of the facial contours—Barbed threads
- Induction of collagen production—Mono PDO threads

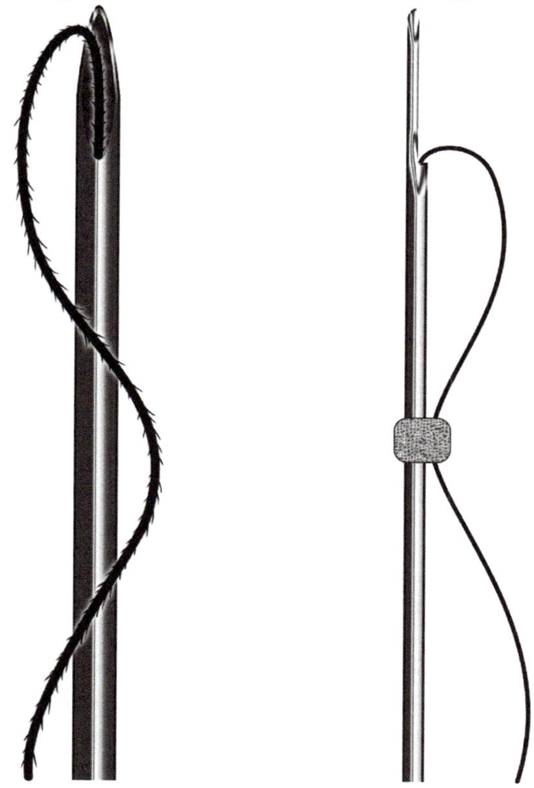


©Association of Oral and Maxillofacial Surgeons of India

**Fig. 32.5** Various types of polydioxanone threads are mono threads for facial rejuvenation and cogs threads for redefining facial contours

(B) Depending on pattern of resorption of implant material:
- Permanent/Non-resorbable threads—Polypropylene threads like Aptos threads, Silhouette lift threads, etc.
- Resorbable threads—Polydioxanone threads like Alfa aqualift, and Poly-L Lactic acid threads like silhouette soft threads, etc.

(C) Depending on mode of Fixation:
- Anchored: Wherein the thread is anchored to a proximal fixed place like the deep temporal facia or mastoid facia.
- Free floating: They are not fixed and cause the pull because of the thread design.

(D) Depending on the surface texture of the thread:
- Barbed
- Non-barbed

The Barbed threads are of 3 types:

- Unidirectional barbed threads—these are anchored on to a fixed point like the deep temporal facia, e.g. Contour thread
- Bidirectional barbed threads—these are placed in the treatment area by a canula and stretch the skin because of the design, e.g. Aptos threads.
- Cogged threads—these can be unidirectional, bidirectional or multidirectional and they lift the skin towards the point of entry once tissues get entangled with the cogs.

The Non-barbed threads can be:

- Plain
- Spiral or spring

### 32.2.3 Mechanism of Action

From a clinical point of view, the barbed sutures simply work by grasping and mechanically pulling the ptotic skin. These barbs get entangled in the subcutaneous tissues and as the thread is pulled backwards, the tissues get squeezed along the barbs and stay there as the thread outside is cut off.

From a histologic aspect, a basic mechanism of mechanical transduction happens when the polydioxanone threads are placed in the tissues. A torrent of intracellular signals in the surrounding cells through which the polydioxanone threads pass is triggered by the mechanical stresses instigated by the threads thus influencing the metabolic responses and encouraging cellular growth and survival and modulating tissue morphology and architecture [14].

There are 2 major types of collagen proteins that are found in our skin. The type 1 collagen or the fibrous collagen makes up about 70% of the total collagen while the type 2 collagen or the reticular collagen makes up to about 5–20%. Both of them provide structural support to the skin. Today, most of the aesthetic procedures are aimed at a phenomenon of biostimulation. The main intention is to improve on the plasticity, resilience, flexibility, firmness and turgor of the skin tissues that are normally lost with ageing due to the loss of proteins like collagen and elastin. This is achieved by penetrating the dermis with substances that would encourage the production of these proteins [15]. The biostimulation caused with PDO threads is due to neocollagenesis, i.e. the production of type 1 collagen which is essentially fibrotic in nature. The PDOs resorb in 6 months and till that time it keeps inducing collagen. The fibrotic collagen exhibits a retracted effect improving the skin appearance. Concurrently, the compaction and stiffening of the collagen fibres also determine the functional damage [16].

### 32.2.4 Indications

There are 2 major indications for the threads treatment:

- Skin rejuvenation
- Elevating the sagging skin

Skin rejuvenation can be done with the use of plain polydioxanone threads. It also increases the volume in certain areas where there is minimal volume loss.

The barbed threads are indicated in areas where there is ptosis of the tissues. The barbs work as cogs and by engaging the tissues along its path, it mechanically pulls the tissues upwards thereby reducing the ptosis.

The plain polydioxanone threads can be used for facial rejuvenation and are mostly utilised for the following indications (Fig. 32.6):

- Fine lines and wrinkles in any part of the face like the periorbital area, malar areas, perioral areas, chin, etc.
- Skin tightening—Under the neck, cheek lifting, lines around and under the mouth.
- Crepey skin
- Acne scar filling
- Outlining of Lips to create a fuller look naturally (Fig. 32.7)

The barbed threads can be used to lift the ptotic skin and hence be utilised in the following areas (Fig. 32.8):

- Nasolabial folds
- Eyebrow lift
- Upper and lower cheeks
- Neck & Jawline
- Marionette lines

### 32.2.5 Treatment Protocol [4]

Choosing the ideal procedure for rejuvenation depends on the grade of skin ageing.

(A) Mild skin ageing
- Rejuvenation—Apply Plain or screwed PDO threads (Fig. 32.9)
- Lifting
  - for a "natural look" lifting—apply PDO cogs along with plain PDO threads.

Fig. 32.6 Various indications of mono polydioxanone threads for facial rejuvenation

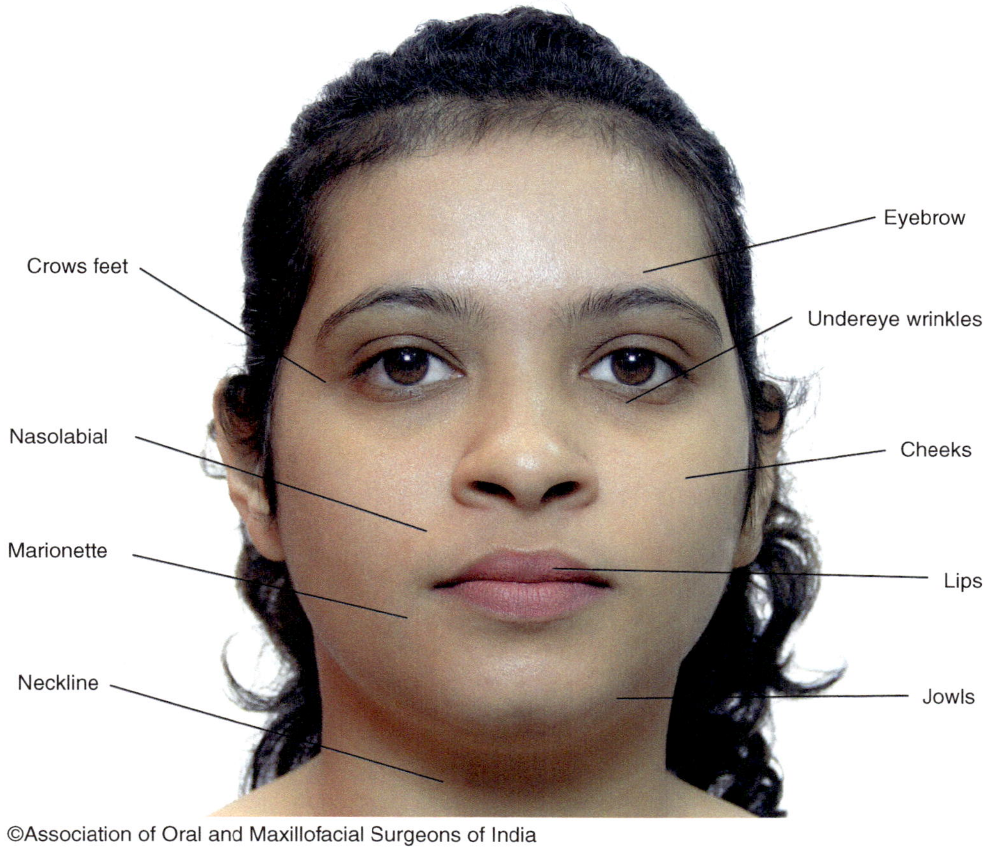


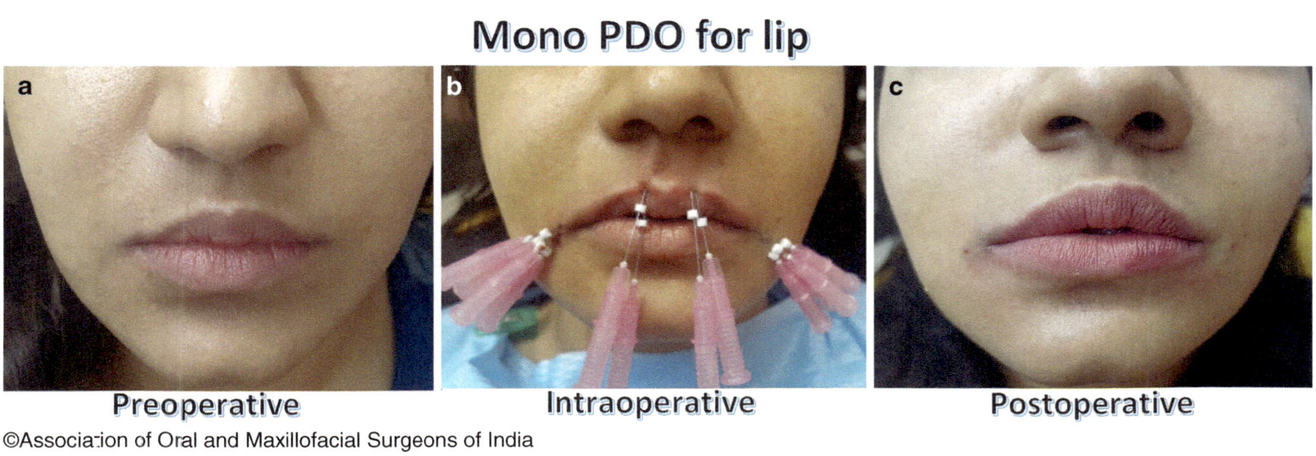


Fig. 32.7 (a, b, c) Mono polydioxanone threads can be used to create the lip borders and also to create a fuller looking lip

- for heavy lifting—apply anchored sutures or long suture technique.

(B) Moderate to severe skin ageing
- Rejuvenation—Apply short PDO cogs along with plain PDO threads (Fig. 32.10).
- Lifting—Not recommended.

### 32.2.6 Procedure

The Polydioxanone thread used in facial rejuvenation are basically of 2 types: Mono PDO thread and Cogs PDO thread

(A) The Mono PDO thread—These are 5-0 or 6-0 suture materials which are essentially monofilament and

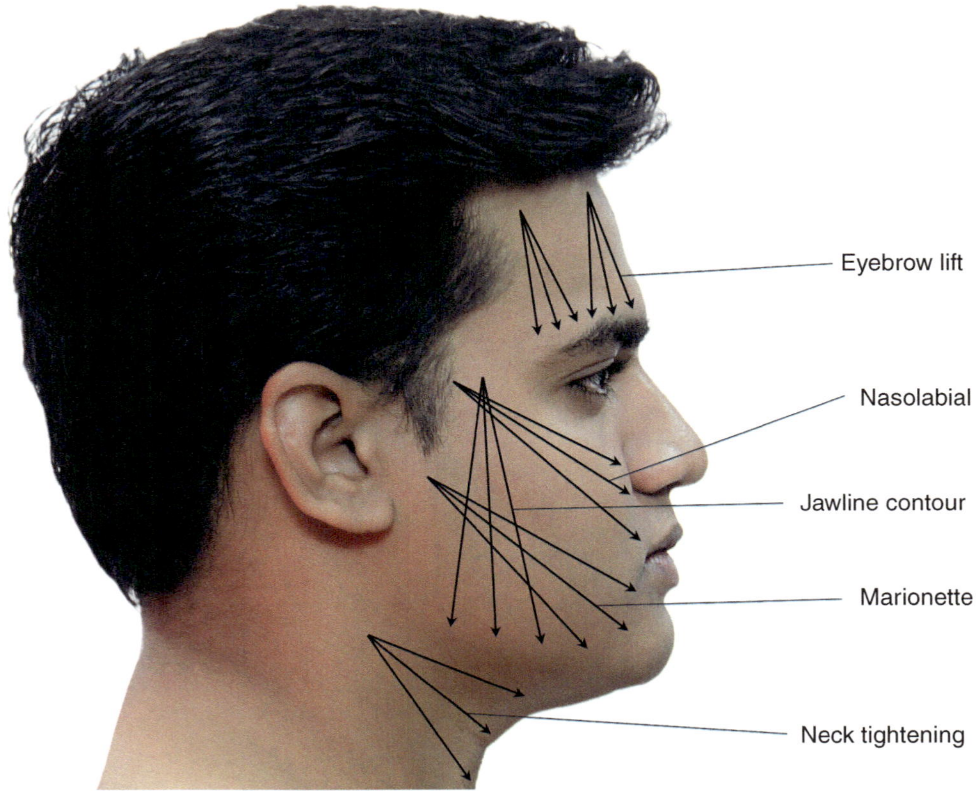




**Fig. 32.8** Various indications of barbed PDO threads for redefining facial contours and lift the ptotic tissues

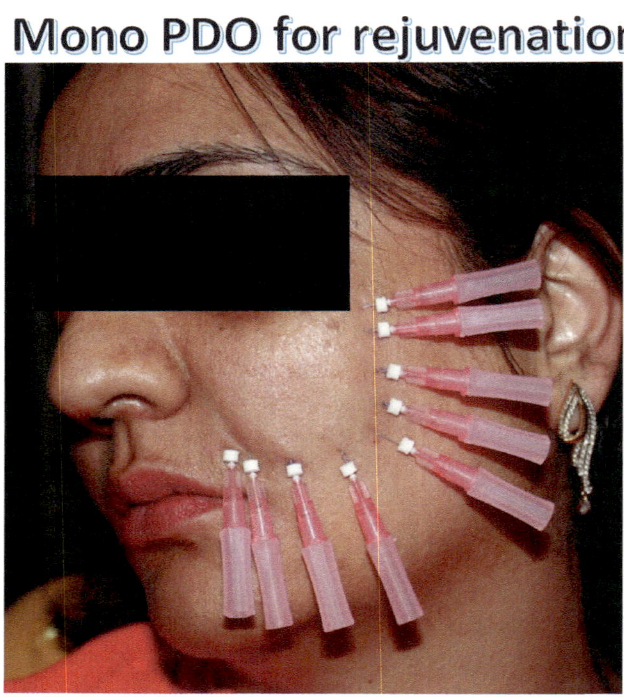




**Fig. 32.9** Mono PDO threads for facial rejuvenation

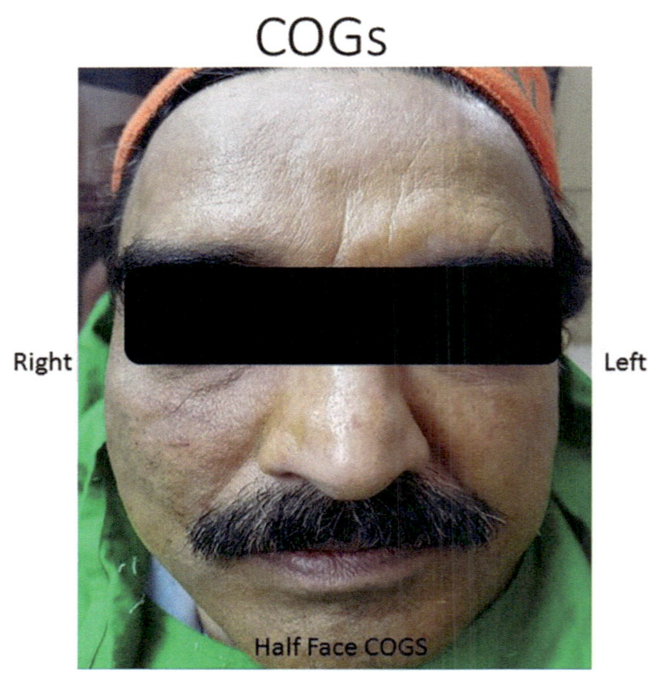




**Fig. 32.10** Cogs thread for lifting nasolabial folds. Note the lifted up right nasolabial fold only as the thread has been applied only on that side. Left side is still untreated

non-barbed. It can also be braided to a spring to provide more tensile strength [17]. The thin suture material forms a V-shape when inserted to a needle of 26–30 g, with one half of the thread inside the calibre of the needle and the other half on the outside. Once the needle with the suture material is inserted into the dermal layer, the thread gets buried into the tissues and at the removal of the needle, the thread stays back intact.

These types of threads are placed in the dermal layer where they cause collagen formation.

EMLA cream must be applied 45 min prior to the procedure. The full face was cleansed with povidone iodine solution. Once ready, the mono PDO threads are placed in the dermal layer making up meshes in the areas of indication. One must keep observing for any threads that stay outside the skin. It must be removed immediately by grasping it with a needle holder so that it doesn't cause any infection or granuloma.

(B) The Cogs PDO thread—Cog PDO thread has small barbs or spikes all along its length, which get engaged to the tissues when inserted and lifts it once pulled back.

Depending on the direction of the spikes, cog PDO thread is classified as unidirectional, bidirectional or multidirectional.

The cog thread is actually 3-0 suture which has barbs and this thread is mounted on an 18 g canula or needle. The canula is considered safer as it does not damage the blood vessels and nerves.

The barbed threads must be placed in the subcutaneous layer so as to prevent any palpability of the implant material.

Local anaesthesia should be given with 2% lidocaine with epinephrine. The full face is cleansed with povidone iodine solution. The path of insertion of the canula is marked on the skin with a sterile marking pen. The vectors are checked by manually stretching the skin upwards. Point of insertion is marked on a line 1.5 cm in the preauricular area. A small opening is made with an 18 g needle for the insertion of the canula. The barbed thread mounted on the canula is then passed along the vector in the subcutaneous plane all the way till the nasolabial fold or the marionette line. Once in place, the end part of the thread gets hooked in the subcutaneous plane, and the canula is pulled back and taken off the skin. The thread stays entangled in the subcutaneous plane. Once all threads are positioned in the skin, the distal part of the suture is held in one hand and the skin is pushed in the opposite direction to fully engage the threads and lift the tissues. The end part of the suture is then cut very close to the skin with help of sharp scissors so that the ends go into the tissues to prevent any future granuloma formation (Figs. 32.11a–d).

Post-operatively, ice packs are applied to minimise edema and bruising. Oral antibiotics are prescribed for 5 days after the procedure.

Anti-inflammatory tablets should be avoided as the more the inflammation at the site, the better would be the results. Patients generally do not require anti-inflammatory drugs post-surgery. Within the first 3 weeks after the procedure, the patients are advised against any strenuous movements of the muscles of midface such as yawning, wide smiling and laughing.

### 32.2.7 Complications and Management

The various complications that could occur with the PDO barbed threads include:

1. Bruising—Bruising is quite common while placing the PDO threads. Post-procedure application of ice prevents further bruise.
2. Pain and Swelling—Thread lift surgery causes very mild to moderate post-operative pain and swelling. Patients are generally asked to apply ice externally to reduce inflammation and pain. If a patient complains of severe pain, anti-inflammatory may be advised. In case of serious swelling, the patient must be evaluated for hematoma and infections.
3. Infection—Proper aseptic protocol needs to be followed to prevent any type of skin infection. However, it is better to prescribe oral antibiotics for 5 days for the thread lift surgery.
4. Palpability of the thread—If the threads are placed too superficial, they become palpable from outside the skin. The barbs or cogs should always be placed in the subcutaneous layer.
5. Hematoma—Since the placement of threads is a blind procedure, the chances of damage to a blood vessel is always there. The patient should always be informed prior to the procedure regarding hematoma. Pressure application and cold compressions should be immediately given. After a period of time, the skin over the hematoma may turn bluish then brown and yellow as the blood is dissolved and absorbed. It may take 1–4 weeks for the hematoma to subside.
6. Nerve damage (Fig. 32.12)—There is always a chance of trauma to the branches of facial nerve since the placement of the threads is in close vicinity to the nerve, especially the marginal mandibular and frontal branches. Thus, the muscles of facial expression can be impaired. Fortunately, the nerve damage resolves soon and motor functions are restored.
7. Asymmetry: Pre-existing asymmetries on the face should be explained to the patient prior to treatment. It's

always a good practice to let the patient seat vertically straight while inserting the barb threads and making the patient participate while retracting the tissues by visualising with a mirror to avoid any potential problems of asymmetry later on.

8. Dimpling: This normally would happen if the depth of the advancing thread is too superficial. A depression or an irregular contour would occur at a portion where the barb is located close to the skin. Most cases normally resolve spontaneously. But remarkable dimples need to be managed by manual reduction at that time itself.
9. Rippling and puckering: The skin would ripple over the thread and cause visible folding if tightened too much while retracting the tissues. This typically resolves itself in a few days if the thread has been placed in the correct tissue plane.
10. Granuloma: Higher incidences of granuloma formation are essentially seen if the threads placed in a more superficial plane and they are not cut very close to the skin.
11. Thread loss: With mono PDO thread, if there is a protruding thread, the end should not be cut as with barbs and cogs, but grasped firmly and removed. It's safer to remove a monofilament thread than leaving it there, thus risking the formation of granuloma. Barbed and cogged threads are very difficult to retrieve and hence excessive care should be taken to place them in the right plane.
12. Thread breakage: This can happen during the tightening of the barbs and cogs just before cutting at the skin level. Hence, careful manipulation should be done to avoid breakage during insertion and tightening.
13. Thread exposure: Repeated inflammation and migration of the thread to superficial layers can cause thread exposure. It can be prevented by placing the threads in proper plane.

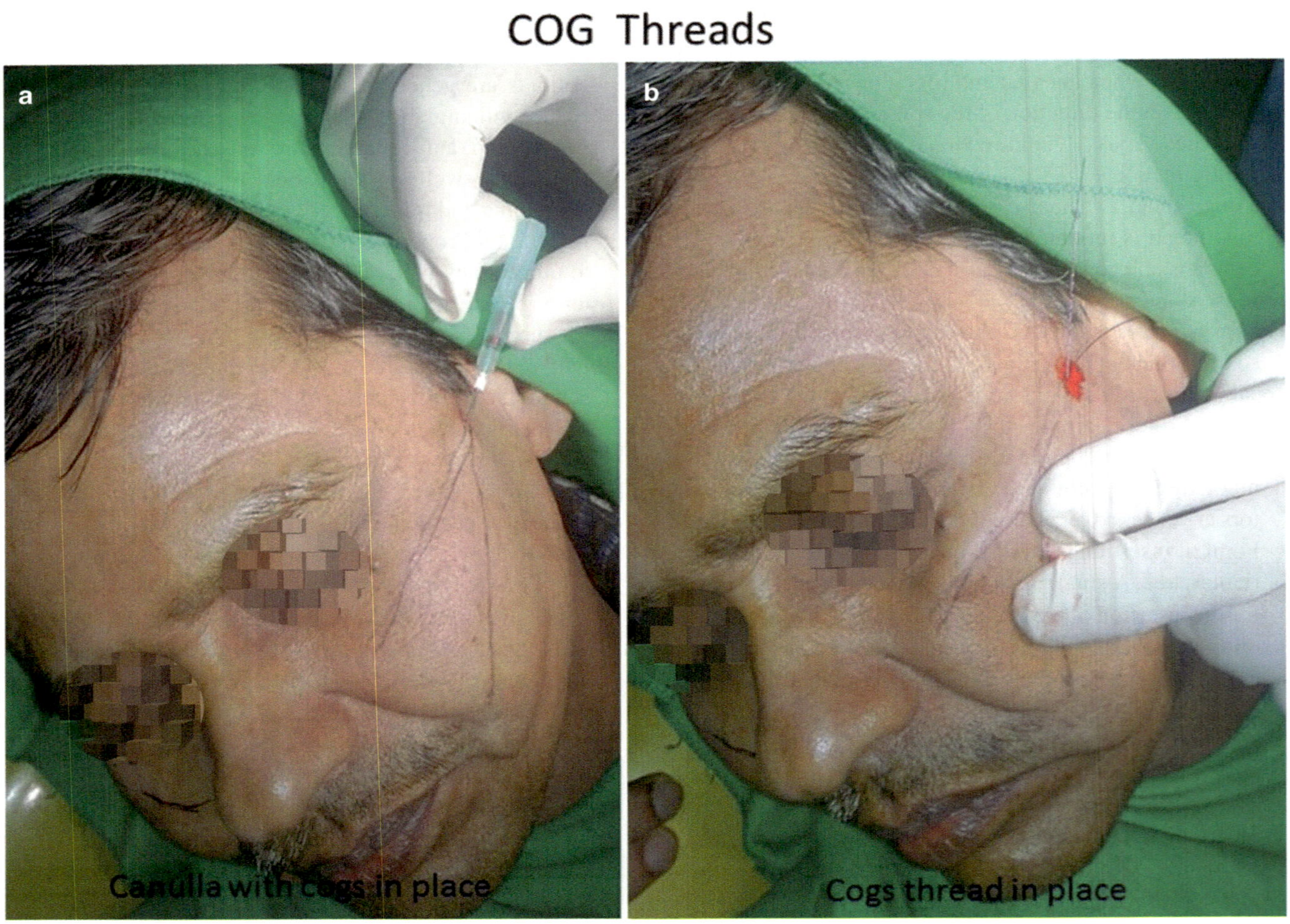




**Fig. 32.11** (**a**, **b**) Placement of cannula with cogs threads along the vectors for nasolabial folds and after removal of cannula the cogs threads in place. (**c**, **d**) Pulling the cogs threads to lift the ptotic nasolabial fold tissues and final twisting and snipping the threads just below the skin level

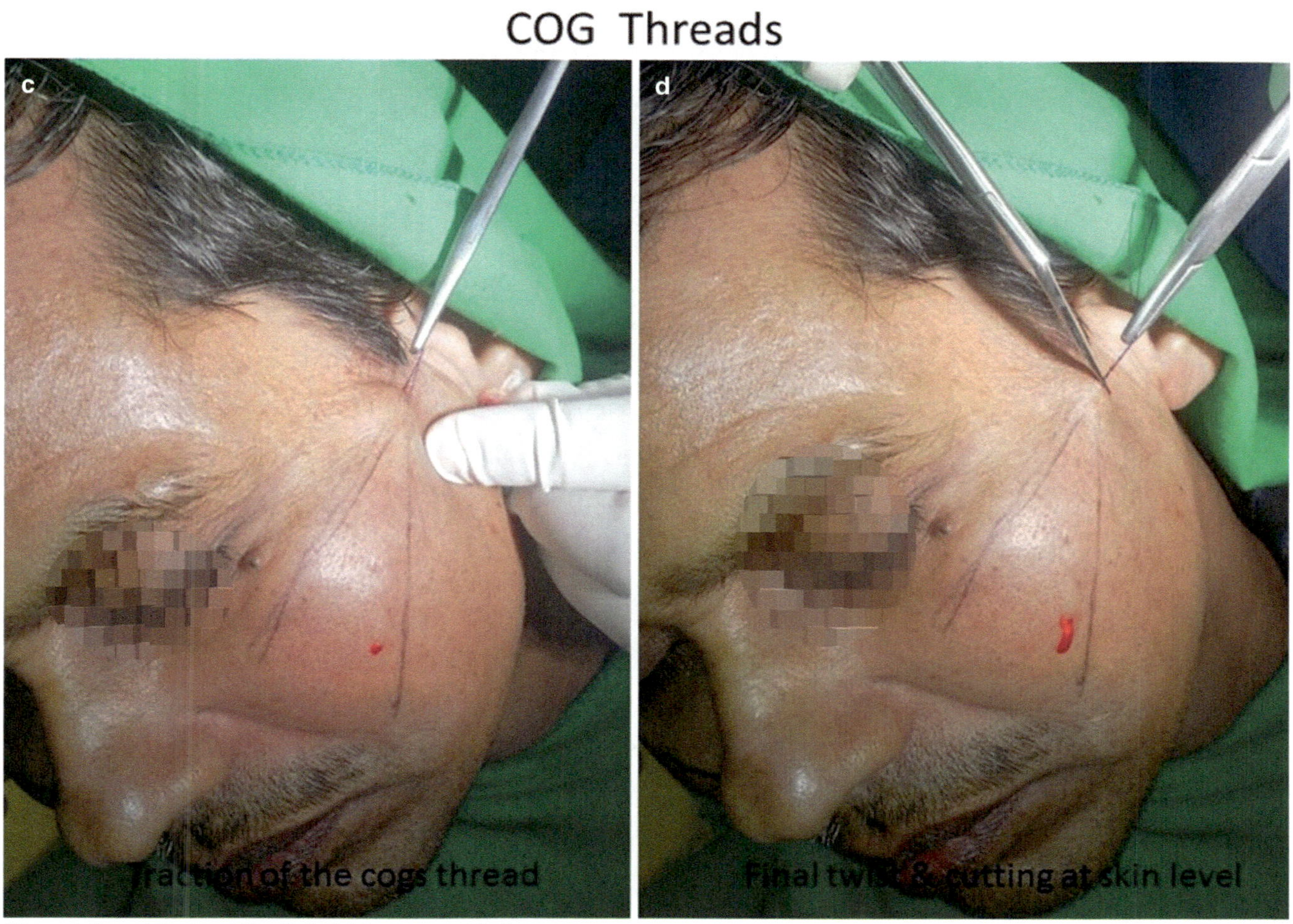


©Association of Oral and Maxillofacial Surgeons of India

**Fig. 32.11** (continued)

### 32.2.8 Conclusion

The PDO thread lift is a non-invasive procedure that actually gives a "lifted effect" of the ptotic skin. It has been widely accepted as a standard procedure for patients who do not want to opt for a more aggressive surgical facelift. Patient selection is of prime importance. Only patients with mild to slightly moderate levels of ptosis should be selected for polydioxanone cogs thread lift. The patient should be given a realistic expectation of the lift of no more than 1 cm. Patients who are too chubby or who are too skinny should not be considered for thread lift. Overall, every aesthetic practitioner should have knowledge of thread lift as it is a simple and versatile anti-ageing procedure.

## 32.3 Biostimulatory Lift with Platelet-Rich Plasma

Today, Platelet-rich plasma (PRP) has been incorporated in many medical specialities including orthopaedics, general surgery, plastic surgery, dental surgery and dermatology because of its healing capabilities. Its usage in aesthetics and trichology has touched newer horizons as we have come to know about the healing cytokines present in the platelets which can be used for antiageing therapies and therapies for regenerative aesthetics.

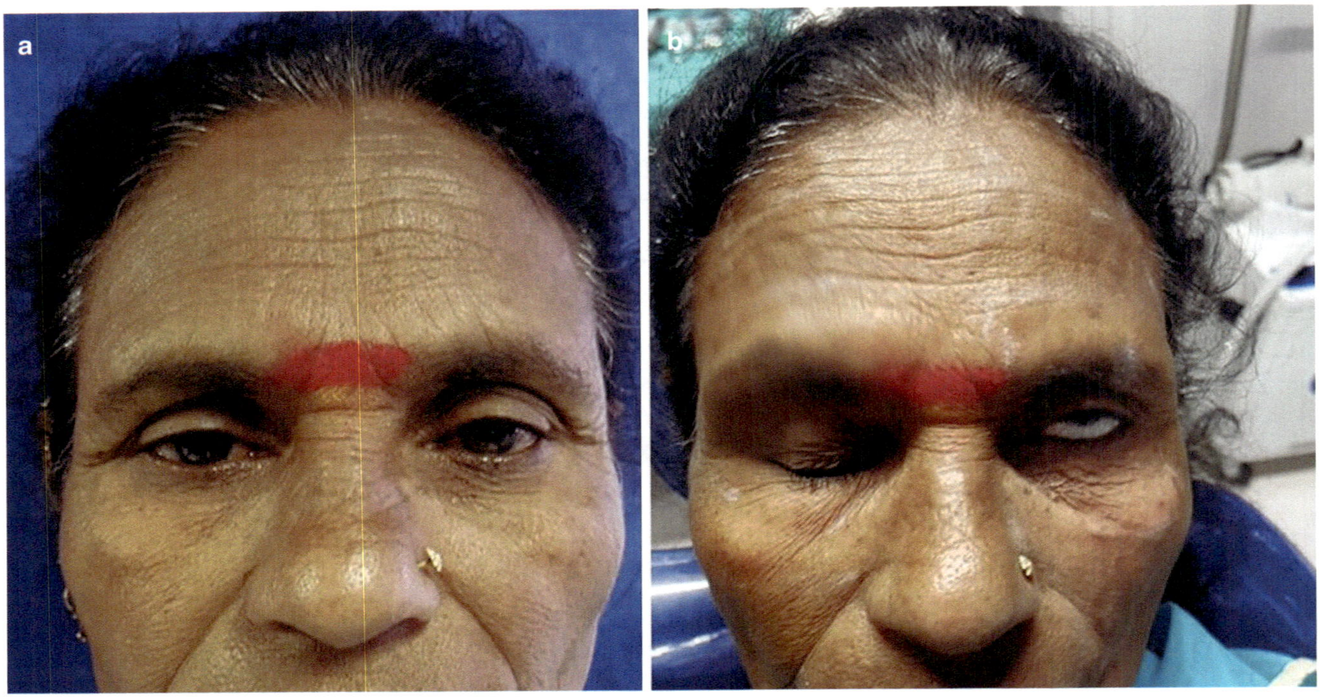




**Fig. 32.12** (**a**, **b**) Damage to frontal branch of the facial nerve during placement of cogs threads

### 32.3.1 Platelets and Platelet Concentrates

Platelets, also called thrombocytes, are enucleated fragments of cytoplasm that are derived from the megakaryocytes of the bone marrow, which are released into the circulation. They have a fundamental role in haemostasis and wound healing.

The platelets contain various secretory granules, namely the alpha granules, dense granules and lysosomes. The alpha granules are the most abundant ones and contain the coagulation factors, growth factors, also called cytokines, adhesion molecules, and a variety of other angiogenic factors which efficiently encourage the proliferation and activation of cells required for wound healing including fibroblasts, mesenchymal stem cells (MSCs) and facilitates angiogenesis [18].

The growth factors along with their function are listed below [19]:

1. PDGF (platelet-derived growth factor)—PDGF plays a role in embryonic development, cell proliferation, cell migration and angiogenesis.
2. TGF-β1 & β2 (transforming growth factor)—TGF is involved in regulating and mediating processes at the cellular level, including cell proliferation, differentiation, motility, adhesion and apoptosis as well as causes wound healing and angiogenesis.
3. VEGF (vascular endothelial growth factor)—Chemotactic and mitogenic for endothelial cells, mediates angiogenesis.
4. EGF (epidermal growth factor)—Mediates angiogenesis, causes proliferation of fibroblasts, endothelial cells and keratinocytes.
5. HGF (hepatocyte growth factor)—Mediates regeneration.
6. FGF (fibroblast growth factor)—Mediates tissue organisation and regeneration.
7. FGF-9—Aids generation of new follicles.

These growth factors or the "cytokines" are proteins, each of about 25,000 Daltons molecular weight. In response to the thrombocyte aggregation, as occurs in injury or surgery, the cell membrane activates the alpha granules which in turn unleash these growth factors via active extrusion through the cell membrane. The active secretion begins within 10 min during which 70% of stored growth factors are released and more than 95% of the presynthesised growth factors are secreted within 1 hour. Platelets then synthesise additional amount of growth factors for about 8 days till they die [20].

Platelet concentrate means plentiful amounts of platelets that are concentrated into a small volume of plasma. There are various types of platelet concentrates which can be formulated, all differing in the way they are made [21]. A general classification takes 2 key parameters into consideration: the presence of a cell content (mostly leukocytes) and the fibrin architecture.

There are 4 major families:

1. P-PRP

   Pure Platelet-rich plasma is a preparation without Leukocytes. It has low-density fibrin network after activation. It is used as liquid solutions or an activated gel form and can be injected. P-PRP is commonly used in sports medicine & aesthetic medicine.
2. L-PRP

   Leukocyte and PRP is a preparation with leukocytes in it. Even this has low-density fibrin network after activation. It is used as liquid solutions or an activated gel form and can be injected. L-PRP is used in aesthetic medicine, sports medicine, orthopaedics, trichology, etc.
3. P-PRF

   Pure Platelet-rich fibrin is a preparation without leukocytes. It has a high-density fibrin network and exists as a strongly activated gel form. It cannot be injected, but can be handled like a real solid material. It has been very commonly used in dentistry & maxillofacial surgery today.
4. L-PRF

Leukocyte and PRF is a preparation with leukocytes. It has a high density of fibrin network and exists as a strongly activated gel form. It cannot be injected and can be handled as a real solid material. It is today used in implant dentistry, periodontal surgeries, oral surgeries, treatment of skin wound ulcers, etc.

## 32.3.2 Mechanism of Action of PRP

PRP can be described as a biologic product derived from autologous blood with the plasma fraction containing platelets at a concentration of more than 3–5 times above baseline.

The scientific evidence suggests that wound healing enhancement is seen using concentrates of 1,000,000 platelets/μl. Any concentration lower than this cannot be depended on to enhance wound healing, and concentrations far more than this has not been scientifically proved to help and enhance healing [22].

So, PRP by virtue of its increased concentration of platelets and thereby an inflated amount of growth factors or cytokines have been theorised to encourage tissue repair and regeneration by neocollagenesis, neoangiogenesis and much more. It has been embraced as a frontline treatment modality for the management of facial ageing, androgenetic alopecia, acne scarring, etc.

## 32.3.3 Indications of PRP Therapy in Aesthetic Medicine

1. Facial rejuvenation.
2. Skin tightening and Antiageing therapy
3. Acne scar management
4. Alopecia
5. Skin lightening
6. Improvement of skin quality in under eye area.

## 32.3.4 Preparation of PRP

PRP is derived from autologous blood by using a centrifuge and can be performed under local anaesthesia under aseptic conditions. An anticoagulant, like citrate dextrose solution formula A (ACD-A) or sodium citrate 3.8%, is used to inhibit platelet aggregation.

**Manual Double Spin Method** (Figs. 32.13, 32.14, 32.15, and 32.16)
Whole blood is collected by venipuncture from antecubital vein in 15 ml polystyrene tubes under sterile conditions containing 3.8% sodium citrate as an anticoagulant. In each tube, 1 ml of sodium citrate is mixed with 12 ml of whole blood. Eight such tubes are taken to make up a volume of 104 ml. The tubes are slowly turned upside down twice to homogeneously mix the whole blood with the anticoagulant. All the 8 tubes are placed in the centrifuge (Remi 8c) and are centrifuged at 1500 rpm for 10 min. This is called the ‘soft spin’ which separates the whole blood into 3 layers. The erythrocytes settle at the bottom of the tube because of the highest specific gravity or density of about 1.090. Just above the erythrocytes, a hazy layer is seen which contains the leucocytes with a specific gravity of 1.060 and platelets with a specific gravity around 1.040. At the top, we find the clear plasma with the lowest concentration of platelets with a specific gravity of around 1.020.

The buffy coat is separated along with some amount of plasma and placed in a separate tube. At this time, if the buffy coat is separated along with the slightest superficial erythrocyte layer, it is referred to as L-PRP (leukocyte-PRP) and if it

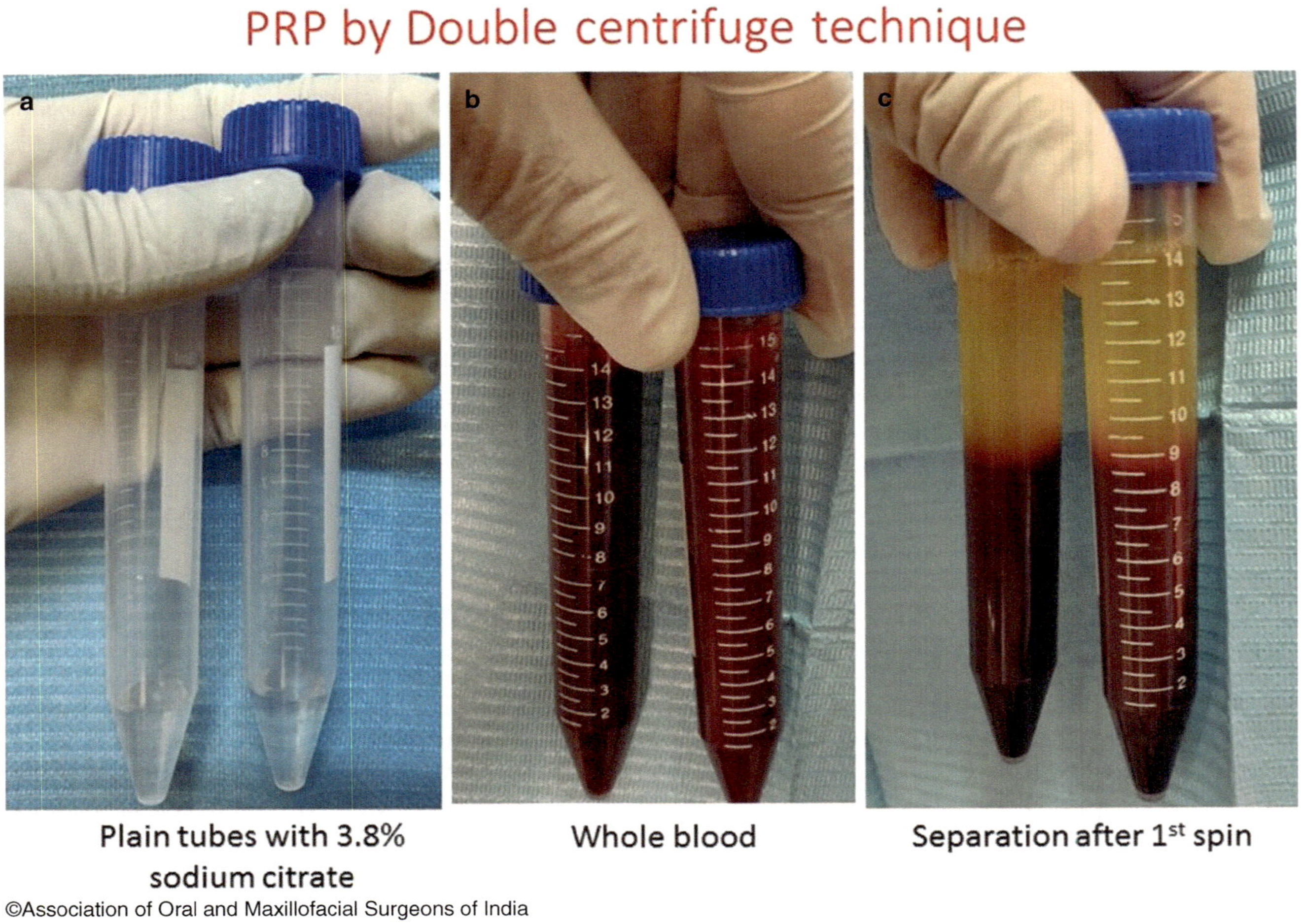


**Fig. 32.13** (**a**, **b**, **c**) Primary separation of erythrocytes during the preparation of platelet-rich plasma using plain tubes containing sodium citrate 3.8%

is taken above the layer of erythrocytes, it is referred to as P-PRP (pure-PRP) depending on the kind of PRP preparation, i.e. with or without leukocytes. About 10 ml of these are taken in 2 tubes and placed in the centrifuge for a second spin called the 'hard spin' at 2500 rpm for 15 min. At the end of the spin, a platelet plug is found at the bottom of the tube. The top 3 quarter of the platelet poor plasma was discarded and the lowest quarter with the platelet plug was mixed and used as the PRP. This gives us a viable platelet count of 5 times the baseline. This was activated by mixing with calcium gluconate at a ratio of 9:1 in an insulin syringe and injected immediately.

**Automated Devices** (Fig. 32.17)
Numerous commercial devices of varying standards are now available for the preparation of PRP. Although time saving, these adapted kits can be quite expensive as compared to the manual process.

In general, a PRP tube typically contains sodium citrate as an anticoagulant along with a separating gel. This gel has a density of about 1.070, which is in between the erythrocytes and platelets.

20 ml of Whole blood is collected by venipuncture and added into two of these PRP tubes. The blood is homogeneously mixed with the anticoagulant by gently turning the tube upside down twice. The tubes are then placed in the centrifuge and spun at 3700 rpm for 9 min. The erythrocytes because of the higher density than the separating gel settle down below the gel, while the plasma along with leucocytes and platelets segregate above the gel. The superficial platelet poor plasma is discarded leaving behind 2–3 ml of plasma above the gel. The tubes can be turned upside down to mix the platelets as they get entangled in the gel. This would give a uniform concentration of platelets throughout. It is now mixed with calcium gluconate as an activator and injected immediately.

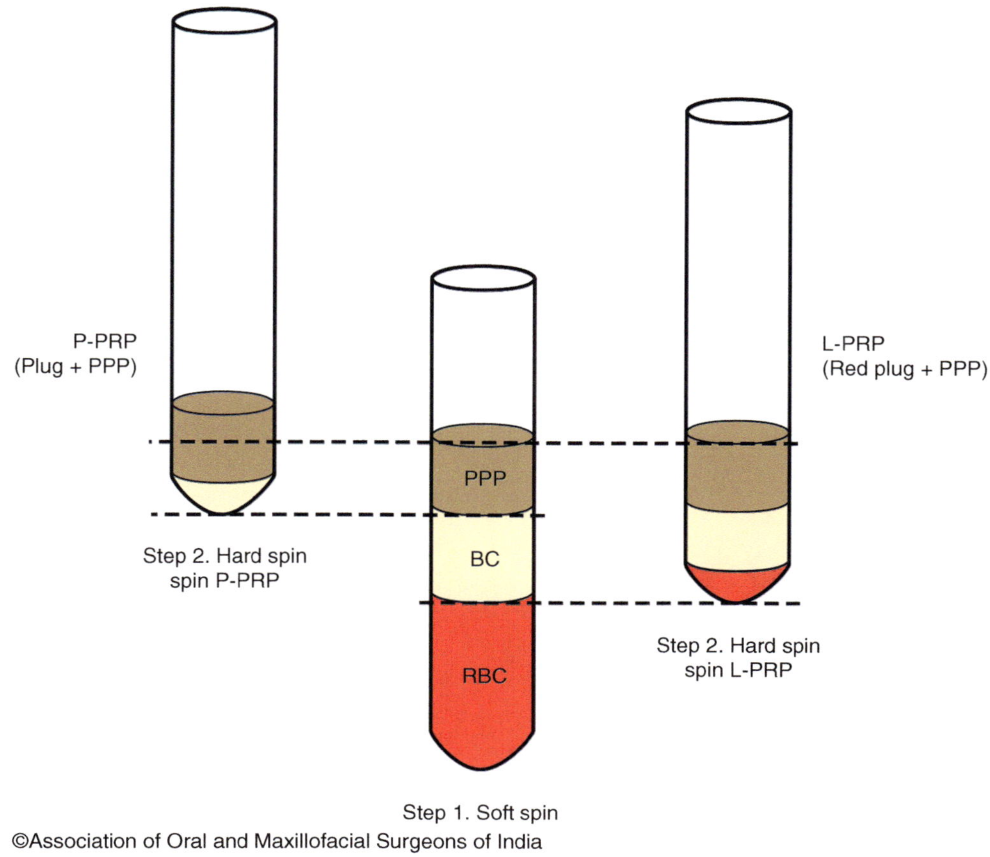


**Fig. 32.14** Difference in preparation of L-PRP and P-PRP

### 32.3.5 PRP Injections for Facial Rejuvenation, Biostimulatory Lift and Acne Scar

Studies have shown that PRP by inducing neocollagenesis through activation of fibroblasts and by removing photodamaged extracellular matrix (ECM) components amplifies dermal elasticity via following molecular mechanisms [23, 24]:

- Encouraging proliferation of human dermal fibroblasts to induce new collagen.
- Increased expression of MMP-1 (matrix metalloproteinase-1) and MMP-3, resulting in the removal of photodamaged ECM.
- Enhanced creation of procollagen type I peptide and expression of collagen type I, alpha-I, resulting in the synthesis of fresh collagen.
- Increases expression of G1 cell cycle regulators resulting in accelerated wound healing.

PRP can be injected using an insulin syringe that has 31 g needle. Local anaesthetic in the form of nerve blocks should be given prior to the session. The facial skin should be cleansed with povidone iodine solution. Multiple intradermal injections of PRP after activating it are given all over the face including the infraorbital area. Three sessions each at a gap of 1 month of PRP therapy along with micro-needling (collagen induction therapy) with derma pen with a needle depth of 0.7–1 mm has been shown to give very good results for rejuvenating the aged skin and acne scars. Histologically, the treated skin showed improved length of dermo-epidermal junction, increased quantity of collagen and fibroblasts.

Post-operatively, patients are advised to apply ice on the face. Sun exposure should be avoided. Patient should be advised not to take anti-inflammatory tablets as the more the inflammation, the better the results are going to be. Most of the times, patients experience very mild post-operative discomfort.

PRP therapy can also be combined with CO2 fractional resurfacing to achieve excellent results in treating acne scars.

PRP has also shown excellent results in infraorbital rejuvenation where the skin is very thin and shows initial signs of ageing [25].

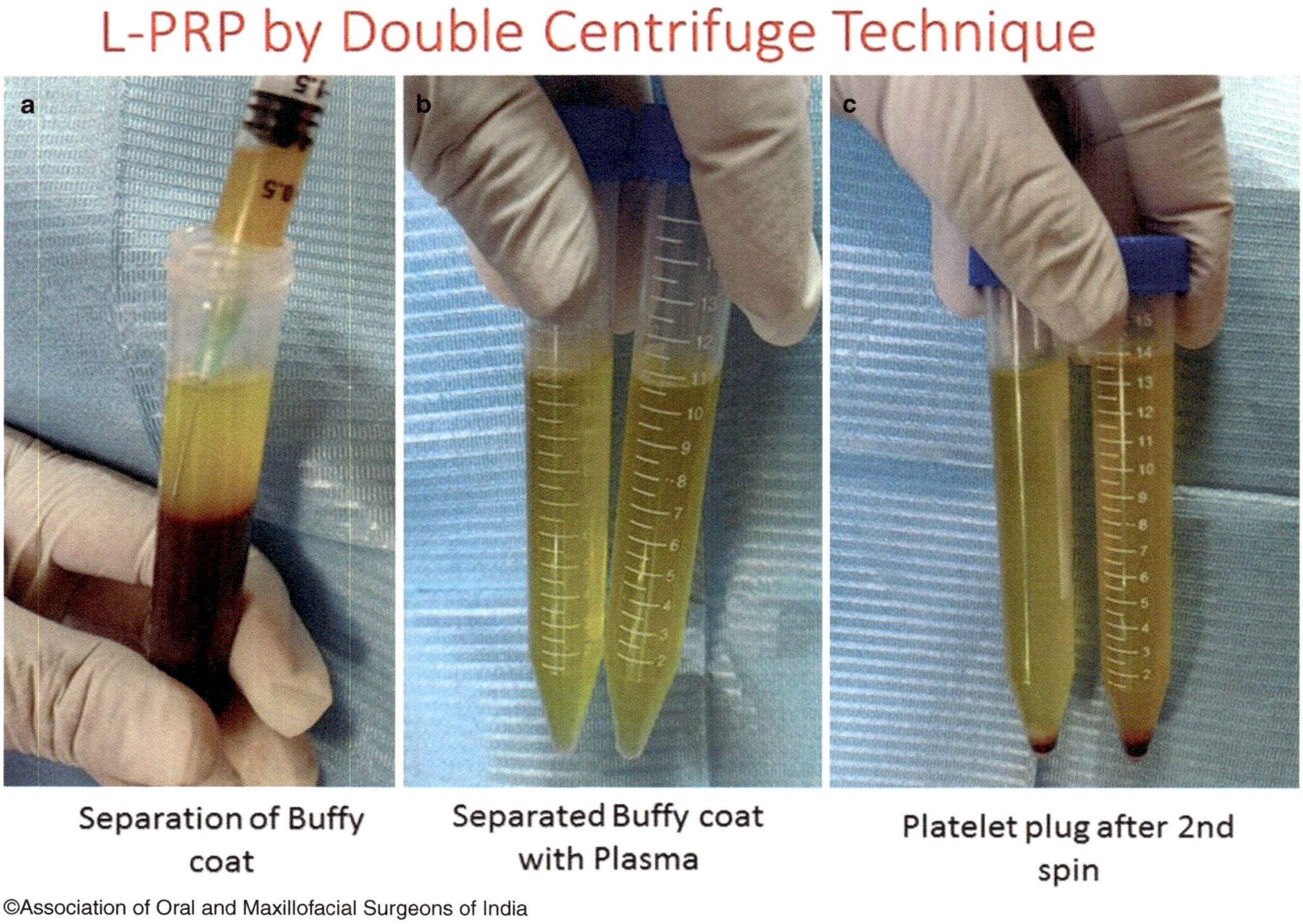


**Fig. 32.15** (**a**, **b**, **c**) Platelet plug formed after the second spin during the preparation of L-PRP

### 32.3.6 Contraindications to PRP Therapy [26]

Absolute contraindications:

- Platelet dysfunctions.
- Thrombocytopenia (low platelet counts).
- Hypofibrinogenemia.
- Local sepsis.
- Hemodynamic instability.
- Septicaemia.
- Patient unwilling to accept risks.
- Patients on long-term anticoagulant therapy (warfarin or heparin).

Relative contraindications:

- Consistent use of NSAIDs and corticosteroids within 15 days
- Recent episode of infections, fever or illness.
- Cancer—especially hematopoietic or of bone.

### 32.3.7 Conclusion

The use of cytokines derived from platelet-rich plasma (PRP) is an effective modality to promote tissue regeneration and hence can be used in regenerative medicine including facial aesthetics and trichology.

PRP therapy is an inexpensive procedure as it does not require complex and voluminous equipment or extensive training for its execution. Furthermore, since the product is primarily autologous in origin, the patient's apprehension regarding the immunogenic reactions or disease transmission is abolished. Over three decades of its application to various fields and the multitude of studies with enormous positive results, PRP therapy today has become a gold standard for facial rejuvenation and hair loss therapy. The release of bioactive cytokines that help in neocollagenesis which takes care of the ageing process of wrinkle formation has made it a versatile tool for many anti-ageing therapies on the face.

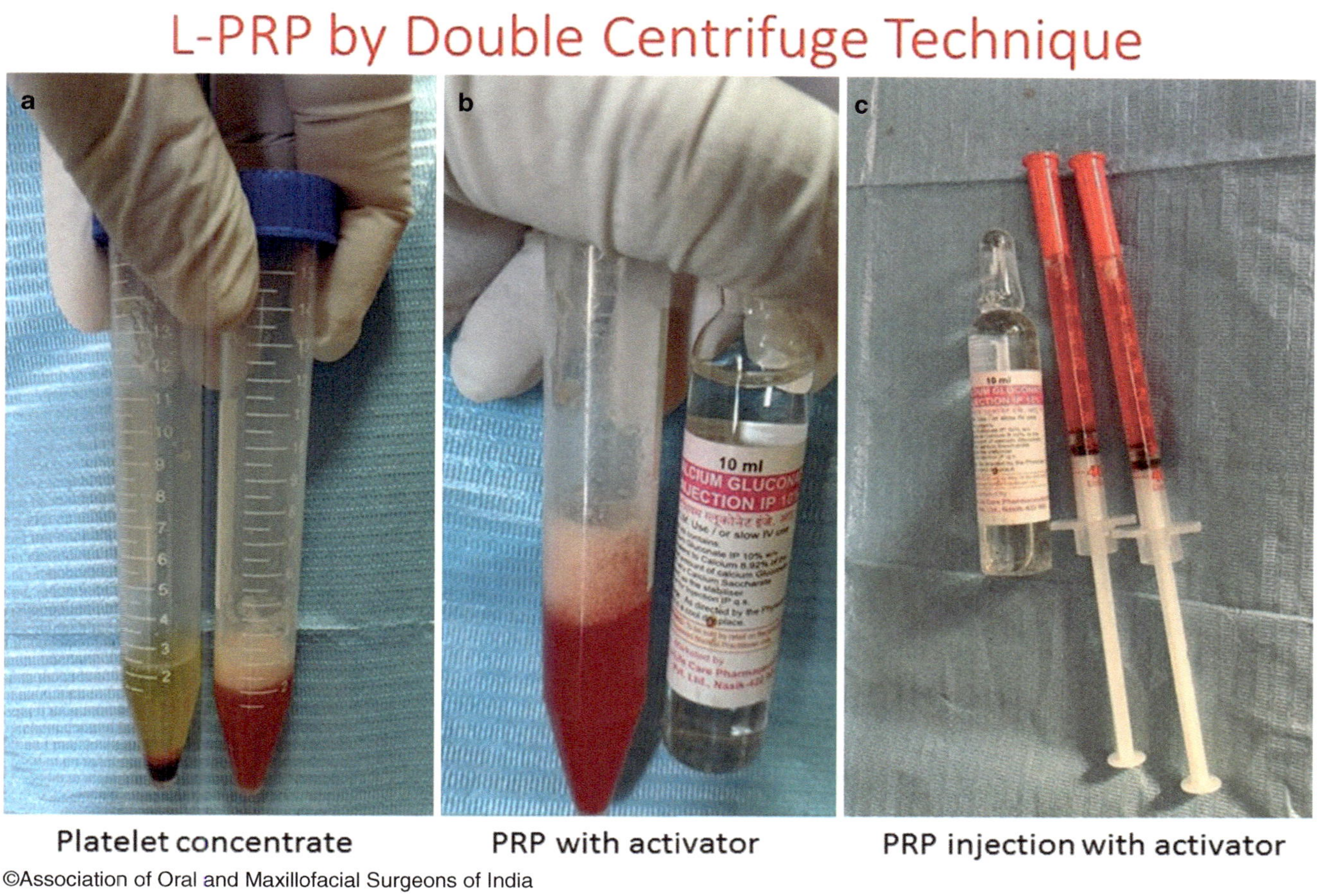


**Fig. 32.16** (**a**, **b**, **c**) Platelet-rich plasma needs to be activated for release of cytokines from the alpha granules

## 32.4 Face Tightening with HIFU (High Intensity Focussed Ultrasound)

Facial wrinkles, reduced elasticity of the facial skin and sagging parts of the face are the most common concerns today an aesthetic surgeon encounters from the patients. In the present social scenario, facial skin laxity is considered highly disgraceful and has a great impact on a person's psychology and quality of life [27]. The natural process of ageing which is inevitable and the other external factors like sun's UV radiations, stress and worry, smoking, unhealthy diet, etc. are the major factors which cause the wrinkles and sagginess. We are aware that the loss of the important proteins viz collagen and elastin, which gives the strength, resilience and elasticity to the skin is the reason behind the loose skin and wrinkles.

Various treatment modalities have been utilised to manage these concerns of the face. Surgical excision of the redundant skin via facelift surgery definitely gives the best results. But with the increasing concerns over the complications and the downtime, the focus of therapeutic modalities is shifting towards non-surgical aspects.

Non-surgical treatment modalities like microdermabrasion, chemical peels, fractional lasers, etc. have been advocated in the past. In recent times, newer modalities like the HIFU and RF have come into limelight due to their non-invasiveness and low or no downtime for the treatment of sagging skin.

### 32.4.1 Introduction to HIFU

Ultrasound was introduced for its diagnostic ability. The capability of the focussed ultrasound energy to cause tissue regression and ablation has been well utilised today as a non-invasive modality to treat solid tumours and also being used to treat both primary and metastatic tumours as these can precisely locate the mass for ablation [28].

More recently this intense focussed ultrasound has also been utilised in many painful conditions including neuropathic pain and musculoskeletal degeneration [29].

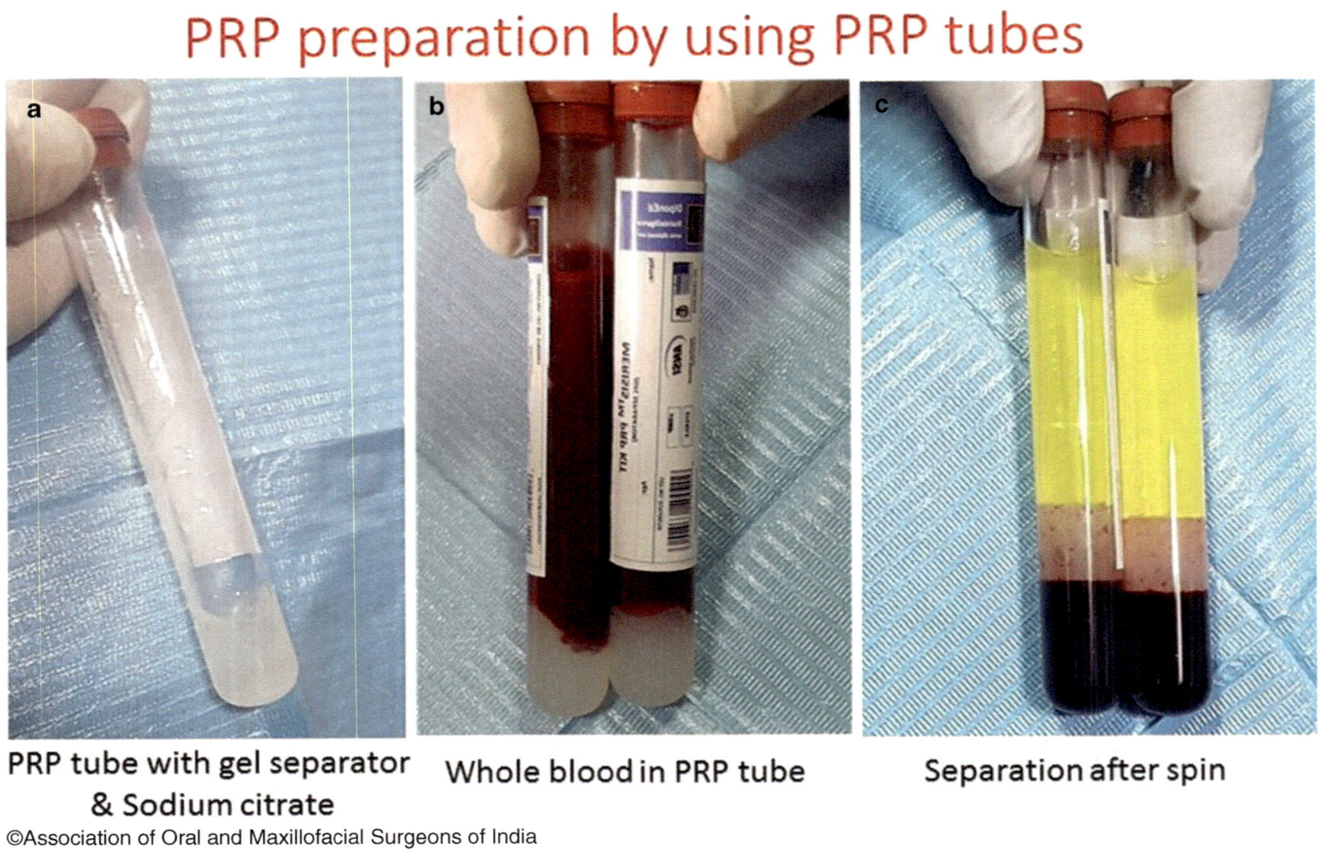


**Fig. 32.17** (**a**, **b**, **c**) Preparation of Platelet-rich plasma with the help of PRP tubes containing anticoagulants and the separating gel

HIFU or high intensity focussed ultrasound was introduced into the field of facial aesthetics very recently to manage the facial wrinkles and periorbital rejuvenation.

FDA in 2009 approved the use of HIFU in brow lifting as the first dermatologic and aesthetic indication following the report by White et al. [30] in 2008. It was later in 2014 cleared as an indication to improve lines and wrinkles of the upper chest and neckline (décolletage). Currently, its use for facial rejuvenation, skin lifting and tightening and body contouring is considered 'off-label'.

### 32.4.2 Mechanism of Action

High intensity focussed ultrasound or HIFU embodies a piezoelectric transducer which produces focussed ultrasound beams. This transducer releases ultrasound waves over a length of around 2.5 cm which are focussed at 1.5, 3 or 4.5 mm depth. The 1.5 mm focusses the superficial or papillary dermis, while the 3 mm focusses the deep or reticular dermis and the 4.5 mm focusses the SMAS layer. Like a magnifying glass, the transducer focusses the ultrasound to the desired depth and at the focal spot, there is a swift rise in temperature to 60–80°C within a very short period (typically 1–20 s). This causes an immediate contraction of native collagen which is subsequently followed by cell injury and tissue shattering due to both coagulation necrosis and protein denaturation. These events occur at the deeper focussed zones, while the superficial tissues are left safe and unaffected [31] (Fig. 32.18).

The focussed ultrasound energy is absorbed by the tissues and this causes the molecules to vibrate rapidly. The friction due to molecular oscillations results in heat generation and a rapid rise of temperature at the focal zone. This thermomechanical process causes tissue injury at the site of focus. Supplemental to this, the ultrasound waves that propagate through the tissues cause continuous compressions and rarefactions that result in powerful shear forces. This microscopic but mighty shearing motion results in frictional heating [32]. Once tissue destruction is done, the inflammatory phase (in first 48 h) sets in wherein the damaged cells are removed and the WBCs, growth factors and enzymes create swelling, heat, pain and redness.

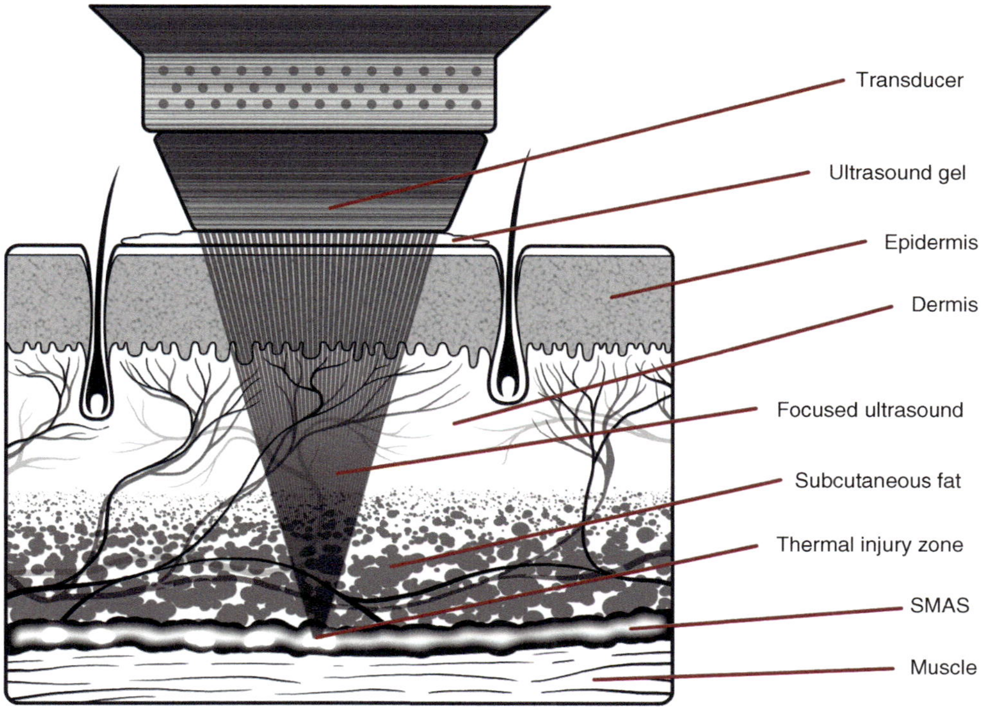


**Fig. 32.18** Mechanism of high-intensity focussed ultrasound. Thermal coagulation zones are created due to the extreme heat produced by the ultrasound focussed to a particular depth

In the next proliferative phase (up to 6 weeks), there is tissue contracture due to the myofibroblasts which are built. New tissues made up of collagen and extracellular matrix are formed.

The last maturation phase (from 3 weeks to 6 months) shows collagen is remodelling from type III to type I. The collagen which was laid down during the proliferative phase is now aligned along the tension lines and also there is cross-linking of the collagen. A histological evaluation post HIFU treatment exhibited significantly regenerated and proliferated quantity of dermal collagen and elastic fibres [33]. This causes skin tightening over a period of time. The results keep improving and the best final results are seen by 6 months.

### 32.4.3 Armamentarium

The HIFU machine basically consists of 2 parts: the body and the transducer (Fig. 32.19).

The screen in the body keeps monitoring the number of shots, depth of shots, length of release of ultrasound waves and the energy of the ultrasound in real time. The transducer releases the focussed ultrasound waves. The following are the 3 transducers usually used on the face:

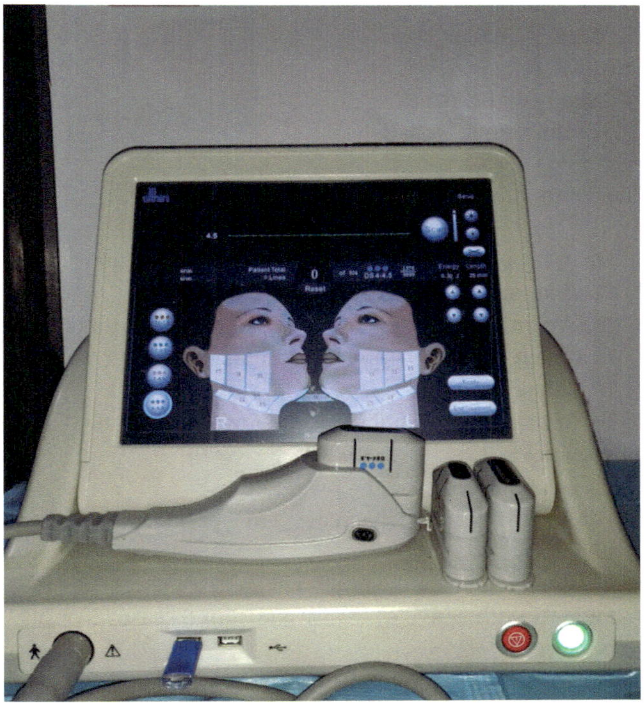


**Fig. 32.19** High-intensity focussed ultrasound device

1. DS-4.5 4—Focussed ultrasound of 4 MHz frequency is transmitted to a depth of 4.5 mm to the SMAS layer, forming "thermal coagulation" spots. It is normally targeted to thicker skin, such as cheeks, etc. and is the most important aspect of midface tightening.
2. DS-3.0 8—High-frequency ultrasound of 8 MHz is focussed to the deep dermis layer at 3.0 mm depth and is responsible for activating the skin's collagen. It effectively reduces the appearance of wrinkles and also ameliorates large pores.
3. DS-1.5 10—Here, 10 MHz frequency ultrasound energy is focussed to the superficial dermis. It is used in thinner tissue in the periorbital area.

### 32.4.4 Indications and Contraindications in Facial Aesthetics

The numerous indications of HIFU are given below.

1. Brow lifting
2. Facial rejuvenation.
3. Fine and deep wrinkles of face.
4. Infraorbital area laxity.
5. Crow's feet.
6. Nasolabial folds (Fig. 32.20).
7. Mentolabial grooves.
8. Jowls.
9. Submental skin.
10. Double chin.

The contraindications are the following;

1. Open facial wounds or lesions in treatment region.
2. Pustular acne in the treatment region.
3. Active implants (e.g. pacemakers or defibrillators) in treatment region (no contraindications to Dental Implants).
4. Perform fillers and threads treatment after the HIFU session.
5. Pregnant or breast-feeding woman.
6. Directly over mechanical and permanent dermal implants.
7. Existing keloids in the treatment area.
8. Patients with active systemic and skin diseases like herpes, etc.
9. Unrealistic expectations of treatment.

### 32.4.5 Procedure for Face Tightening

#### 32.4.5.1 Facial Rejuvenation - HIFU (Video 32.1)

The sequence for HIFU application includes the following:

1. Patient consent and explanation of the procedure, adverse effects and alternatives.
2. Removal of all makeup from face.
3. Cleansing the full face and neck area.
4. Application of local anaesthetics ointment like EMLA, Toplap, etc., and occluding it with plastic sheet for 45 min.
5. Markings of the skin for treatment.
6. Application of ultrasound gel on the skin and face and application of transducer tip at an angle perpendicular to the skin.
7. Start with 4.5 mm transducer, followed by 3 mm and then 1.5 mm with a number of shots and area as mentioned in the figures.
8. Removal of ultrasound gel and explaining post-operative instructions before discharging the patient.
9. Follow up on the next day to assess any complications and at 3 and 6 months to assess the results.

### 32.4.6 Adverse Effects

Severe adverse effects of HIFU are very rare and hence considered a very safe procedure to perform on an outpatient basis. The adverse effects that have been described may be:

- Pain—Transient discomfort may be experiences during the procedure which resolves within 2 h to 2 days. Tenderness is also possible and typically resolves in maximum 2 weeks.
- Erythema—May exhibit immediately after the treatment which resolves in few hours (Fig. 32.21).
- Edema—Skin may exhibit slight edema following treatment which settles in 3–72 h after treatment.
- Motor Nerve paresis—Symptoms of motor nerve paresis can be seen in the first 12 h of the treatment. It normally happens with the marginal mandibular and temporal branches of facial nerve which are pretty superficial. The HIFU could cause inflammation of these nerves and this may lead to disruption of motor function. The frontalis muscle and the muscles of perioral area are affected. The symptoms usually resolve in 2–6 weeks. Anti-inflammatory medications can be prescribed if symptoms of nerve paresis arise.

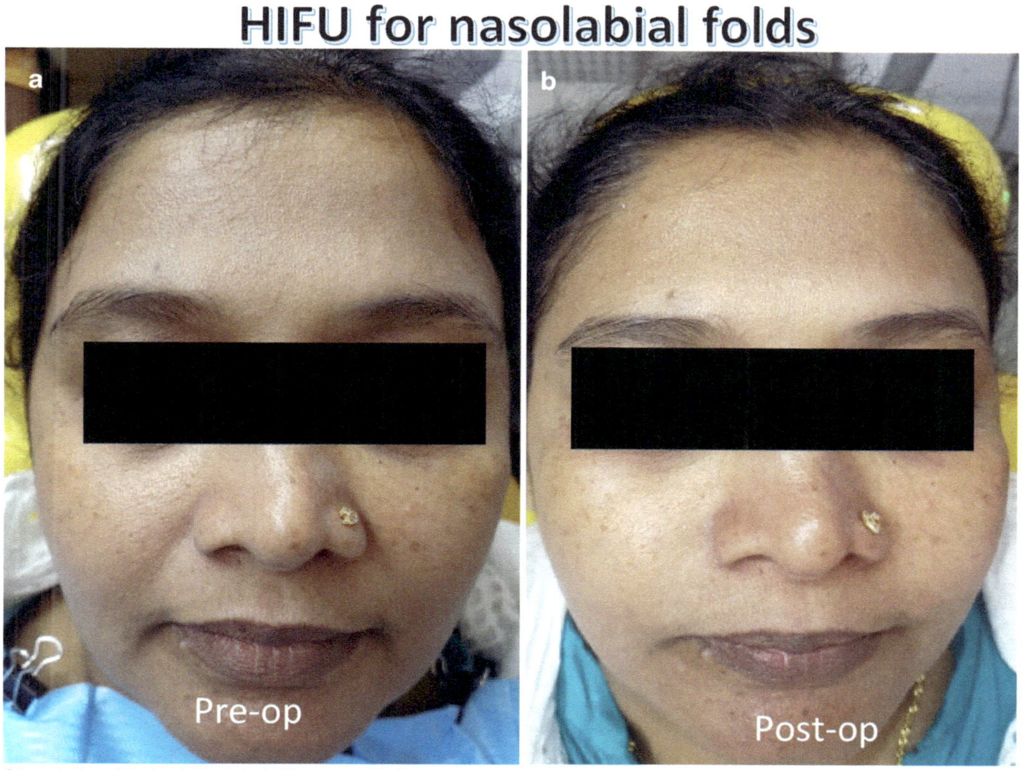




**Fig. 32.20** (a, b) Lifting of nasolabial fold with HIFU

- Skin burns: This happens when inadequate ultrasound gel is not applied between the transducer and the skin. There is thus inadequate acoustic coupling and defocussing of the beam due to air entrapment and deposition of energy at the skin surface leading to skin burn (Fig. 32.21).
- Scarring: Rarely happens if correct treatment protocol and technique is not followed.

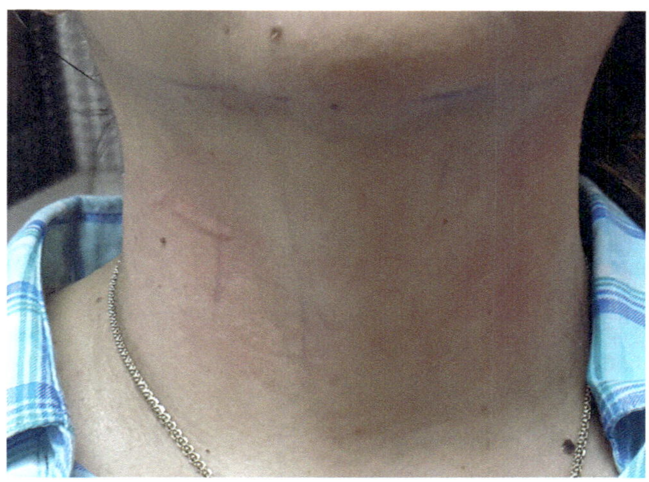



**Fig. 32.21** Complication during HIFU—erythema and skin burn

### 32.4.7 Conclusion

HIFU can be considered as a very effective, non-invasive and safe procedure for tightening the facial skin. The advantages over a surgical facelift are hard to deny. There are no incisions, no scarring and no downtime. Of course, it is much less expensive than a surgical facelift. If patients are chosen carefully, like patients with mild to moderate skin laxity, facial wrinkles, lower eyelid laxity, etc., HIFU can be an excellent option for facial skin tightening.

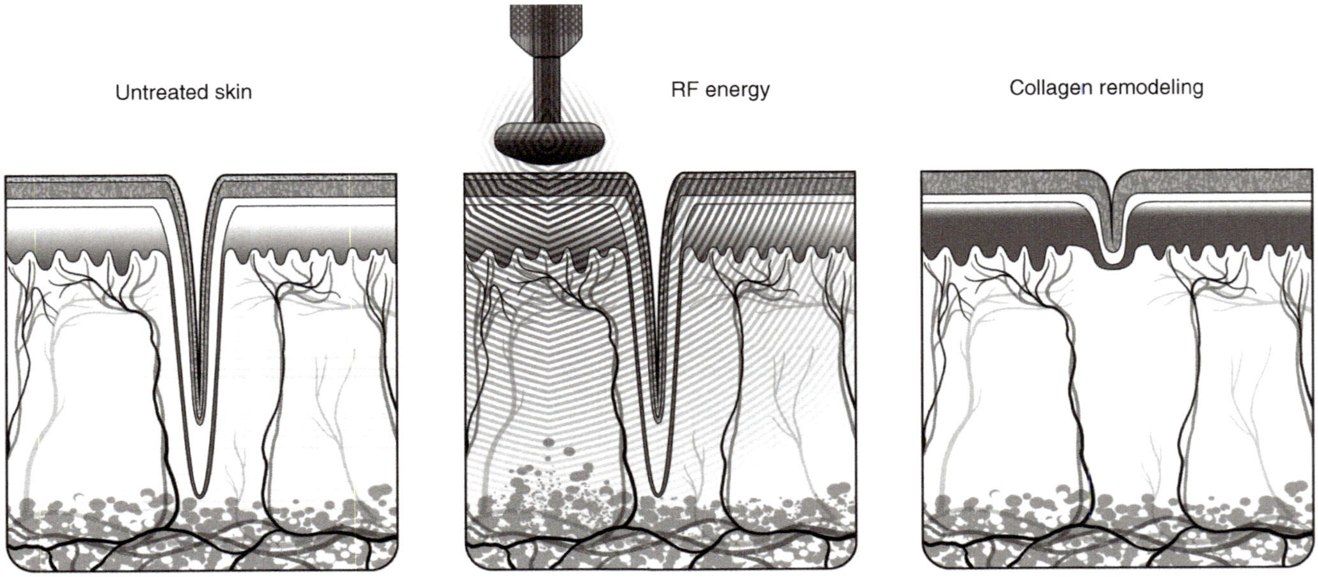




**Fig. 32.22** Mechanism of action of non-ablative radiofrequency. Collagen remodelling takes place because of the heat generated due to the tissue resistance to radiofrequency energy

## 32.5 Skin Tightening with Radiofrequency

Non-ablative radiofrequency or RF is another non-surgical and non-invasive modality of skin tightening. The selective and controlled rise in tissue temperature is because of a high-frequency alternating current (0.3–10 MHz). The amount of energy applied and the tissue resistance determine the amount of temperature and the depth of heating [34].

Since electrical current produces the RF energy, the tissue damage like a laser is minimised and neither is the epidermal melanin compromised to cause hyperpigmentation.

RF therapy was first FDA approved as a non-invasive treatment modality in periorbital rhytids in 2002. Subsequently in 2004 it was cleared for full face. Since then, it has become a very popular non-invasive treatment modality for the facial skin tightening.

### 32.5.1 Principle of Action

High frequency (0.3–10 MHz) alternating current is utilised in a RF therapy. Intrinsic tissue resistance (impedance) to the passage of electrons converts the electric current to thermal energy causing heat generation. Ohm's Law relationships state that:

$$\text{Power}(P) = I^2 \times R \text{ and Energy}(E) = P \times T$$

Hence, Energy $(E) = I^2 \times R \times T$ (where $I$ = current, $R$ = tissue impedance and $T$ = time of application). The level of energy of the alternating current and tissue resistance determines the amount of rise in temperature and the depth of heating. High tissue resistance as demonstrated by subcutaneous fat generate more heat [35]. The thermal damage thus caused stimulates the alterations in collagen configuration and produces neocollagenesis in deep layers of skin and subcutaneous tissue (Fig. 32.22).

Significant results can be observed 2 months post-application of radiofrequency energy. Histological pictures after each session demonstrated expansion of the papillary dermis due to oedema and vascular congestion, followed by accumulation of intercellular substance. Post 2 months treatment histological pictures showed escalated amount of collagen, elastic fibres and mucopolysaccharides [36].

### 32.5.2 Armamentarium

There are 2 major components of the RF machine: the RF generator and the handheld tips (Fig. 32.23). The membrane electrode functions by dispersing energy uniformly across the skin surface by a mechanism termed as capacitive coupling that creates a zone of raised temperature at depths of 3–6 mm [37]. The energy transmitted to the skin is by utilising the capacitive method (bipolar, tripolar or multipolar electrode). Montesi et al. (2007) described the main difference between the inductive and the capacitive method. It depends on the configuration of the electrodes that are applied to the skin that influences the energy transmission in the tissues.

The inductive method (monopolar electrode) uses an active and a passive electrode, in which the passive electrode acts as a grounding electrode. The active electrode transmits power to the tissue via a single point of contact. This enhances the penetration of the generated current.

In the capacitive method (bipolar, tripolar or multipolar electrode), energy alternates between 2 electrodes situated at a short distance from one another. In the tripolar and multipolar devices, bipolar energy switches between different poles at any given point of time. The energy is concentrated at the site of treatment and the achieved depth is half of the distance between the two electrodes [38].

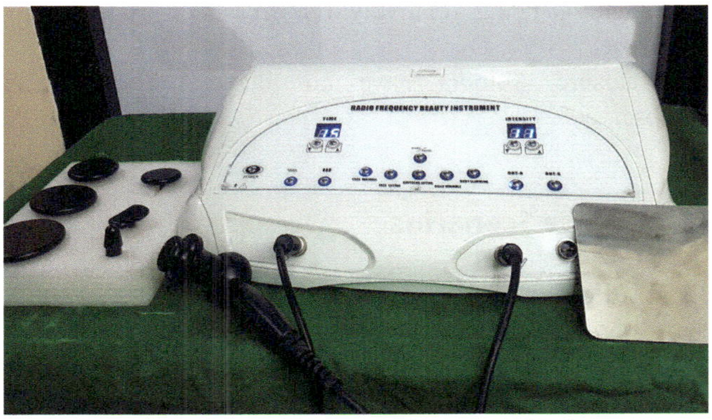



**Fig. 32.23** Non-ablative radiofrequency device

Parameters utilised by the device includes frequency ranging from 1 to 6 MHz and the power ranging from 40 to 240 W. All the parameters can be modified during the treatment. Throughout the procedure, the temperature of epidermis is maintained at 40 °C, whereas that of dermis rises to about 50–75 °C. This heating up of the dermis causes new collagen and elastin production.

### 32.5.3 Indications

The various indications of RF include the following:

1. Complete facial rejuvenation.
2. Wrinkles around eye
3. Fine lines on forehead.
4. Jowls
5. Nasolabial folds (Fig. 32.24)
6. Perioral fine lines
7. Undefined jaw line

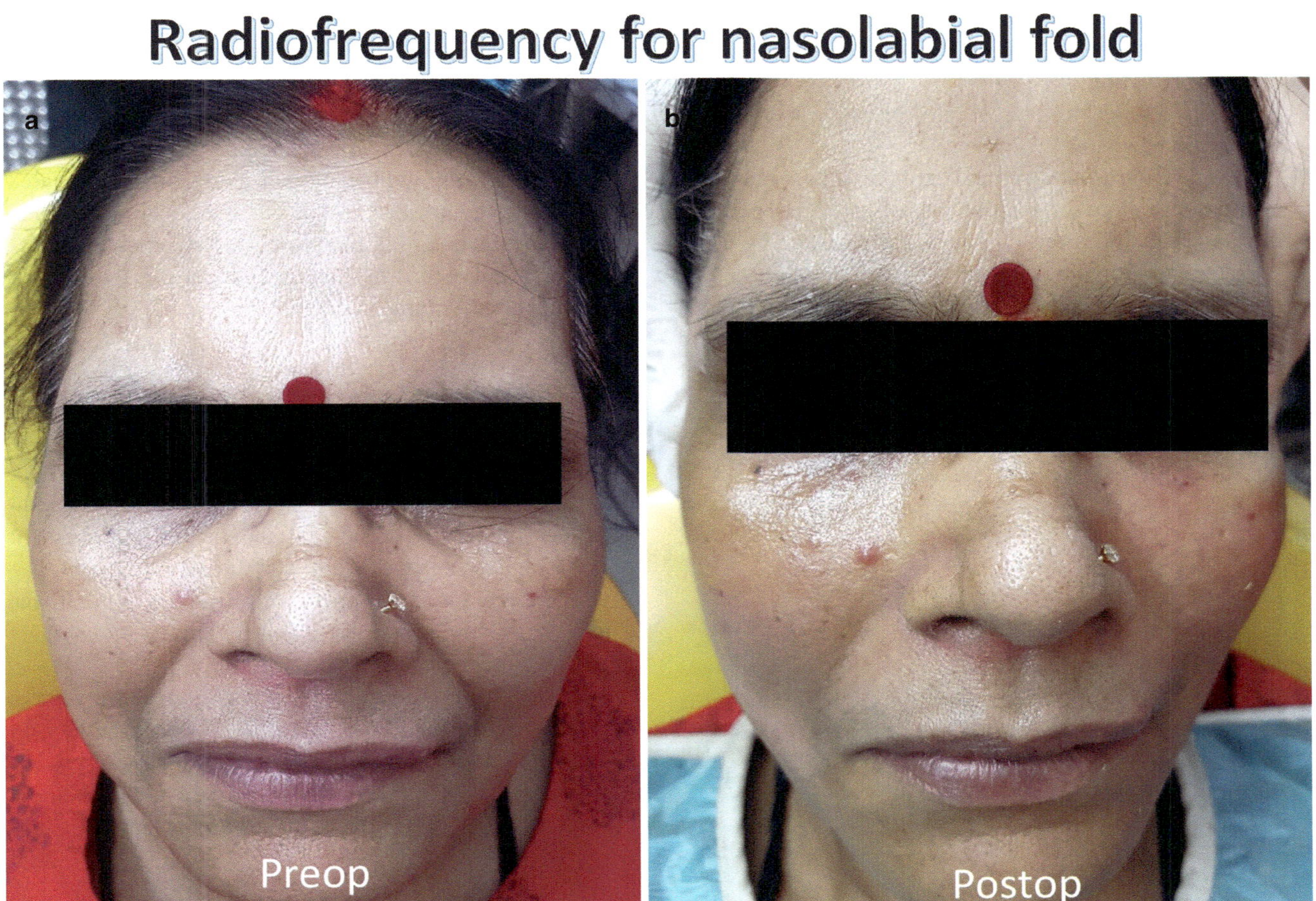




**Fig. 32.24** (**a**, **b**) Nonablative radiofrequency for tightening nasolabial folds

### 32.5.4 Advantages

The biggest advantage of RF is unlike lasers, the energy does not disturb the epidermal melanocytes and thus can be used for all skin types, i.e. type 1–6. The procedure can be performed frequently as per requirement without any adverse effect and different depths of tissue can be treated, allowing for ultimate collagen contraction and production of new collagen.

### 32.5.5 Procedure of RF for Face

Application of RF is done systematically and the various steps involved are mentioned below.

1. Patient consent for the treatment is mandatory after a detailed explanation of the procedure, side effects, benefits and alternatives.
2. Removal of all make-up from face.
3. Cleansing of the full face and neck area.
4. Application of prilocaine and lignocaine skin anaesthetic cream like toplap, prilido, etc.
5. Ultrasound gel is applied generously to the facial skin to establish uniform thermal and electrical contact between the treatment tip and the skin and to enhance proper energy conduction.
6. For each session, a total of 5–8 passes per treatment region can be given.
7. Removal of ultrasound gel and explaining post-operative instructions before discharging the patient. Post-operative instruction includes prevention of sun exposure by using sunscreen to promote healing.
8. Follow up on the next day to assess any complications and at 1, 3, 5 weeks to repeat the procedure and at 3 and 6 months to assess the results. The possible side effects of RF application are found in Box 32.1.

**Box 32.1 Side Effects of RF Treatment**

1. Burns
2. Permanent scarring
3. Skin pigmentations
4. Deeper skin fat loss.
5. Mild swelling of the treated skin.
6. Redness.
7. Sinking of the treated area.
8. Skin sensitivity.

## 32.6 Conclusion

Non-ablative radiofrequency is an effective and non-invasive modality for tightening and rejuvenating wrinkled, photoaged facial skin and contour facial skin laxity. It works on the principle of stimulation repair process by producing new collagen and elastin and by reversing the clinical and the histopathological signs of ageing. The procedure has an added advantage of being relatively risk-free with little or no downtime.

Disclosure Authors have no financial conflicts to disclose.

## 32.7 Case Scenarios

### 32.7.1 Patient 1 (Fig. 32.25a–d)

A 48-year female approached us with complaints of sagging skin. She wasn't happy with her deepening nasolabial folds, loose skin in her neck and the fine wrinkling on her face.

Treatment options included surgical facelift, thread lift therapy and non-invasive therapies like HIFU and RF. The patient consented to undergo non-invasive treatment which included a session of High intensity focussed ultrasound (HIFU).

After cleansing the face, proper markings were made. The treatment was performed with sequential transducers of 4.5, 3 and 1.5 mm with number of shot as recommended, area wise. The patient was evaluated post-operatively and patient's satisfaction was recorded. Post-operative instructions were given before discharging. Patient was recalled for revaluation after 1 month.

### 32.7.2 Patient 2 (Fig. 32.26a–g)

A 52-year male approached us with complaints of loose skin on the face. His main concern was the deepening nasolabial folds and the fine wrinkling on the face. The treatment options included surgical facelift and thread lift therapy. The patient consented to get a thread lift procedure done. It was decided to use 3 COG threads along with 20 mono PDO threads on either side.

After cleansing the face with povidone iodine, vectors were marked to lift the nasolabial folds. Lignocaine with adrenalin was used as local anaesthetic agent. The thread lift procedure with COGS thread was performed with placement of the COGS in the subcutaneous layer for the proper lift and

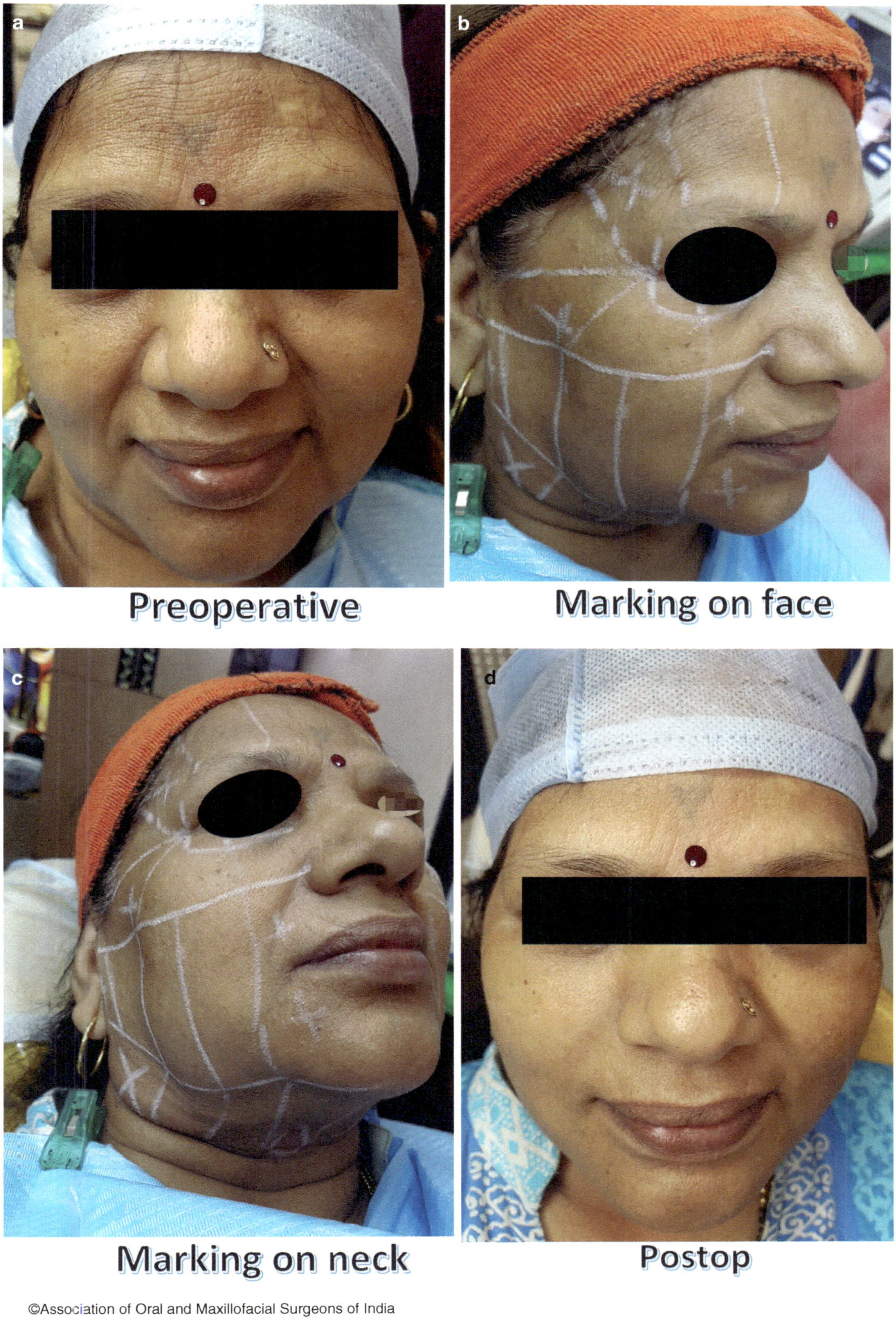


**Fig. 32.25** (**a**–**b**) Case Scenario 1. (**a**) Pre-op photograph. (**b**, **c**) Marking on face and neck, right side. (**d**) Post-op photograph

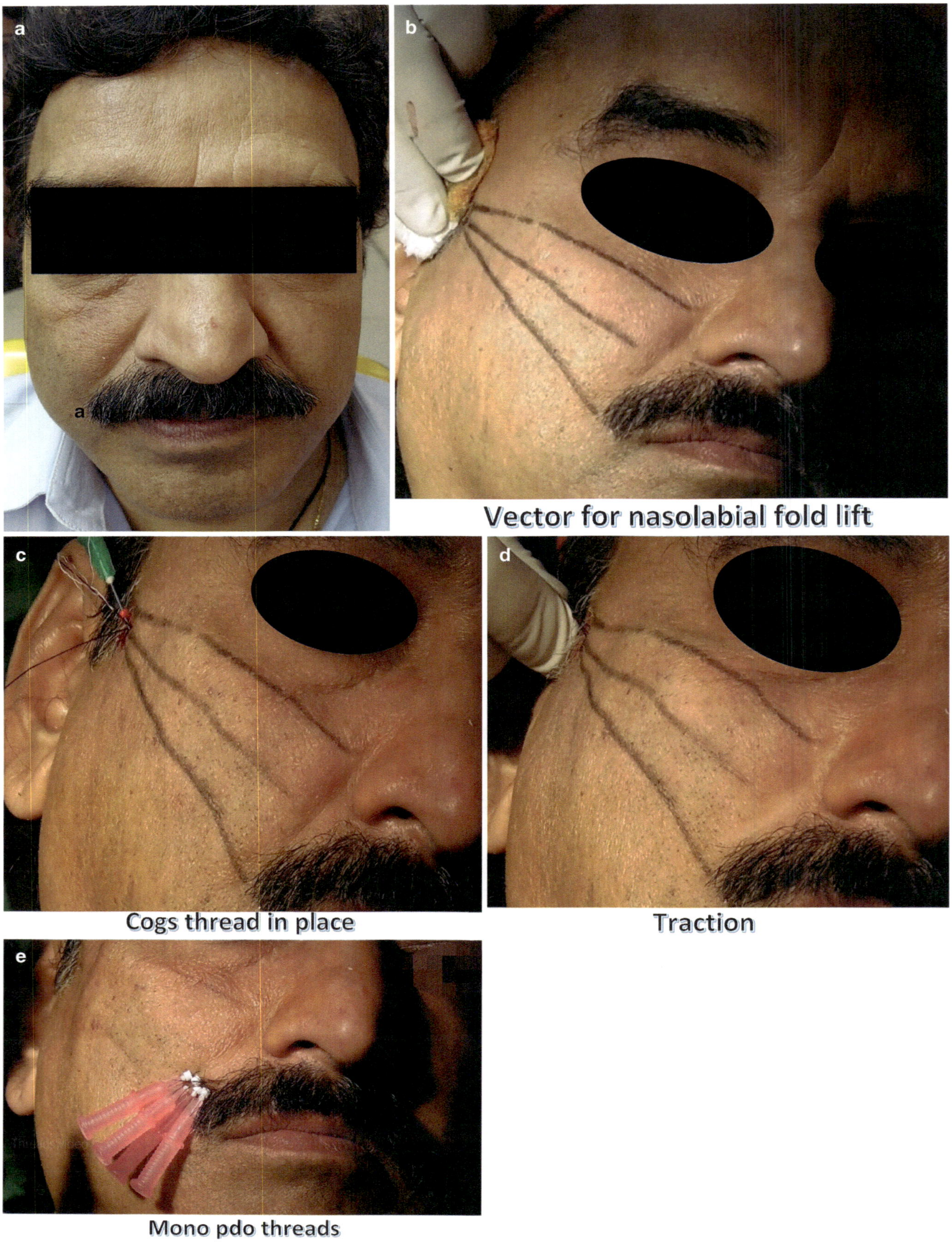


**Fig. 32.26** Case Scenario 2. (**a**) Pre-op photograph. (**b**) Marking of vectors. (**c**) 3 cogs in place at subcutaneous layer. (**d**) The traction on threads lifts the nasolabials. (**e**) Placement of mono PDOS. (**f**, **g**) Post-op photograph (also see Fig. 32.10)

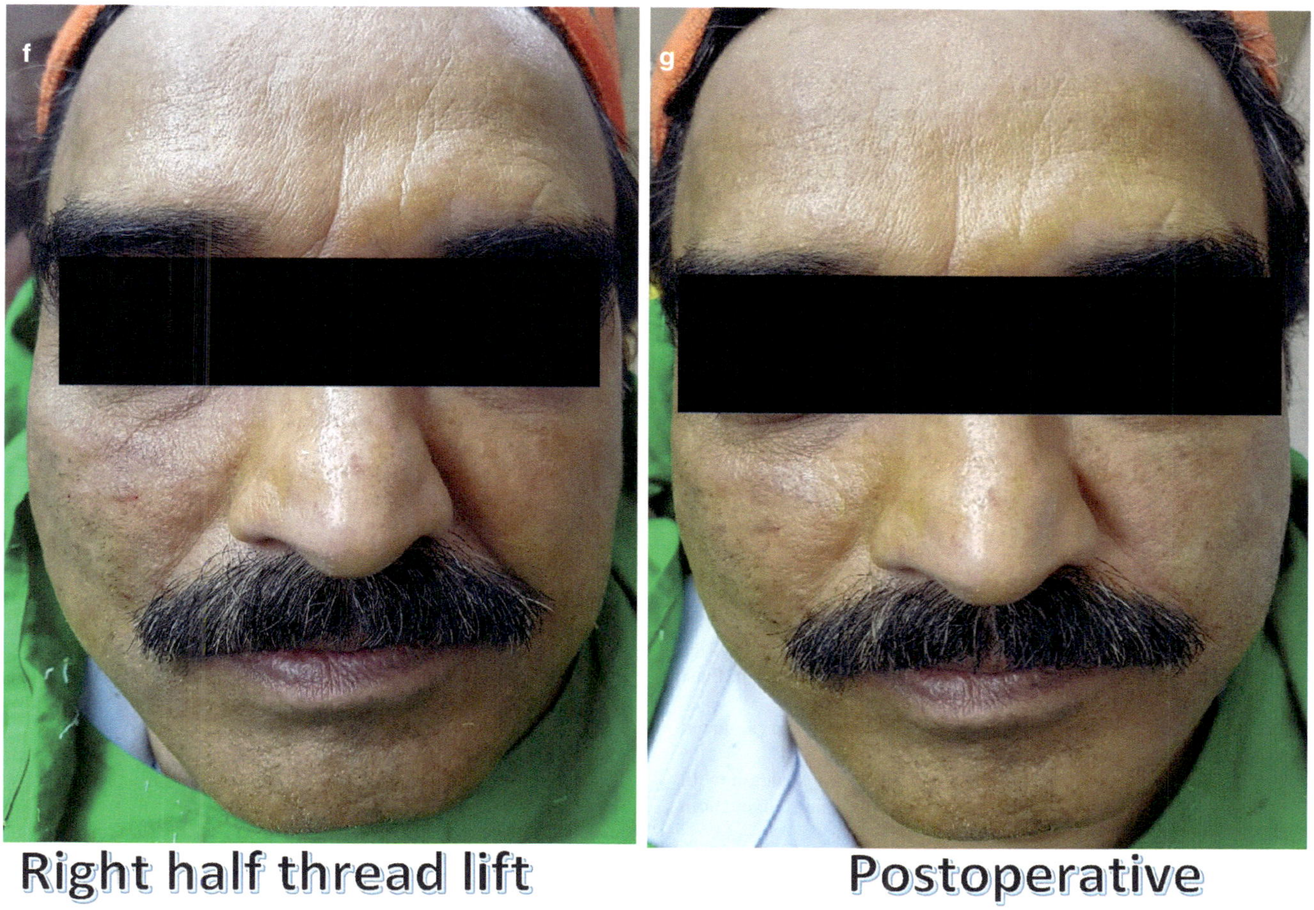




**Fig. 32.26** (continued)

the mono PDO at the dermal layer for rejuvenation and fine lines.

The patient was evaluated post-operatively and patient's satisfaction was recorded. Post-operative instructions were given before discharging. Patient was recalled for revaluation after 3 days and after 1 month.

## References


1. Rohrich RJ, Pessa JE. The fat compartments of the face: anatomy and clinical implications for cosmetic surgery. Plast Reconstr Surg. 2007;119(7):2219–27.
2. Furnas DW. The retaining ligaments of the cheek. Plast Reconstr Surg. 1989;83(1):11–6.
3. Wulc AE, Sharma P, Czyz CN. The anatomic basis of midfacial aging. In: Midfacial rejuvenation. New York, NY: Springer; 2012. p. 15–28.
4. Donofrio LM. Fat distribution: a morphologic study of the aging face. Dermatol Surg. 2000;26(12):1107–12.
5. Lambros V. Observations on periorbital and midface aging. Plast Reconstr Surg. 2007;120(5):1367–76.
6. Gosain AK, Yousif NJ, Madiedo G, Larson DL, Matloub HS, Sanger JR. Surgical anatomy of the SMAS: a reinvestigation. Plast Reconstr Surg. 1993;92(7):1254–63.
7. Owsley JJ. SMAS-platysma facelift. A bidirectional cervicofacial rhytidectomy. Clin Plast Surg. 1983;10(3):429–40.
8. Mendelson B, Wong CH. Changes in the facial skeleton with aging: implications and clinical applications in facial rejuvenation. Aesthet Plast Surg. 2012;36(4):753–60.
9. Mendelson BC, Hartley W, Scott M, McNab A, Granzow JW. Age-related changes of the orbit and midcheek and the implications for facial rejuvenation. Aesthet Plast Surg. 2007;31(5): 419–23.
10. Shaw RB Jr, Kahn DM. Aging of the midface bony elements: a three-dimensional computed tomographic study. Plast Reconstr Surg. 2007;119(2):675–81.
11. Rohrich RJ, Hollier LH Jr, Janis JE, Kim J. Rhinoplasty with advancing age. Plast Reconstr Surg. 2004;114(7):1936–44.
12. Shaw RB Jr, Katzel EB, Koltz PF, Kahn DM, Girotto JA, Langstein HN. Aging of the mandible and its aesthetic implications. Plast Reconstr Surg. 2010;125(1):332–42.
13. Garvey PB, Ricciardelli EJ, Gampper T. Outcomes in threadlift for facial rejuvenation. Ann Plast Surg. 2009;62(5):482–5.
14. Kuang R, Wang Z, Xu Q, Liu S, Zhang W. Influence of mechanical stimulation on human dermal fibroblasts derived from different body sites. Int J Clin Exp Med. 2015;8(5):7641.
15. Amuso D, Amore R, Iorio EL, Dolcemascolo R, Reggiani LB, Leonardi V. Histological evaluation of a biorevitalisation treatment with PDO wires. Union of Aesthetic Medicine–UIME. 2015;1(3): 1–7.
16. World Academy of Science, Engineering and Technology. Int J Med Health Sci. 2016;10(12).
17. Suh DH, Jang HW, Lee SJ, Lee WS, Ryu HJ. Outcomes of polydioxanone knotless thread lifting for facial rejuvenation. Dermatol Surg. 2015;41(6):720–5.
18. Nurden AT. Platelets, inflammation and tissue regeneration. Thromb Haemost. 2011;105(S 06):S13–33.
19. Steed DL. The role of growth factors in wound healing. Surg Clin N Am. 1997;77(3):575–86.
20. Kevy S, Jacobson M, Blasetti L, Fagnant A. Preparation of growth factor enriched autologous platelet gel. In Proceedings of the 27th Annual meeting of Service Biomaterials; 2001 April 26. p. 15–18.
21. Ehrenfest DM, Andia I, Zumstein MA, Zhang CQ, Pinto NR, Bielecki T. Classification of platelet concentrates (Platelet-Rich Plasma-PRP, Platelet-Rich Fibrin-PRF) for topical and infiltrative use in orthopedic and sports medicine: current consensus, clinical implications and perspectives. Muscles Ligaments Tendons J. 2014;4(1):3.
22. Marx RE. Platelet-rich plasma (PRP): what is PRP and what is not PRP? Implant Dent. 2001;10(4):225–8.
23. CHo JW, Kim S, Lee KS. Platelet-rich plasma induces increased expression of G1 cell cycle regulators, type I collagen, and matrix metalloproteinase-1 in human skin fibroblasts. Int J Mol Med. 2012;29(1):32–6.
24. Kim DH, Je YJ, Kim CD, Lee YH, Seo YJ, Lee JH, Lee Y. Can platelet-rich plasma be used for skin rejuvenation? Evaluation of effects of platelet-rich plasma on human dermal fibroblast. Ann Dermatol. 2011;23(4):424–31.
25. Kang B, Lee J, Shin M, Kim N. Infraorbital rejuvenation using PRP (platelet-rich plasma): a prospective, randomized, split-face trial. J Am Acad Dermatol. 2013;1:68(4).
26. International Cellular Medicine Society Guidelines. Section X—uidelines for the Use of Platelet Rich Plasma. Adopted 2011 (Cited 2019, May 20). Available from http://www.cellmedicinesociety.org/icms-guidelines/guidelines
27. Mendonça RD, Rodrigues GB. As principais alterações dermatológicas em pacientes obesos. Arq Bras Cir Dig. 2011;24(1): 68–73.
28. She WH, Cheung TT, Jenkins CR, Irwin MG. Clinical applications of high-intensity focused ultrasound. Hong Kong Med J. 2016;22(4):382–92.
29. Brown MR, Farquhar-Smith P, Williams JE, Ter Haar G, Desouza NM. The use of high-intensity focused ultrasound as a novel treatment for painful conditions—a description and narrative review of the literature. Br J Anaesth. 2015;115(4):520–30.
30. White WM, Makin IR, Barthe PG, Slayton MH, Gliklich RE. Selective creation of thermal injury zones in the superficial musculoaponeurotic system using intense ultrasound therapy: a new target for noninvasive facial rejuvenation. Arch Facial Plast Surg. 2007;9(1):22–9.
31. Jolesz FA, Hynynen K, McDannold N, Tempany C. MR imaging–controlled focused ultrasound ablation: a noninvasive image-guided surgery. Magn Reson Imaging Clin N Am. 2005;13(3): 545–60.
32. Fabi SG. Noninvasive skin tightening: focus on new ultrasound techniques. Clin Cosmet Investig Dermatol. 2015;8:47.
33. Suh DH, Oh YJ, Lee SJ, Rho JH, Song KY, Kim NI, Shin MK. A intense-focused ultrasound tightening for the treatment of infraorbital laxity. J Cosmet Laser Ther. 2012;14(6):290–5.
34. Belenky I, Margulis A, Elman M, Bar-Yosef U, Paun SD. Exploring channeling optimized radiofrequency energy: a review of radiofrequency history and applications in esthetic fields. Adv Ther. 2012;29(3):249–66.
35. Atiyeh BS, Dibo SA. Nonsurgical nonablative treatment of aging skin: radiofrequency technologies between aggressive marketing and evidence-based efficacy. Aesthet Plast Surg. 2009;33(3): 283–94.

36. Alvarez N, Ortiz L, Vicente V, Alcaraz M, Sánchez-Pedreño P. The effects of radiofrequency on skin: experimental study. Lasers Surg Med. 2008;40(2):76–82.
37. Bassichis BA, Dayan S, Thomas JR. Use of a nonablative radiofrequency device to rejuvenate the upper one-third of the face. Otolaryngol Head Neck Surg. 2004;130(4):397–406.
38. Montesi G, Calvieri S, Balzani A, Gold MH. Bipolar radiofrequency in the treatment of dermatologic imperfections: clinicopathological and immunohistochemical aspects. J Drugs Dermatol. 2007;6(9):890–6.

# Botulinum Toxin and Fillers for Maxillofacial Esthetics

# 33

Sainath Matsa

## 33.1 Introduction

### 33.1.1 Facial Aesthetics

The field of cosmetology has steadily progressed over the past decade, and cosmetic procedures are moving towards a new era [1]. People are becoming more aware of the way they look, especially the face and are turning to medical and dental professionals to improve their appearance. Attractive facial aesthetics at any age has social and psychological benefits. Facial skin constitutes a major part in contributing to facial aesthetics. The skin is a reflection of several body characteristics, of which gender is a prominent one [1]. Age, genetic, hormonal and exogenous factors can affect both skin structure and function and are responsible for differences between different men and women. This chapter gives the basics and advances in the field of facial cosmetic and functional correction using Neurotoxins (Botulinum toxin) and Dermal Fillers.

### 33.1.2 Facial Skin Physiology, Muscular Anatomy and Mechanical Properties

In humans, skin including the epidermis and dermis is 1.428 times thicker in men than in women across 5–90 years of age [1]. However, women tend to have thicker subcutaneous fat. It has been found that, in men, it gradually becomes thinner with advancing age (12–93 years), whereas in women, the skin thickness remains constant till the fifth decade, after which it tends to decrease [2].

Gender plays an important role in facial wrinkling. In men, the incidence of forehead wrinkles is higher than in women. However, the incidence of upper eyelid wrinkles does not appear to be influenced by gender. Wrinkles in other parts of the face are found to be greater in men than in women, except above 65 years of age, when the incidence appears to equalise [3]. One study evaluated the skin morphology, elasticity and areas of sagging using photographs and a cutometer. The authors found that these were similar in both genders in the cheek region, but in the lower eyelids, sagging was more severe in males after middle age [4, 5].

### 33.1.3 Facial Muscles and Their Actions (Fig. 33.1)

A good understanding of the action of the various facial muscles is important for precise application of botulinum toxin. The muscles and their actions are tabulated (Table 33.1).

## 33.2 Botulinum Toxin

### 33.2.1 Botulinum Toxin-Type A

Botulinum Toxin type A was first used on the face by Carruthers and Carruthers in the late 1980s [6]. Following studies in the 1990s about its cosmetic use, botulinum toxin was approved by the USA Food and Drug Administration (FDA). This led to a revolution in treating ageing skin in recent years [1].

---

**Electronic Supplementary Material** The online version of this chapter (https://doi.org/10.1007/978-981-15-1346-6_33) contains supplementary material, which is available to authorized users.

S. Matsa (✉)
Praseedha Clinic for Maxillofacial Cosmetic Surgery, Chennai, Tamil Nadu, India



K. Bonanthaya et al. (eds.), *Oral and Maxillofacial Surgery for the Clinician*, https://doi.org/10.1007/978-981-15-1346-6_33

Fig. 33.1 Muscles of facial expression

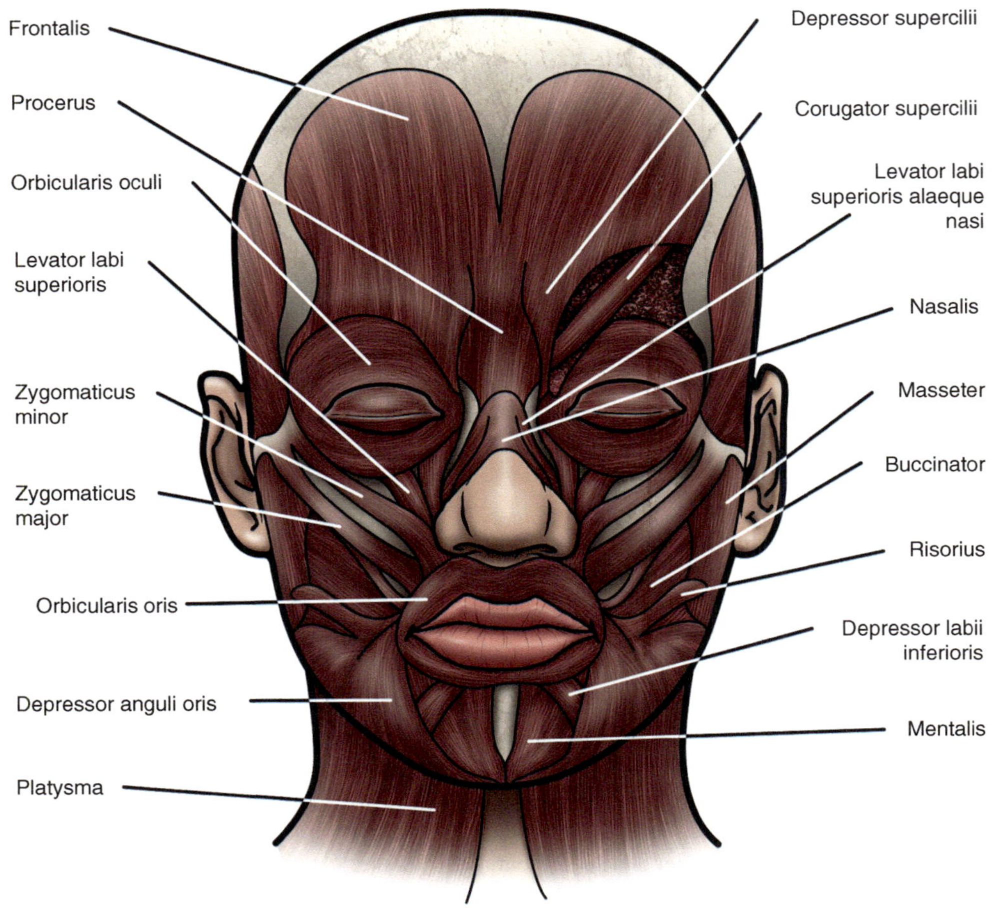


Table 33.1 Facial Muscles and Their Actions

| |
|---|
| *Frontalis*—Raising the eyebrows; transverse wrinkling of the forehead |
| *Corrugator*—Vertical/oblique wrinkling of the forehead; draws the eyebrows together |
| *Procerus*—Pulls the glabellar skin in an inferior direction and causes transverse wrinkles |
| *Depressor Supercilii*—Pulls the eyebrow downwards on the medial canthal region |
| *Orbicularis Oculi*—Controls the sphincter of the eye |
| *Risorius*—Lateral movement of the corner of the mouth |
| *Orbicularis Oris*—Opening and closing of the mouth (sphincter action) |
| *Levator Labii Superioris*—Pulls the upper lip superiorly |
| *Depressor Anguli Oris*—Draws the corner of the mouth inferiorly |
| *Depressor Labii Inferioris*—Pulls the lower lip downwards |
| *Modiolus*—It's a union of muscles, situated lateral to the external commissure of the mouth, allowing symmetrical perioral expression. |

### 33.2.2 Pharmacology and Mechanism of Action

Clostridium botulinum produces an exotoxin. It is an anaerobic gram positive bacillus (Fig. 33.2) which forms spores. It has eight types of strains which are labelled alphabetically: A, B, C, D, E, F, G, and H [7].

Two types of strains, A and B, are available currently. These result from the modification of the protein structure that has been used for a variety of medical and cosmetic purpose. Botulinum Neurotoxin causes denervation of the motor neuron temporarily, in the treated muscle and selectively inactivates the nerve terminals by blocking the release of acetylcholine and the target protein SNAP25, [8] leading to a temporary and reversible blockade of cholinergic transmission. In the neuromuscular junction, the blockade of the release of acetylcholine promotes muscle relaxation to muscular palsy [9] (Fig. 33.3a, b, c).

**Reconstitution, Dilution and Dose:**

Botulinum Toxin Type-A is available as lyophilised powder that must be stored frozen −4 °C or lower. Reconstitution of the powder may be done using 0.9% Normal Saline solution, which is isotonic. Once reconstituted, the solution must be used within 4–8 h, after which the potency of the drug may be lost, and contamination of the vials may occur.

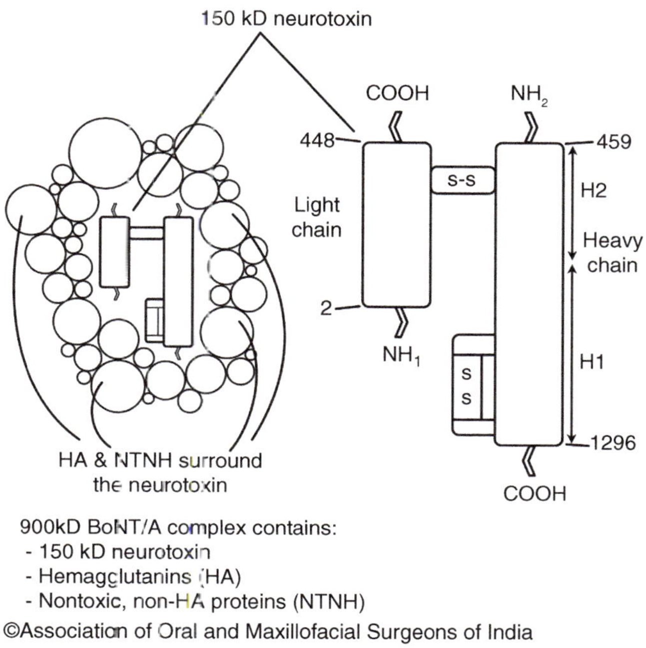


Fig. 33.2 Chemical structure

- Botulinum toxin A is marketed in two vials—50 and 100 U.
- In mice, the *Median Lethal Dose* is 1 U. The *MLD* in humans is estimated at 3000 U.
- For reconstituting 100 U, 2.5 ml of 0.9% Normal Saline may be used, which gives a concentration of 40 U/ml.

Many commercial brands are available for Botulinum Neurotoxin–A, like Siax®, Botox®, Xeomin® and Dysport® and every brand has variation in its dilution.

### 33.2.3 Indications

Botulinum toxin injections may be used in the clinical scenarios highlighted in Box 33.1.

**Box 33.1 Indications of Botulinum Toxin**
- Wrinkling of the face
- Facial rejuvenation of ageing face
- Gingival smile
- Masseteric hypertrophy
- Facial asymmetry
- Platysmal wrinkling and bands
- Hyperhidrotic conditions (excessive sweating)
- Blepharospasm
- Spasmodic torticollis
- Dystonia
  - cranial, lower facial, cervical, oromandibular.

#### 33.2.3.1 Contraindications [10]

The use of Botulinum toxin injections is contraindicated in the following clinical situations:

- Pregnancy and breastfeeding.
- Individuals with an infection in the proposed area of the injection.
- Neuromuscular transmission disorders (myasthenia gravis).
- Individuals under medications that may influence neuromuscular transmission. These include Calcium channel blockers, Penicillamine, Quinine, Aminoglycosides, Pancuronium, Tubocurarine and Succinylcholine.
- Individuals under medications that interfere with coagulation like Acetylsalicylic Acid, Anticoagulants and Vitamin E.

**Patient Selection:**

In the present era, patients have increased awareness and knowledge about their health and skin conditions. They may be very ambitious and optimistic about the procedure and are likely to expect a high level of satisfaction with their personal appearance after the treatment. The goal of treatment is to achieve a better looking and natural appearance. The patients' psychological aspects and expectations should be understood and evaluated prior to the start of any cosmetic treatment.

### 33.2.4 Injection Techniques (Video 33.1)

The following techniques are used for injecting botulinum toxin into various areas of the face.

(a) *Glabellar lines injection technique* (Fig. 33.4a, b): Visualise an imaginary "X" formed by two lines that join the inner brows with the contralateral inner canthus [11]. The injection must be given at the midpoint of the 'X'. Conventionally, the Corrugator Supercilii muscle is visualised by observing the medial part of the eyebrow when the patient frowns. Botulinum Toxin is then slowly injected into the belly [11] of the muscle on either side. The needle must be maintained at 0.5 cm from the upper orbital rim, and lie internal to the mid-pupillary line. The total dose for glabellar line ranges from 10 to 15 U and can be increased to a maximum of 40 U based on the severity of the wrinkles.

(b) *Forehead lines Injection technique* (Fig. 33.5): The frontalis muscle is superficial and may be easily identified by asking the patient to raise and lower the brow. The extent of muscle movement is then assessed. Injections must be done in the superficial subcutaneous tissue, over the entire forehead from medial to lateral. The typical dose ranges from 2 to 3 U in each point of small dots represented on the upper and lower aspects of the forehead or

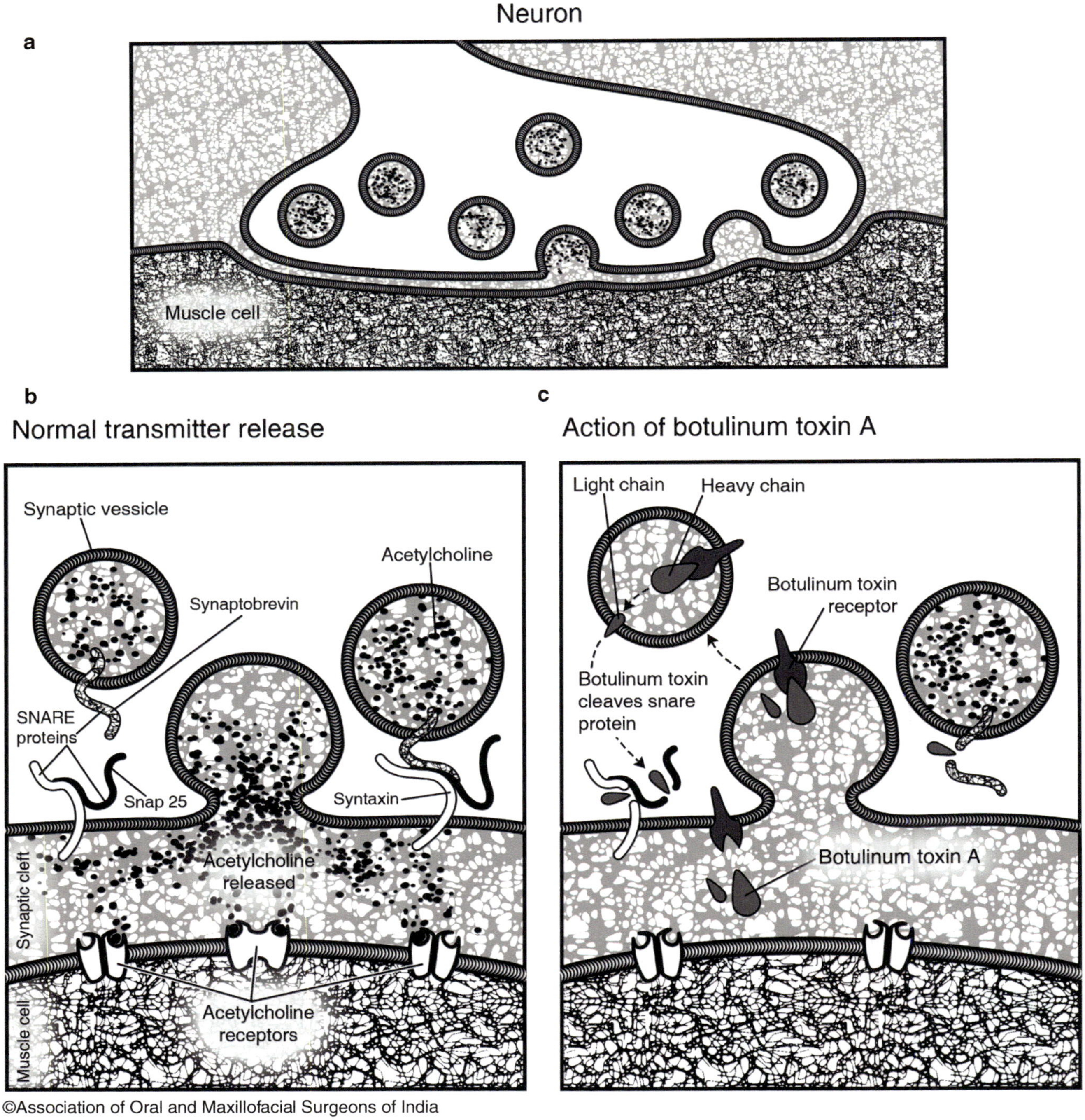


**Fig. 33.3** (**a–c**) Action at the neuromuscular junction

5 U per point of the middle aspect of the muscle, represented in a big dots as given below in the figure. Frontal injections and glabellar injections must preferably be done together, to avoid increased compensatory use of glabellar muscle, which are mainly depressors [12, 13]. The dose of the injections must be kept small enough to just weaken the muscle instead of producing total paralysis. This is because the frontalis is responsible for facial expressiveness, and total paralysis would cause brow ptosis [14, 15]. It is also important to preserve at least some frontal is muscle movement, responsible for facial expression and lift of the eyelids and brows.

(c) *Crow feet wrinkles Injection technique* (Fig. 33.6a, b): Three to four injections of Botulinum toxin-A may be

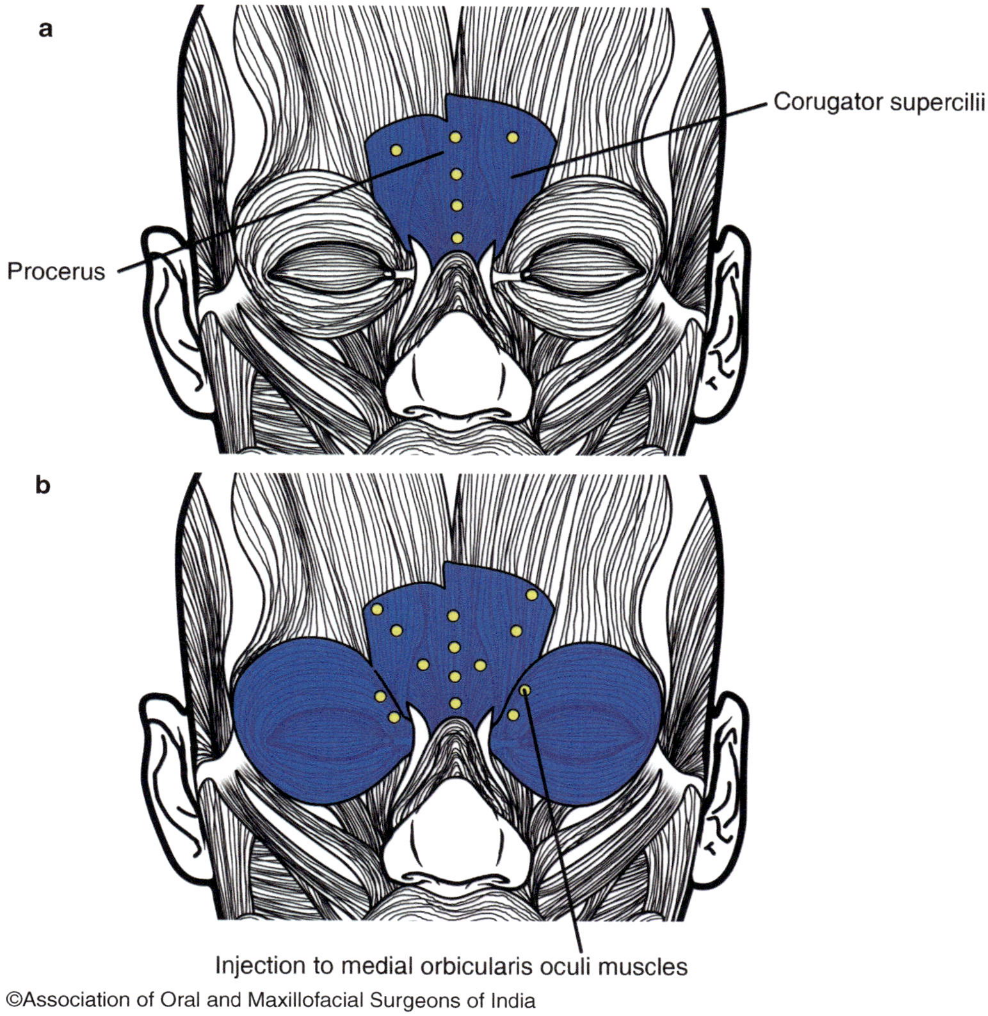


**Fig. 33.4** (**a**, **b**) Glabellar lines injection technique

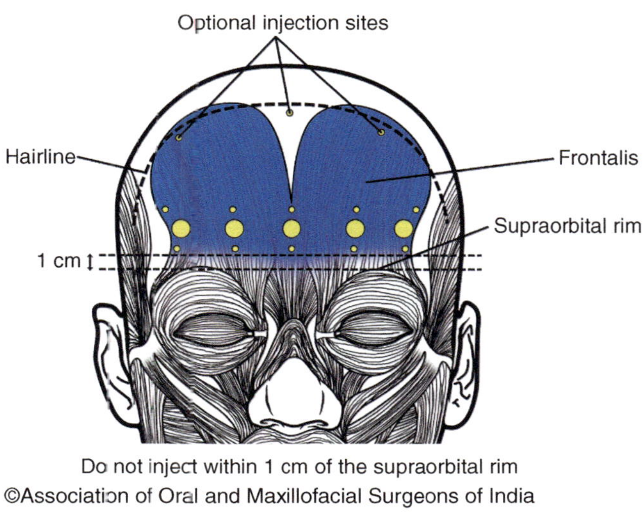


**Fig. 33.5** Forehead lines injection technique

administered lateral to the eye, in the 'crow's feet' region that radiates out from the lateral canthi. Around 8–20 U may be administered on each side [16]. The injection must be placed 1 cm lateral to the orbital rim and must be above the canthal angle, to avoid upper lateral lag. To achieve this, one can place a guiding finger of the other hand at the lateral orbital rim. Owing to the superficial location of the muscle, the needle need not be advanced deep into the subcutaneous tissue. Botulinum Toxin has a wide zone of effect, and therefore a superficial dermal injection will minimise bruising, but will still give good clinical results [16].

(d) *Elevating Oral commissures and Smile line Injection technique* (Fig. 33.7): Depressor anguli oris is the muscle to be elevated for improving the smile lines. It is indicated in patients with inverted smile line (reverse smile line), which is caused by pulling the corner of the mouth inferiorly. To identify the depressor anguli oris muscle, the patient must frown and the muscle must be simultaneously palpated 1 cm lateral and inferior to the oral

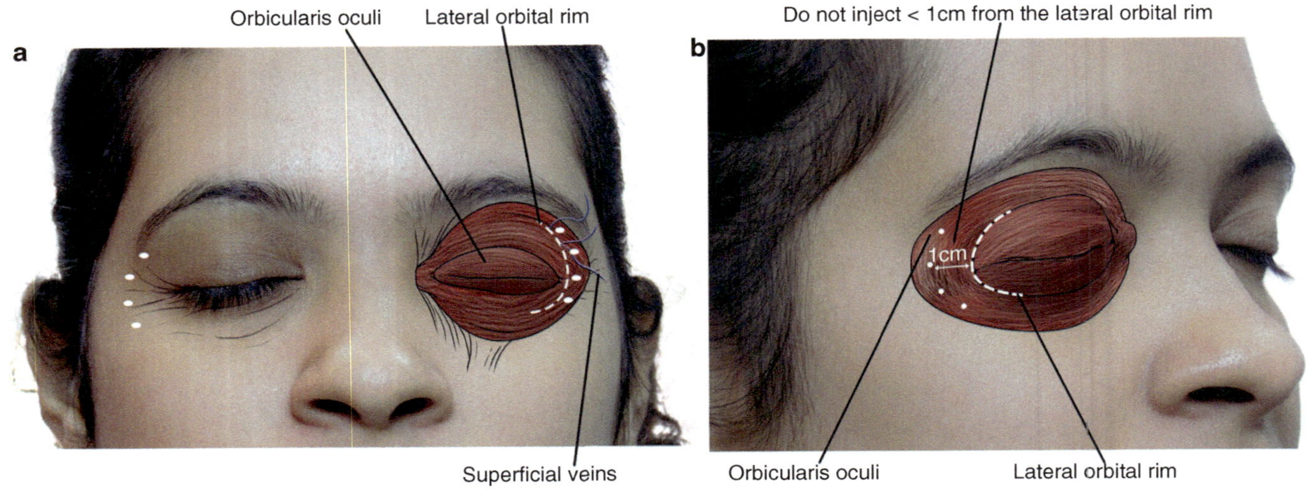




**Fig. 33.6** (**a**, **b**) Crow feet wrinkles injection technique

commissure. Inject approximately 2–5 U deeply into the muscle on either side [16].

(e) *Gummy smile or Gingival show correction Injection technique* (Fig. 33.8): In some patients, while smiling, their upper lip is pulled up, which reveals some amount of gingival tissue. If this is >1 cm, it is referred to as a "*Gummy smile or Gingival Show*". The levator labii superioris alaeque nasi elevates the upper lip during smile. These muscles have their origin on the frontal process of the maxilla, and insert into the skin of the lateral aspect of the nose and upper lip. If only one muscle contracts, it results in a 'snarl', and this muscle has been referred to as the "*Elvis*" muscle [16]. Normally, 1–2 U of the Botulinum neurotoxin is injected on each side in the muscle. Care should be taken because this injection can produce elongation of the upper lip.

(f) *Platysmal wrinkles Injection technique* (Fig. 33.9): The platysma forms horizontal lines or wrinkles. Into every horizontal crease, an intradermal injection of 1–2 U may be injected for every 1.0–1.5 cm [16]. There may be several creases, but each treatment session must not use more than 15–20 U. In these areas, careful injections are absolutely essential, as these muscles are cholinergic, and deep injections may affect swallowing. If the injections are placed at deeper levels, or high volumes are used, a weak or diminished swallow may result.

(g) *Masseteric Hypertrophy Injection technique* (Fig. 33.10): The masseter can give masculine characteristics, such as square jawlines and wide mandibular borders. This is enhanced when the muscle hypertrophies, and may not be attractive in women. Bruxism and clenching of teeth can lead to hypertrophy of the masseter muscle, which in turn increases the horizontal width of the mandible [16]. While injecting into the masseter, one finger may be placed along the lower border of the mandible, one finger along the posterior border and one at mandibular angle. This may be done with the patient clenching, as

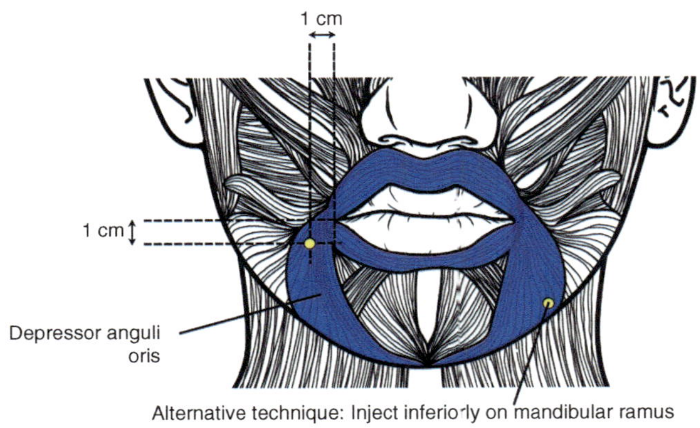




**Fig. 33.7** Smile line correction

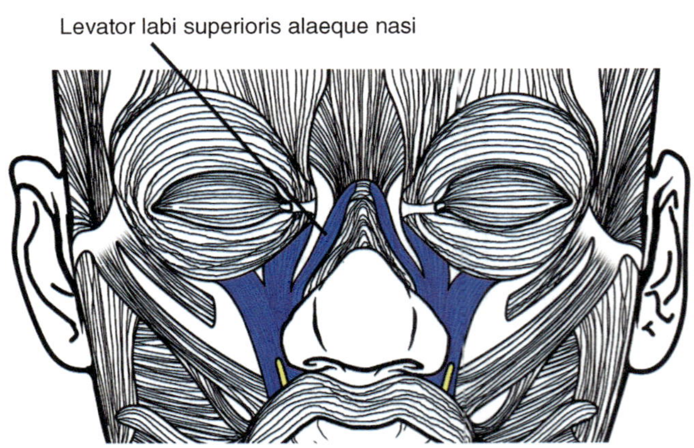




**Fig. 33.8** Gummy smile correction

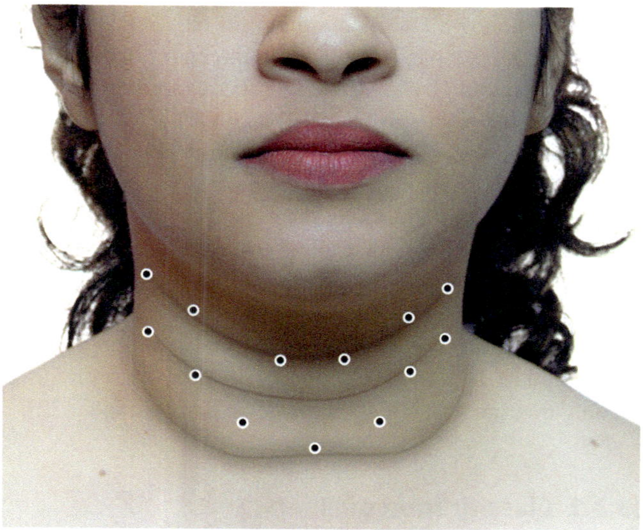

Intradermal injection



**Fig. 33.9** Platysmal banding

this marks the perimeter of the muscle. While injecting bone should be felt by the needle and withdrawn slightly just above the bone and deposit 4–5 U along the marked lines. Depending on the volume of hypertrophy, around 20 U may be injected [16]. Over-injection at the masseter region may result in problems with bite or chewing.

(h) *Frey's Syndrome or Gustatory sweating Injection Technique* (Fig. 33.11): This is a condition in which mild to profuse sweating occurs in the cheek or malar area while eating. A diagnostic test called "*starch-iodine test*" [16] can be performed prior to injection of Botulinum toxin. Povidone iodine is applied over the cheek and corn starch is sprinkled. The patient is advised to eat, to stimulate the salivary gland and left to dry for a few minutes. The corn starch turns black in the area of sweating [16], and a grid is drawn along this area. Once the test is confirmed, usually 30–50 U is injected along the grid as shown. The botulinum toxin blocks acetylcholine, which is the neurotransmitter that stimulates sweating.

### 33.2.5 Complications and Recommendations While Using Botulinum Toxin

- Apply pressure at the site before and after treatment. Cold packs may also be used.
- The use of small syringes and fine-gauge (30 g) needles can reduce pain and bruising at the injected site.
- Using topical anaesthesia (EMLA—Eutectic Mixture of Local Anaesthesia) reduces pain while injecting.

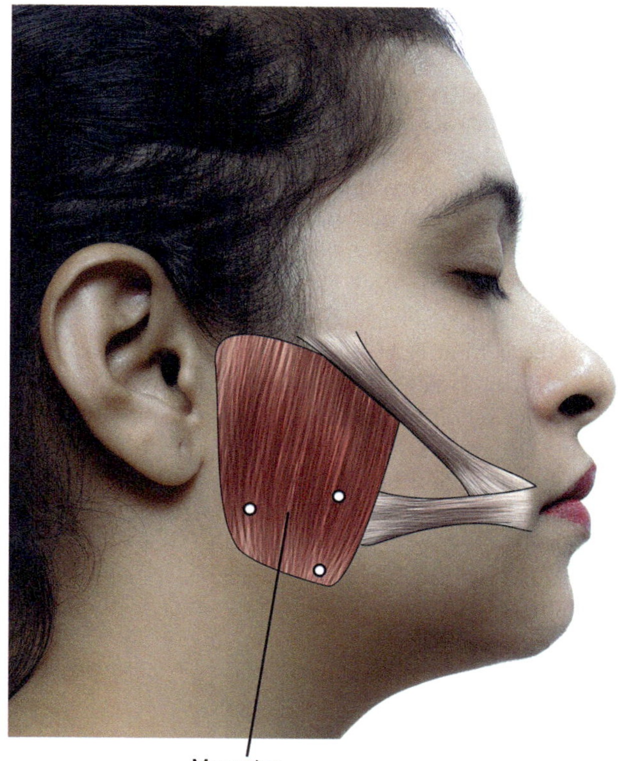





**Fig. 33.10** Masseteric hypertrophy

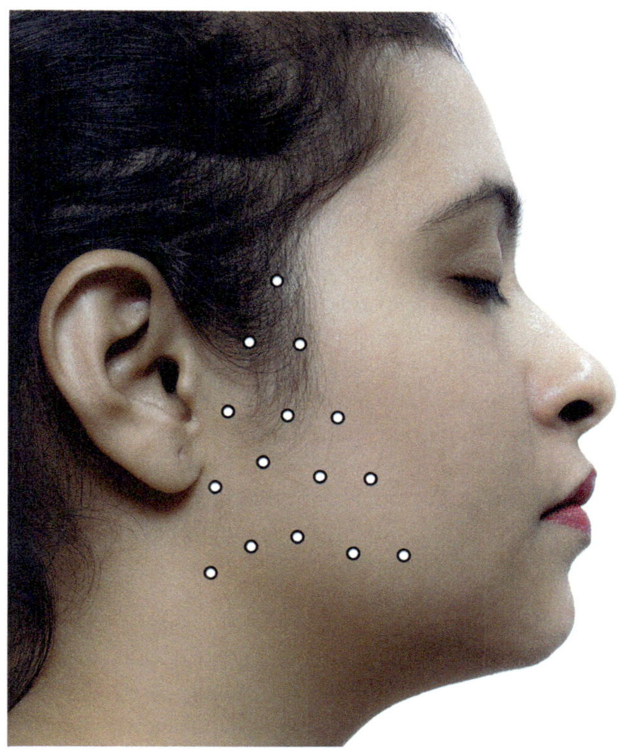



**Fig. 33.11** Frey's Syndrome

- Injections should be symmetrical regarding doses, muscles and areas. This is important for the natural balance of the facial structures and to avoid asymmetries.
- Since the results are expected for 4–6 months, treatments are usually repeated twice a year, for maintenance of the results.
- There are isolated few reports of systemic adverse effects after injections with the use of doses larger than those usually recommended for cosmetic purposes [17].
- The most common injection-related side effects are pain, transient edema at the injected site, erythema, haematomas and ecchymosis [13, 17].
- Common technique-dependent complications include eyelid ptosis, asymmetries and excessive brow elevation.
- In the lower face, complications are related to high doses can cause undesirable paralysis of the musculature, resulting in asymmetric smiling and complications due to the incompetence of the sphincter function of the mouth.
- In the neck, complications can be dysphagia and difficulty in the movements.

## 33.3 Dermal Fillers

### 33.3.1 Role of Fillers in Facial Aesthetics

Throughout the past decades, there have been major changes and advancements in the injectable preparations used for soft tissue augmentation. Introduced by Dr. Arnold Klein [1] in the 1980s, for lip augmentation, collagen has progressed to the broader concept of volumising the face and to correct the subcutaneous atrophy due to ageing and fat loss.

Following extensive clinical trials in the late 1970s, the FDA first approved the use of bovine collagen in 1981, which greatly advanced the field of soft-tissue augmentation. Over the past 10 years, several types of facial fillers have been approved in the United States and Europe, and there is a constantly evolving and expanding assortment of the dermal filler materials and devices for soft tissue augmentation [18].

Hyaluronic Acid (HA), which was introduced as a facial filler in 2003, brought about a much needed change from the allergies being reported due to bovine collagen [18]. Hyaluronic Acid is a member of the glycosaminoglycan family and a natural component of human connective tissue. The HA molecule is identical across all species and lacks a protein component, thus it has little to no potential for immunologic reaction in humans. It is composed of repeating disaccharide units, stabilised with cross-linked hydroxyl groups that bind water to create volume. This gives a plumped appearance to the skin. HA in the skin decreases with age and sun exposure, reducing the skin's water-binding capacity and turgor, ultimately leading to skin wrinkling and sagging [19]. HA can absorb up to 1000 times its molecular weight of water, and Hyaluronic Acid fillers volumise the face by replacing body Hyaluronic Acid and restoring hydration [5]. Studies have shown that hyaluronic acid requires less injection volume as compared to bovine collagen for optimal cosmetic results, and HA is also found to be more effective at maintaining the cosmetic correction [20, 21].

The U.S. Food and Drug Administration (FDA) has now approved various types of Hyaluronic acids, bio-stimulatory products like calcium hydroxyapatite and poly-L lactic acid, as well as polymethylmethacrylate as a substitute for fillers.

Fillers are categorised as permanent, semi-permanent and temporary. The majority of injectable fillers are temporary, lasting from several weeks to several months, although some reportedly last 9–12 months. Many of these processes require ongoing treatment to maintain the desired appearance [22].

### 33.3.2 Classification of Fillers

Based on their duration of action, fillers may be classified as follows:

*Temporary (3–12 Months)* These are mainly used to replace collagen in the skin, which weakens with age and loses its elasticity. Collagen has three main sources—bovine, porcine and human. Bovine collagen is very similar to the human molecule and is widely used. It only has specific differences in the end peptides (telopeptides), which are removed in processing, leaving a core protein similar to that of a humans [23]. Hyaluronic acid is the most commonly used Filler material of this category.

*Semi-Permanent (1–5 Years)* Calcium hydroxyapatite is one of the commonest semi-permanent fillers. It creates a stable scaffold for soft tissues to grow. Calcium hydroxylapatite may be injected into the deep dermis, where the microspheres are held in place until they are resorbed and collagen deposition occurs. This results in formation of non-scar-tissue type of collagen, which provides volume in the area under treatment [24].

*Permanent (>5 Years)* These are mostly synthetic implants, which are made of Polymethylmethacrylate (PMMA) microspheres. PMMA microspheres may be mixed with denatured bovine collagen and lidocaine, and suspended in a phosphate-buffered saline solution. Since PMMA is inert, it is well tolerated by the body and does not induce allergic reactions [25, 26].

**Preparation of the Patient before Injection of Fillers:** The patient's face is washed gently to dry and disinfect the skin. This is done using propanol solution. Since the dermal fillers are very painful while injecting, application of the topical anaesthesia around the area of injection using EMLA (Eutectic Mixture of Local Anaesthesia) for 30–45 min prior or particular branch of Maxillary division or Mandibular division of the trigeminal nerve is anaesthetised using 2% Lignocaine as a local anaesthetic injection.

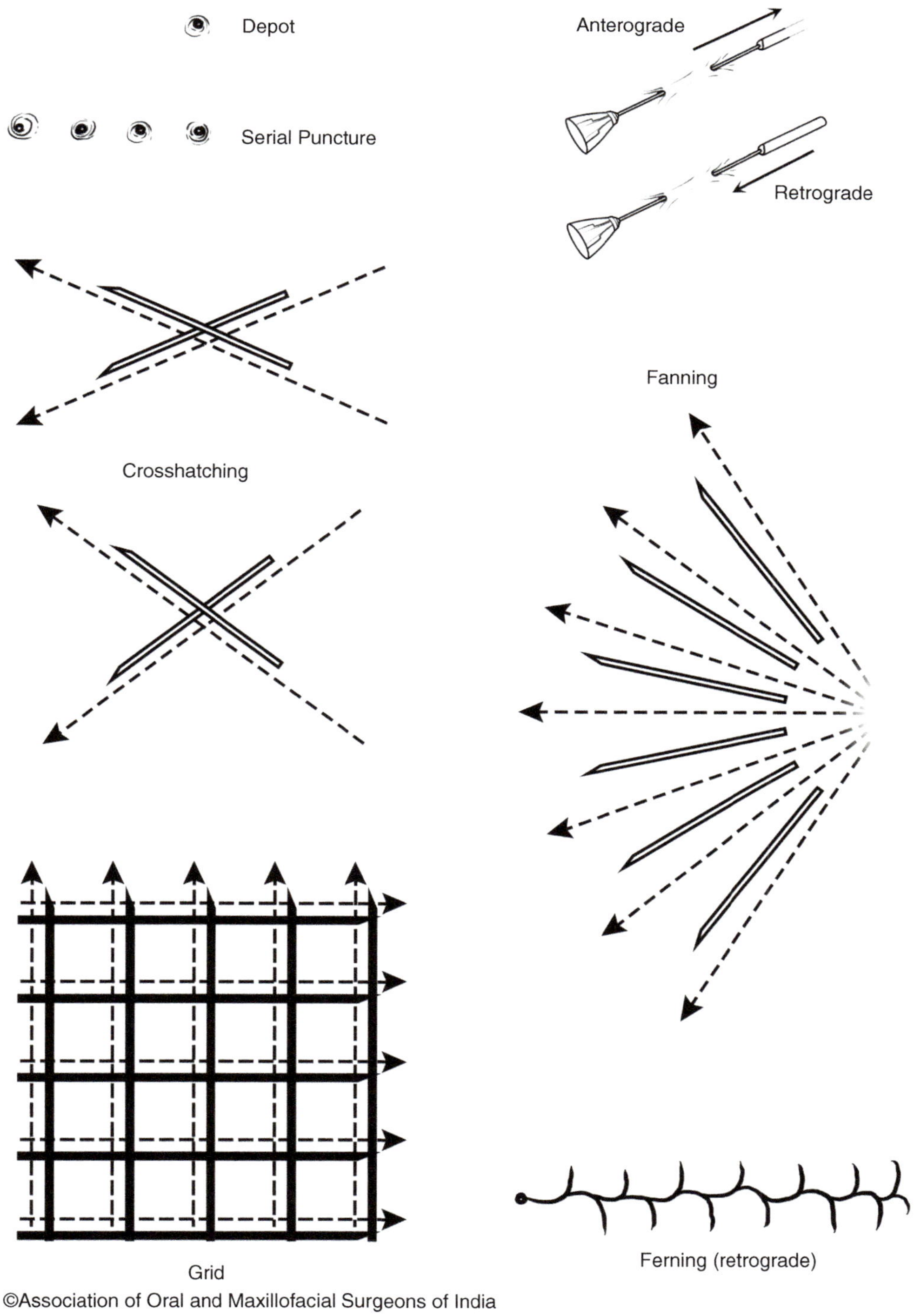


**Fig. 33.12** Various patterns in Injection technique

### 33.3.3 Dermal Filler Injection Methods (Fig. 33.12)

Hyaluronic acid is available in syringes in a sterile packed container. These have 26–30 gauge needle, with a length of 1–1½ inches.

These are injected at the subdermal planes in various fashion which are mentioned in Box 33.2.

The following is a description of various techniques.

**Linear Threading:** In this technique, fillers are injected in a needle and thread fashion. The needle is inserted and withdrawn repeatedly along a straight line. It has two types.

1. *Anterograde Injection:* The filler is injected while the needle is being advanced, and the filler is therefore easily tracked in the front of the needle.

**Box 33.2 Dermal Filler Injection Methods**

- Linear threading,
- Depot injection,
- Fanning method,
- Serial puncture,
- Cross hatching,
- Grid and Ferning

2. *Retrograde Injection:* The filler is not injected simultaneously during needle advancement. Once the needle is slowly withdrawn, the filler is injected.

**Depot:** In this technique, a small amount of the filler is deposited in the correct plane.

**Serial Puncture:** In a single wrinkle or fold, multiple closely spaced depot injections are placed.

**Fanning:** It is done through one point of entry and the needle is rotated like a fan in multiple directions, and the fillers are deposited in a retrograde way. It is important to stop injecting as the needle comes close to the insertion site in order to avoid build-up of fillers at the point of entry.

**Cross Hatching:** Injecting as multiple linear thread deposited in an X-shaped fashion.

**Grid:** It is injected as linear threads intersecting perpendicular to each other point of entry.

**Ferning: [16]** This is similar to retrograde injection. The needle is inserted on either side of the central tract, and the fillers are deposited in a branch-like fashion almost like the branches of a fern.

### 33.3.4 Injection Techniques

(a) *Glabellar and Forehead region* (Fig. 33.13a,b): The Glabellar region is the most prominent site for wrinkling and very well shown even in a mild expression. There are vertical lines of wrinkling, which result from contraction of the corrugator supercilii muscles, and horizontal lines which occur due to contraction of the procerus muscle. Before injecting, the patient should frown the brow and the needle is inserted at the subdermal plane and injected in a linear fashion and it is also deposited deep and parallel to the wrinkle. Small depots or serial puncture fashion of fillers are injected along the line of the wrinkles throughout its entire length. Gentle rub or massaging to be done to distribute the filler uniformly. In the case of bruising, icepacks can be used. Injecting into a vessel must be avoided as this can lead to the formation of emboli.

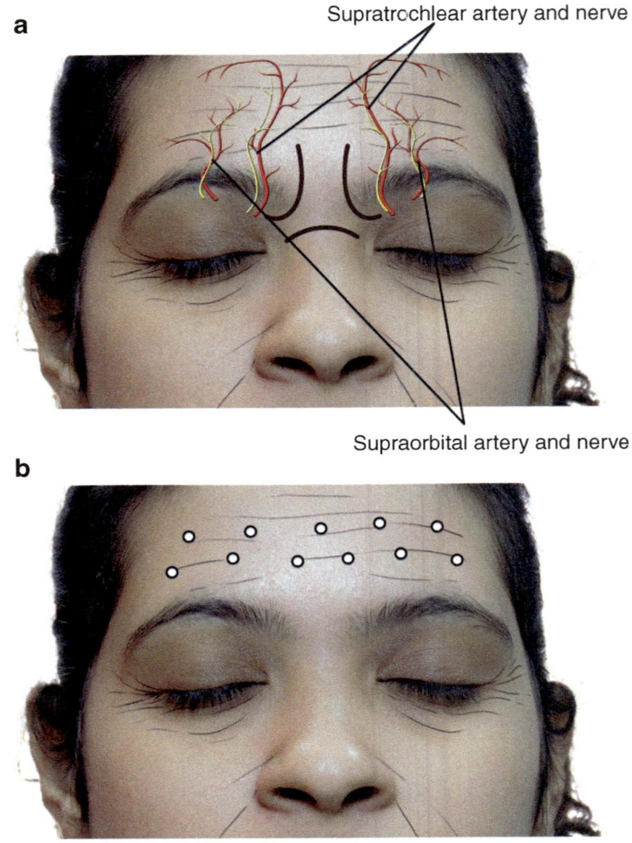




**Fig. 33.13** (**a**, **b**) Glabellar & forehead wrinkles

(b) *Nasolabial Fold* (Fig. 33.14a,b): The nasolabial fold is defined as the groove from corner of the alar base to the margin lateral to the angle of the mouth. The nasolabial groove must never be eliminated completely as this can result in an unaesthetic appearance. Injection may be done using serial puncture, linear threading, cross-hatching, or fanning. Only the medial part of the fold must be augmented, with injections perpendicular to this. This is best done by imagining a tall, thin, triangular deficit in front of the fold that needs to be filled. To prevent bruising, ice and pressure may be applied. Initially, hyaluronic acid swells and may appear as a firm mass on palpation but gradually blends in after the first week.

(c) *Lip Augmentation* (Fig. 33.15): This is one of the most common cosmetic procedures done using Hyaluronic acid filler for augmenting or everting the lips. The areas to be augmented are the outline of the lip, body of the lip or both. There is a potential space in the body of the vermilion, which, if correctly entered, will allow the filler to

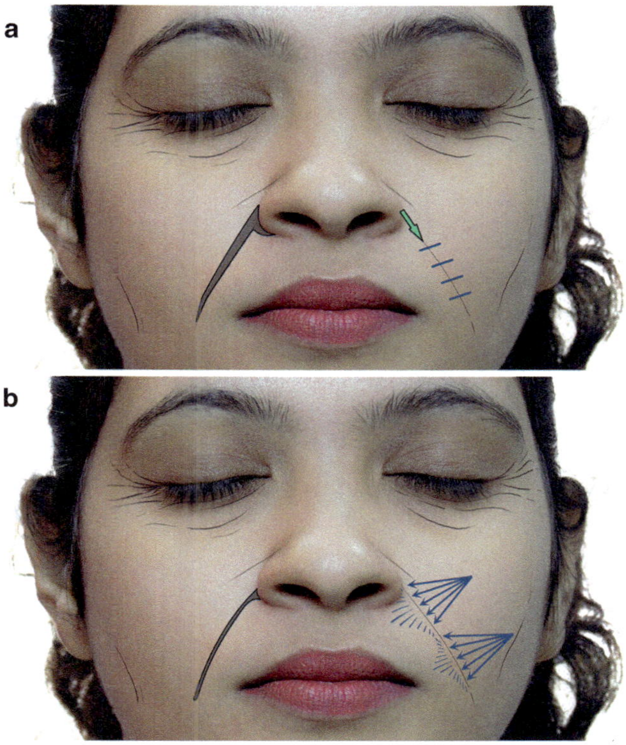



**Fig. 33.14** (**a**, **b**) Nasolabial fold injection technique

move within it along the entire lip margin. Dermal fillers injected in the body of the lips can augment, rejuvenate and improve the symmetry of the lips. Philtral columns can get flattened with age. These can be accentuated by injecting along the border of the vermilion and philtral region to give a more prominent philtrum and cupids bow with eversion of the lip. The philtrum may be pinched after injection to accentuate the ridges. Injections are generally placed superficially in to the subcutaneous plane. Massaging or a gentle rub after injection helps to distribute the filler evenly. Injection may be performed in an anterograde fashion, from lateral to medial, and the filler can be tracked along the vermillion.

(d) *Tear Trough Deformity* (Fig. 33.16): Tear Trough is usually referred to as the crease at the medial segment of the inferior orbital region. As ageing occurs, the infraorbital rim becomes more skeletonised and depressed. To correct this sunken appearance, HA may be injected into the semicircular depression under the eyes. Normally a 30-gauge needle, 2.5 cm long, is used to inject in the dermal layer of the lower eyelid to avoid bruising, as this area is highly vascularised. The needle is then inserted upwards at an angle, till it reaches the top of the orbital rim. The finger of the opposite hand may be used to direct the needle by positioning it at this point. The tip of the needle must touch the bone and its precise location must be verified prior to injection. The filler is injected slowly and deeply into this area. Massaging may be done at the injected area to avoid irregularities. If the HA is deposited too deep, a "*Tyndall effect*" [16] may be observed. Hyaluronic Acid can occasionally increase fluid retention around the periocular area, and lead to infraorbital swelling, edema or discolouration in the medial portion of the orbicularis muscle. If this occurs, subcutaneous hyaluronidase injections may lyse the Hyaluronic Acid and reduce the swelling.

(e) *Injection technique to increase the cheek volume* (Fig. 33.17): In some patients, fat loss or volume deficit can cause cheek hollowing. The loss of buccal pad of fat causes wrinkled cheeks, exaggeration of nasolabial folds and jowling of the skin at the lower border of the mandible. The submalar region (below the zygomatic arch) and buccal region (lateral to the nasolabial fold) are areas that need attention. The injection technique should be administered in a grid or fanning pattern. The injections must be administered at the dermal–subcutaneous plane. Massaging after injection can help smoothen irregularities.

### 33.3.5 Contraindication [22]

Some of the most common conditions to be avoided for fillers include:

- Scarring and collagen/connective tissue disorders
- Diabetes
- Infections—e.g.: Viral Herpes
- Coagulation problems
- Pregnant or Lactating women
- Psychological conditions

## 33.4 Conclusion

Botulinum Toxin Type A and Hyaluronic acid dermal fillers are very safe and effective under a trained physician or surgeon for therapeutic and cosmetic use. Wrinkles especially those which are located in the face and some asymmetries, mainly caused or worsened by the repeated contraction of facial muscles and ageing process can be effectively treated by these methods.

Proper knowledge of the anatomy of facial muscles and proper techniques are important to achieve predictable results and avoid complications. Informed consent for the procedure must be obtained from the patient after explaining the risks and the outcome, before commencing the treatment. Though Botulinum toxin and dermal Fillers give temporary results, they are safe and very effective in achieving aesthetic outcome.

**Disclosure** Author has no financial conflicts to disclose.

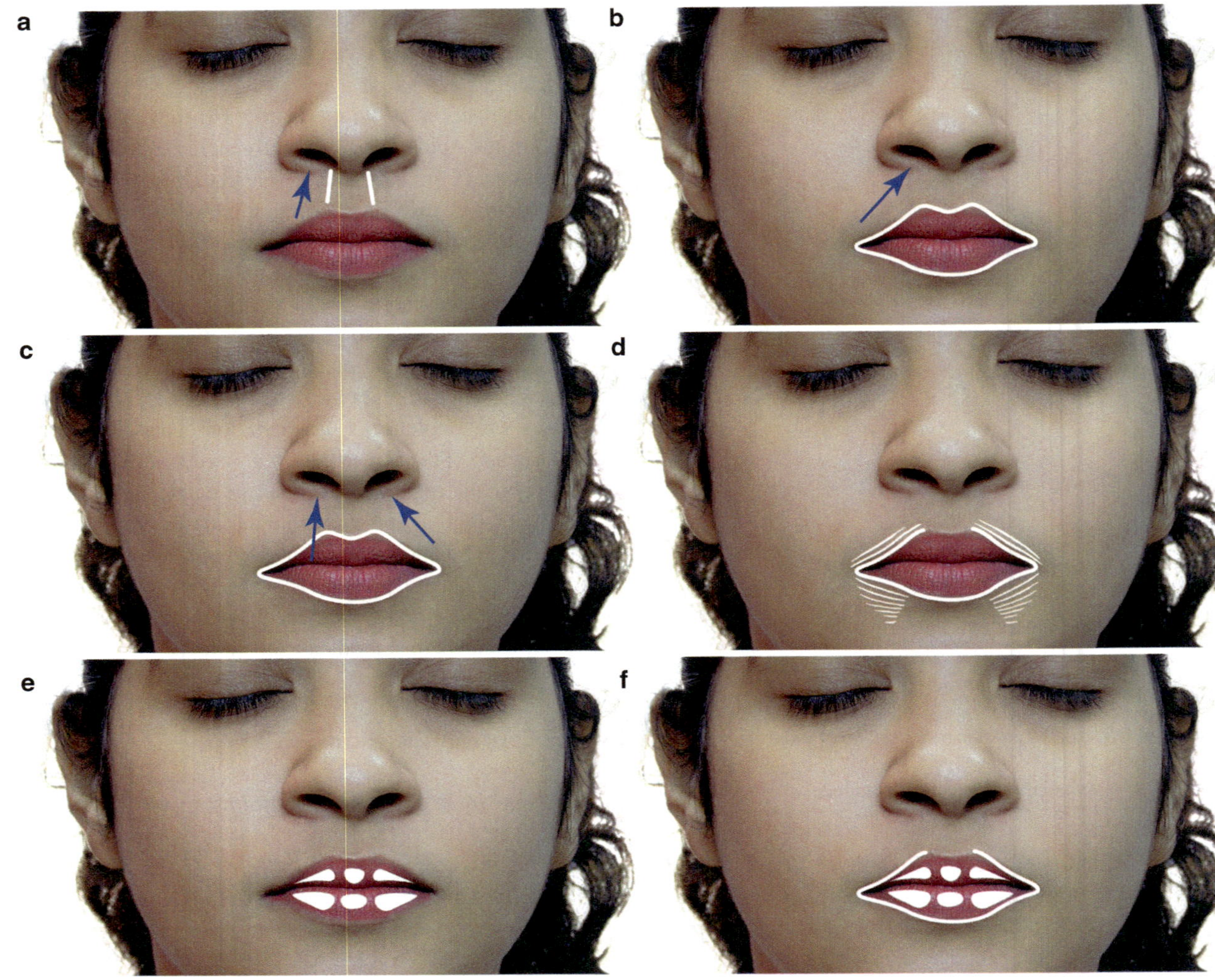




**Fig. 33.15** Injection technique for philtrum, lip line and the body of the lip. (**a**) anterograde filling (**b**) retrograde filling (**c**) both anterograde and retrograde filling (**d**) antero retrograde with fanning if necessary (**e**) depot and serial puncture filling (**f**) anterograde retrograde serial and depot filling

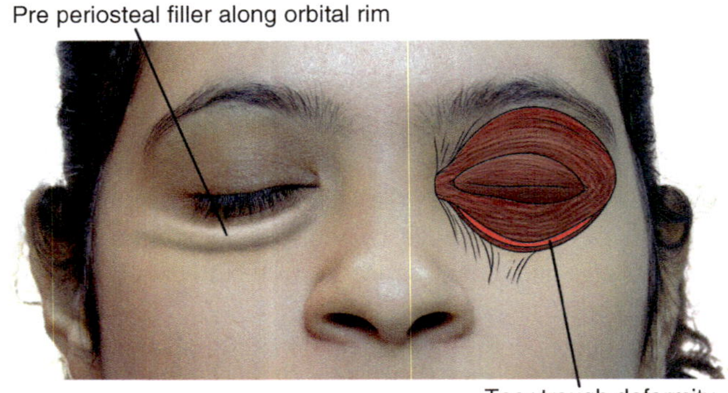




**Fig. 33.16** Tear trough deformity

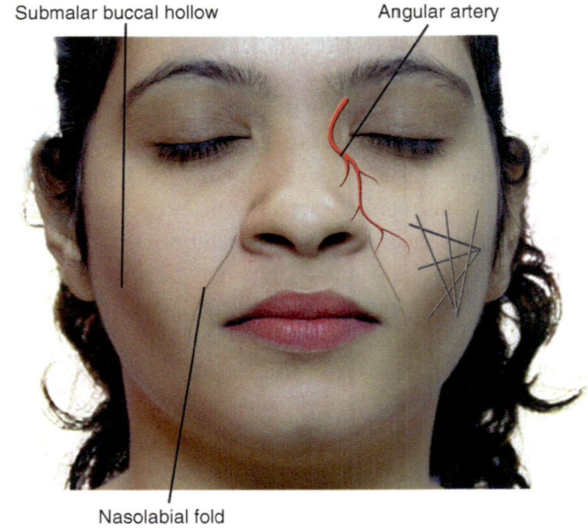




**Fig. 33.17** Injection technique for hollowing cheeks

## Case Scenarios

### Case 1 (Fig. 33.18a,b,c)

A 43-year-old female complaining of excessive tooth and gingival exposure on smiling. Clinical features (Fig. 33.18a): excessive gingival show on smiling normal lip length and normal size of the tooth. Treatment Plan (Fig. 33.18b1, b2, b3 and b4): locating the levator labii superioris muscle and injecting Botulinum toxin Type A with a dose of 5 U on both the sides. The injection point is located at the junction between lip and the ala of the nose. Post-operative findings (Fig. 33.18c): no gingival show on smiling.

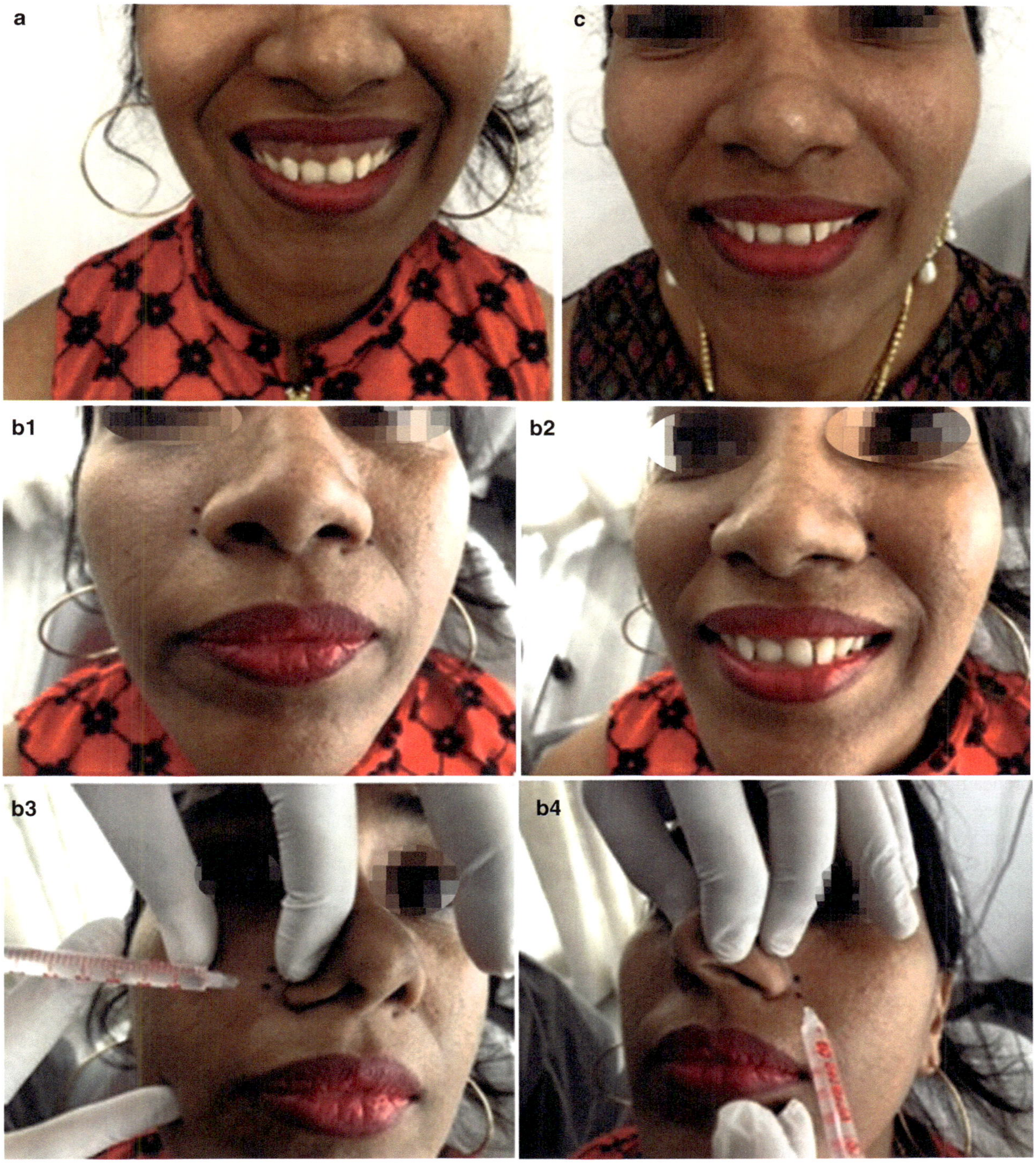


**Fig. 33.18** (**a**) Clinical features with excessive Gingival show. (**b1, b2, b3, b4**) Intraoperative. (**c**) Postoperative, absence of Gingival show

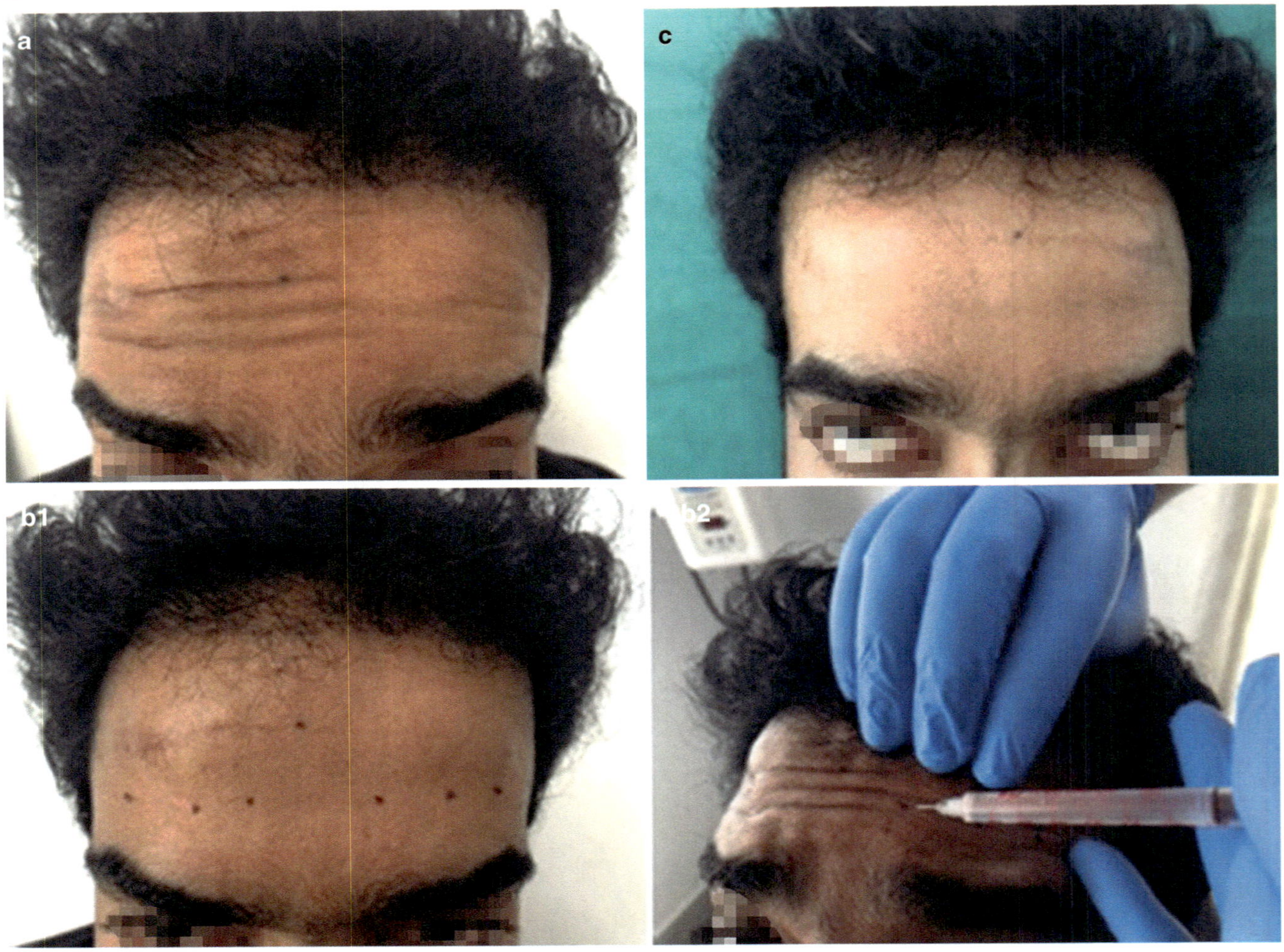


©Association of Oral and Maxillofacial Surgeons of India

**Fig. 33.19** (**a**) Clinical feature with forehead wrinkling. (**b1, b2**) Intraoperative. (**c**) Post-operative, absence of Wrinkling

## **Case 2** (Fig. 33.19a,b,c)

A 47-year-old male, complaining of excessive wrinkling in the forehead on looking upwards and frowning with ageing appearance. Clinical features (Fig. 33.19a): wrinkling and folds found on the forehead on upward starring and frowning. Treatment Plan (Fig. 33.19b1, b2): locating the frontalis muscle and injecting Botulinum toxin Type A with a dose of 5 U on both the sides at 3 different points marked and above 1 cm from the supraorbital margin. The injection point is located midway between supraorbital margin and frontal hairline. Post-operative findings (Fig. 33.19c): absence of wrinkling.

## References

1. Baran R, Maibach HI. DorisHexel Textbook of cosmetic dermatology. 5th edn; Chap 1,50,51—Skin size and Parameters, Botulinum Toxin, Soft tissue Augmentation Chap; Pg – 3,459,473.
2. Shuster S, Black MM, McVitie E. The influence of age and sex on skin thickness, skin collagen and density. Br J Dermatol. 1975;93:639–43.
3. Tsukahara K, Hotta M, Osanai O, et al. Gender-dependent differences in degree of facial wrinkles. Skin Res Technol. 2013;19(1):e65–71.
4. Ezure T, Yagi E, Kunizawa N, et al. Comparison of sagging at the cheek and lower eyelid between male and female faces. Skin Res Technol. 2011;17(4):510–5.
5. Gerhardt LC, Strassle V, Lenz A, et al. Influence of epidermal hydration on the friction of human skin against textiles. J R Soc Interface. 2008;5:1317–28.
6. Carruthers JDA, Carruthers JA. Treatment of glabellar frown lines with C botulinum-A exotoxin. J Dermatol Surg Oncol. 1992;18:17–21.
7. Dover N, Barash JR, Hill KK, Xie G, Arnon SS. Molecular characterization of a novel botulinum neurotoxin type H gene. J Infect Dis. 2014;209:192–202.
8. Lebeda FJ, Hack DC, Gentry MK. Theoretical analyses of the functional regions of the heavy chain of botulinum neurotoxin. In: Jankovic J, Hallet M, editors. Therapy with botulinum toxin. New York: Marcel Dekker; 1994. p. 51–61.
9. Hexsel D, Hexsel CL, Bohn J. Long, mid, and short term effects of botulinum toxin on the musculature. In: Hexsel D, Almeida AT,

editors. Cosmetic use of botulinum toxin. Porto Alegre: AGE; 2002. p. 99–103.
10. Wollina U, Konrad H. Am J Clin Dermatol. 2005;6(3):141–50.
11. Ascher B, Talarico S, Cassuto D, Escobar S, Hexsel D, Jaén P, et al. International consensus recommendations on the aesthetic usage of botulinum toxin type A (Speywood Unit)—part II: wrinkles on the middle and lower face, neck and chest. J Eur Acad Dermatol Venereol. 2010;24(11):1285–95.
12. Carruthers A. Botulinum toxin type A: history and current cosmetic use in the upper face. Dis Mon. 2002;48:299–322.
13. Hexsel D, Mazzuco R, Zechmeister M, Hexsel CL. Complications and adverse effects: diagnosis and treatment. In: Hexsel D, Almeida AT, editors. Cosmetic use of botulinum toxin. Porto Alegre: AGE; 2002. p. 233–9.
14. Benedetto AV. The cosmetic uses of botulinum toxin type A. Int J Dermatol. 1999;38:641–55.
15. Lorenc ZP, Smith S, Nestor M, Nelson D, Moradi A. Understanding the functional anatomy of the frontalis and glabellar complex for optimal aesthetic botulinum toxin type A therapy. Aesthet Plast Surg. 2013;37(5):975–83.
16. Kontis TC, Lacombe VG. Cosmetic injection technique. New York: Thieme; 2013. p. 23–4.
17. Klein AW. Complications with the use of botulinum toxin. Dermatol Clin. 2004;22(2):197–205.
18. Narins RS, et al. A randomized double-blind multicenter comparison of the efficacy and tolerability of Restylane versus Zyplast for the correction of nasolabial folds. Dermatol Surg. 2003;29(6): 588–95.
19. Donofrio L. Fat distribution: a morphologic study of the aging face. Dermatol Surg. 2000;26:1107–12.
20. Guttman C. A generation speaks: dermatology answers growing desire to fight aging skin. Dermatology Times, pp. 56–60; 2004.
21. Guttman C. Advances in anti-aging: new techniques technology should match demand. Dermatology Times; 2004.
22. Burgers CM. Cosmetic dermatology, 2005; Chapter 6—Soft tissue Augmentation; Pg 103.
23. Glogau R, Narins R, Weiss R. Advances in cosmetic procedures. In Fall clinical dermatology conference supplement proceedings. Supplement to skin and aging, pp. 20–27; 2004.
24. Bisaccia D, Scarborough D. The esthetic correction of the aging mouth. Cosmet Dermatol. 1992;11:8–11.
25. Elson M. Soft tissue augmentation techniques: update on available materials. Cosmet Dermatol. 1999:13–5.
26. Lemperle G, Romano JJ, Busso M. Soft tissue augmentation with Artecoll: 10-year history indications techniques and complications. Dermatol Surg. 2003;29(6):573–87.

# Hair Transplantation

# 34

Sreedhar Reddy Pothula and B. S. Jayanth

## 34.1 Introduction

In the past few decades, maxillofacial surgeons have played a pivotal role in enhancing the aesthetic value of the face through many surgical and non-surgical procedures, with hair transplantation being one of the popular choices which has seen an exponential demand in the last decade. Though hair restoration procedures were being performed for many decades ever since Dr. Norman Orentreich in 1959 published them in the annals of the New York Academy of Sciences, there has been many advances to the originally described punch grafting which has become obsolete and has been replaced by the so-called micrografts via the two basic techniques of follicular unit transplantation (FUT) and follicular unit extraction (FUE). The success of the above techniques is in part attributed to the theory of donor dominance which postulates that the hair taken from the donor area of the posterior scalp will continue to grow without getting hit by factors which were responsible for the thinning out of hair in the frontal areas [1].

Apart from hair transplant being a promising procedure for male pattern and female pattern alopecia, it has been applied to other causes of hair loss too; traumatic and burn scars on hair bearing areas, alopecia following surgical procedures (i.e. Craniotomy, rhytidectomy procedures), redo hair transplantation, congenital reasons like cleft lip scenario. Currently the scope for hair transplantation is expanding with the demand from patients who want to strengthen a weak hairline, desire to lower the hairline or fix missing facial hair on the moustache, beard, eyebrow or eyelashes.

As the field of hair transplantation continues to evolve at a breakneck speed with specialists from multiple specialities performing this scientific artistry, it's all the more pertinent that we as maxillofacial surgeons are abreast of the current principles and practice of this hair restorative surgery.

## 34.2 Surgical Anatomy

An understanding of the surgical anatomy of the scalp is necessary to avoid complications and to optimise your performance for hair transplantation.

Scalp consists of five distinct layers with the most superficial layer being the skin which comprises of epidermal and dermal layers. These layers contain hair follicles, sebaceous and sweat glands with rich vascular supply. The second layer of scalp is made up of connective tissue, which is well vascularised and heavily innervated by sensory nerves. The deepest portion of the hair follicle, bulb and papilla, may extend through the skin into this layer (Fig. 34.1a). Thus, when obtaining donor grafts, effort should be made to incorporate the upper part of dermal layer to obtain the entire hair follicle. The third layer also called galea aponeurotica is a tendinous tissue connecting the two bellies of the occipitalis and frontal muscles. Loose areolar connective tissue is the next layer which contains numerous potential spaces, capable of great distension thus allowing for exceptional mobility of scalp. Unfortunately, these spaces are also capable of potential space for haematoma collection and spread of infections. The deepest layer of the scalp defines the pericranium, which is analogous to periosteum throughout the body.

**Electronic Supplementary Material** The online version of this chapter (https://doi.org/10.1007/978-981-15-1346-6_34) contains supplementary material, which is available to authorized users.

S. R. Pothula (✉)
Oral and Maxillofacial Surgery, Pioneer Advanced Hair Transplant Centre, Bengaluru, Karnataka, India

B. S. Jayanth (✉)
ABMSS, Bengaluru, Karnataka, India



K. Bonanthaya et al. (eds.), *Oral and Maxillofacial Surgery for the Clinician*, https://doi.org/10.1007/978-981-15-1346-6_34

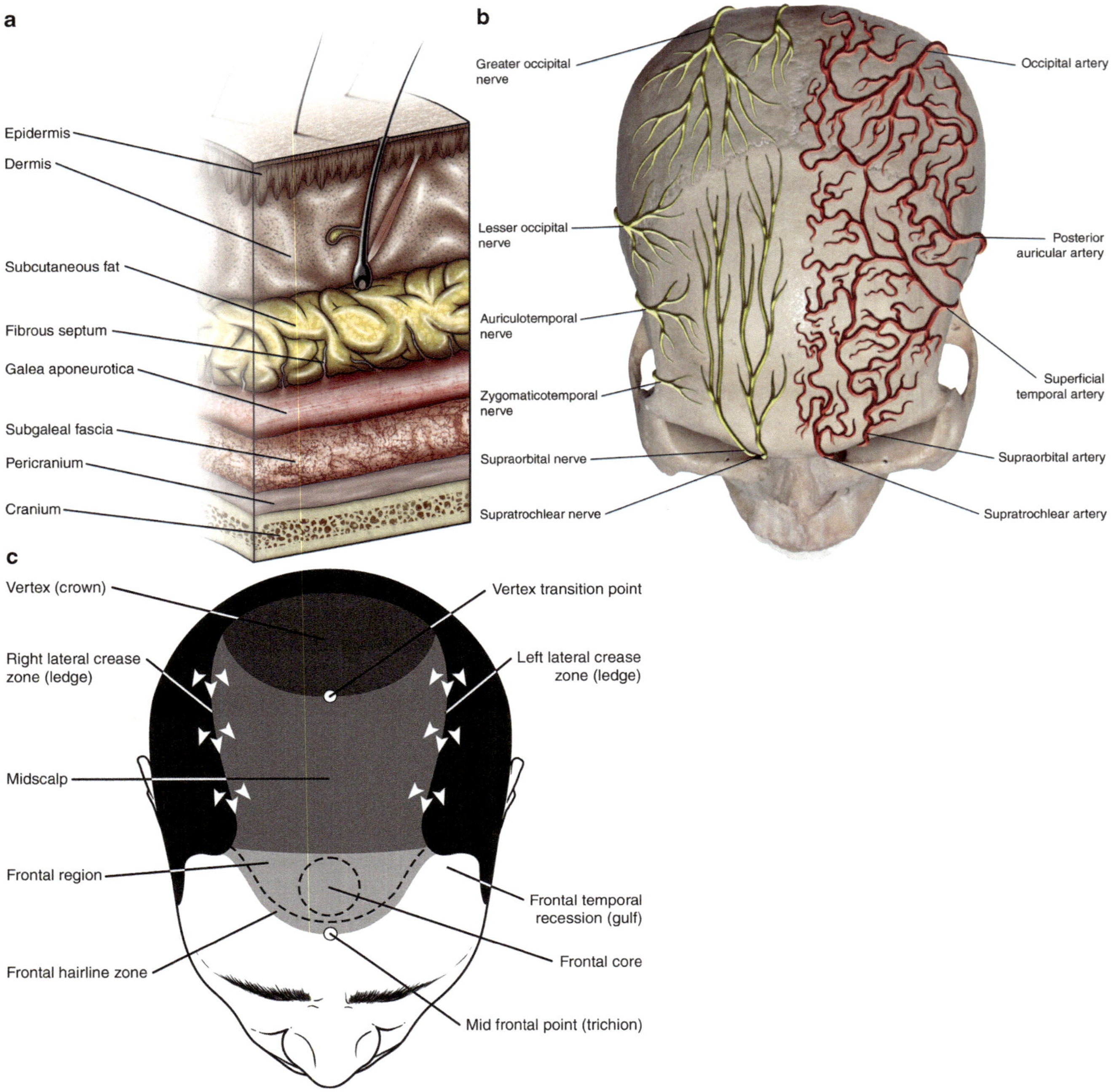




**Fig. 34.1** (**a**) Hair follicle extending into dermis; note the layers of the scalp. (**b**) Arteriovenous supply of the scalp with sensory innervation. (**c**) Zones of the scalp

### 34.2.1 Blood Supply and Sensory Innervation

The arterial supply to the scalp arrives from branches of both external and internal carotid arteries. Branches of the external carotid artery in order from posterior to the anterior include the occipital, posterior auricular and superficial temporal arteries. The supratrochlear and supraorbital arteries are branches of the internal carotid artery. The veins of the scalp follow the same basic network of the arteries and drain into the jugular veins (Fig. 34.1b). All of these vessels freely anastomose in the connective tissue layer of the scalp. Awareness and approximate location of the main branches are very important during the hair transplant surgery not only to avoid haemorrhage or haematoma but also to prevent ischemia to the follicles. Occipital artery which enters the scalp immediately above the external occipital protuberance at the superior nuchal line can easily be injured if depth control is not maintained. If arterial haemorrhage is encountered, electro cautery and suture ligation are adequate to secure homeostasis. Damage to vessels could likely lead to the formation of donor area scar.

Sensory innervation of the scalp arises from all three branches of trigeminal nerve antero-laterally with the forehead getting its supply from the supraorbital and supratrochlear branches of the ophthalmic division, while the anterior temporal scalp is supplied by the maxillary division and the mandibular division goes onto supply the temporoparietal zone of the scalp through its auriculotemporal nerve. The spinal cutaneous nerves of the cervical plexus (c2 and c3) come to supply the area posterior to the auricle via the greater and lesser occipital nerves. These nerves are found in the connective tissue just superior to the galea.

### 34.2.2 Zones of the Scalp

Typically, the areas of male pattern hair loss are horseshoe shaped and are divided into three zones [2] (Fig. 34.1c)

1. Frontal—extends from the hairline to the mid-scalp and is curvilinear. Has a frontal hairline zone anteriorly with the line being irregular like coastline of the sea with mounds and recessions. The follicles in this zone is mainly single hair follicle for the first two to three rows generally blending into multiple follicular units posteriorly giving rise to the density effect known as shingling. The frontal core zone is a small area in the central aspect of the frontal region which is circular to oval and is very important in framing the face receiving the highest density of grafted hairs.
2. The mid-scalp—is at the top of the head. This horizontal area is bordered on both the sides by the temporal parietal fringes and is sandwiched between the frontal zone anteriorly and the vertex posteriorly.
3. Vertex or crown—the most posterior area being rounded and characterised by whorl arrangement of hair is the toughest area to transplant.

The temporal fringe is the lateral hair zone present on the sides of the scalp anterior to the tragus of the ear and posterior to this is the parietal fringe.

The frontotemporal apex is the area usually devoid of hair at the junction of the lateral frontal hairline and temporal fringe. This coincides with the deepest point of the recession on the forehead and is aligned with the lateral canthus of the eye.

### 34.2.3 Microanatomy of Hair

Hair consists of a living part under the skin extending into the dermis known as follicle and a non-living keratinised part above the skin, the so-called hair shaft (Fig. 34.2). The shaft has three further layers namely the outer protective cuticle, inner cortex and in certain cases the medulla forms the core, and they mainly help in protection and anchorage of the hair.

The growing structure of the hair is the follicle with the upper part being constant and consists of the top infundibulum at the opening of sebaceous gland and isthmus in the middle where the piloerector muscle comes to insert. The lower part of the follicle known as the bulb is very vital as it's the one involved with regeneration and most of the stem cells are located here. Hence, while implanting holding, the graft above or beside the bulb is vital to ensure sustenance of regenerative potential.

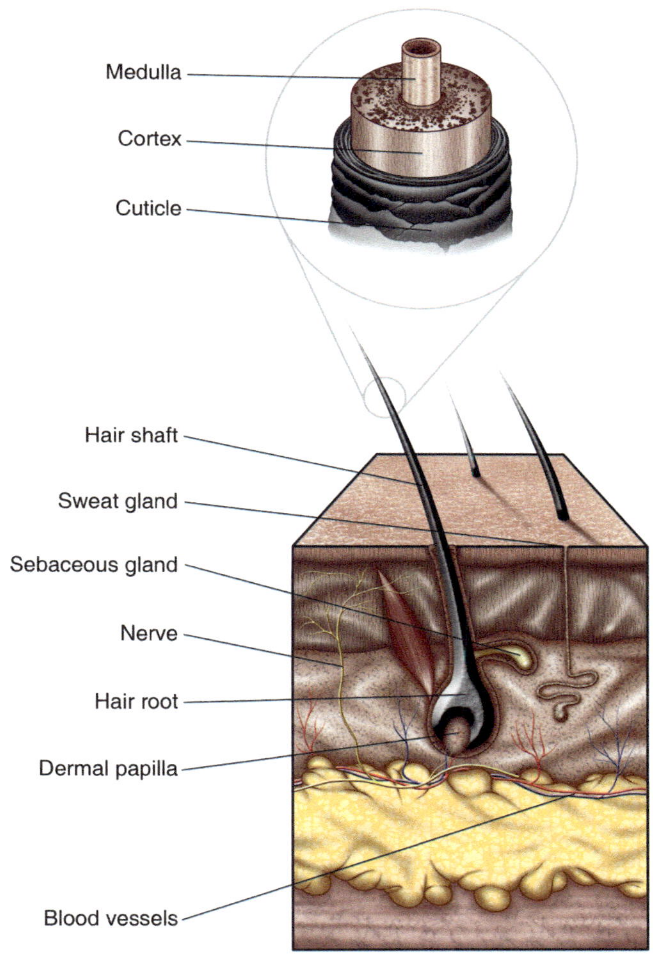




Fig. 34.2 Microanatomy of the hair

## 34.3 Terminology

The unique language of hair transplant surgeons consist of a few common words to communicate within the speciality [3] (Box 34.1).

**Box 34.1 Hair Transplant Surgery: Terminology**

*Follicular unit graft (FU)*: The natural Bundle of hair strands consisting of one, two or three hairs woven within a single unit and held by connective tissue elements as the follicle. The graft containing two or three follicular units becomes a multi follicular unit graft.

*Micrograft*: The follicular unit which has single hair graft within it is referred to as a micrograft, and the same is preferred for frontal hairline implantation.

*Minigraft*: The follicular unit which has more than a single hair graft and houses four to six hair grafts prior to cutting with microscopes are minigrafts.

*Follicular unit density*: It's the number of follicular units per $cm^2$.

*Hair density*: It's the number of hairs per $cm^2$.

*FUT*: The grafts are obtained from the harvested strip through slivering and dissection of individual follicles under magnification.

*FUE*: The grafts are obtained individually in the donor area one at a time utilising a punch and handheld extractor.

*Stick and place implantation*: Refers to implantation made immediately as the recipient site slit is made with a needle or blade.

*Pre slit implantation*: Refers to implantation made after all the recipient site slits are made with a blade or needle.

*Coronal slits*: Refers to slits oriented along coronal from side to side.

*Sagittal slits*: Refers to slits oriented along sagittal plane from front to back.

## 34.4 Growth Cycle and Hair Loss

Hair is cylindrical, outgrowths on the skin made up of keratinous filaments. The normal human scalp contains between 100,000 and 140,000 follicles with hair being arranged in follicular units, small groups of 1–4 hairs each. There are approximately 50,000–60,000 follicular units on the human scalp.

Testosterone is the main regulator of hair growth with the androgens binding to receptors in the dermal papilla influencing the growth. Human hair does not grow constantly and evenly but grows in phases and in cycles which are reproducible. Anagen is the growing phase of hair that accounts for 85% of the hair growth, during which hair grows at 0.5 inch per month for up to 10 cm per year with adequate blood supply providing nutrients and minerals to the hair. This phase lasts for anywhere between 3 and 6 years. As long as this phase persists, the hair stays on the scalp and is genetically determined. Anagen is followed by catagen and the later phase onset signals the end of active hair growth. During this transitional phase which lasts for 1–2 weeks, the production of hair stop and hair follicle start to shrink in size and nearly 2–3% of the hairs are in this phase. Telogen is the final phase of the hair cycle where the aged hair fall out and new ones push themselves out of the skin. This final phase lasts for nearly 3 months with around hundred hairs being shed per day and nearly 10–15% of the hairs are in this phase at any point in time (Fig. 34.3).

People often confuse with hair fall to hair loss. Hair fall is common in every individual. Around 10–20% of total hair will be under shedding process. That hair will grow back in 3 months. On average 80–60 hair strands fall is considered as normal.

Male pattern hair loss or androgenetic alopecia as the word suggests is a result of both androgens and genetic factors which work together causing the clinical effect of baldness [4]. Though there are many reasons for hair loss, androgenetic alopecia is the most common reason and accounts for 95%. Fortunately, it can be treated with hair transplant surgery. The diagnosis of androgenetic alopecia is supported by a family history of hair loss, although a positive history is not always identified. There is a slightly greater incidence of having a positive history on the mother's side but the inheritance of male pattern hair loss can come from either side of the family.

In androgenetic alopecia, there is change of hair from terminal hair to vellus hair. There happens to be a gradual evolution of this pattern, with each subsequent cycle of the new hair being fine and thin leading eventually to various grades of alopecia. It initially starts with the frontal hairline recession and regression, followed by loss of more temporal hair and simultaneous thinning of the vertex hair. Norwood classified approximately 7 different types of male pattern hair loss. Identification of these types is key to an understanding of proper planning of hair transplant surgery.

Testosterone gets converted to dihydrotestosterone (dht) both systemically and in the process of intrafollicular conversion under the influence of the enzyme 5-alpha reductase leading to its binding with androgen receptors of the follicular cells in genetically predisposed men leading to inhibition of protein synthesis by shortening the anagen phase, thereby producing finer hairs with shaft becoming thinner; this stunted hair follicle growth leads to miniaturisation of follicles till they become extinct establishing balding [5].

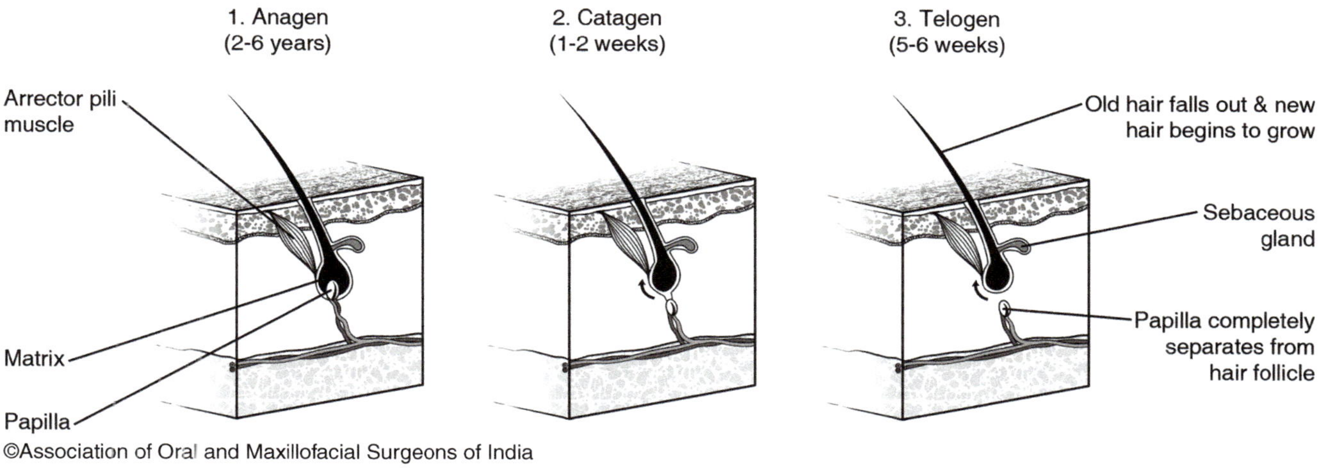


**Fig. 34.3** Hair growth cycle

**Box 34.2 Basic Requirements for Hair Regrowth**

1. Regulating dihydrotestosterone levels in the blood
2. By ensuring normal supply of balanced nutrients to the hair roots
3. Proper blood circulation to carry the nutrients to the roots in the scalp
4. Maintaining good health through general well-being of the individual

Clinical studies have given us an understanding that hair can be grown back if the following four things are ensured (Box 34.2):

Hair loss is not a disease but a condition where anagen or the growth phase reduces and the telogen or fall phase is extended. This forms the basis of hair loss in alopecia conditions other than androgenetic alopecia. The factors leading to hair loss could stem from internal/external factors.

*Internal Factors* There are many factors which internally lead to deficient states harming the hair growth. A few of them which are relevant today are iron deficiency, calcium deficiency, zinc deficiency, general debility, anaemia, hypothyroidism, deficiency of the fat soluble vitamins, thyroid problems, insulin resistance, metabolic disorders like gout and PCOD, prolonged illness, emotional turmoil following surgery and individuals with seborrheic scalp.

*External Factors* The lifestyle and environmental factors do influence the hair health and growth cycle. The common causes are smoking including passive smoking, stress, alcohol intake, lack of sleep, crash dieting, fad diets, high-protein diet, exposure to extremes of heat or cold, less intake of fluids, poor scalp hygiene, dust, pollution, fumes and exposure to endocrine disrupting chemicals.

## 34.5 Classification

The most popular classification of the male pattern hair loss is the Norwood classification system (1975) which is a refined version of the original Hamilton system (1941) [6].

### 34.5.1 Norwood Classification (Fig. 34.4)

Type 1 presents the normal hairline with minimal recession of the frontotemporal area.

Type 2 patients present a symmetrical and mild recession of the frontotemporal area along with thinning of the hair.

Type 3 patients define balding with minimal or no in the frontal areas and a deep recession.

Type 4 patients present with significant recession and loss of both frontal and vertex hair with a bridge of her between the two still retained.

Type 5 category patients present a progression of the type four category with only thin and narrow bridge of hair between the frontotemporal and the vertex areas.

Type 6 represents the loss of hair that separates the frontal and the posterior vertex areas with further progression in lateral and posterior zones.

Type 7 represents the most severe form of balding with only a band of hair remaining in the low occipital and temporal areas with extensive miniaturisation of the hair.

Basically, in the above classification, the two areas of hair loss—a bitemporal recession and thinning crown gradually enlarge and coalesce until the entire front, top and crown of the scalp are bald.

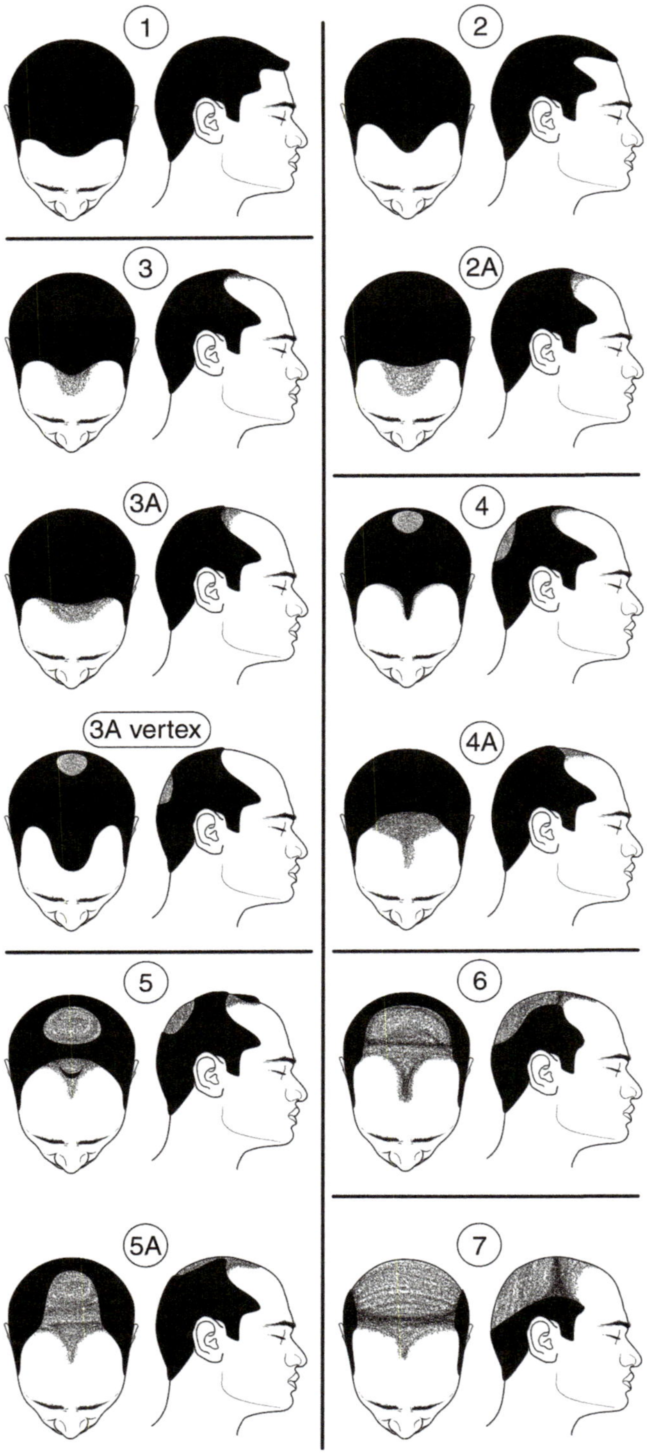



**Fig. 34.4** Norwood classification of male pattern alopecia

To regain the crowning glory, medical treatment gives good results up to type 3 patients while hair transplantation is the only choice for patients between types 4 and 6.

Routinely, clinicians come across variations of the classification which fall outside the Norwood classification, they are as follows: Differential use pattern alopecia, diffuse and patent alopecia.

### 34.5.2 Classification of Hair Loss in Women

The Ludwig classification (1977) uses three stages to describe female pattern genetic hair loss (Fig. 34.5).

Type I (mild), type II (moderate) and type III (extensive). In all three Ludwig stages, there is hair loss on the front and top of the scalp with relative preservation of the frontal hairline. The back and sides may or may not be involved.

In Ludwig type I, there is early thinning that can be easily camouflaged with proper grooming. Type I patients have too little hair loss to consider surgical hair restoration.

Women with type II hair loss have significant widening of the midline part and noticeably decreased volume. Hair transplantation may be indicated if the donor area in the back and sides of the scalp is stable.

In Ludwig type III, there is a thin, see-through look to the top of the scalp. This is often associated with generalised thinning over the entire scalp. Often patients that have progressed to this stage have too little donor hair to make surgical hair restoration worthwhile.

All women experiencing hair loss should have an accurate diagnosis made, preferably by an experienced dermatologist. This is particularly important since the diffuse hair loss that women typically develop, can occasionally be caused by a number of treatable medical conditions. Regardless of the extent or cause of hair loss, only women with stable hair on the back and sides of the scalp are candidates for hair transplantation.

Other infrequent alopecias observed among the patients visiting hair clinics are as follows:

*Alopecia areta*: it's an autoimmune disorder which starts with small round and punched out areas with no hair. Lesion has very smooth skin and not even a single hair is present in the lesion.

*Alopecia totalis*: there is total loss of scalp hair.

*Alopecia universalis*: there is total hair loss in the body including the eyebrows.

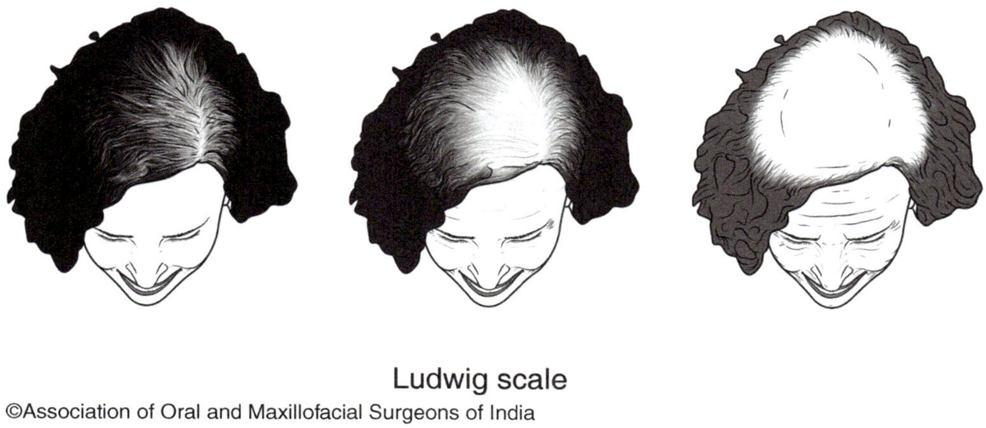


**Fig. 34.5** Ludwig classification for hair loss in women.

*Turban alopecia*: caused due to tight turban usage. It affects frontal and parietal areas mainly and is seen among Sikhs.

*Trichotillomania*: a psychiatric disorder where the individuals deliberately pull their hair every day leading to hair loss in those areas.

## 34.6 Medications for Hair Loss

Only 2 drugs have been approved by FDA and have proven their efficacy in the management of hair loss with good success.

### 34.6.1 Minoxidil

This is a direct hypertrichotic drug, which was initially approved as an antihypertensive agent and was found to have side effect of hypertrichosis. Today, it is available as an over the counter drug with 2% formulation for women and 5–10% formulation for men as topical solution and gel. It improves hair count, weight and growth of hair. Post transplantation too it has been found to decrease the shedding of hair and enhanced the time to onset for hair growth. According to few studies, minoxidil acts as a vasodilator by opening up the potassium channels and thereby enhances the vascularity of the hair bulb which in turn promotes hair growth. However, the exact mechanism is unknown. This topical product needs to be applied to the scalp and not the hair and patients need to be informed about the initial increased shedding of weak hair in the first 4–8 weeks. Further, the patients need to be counselled to apply the product twice a day to maximise the efficacy and to wait for a timeframe of at least 4–5 months prior to seeing the results.

### 34.6.2 Finasteride

Finasteride is a drug which is used only in men for reversal of miniaturised hair follicles. This drug is a competitive inhibitor of the enzyme 5-alpha reductase which blocks the conversion of male hormone testosterone to dihydrotestosterone, and thereby works on the pathogenesis of androgenetic alopecia. It is to be taken orally once a day daily at 1 mg. Finasteride can cause loss of libido and oligospermia in few individuals. However, this side effect is reversible once the drug is discontinued.

Other medicines like Dutasteride though being a potent inhibitor of 5-alpha reductase is not that popular in the market as it has got adverse effects. Few natural products like saw palmatto can be used in young individuals who refuse to take finasteride.

### 34.6.3 Cyclical Therapy

It entails giving vitamins with calcium supplements on a single day, followed by iron and mineral combination product on one other day of the week and finally amino acid blend; the three regiments are also advocated that their intake be on alternative days as different nutrients and the daily dosing is avoided. The basis of this therapy is that hair requires nutritional support during their anagen growth phase and also for its maintenance; without nutrients, hair cannot get support and the stimulated hair growth to demonstrate disappointing outcomes. This therapy is the result of pioneering work on the role of nutritional supplements in hair growth.

Platelet-rich plasma (PRP) is an autologous biological modifier which has many concentrated growth factors in it and has demonstrated good results in reducing hair loss and has shown to enhance hair counts. It is prepared in a three-step process where blood is drawn, processed and injected into the scalp. It is injected into the scalp once every fortnight for 4–6 sittings and this can be combined with the standard therapy.

## 34.7 Clinical Consultation

It is important to begin the consultation by knowing the general health of the patient with a focus on endocrinal conditions affecting hair namely the thyroid disease, any uncontrolled diabetes, polycystic ovarian disease in the case of females and also enquiring specifically about family history of hair loss, past medical management, understanding personal hair care regimen and any past hair transplants done.

The next focus of the clinician during consultations should be on the expectations and motivation levels of the patient trying to drive home the message that it's a progressive condition especially in younger patients who are demanding and want a low hairline. It's important to have a family member during consultation and ensure that they understand that any future hair loss is understood and you are only trying to frame the face. The pattern of the hair loss also needs to be well documented.

The donor site assessment will verify the presence of any white hair, check the elasticity of the scalp, the density of the hair follicles per square centimetre, note the calibre of the hair (thick vs. thin), presence of curly or straight hair, rule out any existing scars and skin pathology including dandruff and infections.

The assessment of the recipient site will focus on the quality and quantity of remaining hair, ascertaining the grade of balding and the pattern of hair loss, previous results of hair transplantation, the skin to hair contrast, direction of the existing hair and existing skin condition. Based on the priorities of the case and having assessed the areas requiring hair transplantation, the number of follicular units required per square centimetre (around $30/cm^2$) is calculated to arrive at the number of follicular units to harvest.

## 34.8 Concept of Hair Transplantation

Hair transplantation as performed today is basically microfollicular unit transplantation and few clinicians call it as hair restoration as there are many methods to achieve the results.

In the early days, hair transplant concept started with flap rotation techniques requiring procedures to be performed under general anaesthesia. These invasive techniques did not gain popularity as the results were not satisfying and the procedures left disfigurement in few individuals. Later on during the evolution of techniques, macro and micrografts being 5–6 mm in size were introduced which were harvested with biopsy punches and the resulting grafts were implanted. These plug like grafts being unnatural in appearance gave a classical doll's hair appearance after growth and got phased out with further refinement of hair transplant procedures.

By around 1963, follicular unit transplantation or strip technique was introduced which became a workhorse of hair transplantation until recently and is still considered to be the gold standard method for hair restoration. In the year 2002, Rossman and Bernstein refined the punch method of harvesting the follicles and named it follicular unit extraction which has seen an exponential growth in the recent years and is today the most popular technique of hair transplantation.

The principle behind hair transplantation is quite simple. The hair that grows on the back and sides of the scalp tends to be permanent in most of the individuals. These occipital and parietal hairs are resistant to androgenic alopecia and are used to implant into the frontal or vertex area which will continue to grow as long as occipital hair grow, but in few individuals with advanced grades even these donor hairs can be miniaturised and lost. That's the reason as to why anticipating the future hair loss is most important factor while planning hair transplant procedure.

Hair transplant as a procedure is successful only when hair loss is stabilised, as it will not stop further hair loss. We as surgeons can only relocate and transfer few strong follicles from donor area to recipient area without increasing any new follicle per se. Many young patients who are frustrated by taking medicines over a period of time will seek hair transplant procedure as a remedy, which is an absolutely wrong decision for the clinicians to encourage. It is imperative on the part of the clinician to stabilise any ongoing hair loss before embarking on the hair transplantation, with individuals below the age of 25 years being denied the scope of the procedure.

Hair transplant surgery demands good planning, great surgical skill and good aesthetic sense on the part of the clinician, as hairs grow in specific direction and angulations for the given area of the scalp, and grafts should be placed in a way which should look natural and cover the scalp gaps thus achieving good density.

Most of the patients would like to know if the results are permanent with guaranteed results. Here, it's the astute clinician who should make all efforts to ensure that patient understands the concept of the hair transplant and the future consequences too, rather than simply promising the results.

The basic concept in hair transplant surgery is one of camouflaging technique which makes them look better rather than taking them back to their crowning glory days of their past during their younger days.

Patient should understand that he may still loose hair further and get worse with his genetic predilection to go bald and it's a progressive process. Hair transplant will only help him to maintain hairs which are aesthetically acceptable for his age and few individuals may require future sessions too.

**Preparation Prior to Hair Transplantation**
Routine blood test consisting of Complete blood count, glycaemic levels, prothrombin time and serology are done for every case. In patients with any underlying medical conditions, further investigations as deemed necessary for the case are done and a medical fitness is obtained from the physician.

All patients are advised to stop topical minoxidil at least a week prior to transplant to avoid bleeding hampering the progress of the case.

Photographs and consent for the procedure are obtained as a part of standard operating procedure for hair transplantation.

Consenting for the procedure should focus on detailed information of the procedure with clarity given on the results that can be obtained explaining the pros and cons of the procedure, their complications and outcomes. Alternative suggestions should also be given including no surgery, use of camouflage techniques and patients being on only medicines. Adequate time should be given to discuss and understand the proposed procedures. Finally, the proposed treatment plan with the fees proposed should be mentioned in the consent along with written preoperative and post-operative instructions.

The treatment plan formulated needs to account for the quantum of hair to be transplanted, the hairline design, the areas of high priority on the scalp, patient commitment and compliance.

## 34.9 Techniques and Description

### 34.9.1 Follicular Unit Transplantation (FUT) (Box 34.3) (Video 34.1)

FUT is also called strip method or stitch method. It's a gold standard method in hair transplant procedures till date though it's an old method [7]. The modern-day FUT is mainly harvesting a single strip, though earlier few doctors practised with multiple blades to obtain multiple strips which are obsolete now.

Strip method includes taking or harvesting a strip of the skin layer from the donor area usually from the occipital area of the head below the occipital protuberance and above the nape of the neck in the so-called safe zone for harvesting.

Strip measurements are variable with 30 cm being the maximum length and 1–2 cm width depending on skin laxity of the patient. However, the length and width are variable according to planning arrived at during the consultation with the patient as per the indication of the case. At times we have to limit strip width to 1 cm if the skin laxity is limited. Usually a strip of 30 cm in length and 1.5 cm in width will give around 2000–3000 grafts depending on the hair density of the individual.

**Box 34.3 FUT**

- Linear scar in donor area.
- Healing time is more in donor area.
- Little post-op discomfort in donor area.
- Difficult in tight scalp, with risk of scarring.
- Can't use in non-scalp hair like beard or body hair.
- Quality of graft is good
- Less time
- No need for shaving entire donor area.
- We can harvest up to 4000 follicular units in a single session.
- Less expensive
- Follicles Transection rate is very less.

#### 34.9.1.1 Assessment of the Donor Hair

Hair transplant outcomes will greatly depend on the donor hair quality and quantity [8]. The important factors that the clinician has to bear in mind are as follows:

1. The number of grafts that are present per square centimetre
   Few individuals have thick density being good or best donors (Fig. 34.6a) while a few have sparse density being poor donors (Fig. 34.6b) with the number of grafts per sq cm varying between 25 and 65 grafts on an average in healthy Indian adults. It further varies from person to person and sometimes from area to area in the same individual. Usually, occipital area has thick density whereas parietal area has less density. Good observation of the grafts in the donor area is most important for the surgeon to achieve good results.
2. Number of follicles present per graft
   This is highly variable with 2, 3 or 4 follicles being present in Indian adults whereas a few have only one or two follicles per graft. The presence of reducing follicles per graft is a sign of the progressive nature of the blading process.
3. Donor skin area
   Few individuals have large donor area as their scalp size is larger while a few individuals have donor bearing area which is smaller (Fig. 34.7a, b). This entity will decide the number of grafts that is available for harvesting.

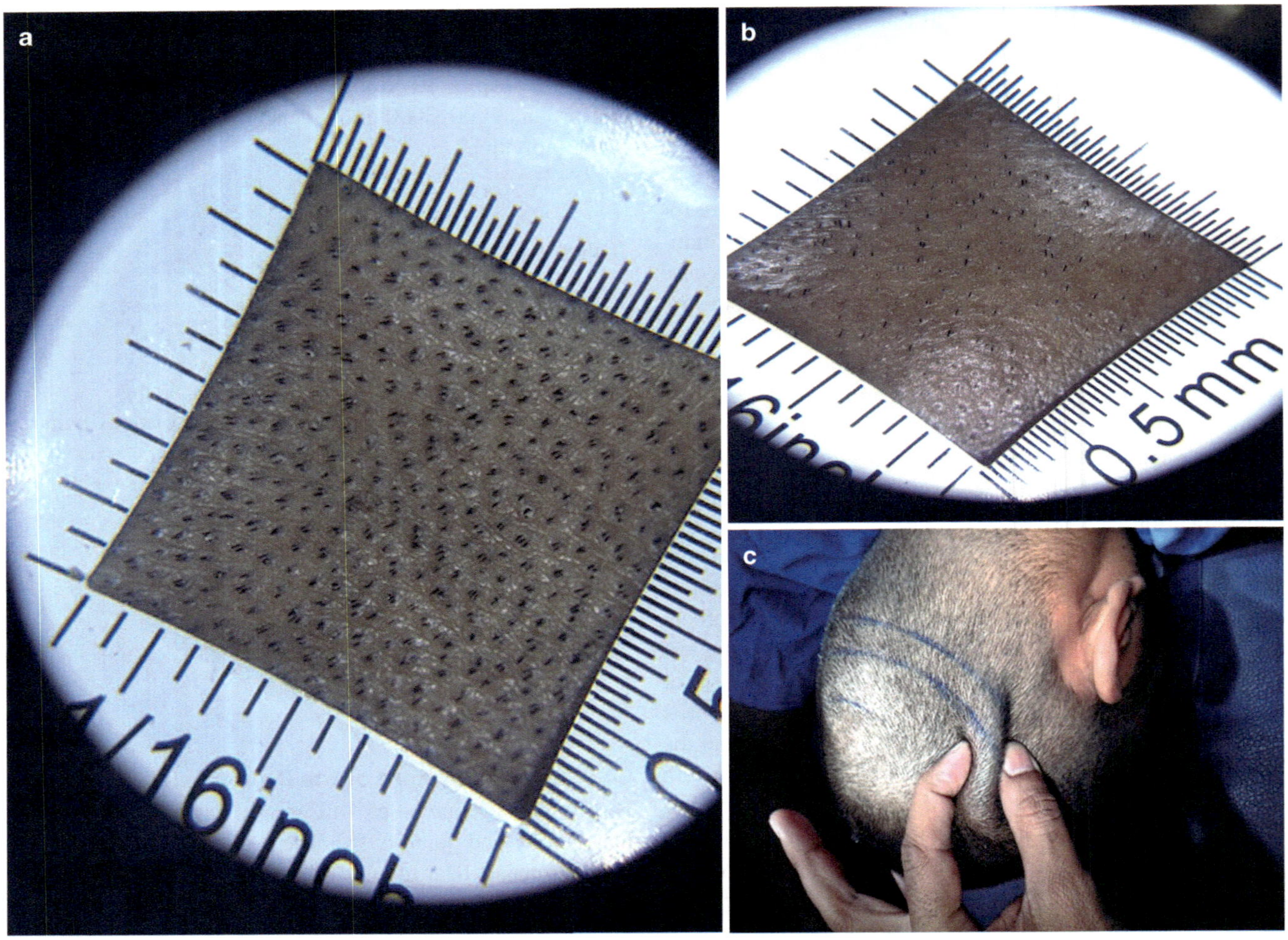




Fig. 34.6 (**a**) Good/best donor area based on hair follicular density. (**b**) Poor donor area based on hair follicular density. (**c**) Donor area skin laxity testing to ascertain the strip width planned for FUT

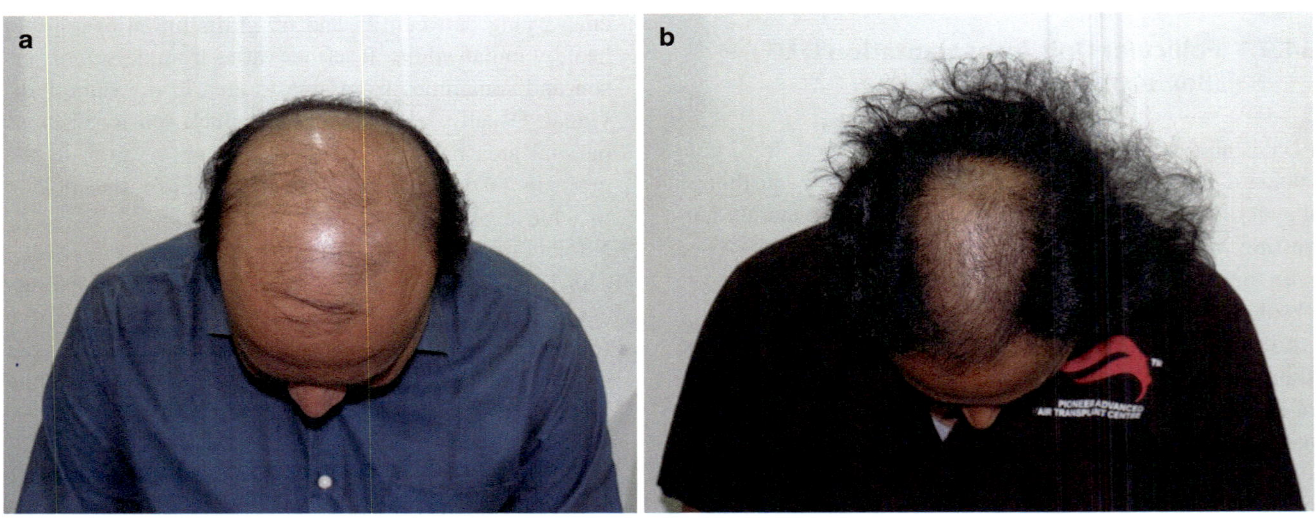




Fig. 34.7 (**a**) Large head with more surface area at donor zone. (**b**) Small head with lesser surface area at donor zone

4. Shaft diameter
   Individuals with thick shaft diameter will have better density and the outcome of the results is enhanced.
5. Skin laxity (Fig. 34.6c)
   In individuals with better skin laxity, we can harvest more grafts by FUT method by going for wider strips in a single session, whereas the same skin laxity may not have any significance with the FUE method.
   Patients who present with straight hair end up optically having less density because light can pass through hair strands and skin becomes visible especially if the hair is black and is contrasting against a fair skin background. Whereas presence of curly and course hair in an individual with dark complexion can give the illusion of thick density.

#### 34.9.1.2 Donor Site Preparation and Anaesthesia

Trimming is essential in the donor site to harvest the strip and the team member in charge of the preparation can ensure trimming the hair to 3 mm all over the scalp. Few surgeons prefer the procedure without trimming so as to reduce the downtime for the patient's social acceptability. But trimming will ensure better visibility and accessibility to the surgeon while performing the suturing with attention to detail to ensure minimal scarring along the strip harvest. Following the trimming, the next step is to wash the scalp with betadine solution. The clinician should ensure that preoperative photos, consent for the procedure, recording of baseline vitals of the patient and his weight is recorded prior to the preparation of the donor site.

The harvesting of the strip is done with the patient in prone posture following the standards of care with an iv line, monitoring of the vitals with a 3 parameter monitor, and following a dose of prophylactic antibiotic under aseptic conditions. Next, the donor area strip length and width to be harvested are marked out based on the skin laxity tests and depending on the individual's follicular density per square cm.

Once the marking is done, local anaesthesia is administered to the donor area, usually preferring field block in that area. Injecting the local anaesthetic in the lower border of the strip would provide sufficient anaesthesia to the field above.

#### 34.9.1.3 Preparation of Local Anaesthesia

Hair transplant procedure is time taking and lasts around 6–8 h. Lidocaine usually is a very safe anaesthetic with a duration of action lasting between 90 and 120 min and therefore we need to add a long-acting drug-like bupivacaine for hair transplant procedure. Combination of the above would work better for 8–10 h and the overall dosage should not exceed the maximum permissible as per the weight of the individual. The local anaesthetic solution used is typically as follows:

Lidocaine 2% 30 ml + bupivacaine 0.5% 4 ml + ns 60 ml.
The above combination gives 64 ml of local anaesthesia, which is of lidocaine 1%.

Tumescence is widely used in hair transplant surgery to raise neurovascular bundles away from the hair follicles which will reduce the trauma to nerves and vessels during the procedure. Another important role for the use of tumescence is in reducing the bleeding during the procedure since scalp bleeds more.

Tumescence solution consists of 500 ml ns + 1 ampule of 1:1000 epinephrine and this is injected into the strip area following the local anaesthesia at least 15 min before the strip harvesting.

#### 34.9.1.4 Instruments for the Strip Procedure

Variscore blade (Fig. 34.8) is useful to have control on the dimensions of the strip and it gives the option to adjust the strip width by adding or reducing the metal spacer plates. Each metal spacer plate comes with thickness of 2 mm and 1 mm and, for example, if we need a strip with width of 1.3 cm, then we need to add 6 plates of 2 mm and 1 plate of 1 mm. The variscore blade has added advantage of depth control while making incision and can accommodate two surgical blades. Usually, for scalp, we can use number 15 surgical blades.

Prior to the incision marking, the strip dimensions are done. Most of the surgeons make straight incision, which may lead to scar. It's always better to follow Langer lines of the skin which ensures less scars with the strip incision looking like a crescent shape with the end tapering off. Strips which are as long as 30 cm (Fig. 34.9) in length run from above one ear to the other ear. It's always recommended to

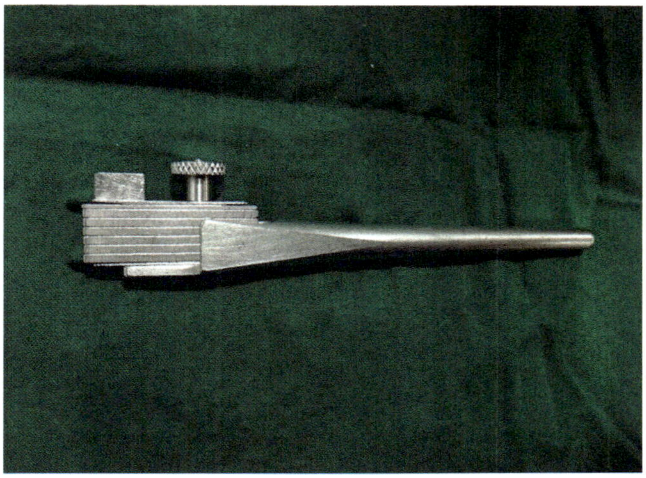



**Fig. 34.8** Variscore blade -popular blade handle for FUT

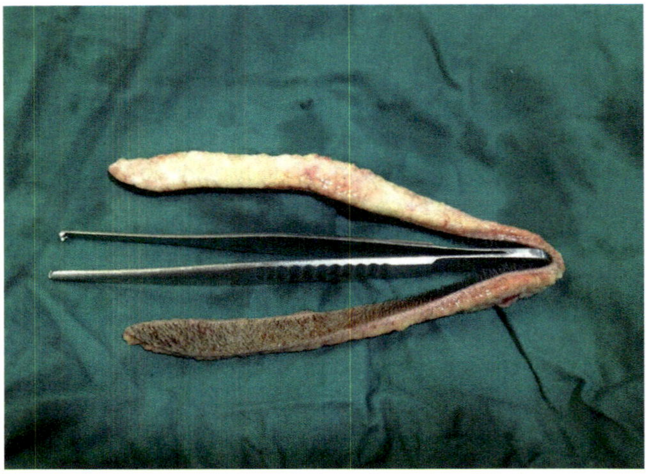



**Fig. 34.9** Strip harvested prior to slivering

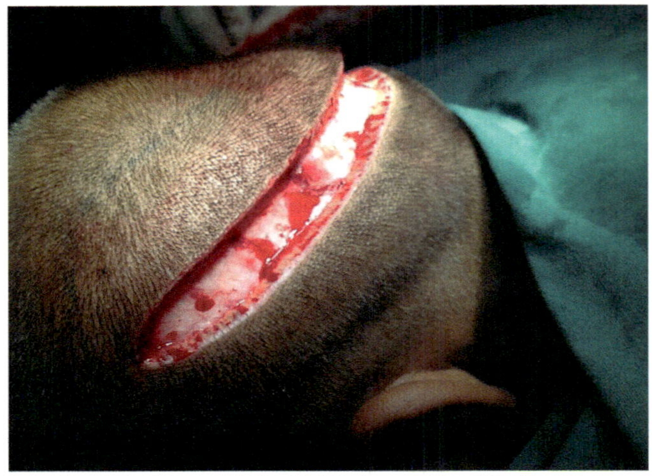



**Fig. 34.10** Wound margins prepared for trichophytic closure

place the incision at or just below the external occiput area as the follicles here are considered permanent. It is indeed not good to go too low below the external occiput as we may end up in big blood vessels. After the initial indentation of the incision is done with variscore blade, it is later followed up by the use of BP blade number 15 and the incisions are made very carefully to reach up to 3 mm beneath the follicular depth with some amount of subcuticular fat around it, while we ensure that we do not cut the galea. While making the incisions, care is taken to prevent slicing of the follicles at the skin margins and the flap is raised from one end to the other using gentle yet deft strokes with the blade.

Good illumination and haemostasis can help to raise strip with minimal damage to both the follicles and vessels in the vicinity. Damage to the vessels is most common if proper tumescence is not attained and can lead to bigger scar and shock loss of hair in the donor area. Any adventure into the galeal layer can lead to haematoma and chances of spreading infections through emissary veins.

Haemostasis is achieved prior to closure by using bipolar diathermy; the scalp wound is irrigated with normal saline and a double layer closure is performed with vicryl 2.0 (TS 2404, 3/8 circle, cutting edge) for the inside and a prolene 3.0 (nw800, 3/8 circle cutting edge) for the outer skin (Fig. 34.11a, b). The strip that is harvested is preserved in cold saline on a petri dish at 4 °C.

#### 34.9.1.5 Trichophytic Closure

Trichophytic closure (Fig. 34.10) involves trimming of the upper and lower edges of the skin which facilitates the hair to emerge through the scar ensuring that we will give aesthetically acceptable scar to the patient (Fig. 34.12b) Wound closure done without the above clinical manoeuvre leads to poor scar (Fig. 34.12a), which is quite obvious.

Post-operative care of the wound is important. Antiseptic creams are optional if the donor site wound is washed with clean water or ns on a daily basis. In our experience, suture removal is recommended on 11th post-operative day to avoid wound gaping or wound dehiscence.

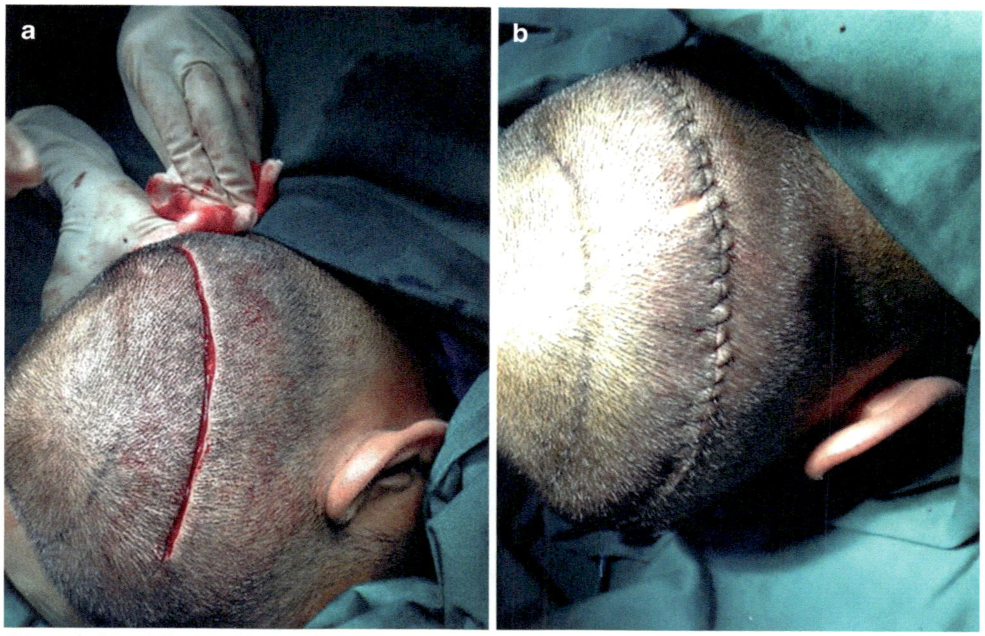




**Fig. 34.11** (**a**, **b**) Wound closure in layers after Haemostasis

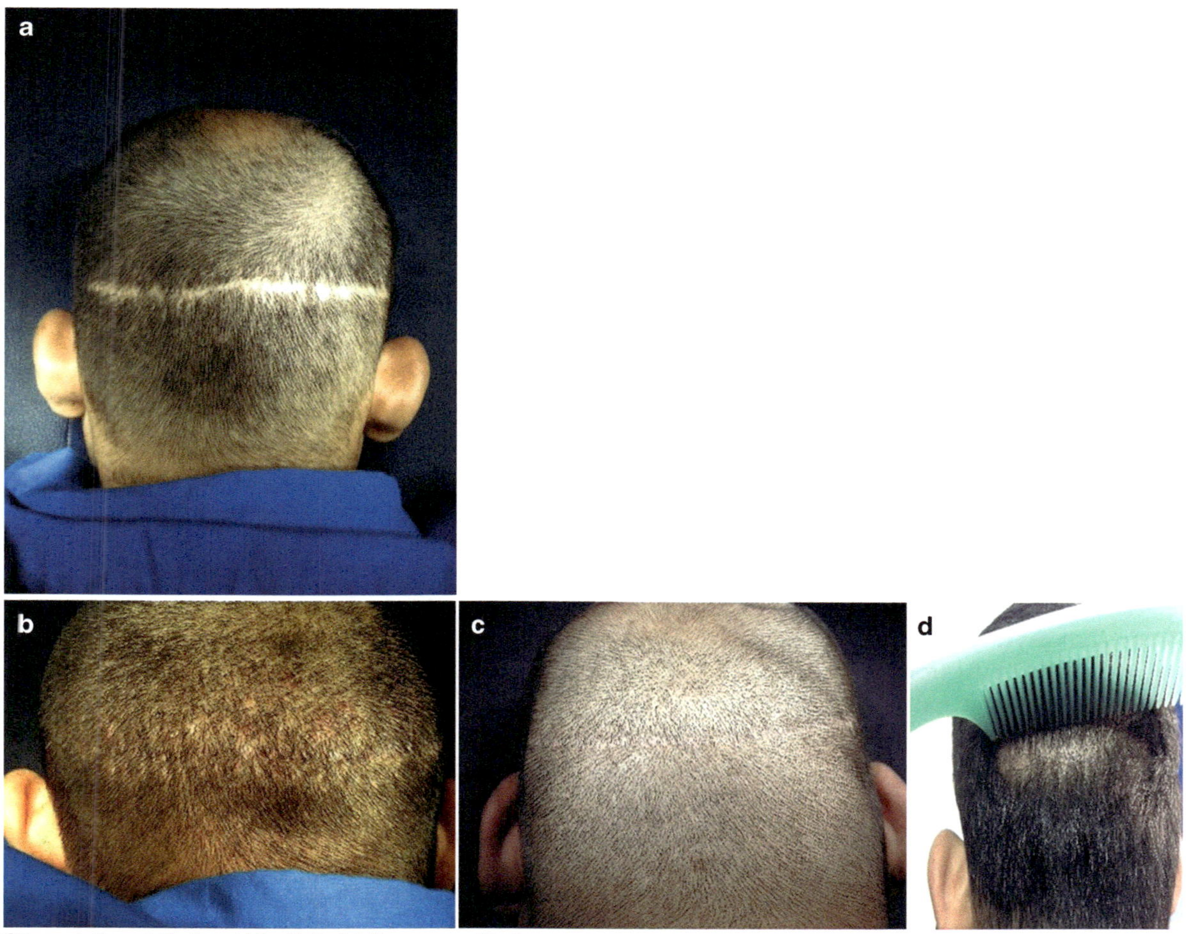




**Fig. 34.12** (**a**) Poor scar resulting from normal wound closure (**b–d**) post operative scar following trichophytic closure

**Variable Strip Technique**

This will help us to get maximum grafts with less tension along the scar leading to a better scar. Most of the individuals have thick density in the occipital area and lesser density in the parietal area and any misjudgement will lead to poor wide scar in the parietal areas. Here, by using variable dimensions of the strip technique (Fig. 34.13), we can target for more grafts with least possible scar. In this technique, the strip width is more in the occipital area than compared to the parietal area as illustrated in the image below.

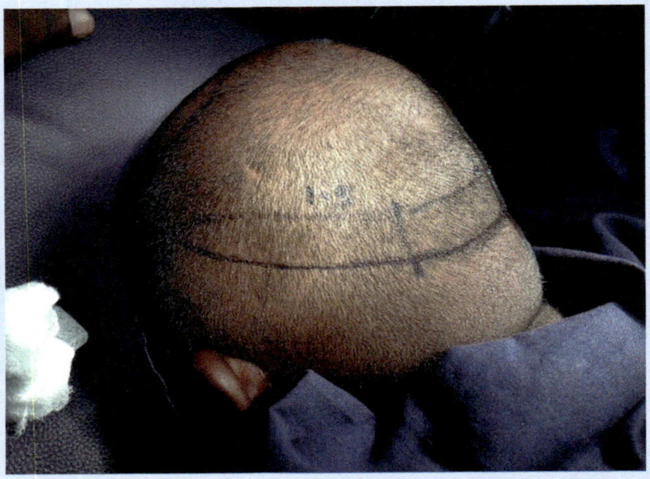



Fig. 34.13 Variable dimensions of the strip marked out for harvesting

#### 34.9.1.6 Slivering

Slivering is a process where the strip is sliced into small bits of tissues with rows of hair follicles in them, through meticulous deft handwork akin to the baker slicing the bread loaf into thin slices. It is the first step of the separation of grafts from the strip while avoiding any transection of the graft. Higher magnifications should be used to perform this important step for which a few clinics are using stereoscopic microscopes while the others manage with normal 10× magnification. It should be done simultaneously while the surgeon performs the wound suturing to save the crucial graft holding time of around 6 h.

At the end of this step, we get slivers which are ready for the separation process (Fig. 34.14). The separation process is separating individual grafts from the sliver. For the separation process, we need more trained technicians as it is cumbersome exercise and needs great attention to detail to avoid any form of trauma to the graft being obtained with an obvious fight against time.

For the separation process, we need to use 3× magnification which can be done on a sterilised wooden spatula or an acrylic illuminated sheet.

Wooden spatula would give us good resistance to cut the grafts whereas acrylic sheets will be slippery. Advantage of the acrylic sheet is we can illuminate from below, which is easy for separating the grafts. The separation process is nothing but getting rid of the excess fat around the grafts and making the grafts slender in a pear shape or tear drop shape. Care is to be taken to ensure that we do not denude the roots and little fat is left behind for survival of the graft through plasma imbibition. All skin has to be trimmed and removed from the graft and finally these prepared grafts are preserved in cold normal saline around 4–8 °C temperature.

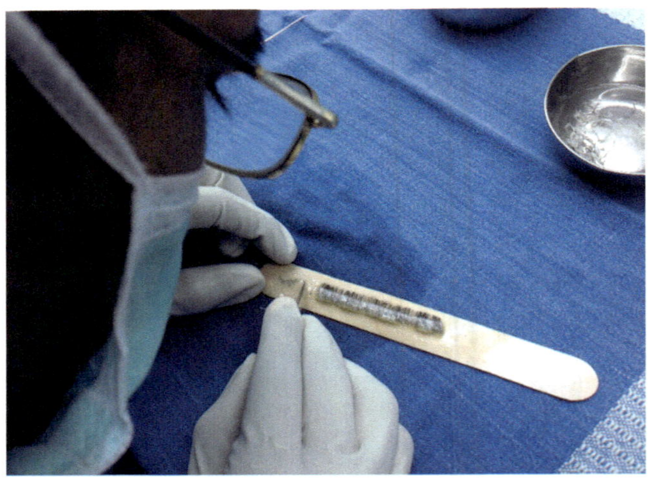



Fig. 34.14 Slivering and separation of grafts from the strip in FUT

While separating the grafts, we would get single, double, triple follicular unit grafts, and care is exercised to maintain the follicular unit (Figs. 34.15 and 34.17a), as it is natural to ensure better survival. These are segregated further in different bowls and are used up for implanting starting with single units for the frontal hairline and progressing onto multiple follicular units as we go posteriorly in a progressive manner.

### 34.9.2 Follicular Unit Extraction (FUE) (Box 34.4) (Video 34.2)

In this technique, we extract the individual follicles one graft at a time with the help of small punches. Also known as no stitch and no cut method, it's minimally invasive procedure compared to the FUT. FUE gained popularity in recent years because of its ease of doing and being less invasive with minimal downtime for the patient. Initially, FUE was introduced with manual punches which was more tedious and time consuming limiting the number of grafts that could be done in a session [9]. Current advances with motorised punch have improved the pace and its effectiveness in harvesting more grafts. Though many different motors and punches are available in the market, normal dental micromotor with straight hand piece would suffice to perform FUE (Fig. 34.16a, b).

Punches are made up of either titanium or stainless steel with the diameter of the punch ranging from 0.6 to 1 mm, with 0.9 mm being suitable for Indian scalp. The advent of FUE has expended the scope of harvesting follicles from other sites of the body wherein 0.6 or 0.7 mm punches are useful for beard site and 0.8 or 0.9 mm punches have been suitable for chest hair harvesting, respectively.

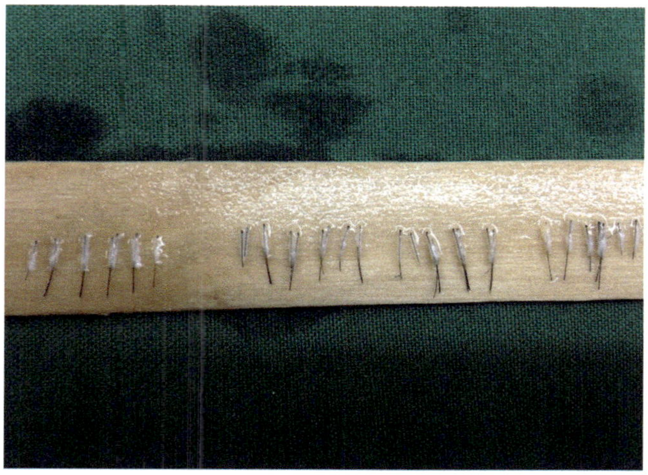



**Fig. 34.15** Separated follicular units

**Box 34.4 FUE**

- No linear scar, small round dots in donor area.
- Decreased healing time in donor area.
- No post-op discomfort in donor area.
- Useful for those with risk of donor scarring. Like young pt, very muscular, very tight scalp.
- Useful in Body hair transplant
- Graft quality is not as good as FUT.
- Procedure is time consuming.
- Large sessions required to shave the entire donor area.
- More expensive.
- Follicles transection rate is more

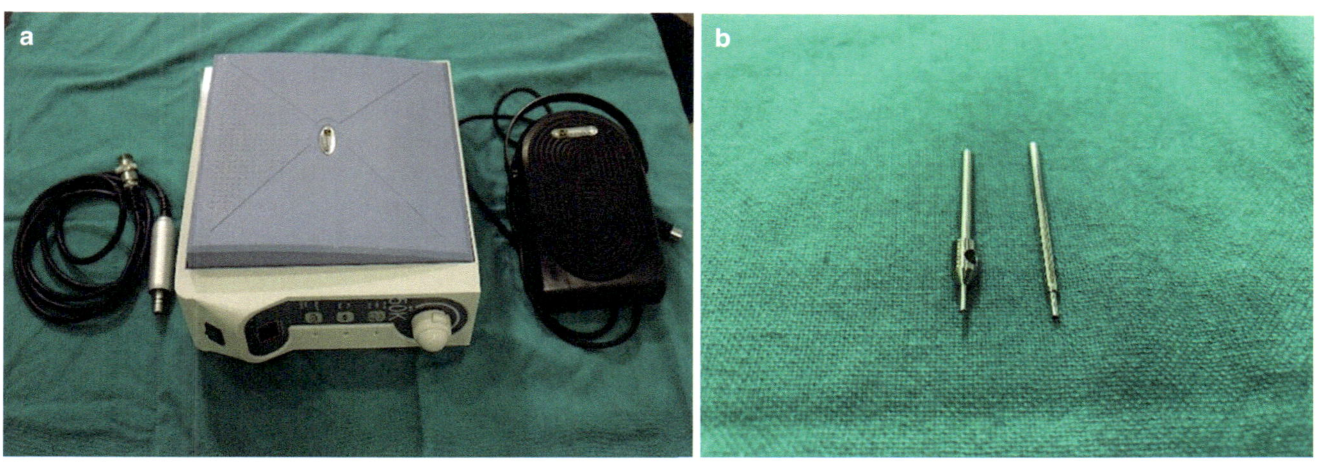




**Fig. 34.16** (**a**, **b**) FUE instruments: micromotor, straight handpiece and punches

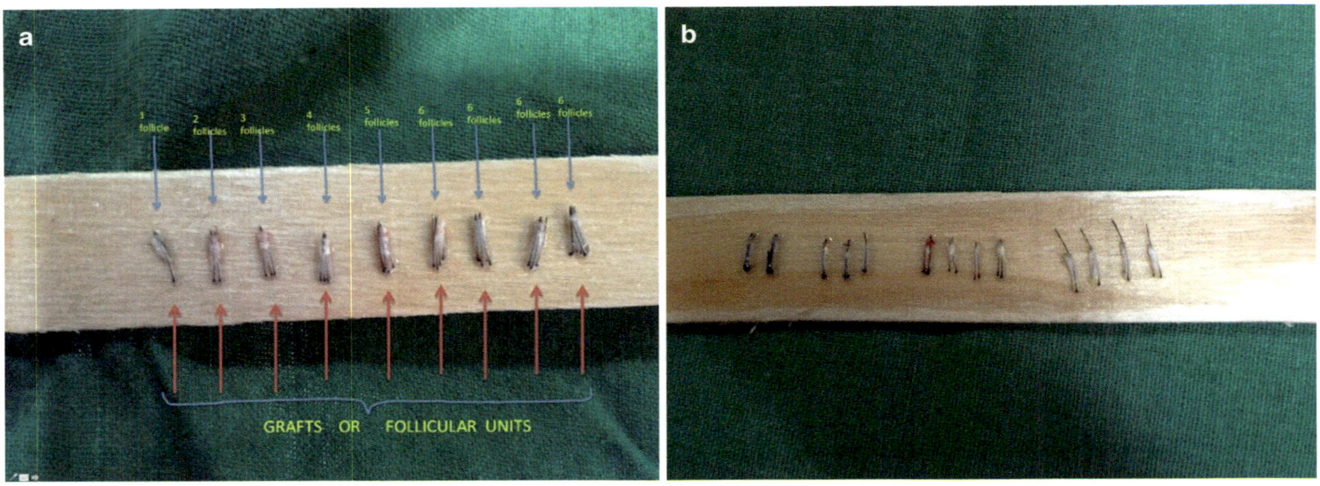




**Fig. 34.17** (**a**) Follicular units and their natural arrangements. (**b**) Comparison – FUE grafts on the left which are lean and slender versus FUT grafts on to the right which are bulkier

Punches are available as dull, sharp, serrated and oscillating type. Normal dull or sharp punched would be sufficient to perform FUE. On an average one punch can be used to harvest around 1000–1500 grafts.

This latest motorised technology has made surgeons' job easy and in experienced hands we can harvest around 800–1000 grafts in 1 h, provided patient's skin is favourable.

Being a blind procedure, this is technique sensitive and is associated with a steep learning curve requiring more concentration. It is performed under 3× magnification controlling the punching around the hair graft while maintaining depth and angulation which is very vital to harvesting the grafts. The punch should get down to epidermis and dermis junction not going beyond 4 mm from the skin. Surgeon should always analyse the angle of exit of the hair and be parallel it prior to the punching. Acute angles of the grafts would lead to difficulty in punching and lead to not only bigger punch holes but higher transaction rates. Most of the Indian skin is favourable for FUE procedure because of thicker skin types. The follicles obtained by FUE are comparatively slender and devoid of extra adventitious tissue in comparison to the FUT follicles (Fig. 34.17b).

#### 34.9.2.1 Blades

They can vary in size and shape from being thin sharp blade to having a pointed chisel as in the case of sp90 which is one of the popular blades for pre slit technique. Today, the surgeons have a choice of customising the blade with commercially available tools and can use a square or tapered blade as per their choice.

#### 34.9.2.2 Needles

Standard 19 gauge hypodermic needle is preferred for making the graft recipient sites while the same can be achieved with solid core needles eliminating epidermal implantation.

#### 34.9.2.3 Limitations of Follicular Unit Extraction

FUE has an important role to play in hair transplant because it can reach the areas where strip cannot reach to harvest grafts. When we plan second session, FUT may not be possible in unyielding skin types. In poor candidates where donor areas of the scalp have poor hair quality, FUE can be used to target beard and body hairs. FUE like any other procedure is associated with a few disadvantages like comparatively more GTR (graft transection rate), especially in curly hair types and in these few cases graft yield is abysmally low wherein the surgeon will have to convert the case to strip technique. Follicular splay is another situation where hair roots are placed apart which causes difficult extraction. In case of scattered grafts too, the punch may tend to damage more grafts while harvesting and would not be an ideal situation to continue harvesting with high graft transection.

#### 34.9.2.4 Hairline (Fig. 34.18a, b)

The hairline design and location are the most critical factors in the success of hair transplantation, for which one should understand the concept of facial thirds. Till the age of third decade of life, the anterior hairline at the midline is located at a distance equal to the middle third height of the face from the glabella, adding additional 1 cm in length to it with each passing decade of life to take the hairline upwards and backwards to give a matured look to face considering the progressive nature of hair loss. The frontotemporal apex is the deepest point of the anterior hairline laterally as it merges with the temporal hairline and is located along the lateral canthus of the eye [10].

It is to be borne in mind that the hairline anteriorly is not a straight line but an irregular one having peaks and troughs making it look like a coastline with the front two rows made

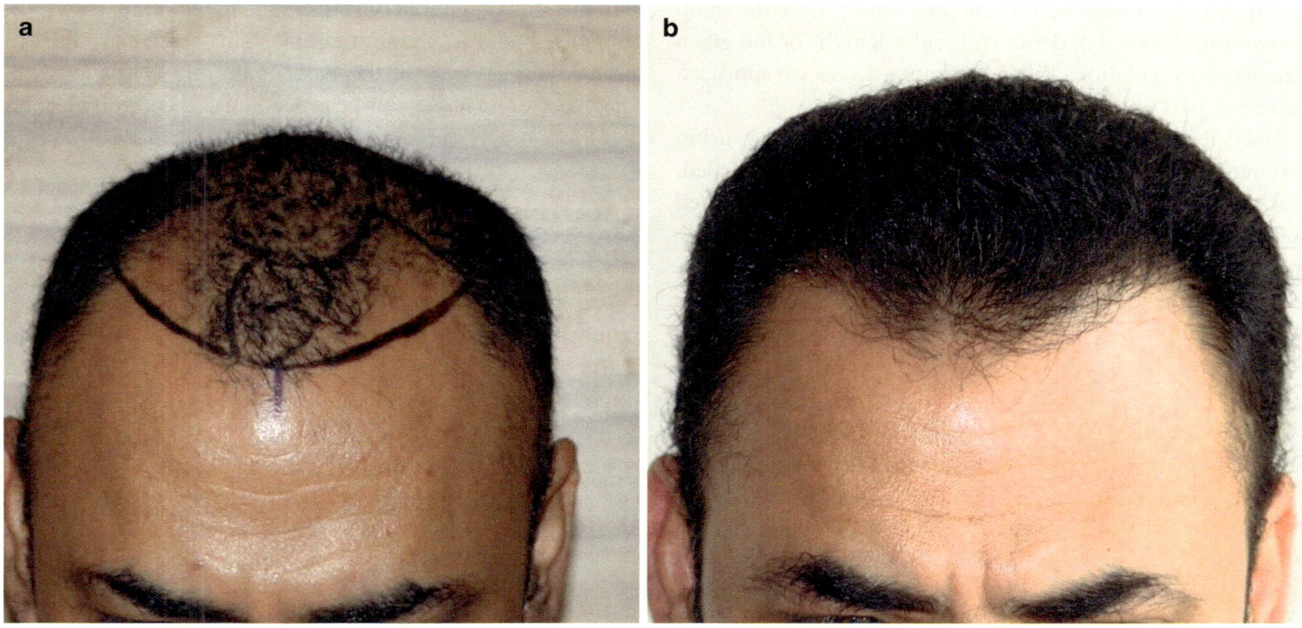


©Association of Oral and Maxillofacial Surgeons of India

**Fig. 34.18** (**a**, **b**) Hairline design and natural looks

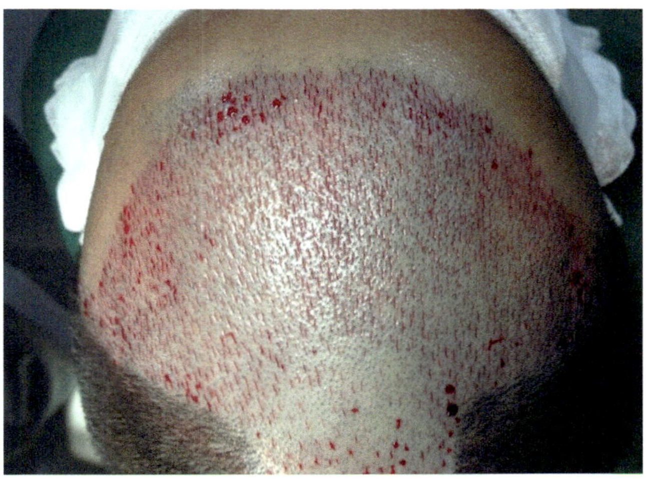

©Association of Oral and Maxillofacial Surgeons of India

**Fig. 34.19** Recipient site slits

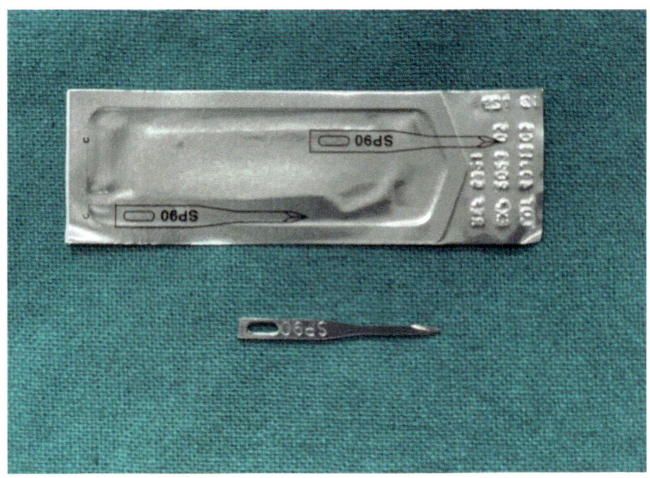

©Association of Oral and Maxillofacial Surgeons of India

**Fig. 34.20** sp 90 blade used for recipient site preparation

up of single follicular units and gradually it progresses to double and triple follicular units to give the density. The central core or frontal tuft area gets the maximum density of hairs implanted to enhance the strength and aesthetic value of the hairline thus created.

#### 34.9.2.5 The Recipient Sites Preparation and Implantation

Recipient sites are prepared (Fig. 34.19) to receive the grafts by making slits in the skin with either 19 gauge hypodermic needles or sp 90 blades (Fig. 34.20) or other microblades which are of 1–1.1 mm in width. This step could be done prior to implantation for all the grafts (pre-slit method) or individually for each graft while simultaneously implanting it (stick and place method).

Slits made with blades tend to give more natural looks when compared to needle implantation (Table 34.1). As a prerequisite to facilitate implantation, the site needs to be trimmed short while the remaining hairs guide us in the direction and angulation of the implantation. Proper tumescence will allow us to expand scalp so that we can place more grafts in the given area while also reducing any damage to the neurovascular bundle and enhances visibility.

The slits are performed in the area with proper direction (converging forwards), depth (follicular length for the given patient) and angulation (15° in the front −45° as we approach the crown part of the scalp).

Once the slits are done, implantation is done by using jeweller's forceps (Fig. 34.21), which are pressure graded. This is also called 2 forceps technique as one forcep is used to locate the slit while the other one is used to implant the graft into the slit. The grafts are to be held above the bulb or beside it where the dermal fat is held.

Implantation of 3000 grafts by forceps would need around 3–3.5 h approximately (Fig. 34.22a).

#### 34.9.2.6 Implanters

Few surgeons use implanters (Fig. 34.22b) which can hold the graft in it and all you have to do is to eject them into the site at the desired direction and angulation. Technicians will preload the graft into the implanter. Implanter can be used with pre slits or without pre slits made in the scalp. However, implanters tend to create a circular slit which may lead to pitting kind of scars at the base of the graft after growth. They need extra hands for the procedure and come at an extra cost too.

**Table 34.1** Advantages and disadvantages of blade versus needle for slit creation

| | Blades | Needle |
|---|---|---|
| Distribution | Uniform | Variable |
| Bleeding | More | Less |
| Direction and angulation control | Better | Possible in few trained hands |
| Time taken | Less | More |
| Aesthetic appearance | More likely | Less likely |
| Healing | Without marks | Leaves pitting/embossed scars |

### 34.9.3 Combi Technique (Fig. 34.23)

This is a combination of FUT and FUE in a single session. Combi technique is recommended when we need more grafts as in anything over and above 3500 follicles in a single session. In this technique, the strip is first harvested

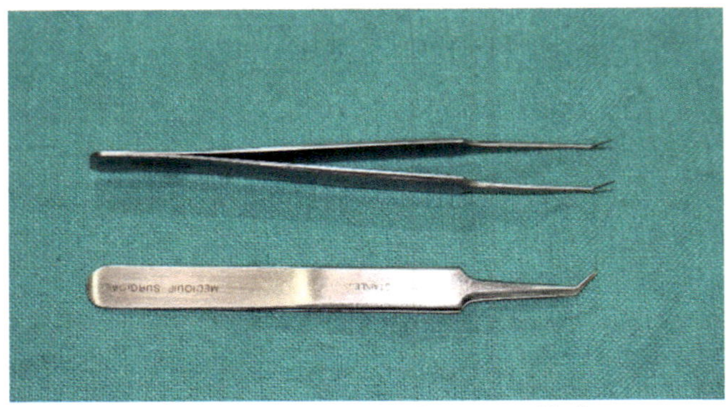



**Fig. 34.21** Jeweller's forceps used for implantation

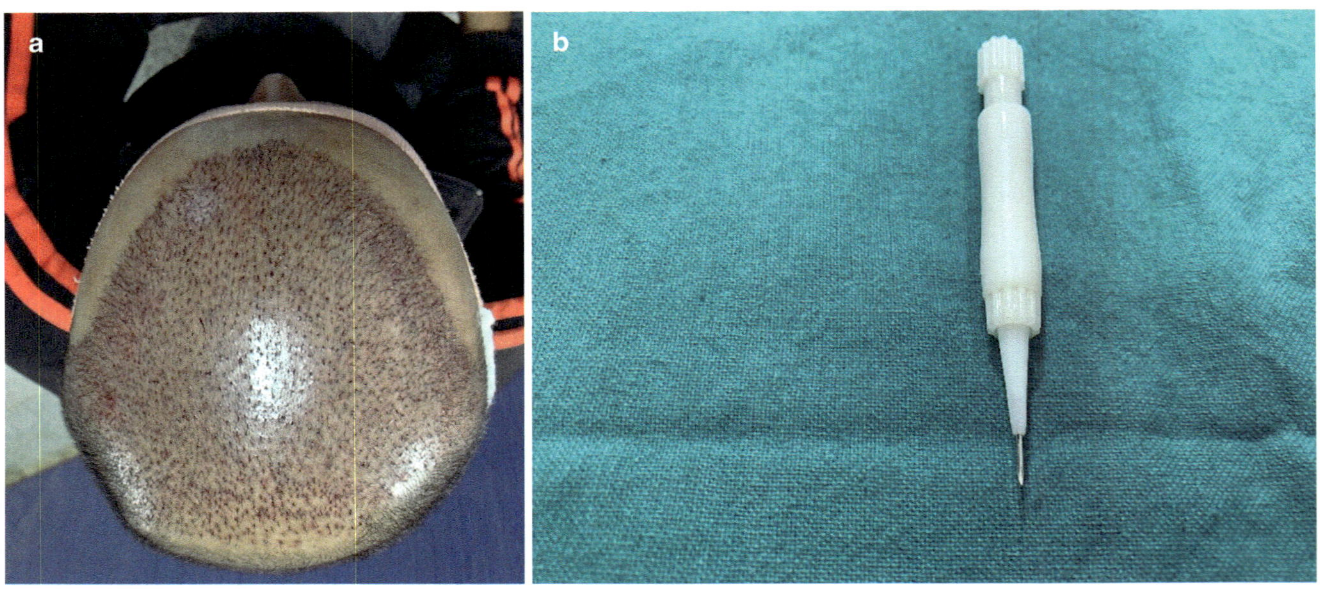




**Fig. 34.22** (**a**) Immediate view of a case post implantation. (**b**) Implanters used for implantation

and then the FUE is performed above and below the strips in the same sitting before implanting. Advantages of this procedure are that the surgeon can reduce the strip length and still can obtain more grafts thereby reducing the strip length and the resulting scar. However, it requires an experienced surgeon and well-trained team to execute the procedure.

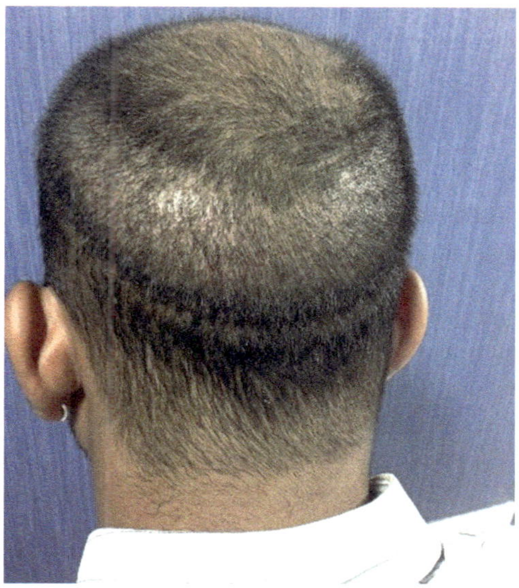



**Fig. 34.23** Combi technique post-operative view

## 34.10 Post-operative Care

Immediately after the procedure, the heaviness, numbness or tightness may be there for a few hours. There is also some swelling on the forehead and temple area due to the tumescence and surgical insult and the resulting swelling is normal. Patients are allowed to sleep on the back or on the sides but are not allowed to sleep on their tummy as otherwise the swelling tends to gravitate onto face and eyes. Patients should be asked to massage the forehead from the middle to the sides for 5 min every hour for first few days. Rarely some patients may feel momentary dizziness especially while standing up from the lying down position on the procedure table.

There is some oozing of blood-stained fluid from grafted site as well as in donor area (both in case of strip or FUE). Bending forward of the neck can stretch the stitches and can initiate some more oozing from the stitches therefore keeping the chin up is recommended.

Patients are restricted to perform any contact sports/gymming for a period of 12 days and should avoid swimming for up to 3 weeks. They should also not get to field work under the sun for first 3 weeks. Patients who ride a bike are allowed to wear a helmet after a period of 4 weeks. Topical minoxidil can be restarted in the transplanted site after a waiting period of about 15 days post-operatively. Patients are also forbidden from riding a bike or driving in an open vehicle for up to 2 weeks.

After the procedure, antibiotics and analgesics are provided for 5 days. The donor and recipient sites may or may not be bandaged. If bandaging is preferred, a non-adhering betadine pad is placed over the operative sites with several layers of flattened gauze sponges over them to hold the betadine pad in place as the scalp is wrapped with clean bandage using to two to three 4-inch gauze rolls. Crepe bandage can

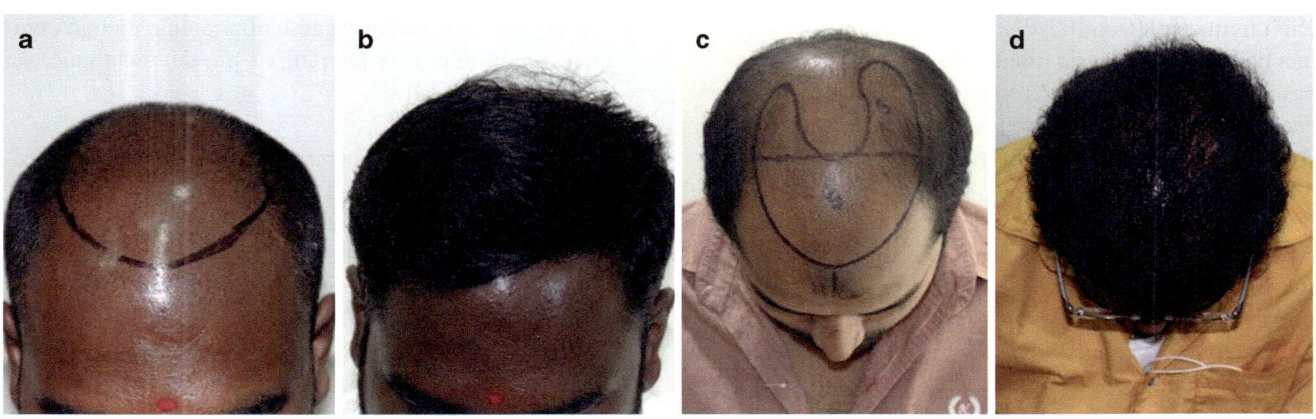





**Fig. 34.24** (**a**–**d**) Outcome following hair transplantation

be used over it. The dressing is removed the following morning, and the scalp and each graft are clean meticulously by gently dabbing with a cotton swab with normal saline. Patients are advised to sprinkle or spray normal saline over the grafts every 3–4 h for 8–10 days. Suture removal is performed on 11th day and is not applicable for FUE. Initially for 10 days the grafted area should be washed without rubbing the grafts. Whereas after the above period, grafted area can be washed and patients can rub the grafts. Most of the grafts will be shed by 12–20 days which is a common phenomenon, one need not to worry about it falling off.

**Regrowth and Results** (Fig. 34.24a–d)
Summary of events following a hair transplant.

Immediate after a hair transplant, there will be mild blood excretion and oozing.

1st day scabs (nothing but dried blood) will form and continue forming for the next few days.

After 4 to 10 days you will notice itching. This is normal, but do not scratch or pick on the transplanted areas.

After 10 days your scalp will be cleared of all scabs.

After 11–20 days your new implanted hair will shed. Now your new follicles are in its dormant (sleeping) stage. It's time to watch and wait.

Pt must be aware that a lag phage exists before hair growth is initiated. After approximately 4 months, the telogen phase to the implanted grafts ends and anagen begins. Complete growth can be seen only after 8 months and hair continue to grow until 12–14 months.

## 34.11 Complications

Able professionals should manage any adverse outcomes by minimising the damage and help achieve the desired outcomes with low morbidity. Fortunately, today the follicular unit hair transplantation is a safe procedure with low rates of complication when performed with care [11].

### 34.11.1 Complications in Preoperative Phase

Overexpectations of the patients are the major cause of complications and arise due to hasty or incomplete consultation and is better addressed with more than one consultation to assimilate the requisite information with the help of informative brochures, websites and discussions with the clinician to arrive at realistic outcomes especially in the younger patients who happen to be unclear and lack maturity for comprehending the results; in such cases, it's better to keep them on medical line of treatment till they become practical in accepting the results. Any individual with body dysmorphic disorder and Norwood vii patients where you would not make much difference would count as poor patient selection by the clinician. In case of ongoing hair loss, the clinicians should not be tempted to promise full coverage or high density influenced by the advent of current medicines as the patients may change their minds and stop the intake of medicines over a long period of time, eventually resulting in inappropriate placement pattern and lack of donor site for harvesting. Clinicians should not be further influenced by the patients' demand for low unaesthetic hairline, or be drawn into performing mega sessions arising out of patients' demand and be careful in choosing the donor material in the middle of the back and sides of the permanent fringe avoiding any slanted scars or scars visible in scanty donor hair bearing areas.

### 34.11.2 Complications in Surgical Phase

1. Pain:
   Patients who are counselled appropriately and are provided with a relaxing ambience generally experience minimal discomfort. In-depth local anaesthesia achieved through precise nerve blocks and ring blocks administered with a long-acting drug-like sensorcaine and taking help of vibrating devices while injecting the solution slowly will go a long way in enhancing the comfort levels. Anxiolytics should be prescribed by the clinicians to patients who are apprehensive about the procedure.
2. Bleeding and popping:
   Optimising the health of the patient prior to the surgery results in blood pressures being within normal limits. Adequate tumescence consisting of saline and epinephrine has to be injected below the dermis to allow the surgical field to be lifted away from the bleed vessels and then the clinician has started the procedure after 15 min will have minimal bleeding. Too much of tumescent in the recipient site can be a cause of popping, though clinician cannot eliminate popping as pre slit technique can minimise the issue.
3. Bad hair direction:
   Clinicians should plan appropriately to maintain the direction and exit angle of the hair that mimics the natural growth. Keeping the grafts with a few millimetres of hair will allow the clinician to ascertain the angle during implantation.
4. Hiccups:
   Due to the irritation of the aberrant branch of the vagus nerve, patients can have hiccups through the procedure.
5. Poor graft quality:
   A good team leader will constantly supervise to ensure proper handling of the follicles, which will minimise trauma to the follicle resulting from transaction, manipulation, desiccation, oxygen starvation and crushing of the graft [12].

### 34.11.3 Post Surgical Complications

1. Donor site effluvium:
   Hair in the growth phase can fall rapidly post transplantation due to temporary lack of oxygen during surgery resulting in loss of hair variably along to suture line when significant blood vessels are cut. Any such hair loss will be noticeable around the third week postoperatively and leads to embarrassment to the surgeon. If the donor area can be raised above the blood vessels with good volume of tumescence, the above complication is rarely encountered.
2. Infection:
   This is a very rare complication seen today given the standard asepsis precautions followed and is rarely encountered where the patients are not given adequate post-operative instructions especially in cases of tight donor area closure and in patients with compromised immunity.
3. Dehiscence:
   A poor surgical technique associated with bad suturing, harvesting wide strips, performing tight closures or resulting infections and necrosis can lead to dehiscence.
4. Dysesthesias:
   Today it's no longer a complication thanks to adequate use of tumescence which will lift the hair follicles above the neurovascular bundles.
5. Scars:
   This unavoidable outcome can be prevented by following the basic principles of surgery with accurate approximation, closure without tension, by using double layered closure, trichophytic technique and avoiding resolvable suture for closing the skin. Donor scars also occur due to improper donor assessment prior to the surgery. Skin laxity test will help us to evaluate the skin laxity so that we can limit the strip width. At times we may need to consider variable width dimension to reduce the tension in the wound, usually where occipital area skin laxity is more and parietal area skin laxity is less. So we can consider more width at occipital area and less width at parietal area. If skin has less laxity, we can consider FUE.
   Any hypertrophic scar can be managed with steroid or injection and later implanting hairs with FUE.
6. Forehead swelling and ecchymosis:
   Based on the laxity of the skin in the frontal area and the trauma induced by the slit making process, swelling occurring at 3–4 days post hair transplantation can be mitigated by including some steroids in the la solution, applying pressure bandage and some digital massage across the forehead.

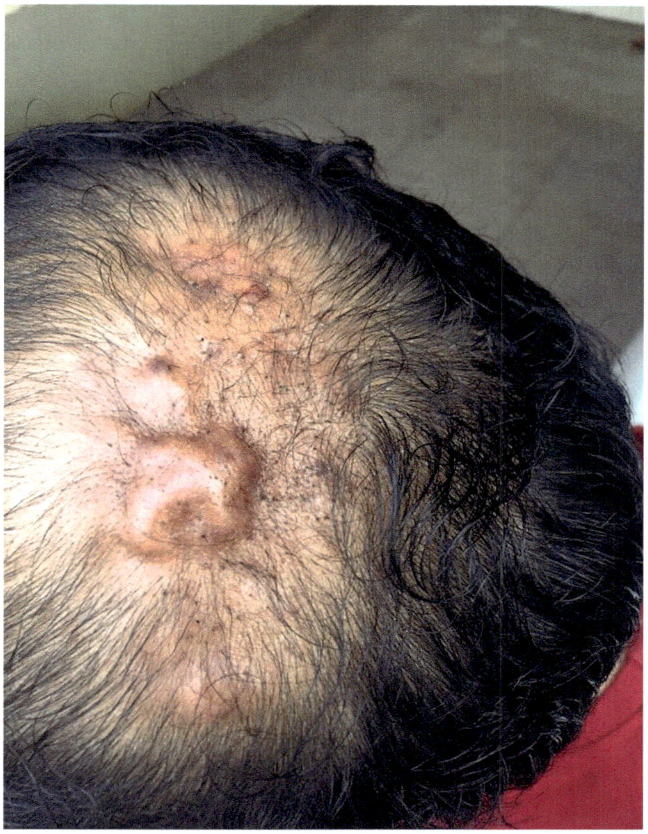



Fig. 34.25 Folliculitis post hair transplantation

7. Surgical effluvium:
   This is similar to the donor site effluvium which results in the anagen hairs going into telogen phase and falling out around the second or third post-operative week and regrowing with the grafts. Preoperative use of minoxidil solution tried 1 month prior to the procedure is recommended to prevent the above complication.
8. Cysts, pustules, pimples and folliculitis: (Fig. 34.25)
   The above sequelae following hair transplantation can be avoided by preventing deep implantation of grafts, transacting hair during site creation and piggybacking of one follicle up on another. Most of them do settle down with time; however, acne like therapy can be offered to resolve the lesions faster.
9. Pitting and tenting:
   It's very important to avoid the above complication in the frontal hairline which could otherwise be unacceptable and are easily preventable by avoiding deep placement of the grafts as in the case of pitting and too superficial placement of the grafts as in the case of tenting.

10. Poor growth:
    This can be attributed to poor handling of the grafts resulting in physical and biological trauma to the grafts associated with dehydration of the follicle, crushing of the follicle during implantation, thermal insult and prolonged holding time outside the body.

The incidence of complications may be reduced by avoiding mistakes by the team in general (Box 34.5) and those related to the technique, specifically graft survival (Box 34.6).

**Box 34.5 Frequently Made Mistakes Made by Team**

- Too much cross talk between team members annoying the patient.
- Members do not address patient by name.
- Grafts prepared either too chubby or skinny.
- Too many single grafts prepared.
- Photography not taken properly.
- Consent not taken properly.
- Grafts allowed to dry.
- Not interested in routine work.

**Box 34.6 Factors Affecting Graft Survival**

- Proper donor tumescence
- Temperature of holding solution
- Dehydration of follicle
- Crush injury of follicle
- Transection of follicle
- Adequate dermis and fat around follicle
- Smoking
- Biological modifiers

## 34.12 Current Advances

Futuristic developments in the field of hair transplant need to focus on the current lacunae in the procedure and revolves around the availability of limited donor supply and the duration of the procedure.

Low-level laser light therapy has been approved by FDA as a device to stimulate the hair growth in the 650–800 nm spectrum. Home-use scalp brush or helmets with laser technology are available which use the pain-free technology to stimulate epidermal stem cells in the hair follicle to move the follicles into anagen phase.

Automation of the FUE process with the use of robotics has shown to reduce the follicular transaction rates and improve the harvest speed, resolving the issue of skills possessed by practitioners. Artas and neo-graft are devices which have glamorised the field by involving robotic technology, but the running expenses and need to create sites and manually implant follicles need to be solved in the coming days.

If hair can be cultured from the scalp biopsy, then the patient would not need to donate hair by going through a painful procedure, by cloning hair we can create unlimited supply of follicles and avoid ration of hair. Current state-of-the-art research promises that the technology would get transferred from bench side to the bedside in a few years from now.

## 34.13 Role of a Maxillofacial Surgeon

A maxillofacial surgeon makes a good hair transplant surgeon as they are well trained in surgical anatomy of the head and neck with a detailed knowledge of flap design and through in-depth working knowledge of the local anaesthesia management. They have a great aesthetic sense with artistic hands and are well versed with cephalometric analysis which comes handy in judging facial proportions and hairline placements, further most of them are very well adapted to handling the rotary handpiece from their formative training. Maxillofacial surgeons are well trained exclusively in head and neck surgery for 3 years and are competent at managing wounds and infections, thus justifying their qualifications to perform hair transplantation alongside plastic surgeons and dermatologists.

## 34.14 Conclusion

Surgeons who deal with aesthetic surgeries on the face need to have a good range of skills to deal with all aspects of beauty which are defined by the individual elements. The most important of them all being framing of the face like a photo frame with hair transplantation which will allow us to focus our vision on the finer elements of the facial beauty be it the nose, lips, eyes, teeth, jawline or a good smile. If surgeons follow the principles of hair transplantation surgery, they will create patients with high degree of satisfaction using the micrografts of FUE or FUT procedure. This sophisticated form of art will bring a sense of gratification to oral and maxillofacial surgeons by embracing it as a tool along with all other tools at his disposal.

## 34.15 Case Scenarios

### Case Scenario 1 (Fig. 34.26)

Figure 34.26: male pattern baldness—Norwood classification 4.

Treatment: FUT method with 2850 plus microfollicular grafts transplanted.

### Case Scenario 2 (Fig. 34.27)

Figure 34.27: male pattern baldness class 5.

Treatment: 4000 follicular units transplantation done through Combi technique involving both FUT and FUE in the same session.

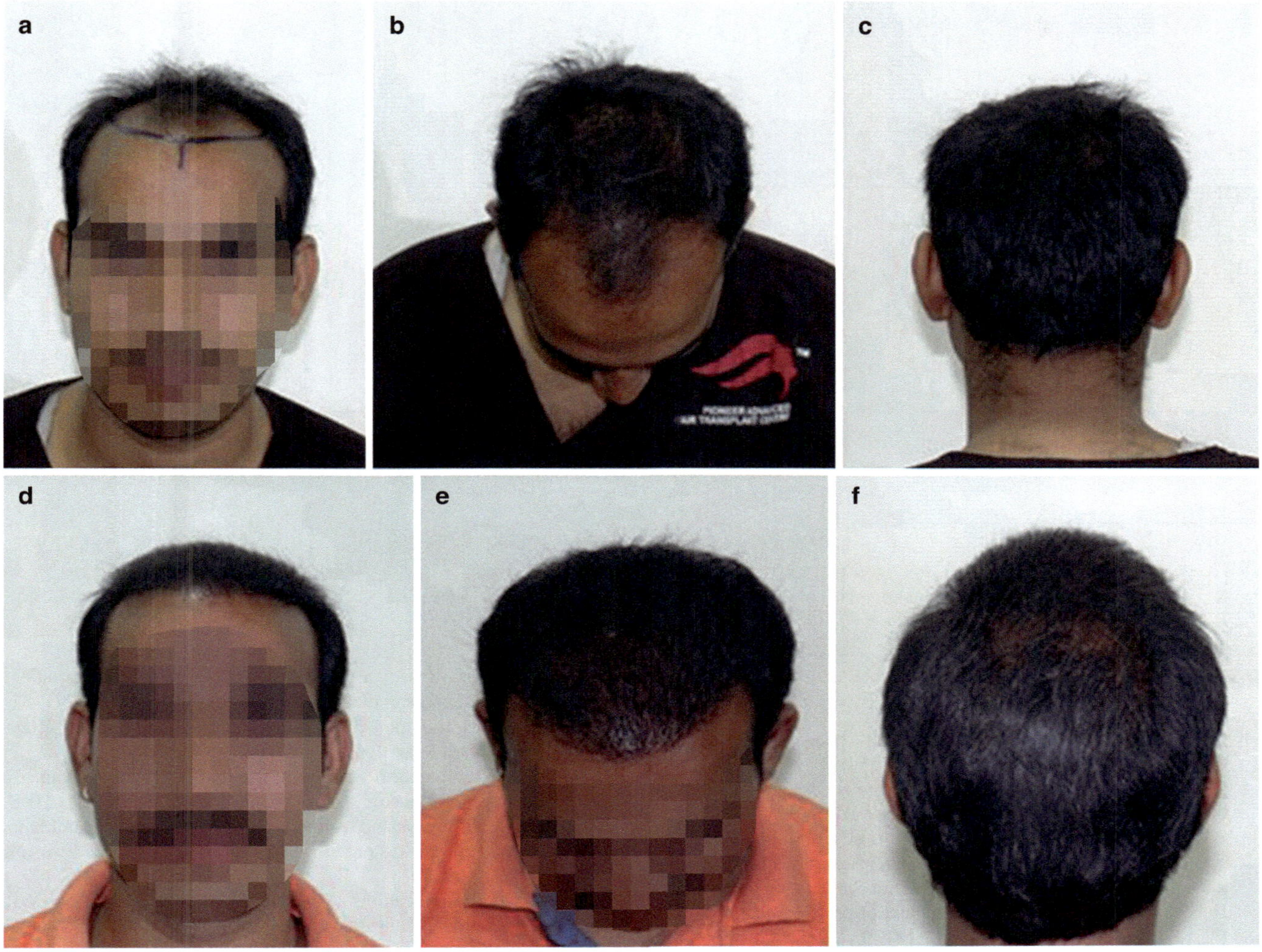



**Fig. 34.26** (**a**–**f**) Case scenario 1

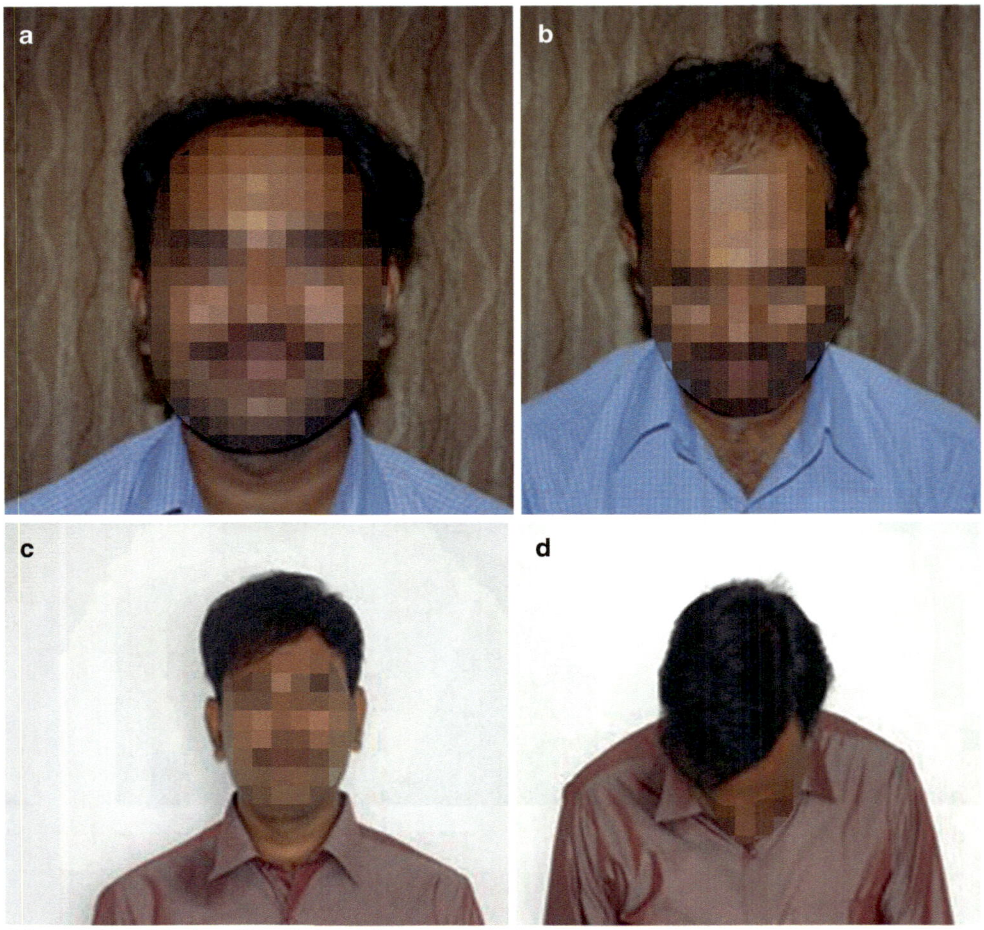


Fig. 34.27 (a–d) Case scenario 2

©Association of Oral and Maxillofacial Surgeons of India

## References

1. Orentreich N. Autografts in alopecias and other selected dermatological conditions. Ann N Y Acad Sci. 1959;83:463–79.
2. Beehner M. Nomenclature proposal for the zones and landmarks of the balding scalp. Dermatol Surg. 2001;27:375–80.
3. Bernstein R, Rassman WR, Seager D, et al. Standardizing the classification and description of follicular unit transplantation and mini-micrografting techniques. Dermatol Surg. 1998;24:957–63.
4. Haber RS. Pharmacologic management of pattern hair loss. Facial Plast Surg Clin North Am. 2004;12:181–9.
5. Price VH. Treatment of hair loss. N Engl J Med. 1999;341:964–73.
6. Unger W, Shapiro R. Hair transplantation. New York: Marcel Dekker; 2004. p. 49–56.
7. Bernstein RM, Rassman WR. Follicular transplantation: patient evaluation and surgical planning. Dermatol Surg. 1997;23:771–84.
8. Bernstein RM, Rassman WR. The logic of follicular unit transplantation. Dermatol Surg. 1999;17:277–95.
9. Rassman WR, Bernstein RM. Follicular unit extraction—minimally invasive surgery for hair transplantation. Dermatol Surg. 2002;28:720–8.
10. Shapiro R. Principles and techniques used to create a natural hairline in surgical hair restoration. Facial Plast Surg Clin North Am. 2004;12:201–17.
11. Cooley JE. Complications of hair transplantation. In: Unger WP, Shapiro R, editors. Hair transplantation. 4th ed. New York: Marcel Dekker; 2004. p. 568–73.
12. Bernstein RM, Rassman WR, Rashid N, Shiell RC. The art of repair in surgical hair restoration. Part 1: basic repair strategies. Dermatol Surg. 2002;28:738–94.

# Ear Reconstruction

# 35

Paritkumar Ladani

## 35.1 Introduction

The human ear is a vital and distinctive feature of the face, and therefore, its deformity confers a significant impact on self-esteem and mental development in affected patients. Microtia is the commonest congenital ear malformation. The management of ear malformations can be challenging, because of its complex 3D structure. To achieve proper reconstructive results, it is first essential to understand the basic anatomy and architecture of the ear [1]. Materials used for reconstruction of the ear include autogenous cartilage, alloplasts like silicone, Medpor, and osseointegrated materials. Surgical reconstruction of the ear with autogenous grafts is a unique marriage of science and art [2]. Good results depend not only on surgical skill but also on conforming to the basics of plastic surgical principles and tissue transfer. The gold standard for external ear reconstruction even today is the use of autogenous cartilage frameworks.

## 35.2 Incidence and Etiology

The incidence of microtia is around 1 in 10,000 live births. It appears to be more frequent at higher altitudes, especially above 2000 m, due to the low oxygen levels. The condition is 2.5 times more common in boys than in girls and more commonly affects the right ear. Unilateral cases are four times as common as bilateral ones. Aural atresia is found with microtia in 75% of cases. Microtia usually occurs if there in an abnormality in the embryologic development of the six auricular hillocks. These develop at 4–12 weeks of gestation. Microtia may be associated with other birth defects. The exact cause behind the abnormal embryologic development remains unknown. However, certain teratogens like isotretinoin and thalidomide have also been implicated in this [3].

Microtia may occur in association with other malformations, including facial nerve weakness, cardiac defects, urogenital defects, hemifacial macrosomia, and spine defects. It has also been associated with syndromes like Goldenhar syndrome and Treacher-Collins syndrome [4].

## 35.3 Surgical Anatomy

It is crucial to understand the external auricular anatomy and architecture before proceeding with reconstruction (Fig. 35.1a). The ear has certain definite structural elements. The overall outline of the ear is oval shaped and is slightly flattened posteroinferiorly. A distinct line can be made out that defines the helical rim, arising from its root and ending at the crus helicis. Another line forms the concha, which consists of the tragus and antitragus. The fossa triangularis is the final defining structure that defines the ear (Fig. 35.1b). A complete understanding of these structures allows the microtia surgeon to use these basic components to reconstruct the complex three-dimensional structure.

When viewed in the horizontal plane, the ear is divided into three parts. The superior portion starts at the top of the helical rim and ends at the helical root at the superior border of the concha cymba. The midportion starts at the upper border of the concha cymba and ends at the upper aspect of the antitragus. The lowest portion extends from the tip of the lobule to the superior border of the antitragus. The length of the ear is defined as the distance between the highest point (supra-aurale) and the lowest point (subaurale). This may vary between patients in accordance with the differences in the shape of the patient's face and their lobule characteristics. For instance, the ear lengths vary from 55 mm to 65 mm, with a

**Electronic Supplementary Material** The online version of this chapter (https://doi.org/10.1007/978-981-15-1346-6_35) contains supplementary material, which is available to authorized users.

P. Ladani (✉)
Oral and Maxillofacial Surgery, Swiss Cleft and Craniofacial Centre, BSES MG Hospital,
Mumbai, India



K. Bonanthaya et al. (eds.), *Oral and Maxillofacial Surgery for the Clinician*, https://doi.org/10.1007/978-981-15-1346-6_35

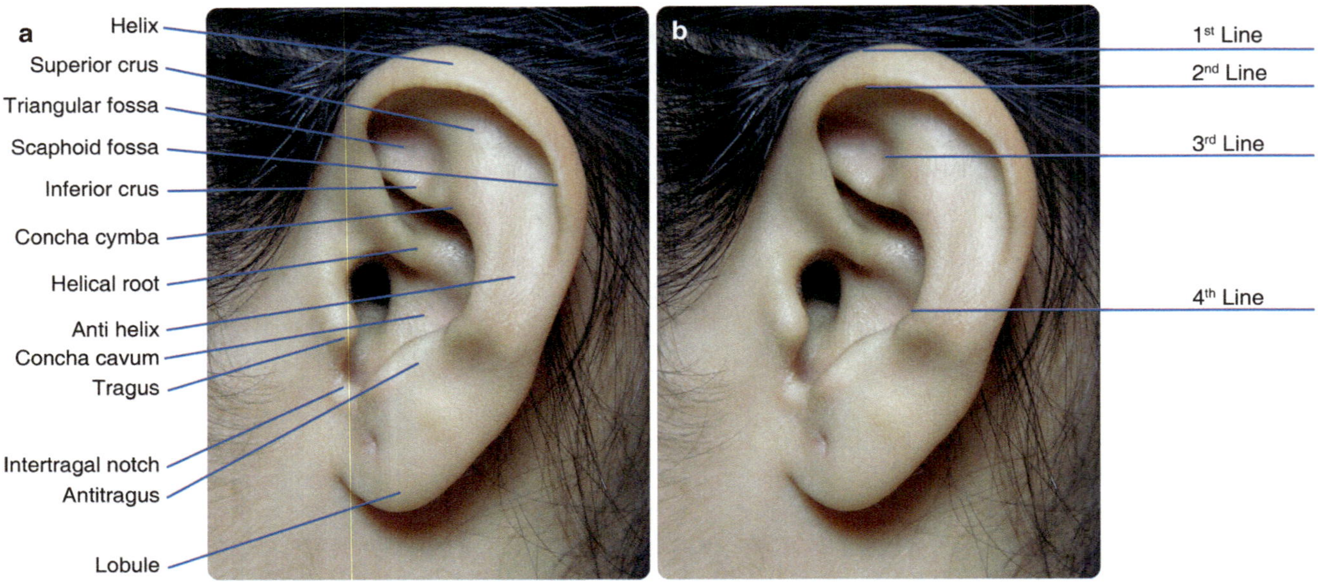




**Fig. 35.1** Normal external auricular anatomy and architecture

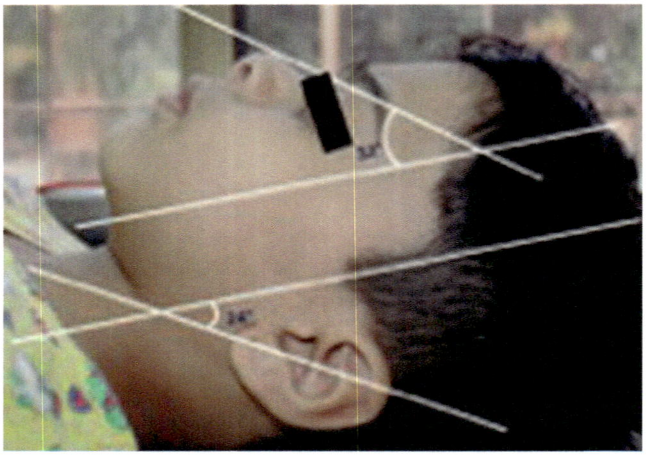



**Fig. 35.2** Relation of ear to nose and facial plane

mean of 62.4 mm in males and a mean of 58.4 mm in females. The width is approximately 55% of the ear length and is around 35.5 mm in males and 33.4 mm in females. The protrusion of the ear, also called the auriculocephalic angle, ranges from 15° to 20°. This is the angle between the mastoid skin and the posterior surface of the auricle. Again, this may show variation between patients. However, this angle should remain the same in both the normal and the reconstructed ears [3]. The angle between the vertical axis of the face and the longitudinal axis of the ear is referred to as the ear inclination. It must be measured with the patient oriented to the Frankfort horizontal position. This is around 24° with the face, but is 32° in relation to the nasal dorsum (Fig. 35.2).

## 35.4 Classification

There are four grades of microtia, depending on the severity. These are as follows:

Grade 1: The ear has anatomically normal characteristics, but may be slightly smaller than normal. An external auditory canal is usually present, but may demonstrate atresia.

Grade 2: The size of the ear is than in grade 1, and it may be less developed. Although a part of the helix may be formed, the triangular fossa, scaphae, and antihelix are under-developed. Atresia of the external auditory canal may or may not be an associated feature.

Grade 3 or classic: This is the commonest grade seen and usually consists of a vertical remnant of skin. There is a superior component that contains the malformed cartilage, and an inferior component that forms the displaced earlobe. This grade is almost always associated with atresia.

Grade 4 or anotia: The outer ear structure is completely absent, and atresia is always present.

There is another simplified classification, in which microtia is divided into the lobular type (ear remnant and lobule

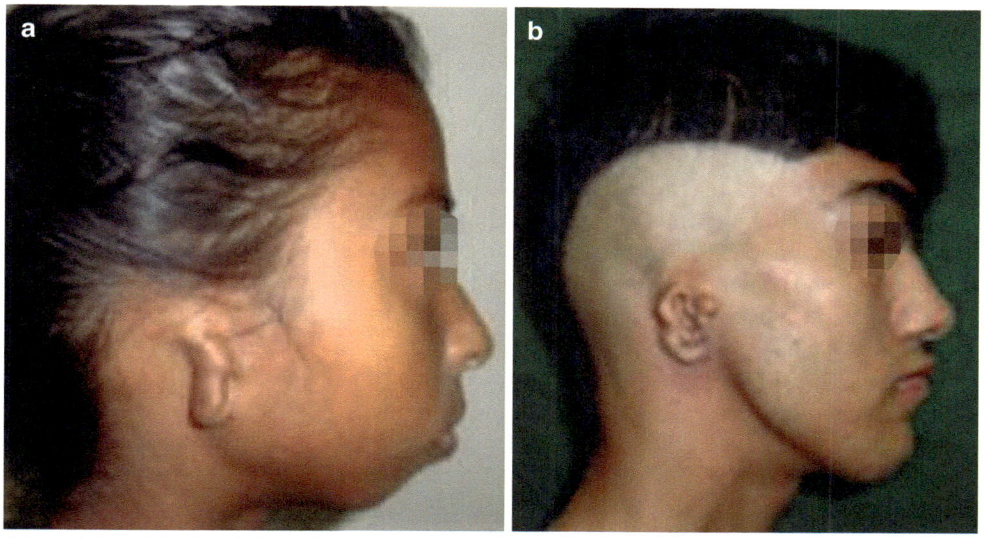


Fig. 35.3 (a) Lobule-type and (b) conchal-type microtia



are present) or conchal type (presence of concha, external canal, and tragus with lobule) (Fig. 35.3).

## 35.5 Evaluation and Management

The management of a child with microtia should ideally be discussed with parents shortly after birth, to reduce parenteral stress and offer them reassurance. The audiologic testing should be performed before discharge. In cases of unilateral microtia, treatment is not urgent because the other side will have normal hearing. Treatment can be thoughtfully planned after consulting with relevant specialists. However, in bilateral cases, brainstem auditory-evoked response testing must be performed as soon as possible so that the child can be fitted with a bone-conduction headband. The microtia surgeon can discuss about all the possible option with the family, including observation, autologous costal cartilage, alloplasts, and prosthetics. Each method of management has a different timing, and therefore, all optins must be discussed at an early stage. In addition, the microtia surgeon must also coordinate ear reconstruction with auditory management, so that the timing of the hearing correction may be optimized [4].

## 35.6 Timing

Timing of repair is governed by both physical growth and psychological consideration. The ears reach much of their mature size by age 7. Generally, by the age of 6, cartilage is sufficiently developed to provide an optimal primary framework. However, the older the child, the more cartilage is available for reconstruction. On the other hand, waiting for cartilage growth must be weighed against the psychological and social effects of the missing ear on the child. Studies show that psychological effects usually manifest only around the age of 7–10. However, by age 6, most children are aware of the problem and want to get it corrected [3]. The timing can also depend on the method of reconstruction chosen. The Brent method, which requires less cartilage, may be performed as early as 6–7 years of age. On the other hand, the Nagata method can be done only after 10 years of age, when the chest measures at least 60 cm at the xiphisternum. This is because it needs larger amounts of cartilage [1].

## 35.7 History

Tanzer et al. first established the technique for total auricular reconstruction. The technique was modified by Brent, who utilized more defined surgical techniques such as fabrication of the framework and reconstruction of the tragus using composite chondrocutaneous grafts. These techniques were three stages and four stages, respectively. Nagata and Park outlined techniques that involved just one or two stages for ear reconstruction [5]. Allolastic implants were tried since the 1960s. Initially, silicone implants were used, but these were associated with complications such as implant failure following minor trauma or abrasions. In 1993, Wellisz reintroduced the prefabricated alloplastic implant for microtia reconstruction. This was constructed from PHDPE [6].

## 35.8 Principle and Planning (Video 35.1)

The Microtia surgeon should begin with proper planning and achievable goals for successful auricular reconstruction. It is important to discuss the details of surgical procedure and limitation of surgical repair with the family during preoperative consultation. The surgeon must prepare the family for multiple stages, long preoperative and postoperative care, and complications. The reconstructed ear will possess some deficits as compared to the normal ear and will be less flexible and elastic. The reconstructed ear can also be prone to complications, including hematoma, poor healing, infection, or skin breakdown. These complications can compromise the definition and contour of the reconstructed ear [3].

If the patient has coexisting anomalies, such as clefts, early surgery must be done first to correct these. For instance, in cases of Treacher Collins syndrome and other first and second branchial arch defects (craniofacial microsomia, Goldenhar's syndrome, etc.), the bone reconstruction must be achieved first, with scars peripheral to the proposed ear [7].

The precise positioning and dimensions of the reconstructed framework will define the end result of the surgery. The reconstruction must be symmetrical to the contralateral ear in the unilateral case. In bilateral cases, the parent's ear is used as a reference. Visual examination may not be reliable, and it is essential to make exact measurements, after properly positioning the patient. For an ideal position, the superior extent of the ear must be placed parallel to the Frankfort's horizontal plane, at the level of the lateral brow (Fig. 35.4). The root of the helix may be positioned at the level of the subnasale, approximately one ear-length behind the lateral brow. Measurements must be taken carefully, particularly from the lower one-third of the face, in cases of facial asymmetry (seen in about 88% of patients with microtia). The asymmetries can range from mild differences in gonial position to full-blown hemifacial macrosomia and can lead to inaccuracies in measurement [3].

The final outcome also depends on the skin quality around the ear area. If the skin is scarred, natural expansion cannot take place, and the final ear may have a poor definition. In such cases, supplemental tissue in the form of flaps (e.g., temporoparietal fascia flap) may be considered to augment the supple skin envelope. In general, skin elasticity varies for each individual, and this can influence the final definition of the ear [8]. In cases of tight skin, a lower-profile 3D framework (1 mm) may be created, to avoid strain on the skin.

## 35.9 Simulation Training

The surgeon must obtain enough training in plastic and reconstructive surgery, including skills such as gentle flap dissection, delicate wound closures, and skin grafting, to achieve optimal outcomes. In addition, surgeons must be familiar with precise carving that is required for forming the 3D framework for the ear. Potato, carrot, or pumpkin can be used to learn and perfect the art of sculpting a framework [8]. Silicone dental impression material provides a convenient replica of costal cartilage, as it has the same consistency and texture. An exact replica of the rib cartilage and a precise template of the ear will allow the simulation to mimic the clinical situation. Creating the framework can be done using wood carving instruments. These techniques aid the novice surgeon in improving their results during the actual surgery [9].

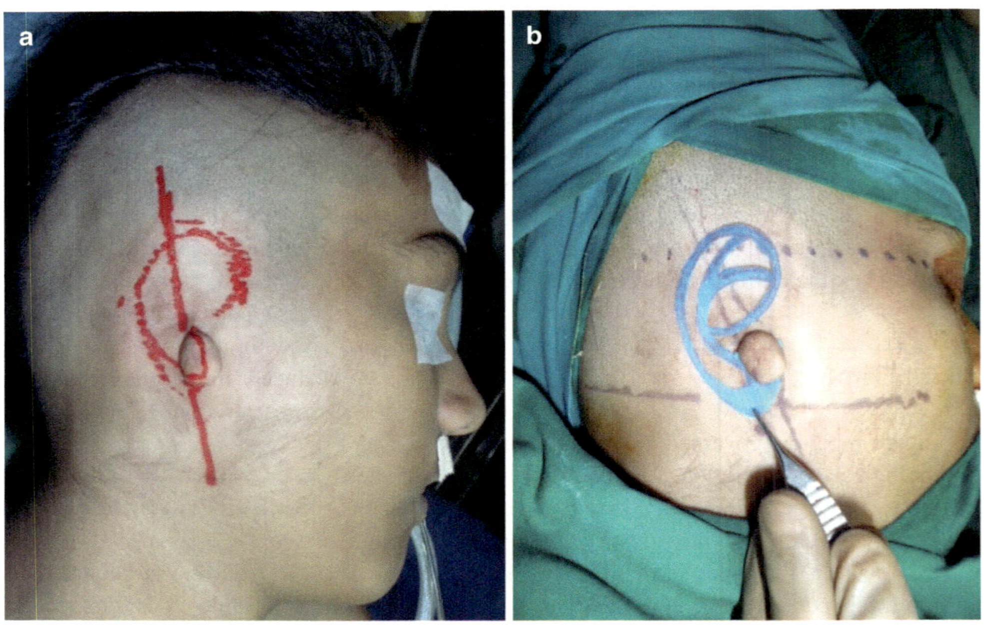




**Fig. 35.4** Future position and size of ear

## 35.10 Template

Preoperative photographs should be obtained, and measurements of the normal ear must be obtained when the patient is awake. The surgical template is prepared from radiograph film using normal ear as a guide. In the beginning, an outline of the helical rim, lobule, antitragus, tragus, and conchal bowl is created from the opposing ear as the first template [3]. This template needs to be reversed to plan the ipsilateral ear. Another mirror image template is created based on the first one, which is smaller in dimension. This would allow for the extra thickness following insertion of cartilage under the skin (Fig. 35.5). The inferior pole on the framework is created much smaller in size, to accommodate the transposition of the earlobe. If the patient does not have usable earlobe tissue, this can be carved into the lower end of the framework. A second template is created, this time minus the helical rim. This template is used as a guide for creating the base of the framework from the sixth and seventh ribs, after which the rim of the helix can be added. The templates must be chemically sterilized prior to intraoperative use. A third template, made along with the first, has markings at the lateral canthus of the eye and commissure of the mouth. This allows ideal framework positioning and orientation. The distances marked on the template must be verified by measuring the distance between the lateral canthus and the root of the helix [3].

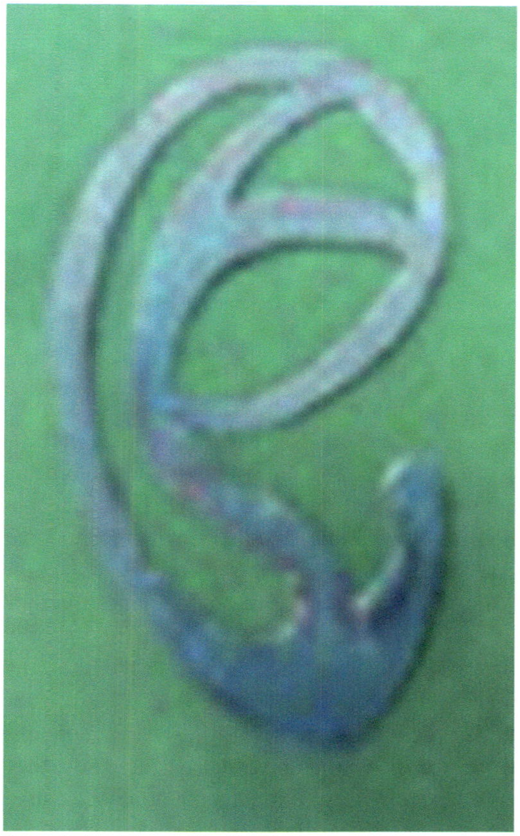



**Fig. 35.5** Final surgical template of ear made from x-ray film

## 35.11 Auricular Reconstruction Using Autologous Rib Cartilage

### 35.11.1 Harvesting Rib Cartilage

For harvesting the rib cartilage, an incision, 4–5 cm long, is placed obliquely on the ipsilateral side, at the level of the synchondrosis of the sixth and seventh ribs [10]. The incision is carried down through the muscle, to expose the costal cartilages. It is safer to harvest the cartilage without perichondrium because leaving the perichondrium behind offers one more layer of protection to pleura. The perichondrium also allows for the regeneration of the cartilage/bone matrix. Removing perichondrium can not only offer less protection but also lead to significant depressive chest deformities [8]. After harvesting is complete, intercostal nerve blocks may be administered. Closure of the muscle and deep fascial layers is done, and a large piece of cartilage may be banked in a subcutaneous pocket for the second stage [10]. Smaller cartilage pieces may be diced and placed inside the sutured perichondrial pocket, where it can aid in cartilage regeneration (Fig. 35.6).

### 35.11.2 Framework

The supporting framework is a living sculpture that serves as the foundation for the repair. Rather than carving the framework to exactly mimic auricular cartilage, the surgeon must make allowances for the abnormal skin coverage that is present. These limitations include skin-volume shortage and greater skin thickness, both of which produce excess skin tension. To prevent the flattening of the ear's rim that this tension might cause, one must carve a somewhat thicker and more substantial helix. This exaggeration of the cartilaginous framework will compensate for the thickness of the overlying skin. The 3D framework must be at least 9.5–10.0 mm high in the case of primary reconstruction and further augmented by 1.0–2.0 mm for secondary reconstruction [8].

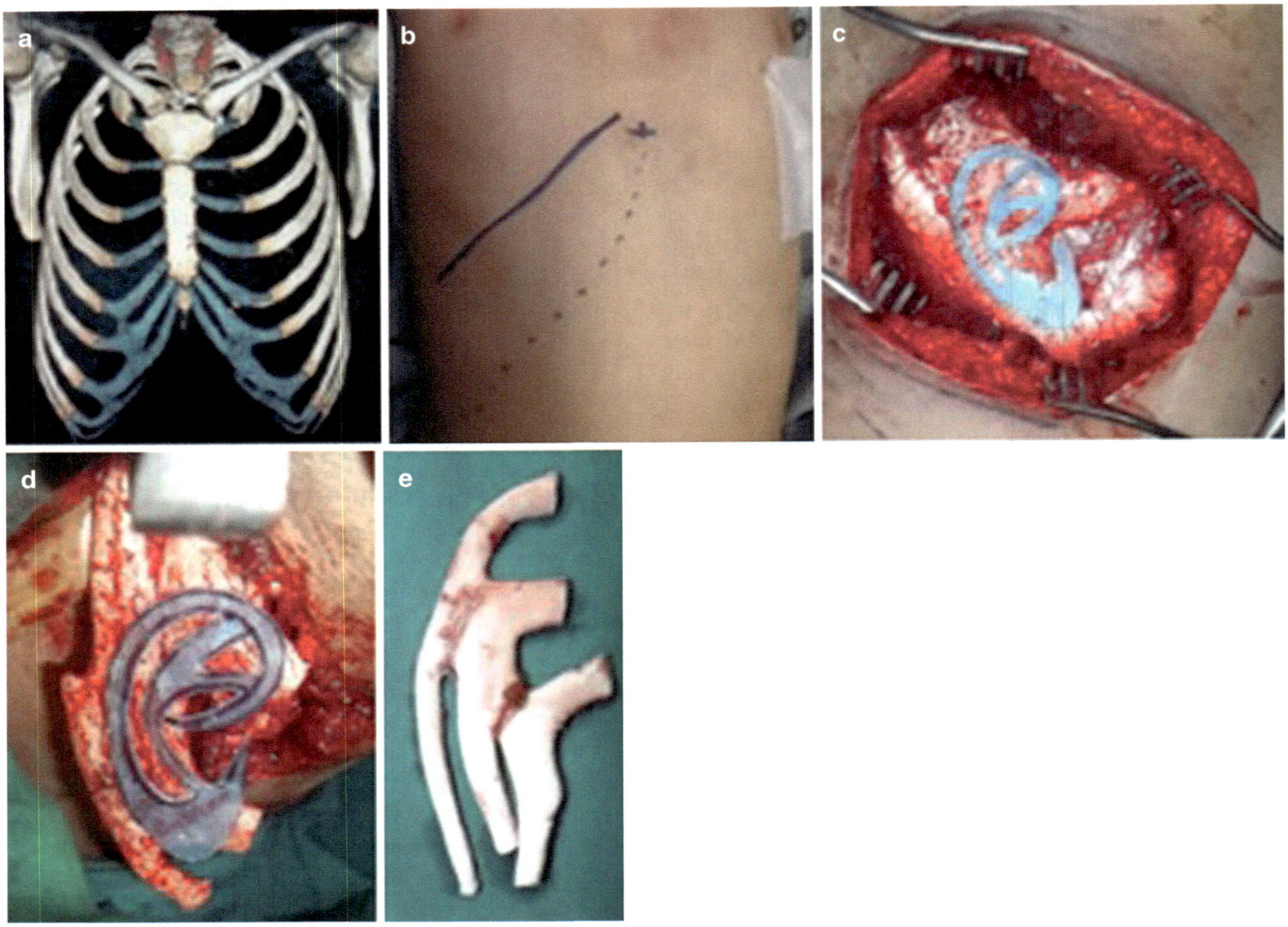




**Fig. 35.6** (**a**) 3D CT scan of Rib cage. (**b**) Incision for cartilage harvest. (**c**) Exposure of rib cartilage. (**d**) Template used to harvest cartilage. (**e**) Harvested cartilage

The cartilaginous framework is constructed from the synchondrosis of the sixth and seventh ribs (Fig. 35.7b, c, d). Cartilage wedges from these ribs are used to create the helical sulcus and the triangular fossa. The helix itself is formed from the eighth rib because it is longer. If additional length is required, the ninth rib can also be harvested (Fig. 35.7e) [10]. While carving the helix, it must be ensured that superior portion is higher than the inferior portion. The part of the helix that will be continuous with the lobule must be trimmed at the lower end, until it is long enough to receive the lobule attachment. The constructed helix is then affixed to the basal cartilage. On doing this, an outward inclination of 10–15° is maintained, at the middle one-third of the ear. The entire length of the lower part of the basal cartilage, at the outer end, is trimmed [5]. The floating rib cartilage that is used to create the helix must be thinned on its outer convex surface. This causes the cartilage to warp in a favorable direction and creates an acute angle that resembles the helix. This cartilage is then fastened to the body of the framework with 5-0 Stainless steel suture. The thickest parts of the remaining segments of cartilage are used to create the rest of the auricle, namely, the antihelix and antitragus-tragus complex, which surround the conchal bowl (Fig. 35.7f). The highest point of the antihelix is the middle, and this slowly tapers down to the helix. The superior and inferior crura are created, at the slope toward the lowest portion of the base frame. Enough space must be secured between the upper helix and superior and inferior crura, in order to accommodate the skin envelope. Otherwise, an effect of continuity between 2 crura and helix is created, which is undesirable [8]. The components of the framework are then assembled and secured together using 5-0 stainless steel wires. To achieve a snug fit, a small incision is placed in the cartilage and the wire is pulled gently toward the incision without burying it [10]. The position of the antihelix within the antitragus must be high, and trimming must be done at a lower level toward the superior and the inferior crura. In order to augment the antihelix, cartilage may be added in a vertical manner near the conchal area.

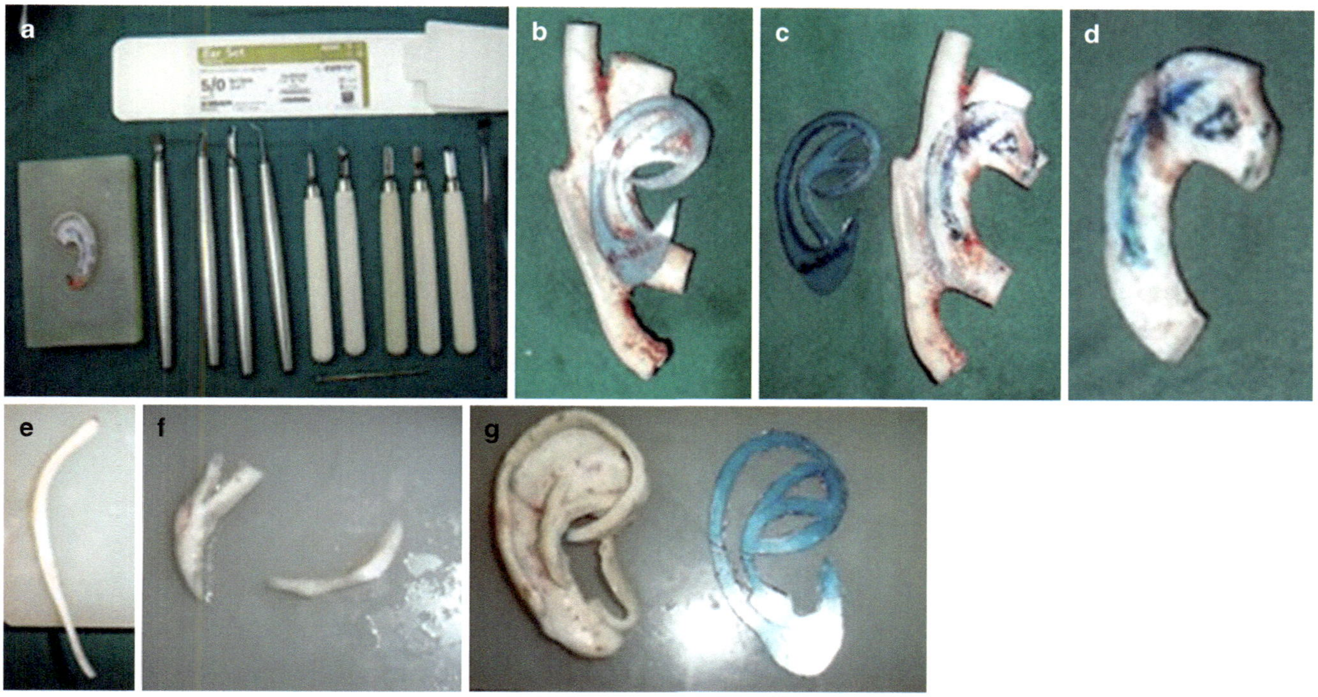




**Fig. 35.7** (**a**) Armamentarium for carving, (**b–d**) preparation of base of the cartilaginous framework from the synchondrosis of the sixth and seventh ribs, (**e**) helix prepared from eighth rib cartilage, (**f**) antihelix and tragus, and (**g**) Final framework

This gives an effect of deepening of the concha. The antihelix is also trimmed in the region of the scaphoid fossa, so that it develops a slight inclination that resembles the natural convolution. Finally, the surfaces of the entire framework must be tapered smoothly tapered, and block-like corners must be removed, to ensure that the covering skin fits on smoothly (Fig. 35.7g). Throughout the process, isotonic saline solution is used to irrigate the cartilaginous framework. This helps preserve chondrocytes. The use of rotary and power tools must be avoided to prevent chondrocyte damage [7].

### 35.11.3 Skin Pocket

A pocket must be created within the skin in a meticulous fashion. This will provide proper vascular covering to receive the framework. As per the level of the lobular remnant, the level of the incision line for rotating the lobule may be determined. A small part of the lobular remnant is transposed posteriorly and separated from the microtic remnant. Then, the lobule is dissected and rotated to create a pocket that will accommodate the caudal end of the cartilage framework. This causes the lobule to be brought down and results in a smooth interface between the lobule and the framework. Creation of the skin pocket preserves the subdermal vascular plexus. The amount of dissection (at least 2 cm beyond the outline) must be wide enough to allow proper draping of the skin flaps over the framework with minimal tension. Any cartilage, if present in the vestigial remnant, is removed. Meticulous hemostasis must be achieved [5]. An incision is placed at the posteroinferior border of the vestigial remnant, and the cartilaginous framework is placed in the subcutaneous pocket. The tail end of the framework is inserted into the lobule first, followed by suturing of the outer incision. In order to let the skin adhere to the framework, two polyethylene drains with multiple perforators must be inserted beneath the framework. These are secured to the skin using 5/0 nylon sutures. A syringe (50-cc) may be connected to the drain. After final suturing of the subcutaneous pocket, the skin flap is approximated, and the piston of the syringe may be fixed in activated position using two wooden tongue depressors (Fig. 35.8) [5]. If skin blanching is noticed at this stage, the pocket must either be enlarged or the framework must be inserted at a lower position. The use of pressure dressings must be avoided as these can compromise the vascular supply. The entire reconstructed ear must be layered in petrolatum gauze, which must be placed loosely and left in place for 3 days [3]. The syringe with the activated piston may be changed frequently in the postoperative perio, ensuring that proper tension is maintained. The drains may be removed on the fourth or fifth postoperative, provided that the volume of fluid drained is less than 1-cc. Petrolatum gauze may be left in place until suture removal, on the sixth postoperative day [5].

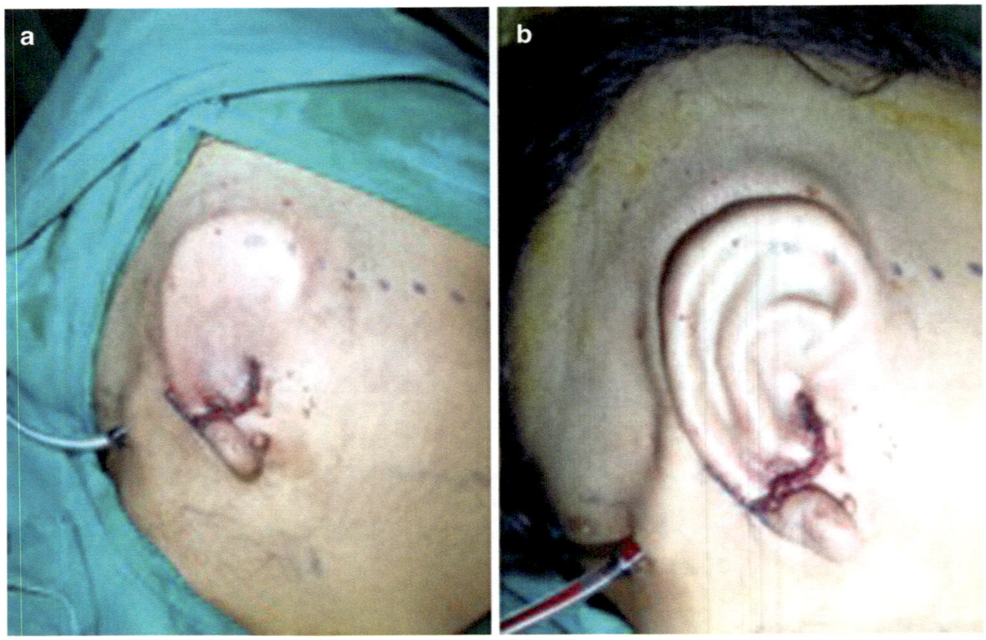


**Fig. 35.8** (**a**) Before activation of suction and (**b**) after activation of suction



### 35.11.4 Second Stage

The second stage of surgery involves elevating the auricle from the head, which creates the auriculocephalic angle. This procedure should ideally be performed 6–9 months following the first stage. In the conventional method, the incision lies several millimeters away from the margin, and reconstructed ear is gently lifted from the base. Care must be taken to preserve connective tissue on the undersurface of the ear, as well as on the bony floor. The posterior part of the auricle and the skin defect overlying the mastoid are grafted with skin. Since the ear lacks skeletal support, it contacts the mastoid skin and is not elevated. This creates a narrow space, which may be difficult for the patient to clean [8].

In the Nagata technique, the second stage is more complex than the conventional one. This involves the following steps: (1) separation of the auricle from the mastoid, (2) The banked subcutaneous rib cartilage or an alloplast is used to create a wedge-shaped block, which is placed underneath the auricle, (3) A temporoparietal fascia (TPF) flap is then harvested to cover the posterior part of the auricle, and (4) A split skin graft harvested from the scalp to cover the fascial flap. Scalp skin is preferred as it has better color match as compared to groin skin (Figs. 35.9 and 35.10) [8].

### 35.11.5 Complications

- During the harvest of Rib Cartilage

The two commonest complications at this stage are pneumothorax and atelectasis. If detected intraoperatively, pneumothorax can be easily treated and may not require chest tube placement. Positive pressure ventilation is used after irrigating the wound to see if there is any leak. If there is no leak, the wound is closed in layers. If a leak is seen, it indicates the presence of pneumothorax. In this case, a red rubber catheter is inserted into the pleural opening to which a syringe is attached to this to evacuate residual air. Following this, the chest may be closed and an intraoperative chest radiograph is asked for to rule out residual pneumothorax. If this is absent, the wound may be closed, the catheter may be removed and follow-up may be done with serial films [3]. Atelectasis is best prevented by frank preoperative preparation of the patient and vigorous postoperative respiratory therapy.

- Skin Flap Necrosis

The first 10 postoperative days are critical to check for any skin flap necrosis. It is essential to achieve a balance between the thickness of the skin flap and the size of the pocket with the contouring of the cartilage framework. To prevent skin necrosis, it is advisable to minimize or completely avoid the use of epinephrine in the flap. The status of vascular supply can be tested by placing the framework in the pocket, activating the suction drain, and observing any for blanching along the rim of the helix. If blanching is present (indicating vascular compromise), the size of the pocket may be enlarged until blanching disappears. If needed, the skin supply may be increased by placing a tissue expander 2 months prior to insertion of the framework and skin adhesion [1]. If skin necrosis is observed, it must be attended to immediately, as it can cause infection of the underlying cartilage

Fig. 35.9 Ear reconstruction in hemifacial microsomia associated with microtia. (a) Preop and (b) Postop

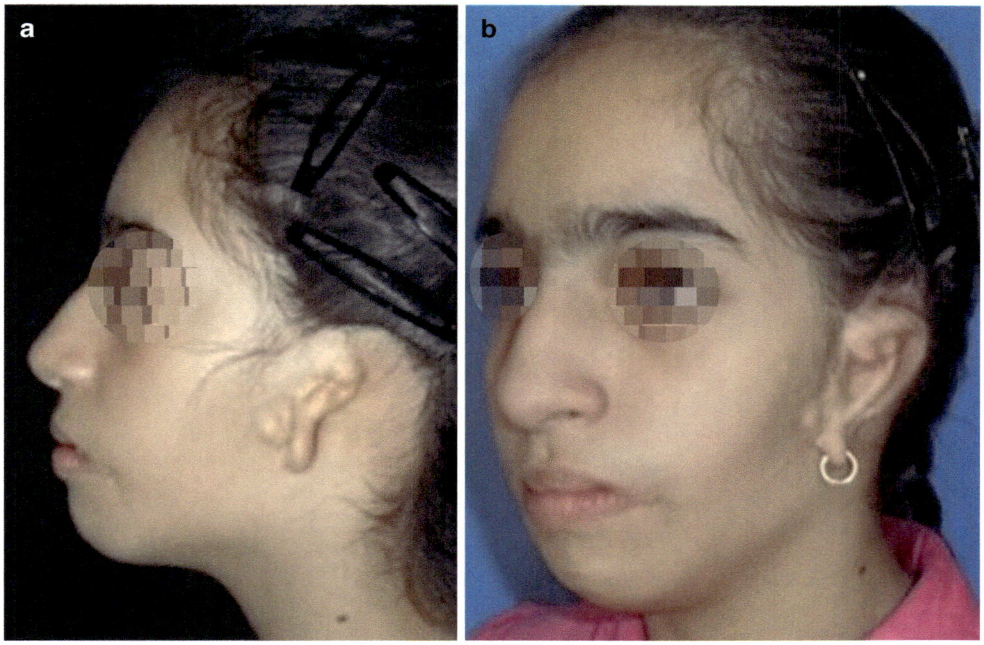




Fig. 35.10 Ear reconstruction after traumatic amputation of upper half of ear. (a) Preop and (a) Post op

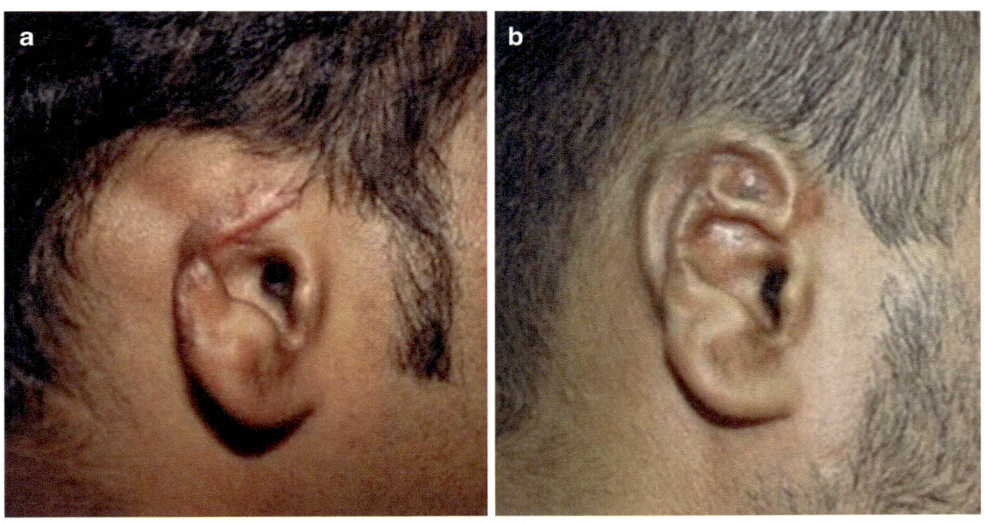




and framework resorption. The damage can be minimized by covering with a local skin flap or fascial flap (Fig. 35.11).

- Infection

This is uncommon in the autologous reconstruction. If it occurs, along with appropriate systemic antibiotics, vigorous irrigation of the surgical site must be done.

- Cartilage Resorption

If there is either ischemia or infection, there are chances that the cartilaginous framework can get resorbed or deformed. This can also occur if the skin envelope is too tight, especially at the hairline border. To avoid this, dissection of the skin pocket around the hairline must be done carefully. Any tight fibrous band that exists along the hairline must be released.

- Wire Extrusion

If any wires extrude from the framework, they can easily be removed at the outpatient facility. It is necessary that the wire must be removed as soon as extrusion is noticed, and the patient/family must be educated accordingly. Otherwise, there are chances that the exposed wires can cause resorption of cartilage around the wire.

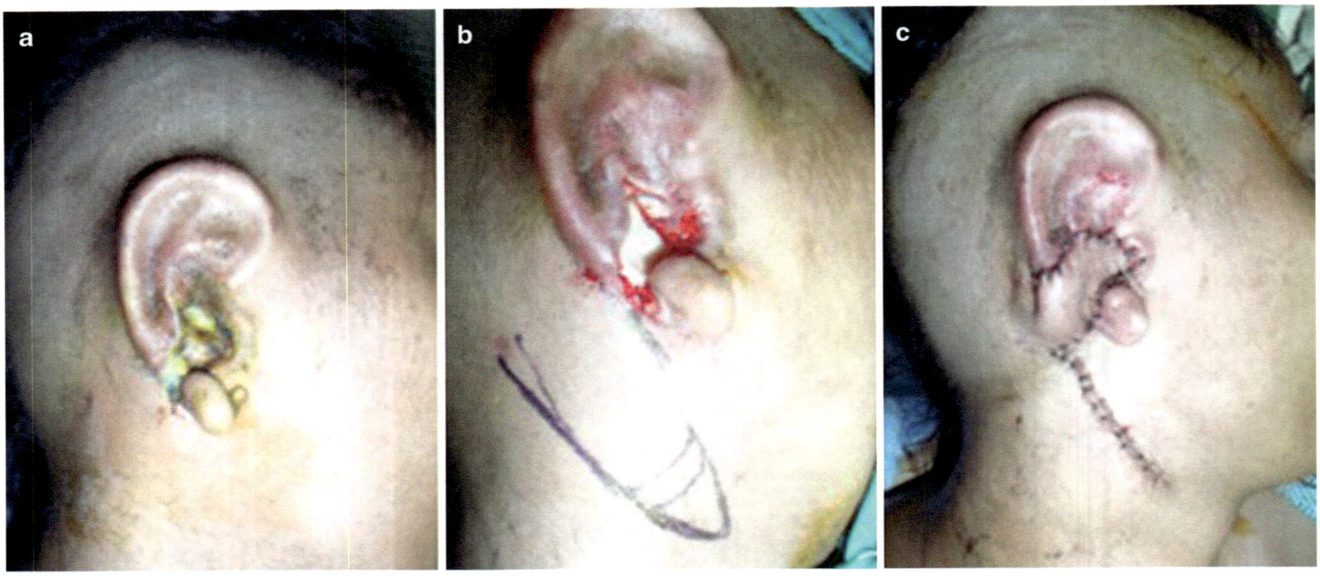



**Fig. 35.11** (**a**) Necrosis of skin at near suture line, (**b**) debridement and marking for local flap, and (**c**) flap in situ

## 35.12 Auricular Reconstruction Using Alloplast

The material used for creating framework has been a subject of debate and research. Autologous costal cartilage is still the most preferred material in microtia repair. However, some surgeons consider using alloplasts because of the following advantages.

1. Donor site morbidity is avoided,
2. Reconstruction can be done at a younger age,
3. Reduction in the number of interventions,
4. More predictable outcome,
5. The structural limitations associated with the use of autologous rib may be avoided
6. The ability to tailor reconstruction to individual patient needs (such as low hairline and bilateral malformations) [11].

The ideal alloplast for auricular reconstruction should have the following features: cost-effectiveness, ability to be implanted safely, ability to resist infection, and capability to undergo customization to resemble the contralateral normal ear. To date, more than 40 different materials have been used for creating the auricular framework. These include ivory, nylon, wire mesh, and silicone. Silicone was thought to show good results since it could mimic the flexibility and form of the native ear cartilage. However, it had a high rejection rate, especially when placed under thin skin flaps. pHDPE (Fig. 35.12) is a modestly flexible, robust enough to withstand microtrauma, and easily shapable and allows soft tissue ingrowth. This permits it to be protected against extrusion and infection. It also allows targeted drug delivery to the implant [11].

### 35.12.1 Technique

It is crucial to assess the age of patient, dimension of contralateral ear in the case of unilateral microtia, and the dimensions of their gender-matched parent's ear preoperatively for achieving equal dimensions between the normal ear and the reconstructed pHDPE ear. The ear created must be adult sized as the alloplast does not increase in size.

The vascular Doppler is used for marking superficial temporal artery. The incision is given in the postauricular area few millimeters behind the new helical rim of the microtic ear to approach TPF flap. Incision is extended in a curvilinear fashion over the TPF flap to improve the exposure and also helps to harvest the distal flap of recommended length. Other approaches may be used, including an Y incision (Fig. 35.13a), which extends superiorly from the mastoid area, and the Z incision, (Fig. 35.13b) which exposes the TPF. These approaches also allow better access to the fascia.

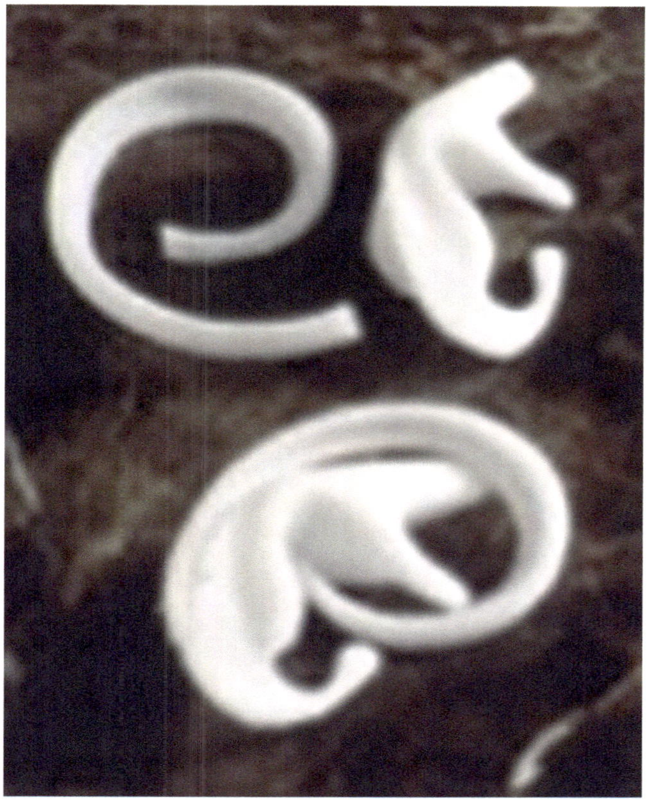


**Fig. 35.12** Porous high-density polyethylene (PHDPE) framework for auricular reconstruction

However, they increase the risk of alopecia at the incision lines and at the apex of a triangular flap.

An anteriorly based skin flap of minimum thickness is elevated meticulously, and microtic cartilage is excised. Usually, the inferior portion of the flap is attached initially to the lobular remnant. If this is malpositioned, this skin flap may be removed and used as a free graft to improve skin coverage. A TPF flap, based inferiorly, of approximately 10.5 by 13.0 cm is raised off the deep temporal fascia and periosteum beneath, superior to the level of the temporal line. The base of the flap is made wide (around 6 cm) to include additional vascular supply (branches of the occipital artery, postauricular artery, and the mastoid emissary vein), and the base of the flap is made wide, around 6 cm. The flap must be made as robust as possible, and loose areolar tissue on the deep surface of the TPF must be included in it. This tissue, which lies deep to the skin graft, allows the skin to slide over the underlying tissue. This resists surface trauma and implant exposure. The pHDPE framework is then sculpted, fused, and matched to contralateral ear. Prior to implant placement, two flat suction drains are inserted through the skin of the mastoid. One drain lies deep to the pHDPE, while the second lies in the posterior part of the donor site on the scalp. The implant is placed over the mastoid area and covered with the TPF flap after checking its anatomic orientation, projection, and axis. The flap is made to wrap tightly around the implant by the negative pressure generated by the first drain. The second drain functions to remove any serous exudate from the donor site. The skin flap, which is based anteriorly, is draped over the TPF. It may also be removed and used as a free skin graft. Sometimes, the skin at the ipsilateral mastoid may not be sufficient to cover the surface of the reconstructed ear entirely. In such cases, a full-thickness skin graft may be harvested from the opposing side postauricular region. A graft taken from this region would provide the best color and texture match. To cover the back of the ear, a larger skin graft may be required, which can be harvested from the inguinal region. After activating the drains, the ear may be coated with a layer of antibiotic cream and the concave regions may be dressed with gauze. The entire ear is then covered in a customized cast made of silicone. This cast prevents seroma, hematoma, or shearing trauma, which may compromise the viability of the skin graft. This cast should not be under pressure. A pressure dressing to prevent seromas can be applied over the donor site. All suction drains may be removed following extubation [11].

### 35.12.2 Complications

The complications of this procedure may be minor, such as a simple wound infection, or major, such as total flap necrosis with exposure of the Medpor framework beneath. In case the implant is exposed or infected, removal may rarely be required. Late complications include traumatic excoriations to the re-constructed ear, which should be managed with good wound toileting or with local skin flaps if required.

## 35.13 Prosthetic Ear

Certain traumatic, congenital, or surgical defects may benefit from auricular prostheses. The choice between surgical and prosthetic reconstruction is controversial, particularly for patients. The ideal age for prosthetic treatment is the same as the age for surgical reconstruction, namely, between 6 and 9 years. The child must be capable of caring for the prosthesis. In cases of unsuccessful surgical outcome, the prosthetic ear is one of the options. Prosthetic ear is a suitable option for the ear defects caused by trauma and disease in adult populations.

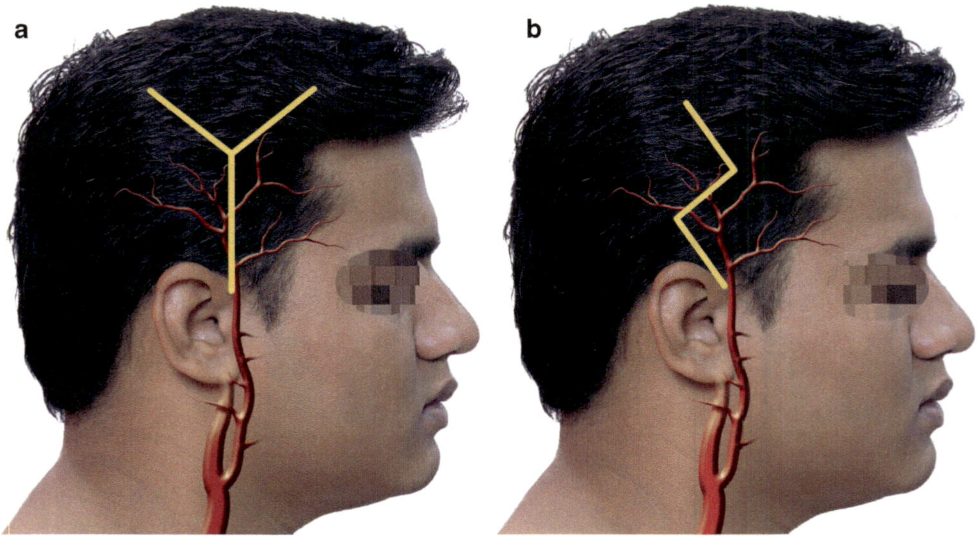


**Fig. 35.13** Approach for temporoparietal flap. (**a**) Y shape Incision. (**b**) Large Z incision



### 35.13.1 Retention of the Prosthesis

Tissue adhesives are used conventionally for ear prosthesis retention because of their low cost and quick results. Tissue adhesive is an old method and causes skin reaction. It is difficult to wear and take off adhesive while bathing and swimming. Osseointegrated implant is superior option for retention, and because of nature sense of prosthesis, ease of use, long lifetime and retention during daily activities, it is accepted by patients. An implant-retained prosthesis is preferred when there is hair on the surface of the defect or when the patient has excessively oily and perspiring skin. The prosthesis may be attached to the implant screws using precision attachments or magnets. Osseointegrated implants are contraindicated during radiation therapy, as the bone is demineralized and prone to hard tissue vasculitis, fibrosis, persistent infections, reduced tissue perfusion, and oxygenation. Osseointegration in such patients is difficult, but may be attained with hyperbaric oxygen treatment [12].

### 35.13.2 Prosthetic Technique

Impressions are made of both the defect and contralateral normal ear. Usually, rubber silicone material is used and plaster models are prepared. The plaster models of contralateral side are used as a reference to sculpt the framework. This is done using wax or clay. Next, a negative mold is obtained when the wax is removed, leaving behind a void. Medical-grade silicone usually of clear shade is mixed with pigments to create the skin colors of the individual patient. This silicone is packed into the void and cured. After removal from the mold, the texture and the color of the skin can be reproduced to match the contralateral side and adjacent skin [12].

## 35.14 Future

Regardless of the method used, ear reconstruction cannot provide an appearance that equals auricular prostheses. Future techniques must focus on emerging tissue engineering technologies that can create bone, cartilage, skin, and blood vessels. This can provide a novel direction for the treatment of patients with microtia. The creation of a natural ear using cultured chondrocytes on a prefabricated cartilaginous framework is an area of active research, but still holds some challenge [1]. Creating functional and durable tissue through tissue engineering can remove the need for donor sites and revolutionize reconstructive surgery.

## 35.15 Conclusion

The human ear is a unique structure that is difficult to replicate owing to its complex cartilaginous structure and thin overlying skin. The ultimate goal of total ear reconstruction should be creation of an auricle that closely matches the normal ear in appearance. Several surgical techniques are available for ear reconstruction. Since microtia is a rare condition, cases are limited, but at the same time, only a high case volume can improve success rates. The learning curve is long and might be at the expense of the patient. Although this learning curve is unavoidable, it is imperative to curtail its steepness. Prior to embarking on ear reconstruction, surgeons must be familiar with the principles and techniques involved. It is important to remember that repetition helps us master the technique.

**Disclosure** Authors have no financial conflicts to disclose.

## 35.16 Case Scenarios

**Case 1** (Fig. 35.14a–g)

24 year-old male with Unilateral Left side Grade 3 or Lobule type microtia. On audiometry testing, hearing was normal with conductive hearing on left side. External auditory meatus is absent. He was planned for auricular reconstruction using autologous costal cartilage. Costal cartilage was harvested from ipsilateral side. Synchondrotic junction and floating rib were harvested from the seventh, eighth, and ninth rib. Framework was prepared as shown in photo (b). Tragal component is added in framework. Skin pocket was prepared, and lobule was transposed posteriorly. Framework was inserted in pocket, and suction was applied for close adaptation of skin to framework. Stage II surgery was done after 1 year. Ear was elevated, and cartilage graft was placed for support. Graft was covered with temporoparietal fascia flap and skin grafting done. 6 months postop shows symmetric projection of both ears.

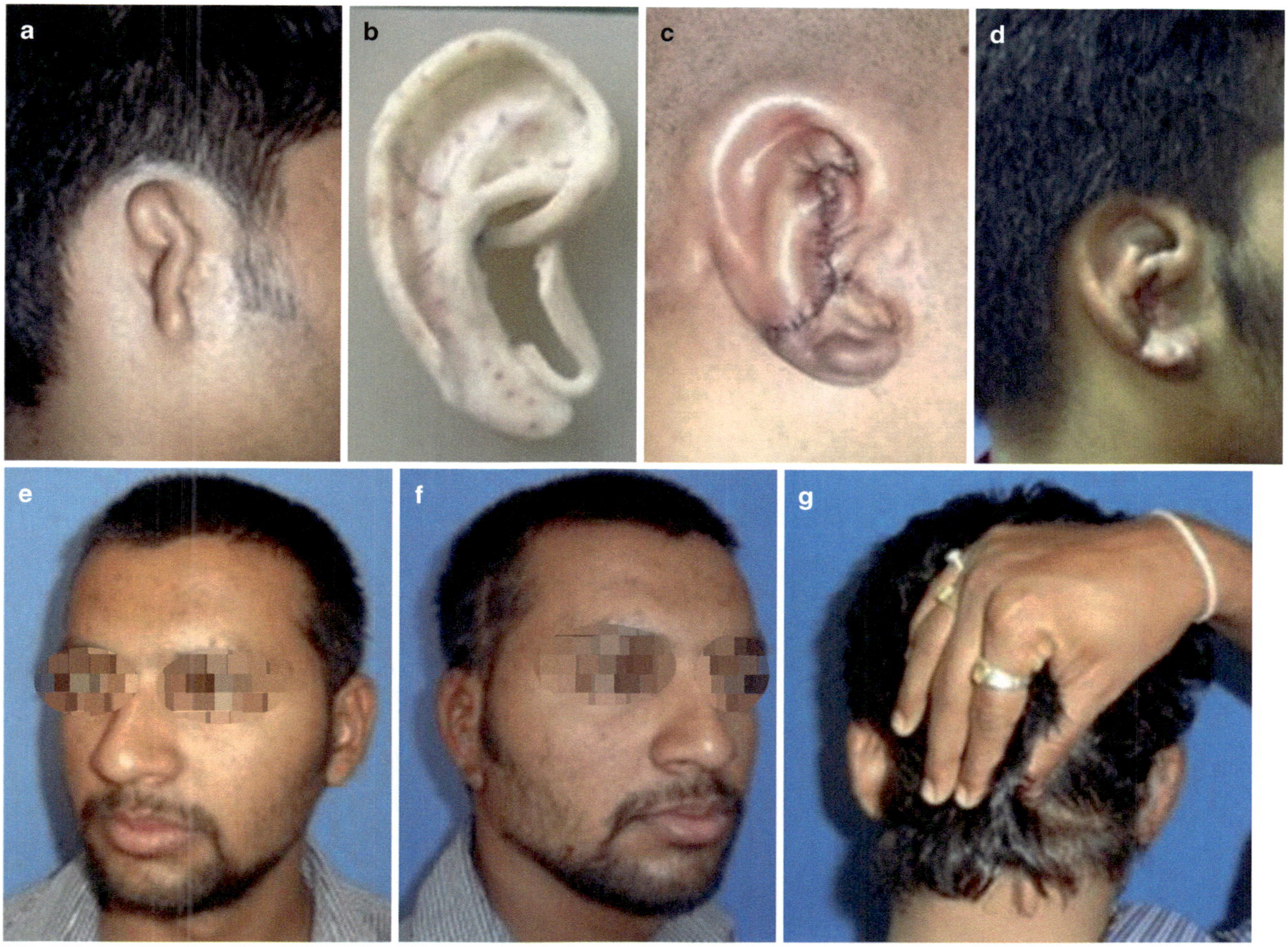




**Fig. 35.14** (**a**) Preop, (**b**) Framework, (**c**) Postop, (**d**) 3 months postop, (**e**) and (**f**) Comparison between normal and reconstructed ear after elevation of ear, and (**g**) Projection of reconstructed ear

**Case 2** (Fig. 35.15a–f)

21 year-old male with Unilateral Left side Grade 4 or Anotia. On audiometry testing, hearing was normal with conductive hearing on left side. He was planned for auricular reconstruction using autologous costal cartilage. Costal cartilage was harvested from ipsilateral side. Synchondrotic junction and floating rib were harvested from seventh, eighth, and ninth rib. Simple Framework was prepared as shown in photo (b). Skin pocket was prepared using Z-plasty incision. Framework was inserted in pocket, and suction was applied for close adaptation of skin to framework. Stage II surgery was done after 1 year. Ear was elevated, and cartilage graft was placed for support. Graft was covered with temporoparietal fascia flap and skin grafting done. 8 months postop shows symmetric projection of both ears.

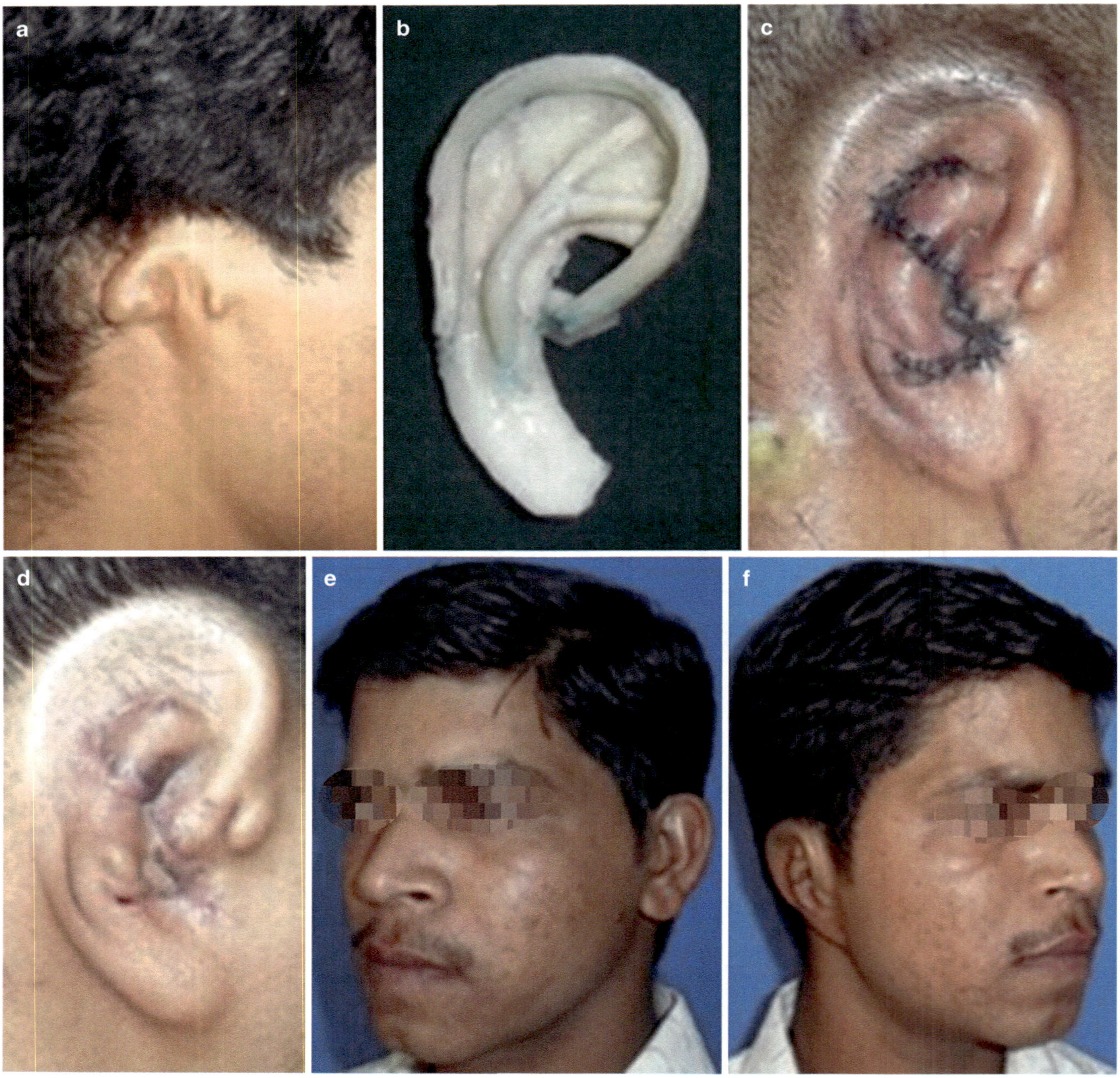




**Fig. 35.15** (**a**) Preop, (**b**) Framework, (**c**) Postop, (**d**) 3 months postop, (**e**) and (**f**) Comparison between normal and reconstructed ear after elevation of ear

## References


1. Tollefson TT. Advances in treatment of microtia. Curr Opin Otolaryngol Head Neck Surg. 2006;14:412–22.
2. Brent B. Microtia repair with rib cartilage grafts. Clin Plast Surg. 2002.
3. Quatela V, Thompson S, Goldman T. Microtia reconstruction. Facial Plast Surg Clin North Am. 2006.
4. Bonilla A. Pediatric microtia reconstruction with autologous rib. Facial Plast Surg Clin North Am. 2018.
5. Cho BC, Kim JY, Byun JS. Two-stage reconstruction of the auricle in congenital microtia using autogenous costal cartilage. J Plast Reconstr Aesthet Surg. 2007;60:998–1006.
6. Wellisz T. Clinical experience with the Medpor porous polyethylene implant. Aesthetic Plast Surg. 1993;17(4):339–44.
7. Kobus K, Szczyt M, Latkowski I, Wojcicki P. Reconstruction of the auricle. Br J Plast Surg. 2002;55:645–51.
8. Yamada A. Autologous rib microtia construction. Facial Plast Surg Clin North Am. 2018.
9. Thadani S, Ladani P. A new method for training of ear framework creation by silicon dental impression material. Indian J Plast Surg. 2012;45(1):134–7.
10. Ladani P, Valand R, Sailer HF. Ear reconstruction using autologous costal cartilage: a steep learning curve. J Maxillofac Oral Surg. 2018.
11. Stephan S, Reinisch J. Auricular reconstruction using porous polyethylene implant technique. Facial Plast Surg Clin North Am. 2018.
12. Tanner PB, Mobley SR. External auricular and facial prosthetics: A collaborative effort of the reconstructive surgeon and anaplastologist. Facial plastic surgery clinics of North America.2006;14(2):137–45.


## Additional Reading


Tanzer RC. Microtia- a long term follow up of 44 reconstructed auricles. Plast Reconstr Surg. 1978;61:161–6.

Brent B. The correction of microtia with autologous cartilage graft: I. The classic deformity. Plast Reconstr Surg. 1980;66:1–12.

Brent B. Technical advances in ear reconstruction with autogenous rib cartilage graft: personal experience with 1200 cases. Plast Reconstr Surg. 1999;104:319–34.

Nagata S. A new method of total reconstruction of the auricle in microtia. Plast Reconstr Surg. 1993;92:187–201.

Nagata S. Secondary reconstruction for unfavourable microtia results utilizing temproparietal and innominate fascia flaps. Plast Reconstr Surg. 1994;94:254–65.

Nagata S. Modification of the stages in total reconstruction of the auricle: part I. Grafting the three-dimensional costal cartilage framework for lobule-type microtia. Plast Reconstr Surg. 1994;93:221–30.

Nagata S. Modification of the stages in total reconstruction of the auricle: part II. Grafting the three-dimensional costal cartilage framework for concha-type microtia. Plast Reconstr Surg. 1994;93:231–42.

Nagata S. Modification of the stages in total reconstruction of the auricle: part III. Grafting the three-dimensional costal cartilage framework for small concha-type microtia. Plast Reconstr Surg. 1994;93:243–53.

Nagata S. Modification of the stages in total reconstruction of the auricle: part IV. Ear elevation for the constructed auricle. Plast Reconstr Surg. 1994;93:254–66.

Firmin F. La reconstruction auriculaire en cas de microtie. Principes, methods et classification. Ann Chir Plast Esthet. 2001;46:447–66.

Firmin F. Ear reconstruction in cases of typical microtia. Personal experience based on 352 microtic ear corrections. Scand J Plast Reconstr Surg Hand Surg. 1998;32:35–47.

# 36 Management of Facial Scars

Velupillai Ilankovan and Anna Sayan

## 36.1 Introduction

When the body sustains injury, the process of wound healing will commence. Scar formation is a part of wound healing. These are described as primary, secondary and tertiary intention processes [1]. In primary, there is close approximation of the wound edges, and in the secondary, the edges could not be approximated. The wound is left open, and the defect is slowly filled with connective tissue. In the tertiary, however, there is infection or contamination and there is a delay until the offending items are removed. This is followed by primary intention healing.

An ideal scar is a thin line or lines in parallel to the relaxed skin tension lines (RSTLs) described by Borges [2]. This should have a natural contour, colour and no distortion of the surrounding structures.

The scar particularly the facial is not aesthetically pleasing and can cause psychological distress to patients, resulting in poor body image, reduced self-esteem, generally loss of confidence and at times certain social stigma.

Prevention of an unsightly scar is primarily important requirement to any Surgeons but particularly important to Facial Plastics and Aesthetic Surgeons.

The origin of the word scar comes from Greek termed "iskharo" and in French "eschori" and interestingly was first used in the English language in the fourteenth century.

The primary aim in the management of scar is to produce an invisible line.

Less than ideal scars demonstrate features that are highlighted in Box 36.1.

Multiple causes can play a role in unsightly scar formation. Non-clear wound edges cannot give an aesthetically pleasing outcome. Nutritional status, co-morbidities such as diabetes, previously radiotherapy field and habits such as smoking have a detrimental effect in wound healing and thus imperfect scars. The most important factor is also the surgical competence of the operator.

**Box 36.1 Characteristics of less than ideal scars**

- wide
- raised
- depressed
- pigmented
- hypo-pigmented
- and erythematous
- may transect natural creases, folds and junctions

## 36.2 Pathophysiology

The pathophysiology of wound healing and scar formation is very complicated [3].

The wound healing is characterised by four separate but overlapping phases (Box 36.2).

Haemostasis and inflammation occur during the first 4–6 days. During the first few minutes after surgery, there are vascular contraction and formation of fibrin clot. The ruptured cell membranes result in the release of inflammatory factors in order to cause vasoconstriction, which will last for 5–10 min, and then the vessel dilatation starts. This process can take up to 20 min. The vessel dilatation is caused by histamine, which, in turns, allows inflammatory cells to arrive at the wound site. The platelets also adhere to the site of injury. Subsequently, the coagulation cascade will be activated. The structure of the clot will be a fibrin protein network filled with platelets and its contents. The main inflammatory mediators released by the platelets are the prostaglandins, leukotrienes, interleukins, growth factors and cytokines. During the inflammatory phase, there is also the arrival of neutrophils, macrophages and lymphocytes. The main function of the neutrophils is the removal

V. Ilankovan (✉) · A. Sayan
Oral and Maxillofacial Surgery, Poole Hospital NHS Foundation Trust, Poole, UK


K. Bonanthaya et al. (eds.), *Oral and Maxillofacial Surgery for the Clinician*, https://doi.org/10.1007/978-981-15-1346-6_36

**Box 36.2 Phases of wound healing**

- haemostasis
- inflammation
- proliferation
- remodelling

of the invading materials such as the microbes and products from the cell death. The macrophages are, however, responsible for inducing and clearing dying cells, which will result in improvement of inflammation. The apoptotic cells are cleaned by the macrophages, and the reparative stage begins. During this stage, there is migration of the epithelial cells usually after 48 hours and this process continues until the tenth day. Fibroblasts promote collagen synthesis. The epidermis is thickened in layers, and the collagen fibres promote dermal strength. The collagen deposition takes 2–3 weeks, and at this time, the remodelling phase begins. The collagen fibres will become rearranged during this period, and the cross-linked will be aligned along the tension lines. Largely, the maturation phase can take up to a year or longer depending on the type and site of wound. Therefore, the inflammatory process plays a major role in scar formation with the resultant fibroblast proliferation migration and differentiation.

The formal scar can be made better by using scar and scar reducing agents such as non-steroidal anti-inflammatory drugs (NSAIDs), minocycline and gene therapy. The main recognised scar reducing agents are transforming growth factor (TGF), TGF beta 3, COX-2 inhibitors and angiotensin receptor blockers [4]. The TGF beta modulating agents are still undergoing phase 2 trials in order to find out ideal scar modulating topical or intralesional agents.

Microfat grafting [5] is a technique with great potential in scar management where fat can be used intralesionally using a small 0.7 mm diameter cannula. It has been shown to be even more effective in placing fat in deep dermal layer of the skin using a 23-gauge needle in a treatment called sharp needle intradermal fat (SNIF) grafting. However, the work carried out by Tonnard et al. [6] in emulsifying the fat filtered until a liquid suspension was obtained, called Nanofat, which is injected using a 27-gauge needle, which conveys excellent outcome.

The ideal scar is an invisible line. There was increased interest in the recent past on intrauterine surgery to improve craniofacial clefts with some success and large failures. The extrauterine scars can present as stretched to depressed, hypertrophic or at times keloid. The stretched and depressed scars are as a result of inadequate primary intention management. The differences between a hypertrophic scar and keloid scar are highlighted in Box 36.3.

**Box 36.3 Hypertrophic scar vs Keloid**

| Hypertrophic scar | Keloid |
|---|---|
| do not grow beyond the boundaries of the original wound | grow horizontally and outgrowing wound boundaries |
| occur when there are skin wounds of any aetiology | can arise from small injuries such as piercing of ears |
| Not genetic | genetic |
| Not related to any race | More in dark skinned |
| Equal sex predilection | More in females |

## 36.3 Scar Management

### 36.3.1 General Principles

Scar management includes prevention, pre-injury treatments during the healing period and definitive treatment once the scar is established.

It is essential to take accurate history about any previous scar formation. If it is known, extra precautions should be taken, patients should be alerted and incisions along the susceptible sites should be omitted.

For example, when doing blepharoplasty with a history of previous hypertrophic scar, we should avoid a subciliary incision and the treatment should be carried out via a transconjunctival approach. Avoidance of treatment should be practised, for example, a patient who had keloid on previous ear-piercing episodes.

Limiting skin stretching during wound healing, facilitating appropriate wound resting and preventive exercises in certain sites such as chest and suprapubic areas are observed. Atkinson et al. [7] reported a randomised control trial of the effect of tape fixation and the prevention of hypertrophic scars post-caesarean section with significant scar reduction.

Therefore, scar reduction therapies are classified into:

- topical,
- intralesional,
- radiation and
- scar revision with Z plasty, local flaps and skin grafts.

The latest progress in scar management includes treatment with lasers to reduce angiogenesis, subcision and intradermal fillers. The emulsified fat (NanoFat) with stromal vascular fraction (SVF) and plasma rich protein (PRP) usage is the current trend in the non-surgical outcome of scar management.

**Box 36.4 Non-surgical remedies**
- *Steroid*
- *5FU*
- *Belonycin*
- *Lasers*
- *Dermabrasion*
- *Subcision*
- *Fillers*
- *Silicone gel sheets*
- *Pressure therapy*
- *Cryotherapy*
- *Radiation*
- *Emulsified fat for scar rejuvenation*

### 36.3.2 Non-surgical Remedies

The non-surgical modalities of scar management are highlighted in Box 36.4, and the description of each is as follows:

- *Steroid*

Triamcinolone is the mostly used steroid for scars. The mode of action when used as an intralesional therapy is in inhibition of the inflammatory mediators, inhibition of fibroblast proliferation, collagen synthesis and inhibition of TGF—BETA 1 and BETA 2—and enhancement of collagen degradation and collagenase action in keratinocytes [8].

The published reports, however, give varying outcomes with dose-dependent side effects such as hypopigmentation, telangiectasia and dermal atrophy [9]. There is an encouraging outcome, however, in combination therapy when the dosage is reduced.

- *5FU*

The suggested mode of action is an inhibition of fibroblast proliferation and TGF-BETA 1-induced collagen synthesis [10]. Anecdotal results are positive; however, trials lack adequate controls. Nonetheless, the effect is encouraging in combination therapy with steroid and pulse dye lasers. Much work is required in controlled studies.

- *Bleomycin*

It is an antibiotic and has been used intralesionally in vascular malformation with good outcome [11].

The mode of action is in reduction of collagen synthesis and increased destruction of collagen by inhibiting Lysyl Oxidase such as TGF-B1 [12]. Much work is needed in its definitive usage.

- *Lasers*

Lasers target three chromophores such as water, melanin and haemoglobin. Laser-induced tissue hypoxia results in the breakdown of disulphide bonds of the collagen fibrils. Pulse Dye Laser (PDL), KTP laser and Nd YAG lasers have affinity to haemoglobin, leading to collagen necrosis, and results in reduction of proliferation of fibroblast and deposition of collagen type 3. Ablative lasers remove the scar layer by layer with minimal thermal injury [13].

- *Dermabrasion*

This technique is still used in treating irregular scars such as ice pick scars of acne. The aim is to abrade up to the reticular dermis, allowing epithelialisation to take place. This treatment causes erythema for a long time, and the symmetrical outcome is not guaranteed.

Microdermabrasion is an advancement where there is high-speed pressurised aspiration-compression system. The benefit is that it minimises deep thermal injury [14].

Carbon Dioxide ($CO_2$) and Erbium laser resurfacing supersedes microdermabrasion with minimal thermal damage. Laser resurfacing acts in a different way compared to the vascular lasers. The vascular laser action is as a non-ablative principle, whereas $CO_2$ and Erbium cause ablation.

Vascular lasers decrease the prominence by destroying the blood vessels and stimulating collagen remodelling, thus softening the scar, whereas the ablative lasers such as $CO_2$ and Erbium ablate or vaporise the excessive tissues. $CO_2$ can induce more collagen remodellation and promote wound contraction [15].

The vascular lasers are used in hypertrophic and keloid scars. $CO_2$ and Erbium are useful in stretched, asymmetric and irregular scars. There is a restriction as it is not effective in all skin types as resurfacing can result in excessive pigmentation in dark, Asian and African skins.

- *Subcision*

It is a technique where depressed scars are elevated, and the controlled trauma can aid in formation of new connective tissue. This is carried out by custom-made subcision knives or 20 gauge needles. It can be combined with autologous fat injection to the subcised areas filling in the space and simultaneous laser resurfacing [16].

- *Fillers*

Synthetic Hyaluronic acid, calcium hydroxylapatite and bovine collagen are used in aesthetic surgery for voluminisation. They can be used in treating depressed scars. However, these agents cannot be used in a larger quantity as they will cause subcutaneous nodules and inflammation, and in bovine collagen, there is 3% incidence of allergic history. There is also a need for repeat injection. Autologous fat has taken over as a material of choice for filling in scar management.

- *Silicone gel sheets*

These sheets are used prophylactically in known patients for bad scars as well as therapeutically. However, the outcome for hypertrophic scars is still questionable and inconclusive.

It appears that controlled studies have shown significant beneficial outcome in scar volume when the silicone sheets are used or not used in mirror image wounds. A Cochrane review of 13 trials involving 559 patients, however, concludes weak evidence in preventing hypertrophic scars in susceptible patients [17].

The mechanism of action is in producing hydration to the scars by occlusion.

- *Pressure therapy*

It is a perceived therapy that there is positive evidence in the literature. The largest randomised trial showed no significant difference in scar reduction with pressure therapy when compared to the controlled group [18].

- *Cryotherapy*

A large uncontrolled study of 135 patients with 166 keloids demonstrated 79.5% response rate with 80% reduction in scar volume. However, the results are not reproducible. This treatment causes atrophic, depressed scars with residual hypopigmentation [19].

Therefore, the usage of cryotherapy particularly on the face should be discouraged as a modality.

- *Radiation*

It is an effective adjuvant to surgical excision particularly to keloid. The effect is caused by inhibition of proliferation

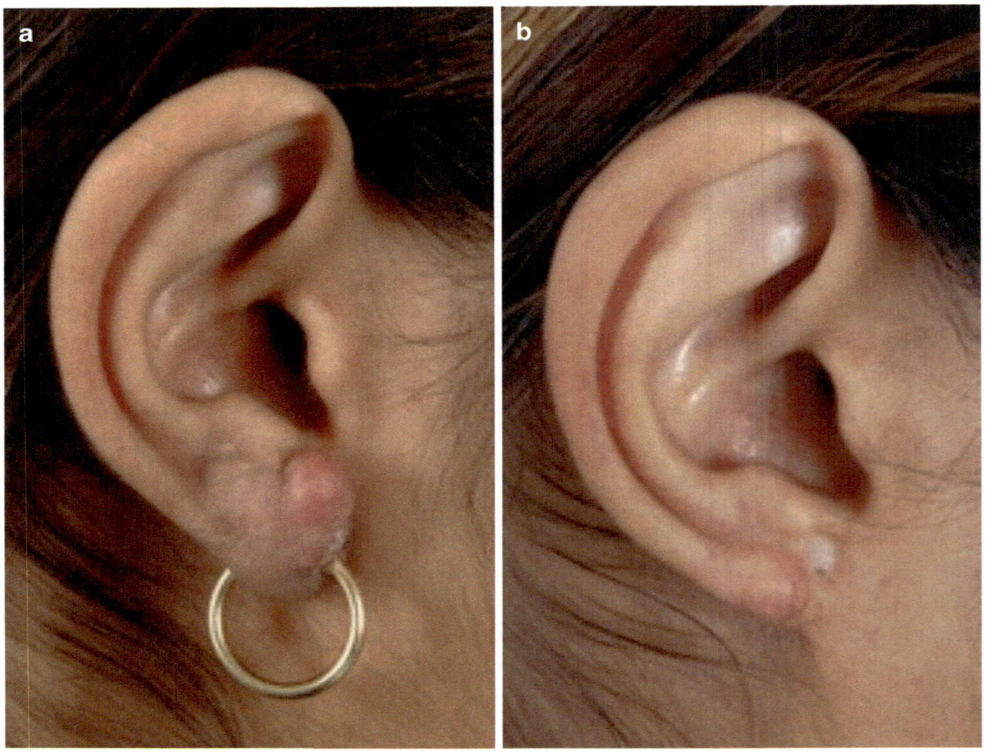




**Fig. 36.1** (**a**) Keloid Scar right ear lobule. (**b**) Post-operative photograph following scar excision and one dose of radiotherapy

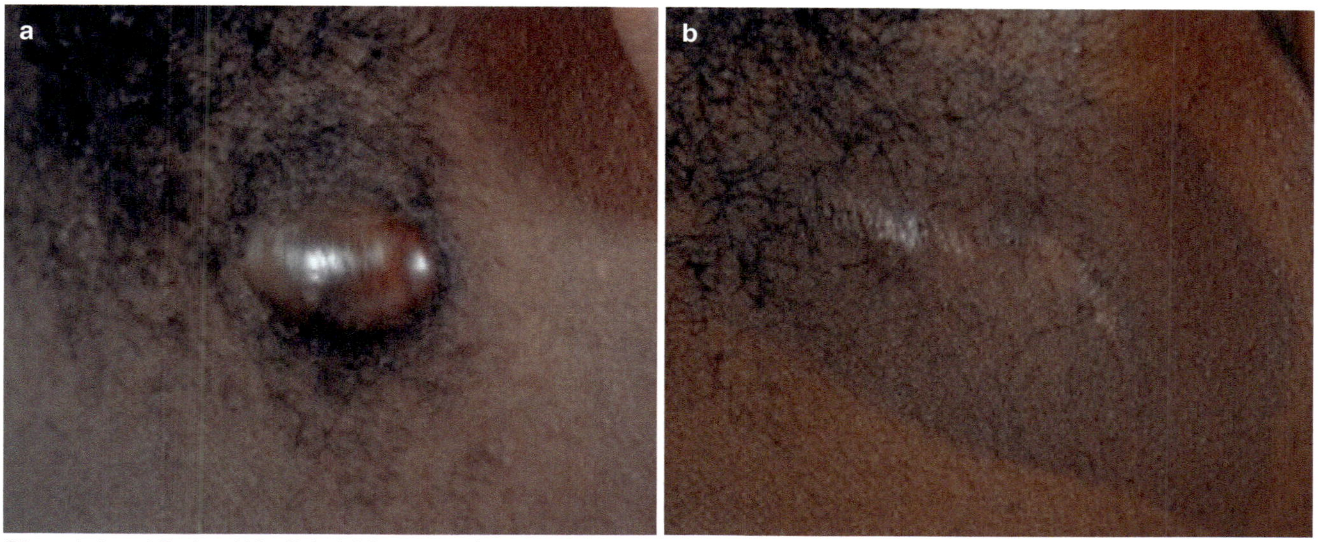




**Fig. 36.2** (**a**) Keloid Scar post-auricular region. (**b**) Post-operative photograph following scar excision and one dose of radiotherapy

of fibroblasts and neo-vascular blood formation, resulting in decreased collagen production [20].

The highest cure rate is described in a single dose within 24 hours after surgical excision; however, further studies are needed to evaluate the dosage and to obtain optimum results (Figs. 36.1 and 36.2).

- *Emulsified fat for scar rejuvenation*

The fat tissue is accepted not only as a simple layer of insulation and as a storage for energy but also as a complex endocrine organ, which is intrinsically involved in metabolism and immunomodulatory activities and can provide multi-source resources for stem cells and other undifferentiated cell population, which is essential for regeneration.

In addition to the adipocytes in the fat tissue, there are other cell groups that are functionally very important such as stromal vascular fraction (SVF) and cell-assisted lipotransfer (CAL). The SVF of adipose tissue is a rich source of epithelial progenitor cells, T cells, B cells and adipose tissue macrophages [21]. Separation of SVF is a time-consuming and expensive process requiring collagenase treatment and centrifugation. The recent clinical results obtained with Nanofat grafting where the cells are emulsified show greater value than the components of SVF used separately.

In Nanografting, a 23 gauge needle is used as a sharp needle for subdermal fat injection technique (SNIF) followed by a 27 gauge needle to superficial layers. In order to do this, the fat should be emulsified and takes the name, thus, Nanofat [6].

This now emerges to the forefront in regenerative medicine due to its ability to differentiate into a variety of different cells of cell lineage and the anti-apoptotic, anti-inflammatory, pro-angiogenic immunomodulators and anti-scarring properties.

Nanofat has shown to improve the aesthetics of hypertrophic and keloid scars by improving the texture of the scars in addition to improving the symptoms of pain and itching [22].

Fat is used in voluminisation initially as foundation micrograft just above the periosteum. The second layer is subdermal graft followed by subcision and lastly Nanofat injection using SNIF technique with 23-gauge needle followed by superficial needle injection using 27-gauge needle. This process is to treat depressed scars. Intralesional Nanofat injection improves hypertrophic and keloid scars. This can be combined with other modalities such as laser resurfacing.

## 36.4 Surgical Scar Management

### 36.4.1 Basic Principles

As described above, an ideal scar should be an imperceptible line parallel to RSTL. The only exception is scar along the lower lid due to the possibility of ectropion, if incisions are made in parallel to RSTL.

The aim of scar revision is to re-orientate the scar to follow the RSTLs and correction of adjacent structure distortion.

Patient understanding, nutrition, expectation and the psychological stability are paramount factors to implement pre-operatively prior to any scar revision exercises particularly in burn scars. The timing of the revision is also important as the remodelling may take up to 12 months.

Nutritional status and the medical history are important pre-operative considerations. It has been described with certain evidence that the use of vitamins A, C and E and zinc have beneficial effects and, at the same time, some herbal supplements such as arnica, garlic, ginseng and saw palmetto can impair wound healing [22]. Systemic conditions such as diabetes and immunosuppression can adversely affect wound healing. Smoking has proven to cause perilous effect on healing and wound repair.

Vitamin E refers to a group of ten lipid soluble compounds that include both Tocotrienols and Tocopherols as a fat soluble antioxidant; it stops the production of reactive oxygen species formed when fat undergoes oxidation [23]. It has been identified that alpha-tocopherol, the most biologically active form of vitamin E, has anti-inflammatory effects by decreasing plasma C-reactive protein (CRP) levels and release of pro-inflammatory cytokines. The CRP, a downstream marker of inflammation in addition to being a risk marker for cardiovascular disease, could contribute to atherosclerosis. Alpha-Tocopherol has been shown to decrease CRP level in patients and has a positive effect in scar reduction. Topical vitamin E application has been practised in managing scar 10 days post-suture removal. Anecdotally, in the last 25 years, good scar outcome has been observed.

### 36.4.2 Surgical Technique

In most circumstances, incisions should be made parallel to the skin surface. A number 11 or 15 blade is ideal. Tissue handling must be atraumatic. The skin flaps should be held with non-toothed forceps, and the tooth forceps should only be used to handle tissues subdermally. Undermining and constant hydration of edges are essential. In stretched scars, preservation of the dermis by de-epithelialisation will provide extra support in correcting the depression. Haemostasis should be achieved using a bipolar diathermy again minimising thermal injury to the surrounding areas.

Suturing is done in layers. In areas where supportive tension is required, resorbable round body needle sutures are useful. Depending on the site and the extent of the scar, short- or long-term resorbable sutures could be selected. With deep suturing as much as possible, the knot should be buried with skin approximation to achieve 'eversion'. Simple-interrupted sutures are preferable in a majority of areas; however, subcutaneous running sutures could be used where only gentle approximation is needed.

1. *Z plasty* (Fig. 36.3)

This is a common technique used in scar revision to either change the direction of the scar or lengthen the scar. Contracted scars can be corrected by plating multiple simultaneous Z plasties.

The Z plasty is created by using the original scar as a central portion, and triangular flaps are raised. Multiple variations are in Z plasty. In the classical Z plasty, all the limbs are of equal length and the angle between the flaps is 60°. The scar will lengthen by 75%. A 30° angle will lengthen by 25%, and 45° will lengthen by 50%. Multiple Z plasties are useful in long scars, which can be divided into separate segments, and the angles are contoured or modified depending on the sites.

2. *W plasty* (Fig. 36.4)

This technique is used to irregularise scars so that dimensions of the scar are not perceived by the naked eye. A series of consecutive triangles are made. It is mirror image on the opposite side. The arm length should be around 5 mm, and the angle in-between the flap should be maximum 90°. One side of the triangle should be in parallel to our RSTL. The

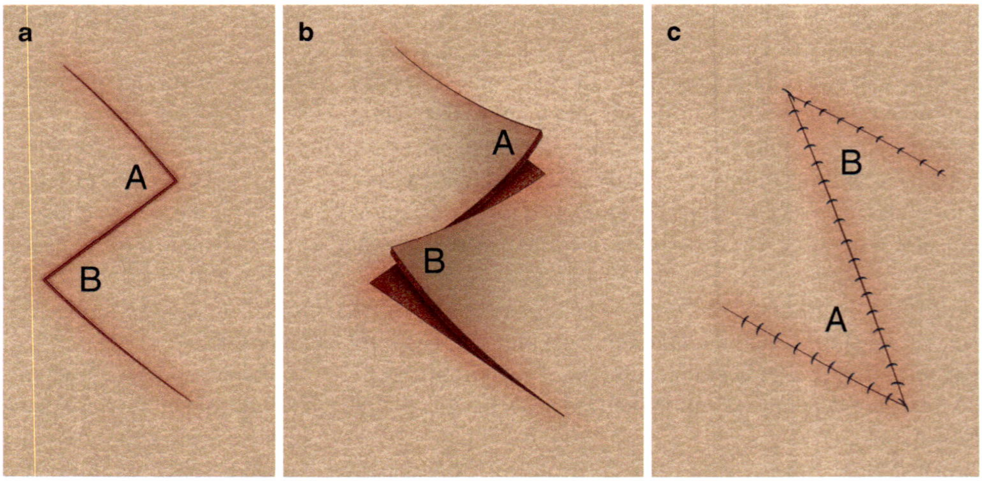


**Fig. 36.3** Z plasty (**a**) scar revision. (**b**) triangular flaps raised. (**c**) interposition of triangular flaps

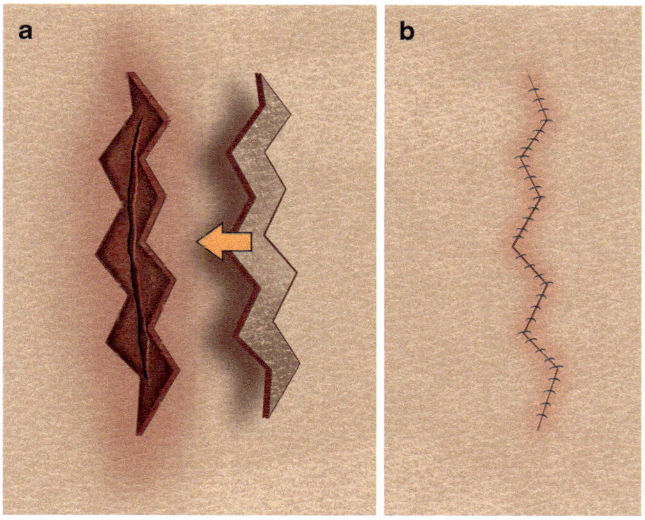




Fig. 36.4 W plasty— (**a**) scar revision. (**b**) post-operative

triangle are excised, undermined and closed with interdigitation. This technique is very useful in correcting unsightly hairline scars such as revision of face lift.

3. *Geometric broken line closure (GBLC)*

This is another technique to minimise the perception of a long scar. Here, random geometric designs are planned with corresponding mirror images. The length of the limbs should be 3–6 mm and at the angle near to 90°, and a W plasty could be done at the end of the design.

4. *V-Y and Y-V advancement*

V-Y scar correction (Fig. 36.5a–c) is utilised when there is an indication on scar lengthening in contracted scars with ‘trap door deformity’. In contrast, Y-V technique is utilised where the scar is shortened, removing the ‘Y ‘extension (Fig. 36.6a–c).

Fig. 36.5 V-Y scar lengthening correction. (**a**) V incision. (**b**) Triangular flaps raised. (**c**) Y closure

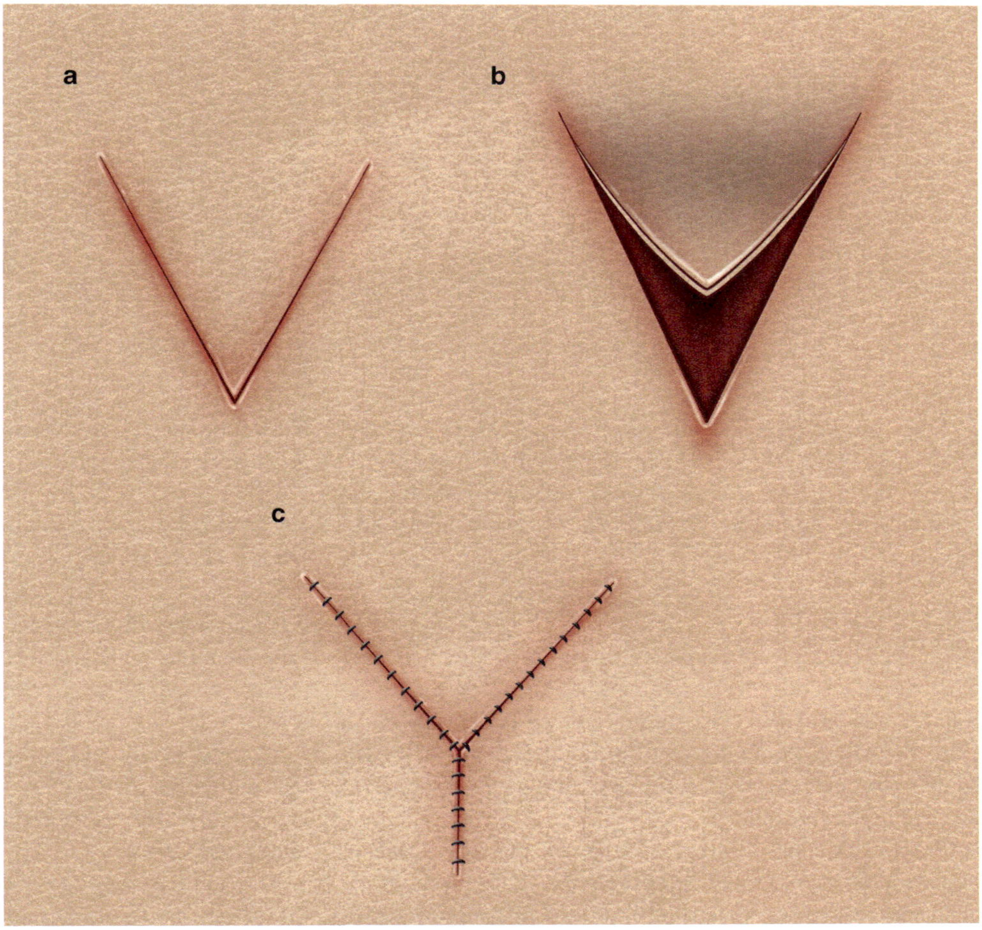

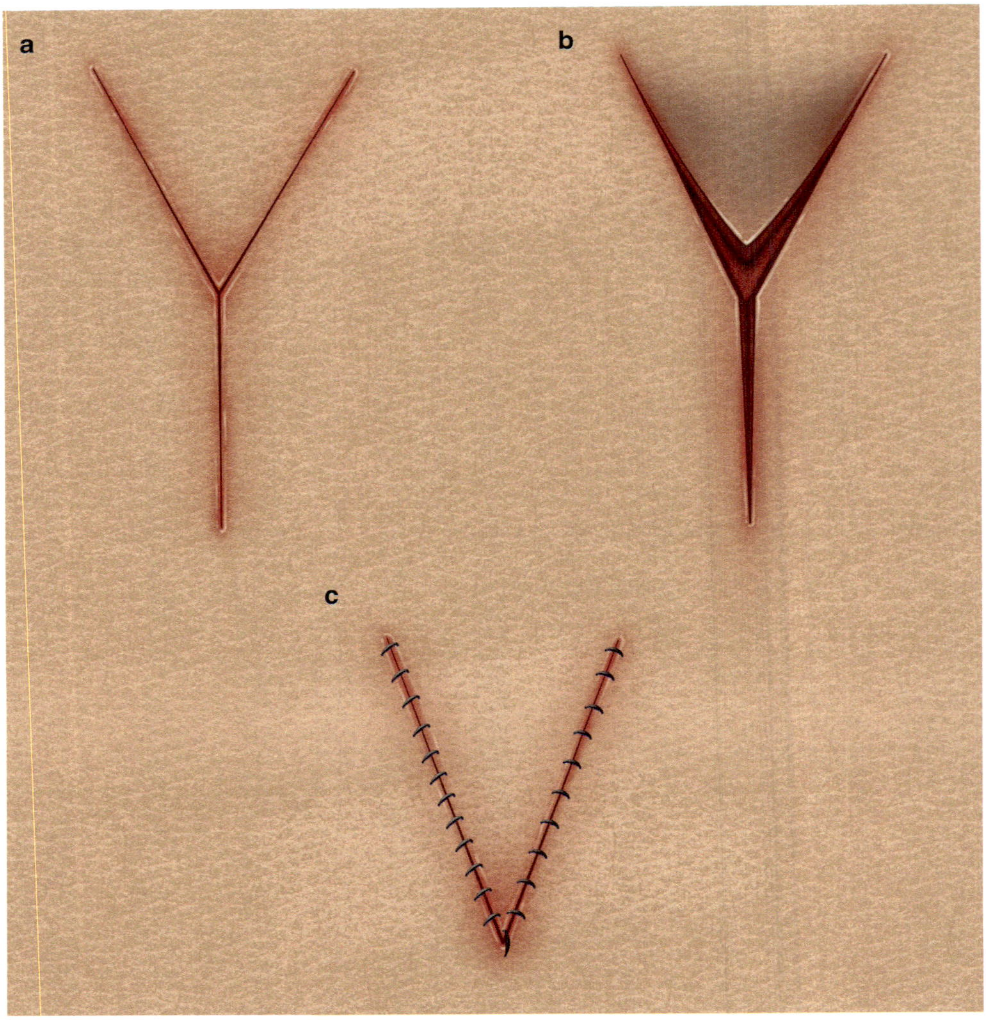


Fig. 36.6 Y-V scar shortening correction. (**a**) Y incision. (**b**) Triangular flaps raised. (**c**) V closure



Flaps can be used to revise large scars. "Doggy ear" and "trap door deformities"could be improved by excising the excess. For passive scar settlement, selective bulking and simultaneous multiple 'Z' and 'W' plasties are useful adjuncts.

**Clinical tip**

When repairing wounds in patients who are prone to develop hypertrophic scars, deep sutures should be placed using round bodied needles. The suture removal is delayed by an extra 3–4 days. Applying steri strips after removal of the sutures adds extra support, and this should be incorporated to achieve the best result.

Prophylactic intralesional steroids in patients prone to hypertrophic scars should be considered. Obliteration of the dead space by appropriate sutures or pressure dressings with or without drains should be considered to prevent haematoma formation. If not, haematoma on its own will spoil the good work of scar revision.

## 36.5 Future

Extrauterine scarless surgery is not possible. Therefore, careful patient factor and scar characteristics should be studied to prevent unsightly scar formation and to correct perceptible scars.

General health and optimising comorbidities are important requirements to achieve good scars. Both non-surgical and surgical options should be available in the armamentarium to the Surgeon.

Nanofat has very positive potential in scar management. The research on gene therapy using adenovirus as a mediator to deliver dermal fibroblast is encouraging [24].

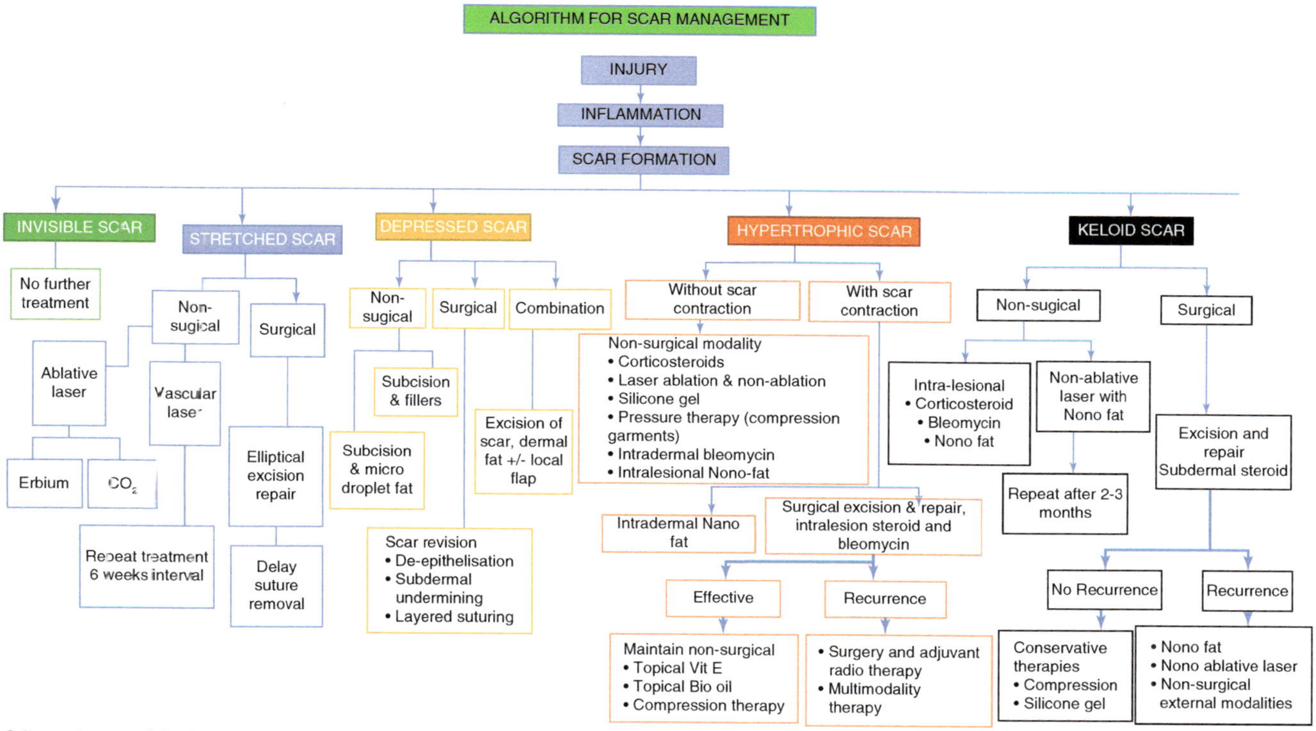




**Fig. 36.7** Algorithm for scar management

Although inflammatory response is traditionally believed to be a key event for wound healing in adult skin, studies of foetal wound healing suggest that a high level of inflammation might prevent good scar formation rather than enhancing the wound healing process. Therefore, further studies are needed to confirm if really inflammation is necessary for wound healing in adult skin. However, at present, we need to follow the inflammatory process and available evidence of therapeutic modulators of scar formation.

Furthermore, it is paramount to consider that there are clinical, histological, biochemical and molecular differences between hypertrophic and keloid scars. There is marked difference in the proliferative and apoptotic cell deaths between the scars, resulting in variable response of different treatments. This should be taken into account in treatment planning process.

It is also essential to avoid excessive movements that can stretch the wound and for avoidance of the scar to direct mechanical forces such as friction and scratching and particularly earlobe wounds, to minimise the contact with pillows and wound hygiene.

Not least the patient's involvement plays a vital role in the management of scars. Variable scales in the literature exist for reliable and reproducible scar management, for both the observer, i.e. surgeon, and the patient. The observer opinion is always influenced by vascularisation, thickness and pigmentation. The patient opinion, on the other hand, is influenced by action of itching sensation and thickness of the scar. Out of the available assessment scales, the patient and observer scar management described by Draaigers L et al. is an informative tool in documentation of the progress in the management of scar, which should be addressed [25].

In summary, a surgeon should have an algorithm to follow on how to manage scars in normal patients as well as patients who are prone for hypertrophic and keloid scars (Fig. 36.7).

## 36.6 Conclusion

Scar formation is a part of wound healing process. Facial scars can be aesthetically detrimental and affect social stigma. As facial surgeons, we need to achieve ideal scars with natural contour, colour and limited distortion. It is paramount to remember that scar management includes prevention, treatments during the healing period and definitive management once the scar has been established. We have, in this chapter, included all the different available treatments separating them into non-surgical remedies and surgical techniques. The algorithm, in this chapter, allows a very easy review process for surgeons who manage stretched,

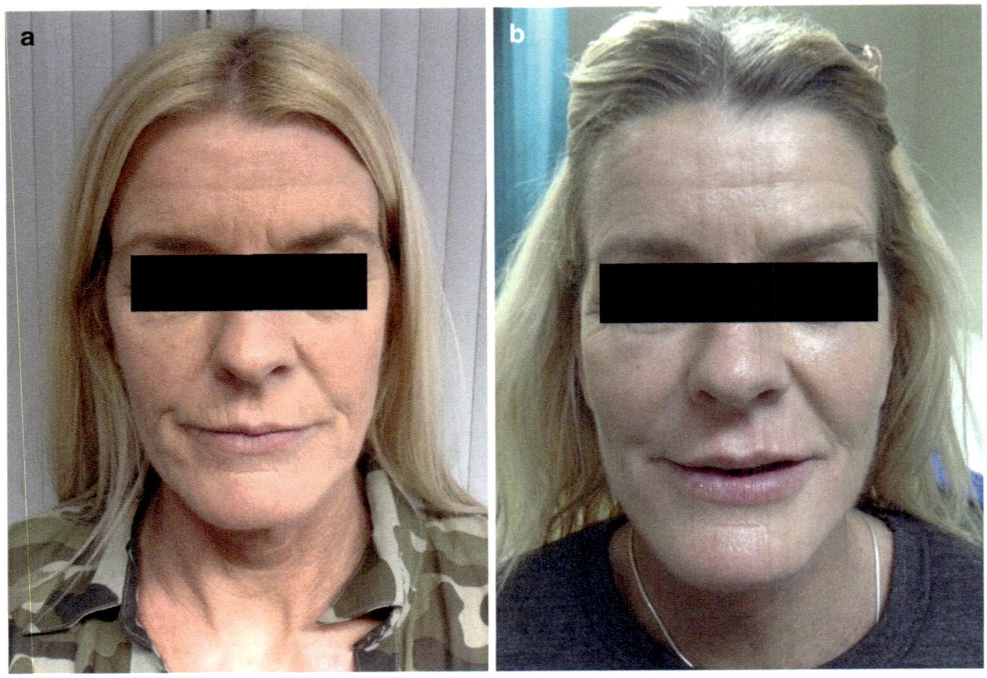


**Fig. 36.8** (**a**) Pre-operative. (**b**) Post-"microfat grafting" and laser resurfacing



depressed, hypertrophic and keloid scars.DisclosureAuthors have no financial conflicts to disclose.

## 36.7 Case Scenarios

### Case Scenario 1 (Fig. 36.1)

A 27-year-old female patient of Asian ethnicity had an extra ear piercing to the right earlobe. Within 4 months, she started to develop a very painful hard lump at the pierced site. Within the following 6 weeks, it developed into an irregular mass involving the whole of the earlobe.

Her medical history was unremarkable, and she was not on any medication.

On examination (Fig. 36.1a), there was an unsightly thick lumpy scar along the right earlobe. A diagnosis of keloid was made.

Under a local anaesthetic, the keloid scar was excised and the earlobe was reconstructed. The next post-operative day she underwent single dose of radiotherapy (10 Gy) as an outpatient.

On review, 6 months post-treatment (Fig. 36.1b), she had no recurrence and on palpation, the skin was soft and non-tender.

### Case Scenario 2 (Fig. 36.8)

A 48-year-old Caucasian patient who had a considerable amount of sun exposure presented with an unhappy peri-oral aesthetics (Fig. 36.8a).

Her medical history was unremarkable, and she was not on any medication.

In one examination, she had loss of volume along the peri-oral site mainly along the upper lip. The vermillion border had lost its definition. She had multiple small vertical subdermal lines, which were crossing the vermillion border. She also had epidermal thinning.

A diagnosis of aging of the peri-oral area, particularly upper lip, was made. She, in fact, had epidermal thinning, subdermal scaring and loss of inter- and intramuscular fat.

She underwent "microfat" grafting to restore the volume, subdermal "emulsified fat" to restore the subdermal structure and an "erbium laser resurfacing" (fluence 500 mJ, mode: SP, spot 3 mm, frequency 20 Hz).

The post-operative appearance 4 months later (Fig. 36.8b) showed excellent volume restoration, much improvement in the subdermal scaring, better vermillion definition and a new regenerative skin.

This combination technique is very useful in burn scar management.

## References


1. Beldon P. Basic science of wound healing. Sci Direct. 2010;28:409–12.
2. Borges AF. Relaxed skin tension lines. Dermatol Clin. 1989;7:169–77.
3. Broughton G, Janis JE, Attinger CE. The basic science of wound healing. Plast Reconstr Surg. 2006;117:12S–34S.
4. Reish RG, Ericksson E. Scars: A review of emerging and currently available therapies. Plast Reconstr Surg. 2008;122:1068–78.
5. Collet C, Laversanne S, Haen P, et al. Micro-re-injection of autologous fat. Rev Stomatol Chir Maxillofac Chir Orale. 2013;114:381–6.
6. Tonnard P, Verpaele A, Peeters G, Hamdi M, Cornelissen M, Declercq H. Nanofat grafting: basic research and clinical applications. Plast Reconstr Surg. 2013;132:1017–26.
7. Atkinson JA, McKenna KT, Barnett AG, et al. A randomised controlled trial to determine the efficacy of paper tape in preventing hypertrophic scar formation in surgical incisions that traverse Langer's skin tension lines. Plast Reconstr Surg. 2005;116:1648–56.
8. Roques C, Teot L. The use of corticosteroids to treat keloids. A review. Int J Lower Extremity Wounds. 2008.
9. Niessen FB, Spauwen PH. On the nature or hypertrophic scars and keloids: a review. Plast Reconstr Surg. 1999;104:1435–58.
10. Fitzpatrick RG. Treatment of inflamed hypertrophic scars using intralesional 5-FU. Dermatol Surg. 1999;25:224.
11. Sindel A, Sayan A, Ilankovan V, et al. Percutaneous treatment of orofacial vascular malformations. Br J Oral Maxillofac Surg. 2018;56:206–11.
12. Crooke ST, Bradner WT. Bleomycin, a review. J Med. 1976;7:333–428.
13. Lupton JR, Alster TS. Laser scar revision. Dermatologic Clin. 2002;20:55–65.
14. Tsai RY, Wang CN, Chan HL. Aluminium oxide crystal microdermabrasion. A new technique for treating facial scarring. Dermatol Surg. 1995;21:539–42.
15. Bowes LE, Nouri K, Bernam B, et al. Treatment of pigmented hypertrophic scars with the 585 nm Pulsed Dye Laser and the 532 nm Frequency Doubled Nd: YAG laser in the Q-Switched and variable pulse modes: a comparative study. Dermatol Surg. 2002;28:714–9.
16. Orientreich DS, Orientreich N. Subcutaneous incisionless (subcision)surgery for the correction of depressed scars and wrinkles. Dermatol Surg. 1995;21:543–9.
17. Neissen FB, Spauwen PH, Robinson PH, Fedler V, Kon M. The use of silicone occlusive sheeting (Sil-K) and silicone occlusive gel (Epiderm) in the prevention of hypertrophic scar formation. Plast Reconstr Surg. 1998;102:1962–98.
18. Chnag P, Laubenthal KN, Lewos R, et al. Prospective, randomized study of the efficacy of pressure garment therapy in patients with burns. J Burn Care Rehabil. 1995;16:473.
19. Rusciani L, Paradisi A, Alfano C, et al. Cryotherapy in the treatment of keloids. J Drugs Dermatol. 2006;5:591.
20. Ragoowansi R, Cornes PG, Moss AL, et al. Treatment of keloids by surgical excision and immediate postoperative single-fraction radiotherapy. Plast Reconstr Surg. 2003;111:1853.
21. Zhu X, Du J, Liu G. The comparison of multilineage differentiation of bone marrow and adipose-derived mesenchymal stem cells. Clin Lab. 2012;58:897–903.
22. Broughton G, Crosby MA, Coleman J, et al. Use of herbal supplements and vitamins in plastic surgery: a practical review. Plast and Reconst Surgery. 2007;119:48–66.
23. Devaraj S, Leonard S, Traber M, Jialal I. Gamma-tocopherol supplementation along and in combination with alpha-tocopherol alters biomarksr of oxidative stress and inflammation in subject with metabolic syndrome. Free Radic Biol Med. 2008;44:1203–8.
24. Liu W, Chua C, Wu X, Want D, Ying D, Cui L. Inhibiting scar formation in rat wounds by Adenovirus-Mediated overexpression of trunated TGF-ß Receptor II. PRS. 2005;115:860–70.
25. Draaijers LJ, Templeman FR, Botman YA, Tuinebreijer WE, Middelkoop E, Kreis RW. The patient and observer scar assessment scale: a reliable and feasible tool for scar evaluation. PRS. 2004;113:1960–5.

# Surgical Facelift

# 37

Velupillai Ilankovan and Tian Ee Seah

## 37.1 Introduction

An ancient Chinese proverb "岁月不饶人" observed that "no one is spared from the ravages of ageing". A combination of age, gravity, physiologic contraction of facial muscles and solar (sun) and chemical (smoking) insults results in intrinsic and extrinsic changes to the skeleton, muscles and skin [1]. Preservation of one's youthful looks has been a goal of humans regardless of cultures and ethnicities. The search for this elixir of youth was found unexpectedly in the hands of cosmetic surgeons. Even with the recent advent of skin peels, botulinum toxin injections, lasers and injectable filler injections, the century-old facelift still possesses the most dramatic improvement to the moderate to severe ageing lower face when done well.

Facelift or rhytidectomy as its name suggests is a procedure to partially eliminate folds, creases and wrinkles (rhytids) caused by gravity and degeneration. In effect, the creation of two large cervicofacial flaps, which, after suspension and trimming, produces an overall tightening of the skin and the fascial envelope of the face and neck, results in restored anatomical structure. Facelift can help to negate some of these gravitational problems and produce some intrinsic improvement.

## 37.2 Historical Perspective

Historically, rhytidectomy was limited to skin elliptical excisions and tightening. The German surgeon, Eugen Höllander, first described being persuaded by his patient to remove excessive skin in the temporal, preauricular and postauricular regions in 1901. With cosmetic surgery frowned upon in those times, he did not report his surgery immediately but only recounted retrospectively that the iatrogenic wounds when approximated resulted in some tightening in 1912 [2]. The initial reports of rhytidectomy were dominated by a slew of American surgeons such as Cantrell (1902), Miller (1907) and German surgeons, Lexer (1906) and Joseph (1912) [3]. The French surgeon Passot wrote an important paper "La chirugie esthétique des rides du visage" in 1919 where he illustrated strategically placed forehead, malar, cheek and submental elliptical incisions to tighten the face for aesthetic purposes, thus heralding the concept of short scar rhytidectomy (Fig. 37.1).

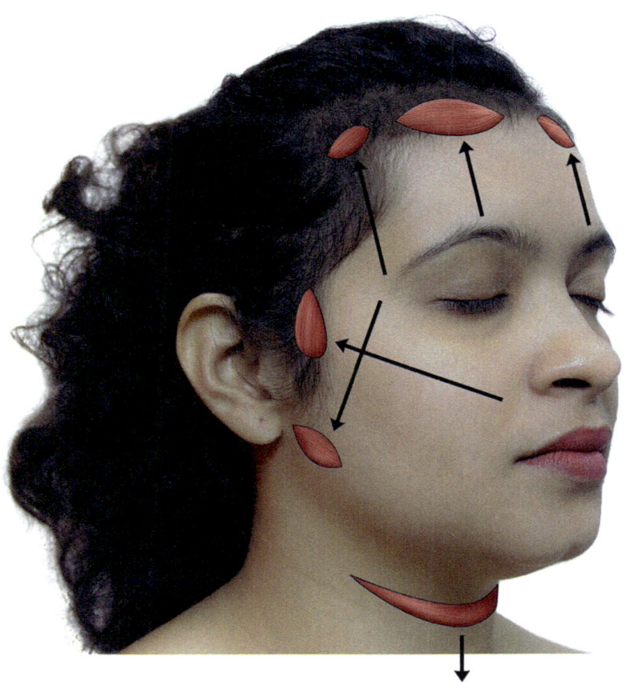

©Association of Oral and Maxillofacial Surgeons of India

Fig. 37.1 Illustration showing Passot's principles on facelift through elliptical excisions

V. Ilankovan (✉)
Oral and Maxillofacial Surgery, Poole Hospital NHS Foundation Trust, Poole, UK

T. E. Seah
TES Clinic for Face and Jaw, Singapore, Singapore


K. Bonanthaya et al. (eds.), *Oral and Maxillofacial Surgery for the Clinician*, https://doi.org/10.1007/978-981-15-1346-6_37

However, with limited undermining, wounds were closed under tension, resulting in unsightly scarring. To circumvent this problem, skin flap only procedures during which only the skin was raised, undermined for a short distance and tightened were introduced (Bames 1927) [4].

The results of skin flap only facelift were short term with limited correction of the ageing face, forcing surgeons to search for better alternatives. In 1974, Tord Skoog, a Swedish surgeon, revolutionized facelift concepts by describing the dissection, elevation and tightening of the superficial fascia of the face in addition to removing excess skin. He expounded the importance of retro-positioning the "buccal fascia" and the platysma for better results. The importance of this technique was later cemented when the superficial fascia of the face was clarified as the "superficial muscular aponeurotic system" (SMAS) by Mitz and Peyronie in a landmark paper in 1976 [5]. Manipulation of the SMAS layer in a superior or supero-lateral vector became an important part of modern facelift. Soon, a flurry of papers on the modifications to facelift procedures concentrated on the management of the SMAS.

Treatment of the SMAS layer could be broadly categorized into three methods. They were plication, elevation, imbrication and SMASectomy [6]. The most conservative of these methods was plication of the SMAS layer, as it did not actually involve dissecting the SMAS layer but instead used sutures to fold the SMAS and achieve a tightening effect [7]. More aggressive management of the SMAS included imbrication, which involved the elevation and repositioning of the SMAS in a superior or superolateral vector [8]. In standard SMAS elevation, the SMAS was dissected, lifted off the parotid fascia and secured to the underlying zygomatic soft tissues or the deep temporal fascia (Fig. 37.2).

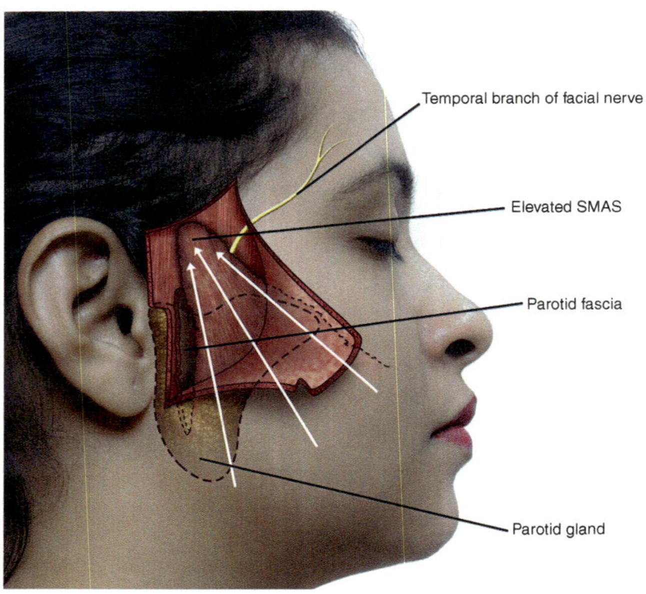




**Fig. 37.2** SMAS imbrication

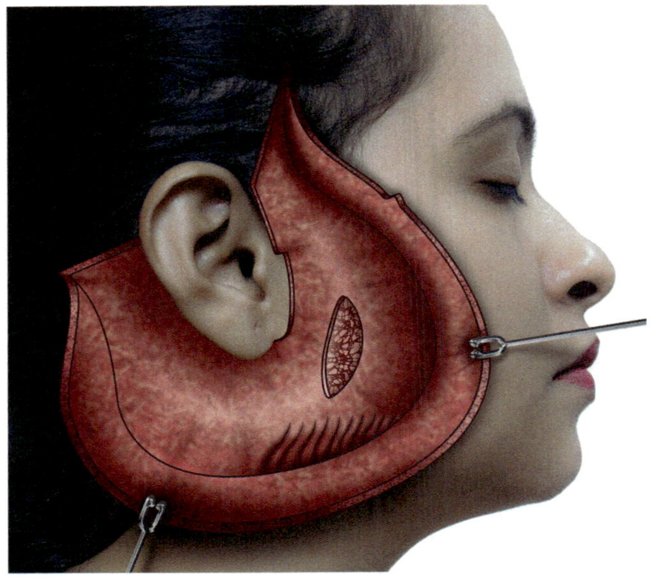



**Fig. 37.3** SMASectomy. 1–2 cm of the SMAS is excised superficial to the anterior border of the parotid

SMASectomy was later described [9]. This required excision of approximately 1–2 cm strip of the SMAS, superficial to the underlying parotid fascia, and then tightening were carried out by suturing the opposing two cut SMAS margins [6] (Fig. 37.3).

It soon became obvious to the surgeons that skin excision and SMAS manipulation were only effective in treating the lower face but not as effective in treating midface ageing. In particular, the nasolabial fold proved to be a stubborn adversary. The spotlight turned towards the high density, retaining ligaments such as the zygomatic retaining ligaments, which prevent effective rejuvenation of the midface using the aforementioned procedures.

The deep plane facelift was described by Hamra to include the malar fat pad [10]. In this, the dissection and elevation of the SMAS layer were carried out further to release the zygomatic retaining ligaments so that more traction could be obtained from the midface. The orbicularis oculi and later septal reset were included to improve midface aesthetics, and the term composite facelift was coined by Hamra [11].

As the facelift landscape progressed, efforts turned almost full circle towards smaller incisions. Comparisons of different published facelifts were unable to reveal an optimal technique [12] although complications were significant higher in extensive SMAS procedures.

Attention turned towards having minimal excision, limited dissection and SMASectomy with imbrication, and in 2001, Saylon and later Fulton et al. described the S-lift [13]. In this technique, the preauricular skin was excised in a predetermined S-shape followed by purse-string plication of the mobile SMAS using a U-shaped purse string suture and an O-shaped purse string suture. Both sutures were anchored into the periosteum of the zygoma.

Tonard et al. later introduced the minimal access cranial suspension (MACS) as a modification to the S-lift [14] (Fig. 37.4).

In this procedure, he described suspending the sagging SMAS tissues with cranially directed purse string sutures via limited incisions that extend from the sideburn to the inferior helical attachment. Four main differences lie between the "S" lift and the 'MACS' lift. First, the S-Lift pre-empted the amount of excess skin and excised it via an S-shaped incision. The MAC lift redraped the excessive skin and removed it according to the margin. The second difference lies between point of anchorage as the 'S-lift' anchored to the periosteum of the zygoma, while the 'MACS lift' anchors to the superficial layer of the deep temporal fascia. Third, during the S-lift, SMASectomy and imbrication were carried out, while during the MACS lift, only plication was performed. Fourth, besides the two O and U-shaped sutures, the MACS lift utilizes a third vertical suspension suture that suspended the malar fat pad, thus reducing the depth of the nasolabial fold. This area is accessed by extending the temporal hairline incision, and Tonard and Verpaele called this the extended MACS lift.

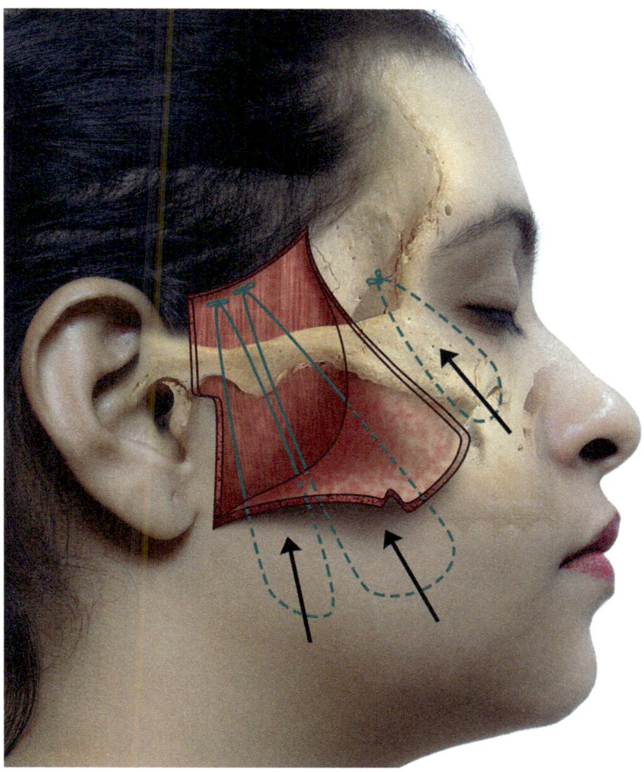



Fig. 37.4 MACS Lift

## 37.3 Anatomy of Ageing Face

Some of the gravitational changes include lateral brow ptosis, tear trough, malar palpebral groove, SOOF descent, malar fat descent, deepening of the nasolabial groove, buccal fat pad herniation, marionette lines, jowls, loss of neck definition, submental fat and excess skin [1].

With ageing, a combination of gravitational forces, laxity of the skin due to loss of elasticity, decreased dermal thickness and loss of dermal appendages results in ptotic, hanging skin.

The mid cheek's fat is divided into three compartments [15] (Fig. 37.5). It is thinnest at the lid-cheek segment and is thickest in the nasolabial region. The malar fat is also moderately thick although not as thick as the nasolabial region.

Accumulation of fat in the cervical region results in loss of neck definition and submental fat.

Superficial fat and deep fat are separated by SMAS layer. The superficial fat is separated into five compartments, namely, the nasolabial, medial cheek, middle cheek,

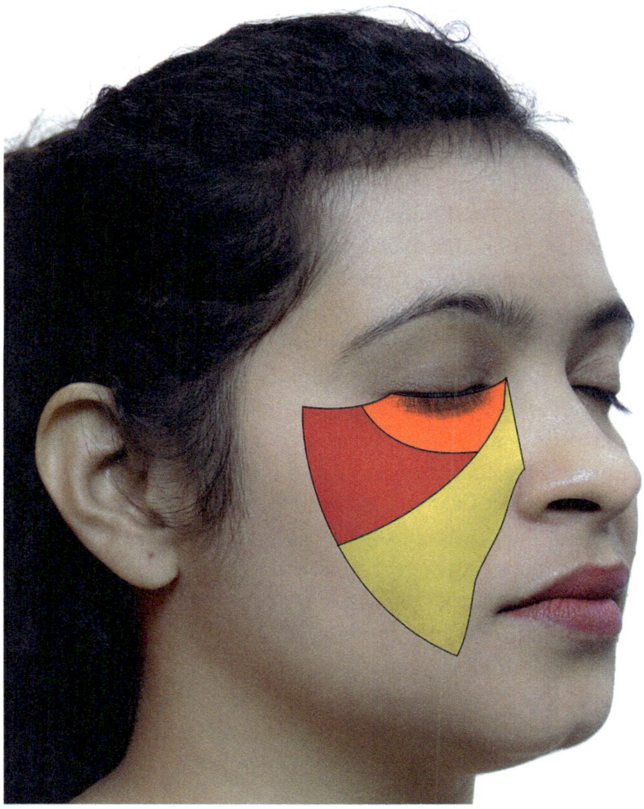



Fig. 37.5 Cheek fat is divided into three compartments. They are lid-cheek segment (Orange), Malar segment (red) and nasolabial region (yellow). (Figure adapted and redrawn from Aesthetic Plastic Surgery 2009, Chapter 6 by Mendelson BC)

lateral temporoparietal and inferior orbital fat. Deep fat is divided into the deep medial fat and suborbicularis oculi fat (SOOF) [16].

The superficial musculoaponeurotic system (SMAS) is a fibrous sheath, which was described in a classical paper by Mitz and Peyronie [5] in 1976, and starts from the galea superiorly. Superolaterally, it is continuous with the superficial temporal fascia also known as the temporoparietal fascia. In the central upper face, deep into the superficial fat, the SMAS layer is invested by the muscles of facial expression, derived from the embryonic second branchial arch: frontalis, orbicularis oculi, corrugator supercilii, depressor supercilii and the procerus. In the middle third, the SMAS is invested by the nasalis muscles, zygomaticus major, minor, levator labii superioris alaeque nasi and levator labii superioris. Laterally, the SMAS is superficial to the parotid fascia and extends inferiorly to include the platysma muscles. Inferomedial, the SMAS is invested by the orbicularis oris, risorius, depressor anguli oris, depressor labii inferioris and mentalis and is continuous with the platysma.

With the exception of the levator anguli oris and mentalis, the facial nerve travels deep into the SMAS layer and innervates the muscles of facial expression, making dissection above the SMAS during facelift safe [16].

An analogy of the retaining ligaments is that they are rooted in a tree into the periosteum and deep fascial thickening, and as it approaches the SMAS, it divides into numerous branches and inserts into the dermis called retinacular cutis [15] (Fig. 37.6).

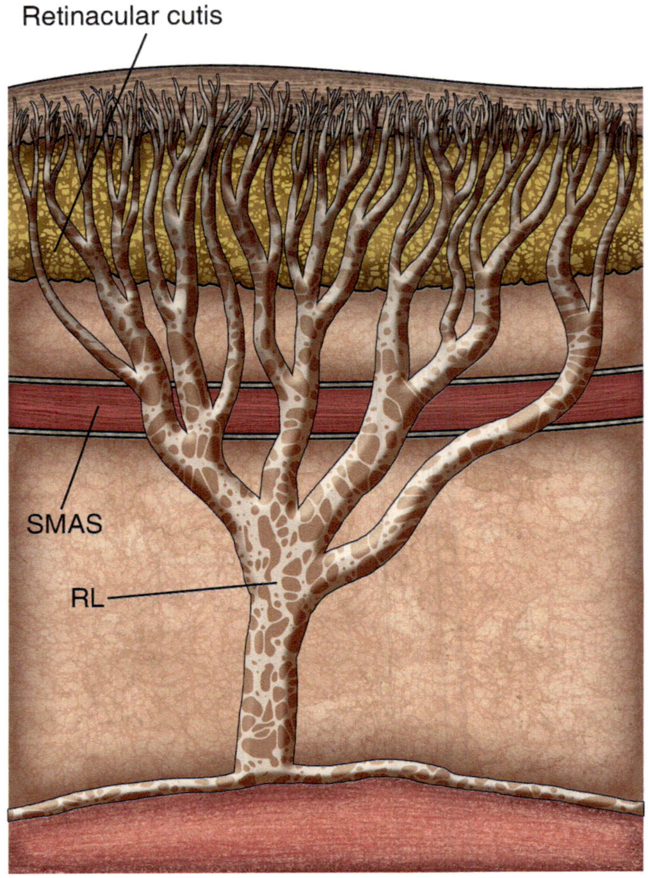


Fig. 37.6 Retaining ligaments (RLs) insert into the subcutaneous layer as retinacular cutis. It is likened to a tree by Mendelson BC [15]. (Figure adapted and redrawn from Aesthetic Plastic Surgery 2009, Chapter 6 by Mendelson BC)

Stuzin [17] and Furnas et al. [18] described the retaining ligaments [17]. The partitioning of separate fascial spaces and compartments is caused by these retaining ligaments, which are classified into osteocutaneous and fasciocutaneous retaining ligaments.

Osteocutaneous retaining ligaments originate from the periosteum and include the zygomatic and mandibular cutaneous ligaments. Stout zygomatic retaining ligaments originate from the inferior border of the zygomatic arch towards the junction between the arch and the body and insert into the dermis of the skin as fibrous septa. It is posterior to the zygomaticus major muscle, approximately 3 mm in width, 0.5 mm in thickness and 4.5 cm anterior to the tragus [18]. Loss of support results in malar fat descent.

The mandibular ligament originates from the periosteum 10 mm above the mandibular border, extends along the anterior one third of the mandibular body and inserts into the dermis [19] (Fig. 37.7). It coincides with the anterior margin of the jowl.

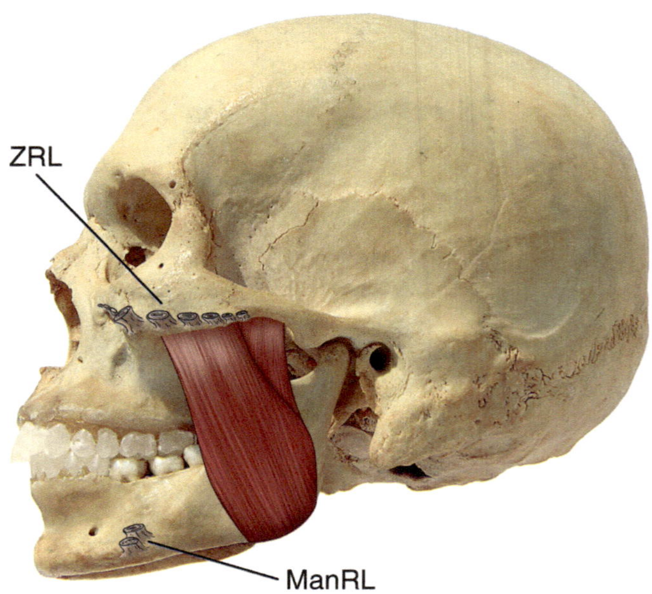


©Association of Oral and Maxillofacial Surgeons of India

Fig. 37.7 Osteocutaneous ligaments comprising the zygomatic retaining ligaments (ZRLs) and the mandibular retaining ligaments (MRLs)

Fasciocutaneous retaining ligaments include the masseteric and parotid cutaneous ligaments also known as the platysma auricular ligament and coalesce between the superficial and deep fascia of the face [1].

Masseteric ligaments originate from the parotidomasseteric cutaneous ligaments, and loss of support results in

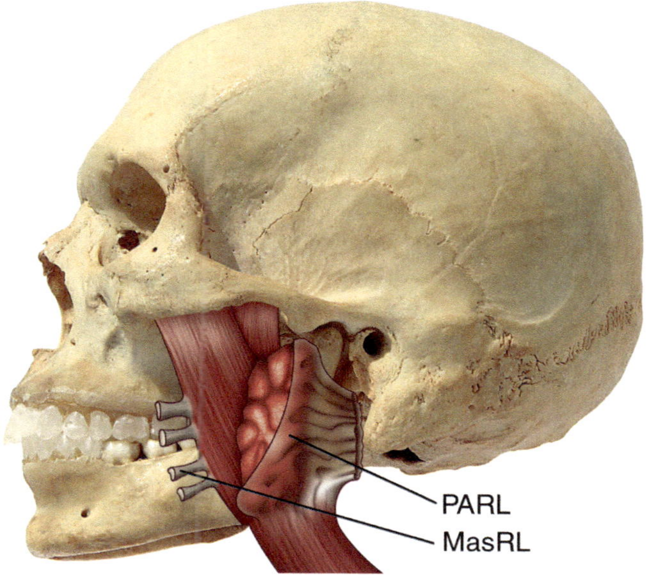


©Association of Oral and Maxillofacial Surgeons of India

**Fig. 37.8** Fasciocutaneous retaining ligaments comprising the masseteric retaining ligaments (MasRLs) and the parotid cutaneous ligaments also known as platysma auricular retaining ligaments (PARLs)

facial jowling. Parotid cutaneous ligaments are formed by the posterior border of the platysma, which had receded into fascial condensation. It is fused with the parotid fascia, is attached to the overlying skin and provides firm anchorage between the platysma and the dermis in the inferior auricular region (Fig. 37.8).

## 37.4 Standard Facelift

Surgery can be carried out either under general anaesthesia or under local anaesthetic with or without sedation.

Local anaesthesia comprising Lidocaine 2% with adrenaline 1:80,000 is infiltrated in the zygomaticofacial region, infraorbital, mental, greater auricular (Fig. 37.9) and the lesser occipital nerves.

Tumescent solution reconstituted with 1 L of saline, 50 mL of 1% lidocaine, 1 mL of adrenaline 1:1000 and 6 mL of 8.4% Sodium Bicarbonate is then injected subcutaneously after stab incisions are placed in the temporal, preauricular, postauricular and submental regions. Approximately 300 mL of tumescent solution in all is injected.

In both approaches, infiltration of Tumescent solution in a subcutaneous plane is essential to carry out atraumatic dissection. In our practice, 95% of standard facelift are carried out with simultaneous neck lift, as we feel it would be impossible to mobilize the attenuated soft tissue to achieve symmetry and an unoperated look of the midface without bringing attention to the neck aesthetics.

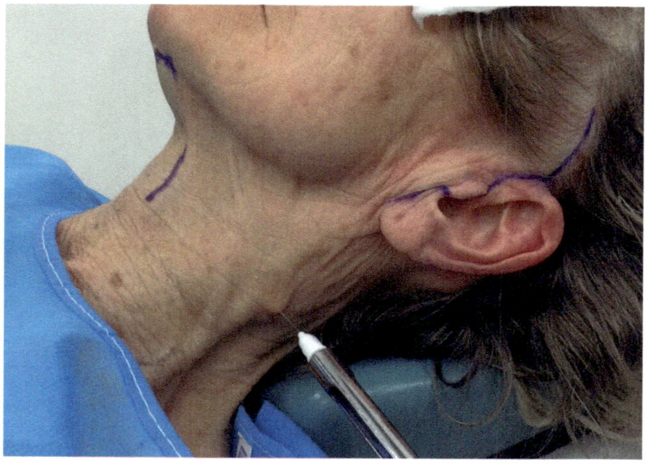

©Association of Oral and Maxillofacial Surgeons of India

**Fig. 37.9** Greater auricular nerve block

### 37.4.1 Incision

The incision lines are divided into four sections: temporal, preauricular, postauricular and scalp extension. The temporal component is either into the hairline or just at the hairline/sideburn border. The latter has the advantage of not moving the sideburn position; however, it would give a telltale sign of a visible scar. In the former approach, the sideburn area may get lifted into the temporal area and the scar will be hidden. This position should be made in conjunction with discussion with the patient, and suitability of the incision should be selected.

The preauricular marking could be a pre-tragal, intra-tragal or post-tragal. The latter can distort the tragal projection, and the pre-tragal will give a visible scar. We prefer an intra-tragal approach and obtain the tragal projection by placing a subcutaneous anchor suture before the final closure in order to maintain the natural concavity and simultaneously achieve an invisible scar (Figs. 37.10 and 37.11).

The postauricular incision should be a few millimetres into the postauricular area from the sulcus so that postoperatively the scar will settle down comfortably into the sulcus. The scalp extension is carried out by multiple W or Z plasty type incisions in a trichophytic fashion to minimize hair loss and to have an invisible scar (Fig. 37.12).

A 2.5 cm curvilinear incision parallel to the mandibular contour is the submental incision to the neck lift section in order to expose the anterior border of the platysma and the platysmal dissection.

### 37.4.2 Dissection

The submental flap dissection is carried out at first to expose the platysma muscle as much as possible (Fig. 37.13).

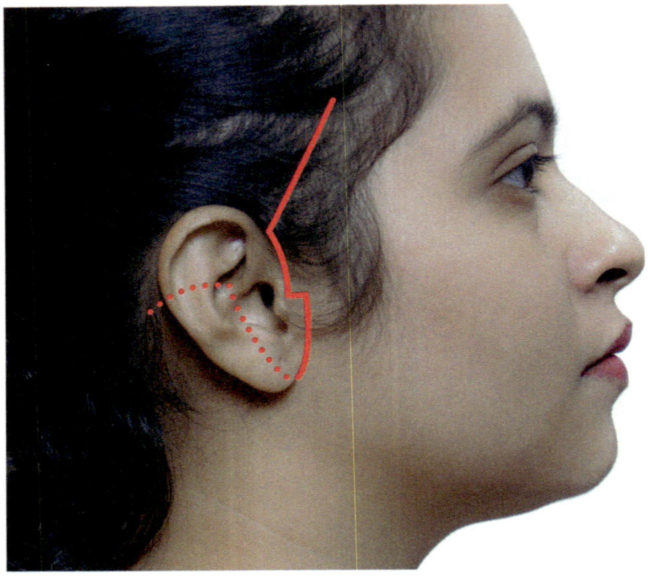



**Fig. 37.10** Temporal to preauricular incision (red). Occipital or scalp extension (broken line)

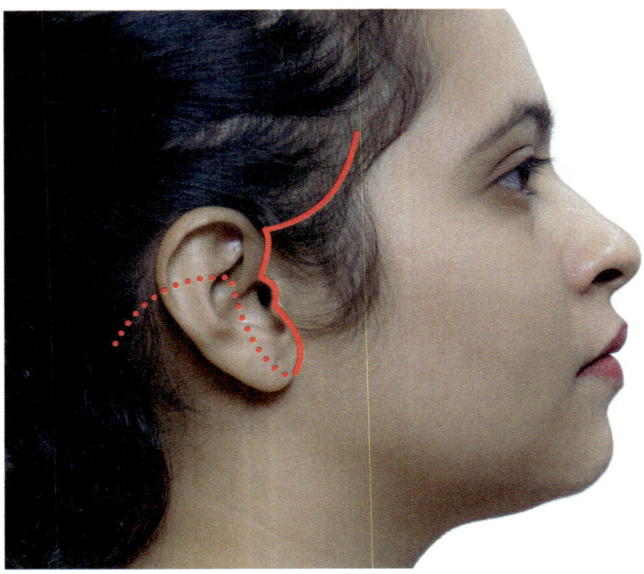



**Fig. 37.11** Hairline to tragal incision (red). Occipital or scalp extension (broken line)

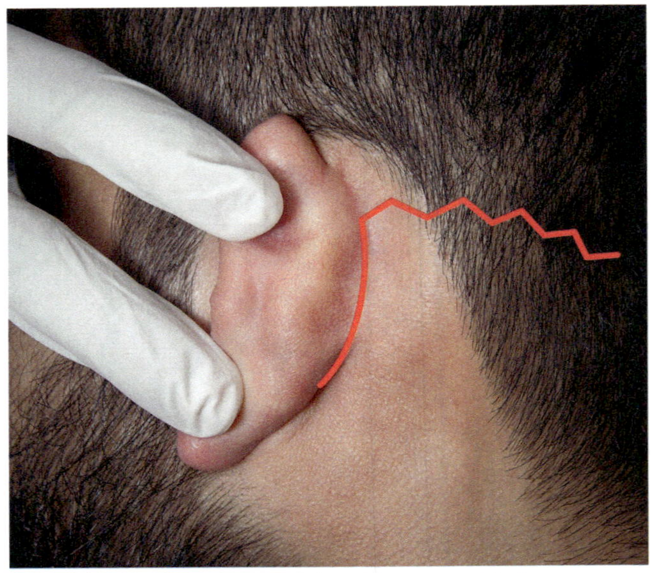



**Fig. 37.12** Illustration showing the postauricular and occipital or scalp extension

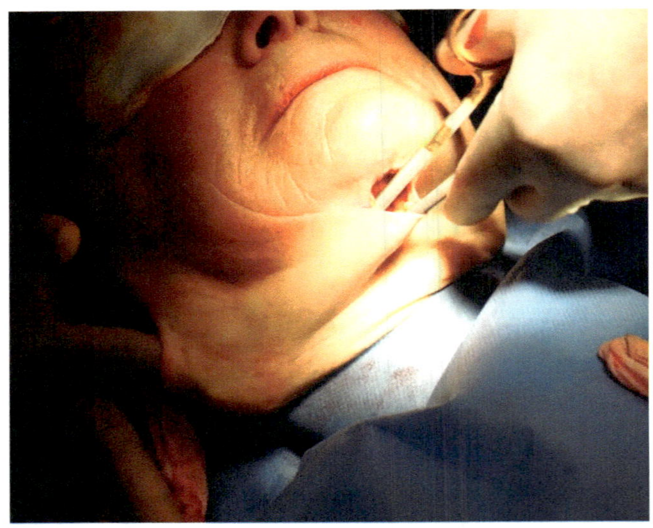



**Fig. 37.13** Dissection is in the supraplatysma plane

Next, the scalp and postauricular dissection is carried out. The anterior border of the sternocleidomastoid muscle and posterior border of the platysma are exposed, and a cavity of the neck is connected anteriorly and posteriorly (Fig. 37.14). The next step is to focus on the temporal and preauricular dissection. In the temporal, the deep part of deep temporal fascia is exposed, which we use as an anchor point to the SMAS suturing (Fig. 37.15). The preauricular dissection will expose the zygomatic ligaments, lateral end of the orbicularis oculi and the anterior border of the parotid–masseteric fascia with careful attention towards the buccal branch of the facial nerve (Fig. 37.16).

The preauricular, neck and postauricular dissection should now be in one cavity.

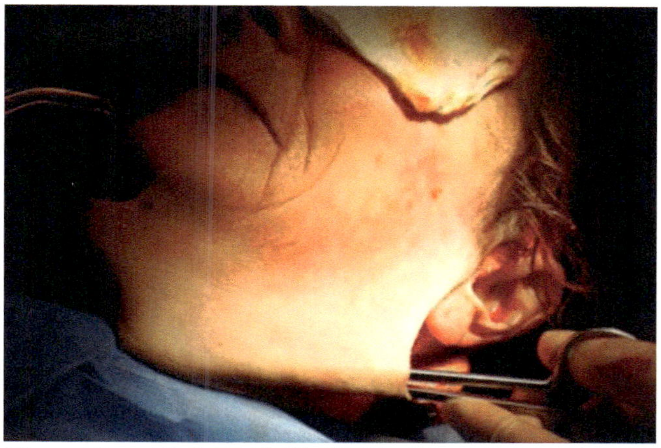

©Association of Oral and Maxillofacial Surgeons of India

Fig. 37.14 The postauricular flap is then connected to the cervical flap and the submental region made previously

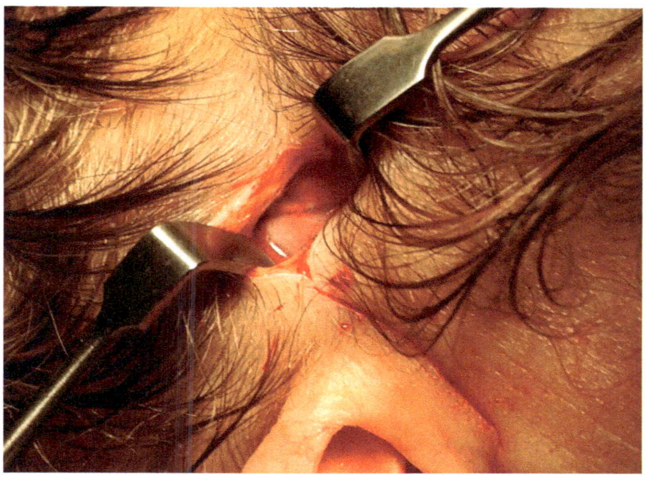

©Association of Oral and Maxillofacial Surgeons of India

Fig. 37.15 Deep layer of the deep temporal fascia exposed

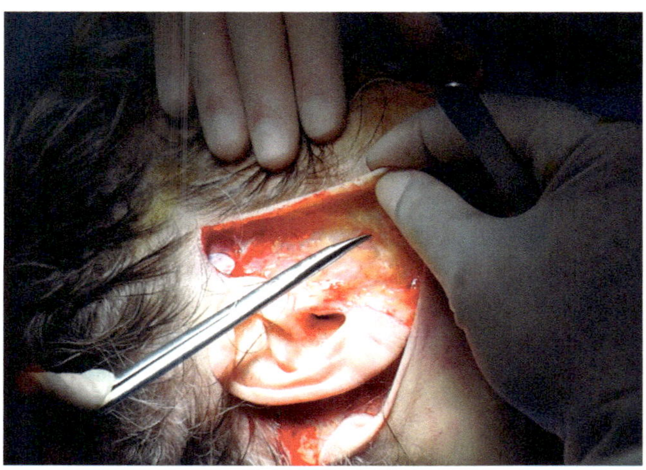

©Association of Oral and Maxillofacial Surgeons of India

Fig. 37.16 After the deep temporal fascia is exposed, dissection is carried out in a different plane subcutaneously to raise a skin flap

### 37.4.3 SMAS and Platysmal Elevation and Plication

SMAS elevation and management are carried out in various forms. We elevate the SMAS in an inverted L fashion (Fig. 37.17) starting at the preauricular plane, and the superior limit is at the lateral end of the zygomatic arch. The anterior dissection passes to the parotid-masseteric fascia (Fig. 37.18). The inferior dissection is to join the subplatys-

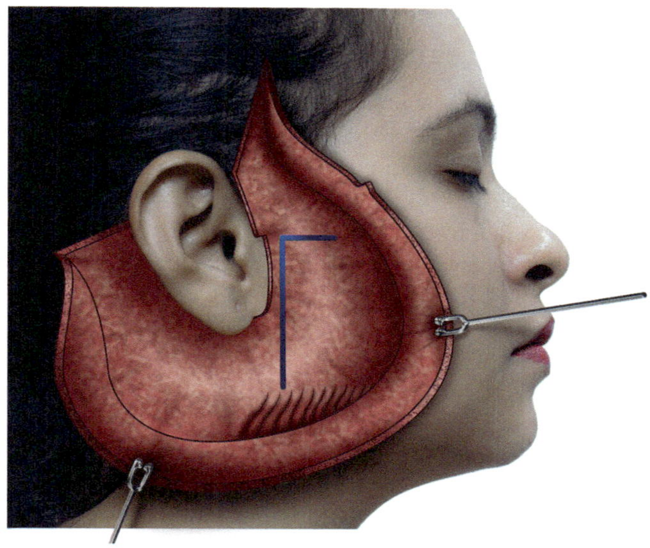

©Association of Oral and Maxillofacial Surgeons of India

Fig. 37.17 An inverted L shape incision (blue lines) is made on the SMAS stopping short of the parotid fascia. The shorter limb is just below the zygomatic arch, while the longer limb is in the preauricular region

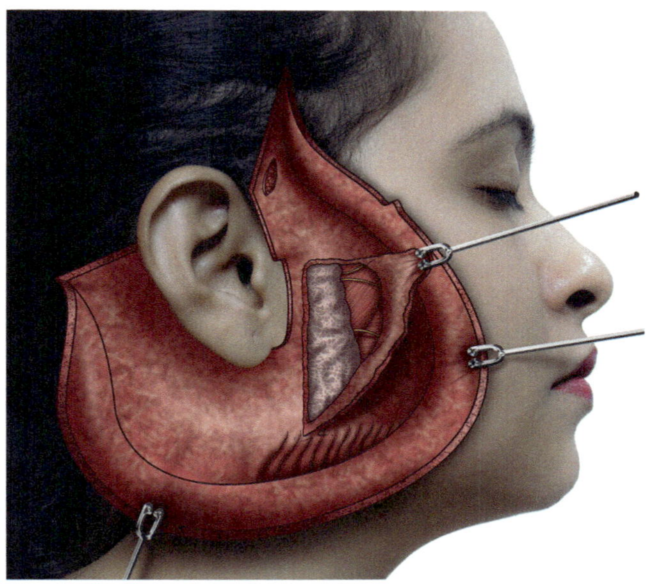

©Association of Oral and Maxillofacial Surgeons of India

Fig. 37.18 Cut SMAS peeled anteriorly to show underlying parotid. Facial nerve exits the parotid deep into the SMAS. Deep into these are the masseter muscles followed by the buccinator muscles with horizontal muscle striations mal plane at the angle of the jaw with consideration to avoid damage to the two or three cervical branches. In our practice, the elevated SMAS is anchored in a superior direction to the deep part of the deep temporal fascia (Fig. 37.19).

Our platysma dissection and plication are in four steps. The anterior border of the platysma is sutured in the midline [20] (Fig. 37.20). In some patients with short neck, the platysmal suturing needs to be hitched to the body of the hyloid bone. In some patients, a release of the inferior border of the platysma muscle at this area could also be considered. Then,

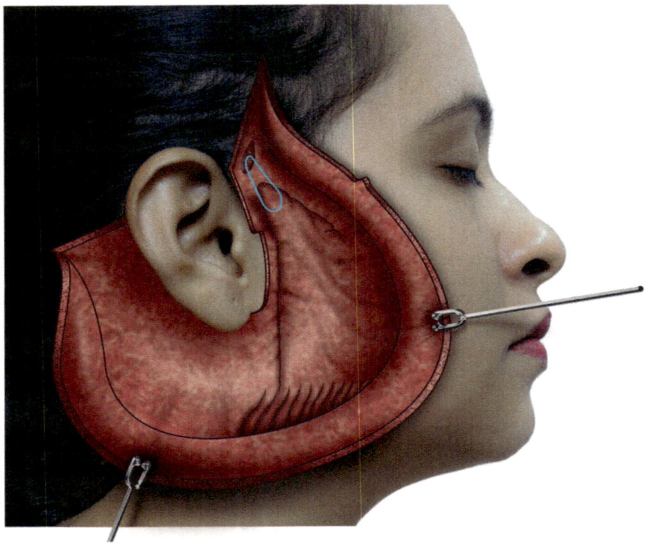

©Association of Oral and Maxillofacial Surgeons of India

**Fig. 37.19** The cut SMAS is then advanced superiorly and sutured to the deep temporal fascia with 3/0 Polygluconate (Maxon, Tyco Health UK Ltd., Gosport PO130AS, UK) (blue line)

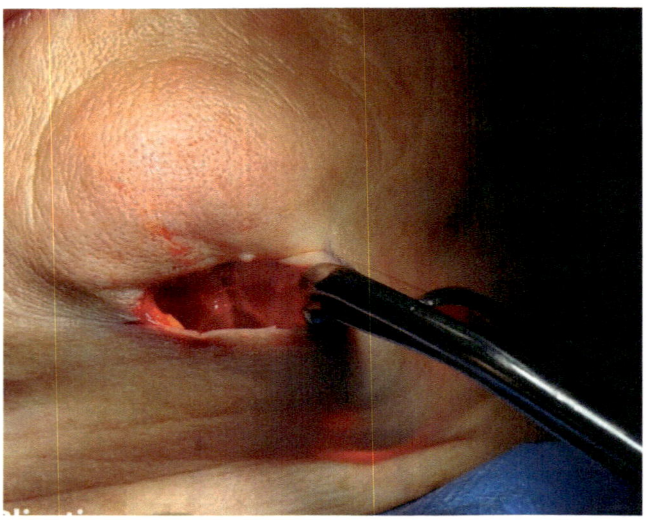

©Association of Oral and Maxillofacial Surgeons of India

**Fig. 37.20** The medial edges of the platysma are sutured to each other at the midline in a corset manner

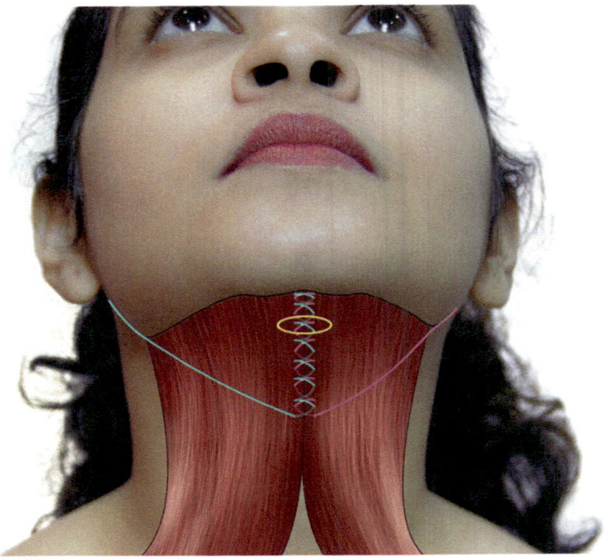

©Association of Oral and Maxillofacial Surgeons of India

**Fig. 37.21** A submental incision is made (white outline). Corset sutures are done twice, and the suture is plicated to the mastoid fascia on both sides

the lateral border of the platysma muscle is sutured to the anterior border of the sternocleidomastoid muscle. The third step ~~is~~ in platysmal plication is placing a cinch suture, which is placed joining the two anterior borders of the muscles in the midline and, after catching the platysma muscle in two or three areas, hitched the sternocleidomastoid muscle and the final anchor into the mastoid periosteum (Fig. 37.21). Depending on the neck anatomy, we sometimes place a second cinch suture about 5–6 mm below the first to avoid bulging of the submandibular gland.

### 37.4.4 Closure

Meticulous haemostasis is done with bipolar electrocautery throughout the procedure. The cervicofacial flaps are draped over the margins in a superolateral vector with much emphasis on the superior than the lateral direction (Fig. 37.22). Final anchoring is done with two key sutures that are placed along the helical attachment and the superior aspect of the postauricular incision. Cuts are made on the excess skin, perpendicular to the flap margin, stopping just short of it (Fig. 37.23). This allows the margins to be visualized when trimming the excess skin. If a tragal incision was made, the skin can be thinned and trimmed to mimic tragal shape and skin during closure at the tragus. Dog ears are preferably removed at the apex rather than in the ear lobe region. The ear lobe is then replaced 15° posterior to the vertical position to reduce the telltale signs of facelift procedures. Layered repaired is then carried out in the final closure.

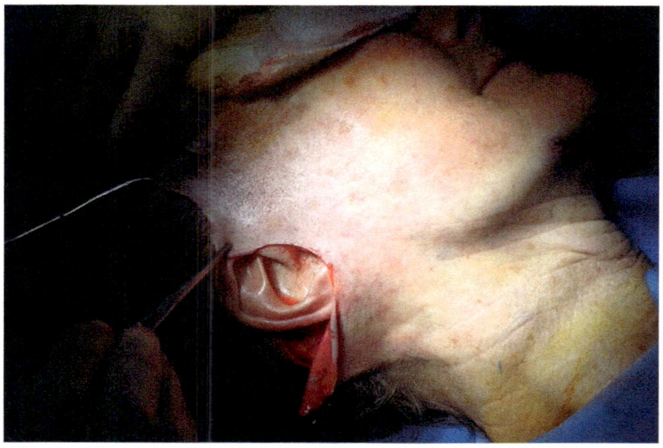

©Association of Oral and Maxillofacial Surgeons of India

**Fig. 37.22** Excess skin is draped in a superolateral vector over the margins and excised

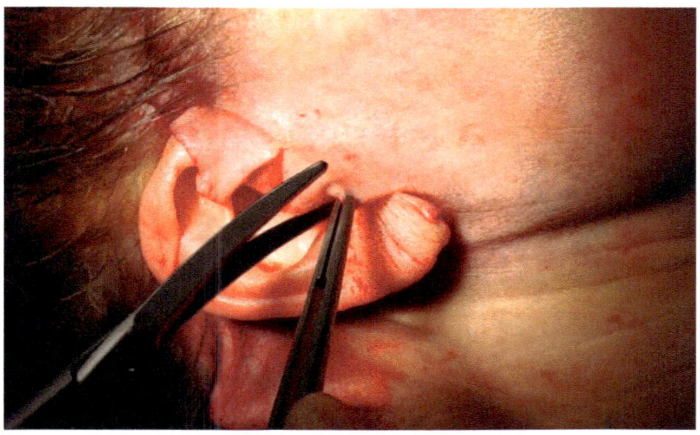

©Association of Oral and Maxillofacial Surgeons of India

**Fig. 37.23** Cuts are made perpendicular to the flap margin stopping short of the margins and then excised accordingly

### 37.4.5 Support Dressings

There are different ways of providing this final exercise. We apply antibiotic topical ointment followed by non-sticky dressing to the pre- and postauricular area and an adjustable Velcro band. In the literature, however, various pressure dressings are applied.

## 37.5 Post-operative Management

Velcro bands are removed on a daily fashion. Wounds are cleaned followed by topical ointment and reapplication of the Velcro band.

The medications are taken on a prescribed fashion.

The patient is placed on antibiotics and painkillers for a week. Sleeping is done with the head elevated by 2–3 pillows. The patient is seen on the day after the surgery to ensure that there is no haematoma. If drains are placed, they are removed during this time.

Facial bandages are placed between 2 and 5 days. Sutures are removed 7–10 days later. The wounds are kept moist with antibiotic ointment such as Tetracycline 3% or Mupirocin ointment 2% (Figs. 37.24a, b and 37.25a, b).

## 37.6 Complications and Management

Post-operative complications of facelifts include post-operative haematoma, skin necrosis, sensory and motor disturbances, obvious scarring, seroma, alopecia, auricular deformity and dyspigmentation [21]. Detailed informed consent should be obtained from patients prior to the surgery.

### 37.6.1 Haematoma

A thorough medical history is needed prior to surgery. Antiplatelet medications such as Aspirin, Clopidogrel, Dipyridamole and powerful anticoagulation drugs such as warfarin will have to be stopped after consultation with the patient's prescribing physicians. Patients on herbal or traditional Chinese medications such as ginkgo biloba and Cordyceps will also need to be stopped before surgery.

Haematoma formation is by far the most common complication with some papers reporting up to 15% [21]. Expanding haematoma usually happens in the first 24 hours and must be evacuated. Smaller haematoma can be aspirated, and pressure bandage is placed for pressure haemostasis. Meticulous haemostasis with bipolar diathermy is mandatory for facelift procedures. The flap and the underlying bed should be scrutinized for bleeding spots with a good head light or fibre optic light attached to a retractor. Brisk bleeding from larger vessels should be ligated. Adjunctive measures including fibrin glue [22, 23] and platelet gel and facelift bandages have been explored.

Large haematoma are a cause for concern and need to be evacuated. They can cause problems in healing including skin ischaemia.

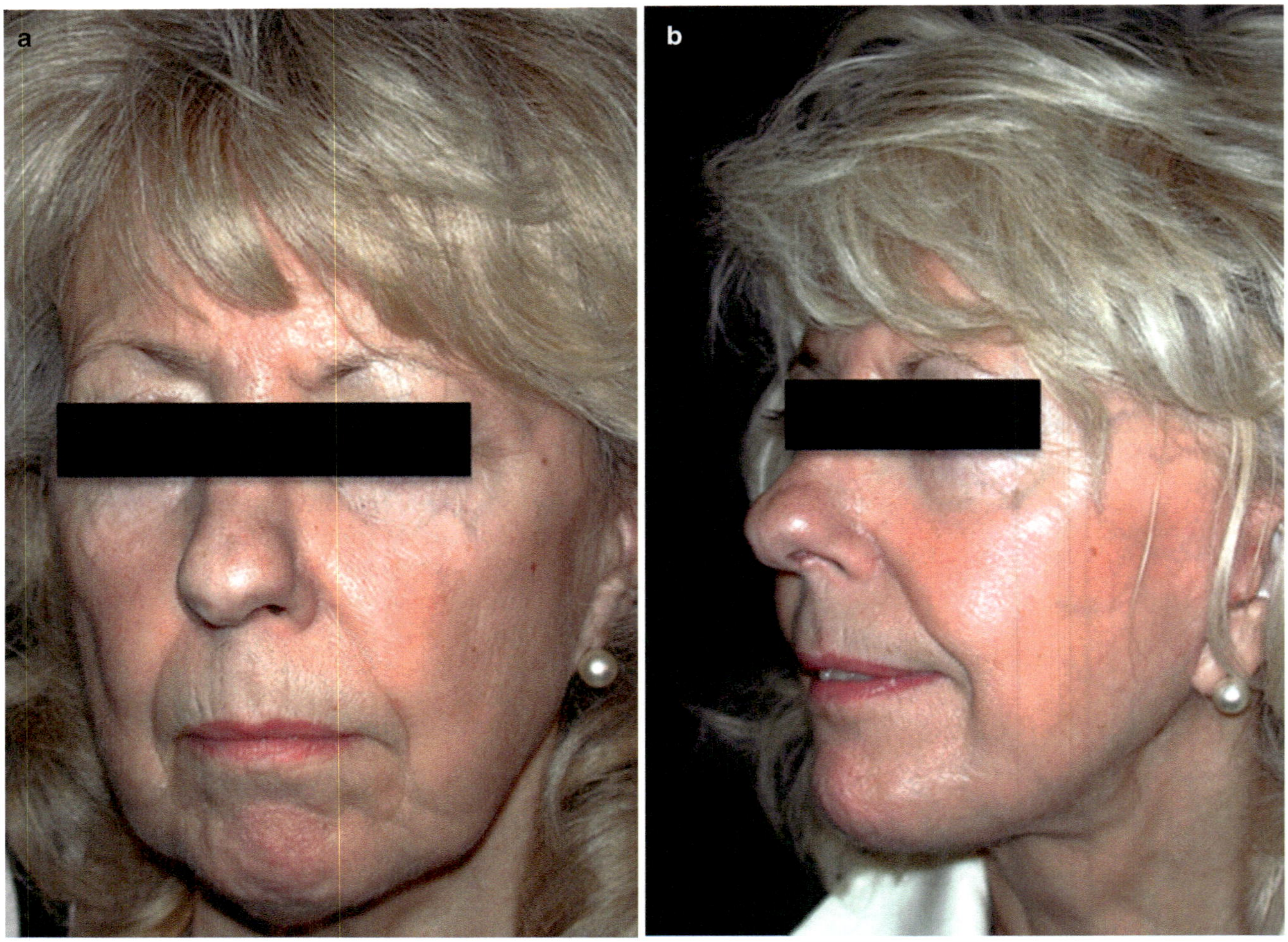




**Fig. 37.24** (**a**) Pre-operative profile view showing excess loose skin, jowling, submental fat and deep nasolabial fold. (**b**) Post-operative profile view after facelift and platysma plication. Excessive skin had been resected, jowls had been corrected and there was improved cervicomental definition

### 37.6.2 Skin Ischaemia and Necrosis

Ischaemic changes and flap necrosis can occur due to circulatory disturbances. This can happen when the flap is too thin or had underwent extensive undermining and exuberant cautery, closed under excessive tension or compromised by excessively tight bandage compression. The incidence ranges between 1.1 and 3% [24]. Venous congestion or arterial obstruction can result in skin ischaemia and necrosis. Large unevacuated haematoma separates the flap off the underlying bed during which perfusion is only by the vessels supplying the flap. This causes the areas furthest away from the perfusing vessels to be at risk of ischaemia.

Necrosis of the skin is more common in the postauricular than the preauricular region.

Application of nitroglycerin paste may help to encourage vasodilation when done in the early stages [25]. Conservative treatment to allow healing via secondary intention followed by laser, excision of the scar with repair via rotation flaps can be carried out at a later stage.

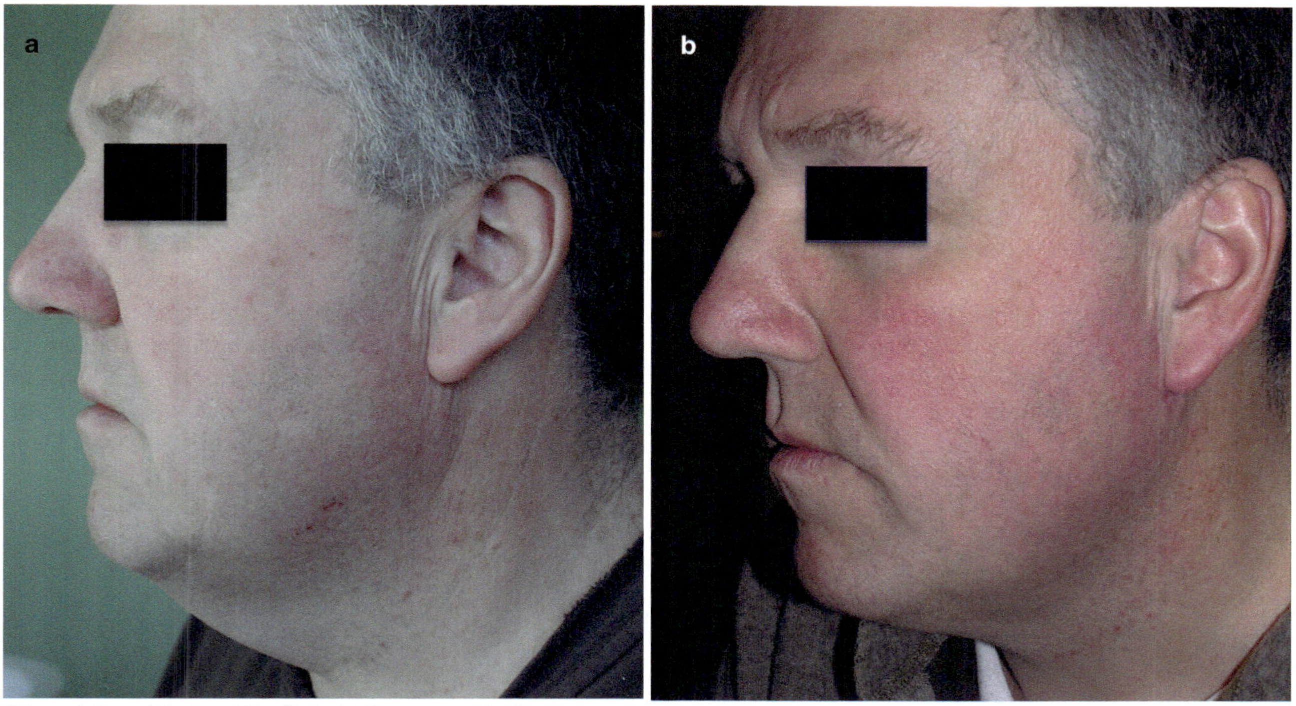




**Fig. 37.25** (a) Pre-operative profile view showing excess skin, slight jowling, submental fat and severe loss of neck definition. (**b**) Post-operative profile view after facelift and platysma plication

### 37.6.3 Obvious Scarring

Scarring can occur when the wounds are closed under excessive tension or if the incisions are placed at an inappropriate position due to poor design. Skin slough and necrosis of the flap can lead to severe scarring. Patients who are more prone to hypertrophic scarring or keloids should be warned. Wound tension can develop and cause scarring if there is excessive removal of skin or if undermining of the flap is inadequate.

Treatment of scarring includes conservative treatment with antibiotic ointment such as Tetracycline cream 3% or Bactroban cream. This is followed by steroid injections such as triamcinolone acetate, application of silicone sheet or gel dressing. As the scar improves and stabilizes, it can be lasered, excised and revised.

### 37.6.4 Sensory Disturbances

Sensory disturbances occur invariably due to the dissection and separation of the facial planes during the facelift procedure, but this usually occurs temporarily and resolves in 1 year.

The most common sensory disturbance occurs to the great auricular nerve. The greater auricular nerve crosses the sternocleidomastoid muscle at approximately 6.5 cm inferior to the external auditory meatus and travels superiorly to supply the postauricular region.

Injury to this nerve can be temporary or permanent due to dissection over the postauricular, mastoid region and to a lesser extent in the cervical region. This results in numbness of the ear lobe and postauricular area.

Other forms of numbness can be found in preauricular region.

### 37.6.5 Motor Nerve Disturbances

Keeping away from the planes that the facial nerve travels in is the safest method to avoid motor nerve problems. The facial nerve branches course through the parotid gland and exits the parotid gland to travel deep to the SMAS layer before innervating the muscles of facial expression. Care should be taken when dissecting beyond the parotid or when dissecting deep into the SMAS layer.

Facial nerve injury ranges from 0.4 to 2.6% [21]. The most common motor nerve damage is the marginal mandibular nerve followed by the temporal nerve and then the buccal branch. Neuropraxia from exuberant retraction, cautery heat and compression can result in temporary or permanent loss of the motor function. The marginal mandibular branch courses in the superficial layer of the deep cervical fascia, deep into the platysmal layer, and may be damaged when dissecting in this region. The temporal branch of the facial nerve courses just deep to the superficial temporal fascia and travels 0.5 cm anterior to the tragus and then obliquely to 1.5 cm above the lateral edge of the eyebrows.

### 37.6.6 Ear Lobe Irregularities

"Pixie or elf-like" ear is a stigma of facelift. The ear lobe should be repositioned in a tensionless fashion, and the ear lobe should be placed 15° posterior to the vertical axis of the pinna [6]. Over resection of the flap at the base of the auricle as well as failure to place subcutaneous stay sutures on the facial flap at the ear base can result in the ear being pulled inferiorly.

Pixie ears can be revised by releasing the base of the auricle and creating a new ear lobe.

## 37.7 Conclusion

The facelift remains the single most powerful method in facial rejuvenation for the moderate to advanced ageing face. It has developed from small elliptical incisions and closure to full facelift with simultaneous neck lift. A variety of techniques have been described contributing to its evolution including SMAS layer management, standard facelifts, composite facelifts, platysmal plication and smaller flaps such as the MACS lift and S-lifts. The standard face and simultaneous neck lift can treat most of the problems of the mid and lower face as well as the neck. An intimate understanding of the anatomy of the face, appropriate choice of the facelift design and meticulous execution are paramount in giving the patient an ideal outcome while avoiding the possible complications.

**Disclosure** Authors have no financial conflicts to disclose.

## 37.8 Case Scenarios

### Case Scenario 1 (Fig. 37.26)

A 67-year-old Caucasian lady presented with unhappy aesthetics of her face. She had had a considerable amount of sun exposure over the years. Her medical history was unremarkable.

Clinical features:

On examination she had multiple minor and major wrinkles on her face. On examination of the mid face, she showed descending SOOF and malar fat pads. She had prominent folding of the nasolabial fold and loss of mandibular border definition. Her neck was a good shape for her age (Fig. 37.26a, b).

Treatment:

She underwent a standard facelift without a neck lift and simultaneous autologous fat augmentation malar, chin and perioral areas.

Post-operative findings:

The post-operative profile shows aesthetically pleasing contour with an unoperated look (Fig. 37.26c, d). A majority of ageing changes have been removed. She ideally should undergo perioral laser resurfacing to improve the skin quality.

### Case Scenario 2 (Fig. 37.27)

A 73-old lady presented with ageing changes and was unhappy with the mid and lower face. She was concerned about the aesthetics of her neck (Fig. 37.27a, b).

She is an insulin-dependent diabetic and takes medication for hypertension.

Clinical features:

On examination, the mid face showed malar fat descent with prominent nasolabial fold. She had marked marionette lines, pre-jowl sulcus and prominent jowls. Examination of the lower face showed platysmal bands and loss of mandibular neck definition with submental fat projection.

Treatment:

She underwent a standard face and neck lift with platysmal and SMAS plication.

Post-operative findings:

Three month post-operative photograph shows correction for the ageing changes and a pleasing facial and neck profile (Fig. 37.27c, d).

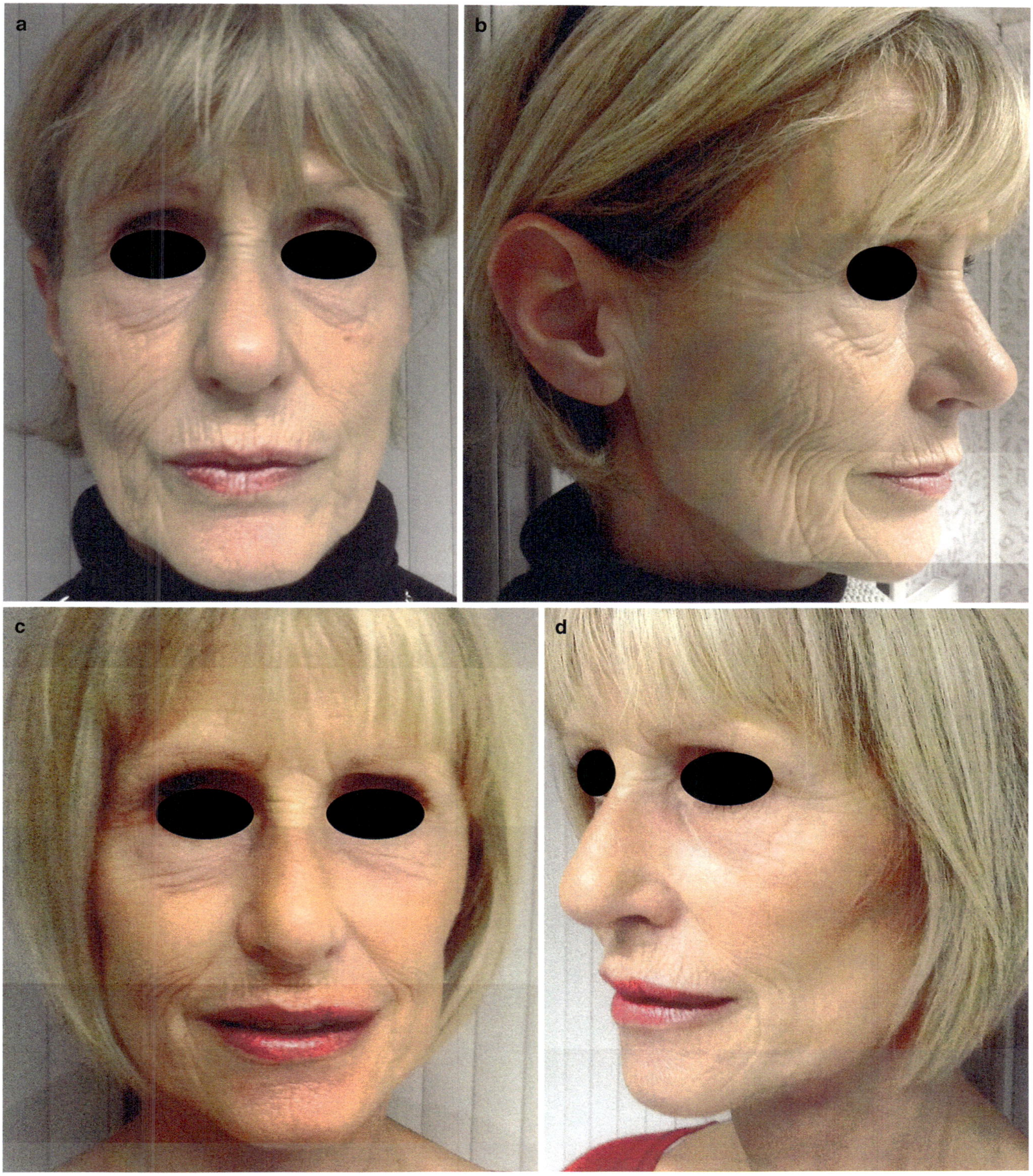




**Fig. 37.26** Standard face and neck lift with platysmal and SMAS plication. (**a**, **b**) Pre-operative appearance demonstrating wrinkles in frontal and profile view. (**c**, **d**) Post-operative appearance demonstrating wrinkles in frontal and profile view

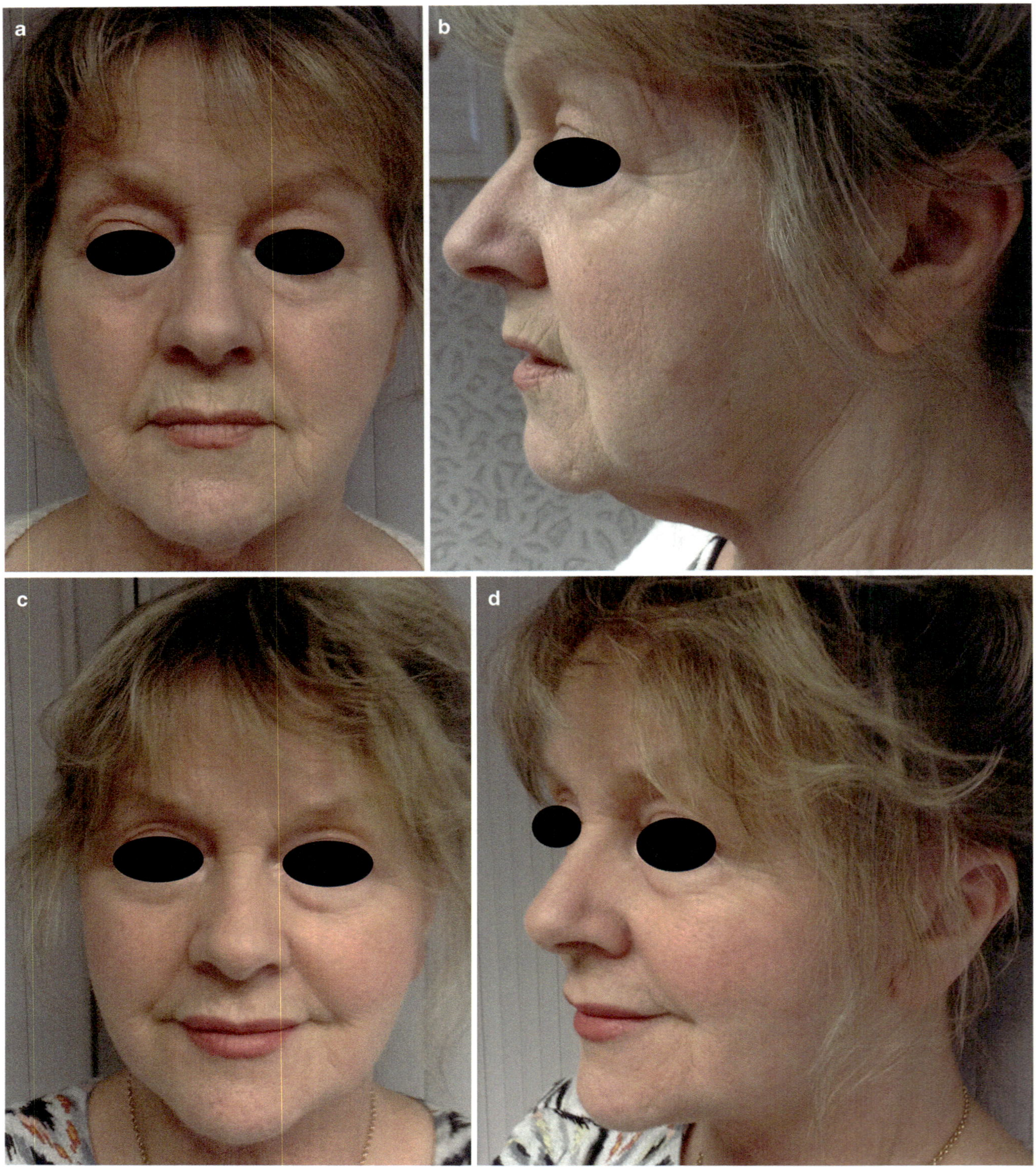




**Fig. 37.27** Standard face and neck lift with platysmal and SMAS plication. (**a**, **b**) Pre-operative appearance demonstrating wrinkles in frontal and profile view. (**c**, **d**) Post-operative appearance demonstrating wrinkles in frontal and profile view

## References


1. Ilankovan V. Anatomy of the aging face. Br J Oral Maxillofac Surg. 2014;52:195–202.
2. Hollander E. Die kosmetische chirurgie. In: Joseph M, editor. Handbuch der Kosmetik. Leipzig: Von Veit; 1912. p. 688.
3. Mangat DS, Frankel JK. The history of rhytidectomy. Facial Plast Surg. 2017;33(3):247–9. Epub 2017 Jun 1.
4. Tonnard PL, Verpaele AM. The MACS-lift short-scar rhytidectomy. Quality Medical Publishing; 2004. p. 4.
5. Mitz V, Peyronie M. The superficial musculoaponeurotic system (SMAS) in the parotid and cheek area. Plast Reconstr Surg. 1976;58(1):80–6.
6. Ilankovan V. Recent advances in face lift to achieve facial balance. J Maxillofac Oral Surg. 2017;16(1):3–12.
7. Webster RC, Smith RC, Papsidero MJ, Karolow WW, Smith KF. Comparison of SMAS plication with SMAS imbrication in face lifting. Laryngoscope. 1982;92(8):901–12.
8. Lemmon ML, Hamra ST. Skoog rhytidectomy: a five year experience with 577 patients. Plast Reconst Surg. 1980;65:283–97.
9. Baker DC. Lateral SMASectomy. Plast Reconstr Surg. 1997;100:509–13.
10. Hamra ST. Approaches to rejuvenation of the upper face. Aesthet Surg J. 2000;20(1):47–52.
11. Hamra ST. The role of the septal rest in creating a youthful eyelid-cheek complex in facial rejuvenation. Plast Reconstr Surg. 2004;113(7):2124–41.
12. Antell DE, Orseck MJ. A comparison of face lift techniques in eight consecutive sets of identical twins. Plast Reconstr Surg. 2007;120:1667–73.
13. Fulton JE, et al. The S-Lift facelift featuring the U-Suture and O-Suture combined with skin resurfacing. Dermatol Surg. 2001;27(1):18–22.
14. Tonnard P, et al. Minimal access cranial suspension lift: a modified S-Lift. Plas Reconstr Surg. 2002;109(6):2075–86.
15. Mendelson BC. Aesthetic plastic surgery. Saunders Elsevier; 2009. Chapter 6, pp. 53–71.
16. Warren RJ, et al. Face lift. Plast Reconstr Surg. 2011;128:747e–64e.
17. Stuzin JM, Baker TJ, Gordon HL, Baker TM. Extended SMAS dissection as an approach to midface rejuvenation. Clin Plast Surg. 1995;22(2):295–311.
18. Furnas DW. The retaining ligaments of the cheek. Plast Reconstr Surg. 1989;83:11–6.
19. Alghoul M, Codner MA. Retaining ligaments of the face: review of anatomy and clinical applications. Aesth Surg J. 2013;33(6):769–82.
20. Sebasan T, Ilankovan V. Plication of the platysma. Br J Oral Maxillofac Surg. 2006;44(4):325.
21. Bloom JD, et al. Face-lift complications. Facial Plast Surg. 2012;28:260–72.
22. Griffin JE, Jo C. Complications after superficial plane cervicofacial rhytidectomy: a retrospective analysis of 178 consecutive facelifts and review of the literature. J Oral Maxillofac Surg. 2007;65(11):2227–34.
23. Zoumalan R, Rizk SS. Hematoma rates I drainless deep-plane facelift surgery with and without the use of fibrin-glue. Arch Facial Plast Surg. 2008;10:103–7.
24. Baker DC. Complications of cervicofacial rhytidectomy. Clin Plast Surg. 1983;10:543–62.
25. Niamtu J. Cosmetic facial surgery: Elsevier Mosby; 2011. p. 354.

# Rhinoplasty

# 38

Nasir A. Nasser

## 38.1 Introduction

The nose occupies the centre of the face and receives enormous attention as a key aesthetic element. It is also an important organ contributing to vital functions of breathing and olfaction. A nose with ideal proportions creates a harmonious balance of aesthetic and psychological wellness. Whilst a rhinoplasty can significantly improve the quality of life of patients, there may be associated complications and undesirable outcomes. It is imperative that the surgeon desiring to practise the art and science of rhinoplasty should be familiar with the essential basics before embarking on this journey.

The aim of this chapter is to provide a clinical overview of the spectrum of rhinoplasty in an easily comprehensible manner. The primary section is focussed on the key elements of anatomy, diagnosis and documentation prior to any surgical procedure on the nose. Basic operative techniques including approaches, septoplasty, osteotomies and grafts are described in the next section. The management of most common nasal deformities is covered in the last section.

## 38.2 Surgical Anatomy of the Nose

The nose is a complex anatomic unit composed of skin, subcutaneous tissue and fibro-fatty tissue draped over a complex osteocartilaginous framework [1]. Understanding its overall morphology along with other characteristics helps in accurate diagnosis and management of various deformities. Based on the framework, the nose can be divided into external nose and internal nose. The important landmarks (Figs. 38.1A, B and 38.2) related to nasal anatomy are highlighted in Box 38.1.

### 38.2.1 External Nose

A. **Skin and underlying tissues**: The features of nasal skin including color, consistency and thickness can vary between patients and are important determinants of outcome of rhinoplasty. Skin thickness varies in different parts of the nose and at different stages of life. The average skin thickness is the greatest at the radix (measuring 1.25 mm) and the least at the Rhinion (0.6 mm) [2]. The supratip area has abundant sebaceous glands especially in adolescent males. Skin thickness is reduced in the columella and mid-alar area and increased in the alar base area. Both the thickness of the skin and the presence of sebaceous glands in the caudal half of the nose make it difficult to achieve an ideal result in a predictable manner.

   Beneath the skin and above the underlying osseocartilaginous framework are the layers of the superficial musculoaponeurotic system (SMAS), fibromuscular layer, deep fatty layer, and periosteum/perichondrium [3]. The SMAS of the nose is the continuation of the sheath that extends across the entire upper half of the face with adipose tissues, vertical fibres and septi, extending to the skin. Under the SMAS is a layer of thin fibrofatty tissue that divides the superficial and deep muscles of the nose [4]. The deep fatty layer separates the fibromuscular layer from the underlying nasal framework. Major blood vessels, lymphatics and nerves run within it. Deep to this layer is the periosteum of the nasal bones and the perichondrium of the cartilaginous frame. The avascular plane of dissection is in the supra perichondrial plane just below the fibrofatty SMAS layer.

**Electronic Supplementary Material** The online version of this chapter (https://doi.org/10.1007/978-981-15-1346-6_38) contains supplementary material, which is available to authorized users.

N. A. Nasser (✉)
Barts & London NHS Trust, Whipps Cross University Hospital, London, UK


K. Bonanthaya et al. (eds.), *Oral and Maxillofacial Surgery for the Clinician*, https://doi.org/10.1007/978-981-15-1346-6_38

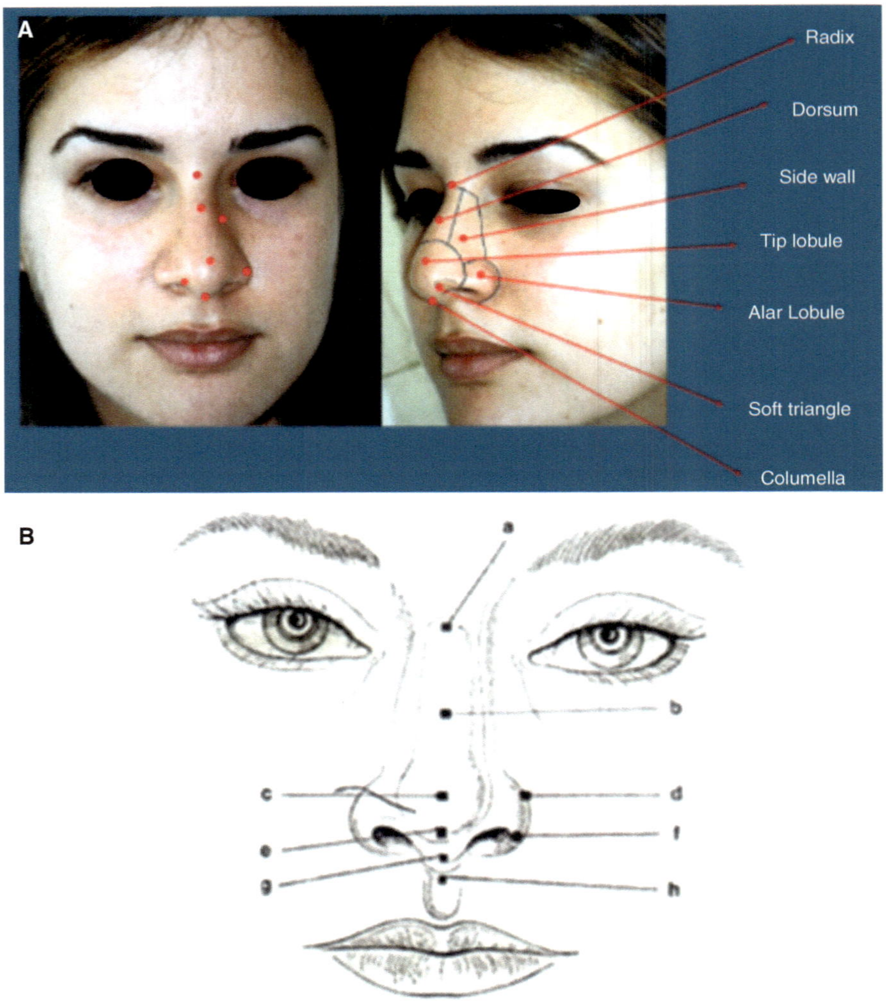




**Fig. 38.1** Nasal anatomy landmarks—frontal view. (**A**) Clinical picture, (**B**) Line diagram: (**a**) Radix, (**b**) Dorsum, (**c**) Tip lobule, (**d**) Alar lobule, (**e**) Tip, (**f**) Alar base, (**g**) Columella, (**h**) Philtrum

B. **External Vault**

The nose is divided topographically into thirds as shown in Figs. 38.3 and 38.4.

*Upper third:* The nasal bones constitute the upper one third. This part of the nose is pyramidal in shape, the narrowest portion being at the intercanthal line. Nasal bones vary in length and become thinner as they extend caudally toward the Rhinion. The nasal bones are attached to the frontal bone above at the radix which forms the frontonasal angle. They articulate with the ascending process of the maxilla. Caudally, the nasal bones overlap the upper lateral cartilages [Keystone area] [5].

*Middle third:* This contains the paired upper lateral cartilages (ULCs) and is referred to as the cartilaginous vault. The ULCs are fixed above to the under-surface of the nasal bones and fused with the septum, and they separate from the septum as they extend inferiorly. An important surface landmark in this region is the external lateral triangle; bounded above by the upper lateral cartilages, laterally by the frontal process of the maxilla, and caudally the cephalic border of the lower lateral cartilage. The angle between the caudal border of the upper lateral cartilage and the septum is usually 10–15° and constitutes the internal nasal valve (Fig. 38.5a, b).

*Lower Third:* The lower third or lobule of the nose is further subdivided into the tip, supra tip and infra tip regions. These specific areas of the lobule are formed by variations in the shape, size, and angles of the lower lateral cartilages (LLCs). The form of the lobule is defined by the tip or apex of the nose. The area defining the overlap of the LLC and the caudal aspect of the ULC is called the "scroll" area and has a fibrous attachment. The size of the scroll area along with the slope of the lateral crus contributes to the bulbosity of the lobule.

The lower lateral cartilages have four essential components: the medial crus, intermediate crus, dome and the lateral crus (Fig. 38.6a, b, c): The cephalic edge of the domal segment of the intermediate crus is responsible for the aesthetic point known as the pronasale. The supra tip is immediately cephalic to the pronasale. The infra tip is located between the pronasale and the apex of the nostrils. The infra tip region should have a gentle curve that

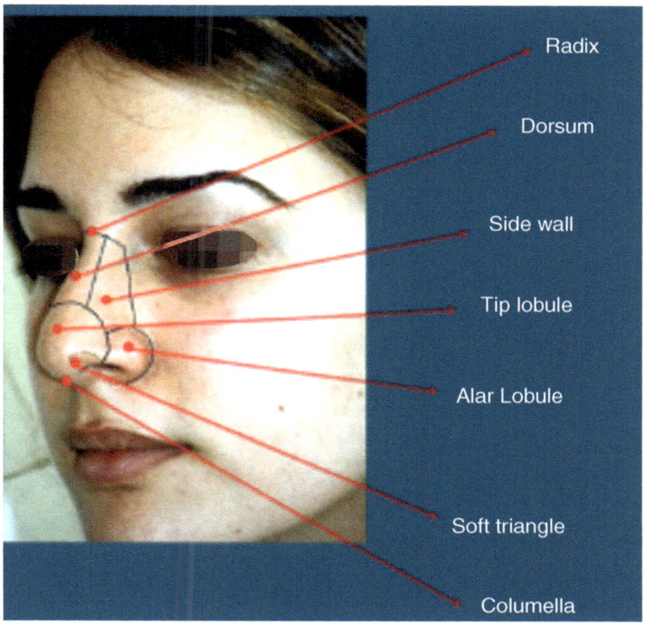




**Fig. 38.2** Nasal anatomy landmarks—lateral view

**Box 38.1 Rhinoplasty landmarks**

| Landmark | Definition |
|---|---|
| 1. Nasion | Depression at the junction of the nose with the forehead<br>Deepest point at the root of the nose |
| 2. Radix | Area centred around the nasion. |
| 3. Nasal pyramid | Part of the nasal frame made up of the bilateral nasal bone and frontal process of the maxilla |
| 4. Keystone area | Junction of the perpendicular plate of the ethmoid with the septal cartilage at the dorsum of the nose |
| 5. Rhinion | The point located at the osseocartilaginous junction over the dorsum of the nose |
| 6. Nasal tip lobule | Caudal part of the nose bounded posteriorly by the anterior nostril edge, superiorly by the supra tip area and laterally by the alar grooves |
| 7. Nasal tip | The most anterior point of the lobule |
| 8. Anatomic dome | Most anterior projected portion of the lower lateral cartilages between the medial and lateral crus |
| 9. Tip defining points (TDP) | Summit of the domes. Most projecting area on each side of the tip that produces external light reflection |
| 10. Supratip area | Area just cephalad to the nasal tip at the caudal portion of the nasal dorsum |
| 11. Infratip lobule | Portion of the tip between the tip defining points and apex of nostrils |
| 12. Tip projection | Distance from the most projected portion of the tip to the most posterior point of the nasal–cheek junction |
| 13. Alar groove | Oblique skin depression between the tip and the ala |
| 14. Supra-alar crease | Groove immediately cephalad to the alar crease |
| 15. Sub-nasale | Junction of columella with the lip |

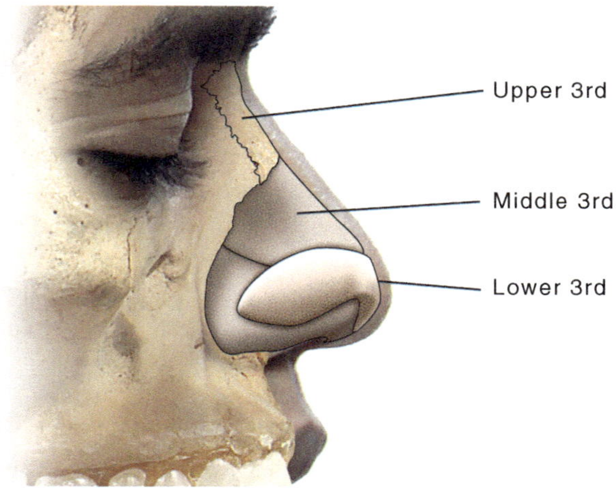




**Fig. 38.3** External vault—lateral view

slightly projects inferiorly to the alar margins. The medial-lateral crura complex forms a tripod that is an essential concept to understand for correction of tip deformities. The lateral crura form the two cephalic lateral legs while the medial along with the intermediate crus form the caudal leg of the tripod (Fig. 38.7a, b, c).

*Medial crus:* The medial crus has two distinct segments: the footplate and the columella. The footplate varies in size and in the degree of lateral angulation, which governs the width of the columellar base.

*Intermediate crus:* It extends between the medial crus and the lateral crus. The length and width of the intermediate crus control the configuration of the infra-tip lobule.

*Dome:* The domal segment is the narrowest and thinnest portion of the lower lateral cartilage, yet is the most important in relation to the tip shape. In an ideal nose, the cephalic edges of the paradomal segments are in close approximation and the caudal portions are divergent. Whenever the cephalic margins diverge, they result in widening of the nasal tip. A wide domal angle with increased interdomal width results in a boxy tip.

*Lateral Crus:* It constitutes the larger component of the nasal lobule. It is narrow anteriorly, widens in the mid-portion and narrows again laterally. The anterior portion of this cartilage can curve with different angulations and controls the convexity of the ala. The lateral crus also provides support to the anterior half of the alar rim. This cartilage is usually oriented at a 45° angle to the vertical facial plane. Narrowing of the angle between the dorsum and the long axis of the lower lateral cartilage

**Fig. 38.4** External vault—lateral view. Line diagram showing the three divisions

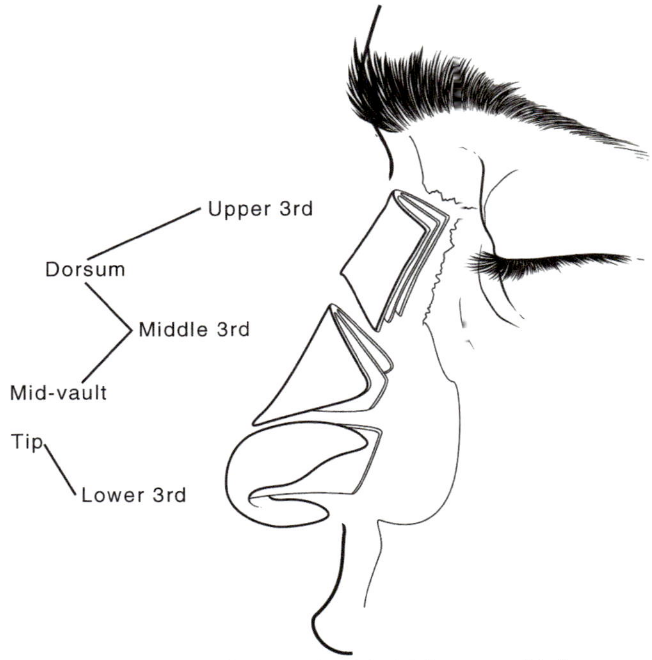


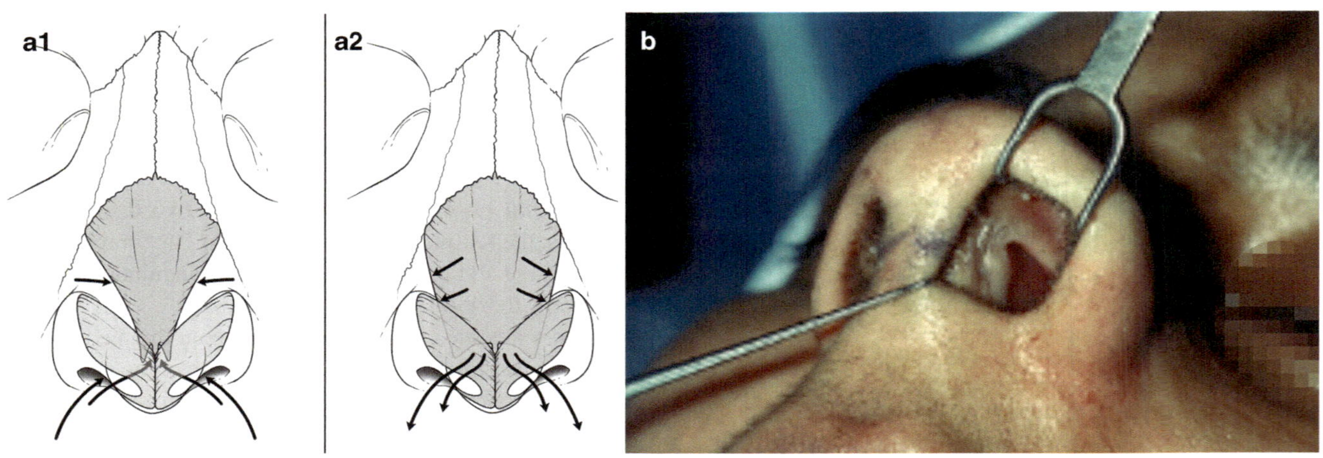


**Fig. 38.5** Nasal valve; (**a1**, **a2**) line diagram, (**b**) clinical photograph

may cause dysmorphology of the tip called cephalic malposition or 'parenthesis deformity'.

Several fibrous attachments exist joining the cartilages to each other, namely, lower lateral cartilages to the upper lateral cartilage, from one lateral crus to the opposite in the supratip area (the Pitanguy ligament), dense fibrous bands between the caudal septum & the medial crura and between the medial crura themselves [6].

**Muscles** (Fig. 38.8): The muscles of the nose are divided by their functions into four categories; elevators, depressors, compressors, and dilators. The procerus, levator labii superioris alaeque nasi, elevates and shortens the nose. These muscles are important because they assist in opening the nasal valves. The depressor muscles consist of the nasalis and depressor septi. On contraction, this group of muscles adversely affect the tip rotation by displacing it inferiorly and elevating the lip superiorly [5]. The transverse nasalis muscle forms the compressor, while the dilator naris has the opposite function.

**Blood Supply and innervation**: Both external and internal carotid arteries contribute to the vasculature of the external nose (Fig. 38.9). The major blood supply is from

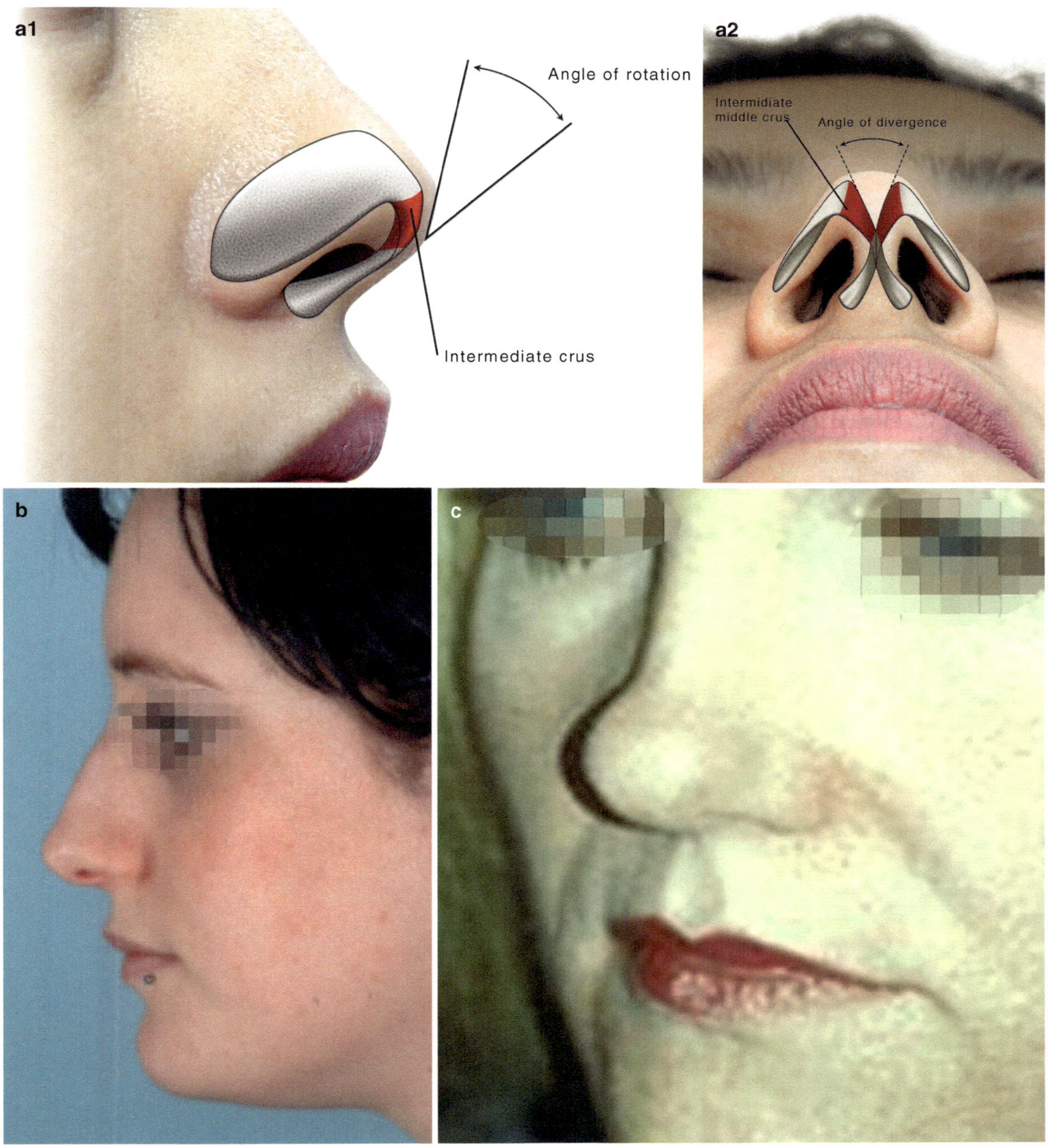




**Fig. 38.6** Lower lateral cartilage (**a1**, **a2**) Diagrammatic representation and (**b**, **c**) clinical pictures

three vessels: the dorsal nasal artery—a terminal branch of the ophthalmic artery, the angular and superior labial arteries from the facial artery. The lateral nasal artery (branch of the angular artery) forms a plexus with the dorsal nasal artery, branches of infra-trochlear artery, and the external branches of the anterior ethmoidal artery. A small contribution is also received from the lateral branches of the infra-orbital artery.

Sensory innervation to the nose is provided by the maxillary and ophthalmic branches of the fifth cranial nerve [7].

### 38.2.2 Internal Anatomy

The internal nose is divided by the "midline" nasal septum. Anteriorly, the septum forms the medial boundary of the nasal vestibule whose lateral wall is formed by the lower lateral cartilages and their attachment to the pyriform rim.

The deeper part of the nasal cavity is bounded laterally by the medial wall of the antrum, medially by the osseocartilaginous septum, superiorly by the ethmoid and the sphenoid bones and inferiorly by the palatal process of the maxilla and

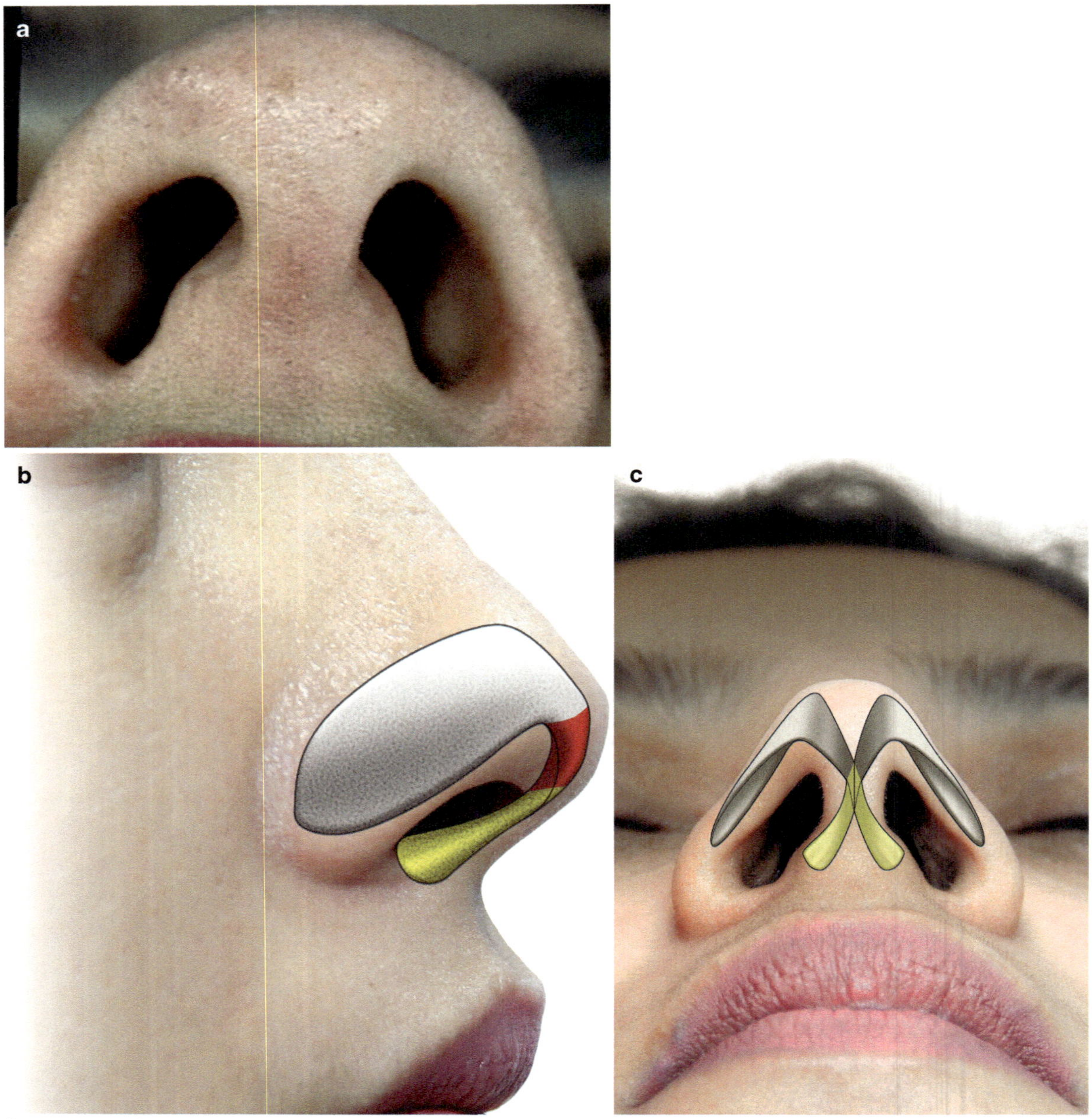




Fig. 38.7 Nasal tripod; (**a**) clinical photograph, (**b**) line diagram showing medial crus (yellow), intermediate crus (red) and lateral crus (grey) (**c**) line diagram showing basal view

the palatine bones. There are thin, curved, bony prominences in the lateral wall called the inferior, middle, and superior concha. The cephalic portion of the lateral nasal wall is bound with the ethmoid cells, interposed between the lateral wall of the nasal cavity and the medial wall of the orbit.

### 38.2.3 Nasal Septum

The septum is partly cartilaginous and partly bony. The ethmoid perpendicular plate forms the upper bony septum and is continuous with the frontal bone and the cribriform plate. The lower bony septum is composed of the vomer and nasal crest of the maxilla (Fig. 38.10a, b).

The cartilaginous septum is formed by the quadrangular cartilage that extends from Rhinion to the supratip area and supports the dorsum and the tip complex. Inferiorly, the cartilagenous septum is attached firmly to the anterior nasal spine and the maxillary crest. The junction between the dorsal and caudal portion of the cartilaginous septum is called the "anterior septal angle". There is tenuous attachment of the perichondrium and periosteum at the junction of the bony and cartilaginous septum. The membranous septum lies above the cephalic margins of the paired medial crura. It encases fibrous bands between two layers of soft tissue covering and the depressor septi muscle.

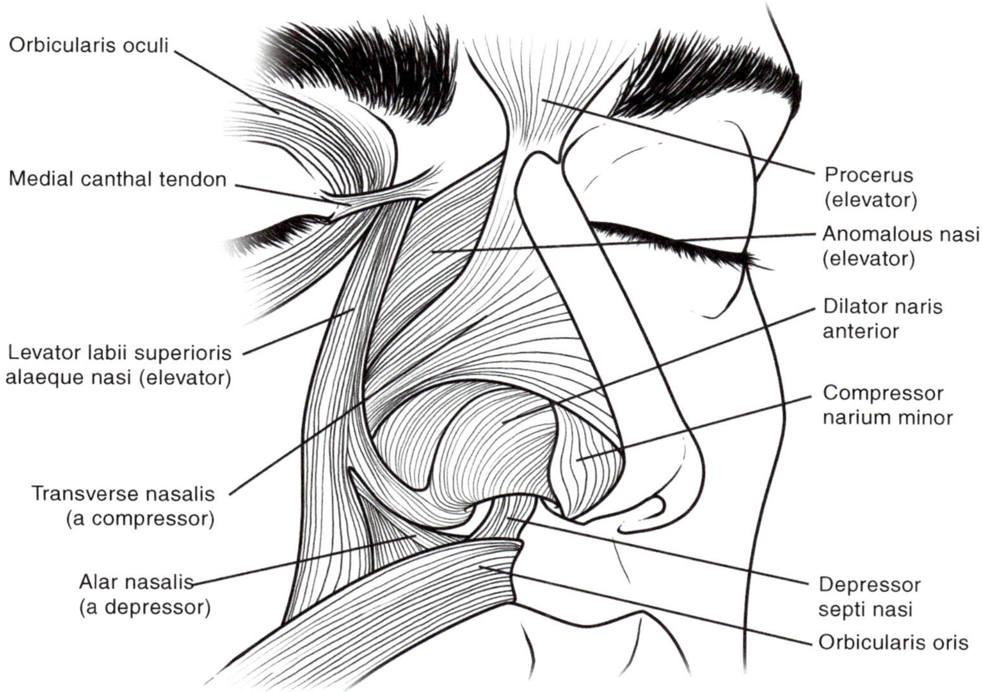




**Fig. 38.8** Muscles of the nose

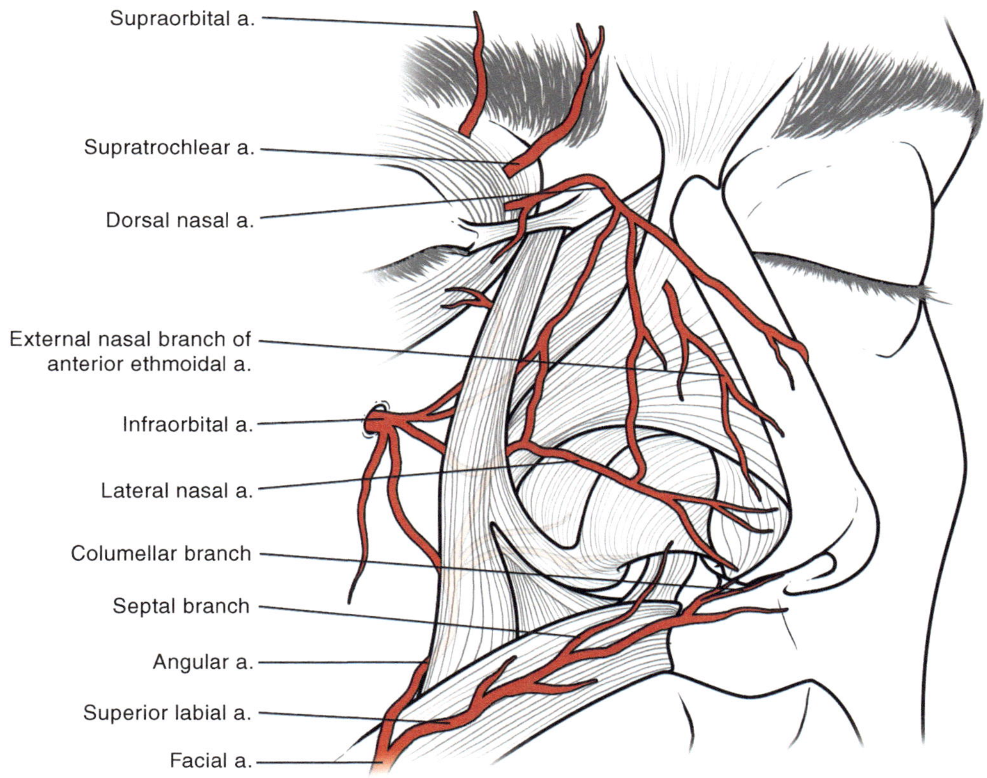




**Fig. 38.9** Vascularity of the nose

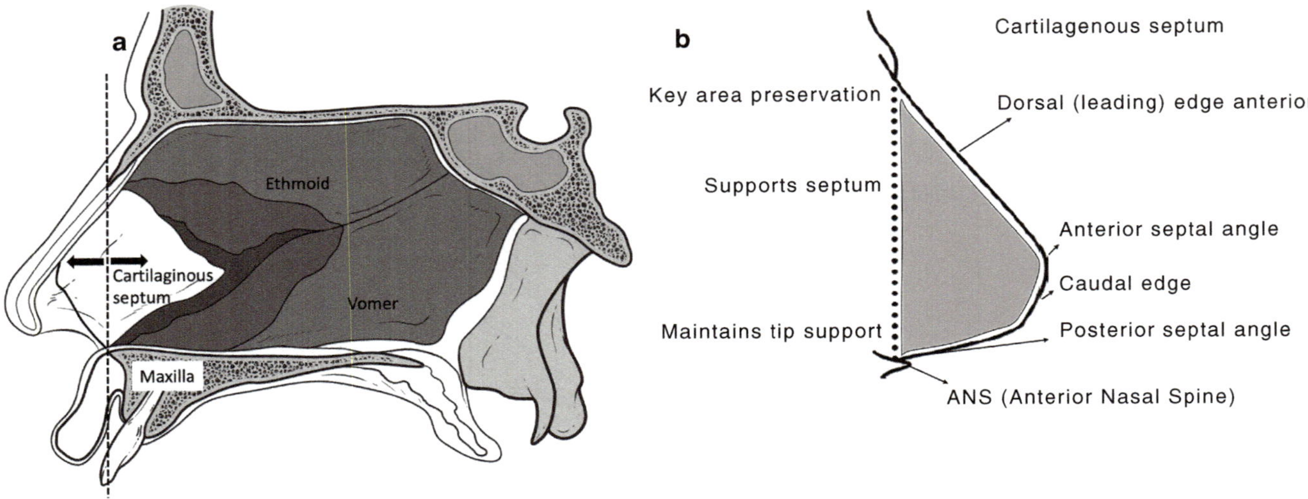




**Fig. 38.10** (**a**) Anatomy of nasal septum, (**b**) line diagram with landmarks

**Box 38.2 Clinical examination for Rhinoplasty**

| | Local | |
|---|---|---|
| **General/Systemic** | **Facial** | **Nose** |
| Airway/breathing<br>Mouth breathing | Intercanthal distance | Skin quality |
| Bleeding disorders | Inter-eyebrow distance | Nasal bone—width, length and symmetry |
| Hypertension | Frontal-bossing/glabellar projection | ULC (Upper Lateral Cartilage)—width and symmetry |
| Diabetes/ immunosuppression | Upper lip position | LLC (Lower Lateral Cartilage)<br>• Cephalic malposition<br>• Interdomal distance<br>• Asymmetry of light reflecting points<br>• Lobule position<br>• Nostril-columellar relation |
| Psychological assessment | Chin position | Alar base<br>• Vertical and horizontal position (in repose and smile)<br>• Inter alar distance (should be 2 mm wider than intercanthal distance)<br>• Insertion of the alar base |

### 38.2.4 Lateral Nasal Wall

The lateral aspect of the nasal cavity is composed of three anatomic structures: the inferior, middle, and superior turbinates. The inferior turbinate forms a boundary of the internal nasal valve, where its specially adapted erectile tissues regulate the air flow and facilitate heat and moisture exchange.

Branches of the anterior ethmoidal artery accompany the external nasal branch of the anterior ethmoid nerve, passing between the nasal bone and upper lateral cartilages, and supply the soft tissues of the dorsum and tip of the nose. The posterior ethmoidal branches supply the smaller area above the superior concha on the lateral wall and a corresponding area high on the septum [8]. The posterior part of the internal nose is supplied by branches of the sphenopalatine ganglion of the second division of the trigeminal nerve (the long sphenopalatine, the nasopalatine and part of the greater palatine nerves).

## 38.3 Clinical Examination

Clinical examination should be comprehensive and include the assessment of systemic diseases (Box 38.2) [9].

General examination would include ruling out any syndromic deformities [9]. Obtaining correct history of systemic disease and bleeding disorders are of paramount importance. The extensive vascular network in the nose, in the presence of a coagulation disorder, may predispose the patient to severe haemorrhage in the intra- or post-operative period.

Existing breathing difficulty or any allergy-related symptoms such as rhinorrhea, sneezing, watery eyes, itching and loss of sense of smell and taste are observed. Majority of successful rhinoplasties are reductive in nature; an undetected or uncorrected underlying airway compromise may cause further deterioration and convert an aesthetic concern to a functional predicament. If the presence of any sinus infections and headaches is not recorded preoperatively, the patient may attribute these conditions to rhinoplasty [10].

### 38.3.1 Examination of the Face

The face in the frontal view is divided into thirds and fifths for assessment of proportion and harmony of various structures (Fig. 38.11a, b, c). In the upper third, the intercanthal distance and interpupillary distance is important in assessing the nasal bones, dorsum and radix. For a proper facial balance, the malar bone, maxilla, mandible and the nasal bones should be in an optimum spatial relationship. The length of the upper lip, its position during rest and smile, upper incisor show and its proportion in relation to the rest of the face are also assessed. The nose and chin may have a paradoxical relationship whereby a patient may have an overprojected nose and at the same time an underprojected chin and vice versa.

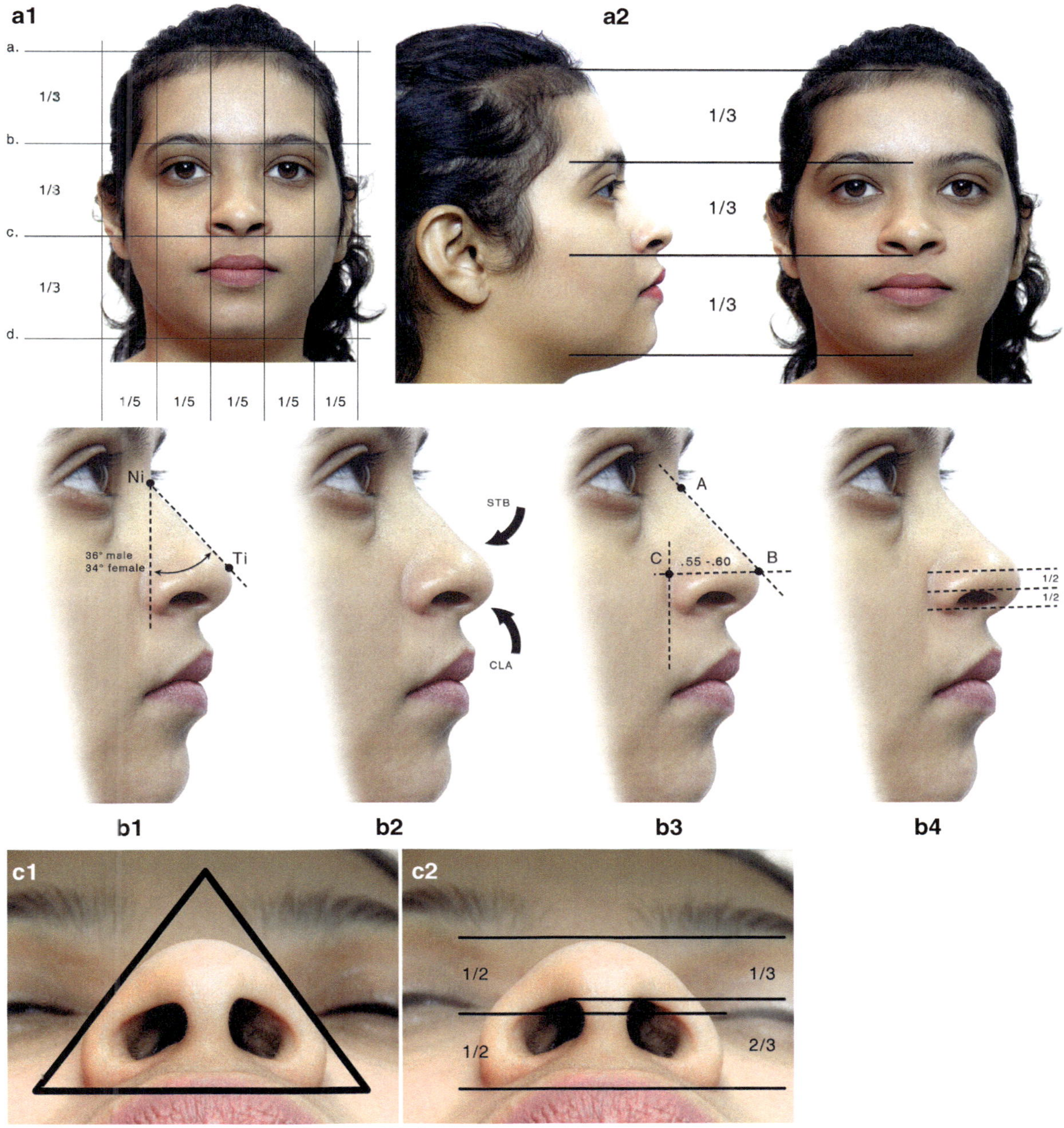




**Fig. 38.11** (**a**)–(**c**) Examination of face and nose; frontal, lateral, basal. (**b1**) Ni - Ideal nasion, Ti Ideal tip. (**b2**) STB - Supra Tip Break, CLA - Columella Labial Angle. (**b3**) Nasal Length is measured from nasal radix to nasal tip (A–B), Nasal projection (C–B) is length from Naso-labial junction to nasal tip. The ratio between AB and CB (Goode's Ratio) should be ideally 0.55 to 0.60

### 38.3.2 Examination of the Nose

Visual analysis of the nose along with careful palpation allows the surgeon to assess the morphology and thickness of the skin and soft tissue envelope.

Frontal, profile and basal views should be used to assess the various components of the nose discussed above, individually.

### 38.3.3 Photographic Assessment

Patient's photographs are an important component of preoperative analysis and planning of the procedure. In addition, pre- and post-operative photographs are crucial for outcome monitoring and are indispensable from a medicolegal point of view [11]. With the advent of 3D imaging, image fusion and photogrammetry, preoperative and postoperative features can be compared in all dimensions [12].

There are four important photographic views that are used for analysis of the nose, namely, frontal, basal, lateral (at rest and smiling) and oblique views (Fig. 38.12). Photographs are standardised in relation to the Frankfurt horizontal plane. All four views are evaluated for the assessment of the facial horizontal thirds and vertical fifths. The quality of skin (thickness and Fitzpatrick type) and facial symmetry are also studied using all the views. The basic focus lies in the study of the loco-regional anatomy and the inter-relationships of the structures. The pictures are evaluated to assess any discrepancies in size, deviations or dorsal hump that may be immediately evident and recordable.

- **Frontal view**

  The length, width and the tip characteristics are well observed on the frontal views. The width is individually assessed in the upper, middle and lower thirds of the nose. Frontal views also show a straight or a crooked nose. The presence of a dorsal hump or a saddle deformity is noted as these may provide an illusion of the nose being narrow or wide, respectively. The presence of a truly wide nose may also demonstrate features of pseudo/true hypertelorism.

  The dorsal aesthetic lines should be studied in detail. They follow the eyebrows across the radix and along the dorsum to end at the tip defining points on either side.

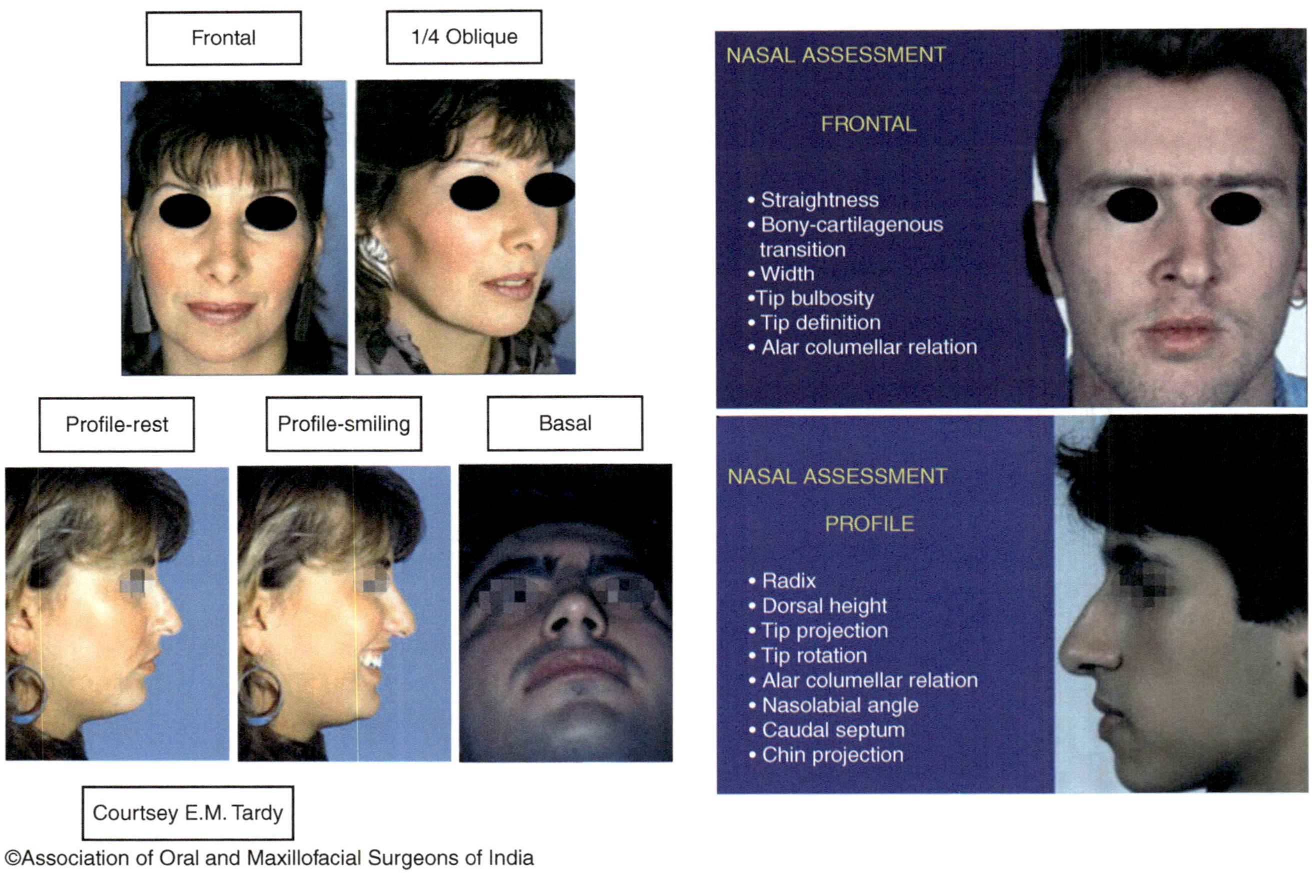


**Fig. 38.12** Photographic analysis

The lines should be almost parallel with a smooth divergence at the brow but without any visible or perceptible breaks.

The nasal tip is assessed for symmetry and definition. The tip is also assessed for features of boxy appearance, bulbosity or bifidity. The alar base, ala and columella are also evaluated. The formation of a gentle "gull in flight" form should be appreciated for the relationship of the ala and the infratip lobule. An exaggerated curve may be indicative of a retracted ala or a plunging lobule. The position and insertion of both ala and their symmetry and direction are also noted.

- **Basal view**
  Assessment should include the study of lobule, columella, ala and the alar base. Emphasis should be placed on the evaluation of the triangular shape of the nasal base, symmetry and the ratios, namely, the columella/lobule ratio and the lobule to ala ratios. The nasal base should present as an isosceles triangle with a rounded apex. The alar sidewalls should demonstrate a gentle flare. Poor triangular form or a trapezoidal form is indicative of a broad dome. Nostril symmetry and the angulations are studied next. The nostrils are angulated at 30–45° to the midline and are pear shaped. The caudal septum is assessed for straightness and its position in relation to the maxillary crest and anterior nasal spine. The alar base width, flare and insertions are also assessed in this view.

- **Profile view**
  Key points that need to be evaluated from the lateral view include (1) a dorsal profile that may demonstrate a saddle/hump and the supratip break, (2) evaluation of the chin and mentolabial sulcus, (3) projection and rotation of the nasal tip, (4) nasal length, (5) assessment of the radix and (6) columellar show with double break.

  The ratio of nasal projection is evaluated by the method of Goode. The ideal ratio between the line joining the tip defining point and alar-facial groove tangent, to the line dropped from the nasion to the alar facial groove should be between 0.55 and 0.60. Rotation of the nasal tip is approximately considered 90° in Caucasian males and between 90 and 95° in Caucasian females.

  The length of the nose is relative to the person's facial profile and general stature. It may be categorized as the central nose length from the nasion to the nasal tip and lateral length from the nasion to the alar rims. A short or long lateral length may reflect as retracted or hooded ala, respectively. The nose may also show a relative increase or decrease in length depending on the depth of the radix. A deep radix may make the nose look short while a shallow radix makes the nose appear long.

  The columella is also assessed for over- and undervisibility with the evaluation of a columellar double break that is formed by the junction of the medial and intermediate crus.

- **Oblique view assesses the volume of the tip lobule and Brow tip aesthetic line.**
  Assessment of the oblique view may not provide objective details. However, the nose is most viewed at this angle thus making it an important view to assess the aesthetic balance of the face and nose. Important features that need to be assessed in this view include soft tissue facets, lateral aspect of the nasal bones, nasal length, dorsal contour and tip projection.

### 38.3.4 Investigations

- Inspection with speculum will demonstrate any septal curvatures, angulations or spurs.
- *Computed tomography* is helpful if sinus pathology is suspected.
- *Endoscopy* of the middle meatus should be done to rule out clinical evidence of sinus disease.
- *Tests for functions of internal nasal and external nasal valves* should be done. Careful observation of the nasal valves while the patient is asked to inspire will provide a significant amount of information. A speculum or Q tip facilitates proper examination. Cottle's Maneuver helps in localizing obstruction due to nasal valve dysfunction.
- *Acoustic rhinometry* is a recently developed objective technique for assessment of geometry of the nasal cavity. The technique is based on the analysis of sound waves reflected from the nasal cavities. It measures cross-sectional areas and nasal volume.
- *Rhinomanometry* has also been widely accepted and used as an objective method to assess nasal patency. However, these tools may not necessarily show clinical correlation [13].

## 38.4 General Operative Techniques

### 38.4.1 Surgical Approaches for Rhinoplasty

Rhinoplastic approaches: (1) open approach or the open structure rhinoplasty approach and (2) closed or the endonasal approach.

Open approach involves an external cutaneous incision while the closed approach involves intranasal incisions only (Fig. 38.13a, b).

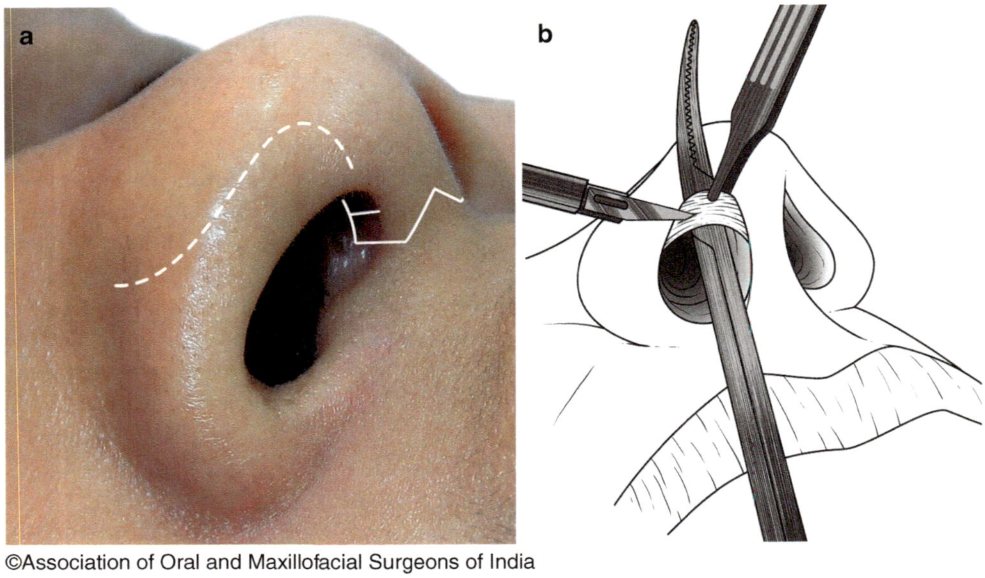


**Fig. 38.13** Open (**a**) Vs Closed (**b**) approach

Choice of incision is based on the clinical problem to be corrected and the exposure required. The ideal incision must enable adequate and easy access to the nasal architecture without compromising the nasal structures. The differences between the different types of incisions are highlighted in Table 38.1.

A. **Open structure rhinoplasty**

The open structure approach is employed when extensive reconstruction is required. There is more emphasis on the preservation and realignment of structures of the lower third of the nose and also achieving balance of the nasal "tripod".

The open approach involves the use of a marginal and mid-columellar incision (Fig. 38.14b)

- *Marginal incision*
- The incision is placed along the caudal margins of the LLC, starting at the caudal margin of the medial crus, running along the entire dome and extended laterally along the caudal margin of the lateral crus.
- *Columellar incision*
- This is a transverse mid-columellar incision extending across to connect the marginal incisions on either side. Numerous modifications of the columellar incision have evolved over a long period (Fig. 38.15a, b, c).
  - Rethi transcolumellar incision 1931 (across the apex of the nostril aperture)
  - Sercer "nasal decortication" approach—1957
  - Bardach columellar base incision extending into prolabium (reserved for cleft rhinoplasty)
  - Goodman modification mid columellar 'V' facing upwards 1952
  - Johnson & Toriumi inverted 'V' midcolumellar incision
  - Stair-step mid columellar incision (Bahman Guyuron)

The **indications** for the open structure approach are highlighted in Box 38.3.

B. **The endonasal approach** (Fig. 38.14a)

Nondelivery/Partial delivery and delivery approaches (Fig. 38.16a, b).

1. **Nondelivery approaches are employed when** minimal reduction of the lateral crus or mild cephalic rotation of the tip complex is indicated.

   The technique in turn may involve either the cartilage splitting approach or the retrograde eversion approach.

- The *cartilage splitting method* involves a trans-cartilaginous incision through the most cephalic portion of the lower lateral cartilage that needs to be resected. However, extreme care is taken to preserve at least 8 mm of sound LLC to prevent structural compromise.
- The *retrograde eversion method* is difficult for beginners and hence not favoured in current practise, and most surgeons today prefer to use the delivery method.

2. The technique for the **delivery method** encompasses two incisions: the first inter-cartilaginous incision and the subsequent marginal incision to mark the chondrocutaneous unit of the LLC. The nonvestibular side of the LLC is

**Table 38.1** Differences between the different types of incisions

| | | Closed/endonasal | |
|---|---|---|---|
| | Open/external | Nondelivery<br>Cartilage splitting<br>Retrograde eversion | Delivery |
| Incision | • Marginal<br>• External (columellar) | • Transcartilaginous (Cartilage splitting)<br>or<br>• Intercartilaginous<br>(Retrograde eversion) | • Marginal<br>• Intercartilaginous |
| Exposure | Extensive | More of LLC exposure<br>Less of tip exposure | Increased dome and interdomal visibility |
| Indications | Marked asymmetry<br>Secondary rhinoplasty<br>Need for structural grafting<br>Post traumatic nasal deformity<br>Nasal valve correction | Minimal tip correction<br>Access to dorsum and middle vault<br>Volume reduction of LLC<br>Septal surgery<br>Bony and cartilaginous hump removal | Allows more delicate tip work than the nondelivery approach septal surgery |
| Advantages | • Excellent visual control of entire nasal framework<br>• Enhanced surgical access<br>• Accurate structural grafting under direct vision<br>• Ideal for demonstration and teaching<br>• Predictable results | Less invasive<br>Less disruption of support mechanisms of nasal tip<br>May be used for septal cartilage harvesting | |
| Limitations | • External (transcolumellar) scar<br>• Destabilization of tip support<br>• Protracted edema<br>• Risk of columellar necrosis (poor operative technique)<br>• Sensory disturbances at the tip area | Steep learning curve<br>No binocular vision<br>Essential ENT experience<br>Limits assistant's view of exposure<br>Difficult to perform complex nasal tip surgery<br>Spreader-grafts are difficult/impossible | |

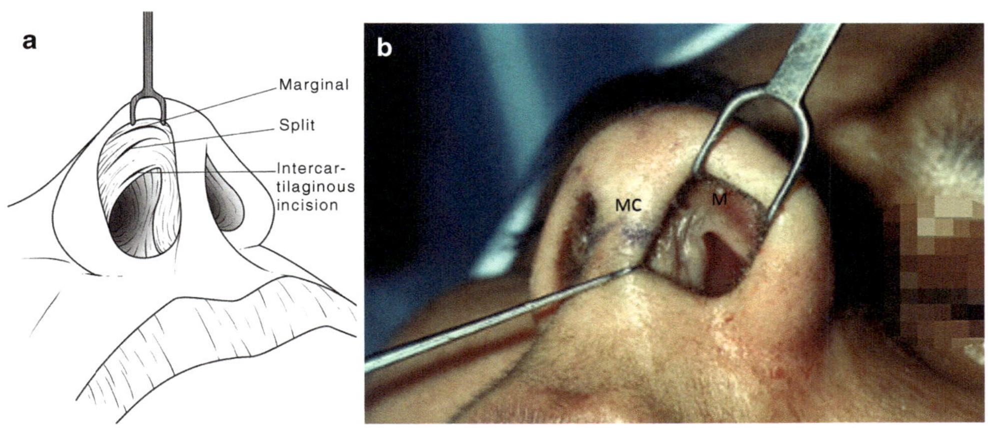


**Fig. 38.14** Incisions for rhinoplasty: (**a**) closed and (**b**) open approach (MC- mid columellar, M- Marginal)



then dissected off the overlying SSTE permitting the delivery of the LLC chondrocutaneous unit as a bipedicled flap. Improperly positioned intercartilaginous incision may predispose to scarring at the valve area.

**Incisions for the endonasal approach**

- Intercartilaginous (limen-vestibular) incision
- Intracartilaginous (trans-cartilaginous/cartilage splitting) incision
- Infracartilaginous (alar marginal) incision
- Septal transfixion incision
  - Hemi-transfixion
  - Bilateral transfixion—partial/full
- Pyriform rim incisions for access to the lateral nasal wall
- Lateral nasal vestibular incisions for access to the paranasal premaxillary area
- Endonasal transmucosal medial osteotomy facilitated high up in the nasal vault.

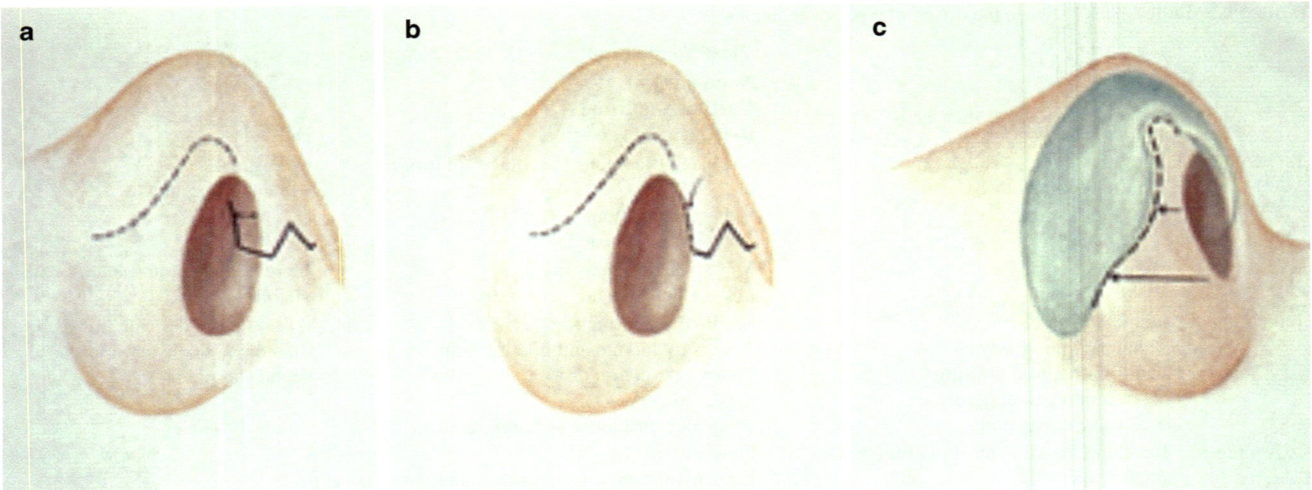


Courtesy Rollin Daniel



**Fig. 38.15** (**a**–**c**) Modifications of columellar incision

**Box 38.3 Indications for open Rhinoplasty**

- Secondary/revision rhinoplasty
- Post-traumatic nasal deformity
- Cleft nasal deformity
- Need for structural grafting
- Septal reconstruction
- Nasal valve surgery
- Dermoid cyst excision

**Indications for the endonasal approach**

- Symmetrical anatomy
- Good size nostrils
- Principal deformity at the nasal vault
- Ability to insert cartilage grafts

The endonasal approach is, however, unsuited for the novice surgeon and does depend on the surgeon's experience and prior training in Rhinoplasty for optimal outcomes.

## 38.4.2 Grafting in Rhinoplasty

Reduction rhinoplasty can weaken the underlying nasal tip framework with subsequent buckling and late structural deformity. Cartilage grafting during primary and revision procedures helps to prevent such a secondary deformity [14–17]. An open technique is preferred as it offers better visualization for placement of grafts. The grafts used in rhinoplasty can be summarised as follows (Fig. 38.17a, b) (Tables 38.2 and 38.3):

## 38.4.3 Septoplasty

### 38.4.3.1 Deformities of Nasal Septum

Deformities of the nasal septum may either be congenital or acquired. They are classified as shown in Box 38.4.

Septal deformities depend on alterations in the growth and direction of growth of the septal cartilage.

Deformities of the nasal septum may present clinically (Fig. 38.18a, b).

1. Dorsal excess may present as a tension nose
2. Dorsal deficiency causes concave or Saddle nose
3. Caudal excess causes increased columellar show
4. Caudal deficiency leads to columellar retraction
5. Lateral angulation of the septum is seen as a bent nose
6. Both lateral & AP curvatures give a twisted nose/ crooked nose
7. Septal perforations and collapse may lead to a variety of deformities

**Fig. 38.16** (**a**, **b**) Nondelivery vs. delivery method

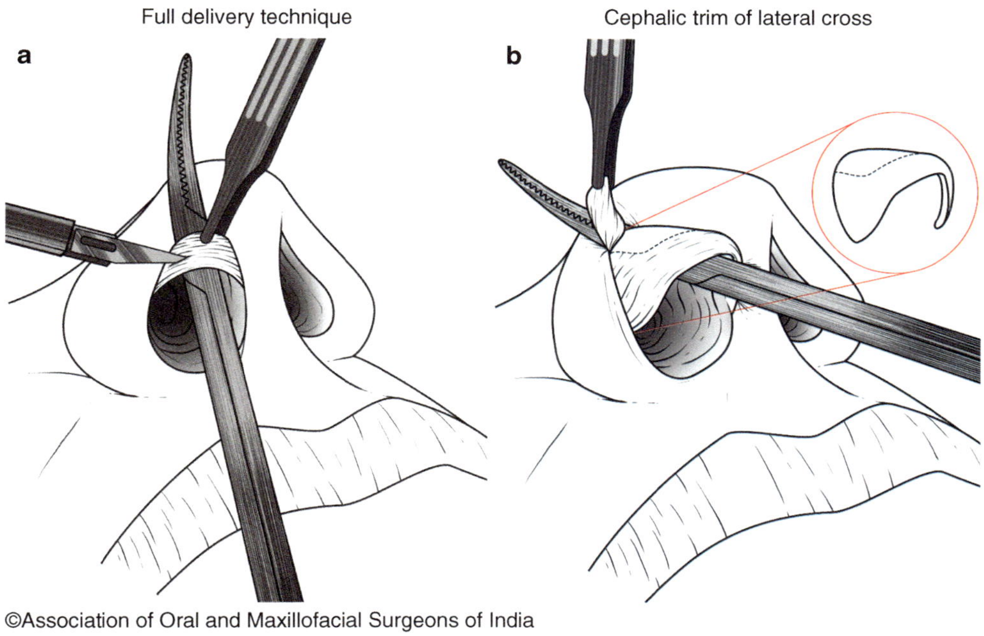


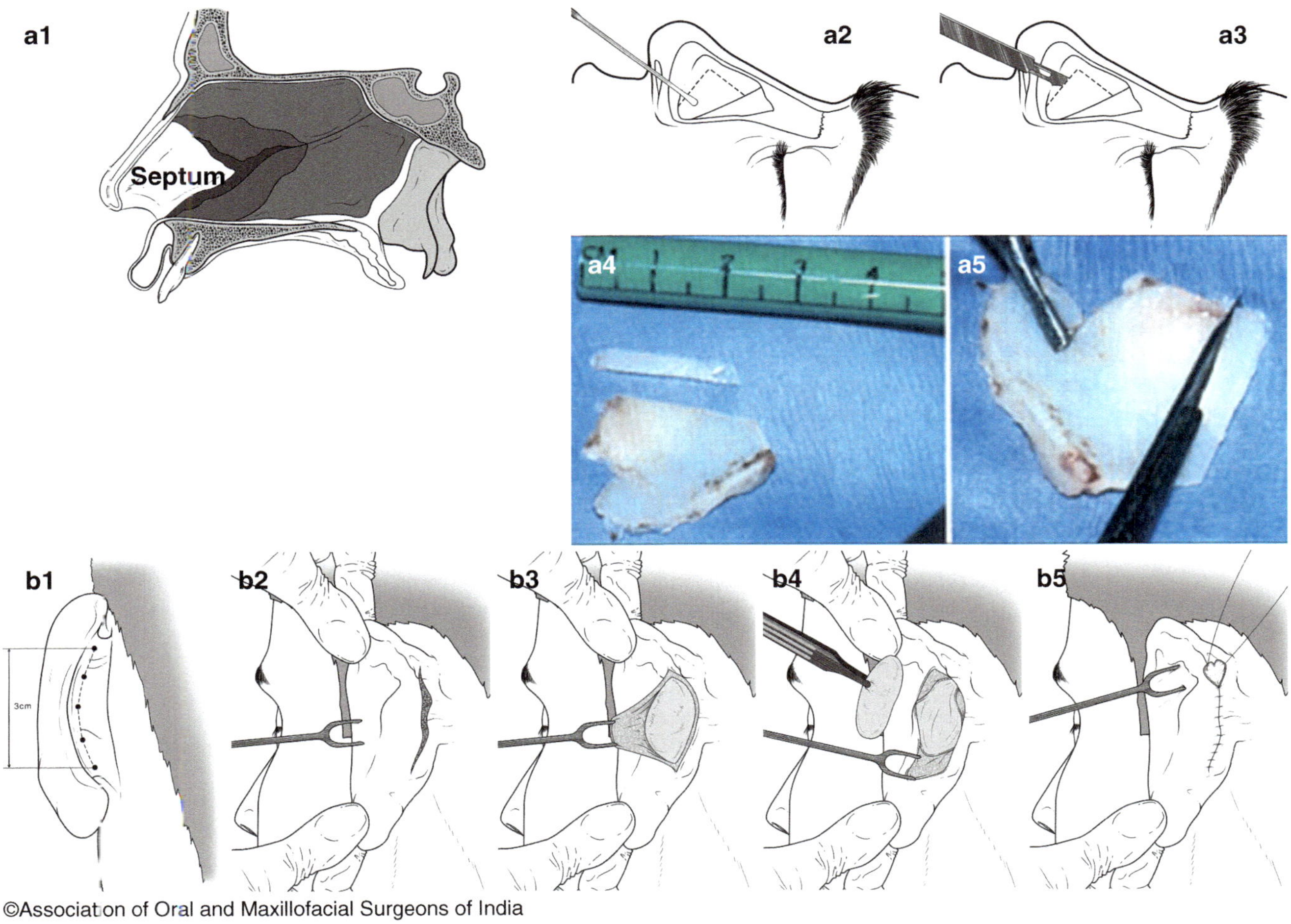


**Fig. 38.17** Sources of cartilage graft; (**a**) septal cartilage graft (**a1**) anatomy of septum (**a2**) marking for cartilage harvest preserving L shaped dorsal strut (**a3**) incision for cartilage harvest (**a4**) harvested cartilage (**a5**) carving of harvested cartilage and (**b**) Harvest of auricular cartilage; (**b**)- marking on the ear (**b2**)- incision (**b3**)- reflection of sub perichondrial flap to expose cartilage (**b4**) cartilage harvest (**b5**) closure of donor site

Table 38.2 Autologous graft materials

| | |
|---|---|
| *Autogenous grafts*—Donor site morbidity, increased operating time, predictable long-term results, minimal risk for extrusion and infection | |
| Nasal septal cartilage | Considered to the best grafting material as it is easy to harvest and contour |
| | Intrinsic anatomy of septal cartilage [firmness, resiliency, flatness] provides optimal aesthetic results |
| | Sufficient rigidity to provide structural support |
| | No donor site morbidity with excellent long-term results |
| | Insufficient when large volumes are needed/previous septal surgery |
| Auricular/conchal cartilage | Easy to harvest but difficult to contour due to its brittle nature |
| | Low strength and hence provides poor structural support |
| | Low donor site morbidity and with good long-term results |
| | Intrinsic anatomy [curved shape with elastic memory] of auricular cartilage makes it difficult to provide optimal aesthetic results |
| | Used if nasal septal cartilage is not adequate e.g. extensive revision cases and simultaneous multiple grafting procedures |
| | Useful when elasticity is needed e.g. lateral crus reconstruction |
| | Insufficient when large volumes are needed |
| Costochondral grafts | Abundant supply |
| | Sufficient rigidity to provide structural support |
| | Can be reharvested |
| Temporalis fascia | Used for cartilage-fascia grafts in primary and revision rhinoplasty. For smoothening contour defects and irregularities on the nasal dorsum. |
| | Easy to harvest |
| | Adequate size available |
| | Shows minimal resorption and is stable in followup |
| Perichondrium over rib | Used for repair of septal perforations and for smoothening irregularities over the dorsum |
| | Easily available and harvested contiguous with rib cartilage which is a commonly used graft in rhinoplasty |

Table 38.3 Alloplastic graft materials

| | |
|---|---|
| *Alloplastic grafts*—No donor site morbidity, reduced operating time, unpredictable long-term results and increased risk of extrusion and infection | |
| Silicone | Pliable, elastic solid that causes little tissue reaction |
| | Easy to handle, comes in prefabricated shapes—most commonly used alloplastic graft material |
| | Increased risk of displacement/extrusion as its nonporous nature prevents surrounding tissue in-growth, instead, leading to the formation of a fibrous capsule |
| | Easy to remove even after a long time as a fibrous capsule will form around the implant, without ingrowth in to the graft |
| | Asymmetric contracture of the capsule around the implant can deform the implant over time |
| | Low strength and hence provides poor structural support |
| | Preferred in Asians with thicker dorsal nasal skin |
| Medpor [high density polyethylene] | Easy to carve and bend due to thermoplastic property |
| | Poor aesthetic results and comfort due to its stiffness |
| | Sufficient rigidity to provide structural support |
| | Minimal risk for displacement due to its porous nature with subsequent ingrowth of surrounding fibrovascular tissue |
| | Difficult to remove in the long term as there will be extensive tissue ingrowth |
| | Tends to shed particles, when implanted in stress-bearing and mobile areas may cause a chronic inflammatory response |
| Gore-tex [expanded poly-tetra-fluoro-ethylene (PTFE)] | Porous implant composed of carbon and fluorine molecules with pores |
| | Second most widely used alloplastic implant, after silicone |
| | Better comfort and aesthetics due to its softness |
| | Minimal risk for displacement due to its porous nature with subsequent ingrowth of surrounding fibrovascular tissue |
| | Poor long-term aesthetics as it decreases in volume over time |
| | Difficult to remove in long term owing to extensive tissue ingrowth |
| | Low strength and hence provides poor structural support |
| *Injectable filler materials*—No donor site morbidity; reduced operating time; unpredictable long-term results and increased risk of extrusion, infection and embolization | |
| Bovine collagen, human-derived collagen, hydroxyapatite microspheres, hyaluronic acid | Mainly used for minor augmentations |
| | Necessary to overaugment by 20–30% to compensate for long-term absorption |
| | Provides poor structural support |
| | High complication rate including persistent redness, contour irregularity, swelling and necrosis of surrounding dermis or soft tissue, hypersensitivity reactions, extrusion |
| | Patients may object on religious grounds |

**Box 38.4 Classification of septal deformites**
**Congenital:**

- Syndromic
  - Cleft lip and palate
- Congenital syphilis

**Acquired:**

- Developmental: midline dermoid cyst, short nose/long nose
- Post traumatic: bent nose/crooked nose
- Iatrogenic
  - Incorrect or aggressive rhino/septal surgery.
  Lefort I maxillary impaction with inadequate trimming of septum
- Cocaine misuse: destruction of cartilage and bony septum

#### 38.4.3.2 Sequencing for Treatment

The sequence to be followed for planning a proper septoplasty includes

1. Establishing an accurate diagnosis. Apply Mladini classification for septal deformities (See additional Reading)
2. A thorough external and internal examination of the nose
3. Internal examination should include (1) anterior rhinoscopy and (2) nasendoscopy
4. Imaging of the nose, septum and the paranasal sinuses is mandatory. This should include CT scans with both soft tissue and bony windows [18].
5. It is preferable to perform the surgery "in conjunction with ENT colleagues"
6. Gross iatrogenic nasal deformities need careful evaluation of previous surgical records before treatment planning
7. Informed consents to be obtained for the harvest and use of grafts (Septum, Concha or Rib cartilage)
8. Care should be exercised to preserve the integrity of the turbinates and the internal nasal valve.

#### 38.4.3.3 Surgical Approaches

Septoplasty may be performed in conjunction with a formal rhinoplasty using an open or closed approach.

Closed approaches for septoplasty include;

1. Endonasal caudal vestibular access via a right or a left hemi-transfixion incision or
2. Bilateral septal transfixion incision [19, 20].

#### 38.4.3.4 Surgical Technique (Fig. 38.19a, b, c)

The local anaesthetic solution is infiltrated with adrenaline for optimal haemostasis. This not only provides a clear field for surgery but also aids in developing planes by the process of hydrodissection. An incision is made at the caudal margin of the septal cartilage, which may be unilateral or bilateral. Cautious, careful, unhurried dissection in the correct anatomical plane is done, using sharp precise instrumentation (Cottle/Masing, Freer or Joseph's elevator). It is imperative to identify and stay in a bloodless sub-mucoperichondrial plane. The light blue colour of the septal cartilage ensures the correct plane of dissection. An anterior tunnel is first made, followed by an inferior tunnel to expose the entire septum. The plane is then expanded and separated further with a Killian forceps. This offers bilateral exposure of the dissected tunnel and the septum. Sharp curvatures, angles and fracture lines are negotiated carefully also bearing in mind that the transition zone between the mucoperichondrium and the mucoperiosteum is an area vulnerable to tears. Tears over the mucoperichondrium require careful repair with vicryl sutures on a round body needle. However, tears in the inferior tunnel overlying bone need not be sutured and may act as drains. The flap elevation is extended posterior to chondrovomerine and chondroethmoid junctions for complete exposure of the bony septum.

Bony spurs or angulations and bends are identified, which may contribute to airway block. The osteocartilaginous junction is then separated to free the septum in the posterior aspect. Takayashu forceps are used to nibble away any bony/cartilage spurs. This may also be performed using thin chisels and osteotomes. Buckling of the septum may be corrected by resection of overhanging cartilage in the caudal aspect. Adequate relief thus allows the passive return of the septum to midline. Measures such as scoring, suturing or the use of PDS sheets/cartilage grafts may be required to correct and straighten residual curvatures. Harvest of septal cartilage may be performed at this juncture and should be done posterior to the key area (imaginary vertical line joining the tip of the nasal bone and the anterior nasal spine). Stabilisation to the midline is achieved by the use of a PDS suture anchoring the dissected septum to the anterior nasal spine. The flaps are reapposed with one or two transfixion sutures to prevent septal haematoma. Nasal packing is outdated and has been replaced by silastic sheets and intra-operative control with Merocel packs.

Advantages of the endonasal approach include

1. Minimal trauma to local tissues
2. Reduced post-surgical oedema and
3. A-faster-recovery-to-normalcy

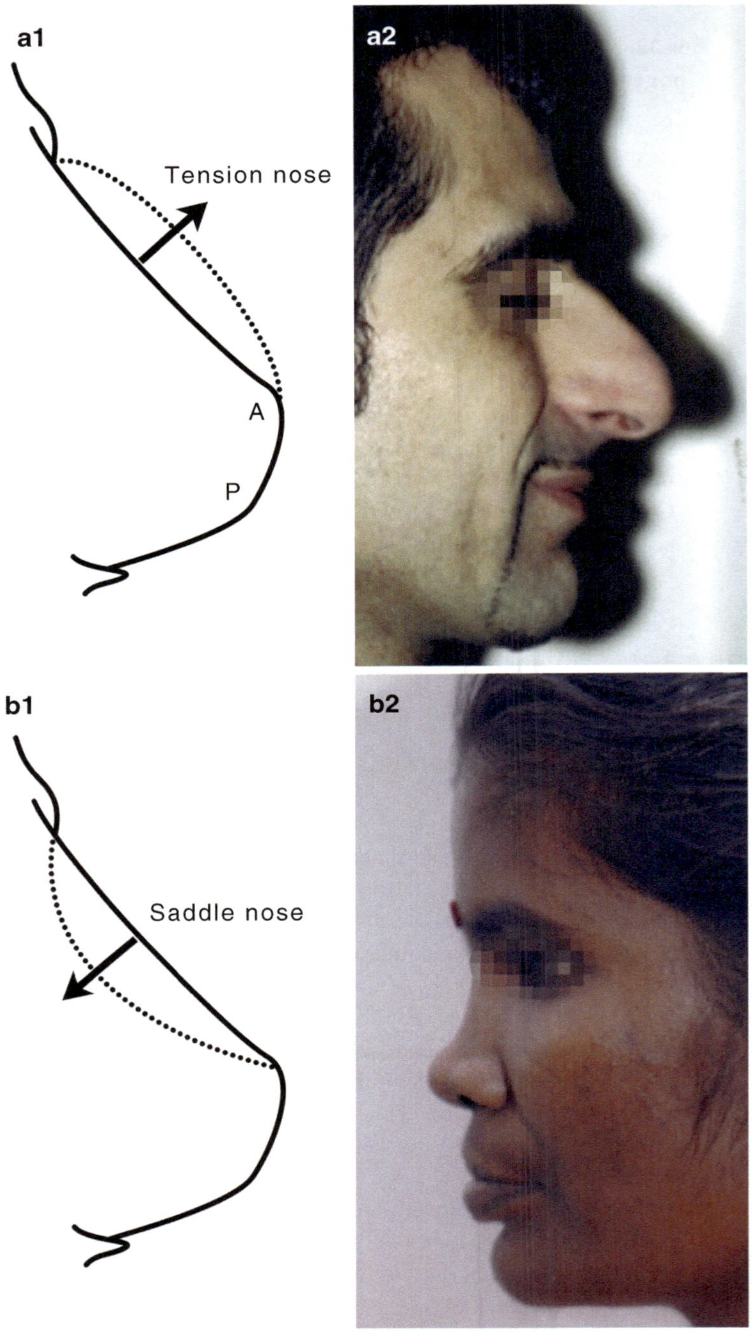


**Fig. 38.18** Deformities of nasal septum; (**a**) tension nose and (**b**) saddle nose



Disadvantages of the endonasal approach are

1. Steep learning curve
2. Limited exposure & visualisation (headlight required)
3. Limited visualisation for the assistant
4. Difficult to place spreader grafts
5. Contour irregularities at the dorsal edge
6. Septal malposition/perforation
7. Increased risk for secondary deformities like saddling

### 38.4.4 Nasal Osteotomies

Nasal osteotomies are often required during correction of deformities of the nose as well as an adjunct to procedures which involve correction of the osseocartilaginous vault.

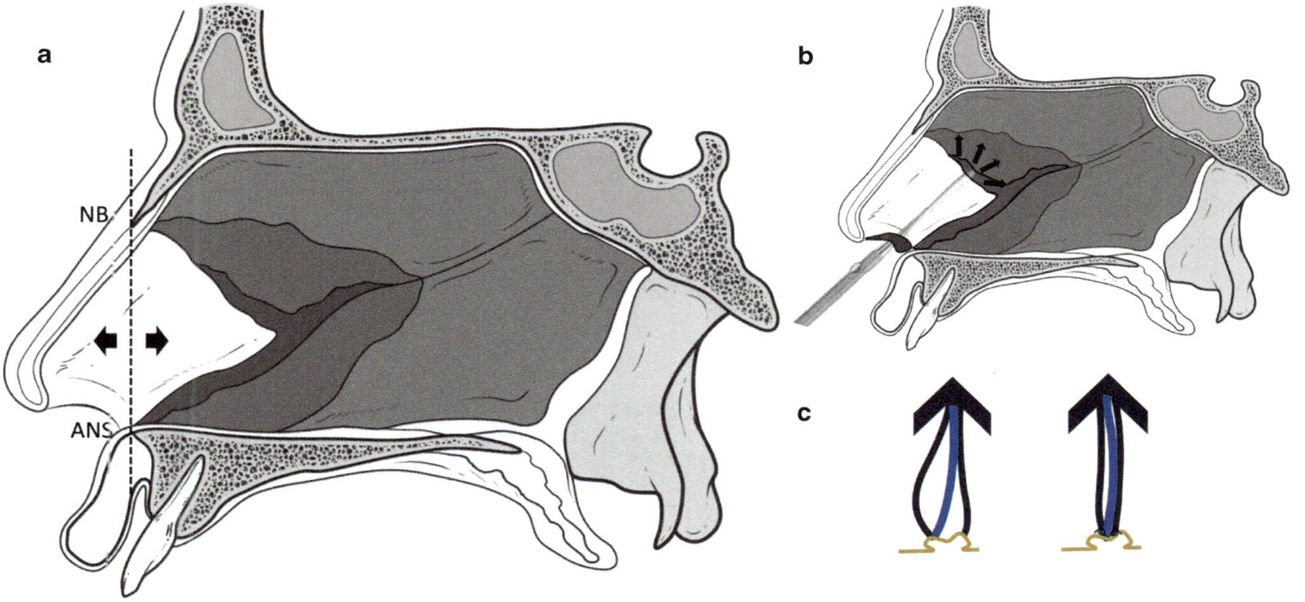




**Fig. 38.19** Septoplasty intra-operative steps. (**a**) the part of the septum anterior to the line dropped from the tip of nasal bone (NB) to the anterior nasal spine (ANS) has tobe preserved. (**b**) Dysjunction of the cartilaginous septum from the bony septum. (**c**) Septal repositioning with sutures to the midline crest of the maxilla

#### 38.4.4.1 Indications for Nasal Osteotomies

1. Close an open roof after dorsal hump removal
2. Correction of a deviated bony nasal vault (crooked nose/bent nose)
3. Correction of concave or convex nasal bones
4. Reduce or narrow bony base width
5. Mobilise malunited fractured nasal bones prior to reduction

Different types of nasal osteotomies (Fig. 38.20a, b) are utilised for a variety of clinical indications [21, 22]. They are enumerated in Box 38.5.

#### 38.4.4.2 Armamentarium for Nasal Osteotomies

- Chisels/Osteotomes
  - Straight osteotomes—2 mm microosteotome
  - Curved osteotomes
  - Guarded osteotomes—Nievert, Silver
  - Angled blade osteotomes—Murray-Parkes
  - Notched osteotomes—Walter
- Power instruments
  - Oscillating/reciprocating saws
  - Piezo saw

#### 38.4.4.3 Surgical Technique

The different techniques for performing nasal osteotomies are (1) endonasal, (2) percutaneous, (3) endoral and (4) nasofrontal

**Percutaneous technique** (Fig. 38.21a, b, c)

The percutaneous technique involves the completion of a lateral osteotomy and a transverse root(superior) osteotomy. The local anaesthetic solution is infiltrated with adrenaline 10–15 min earlier for good haemostasis.

The sites of the lateral and superior osteotomies are marked on the skin. The cephalic end of the cross-over of these two osteotomies should be kept no higher than the level of the intercanthal line.

A small 2–3 mm stab incision is made on the skin at the middle of the lateral osteotomy marking. The incision is deepened down and to bone. The osteotome is swept along the entire length of the marking to provide good release of the skin and subcutaneous tissue and keep the angular artery away from the line of osteotomy. The osteotome is then positioned supraperiosteally at 2 mm intervals and struck with a mallet to produce an interrupted line of punch holes. The osteotomies are started at the pyriform rim and continued superiorly to the nasofrontal junction. The same technique is followed for the transverse root(superior) osteotomy. The contra-lateral nasal wall is osteotomised in a similar

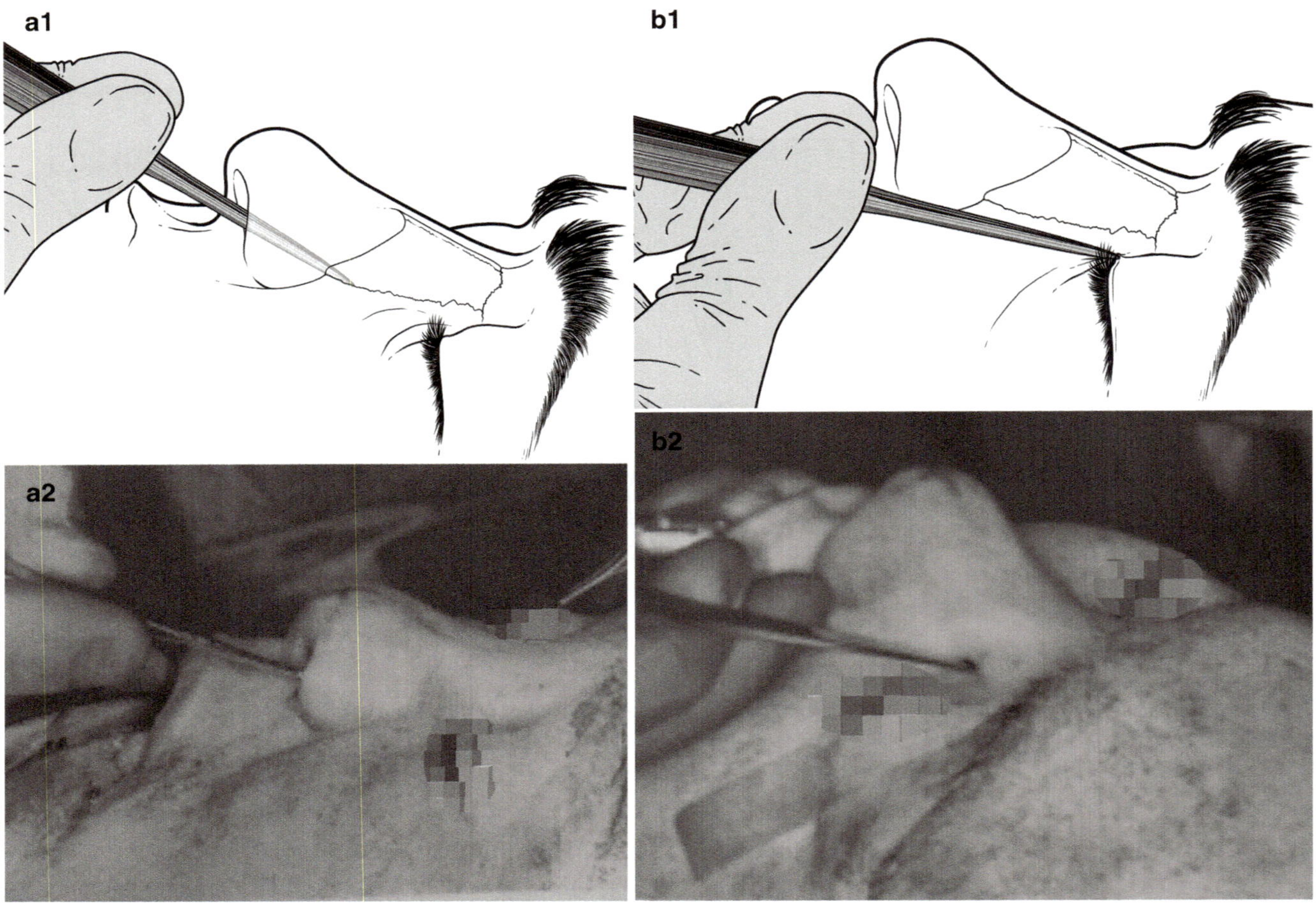




Fig. 38.20 Types of osteotomies. (**a**) Endonasal and (**b**) Percutaneous

**Box 38.5 Osteotomies types**

- Lateral osteotomy
  - Low to high
  - Low to low
- Medial osteotomy
  - Fading paramedian
  - True median
- Superior osteotomy
  - Transverse root
- Intermediate osteotomy
  - Vertical
  - Horizontal
- Fragmentation/comminution (largely outdated)

fashion. Once this is completed, the nasal bones are held with firm/controlled pressure between the thumb and the fore-fingers of both hands over a gauze square and then fractured along the already osteotomised punch holes. Moderate pressure over the wound helps with haemostasis and prevention of ecchymosis. No sutures are required and the skin is dressed with a Steri-Strip.

**Complications** include comminution, unpredictable fracture line, loss of lateral wall support, avulsion/displacement of upper laterals, step deformity, residual deformity and failure to in fracture/mobilise nasal bones.

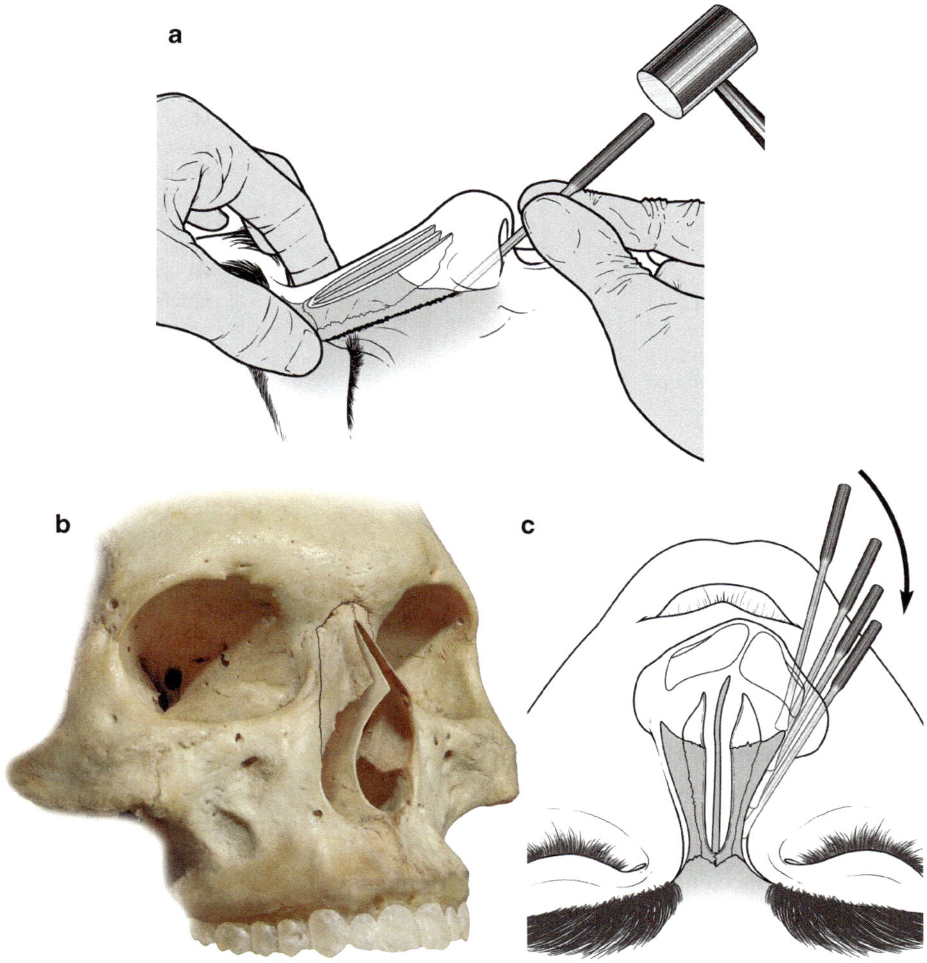




**Fig. 38.21** Steps in nasal osteotomy. (**a**) Start of the lateral osteotomy. (**b**) Osteotomy marking on skull. (**c**) Movement of the osteotome for lateral osteotomy

## 38.5 Surgical Management of Basic Nasal Deformities

### 38.5.1 Dorsal Hump Deformity

The dorsal hump is the most common problem for which a patient may seek rhinoplasty. Based on the anatomical units involved, three main types of dorsal hump may be identified [23, 24];

1. Osseous/bony hump that exclusively involves the bony vault,
2. cartilaginous hump that involves the cartilaginous middle vault with septal and upper lateral cartilages and
3. the osseocartilagenous hump that is a combination of the two.

#### 38.5.1.1 Types of Dorsal Humps

Dorsal humps can also be categorised as true and pseudohumps. True humps may occur isolated or may occur in conjunction with other nasal deformities. The pseudohump may produce a relative appearance of a dorsal hump, while in reality, the appearance may be due to a high anterior septal angle, supratip prominence or tip ptosis (Box 38.6).

#### 38.5.1.2 Clinical Assessment of a Dorsal Hump (Fig. 38.22a–d)

- Palpation of nasal bones, normal, long or short
- Ascertain area of hump requiring reduction
- Dorsal line—imaginary line from the radix extended along the nasal dorsum
- Assess if tip projection is adequate; reduced or increased, prior to hump reduction
- Assess if tip support is adequate; weak or strong, prior to hump reduction

#### 38.5.1.3 Armamentarium for Dorsal Hump Reduction

The armamentarium required for dorsal hump reduction are shown in Box 38.7.

**Box 38.6. True vs. Pseudo humps**

| True dorsal hump | Pseudo hump |
|---|---|
| Hump associated with the following clinical situations<br>• high dorsum<br>• low dorsum<br>• short nasal bones<br>• wide bony base<br>• narrow bony base<br>• deviated nasal bones<br>• cleft nose deformity<br>• under-projected nasal tip<br>• over-projected nasal tip<br>• short nose<br>• long nose | • High anterior septal angle<br>• Supra-tip prominence<br>• Loss of tip projection |

**Box 38.7. Bony vs. Cartilaginous hump, (Armamentarium)**

| Bony hump | Cartilagenous hump |
|---|---|
| Manual nasal saw.<br>• Joseph saw<br>• Bull saw (guarded tip)<br>Osteotomes.<br>• Rubin (dorsal fin)<br>• Cinnelli (guarded edges)<br>• Aiach (wire guide)<br>• McIndoe grooved chisel (not recommended)<br>Bone cutters/nibblers<br>• Sulsenti<br>• Heanley<br>Rasps<br>• Graded two way tungsten carbide rasps (Rees)<br>• Pull rasp/push rasp (Daniel)<br>• Diamond rasps<br>Power saw<br>• Rhinobur (Toriumi)<br>• Piezoelectric saw | • Scalpel (11 bard Parker)<br>• Fomon scissors (angled on flat)<br>• Turbinate scissors (angled on side)<br>• Kaplan scissors (double action)<br>• Cautious, conservative reduction at osteocartilaginous junction only<br>• Preserve leading edges of ULC to create spreader flaps (prevent middle vault narrowing) |

#### 38.5.1.4 Dorsal Hump Reduction (Profile Lowering)

The procedure for dorsal hump reduction (profile lowering) is facilitated by two important steps, namely, (1) bony hump removal and (2) cartilaginous hump removal.

**Bony hump removal** (Fig. 38.23A–K)
En-bloc bony or cartilaginous hump removal requires experience as there is a high risk of excessive reduction when the surgeon may be inexperienced. The procedure begins with infiltration of lidocaine 2% with 1 in 100,000 adrenaline.

After exposure of the osteocartilaginous vault is completed, the osteotome is engaged at the caudal edge of the nasal hump (osteocartilaginous junction) and the bone is removed using an osteotome and mallet (18 oz Heath mallet) with firm blows to follow a careful alignment. It is better to always under-reduce, rather than over-reduce as it may cause severely compromised results. The dorsal edges can then be rasped down to the desired extent. Care is taken not to rasp the cartilage as it may produce irregularities, tears or avulsions.

When separation of a large hump is desired, placement of a superior stop-cut as described by Tardy allows precise and clear separation at the desired level. Diamond rasps are used to smooth irregularities at the dorsal edge of the nasal bones. Removal of an osteocartilagenous hump results in an open roof deformity of the nasal dorsum, which needs to be closed with an osteotomy [23].

#### 38.5.1.5 Complications

- Unpredictable hump reduction
- Avulsion of upper lateral cartilages
- Fenestration of the skin envelope
- Residual irregularities
- Excessive overzealous hump reduction
  - Bony saddle
  - Loss of support to ULC
  - Loss of key area support to septum
- Inadequate hump reduction
  - Residual hump
  - Failure to follow dorsal line: superior bony spur

#### 38.5.1.6 Preservation Technique of Hump Removal (Regnault & Daniel)

This technique advocates aggressive removal of the large hump with osteotome. The under-surface of the hump is then reduced extracorporeally with a bur. The reduced hump is replaced in the dorsal defect. This obviates the need for nasal osteotomy and provides optimal results of a corrected dorsum.

### 38.5.2 Saddle Nose Deformity

A saddle nose deformity is defined as a wide and flat nose with a concavity on the nasal dorsum.

Classical clinical presenting features of this deformity are

- Loss of height of the nasal dorsum (appearance of a shortened nose)
- Increased width of the nasal dorsum (wide nose)
- Underprojected tip due to inadequate septal support to the tip complex

#### 38.5.2.1 Classification

Saddle nose deformity can be classified based on the underlying structural problem into

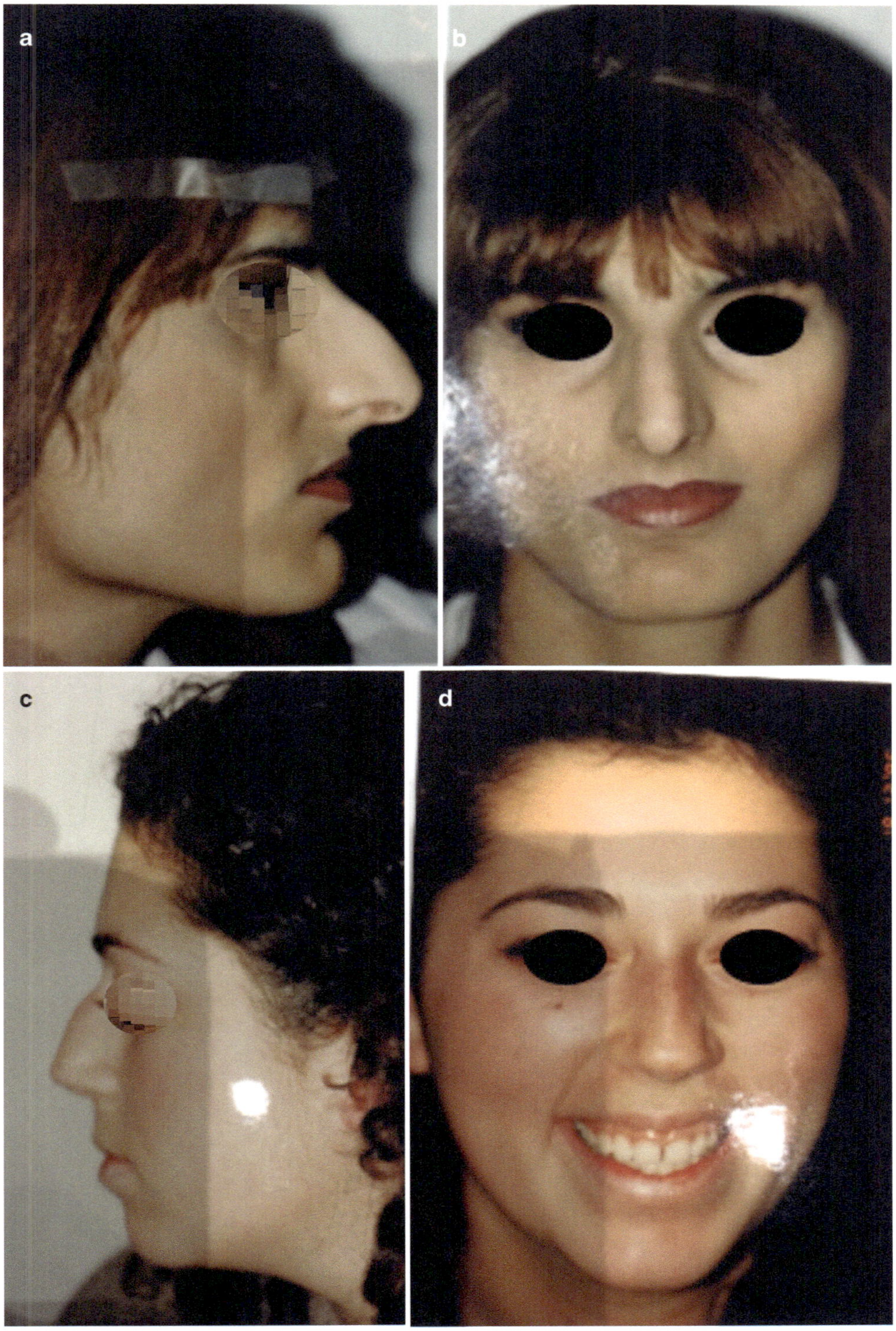




**Fig. 38.22** Dorsal hump - clinical presentation. (**a**) Profile and (**b**) frontal pictures of patient 1. (**c**) Profile and (**d**) frontal pictures of patient 2

1. Bony saddle
2. Cartilaginous saddle
3. Combination of bony and cartilaginous elements

The causes responsible for saddle nose deformity are many, namely, septal hematoma following trauma, iatrogenic—inappropriate surgery to the septum, bony vault &

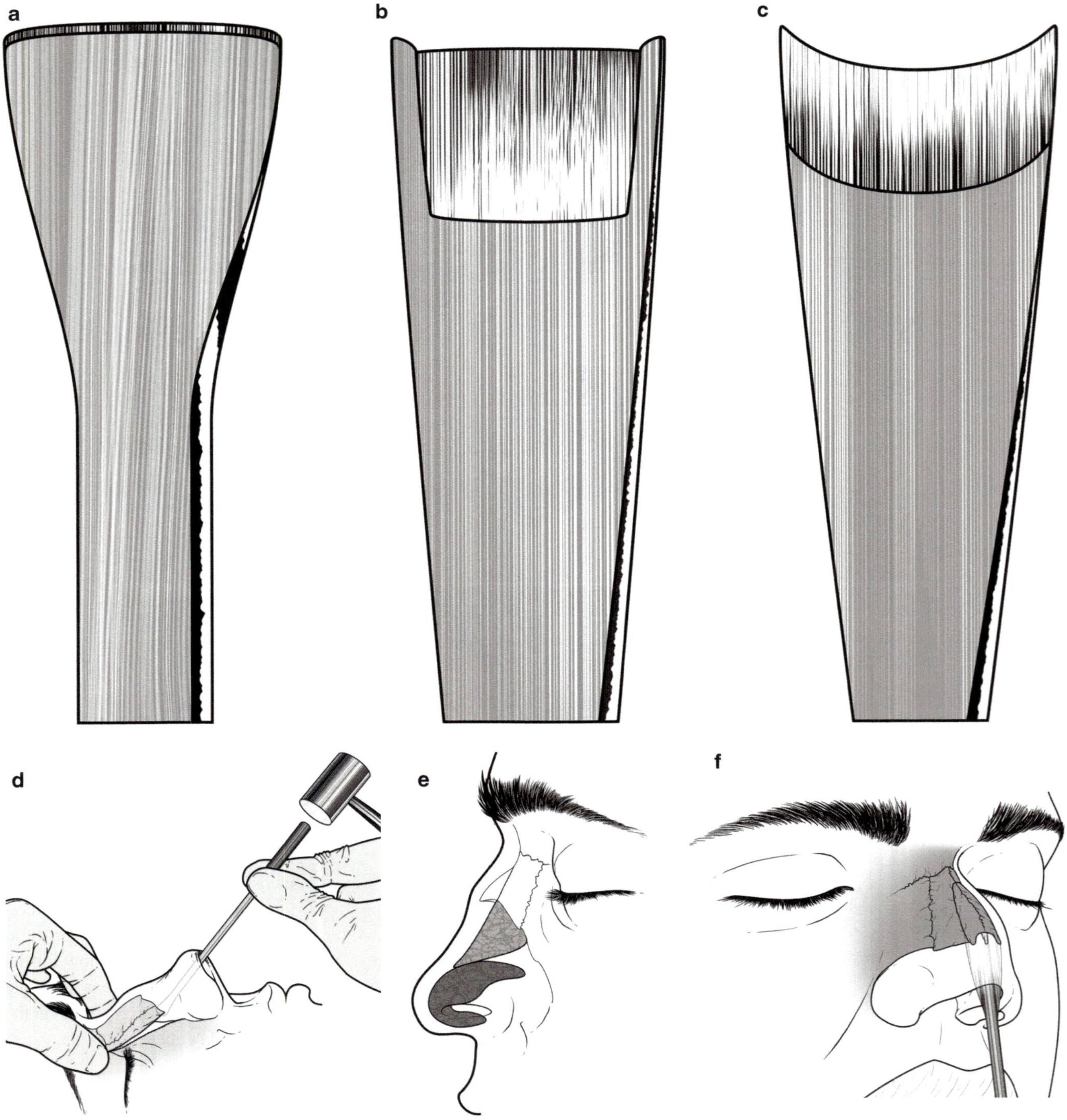




**Fig. 38.23** Hump reduction technique: Armamentarium (**A**, **B** & **C**). Surgical technique (**D**, **E** & **F**) Removal of the dorsal hump with the osteotome, (**G–K**) Preparation of the "open roof" deformity for closure

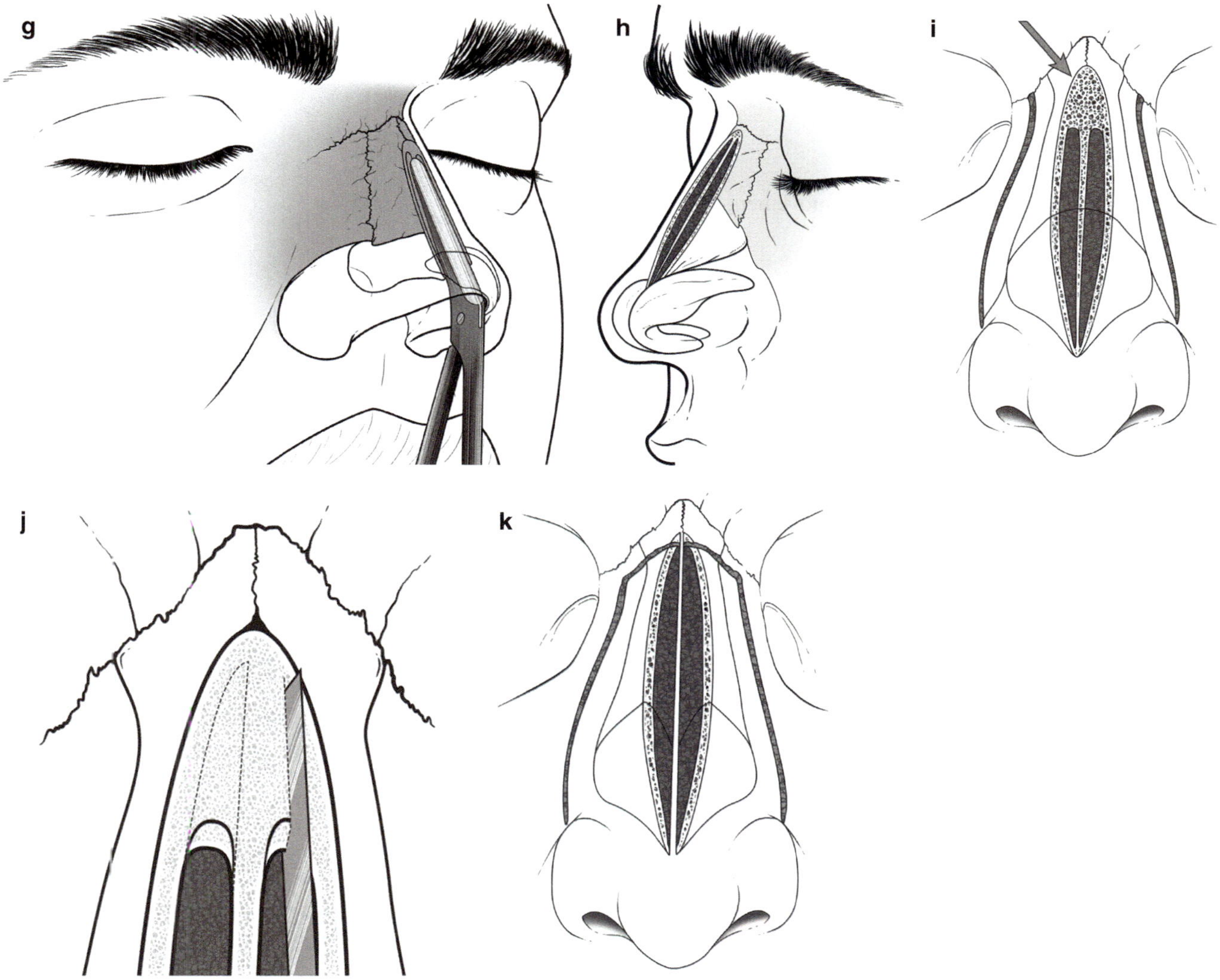




Fig. 38.23 (Continued)

middle vault and substance abuse (cocaine), diseases like congenital syphilis/leprosy and racial predisposition—African, Afro-American, and Asian.

#### 38.5.2.2 Clinical Features

The salient features (Fig. 38.24) demonstrable on a patient with saddle nose deformity are enumerated in Box 38.8.

The septum may exhibit deformity with twisting/deficiency or at times may be totally absent.

The skin and soft tissue envelope may show a "concertina" effect due to loss of structural support.

#### 38.5.2.3 Surgical Management (Fig. 38.25a, b)

Surgery for the correction of saddle nose deformity may be planned in a staged manner with the first stage involving the correction of the foundation of the nose and the second stage involving the aesthetic makeover [25, 26]. The aim of the procedure is to re-establish the tension between the nasal tip

**Box 38.8 Features of saddle nose deformity**

**Frontal:**

- Wide nasal dorsum
- Loss of dorsal lines
- Epicanthal folds due to the lateral movement of dorsal skin
- Loss of tip definition
- Increased tip width
- Presence of a flat alar-columellar line

**Profile:**

- Loss of dorsal height
- Marked concavity of the nasal dorsum
- Loss of tip support and projection
- Tip rotation may be increased or decreased
- Retraction of the columella
- Relative increase of the upper lip length (columellar skin migrates downward)

**Basal:**

- Wide alar base
- Shortened and deformed columella
- Loss of nostril orientation
- Ballooning of the internal nasal valve

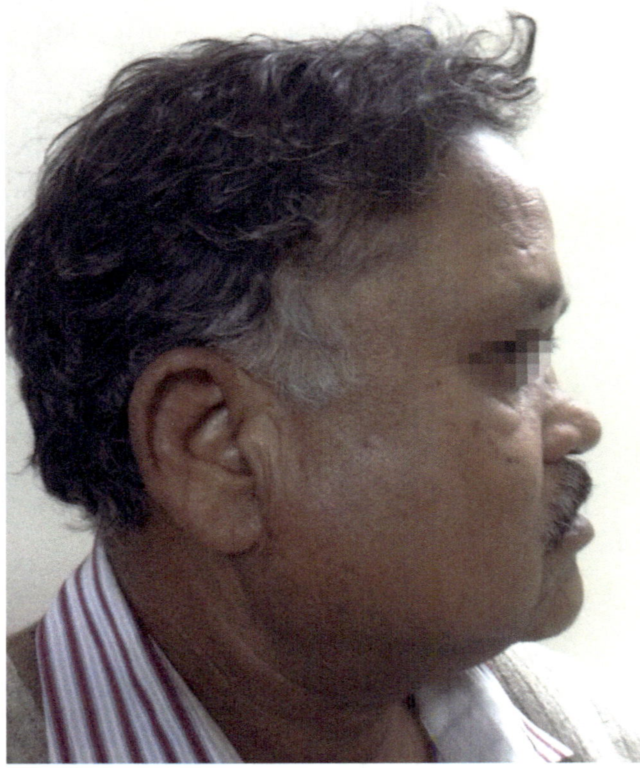



Fig. 38.24 Saddle nose clinical photo

complex and the dorsum, which has been lost due to the concertina effect.

Surgical correction involves three essential steps that are independent of each other.

- Establish the height and length of the septum to restore structural support to the entire nose. This involves the use of a robust septal extension graft, fashioned from harvested rib cartilage (preferably the eighth rib).
- Correction of the dorsal deficiency using a dorsal strut graft that extends from nasion to under the domes.
- Provision of support for the tip complex. This is achieved with the use of a columellar strut graft to restore tip projection.

This procedure involves the use of strong and robust cartilage grafts. The eighth rib provides an adequate amount of cartilage which is ideal for this situation. Ear cartilage lacks rigidity, while banked cartilage tends to undergo resorption.

### 38.5.3 Correction of the Deviated Nose

Deviated noses can be of two types

1. "Bent" nose where the nasal bones and the upper lateral cartilages point to the same side, and
2. "Crooked" nose where the nasal bones and the upper laterals face in opposite directions

#### 38.5.3.1 Aetiology

The most common causes of a deviated nose

1. Developmental—unilateral cleft nasal deformity
2. Post trauma to the face and nose—following road traffic accidents, sports injuries or interpersonal violence
3. Iatrogenic—as a result of earlier surgical procedures; Maxillary impaction by a LeFort 1 osteotomy without addressing the septum or septoplasty with excessive scoring, resection and weakening

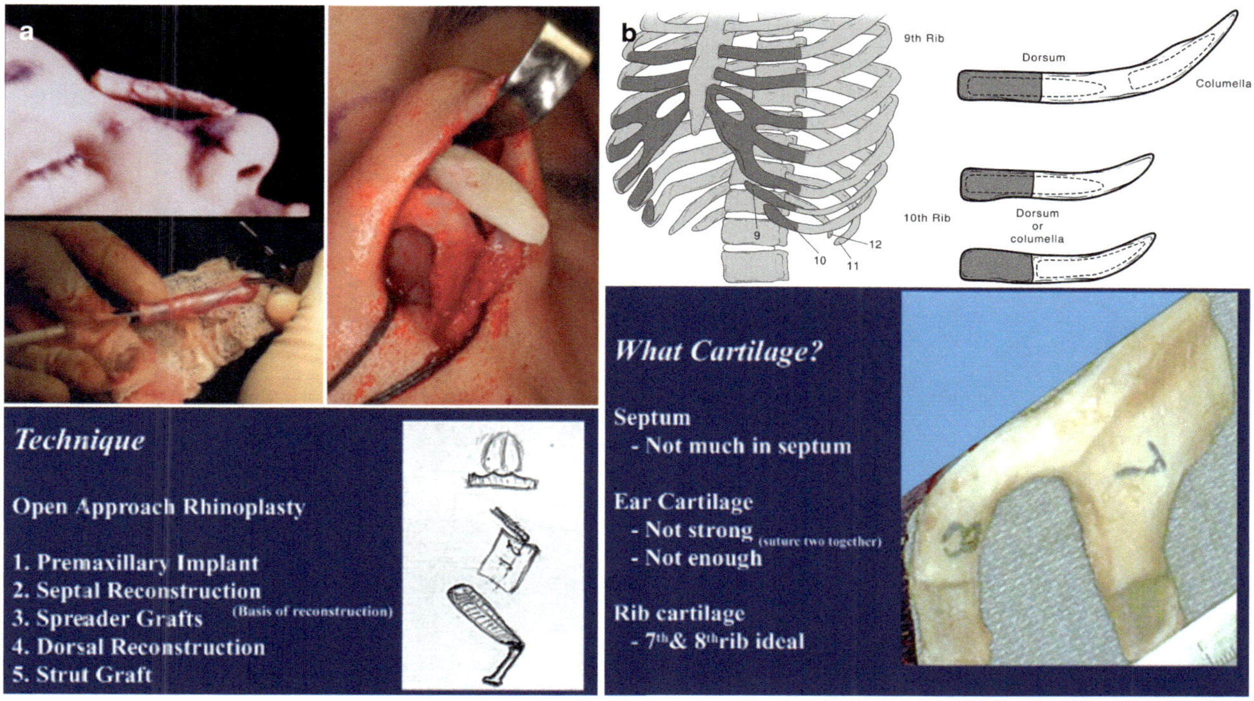



**Fig. 38.25** Saddle nose-intra op. (**a**) intra-operative pictures demonstrating use of rib cartilage for dorsal nasal reconstruction. (**b**) Landmarks for rib harvest

#### 38.5.3.2 Clinical Features

Clinical features of a deviated, bent or crooked nose include both functional and aesthetic issues

1. Blockage of the nasal airway, unilateral or bilateral
2. Visible deformities affecting the upper, middle and lower thirds of the nose
   (a) Frontal
   - Deformity of the nasal pyramid
   - Twisting or angulation of the nose
   - Constriction or bulge at the middle vault
   - Bending of the nose showing midline discrepancy
   - Unequal height of the nasal bones
   - Tip deformity secondary to the loss of septal support/angulation

   (b) Profile
   - Patient may present with a dorsal hump or a saddle deformity
   - Loss of tip projection
   - Nasal tip ptosis
   - Retraction of the columella

   (c) Basal
   - Deviation of the nasal tip or middle vault
   - Angulation or shortening of columella
   - Displacement of the caudal septum from the maxillary crest into the nasal vestibule
   - Nasal valve obstructions

   (d) Varied presentations of septal deformities (Mladini classification)

#### 38.5.3.3 Treatment (Fig. 38.26a–g)

Septorhinoplasty is required to correct the deformity. Some prefer single-stage correction, while others may choose staged procedures (first stage septoplasty followed by a second stage external deformity correction). However, a single-stage correction is preferred. This is usually performed using an open structure approach with exposure and separation of the septum from the upper lateral cartilages. Straightening of the septal cartilage is performed by excision and/or partial division of the cartilage and may be followed by scoring or sutures as indicated. Some surgeons prefer the use of a PDS sheet to splint the corrected septum. However, costal cartilage may be harvested for reinforcement of the straightening

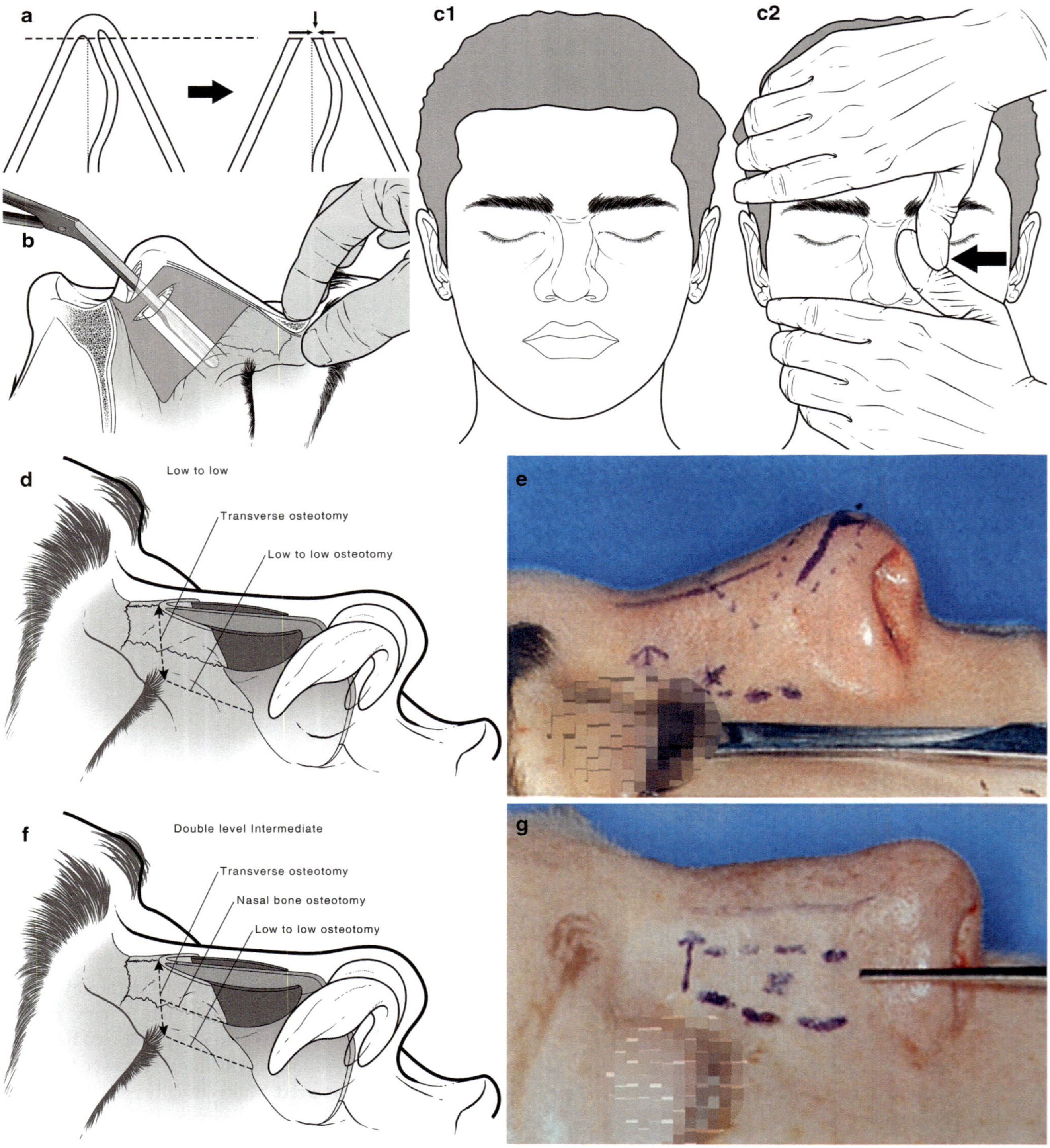




**Fig. 38.26** Techniques of reduction of crooked nose deformity with twisting/angulation of septum, (**a**) differential reduction of hump prior to ostetotomy, (**b**) septal repositioning, (**c**) digital reduction/manipulation after osteotomy, (**d**) line diagram of "low-to-low" osteotomy, (**e**) intra-operative picture with osteotome positioning (low-to-low), (**f**) line diagram of "nasal bone osteotomy", (**g**) intra-operative picture with osteotome positioning (nasal bone osteotomy)

and to provide a spreader effect to correct the nasal valve simultaneously. Osteotomy of the nasal bones is often required to correct the angular deformity of the bony vault. A tip plasty may be necessary in most cases to correct the nasal tip tripod deformity secondary to nasal deviation.

It is to be borne in mind that the results for the correction of deviated noses are not always satisfactory. There is a possibility of residual deformity, recurrent deformity, loss of tip support and saddling.

### 38.5.4 Tip Plasty

The nasal tip is the centre of focus for both nasal anatomy and aesthetics. It is a very important anatomical subunit and can be most challenging to refine surgically.

Nasal tip deformities may show varied morphology and diverse clinical presentations (Fig. 38.27a–f). They may occur in isolation or concomitant with deformities of the dorsum or septum.

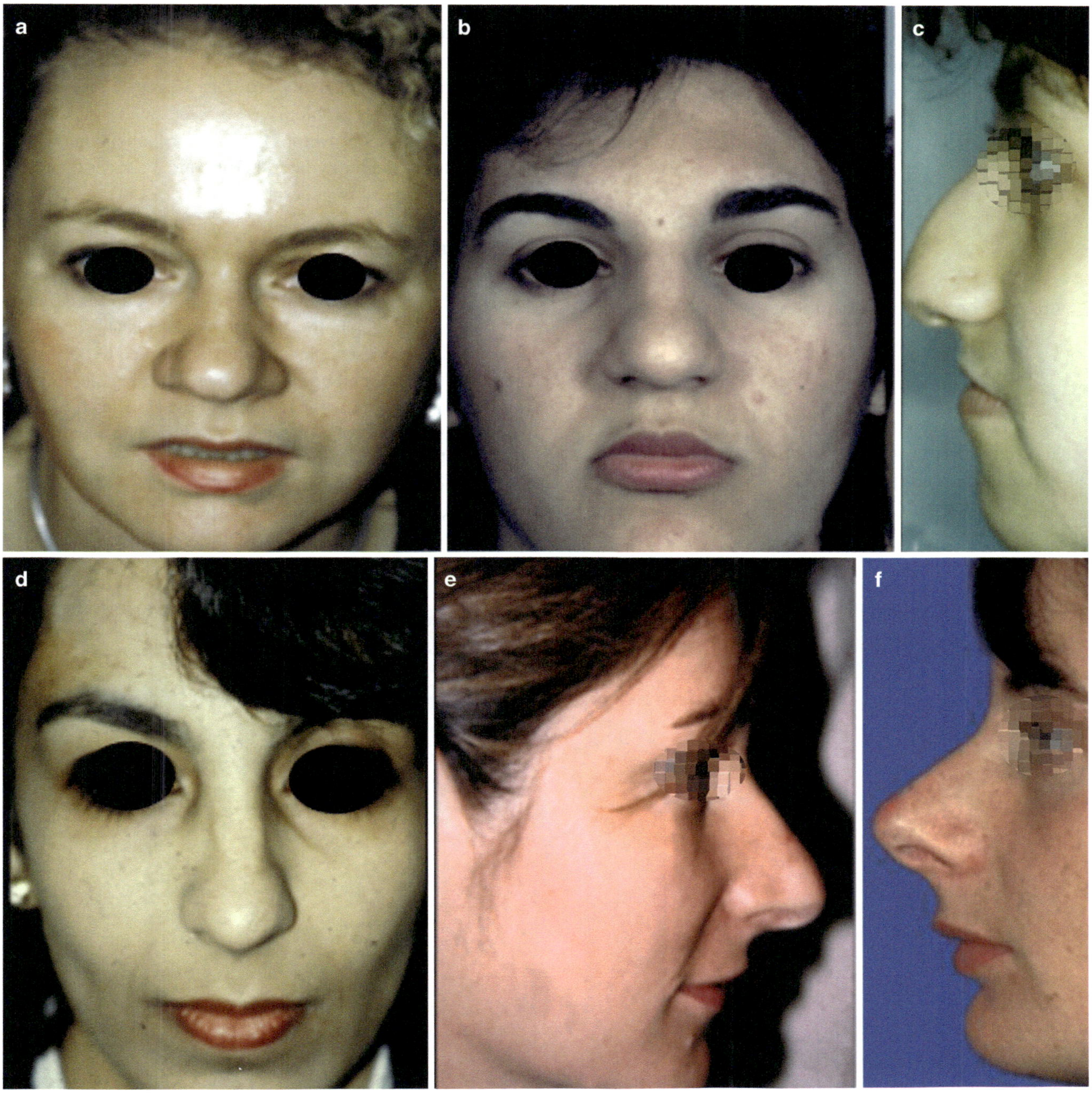




Fig. 38.27 Types of tip deformity. (**a**) Wide bulbous tip, (**b**) ball-ended amorphous tip, (**c**) plunging infra-tip lobule, (**d**) amorphous bulbous tip with deviation and constriction of right lower middle vault, (**e**) over-projection of nasal tip owing to prominent ANS & overtly long lower lateral cartilage with normal naso-labial angle, and (**f**) nasal tip over-projection with upward over-rotation

Tip deformities can be enumerated as follows as in Box 38.9.

### 38.5.4.1 Wide Nasal Tip

A tip is considered abnormally wide when the width of the tip is greater than the width of the dorsum. Normally, the tip width is equal to the width of the dorsum.

This can be further subclassified as mild, moderate or severe.

A wide nasal tip may be caused due to three morphological alterations:

1. increased interdomal width (wide interdomal angle)
2. increased intradomal width, where the domal angle is wide, and
3. increase in both intradomal width and interdomal width

**Box 38.9 Types of tip deformities**

- Wide
- Bulbous
- Over projected
- Under projected
- Over-rotated (piggy nose/toffee nose)
- Under-rotated (ptotic tip)
- Asymmetric

**Surgical management**

Surgery for the nasal tip can be performed either through a closed or open structure rhinoplasty approach. This may depend on the clinical indications involved as well as the skill and experience of the operating surgeon. Steps for correction of a wide nasal tip include reduction of the interdomal width by placing a permanent interdomal suture with 5-0 prolene or 5-0 PDS (semipermanent). This is followed by the creation of a new domal angle (transdomal suture followed by the interdomal suture). One should also consider surgical removal/excision of a segment of the intermediate crus for better tip definition (Fig. 38.28a, b).

### 38.5.4.2 Bulbous/Boxy Tip (Fig. 38.29)

Bulbous tips have problems associated with thick SSTE (skin & soft tissue envelope), excessive subcutaneous fat, strong convex and bulky lateral crura and a concertina effect of a shortened nose in general.

**Surgical management**

This involves careful degloving of the SSTE leaving the subcutaneous fibrofatty tissue on the lateral crura. Careful defattening and thinning of the subcutaneous plane should be performed. A modest cephalic trim is performed to correct the large and bulky lateral crura. As this is a more general deformity involving not only the tip but also the associated SSTE, a careful distribution of volume to produce balance may be required. This helps camouflage the deformity to a great extent while improving outcomes.

Excessive or injudicious defattening of the nasal tip may cause ischemia/necrosis of the skin of the nasal tip,

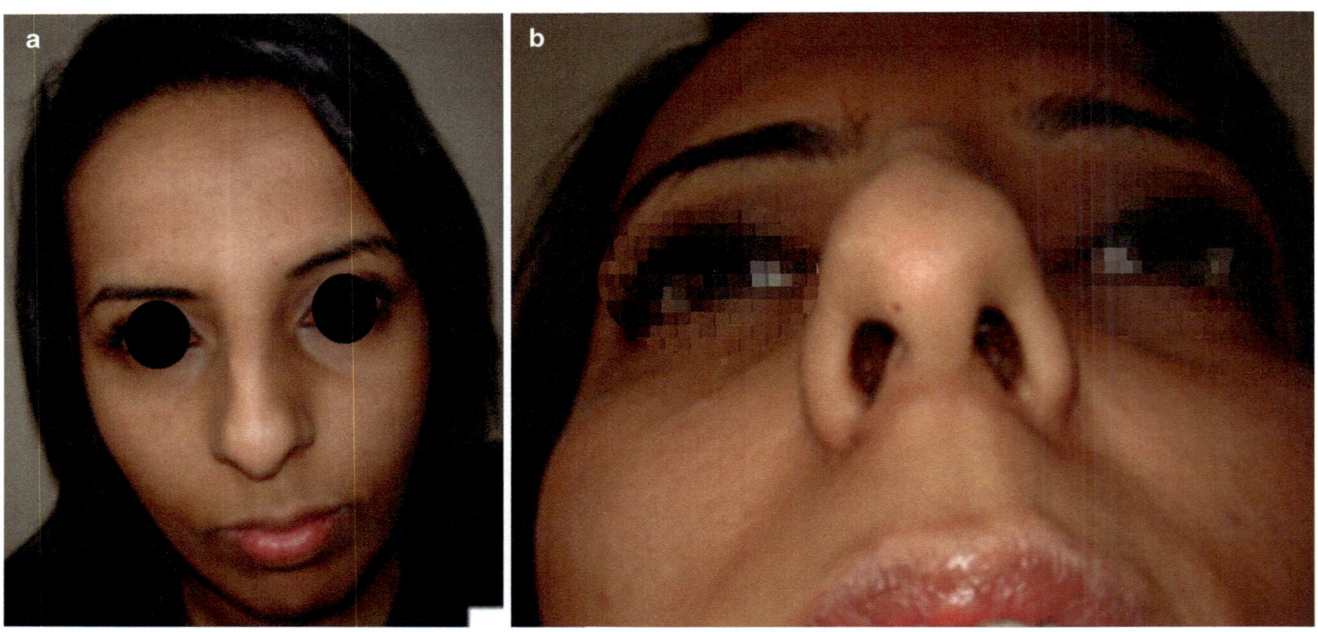




Fig. 38.28 (**a**, **b**) Wide nasal tip clinical

blanching of the tip skin with exposure to cold, contour irregularities of the underlying cartilage to become visible and may also lead to the skin pores communicating to the underlying tissues.

#### 38.5.4.3 Overprojected Nasal Tip (Fig. 38.30a–c)

Nasal projection is defined as the distance along a perpendicular line from the vertical facial plane to the anterior most point on the nasal tip. The nose when not in normal facial balance can either be overprojected or underprojected.

The key to correction of the overprojected nasal tip is to establish the cause. This may be due to the increased length of the anterior nasal spine, excess caudal septal height or overtly long alar cartilages.

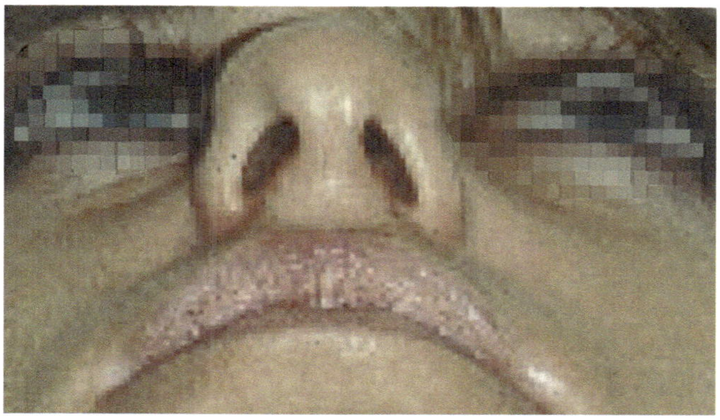

©Association of Oral and Maxillofacial Surgeons of India

Fig. 38.29 Bulbous tip clinical

**Surgical management**

Surgery for the overprojected nose should be performed through a full bilateral septal transfixion incision with the aim of deprojecting the nose by 4–5 mm. The anterior nasal spine is reduced judiciously followed by the resuspension of the upper lip to the ANS. The anterior septal angle is lowered to achieve further deprojection. Deformities of the alar cartilage may be varied and may require division and overlap of the medial crura, division or resection of the medial footplates. A lateral crural overlap with resection of a segment is performed 1 cm from the dome. Domal resections are to be avoided as they may produce secondary deformities: irregularities, angulation, and bossa formation. They may produce a sharp angulation with a pointed tip (pinched nose), which may require a shield graft for tip camouflage. Care should be taken to avoid/prevent loss of tip support during these manoeuvres.

#### 38.5.4.4 Underprojected Tip (Fig. 38.31a, b)

It is important to establish the cause for underprojection prior to treatment. Causes of underprojection may include

- Short medial crura (short columella)
- Underdeveloped lower lateral cartilages e.g. binders
- Deficient height of caudal septum

Fig. 38.30 Overprojected nasal tip (**a**) profile of patient 1, (**b**) profile of paitent 2 at repose and (**c**) profile of patient 2, smiling

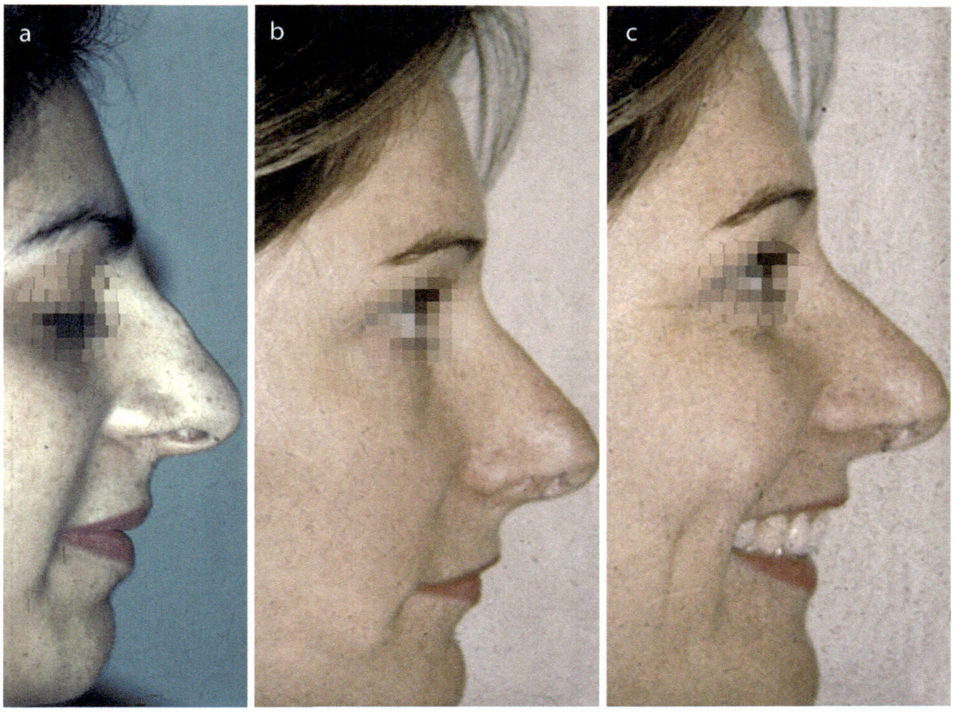


©Association of Oral and Maxillofacial Surgeons of India

- Deficient or absent anterior nasal spine/premaxilla
- Bilateral cleft lip nose

**Surgical management**

Surgery for the underprojected nose should follow the sequence provided below: the columella is strengthened with a strut graft, a transdomal suture is placed to project the dome. A shield, cap or an umbrella graft may be used to increase tip projection. A caudal septal extension graft is added to strengthen the septal support and increase projection. Finally, a transcolumellar suture is performed through the medial foot-plates. In patients with the deficiency of the premaxilla or the total bony maxilla (cleft maxillary hypoplasia) where loss of bone support contributes to the loss of nasal projection, advancement of the maxilla or Onlay grafting of the premaxillary segment may offer the correct solutions.

#### 38.5.4.5 Over-Rotated Tip (Piggy Nose) (Fig. 38.32b)

Tip rotation denotes the angle formed by the columella to the upper lip. The point of reference here is the nasolabial angle. Deformities of the nasal tip related to the rotation can be either over-rotation or under-rotation (ptotic nose).

Over-rotation of the nose may arise due to various causes: post-traumatic (caudocephalic impact to the nose) or an inherently short nose. Over-rotation may also be a complication of prior rhinoplastic procedures due to overzealous caudal septal reduction, excessive cephalic trim of the lateral crura or injudicious lowering of the anterior septal angle.

**Surgical management**

Surgery for the correction of over-rotation of the nasal tip should include techniques for de-rotation of the nose like placement of a caudal septal extension graft and/or extension of the dorsal graft beyond the domes. These procedures require extensive cartilage grafting to lengthen the shortened nose.

#### 38.5.4.6 Under-Rotated Tip (Ptotic Nasal Tip) (Fig. 38.32a)

Under-rotation denotes cephalocaudal rotation of the nasal tip, which makes the tip point downward. This needs to be differentiated from an underprojected tip. However, occasionally both problems may co-exist. It is also important to identify the presence of pseudo-ptosis in which the tip is normal but a more prominent anterior septal angle makes the tip appear ptotic.

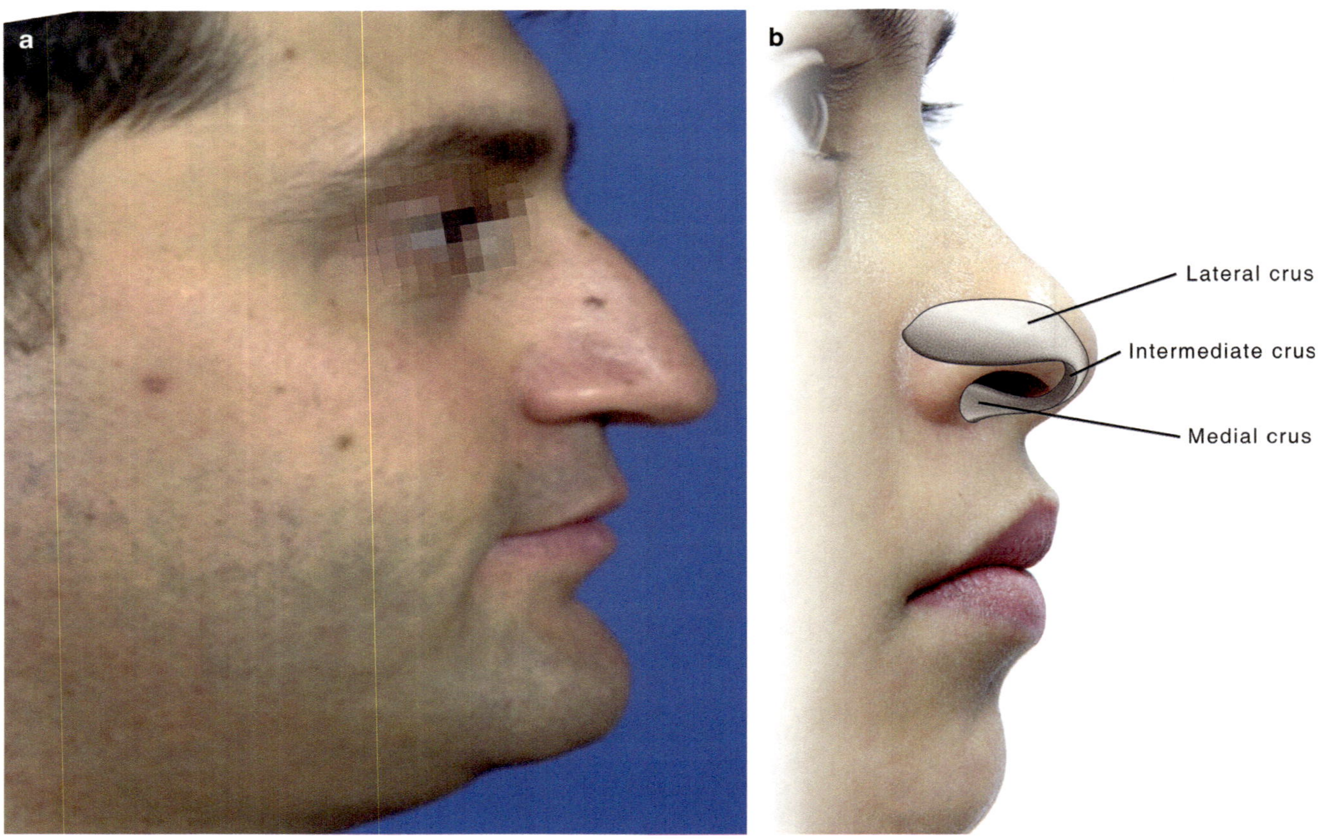




**Fig. 38.31** Underprojected tip. (**a**) Clinical picture and (**b**) diagrammatic representation

Ptotic tips need to be examined both at rest and dynamically. The dynamic inferior movement of the nasal tip may occur due to the downward pull of a strong depressor septi muscle. Care should also be taken to look for any other associated deformities.

Causes for an under-rotated or ptotic tip may be hereditary as in the noses of people from the Mediterranean countries, developmental due to heavy SSTE and weak cartilages or the presence of excessive skin in the membranous columella. Patients with bilateral cleft lip deformities are predisposed to have underprojected and under-rotated noses due to columellar deficiency.

Iatrogenic causes for tip ptosis include: poorly planned and executed septorhinoplasty with loss of septal support, inadequate maintenance of tip support or reattachment of the tip support structures. It may also be a complication following (1) prolonged intubation with the nasotracheal tube not anchored well and (2) tumour ablations with inadequate reconstruction.

**Surgical management**

Correction of the ptotic tip should be based on the anatomy involved. It is best to follow an algorithm for planning the surgical procedure. The structures contributing will enable us to plan and perform the correct procedure.

- An elongated septum producing the ptosis is corrected by a wedge excision of the excessive septum and the overlying mucosa (Fred technique).
- Elongated lower lateral cartilages can be managed by two methods depending on the tip projection; in underprojected tips, a columellar strut is provided for enhancing support and augmented with the tip rotation suture, while in the case of an overprojected tip, transection of the LLC is performed with overlapping and suturing. The tip rotation suture may be optional depending on the clinical indication.
- In the case of a shortened medial crura, a columellar strut or a medial crural anchor suture is placed with the tip rotation suture again being optional.

### 38.5.5 Managing the Wide Ala

The normal width of the ala falls within or just beyond an imaginary vertical line dropped from the medial canthus to the upper lip. The ala may be either narrow or wide. A wide

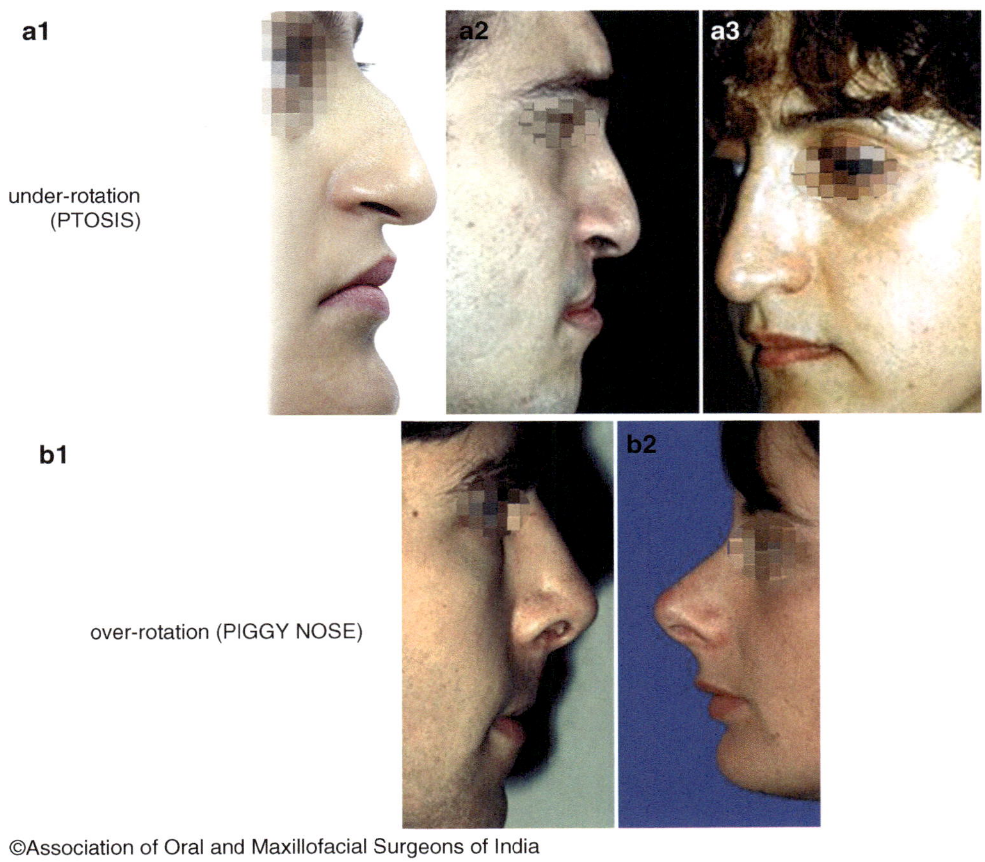


**Fig. 38.32** Nasal tip rotations clinical. (**a1**, **a2**, **a3**) Under-rotation of tip and (**b1**, **b2**) Over-rotation of tip

ala compromises facial aesthetics and is often a complaint for which the patient seeks help.

#### 38.5.5.1 Causes of Variations in Alar Base Width

A wide alar base may be a characteristic of racial variations, for example, African and Asian races exhibit increased width of the alar base. It may also be wide in patients with congenital anomalies like cleft lip and palate. Wide alar base may also be due to iatrogenic causes like

1. after a Le Fort 1 maxillary advancement or impaction surgery,
2. injudicious rhinoplasty with loss of tip projection due to loss of septal support

#### 38.5.5.2 Clinical Features

Patients with a wide alar base exhibit a nose that looks flat and broad; the alar columellar line may be straight and they may have an associated wide nasal tip. In the basal view, the nose presents with reduced tip projection and short or distorted columella. The alar side walls show increased bulk and increased flare, and the alar insertion into the nasolabial area may be horizontal or oblique. The alar sill width may also show an increase. The premaxillary base that supports the alar complex may be normal, deficient or asymmetric.

#### 38.5.5.3 Evaluation

The nose should be evaluated for the cause of alar widening. This is the basis on which the treatment may be planned. When there is a doubt regarding the width of the ala, it may be wise to abandon the idea during a primary rhinoplasty and perform the alar correction as an isolated secondary procedure.

#### 38.5.5.4 Surgical Treatment (Fig. 38.33a, b)

Surgery for the wide ala needs to be sequenced after assessment of the cause; this may be a wide ala demonstrating

1. significant flaring,
2. flaring with increased sill width,
3. rarely isolated increase of sill width and
4. presence of a lateral insertion of ala on the face.

- The treatment of choice for the flaring ala is wedge excision (Weir) (Fig. 38.34), which helps to preserve the natural contour of the ala as well as provide a good camouflage

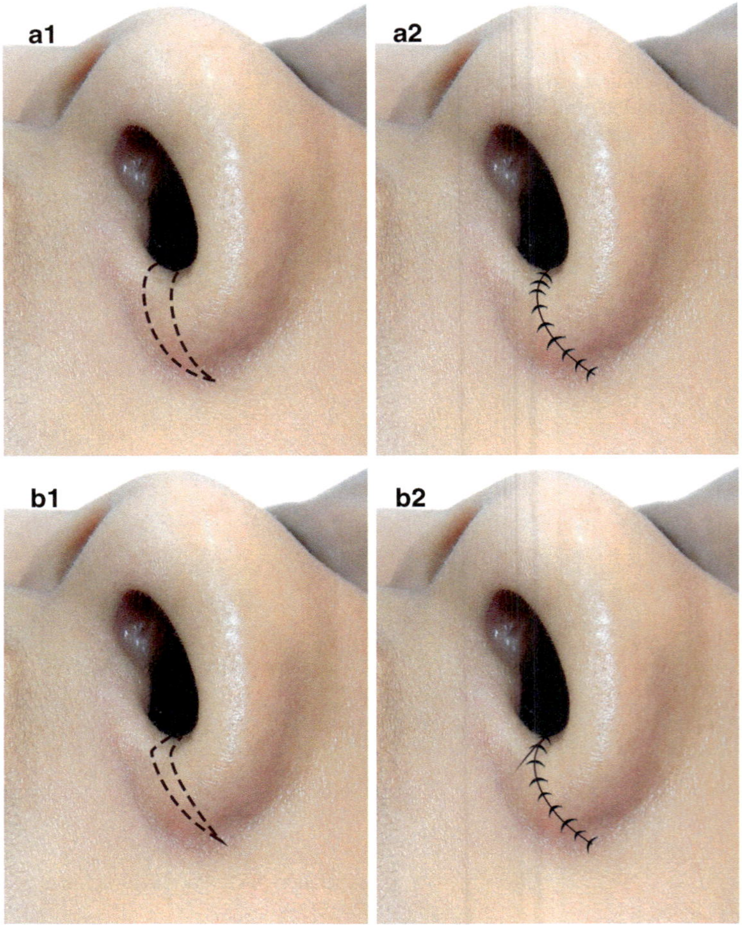




**Fig. 38.33** Wide ala surgery techniques. (**a**) Traditional Weir excision (leaves a notch deformity) and (**b**) modified excision incorporating a lateral advancement which prevents notch deformity and restores continuity of alar rim

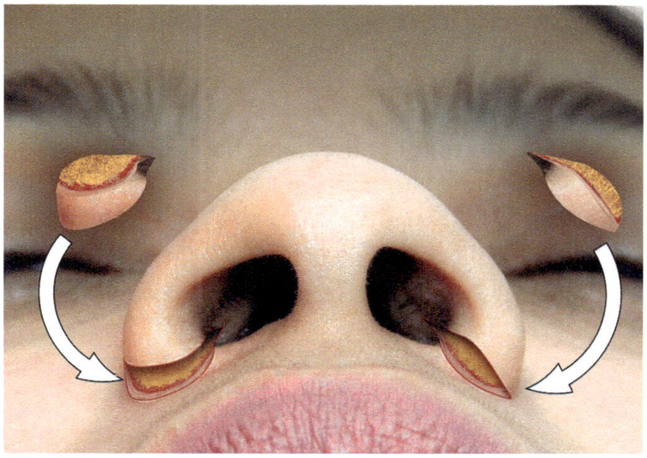



Fig. 38.34 Wedge technique for alar base reduction

of the scar. A medial flap excision technique as described by Sheen may also be a good alternative to this. The decision regarding medial repositioning of the alar base should be in accordance with Sheen, who recommends it only in cases of extreme lateral divergence.

- When flaring is associated with a wide sill then a wedge with a sill excision may be preferred to correct the deformity. In rare instances an isolated sill excision may be indicated for a problem of increased sill width alone.
- When the nose demonstrates a lateral insertion of the alar base on to the face, then a "V to Y" plasty is performed as described by Bernstein, which helps relocate the alar base medially.

## 38.5.6 Septal Perforations

Septal perforations are pathological defects in the nasal septum which form communications between the right and the left sides of the nasal cavity. These may present as anterior, mid-septal or posterior perforations (Fig. 38.35a, b).

The most common aetiological factors producing septal perforations are

1. Cocaine misuse
2. Trauma to the face and nose—e.g. NOE fractures
3. Iatrogenic—injudicious septal surgery or poor techniques during septorhinoplasty
4. Self induced—obsessional nasal toileting or habitual nose picking
5. Granulomatous diseases
6. Malignancy

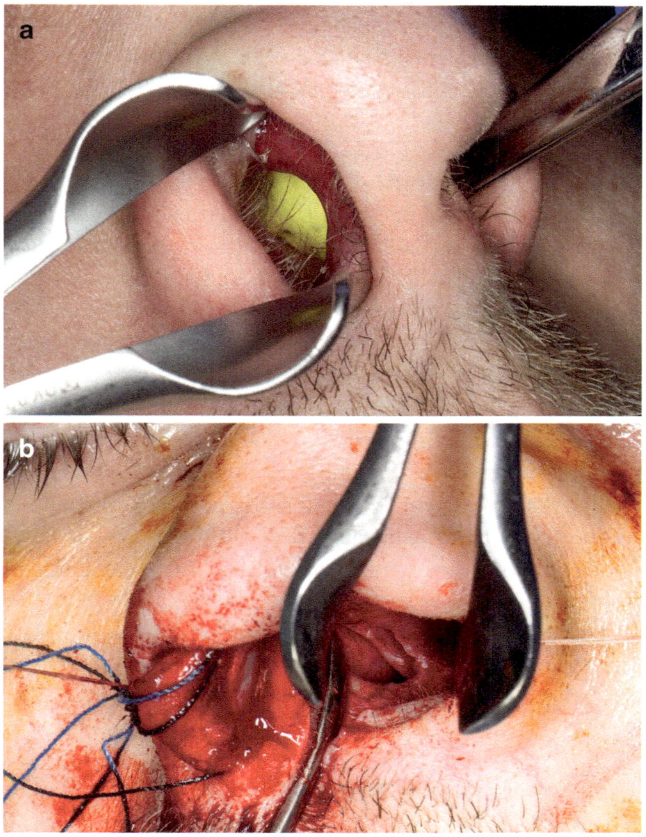



Fig. 38.35 Septal perforation; (**a**) clinical presentation, (**b**) intra-operative picture

### 38.5.6.1 Clinical Features

The occurrence of septal perforations also leads to a variety of sequelae that produce secondary deformities of not only the nose but also significantly affect the face and the oral structures. The nose may show a saddle deformity, columellar retraction and narrowing of the nasal valve. Furthermore, the loss of nasal cartilage and bony framework may lead to a concertina deformity of the skin envelope. Perforations may expand in an inferior direction with associated necrosis of the vomer and maxillary crest, thus causing a palatal fistula. Other symptoms include nasal airway block, nasal discharge, crusting, epistaxis, midfacial pain, and a characteristic whistling noise.

### 38.5.6.2 Investigations

Investigations for perforations of the nasal septum include a thorough clinical evaluation of the nasal cavity, oral cavity and the face for accurate diagnosis. The patient is also subjected to a rhinoscopy and a nasendoscopy for assessment of the intranasal deformity. This is followed by a biopsy from the margins of the perforation. A swab may also be performed for culture and sensitivity when there are signs of acute infection of the region.

#### 38.5.6.3 Treatment

Treatment is initiated in a conservative form with counselling, wound care and topical medication. This involves abstinence from cocaine use with rehabilitation under supervised care. Regular inspection of the nasal cavity and nasal toileting with seawater douches. Topical administration of Naseptin cream alternating every 2 weeks with Bactroban (Mupirocin) ointment is mandatory prior to surgical intervention.

Surgical management (Fig. 38.36a, b, c) for septal perforations is extremely challenging and often give disappointing results. Any treatment is bound to be compromised due to resurgence of the cocaine addiction and poor vascular status of the involved anatomy resulting in a high incidence of residual defects after surgery.

There are also risks of total failure of procedures with secondary donor site deformities, adding to the post-surgical morbidity in these patients.

### 38.5.7 Nasal Valve Problems

To understand the problems associated with the nasal valve, it is important to see the distinction between the "nasal valve area" or the internal nasal valve, the "nasal valve" and the external nasal valve: The nasal valve area is the empty triangular space that is bounded medially by the nasal septum, laterally and superiorly by the caudal margin of the upper lateral cartilage and its attachment to the pyriform rim and inferiorly by the bony nasal floor. The nasal valve specifically denotes the slit that is seen between the caudal end of the upper lateral cartilage and the nasal septum. Physiologically, the internal nasal valve is the area offering the highest resistance to airflow, and any deformities of this region may compromise the air-flow dynamics.

#### 38.5.7.1 Anatomy of the Nasal Valves

The components of internal and external valves are projected in Box 38.10.

The aetiology of nasal valve problems are enumerated in Table 38.4.

**Box 38.10. Components of nasal valves**

| Components of the external nasal valve | Components of the internal nasal valve |
|---|---|
| • Alar rim and alar side wall<br>• Columella<br>• Caudal septal margin<br>• Nasal sill | • Caudal septum<br>• Caudal margin of the upper lateral cartilage<br>• Floor of the nose<br>• Head of the inferior turbinate |

**Table 38.4** Etiology of nasal valve problems

| External nasal valve | Internal nasal valve |
|---|---|
| • Inherently weak alar sidewall (collapsing on inspiration)<br>• Caudal septal deflection<br>• Deviated footplate of the medial crus<br>• Narrow/scarred nasal sill<br>• Wide columellar base<br>• Iatrogenic causes (knock-knee deformity of the alar sidewall due to excessive cephalic trim)<br>• Medialisation of lateral crus following domal suture | • Caudal septal deviation<br>• Mid-septal bulge impinging on the upper lateral cartilage<br>• Inferior turbinate hypertrophy<br>• Iatrogenic causes<br>– Misplaced intercartilagenous incisions<br>– Medialisation of the inferior turbinate due to an injudicious lateral osteotomy<br>– Narrowing of the middle vault due to closing of an open roof deformity |

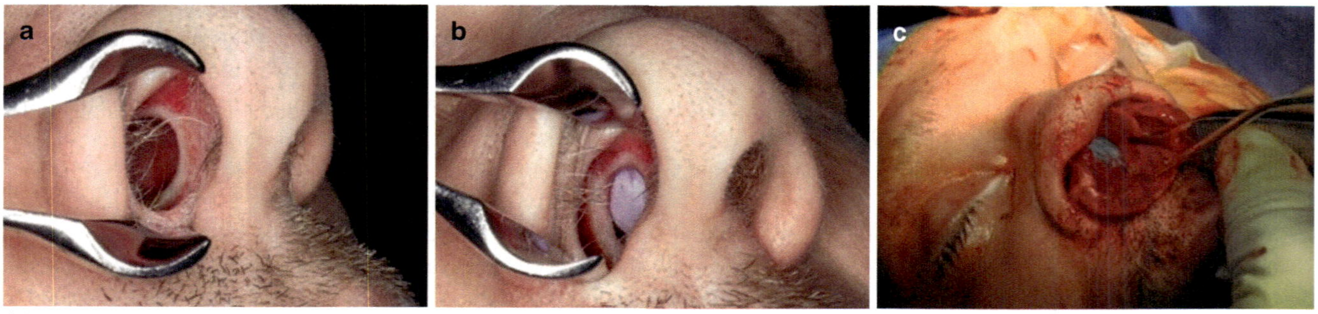




**Fig. 38.36** (a–c) Septal perforation surgical technique

#### 38.5.7.2 Clinical Examination of Nasal Valve Problems

It is extremely important to identify the exact location of the nasal obstruction to obtain the best surgical outcomes. This can be accomplished using

1. Clinical testing using "Cottle's sign"
2. Endonasal examination and rhinoscopy
3. Dynamic photographs or video recordings of the "external valve flutter"
4. Air-flow studies using CT scans and computer simulation models

#### 38.5.7.3 Surgical Management

Sequencing of treatment for the management of nasal valve problems should include certain empirical steps. The first step is to perform an optimal septoplasty to relocate the septum to the midline. This is followed by straightening and strengthening of the alar sidewall using alar batten grafts and rim grafts. Narrowing of the columellar base may be performed in cases of true columellar widening. Collapse of the nasal valve can be corrected by the use of spreader grafts that help in widening. In certain cases, there may be webbing or scarring along the nasal valve area. This may need a "Z" plasty for release and correction. Finally, judicious removal of the inferior turbinate may be contemplated in indicated patients after due consultation with the ENT surgeon.

## 38.6 Complications Following Rhinoplasty

A sequela may be defined as a natural consequence following a disease process or a surgical procedure while a complication implies undesirable sequelae or process following surgery.

This section with dwell on the common sequelae and complications that may occur following rhinoplasty and will help providing tips for reducing or preventing complications.

Common sequelae following rhinoplasty may be tabulated as early and late in Box 38.11.

**Box 38.11. Complications of Rhinoplasty**

| Early sequelae | Late sequelae |
|---|---|
| Swelling | Infra-orbital discoloration |
| Bruising | Loss of tip-lobule definition |
| Paraesthesia | Lateral shortening |
| Swelling of the tip and supratip area | False "polly-beak" deformity |

Most sequelae are self-limiting and may not require any active intervention. However, it is imperative to follow certain steps to minimise or avoid complications as discussed below.

The key to minimising or preventing unfavourable outcomes depends on proper case selection after a thorough evaluation of the patient both physically and psychologically (perceived complaint vs objective deformity). A good clinical examination should follow with optimal documentation (clinical analysis and photographs). The subsequent consultation should include obtaining informed consent from the patients after discussion of the indications and anticipated complications associated with the surgical procedure. It is important to understand our limitations and accept them while not refraining from seeking professional help/support when needed.

Complications in rhinoplasty may depend on the area of surgery and the procedure performed as indicated below:

1. *Complications associated with the nasal dorsum* include loss of dorsal height, concavity or saddle deformity (due to over-resection), residual hump, supratip prominence or a true "polly-beak" deformity due to under-resection. There may be bony or cartilaginous irregularities (inadequate removal). An open roof deformity may present if the nasal bones are not infractured after hump reduction. An incomplete lateral osteotomy may result in a lateral wall step deformity, while medialisation of the upper lateral cartilages may result in an inverted "v" deformity. Another complication is the appearance of a visible dorsal septal edge.
2. *Complication of tip deformities* may present as a "pinched tip" or a "knock-knee" alar deformity (over-resection of the lateral crus). It may also show tip changes like "button-tip" deformity, tip/domal asymmetry, supra-alar concavity or alar retraction. Loss of tip support produces ptosis of the tip, loss of tip projection may produce infratip slip below the anterior septal angle and excess resection of the caudal septum may lead to over-rotation of the tip complex.
3. *Alar base reduction complications* may include narrowing of the nostril circumference, which may contribute to increased nasal airway pressure. The surgery by itself may cause a web scar at the alar-facial junction. It may also result in distortion and secondary deformity of the nose, cheek and lips.
4. *Complications following septal surgery* include failure to straighten, midline deviation, tip deviation secondary to caudal septal displacement and septal collapse leading to a saddle nose deformity. The columella may develop retraction or scarring and rarely necrosis.

   The skin and soft tissue envelope may also show scarring, ischemia/discolouration and at times telangiectasia.

Management of complications may be necessary when the deformity is visible to both the surgeon and the patient. This necessitates revision or secondary surgery which may be indicated in about 5–8% of the patients. Even when indicated, it is better to wait for a year prior to attempting revisions or secondary interventions. This is to facilitate a careful assessment of long-term changes following the procedure and the final outcome prior to intervention.

## 38.7 Conclusion

Rhinoplasty in most realms is considered as the epitome of aesthetic surgical skill. This burdens the surgeon with the responsibility of performing the surgery with accurate planning and prediction of outcomes. It is also important for both the young surgeon and the patient to understand that the final outcome of the surgery is not in the immediate future but is a culmination of all the surgical manoeuvres and their response over a period of time. This is the same fact that makes rhinoplasty among the most difficult to master. Rhinoplasty has transgressed from the early procedures of sole nasal reduction to encompassing not only the aesthetics of the nasal complex but also improvement of the function and establishing a balance for today's patient. This chapter is aimed to provide the reader with the basics of surgical techniques. Perhaps, this is one surgical skill where the surgeon still holds all the cards while the others are losing the battle to technology.

## References


1. Oneal RM, Beil RJ. Surgical anatomy of the nose. Clin Plast Surg. 2010;37(2):191–211.
2. Lessard ML, Daniel RK. Surgical anatomy of septorhinoplasty. Arch Otolaryngol. 1985;111(1):25–9.
3. Gonzalez-Ulloa M, Castillo A, Stevens E, et al. Preliminary study of the total restoration of the facial skin. Plast Reconstr Surg (1946). 1954;13(3):151–61.
4. Letourneau A, Daniel RK. Superficial musculoaponeurotic system of the nose. Plast Reconstr Surg. 1988;82(1):48–57.
5. Wright WK. Surgery of the bony and cartilaginous dorsum. Otolaryngol Clin North Am. 1975;8(3):575–98.
6. Pitanguy I. Surgical importance of a dermocartilaginous ligament in bulbous noses. Plast Reconstr Surg. 1965;36:247–53.
7. Guyuron B. Soft tissue functional anatomy of the nose. Aesthetic Surg J. 2006;26(6):733–5.
8. Hollingshead WH, editor. Anatomy for surgeons, vol. 1. 3rd ed. Philadelphia, PA: Harper and Row; 1982.
9. Khan HA. Rhinoplasty: initial consultation and examination. Oral Maxillofac Surg Clin North Am. 2012;24(1):11–24. Review.
10. Patient assessment for Rhinoplasty. In: Guyuron B, editor. Rhinoplasty. Edinburgh: Elsevier/Saunders; 2012.
11. Guyuron B. Precision rhinoplasty. Part I: The role of life-size photographs and soft tissue cephalometric analysis. Plast Reconstr Surg. 1988;81(4):489–99.
12. Moscatiello F, Herrero J, González Ballester MÁ, Carreño Hernández E, Piombino P, Califano L. Preoperative digital three-dimensional planning for rhinoplasty. Aesthet Plast Surg. 2010;34:232–8.
13. Andre RF, Vuyk HD, Ahmed A, Graamans K, Nolst Trenite GJ. Correlation between subjective and objective evaluation of the nasal airway. A systematic review of the highest level of evidence. Clini Otolaryngol. 2009;34(6):518–25.
14. Sajjadian A, Naghshineh N, Rubinstein R. Current status of grafts and implants in rhinoplasty: Part II. Homologous grafts and allogenic implants. Plast Reconstr Surg. 2010;125(3):99e–109e.
15. Sajjadian A, Rubinstein R, Naghshineh N. Current status of grafts and implants in rhinoplasty: Part I. Autologous grafts. Plast Reconstr Surg. 2010;125(2):40–9.
16. Koehler J, McLain L. Grafting in cosmetic rhinoplasty. Oral Maxillofac Surg Clin North Am. 2012;24(1):59–66.
17. Jang YJ, Moon BJ. State of the art in augmentation rhinoplasty: implant or graft? Curr Opin Otolaryngol Head Neck Surg. 2012;20(4):280–6.
18. Wotman M, Kacker A. What are the indications for the use of computed tomography before septoplasty? Laryngoscope. 2016;126(6):1268–70.
19. Shah J, Roxbury CR, Sindwani R. Techniques in septoplasty: traditional versus endoscopic approaches. Otolaryngol Clin North Am. 2018;51(5):909–17.
20. Most SP, Rudy SF. Septoplasty: basic and advanced techniques. Facial Plast Surg Clin North Am. 2017;25(2):161–9.
21. VanKoevering KK, Rosko AJ, Moyer JS. Osteotomies demystified. Facial Plast Surg Clin North Am. 2017;25(2):201–10.
22. Wayne I. Osteotomies in rhinoplasty surgery. Curr Opin Otolaryngol Head Neck Surg. 2013;21(4):379–83.
23. Bohluli B, Moharamnejad N, Bayat M. Dorsal hump surgery and lateral osteotomy. Oral Maxillofac Surg Clin North Am. 2012 Feb;24(1):75–86.
24. Barrett DM, Casanueva F, Wang T. Understanding approaches to the dorsal hump. Facial Plast Surg. 2017;33(2):125–32.
25. Suh MK. Dorsal augmentation using autogenous tissues. Facial Plast Surg Clin North Am. 2018;26(3):295–310.
26. Kim CH, Park SC. Homologous tissue for dorsal augmentation. Facial Plast Surg Clin North Am. 2018;26(3):311–21.


## Additional Reading


Mladina R. The role of maxillar morphology in the development of pathological septal deformities. Rhinology. 1987;25(3):199–205.

# Part XIII

# Advances in Oral and Maxillofacial Surgery

# Lasers in Oral and Maxillofacial Surgery

# 39

Shravan Renapurkar and Robert A. Strauss

## 39.1 Introduction

The first successful demonstration of laser was performed by Maiman in 1960 who also predicted one of its uses to be in medical science [1, 2]. Decades after the first medical use in the oral cavity and face, lasers are not just an adjunctive tool today but are an integral part of an Oral and Maxillofacial Surgeon's (OMS) armamentarium. Although $CO_2$ laser has been the traditional workhorse for an OMS, advancement in the capabilities of $CO_2$ lasers, as well as the development of other types of lasers, has helped grow their utility. Increasing use of lasers in turn has created greater evidence of its efficacy and safety record. Use of lasers has not only added advantages to conventional OMS procedures, as opposed to a scalpel, it has also given rise to newer procedures, which were not possible with conventional tissue-cutting tools.

## 39.2 Laser Physics

Modern lasers are simple to use but a lack of knowledge on the physics of lasers, inadequate training and caution in handling lasers, can give rise to potential adverse outcomes and unwanted complications. The term "laser" stands for light amplification by stimulated emission of radiation and was first used by Gordon Gould in 1957 [3]. The laser, as opposed to a regular light source, is composed of monochromatic, coherent and collimated beams, which, when they strike a suitable target, create photoacoustic, photochemical, photoablative, and photothermal effects. Laser light energy can undergo absorption, reflection, transmission, and scattering based on the optical properties of the target tissue or matter. For surgeons, the most desirable action is absorption into the tissue, which creates the predictable photothermal outcome of coagulation and then vaporization of tissues [4].

The basic component of a laser unit includes a "laser cavity" where the laser beam is produced via the phenomenon of stimulated emission as postulated by Albert Einstein. The laser cavity is composed of an active medium, an excitation source acting as a pumping mechanism, and an optical resonator (Fig. 39.1). The active medium is the chemical (gas/liquid/solid) that the type of laser is named after and is the material that undergoes stimulated emission. The photons of energy produced are collimated and amplified to produce the laser beam, which is then delivered to the target tissues via an appropriate delivery mechanism, either a flexible fiberoptic system, semiflexible hollow waveguides, or articulated mirrored arms (Fig. 39.2a–c). Lenses focus the active laser beam to create a "focal point," the point at which the energy is condensed to the smallest area to create the maximum effect. Some fiberoptic laser systems utilize a quartz or sapphire crystal at the tip of the fiber to enable the beam to be absorbed by this crystal and allow contact with tissues at the tip of the fiber, while others are used in a noncontact mode. A laser beam is an electromagnetic beam of radiation, which can fall anywhere in the spectrum of visible or invisible light. Nd:YAG, $CO_2$, and erbium lasers fall into the infrared invisible spectrum; hence, they are often accompanied by a visible aiming beam, which helps the surgeon to know the point in the tissues where laser beam hits the target tissues. Aiming beams can be another low power laser or a regular light source [4] (Fig. 39.3).

The factors related to the use of lasers that are under control of the surgeon include the spot size, power, and time on target. The spot size of the laser is the width of the laser beam on target. At the focal point, the maximum energy is focused to produce the smallest spot size or the thinnest possible incision but to the greatest depth. When the tip of the laser delivery system is moved away from the tissues, the laser beam diverges causing a bigger spot size and the energy is then distributed over a larger area and the related depth is

S. Renapurkar (✉) · R. A. Strauss
Department of Oral and Maxillofacial Surgery, Virginia Commonwealth University Medical Center, Richmond, VA, USA
e-mail: srenapurkar@vcu.edu; rastrauss@vcu.edu


K. Bonanthaya et al. (eds.), *Oral and Maxillofacial Surgery for the Clinician*, https://doi.org/10.1007/978-981-15-1346-6_39

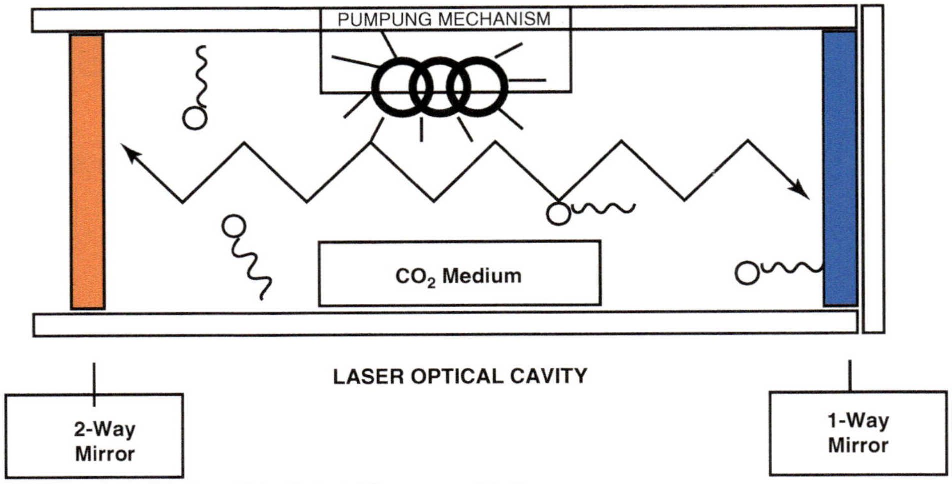


**Fig. 39.1** Components of laser tube

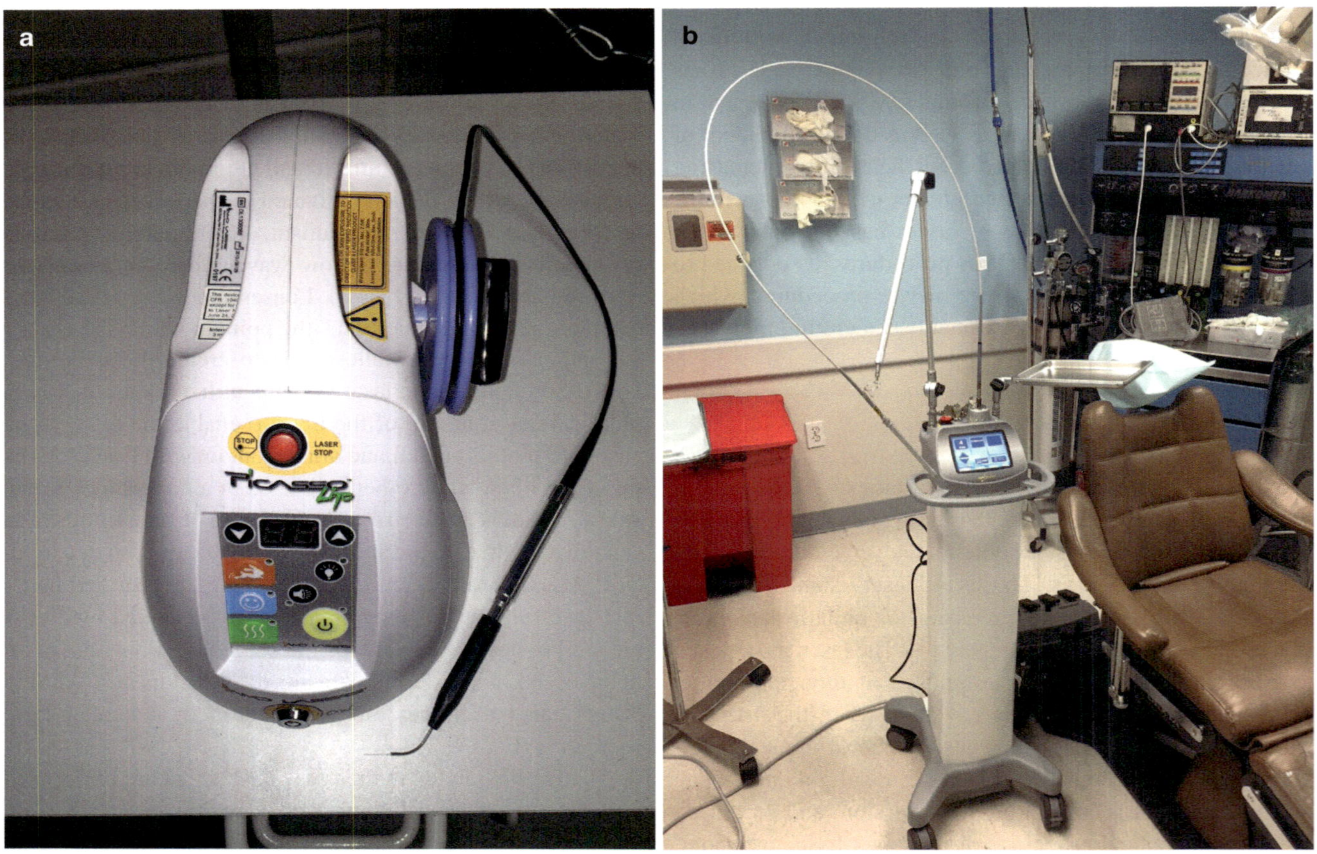


**Fig. 39.2** (**a**) Fiberoptic laser. (**b**) Hollow waveguide laser. (**c**) Articulated arm laser

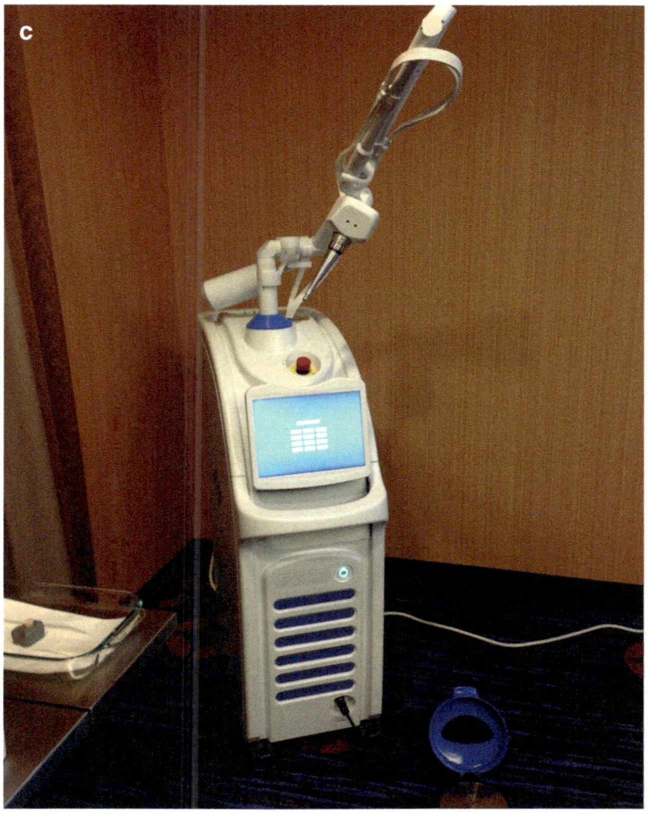


©Association of Oral and Maxillofacial Surgeons of India

Fig. 39.2 (continued)

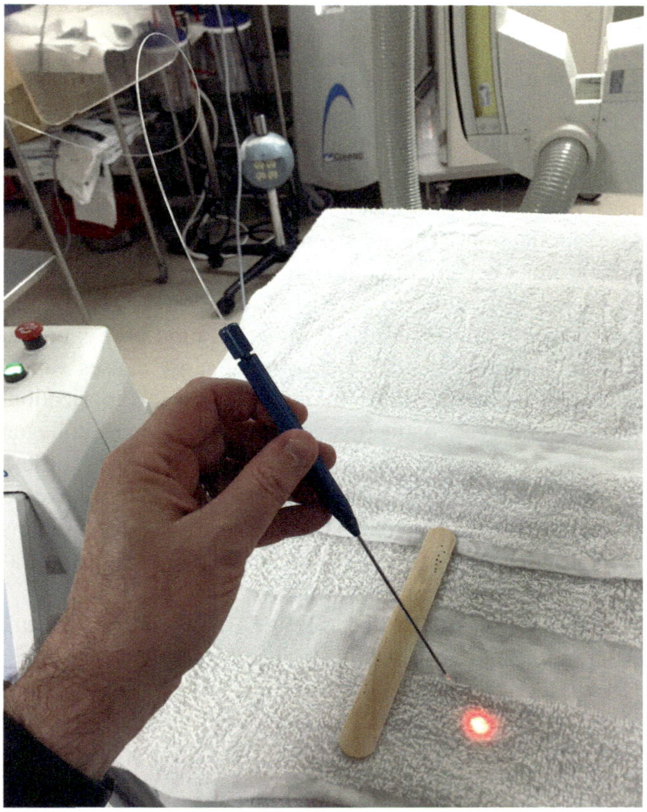

©Association of Oral and Maxillofacial Surgeons of India

Fig. 39.3 Low-level laser-aiming beam

decreased [5]. Laser emission modes and the surgeon's hand speed can affect the temperature rise and effect in the tissues. Lasers can be emitted in "continuous-wave" mode or in a "pulsed mode." Lasers used in pulsed mode allow time for tissues to cool before the next pulse of laser radiation is started while continuous wave mode of laser must be stopped manually to allow the tissues to cool. The time between pulses can help avoid thermal effects on surrounding tissues or excessive thermal effect on target tissues. The lasers with pulsed mode of emission can be of two types, "gated pulsed" or "true pulsed." True-pulsed lasers are pulsed by a mechanism within the laser cavity, while the gated-pulsed lasers have a shutter-like mechanism outside the laser cavity [4].

### 39.2.1 Advantages of Laser

Lasers have obvious advantages, which make them superior to conventional cutting tools. An ability to provide better hemostasis is a great advantage for surgeons to maintain visibility and reduce blood loss. Since spot size, power, and time on target are regulated by the surgeon, lasers provide better control of desired tissue changes, which enhances the precision of surgery. Increased precision of the depth of tissue damage along with fewer myofibroblasts in laser wounds compared to scalpel wounds, allow for improved tissue healing and decreased scarring. The mentioned advantages are presumed to decrease postoperative pain with the use of lasers, although the pathophysiology for this effect is not well understood.

### 39.2.2 Disadvantages of Laser

Despite several advantages of lasers in surgery, the provider should make sure the benefits outweigh the risks and disadvantages. Hard-tissue lasers such as Er:YAG and Er:CR:YSGG do not match the speed of bone or tooth cutting as do conventional tools such as burs or saws. Soft-tissue healing after laser-assisted incision or excision is slower (although with decreased scarring) than tissue healing using scalpels. The associated learning curve and costs of the laser equipment add to the drawbacks of using lasers.

## 39.3 Selection of Lasers

The type of laser to be used is based on the laser's physical characteristics, interaction with the target tissues, and the goals of the procedure. For example, $CO_2$ laser's excellent affinity for water, which is the main component of soft tissues, makes it the most widely used laser for soft-tissue surgical applications. The most commonly used $CO_2$ laser is the 10,600-nm wavelength, although 9600-nm and other wavelength variants of this laser exist. The $CO_2$ laser is currently the most ideal laser used for most intraoral and extraoral soft-tissue procedures. The absorbed energy causes vaporization of the intracellular fluid causing tissue vaporization, while lateral heat conduction causes contraction of collagen and closure of blood vessels of approximately 500 μ or less in diameter. High-power $CO_2$ lasers are generally delivered via articulating arms, but new hollow waveguide systems suitable for office use provide increased accessibility intraorally along with their ease of use [6, 7].

Other lasers include the Nd:YAG (a crystal of Ytrrium, Aluminum, and Garnet doped with the rare earth element Neodymium) laser, which functions in the near-infrared electromagnetic spectrum at 1064 nm, and has minimal water and superficial tissue absorption leading to deeper tissue penetration. Hence, the Nd:YAG can be used for coagulation of deeper and larger (2–3 mm) diameter vessels. These qualities of Nd:YAG have led to its use in treating angiomatous or vascular tissue lesions, although this same lack of water absorption limits its utility for the OMS. Depending on the desired effect, the Nd:YAG laser can be used both in contact and noncontact modes [8–10].

The Er:YAG laser works at a 2940-nm wavelength and is even more highly absorbed in water than the $CO_2$ laser leading to rapid absorption by the superficial layers of tissue and minimal penetration. This can be an advantage in some cases but also means that this laser is less effective on tissue than the $CO_2$ laser. As an example, when used for cosmetic skin resurfacing it shows much more superficial effects, which heal quite quickly, but also shows much less of a result than $CO_2$ laser does. For this reason, it has fallen somewhat out of favor for this purpose [11–15]. Owing to limitation of its thermal effects mostly in superficial layers of soft and hard tissue, Er:YAG laser has become popular in implant dentistry. It can be used on both soft and hard tissues and finds its application in bone preparation, second-stage surgery, treatment of peri-implantitis. Being reflected off the surface, it has minimal or no apparent adverse effects on dental implants [16].

The Holmium:YAG laser is generated at a 2100-nm wavelength, which enables it to be delivered in contact mode via fiberoptic cable also demonstrates very little water absorption but is well absorbed by other tissue components [17]. This allows it to be transmitted through water-rich environments while having similar tissue effects as the $CO_2$. Minimal lateral thermal damage, precise depth of cut, and good coagulation combined with its ability to be used in presence of saline/lactated Ringer's solution makes it the preferred laser for operative TMJ arthroscopy [18].

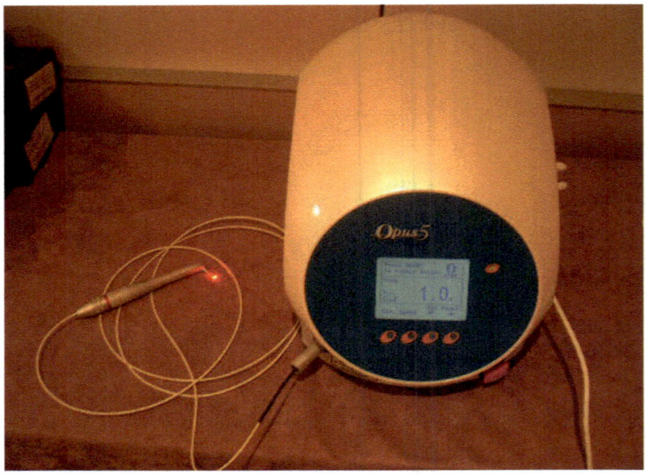


©Association of Oral and Maxillofacial Surgeons of India

**Fig. 39.4** Diode laser

Diode lasers at wavelengths between 805 and 980 nm have been reported to be compact, inexpensive, and easy to use in OMS procedures (Fig. 39.4). These can be used in continuous or pulse modes with contact or noncontact handpieces. However, it should be understood that these wavelengths are not well absorbed by soft tissues (although pigmented tissue will absorb it the most), the use of this laser wavelength would lead to very limited effects on surface tissue and very deep, poorly controlled, and undesirable tissue penetration. This is bypassed by using a material on the tip of the fiber that absorbs these wavelengths (either pigmented material such as ink paper or a suitable crystal material) and creates a red hot thermal tip, which is then used in surgery. In reality, the laser wavelength produced is not actually used for surgery; it is only absorbed by the fiber tip to essentially produce a thermal cautery. Although diodes are cheap and easy to use due to their fiberoptic contact tip, this thermal cautery effect rather than the use of the actual laser beam is very inefficient for surgery and severely limits its use by the OMS [19].

## 39.4 Applications of Lasers in Oral and Maxillofacial Surgery

Three basic categories of application of lasers in OMS can be classified as follows:

1. Incisional/excisional procedures
2. Vaporization (tissue ablation)-based procedures
3. Surgical hemostasis

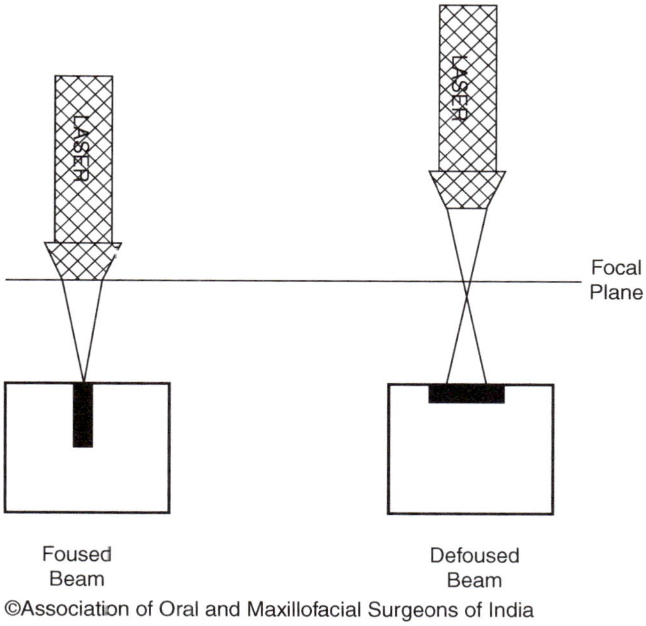


**Fig. 39.5** Focused vs. defocused beam

Incisional procedures require a precise thin cut with careful control of the depth of the cut. The thickness or thinness of the cut with a laser is controlled by the spot size (usually 0.1–0.4 mm). The laser beam's focal length is usually between 1 mm and 1 cm, depending on the delivery system, and is where the smallest spot size can be achieved with maximum power density. This is called "focused mode" (Fig. 39.5). The laser can be controlled by a foot pedal, but it is often useful to limit time on tissue to speeds faster than a foot control allows. Hence, a "gated/pulsed mode" can be used to generate 2–20 pulses per second to create or mark a dotted outline with lesser depth and allow careful delineation of the margins of the excision. This is then followed by a continuous mode (using the foot pedal) to "connect the dots" and complete the excision. The settings to obtain a desired depth of cut vary from one tissue to another due their different water content and absorption coupled with the surgeon-controlled factors as mentioned earlier. It is not possible to have standard laser parameters for all types of tissues or lesions. The smallest spot size possible with 4–10 W power can be a good initial setting. The initial cut then gives the surgeon ability to observe the clinical effect and depth of incision, which then can be used to lead to adjustments of the power and time on target to achieve the desired changes. Common soft-tissue lesions that can be incised or excised using lasers include fibromas, mucoceles, epulis fissuratum, mucosal or gingival lesions, papillomas, etc. Wound closure after a laser-assisted incisional biopsy or excisional procedure is often unnecessary due to the limited scarring and excellent hemostasis and is up to the surgeon's discretion, as healing is excellent regardless of closure. Closure does not usually effect hemostasis or pain relief (Fig. 39.6a–c) [5].

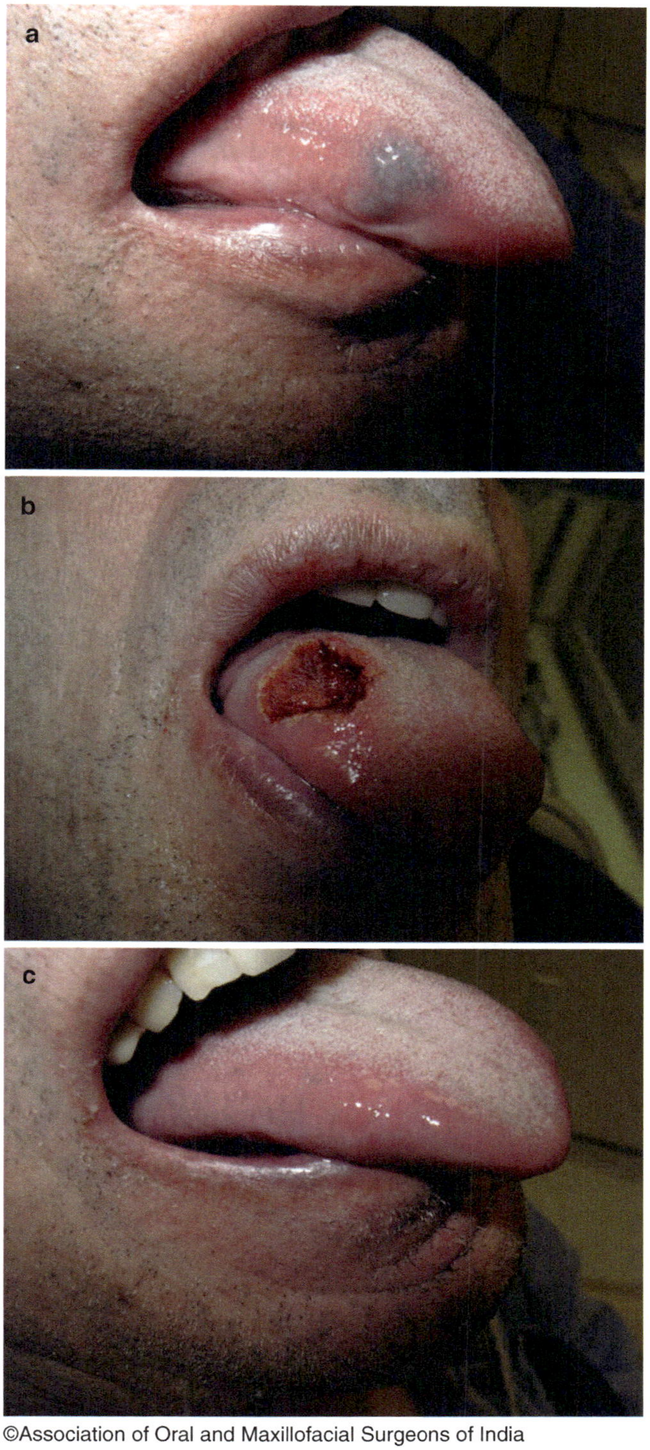


**Fig. 39.6** (**a**) Lesion of tongue. (**b**) Tongue after laser excision with no closure. (**c**) Excellent healing

Ablative or vaporization procedures are done when the surgeon wants to remove only a superficial layer of the tissue. Lasers, cryotherapy, chemical peeling, and scalpel can be used for this purpose, but the precision of cut and control of the depth of tissue changes along with excellent hemostasis make lasers the preferred tool for vaporization procedures. Lasers, when used for vaporization procedures, are used defocused so as to decrease the power density (the energy per unit area) and limit the depth of effect while increasing the area of the tissue ablation. The spot size used for vaporization ranges from 1.5 to 3 mm and allows large surface areas to be removed very superficially (literally cell layers at a time if desired). This is ideal for large but flat and superficial lesions such as hyperkeratosis, dysplasia, lichen planus, etc. The laser is again used in gated mode to carefully and precisely outline the margins. This is followed by passing the laser in overlapping "U"-shaped patterns to cover the entire area. The parameters can be adjusted by the surgeon, just as in incision cases, after the first pass is done at 4–10 W power. As implied by vaporization, there is no tissue available for biopsy in these cases. Hence, a definitive diagnosis should be established prior to performing ablative or vaporization procedures on mucosal lesions (Fig. 39.7a–c).

Due to the ability of $CO_2$ lasers to constrict blood vessels rather than coagulate blood, it can be an excellent tool to obtain hemostasis in most surgical wounds where the vessels are smaller than the thermal effect of the laser in tissue (about 500 μ). The lateral thermal effect of the laser beam should be equal to or greater than the diameter of the bleeding vessels. If the vessel is of larger diameter, conventional hemostatic techniques should be used. For small superficial vascular lesions, the $CO_2$ laser can be used to excise the lesion (since the feeding vessels are usually smaller than 500 μ), while deeper or larger vascular lesions are best treated using lasers that are specifically absorbed by hemoglobin, leading to true coagulation of the lesion itself [6].

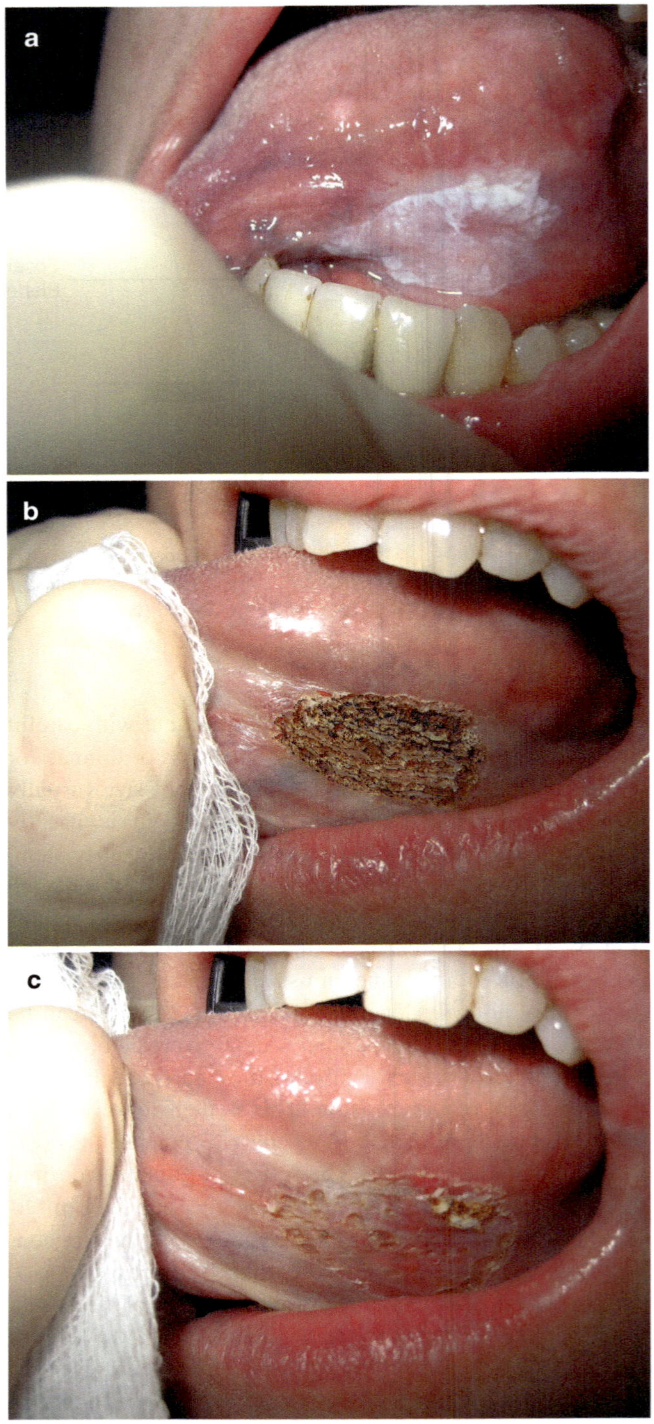




**Fig. 39.7** (**a**) Hyperkeratosis of lateral tongue. (**b**) Laser ablation of tongue. (**c**) Healing after laser ablation

## 39.5 Specific Examples of Application of Lasers in Oral and Maxillofacial Surgery

1. ***Cosmetic facial surgery:***

   The use of lasers in cosmetic surgery has changed these procedures significantly over the years. The advantages of lasers as previously described, including the capability of lasers to only affect the superficial layers of skin with precise depth control, turned out to be its critical advantage. Lasers in cosmetic facial surgery can be used both for incisional or ablation procedures based on indication [20].

   Lasers used for laser skin resurfacing (removal of superficial skin wrinkles from the face) are an example of ablation or vaporization procedure. In skin resurfacing procedures, the superficial layers of the epidermis and papillary dermis are removed while leaving behind the reticular layer of the dermis with its adnexal structures. This layer, if intact, provides epithelial cells that are required for rapid re-epithelialization of skin in a uniform

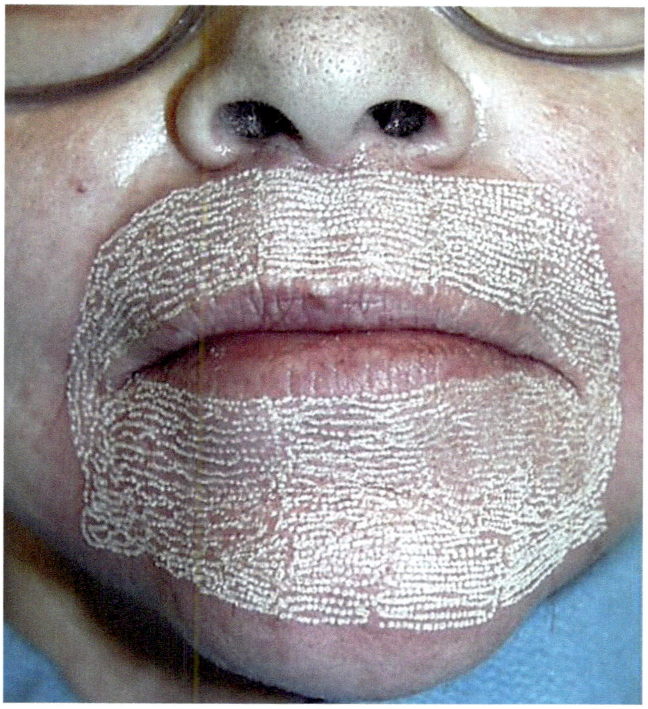



Fig. 39.8 Laser cosmetic skin resurfacing of face

manner. As opposed to chemical peels or dermabrasion, lasers offer more precise depth control, which is crucial in uniform healing and improved outcomes. $CO_2$ and the Er:YAG are the commonly used lasers for skin resurfacing, although recent improvements in the way $CO_2$ is used to improve results with lessened postoperative healing time, have severely diminished the use of the Er:YAG. Although the $CO_2$ laser is most commonly used and is more effective, it can be associated with long-term erythema and greater risk of scarring if exposure is done too deeply. Since $CO_2$ is a continuous-wave beam, which means that even at a short "pulse" the laser would be on tissue too long and lead to scarring, it must be electronically "pseudopulsed" at high powers to obtain the short times needed to reduce risk from lateral thermal damage to the unintended underlying dermis (roughly less than 1000 μs). On the contrary, the Er:YAG laser has less penetration in skin owing to its higher affinity to water in tissue. It is also a true pulsed laser and hence it allows higher power with shorter pulse duration. Although this is an advantage of Er:YAG laser, which helps reduce risk of excessive ablation and scarring, as mentioned before, it also decreases the effectiveness and results of the Er:YAG laser and most surgeons have abandoned its use in favor of newer $CO_2$ lasers that create very deep but thin vertical columns in the skin, allowing for tissue contraction with quick healing and less chance of scarring [21].

In skin resurfacing, as opposed to ablation of intraoral mucosal pathology, the passes of laser should not be overlapping to avoid excessive tissue ablation (Fig. 39.8). Computer pattern generator handpieces (CPG) can be used, which automatically create a uniform pattern of coverage on the skin (Fig. 39.9a, b) [22].

Skin resurfacing principles are also used in scar revision procedures. The prominence or visibility of a scar is mainly affected by the surface depression or elevation. The $CO_2$ and Er:YAG lasers can be used to reduce the elevation of the scar tissue or decrease the elevation of the surrounding skin to make a depressed scar tissue blend well with it (Fig. 39.10a–c). Healing scars can also have hypervascularity as evidence by prolonged erythema. This can be managed by decreasing the vascularity within the scar by use of vascular-specific lasers such as 532-nm KTP:YAG or Pulsed Dye Lasers (PDL) lasers [23].

In blepharoplasty, the $CO_2$ laser can be used to make a transconjunctival incision on the lower eyelid as well as the skin incision for the upper eyelid blepharoplasty. The use of laser to then excise muscle or fat with excellent hemostasis provides great visualization and tissue control (Fig. 39.11).

In endoscopic brow lift techniques, lasers are passed through either flexible fiberoptic cables or through small diameter hollow waveguide extensions in order to be used for incisions made within the optic cavity. The advantage of using lasers in endoscopic procedures is to provide precise incisions with excellent hemostasis, which aids in better visualization. Laser is used to incise the periosteum and/or muscle attachments. $CO_2$ laser is a commonly used laser for this purpose.

2. ***Intraoral mucosal surgery:***

Lasers have been extensively used in intraoral mucosal surgeries. Common applications include incisional/excisional biopsy of intraoral soft-tissue lesions (Fig. 39.12a–c), frenectomy (Fig. 39.13a, b), ablation of premalignant lesions, preprosthetic procedures such as vestibuloplasty and excision of epulis fissuratum (Fig. 39.14a–d). As mentioned previously in this chapter, advantages of lasers stand superior compared to traditional scalpels in terms of wound healing, tissue handling, and hemostasis, which ultimately help improve patient experience when used for intraoral procedures as well. Vaporization or ablation of tissues intraorally is usually performed on premalignant lesions, commonly for white lesions such as hyperkeratosis or mild epithelial dysplasia. More severe dysplasias are best excised with the laser to allow for margin control. Definitive diagnosis with the help of a biopsy is a precursor for management of premalignant lesions with laser vaporization since there will be no specimen to biopsy [24].

Although diode, ND:YAG, Er:YAG and $CO_2$ lasers can be used for intraoral mucosal surgeries $CO_2$ lasers stand out as the workhorse and most studied laser over the

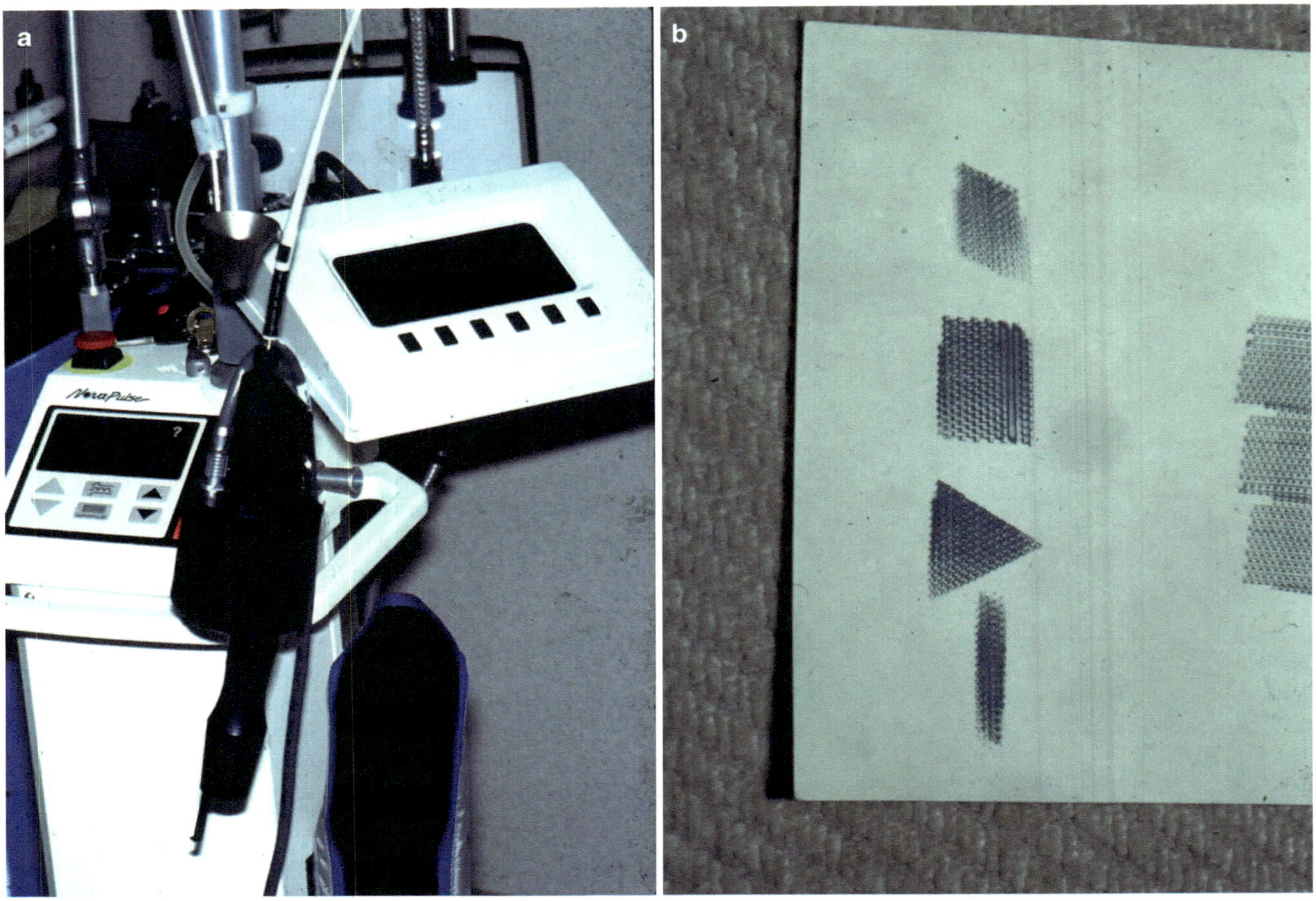




**Fig. 39.9** (**a**) Computerized pattern generator (CPG) for laser skin resurfacing. (**b**) Optional patterns for CPG

past four decades. When using lasers intraorally on intended soft tissues, care must be exercised to protect adjacent hard/soft tissue from inadvertent damage or devitalization due to pulpal damage. This is done with either a moist gauze, a mouth guard, a wet tongue blade, or nonreflective plastic instrumentation [25]. The use of lasers as compared to scalpel is presumed to also provide a decreased chance for lymphatic and hematogenous seeding as an added advantage in the management of premalignant or malignant lesions. Principles and technique of incision and ablation have been detailed elsewhere in the chapter.

3. ***Implant surgery:***

   Lasers are also useful in the management of peri-implant soft tissues. 10,600-nm wavelength $CO_2$ laser and 980-nm diode are the commonly used soft-tissue lasers in implant surgery. ND:YAG laser, due to its inherent high depth of penetration and risk for damage to adjacent tissue and implant surface, is considered unsafe for use on implants. Er:YAG laser, which has been approved for use on hard tissues, has been used in uncovering a thin layer of bone in second-stage implant uncovering and initiating the implant osteotomy, but there is need for further data on the use of Er:YAG for complete preparation of implant osteotomy. 9300-nm $CO_2$ laser has been used for hard-tissue applications, but more data on its safety and efficacy are needed. Advantages of using lasers in implant surgery include the precision, atraumatic tissue handling, bloodless field of view, and decreased bacterial contamination. Lasers have been used for several indications in implant surgery, including implant site preparation procedures such as the release of frenal attachment, excision of redundant tissue, and incision placement prior to bony osteotomy. Placement of incisions with lasers as opposed to scalpel creates less inflammation, swelling, and post-operative discomfort to the patient as well as added property of tissue sterilization from antibacterial effect. They can also be used for second-stage surgery, including removal of soft tissue and, in the case of Erbium lasers and 9300 nm $CO_2$ lasers, bone covering the implant [26].

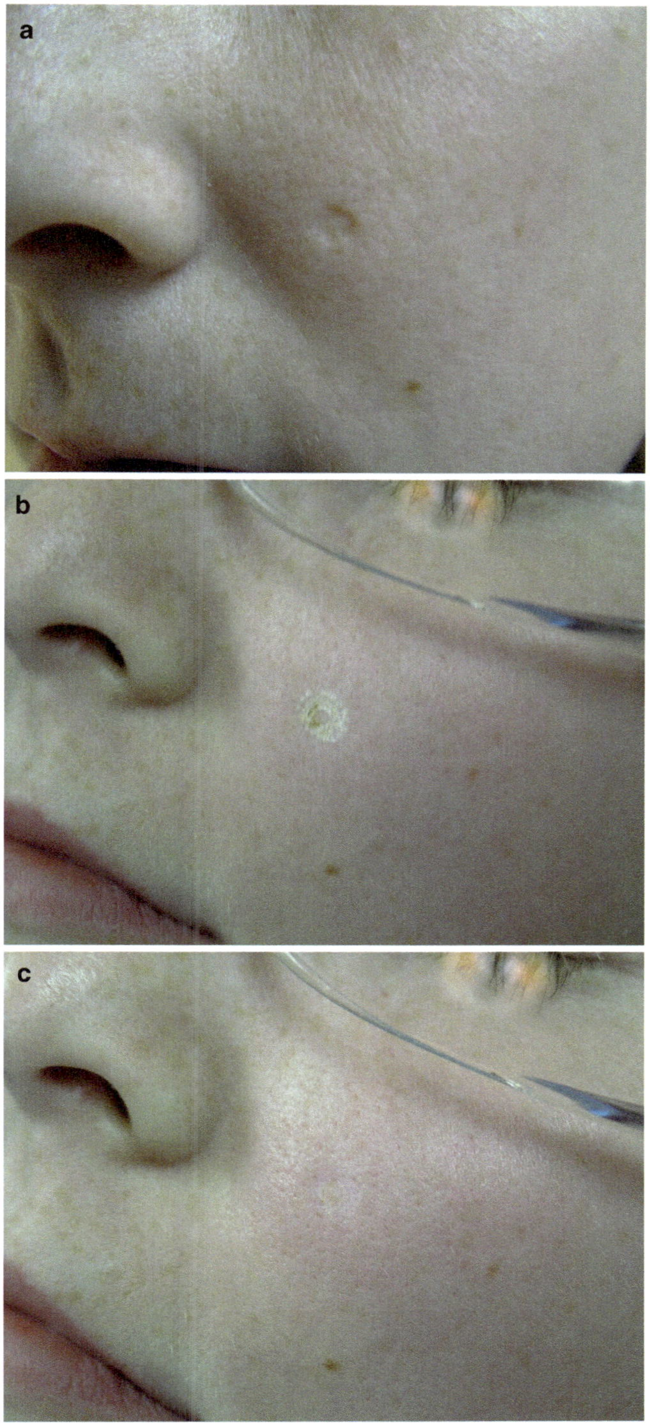




**Fig. 39.10** (**a**) Depressed scar of face. (**b**) Blending of scar using $CO_2$ laser. (**c**) Results of laser scar revision

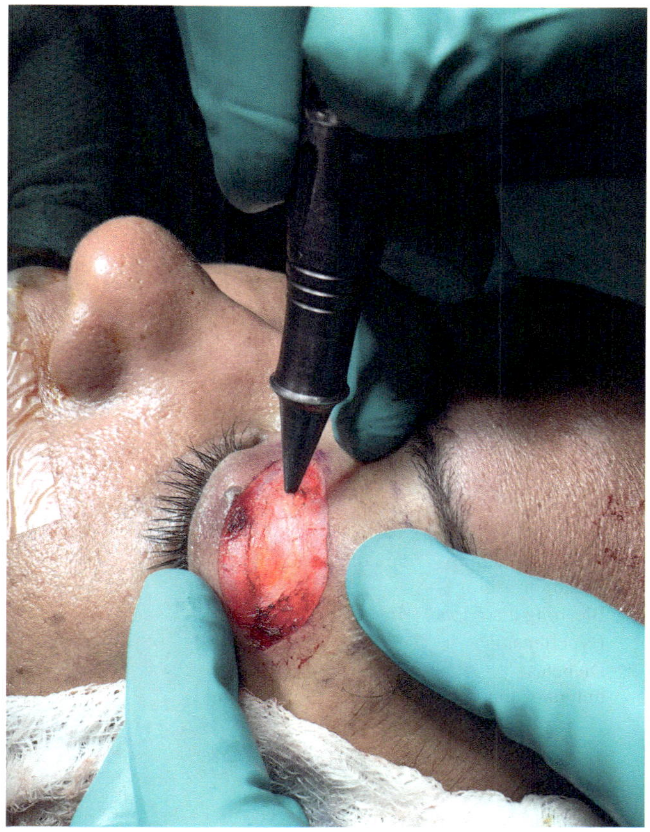



**Fig. 39.11** Laser blepharoplasty

Treatment of mucositis and peri-implantitis around implants is a challenging problem in implant surgery with limited efficacy when managed via conventional treatment protocols. If an implant with signs of peri-implantitis is deemed stable without severe bone loss and/or mobility, then treatment is attempted to salvage. Treatment of choice includes debridement of the granulation tissue accompanied by the administration of antibiotics around the implant for the eradication of as much bacteria as possible followed by bone graft of any defect created. Traditional tools include plastic instruments, citric acid, chlorhexidine, and topical Tetracycline. A laser-assisted algorithm for management of peri-implantitis includes obtaining access to the implant in question via a laser incision and reflection of flap leading to exposure of implant and surrounding bone. Then, the pathologic tissue is vaporized by laser energy and the implant surface and bony defect are decontaminated by the laser, which is accomplished by ablating the surface at low energies to kill off any bacteria on the surface as well as any attached soft tissue. Bone grafting, if necessary, can then be performed. Data have shown significantly better outcomes in cases of peri-implantitis as compared to conventional tools. As in other laser-assisted surgeries, healing is enhanced because of reduced inflammation and decreased postoperative pain as opposed to conventional tools [26] (Fig. 39.15a, b).

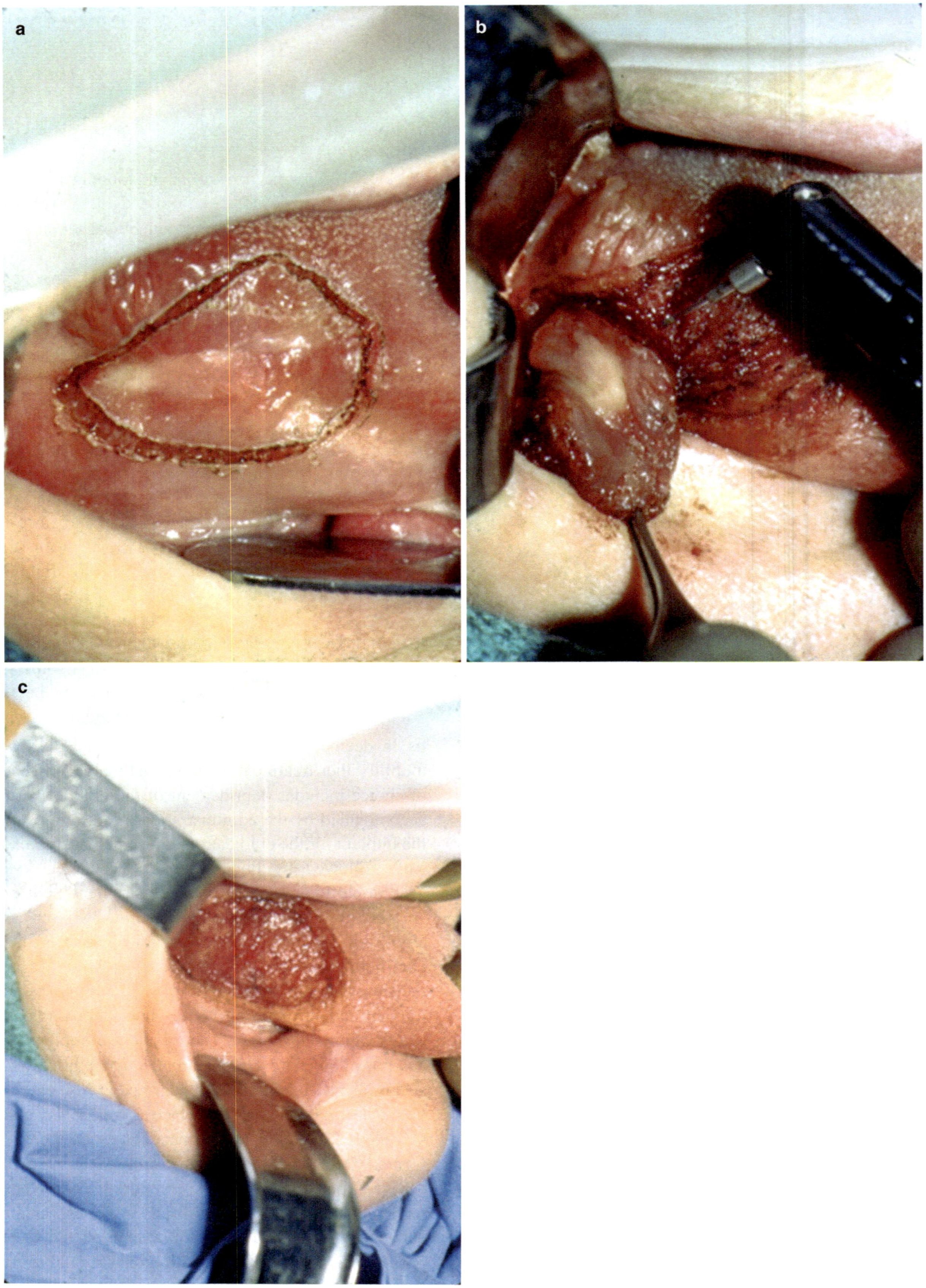




Fig. 39.12 (**a**) Outlining a small tongue cancer for laser excision. (**b**) Excision of lesion with $CO_2$ laser. (**c**) Lesion excised and allowed to heal with no closure

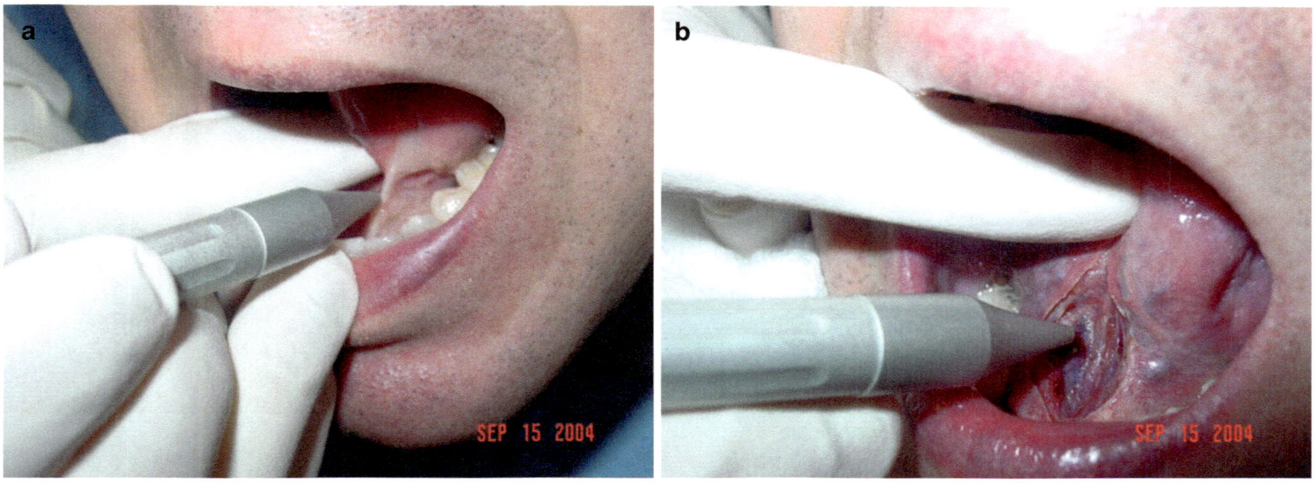




**Fig. 39.13** (**a**) Laser frenectomy with $CO_2$ laser. (**b**) After laser frenectomy

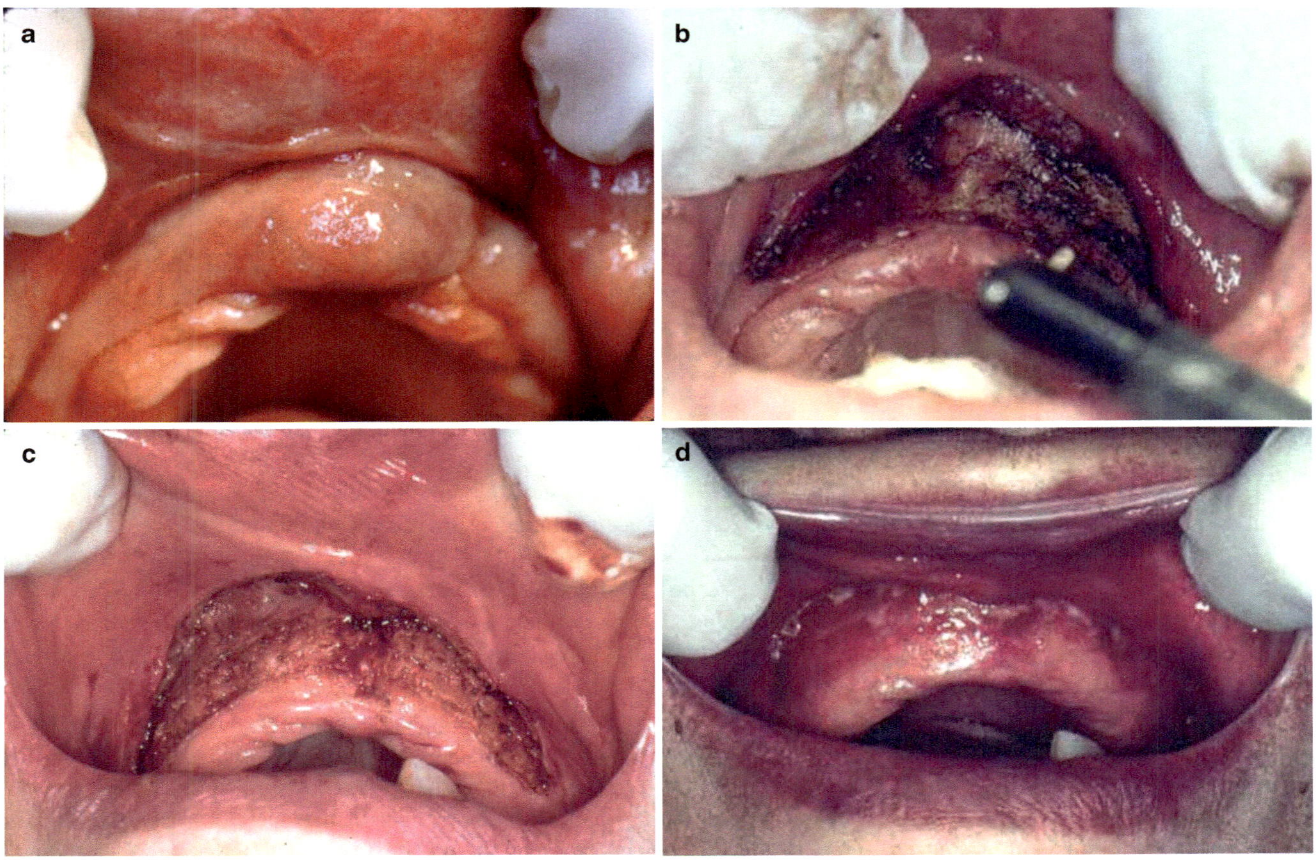




**Fig. 39.14** (**a**) Epulis fissuratum of maxilla. (**b**) Excision of epulis with $CO_2$ laser. (**c**, **d**) Supraperiosteal dissection allowed to secondary heal

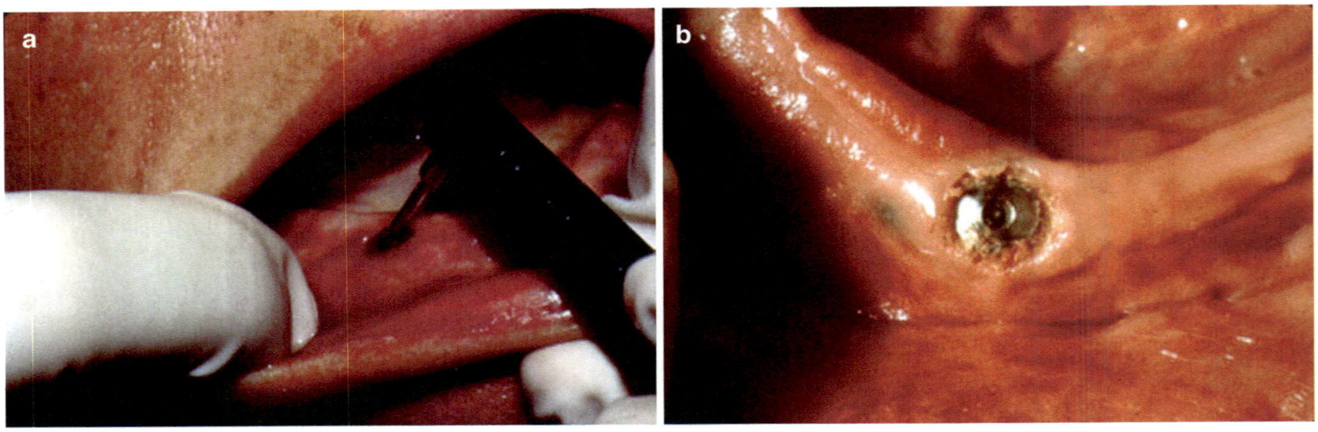




**Fig. 39.15** (**a**, **b**) Implant uncovering with $CO_2$ laser

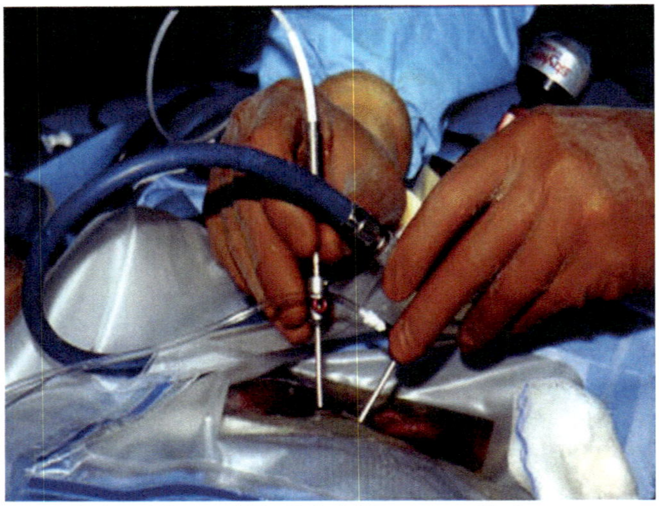



**Fig. 39.16** TMJ arthoscopy with Holmium YAG laser

4. ***Temporomandibular joint surgery (TMJ):***
   Arthroscopic TMJ surgeries have been proven to be efficacious, minimally invasive, and efficient procedures to treat and manage several aspects of temporomandibular joint disorders. Arthroscopic surgery utilizes various modified cutting instruments, which are passed through a narrow trocar to be able to release the disc attachments, remove redundant inflamed tissues, and/or perform synovial biopsies. These conventional cutting tools are difficult to maneuver, increase the risk of bleeding, which creates a poor visual field and a higher risk of complications. Use of lasers administered via narrow-diameter fiberoptic cables adds advantages in maneuverability, which makes it easier to sweep through the small-sized TMJ and make precise incisions and ablation with better hemostasis in a noncontact mode. Due to their high water absorption, $CO_2$ and Er:YAG lasers cannot be used for this purpose. Ho:YAG is the commonly used laser for the purpose of TMJ arthroscopy. With low water absorption, it is less affected by the presence of the synovial and lavage fluids, while low penetration (~0.5 mm) decreases the risk of damage to adjacent tissues. Other TMJ procedures such as disk repositioning and removal have been described with the use of arthroscopic techniques and laser assistance with significant success (Fig. 39.16) [17, 18].

## 39.6 Safety Concerns with Use of Lasers

Efficient and safe use of lasers starts with operator's familiarity with details of the laser system in use. All laser systems come with a user's manual, which lists all required technical details as well as recommended indications for use of that laser system. Common safety issues with lasers happen with accidental exposure of surrounding tissues.

1. ***Personnel protection:***
   Patients, providers, and the assistants are all at risk of inadvertent irradiation with lasers. Any reflective surface in the area of laser target can divert the beam away from the intended area and potentially cause harm. Use of special protective glasses (that are matched to the specific wavelength of the laser) can help avoid injury to eyes of patients or personnel in the operatory. Everyone in the operatory should be familiar with the basic functioning of the laser equipment and nonreflective tools should be used and reflective surfaces intraorally such as crowns be protected with a wet sponge or nonreflective retractors. Posting a "danger" sign for use of laser on the door of the operatory in order to avoid unprotected personnel from entering the room, while laser is in use could avoid accidental injuries as well (Fig. 39.17a, b) [6].

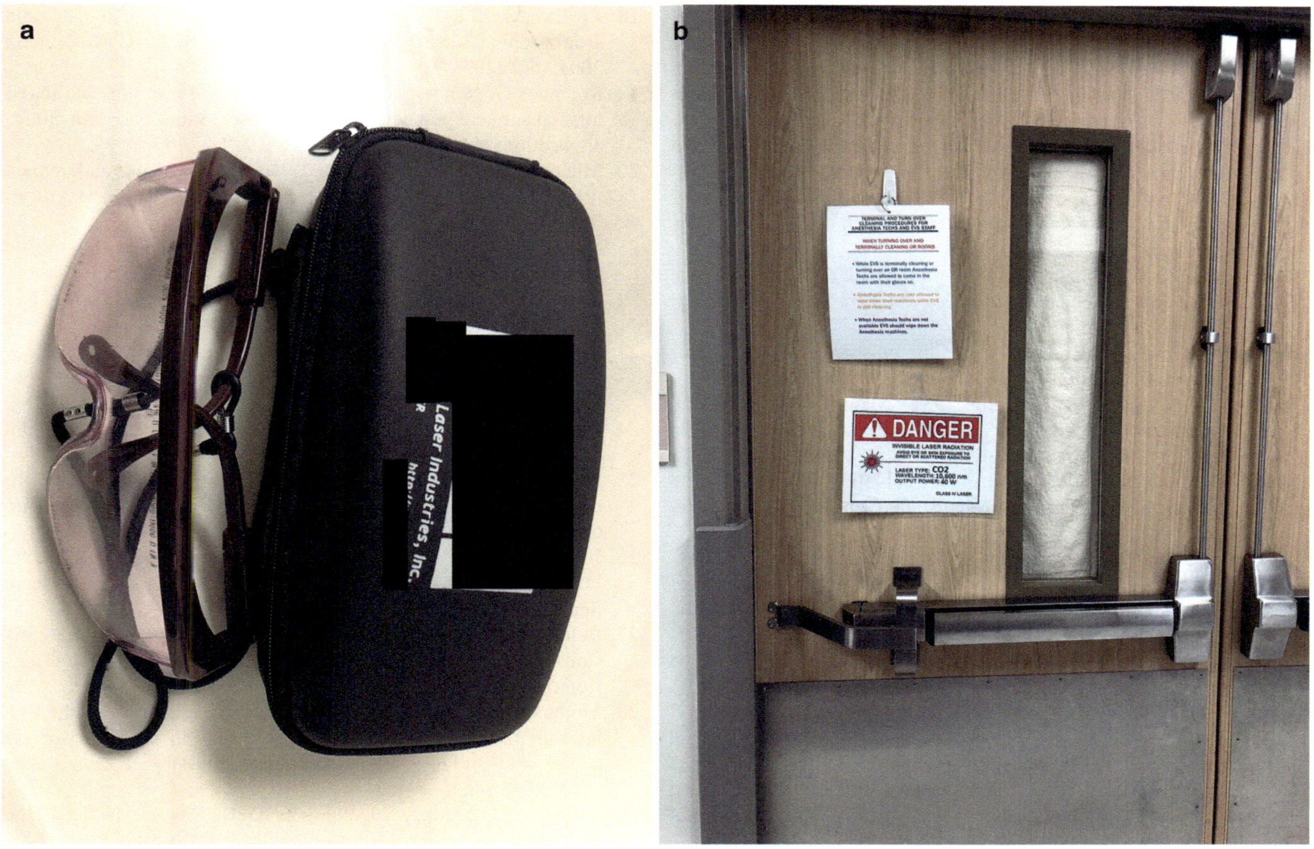




**Fig. 39.17** (**a**) Wavelength-specific eyewear for protection of operator, patient, and assistants. (**b**) "Danger" sign outside the operatory along with closure of any see-through glass panels on the door

2. ***Fire hazard:***

   Lasers in an oxygen-rich environmental such as the oral cavity of a patient being provided supplemental oxygen, or inside an endotracheal tube, can pose a significant fire risk. To avoid fire, supplemental $O_2$ concentration should be kept to a minimum required level or use of room air is recommended. For endotracheal tubes, compressed air can be substituted for oxygen to keep the inspired concentrations of oxygen to below 30% [6].

3. ***Laser plume:***

   When a laser is used for incision or vaporization procedures, the tissue that is being handled will create a "plume," which consists of potentially hazardous particulate debris, which is considered infectious. There are studies, which showed the presence of viral DNA in the plume, but to date there hasn't been any clinical significance or transmission proven. Nevertheless, for protection of the provider/staff, high flow suction made of a nonreflective material such as plastic should be used to remove the plume. Wearing masks and other personal protective barriers such as eyeglasses will help avoid infection transmission as well [27–29].

## 39.7 Conclusion

Lasers have changed the OMS practice significantly to a point that it is today an essential surgical tool in many ways. Development of lasers in future may overcome current disadvantages and increase utility and safety. Use of lasers in hard tissue is still somewhat limited in comparison to soft-tissue applications. Further research and development could help improve this aspect of laser.DisclosureAuthors have no financial conflicts to disclose.

## References


1. Hecht J. Beam the race to make the laser. Oxford: Oxford University Press; 2005.
2. Maiman T. Comments on his precocious five-year-old [editorial]. Laser Focus. 1965;1:2–4.
3. Sulewski JG. Einstein's "Splendid Light": origins and dental applications. In: Convissar R, editor. Principles and practice of laser dentistry. 2nd ed: Elsevier Health Sciences; 2016. p. 1–11.
4. Coluzzi DJ, Convissar RA, Roshkind DM. Laser fundamentals. In: Convissar R, editor. Principles and practice of laser dentistry. 2nd ed: Elsevier Health Sciences; 2016. p. 12–26.

5. Strauss RA, Fallon SD. Lasers in contemporary oral and maxillofacial surgery. Dent Clin N Am. 2004;48(4):861–88.
6. Strauss RA, Coleman M. Lasers in major oral and maxillofacial surgery. In: Convissar R, editor. Principles and practice of laser dentistry. 2nd ed: Elsevier Health Sciences; 2016. p. 234–50.
7. Barak S, Kaplan I, Rosenblum I. The use of the CO2 laser in oral and maxillofacial surgery. J Clin Laser Med Surg. 1990;10:69–70.
8. Bradley P. A review of the use of the neodymium YAG laser in oral and maxillofacial surgery. Br J Oral Maxillofac Surg. 1997;35(1):26–35.
9. Romanos G. Clinical applications of the Nd:YAG laser in oral soft tissue surgery and periodontology. J Clin Laser Med Surg. 1994;12:103–8.
10. White J, Goodis H, Rose C. Use of the pulsed Nd:YAG laser for intraoral soft tissue surgery. Lasers Surg Med. 1991;11:455–61.
11. Khatri KA, Ross V, Grevelink JM, Magro CM, Anderson RR. Comparison of erbium:YAG and carbon dioxide lasers in resurfacing of facial rhytides. Arch Dermatol. 1999;135:391–7.
12. Li Z, Reinisch L, Van de Merwe W. Bone ablation with Er:YAG and CO2 laser: study of thermal and acoustic effects. Lasers Surg Med. 1992;12:79–85.
13. Arnabat-Dominguez J, Espana-Tost AJ, Berini-Aytes L, Gay-Escoda C. Erbium:YAGlaser application in the second phase of implant surgery: a pilot study in 20 patients. Int J Oral Maxillofac Implants. 2003;18:104–12.
14. El-Montaser M, Devlin H, Dickinson MR, Sloam P, Lloyd RE. Osseointegration of titanium metal implants in erbium-YAG laser-prepared bone. Implant Dent. 1999;8:79–85.
15. Walsh L. The use of lasers in implantology: an overview. J Oral Implantol. 1992;18:335–40.
16. Kreisler M, Kohnen W, Marinello C, Gote H, Duschner H, Jansen B, dHoedt B. Bactericidal effect of the Er:YAG laser on dental implant surfaces: an in vitro study. J Periodontol. 2002;73:1292–7.
17. Hendler BH, Gateno J, Mooar P, Sherk HH. Holmium:YAG laser arthroscopy of the temporomandibular joint. J Oral Maxillofac Surg. 1992;50:931–4.
18. Koslin M. Laser applications in temporomandibular joint arthroscopic surgery. Oral Maxillofac Surg Clin N Am. 2004;16(2):269–75.
19. Romanos G, Nentwig G. Diode laser (980 nm) in oral and maxillofacial surgical procedures: clinical observations based on clinical applications. J Clin Laser Med Surg. 1999;17:193–7.
20. Mitchell O, Blackhall K, Lister T, Downie I. The use and application of lasers in oral and maxillofacial surgery. Br J Oral Maxillofac Surg. 2017;55(10):E155.
21. Guttenberg SA, Emery RW III. Laser physics and tissue interaction. Oral Maxillofac Surg Clin N Am. 2004;16(2):143–7.
22. Watson SW, Sawisch TJ. Cosmetic ablative skin resurfacing. Oral Maxillofac Surg Clin N Am. 2004;16(2):215–30.
23. Boyden DK. A brief overview of noninvasive lasers in cosmetic maxillofacial surgery. Oral Maxillofac Surg Clin N Am. 2004;16(2):231–7.
24. Wlodawsky RN, Strauss RA. Intraoral laser surgery. Oral Maxillofac Surg Clin N Am. 2004;16(2):149–63.
25. Stephen Brandon M, Strauss RA. Complications of CO2 laser procedures in oral and maxillofacial surgery. Oral Maxillofac Surg Clin N Am. 2004;16(2):289–99.
26. Julian J. Lasers in implant dentistry. In: Convissar R, editor. Principles and practice of laser dentistry. 2nd ed: Elsevier Health Sciences; 2016. p. 107–30.
27. Bellina JH, Stjernholm RL, Kurpel JE. Analysis of plume emissions after papovavirus irradiation with the carbon dioxide laser. J Reprod Med. 1982;27:268–70.
28. Mullarky MB, Norris CW, Goldberg ID. The efficacy of the CO2 laser in the sterilization of skin seeded with bacteria: survival at the skin surface and in the plume emission. Laryngoscope. 1985;95:186–7.
29. Walker NPJ, Matthews J, Newson SWB. Possible hazards from irradiation with the carbon dioxide laser. Lasers Surg Med. 1986;6:84–6.

# Piezosurgery in Oral and Maxillofacial Surgery

# 40

Shravan Renapurkar and Sowjanya Nagamalla

## 40.1 Introduction

The term "piezo" has been derived from the word "Piezien," which implies pressure in the Greek language. Piezoelectric effect was first described by Jacques and Pierre Curie in 1880 and involves the appearance of an electric charge across certain crystals when they are under mechanical pressure. Inversely, when an electric current is applied across them, they deform. This phenomenon of deformation when under alternating current creates microvibrations or oscillations of ultrasonic frequency [1]. Although ultrasonic microvibration technology was experimentally used earlier, it was in 1988 that Italian oral surgeon Tomaso Vercellotti developed the first commercially available Mectron® piezoelectric bone surgery unit to cut bone tissue while minimizing the limitations of conventional tools [2, 3]. The first use of piezoelectric surgery was for osteotomies by oral and maxillofacial surgeons and later on used for neurosurgical and orthopedic procedures. This revolutionary tool not only lowers the chance of damage to adjacent vital soft-tissue structures such as nerves and vessels during osteotomies, but also preserves osteocytes, which in turn complements bone healing [4, 5].

## 40.2 Equipment and Principles of Use

Piezoelectric surgery devices are generally small portable units comprising a handpiece with a working tip and a foot control switch, which are connected to the main power-generating unit. The main power unit also features holders for the handpiece and irrigating/cooling fluid (Fig. 40.1a–c). The handpiece is the critical part of this device, containing within it the ceramic chips where the microvibrations are created and later transmitted to the working tip. Commonly used ceramic chips in Piezoelectric surgery units are Barium Titanate or an equivalent material. The amount of deformation in the crystals within the handpiece and resultant vibrations in the insert depend on the power applied [6].

The working tips of a piezoelectric system used for surgical purposes are interchangeable inserts, which can be of different shapes, sizes, and cutting edges based on the intended clinical applications. These inserts can be made of different materials and be coated with titanium or a diamond layer to improve the cutting efficiency. To create a cutting effect rather than a debriding effect, the vibrations of the insert enter into a resonance with the ceramic chips, which increases the energy output. This, combined with the form of the insert, acts like a micrometric oscillating saw. The main energy unit has an interactive touchpad, which allows the operator to control the frequency of vibrations, power of the unit, and the amount of irrigating or coolant fluid. The pressure applied on the insert can also be manually controlled by the operator and can affect the frequency delivered to the target tissue, which in turn affects the cutting efficiency. When higher pressure is applied at the tip, it impedes the cutting efficiency of the insert and releases the energy as heat, which is detrimental to the bone as well as adjacent soft tissue [6, 7].

The Piezoelectric unit also allows for election of modes of operation, which are preset power modes with varying frequencies to match the clinical application. The frequency is usually set between 25 and 29 kHz, which can create micro-oscillations of 60–210 μm amplitude, providing the handpiece with power exceeding 5 W. The vibrations produced in the "Low mode" result from average ultrasonic powers, without frequency overmodulation, and allow the operator to perform endodontic procedures. On the contrary side, the "high mode" and the "boosted mode" are characterized by vibrations with higher ultrasonic power and frequency overmodulation, which allows cutting of mineralized tissue. The "boosted mode" has frequency overmodulation with an increased rate that is most efficient for osteotomy and osteoplasties in surgical procedures, while the "high mode" is less

S. Renapurkar (✉) · S. Nagamalla
Department of Oral and Maxillofacial Surgery, Virginia Commonwealth University Medical Center, Richmond, VA, USA
e-mail: srenapurkar@vcu.edu; nagamallas@vcu.edu


K. Bonanthaya et al. (eds.), *Oral and Maxillofacial Surgery for the Clinician*, https://doi.org/10.1007/978-981-15-1346-6_40

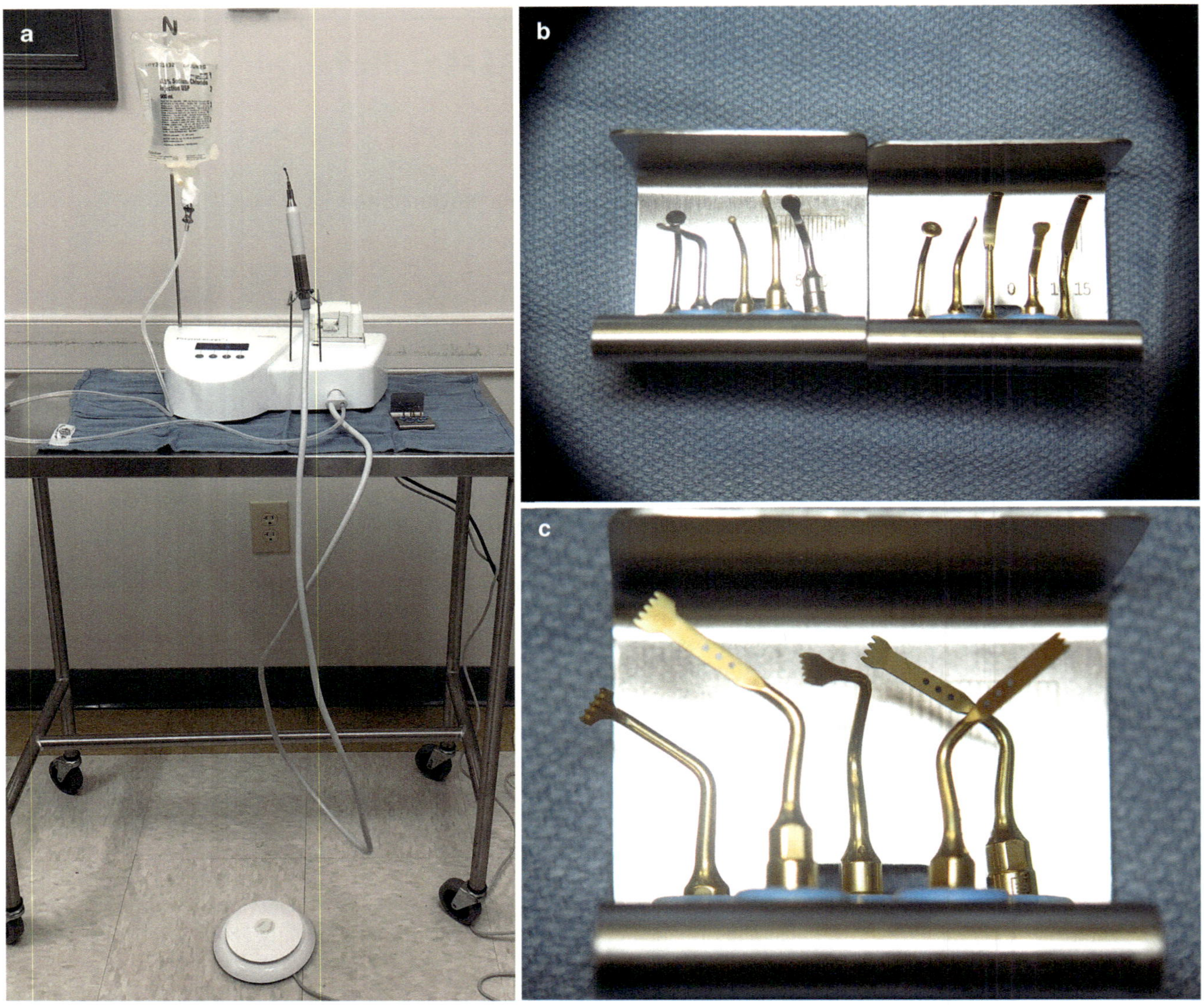



**Fig. 40.1** (**a**) The Piezosurgery® unit from Mectron® is made of a power supply unit, a handpiece, its holder, an irrigant solution holder, foot control switch. (**b, c**) Inserts or working tips of a piezosurgery unit. (**b**) shows working tips for Sinus lift and (**c**) shows osteotomy tips

efficient but more helpful in periodontal procedures and bone smoothening [6–8].

The device includes an irrigating system for cooling that creates an adjustable jet of coolant solution through a peristaltic pump at rates between 0 and 60 ml/min and helps remove debris from the cut surface and helps maintain hemostasis because of its cavitation effect. This enhances visibility, particularly in difficult-to-reach anatomical zones, by scattering coolant liquid as an aerosol. The irrigation liquid should be refrigerated at 4 °C for effectual cooling [6, 8, 9].

For optimal use and maximum efficiency, the operator could select the proper power based on the surgical tissue, apply light pressure with the tip, and adjust the rate of delivery of the irrigating solution to avoid overheating the tissue and decrease the chance of damage to soft tissues. Although the device has a safe frequency range along with the cooling irrigation liquid, there is a possibility of damage to soft tissues due to high pressure and overheating [10].

## 40.3 Advantages

Used in many therapeutic surgical procedures, piezosurgery has several advantages when compared to traditional methods of surgical instrumentation used for osteotomies or osteoplasty. These are as follows:

- *Decreased risk of damage to adjacent soft tissues*: This is the major advantage with use of a piezoelectric surgical unit. When used as recommended, at the appropriate frequency, the micrometric oscillating motion decreases the chance of damage or cutting of adjacent soft tissue while cutting through hard tissues. For example, it allows improved Schneiderian membrane preservation during osteotomy of the maxillary lateral wall during a sinus lift and preservation of the inferior alveolar nerve (IAN) during mandibular osteotomy.
- *Improved visibility*: With use of piezosurgery, better visibility is secondary to the decreased amount of bleeding and the phenomenon of cavitation. Cavitation refers to the phenomenon of "microboiling" occurring in liquids in a solid-liquid interface at intermediate frequencies of vibration secondary to the creation of imploding bubbles when the irrigating solution contacts the insert. Improved visibility helps the operator to place the osteotomy in the preferred location with increased accuracy [6].
- *Increased patient comfort:* Due to the micrometric nature of the vibrations and decreased noise, use of a piezosurgery device improves patient comfort and decreases anxiety during procedures done under local anesthesia. When used for bone harvesting, it also reduces the need for use of chisels, which can help improve the patient experience and reduce stress.
- *Improved survival of osteocytes:* Bone harvested with various techniques, including rotary instruments, chisels, rongeurs, and a piezosurgery device, was studied with histomorphometry evaluation by Berengo et al. The piezosurgery device was shown to be one of the best methods of harvesting bone along with gouge chisels, back action chisels, and rongeurs in terms of the viability of the harvested bone and number of osteocytes. Bone harvested with rotary instruments, including burs and safe scrapers, was noted to be completely nonvital with an absence of osteocytes. In another histomorphological study done with the placement of porous titanium implants in minipig tibias, neo-osteogenesis was noted to be consistently more active in bony samples from implant sites that were prepared using piezoelectric surgery, and there was an earlier increase in BMP-4 and TGF-2 proteins and fewer proinflammatory cytokines in bone around the implants [5, 11].

## 40.4 Disadvantages/Limitations

Although piezosurgery has numerous advantages as listed here, it is associated with some drawbacks as follows:

- *Low efficiency/increased operating time*: One of the major drawbacks with ultrasonic/piezo surgery osteotomes is the increased time required for the procedure. The cutting efficiency of a piezosurgery device has been reported to be 3–4 times less than that of conventional osteotomes for some procedures [12, 13]. For example, in a randomized prospective crossover clinical study done by Stefano Sivolella, piezoelectric osteotomy of a lower third molar took 9.4 min longer than rotary tools to complete [14].
- *Expense*: The cost of equipment is sometimes an additional burden to the provider. Each individual cutting tip in a piezosurgery equipment setup is generally more expensive than traditional cutting tools such as burs, chisels, or saw blades. These tips can also potentially break or fracture when improperly used, which can again increase the need for more equipment.
- *Learning curve*: Use of piezo requires a short learning curve to attain maximum efficacy, which could be frustrating to the operator. The digital pressure applied by the surgeon while using conventional tools such as saws and drills is quite different from piezoelectric surgery as it mandates less pressure and failing to calculate the pressure according to the speed of the insert prevents microvibrations of the insert. When the microvibrations are prevented due to excessive pressure on the working tip, energy not used for cutting will be transformed into heat, which, if it continues for long time, would damage the tissue.
- *Pacemakers and defibrillators*: Piezosurgery is *relatively* contraindicated for use in patients with pacemakers, although there is no evidence of electromagnetic interactions produced by piezoelectric devices according to one in vitro study [15].

## 40.5 Applications for Piezosurgery

### 40.5.1 Dentoalveolar Procedures

Piezosurgery can be applied toward multiple dentoalveolar procedures where there is a requirement for meticulous bone preparation, atraumatic tooth extraction/exposure, and when the location of the surgical site is in proximity to vital anatomical structures. Example of applications in dentoalveolar surgery include ankylotic tooth root extraction, impacted third molar extraction, surgical exposure of impacted teeth, and extractions in patients with a thin periodontal biotype. In all of these indications, piezosurgery has the potential to limit bone loss and maximize maintenance of alveolar bone integrity, especially when the alveolar bone is thin and the procedure requires a high degree of precision. A split-mouth design, randomized, clinical trial conducted by Mantovani et al. studied differences in postoperative pain, orofacial swelling and duration of the procedure when using a rotary bur for third molar ostectomy versus a piezosurgery device. They found that, although the duration of the procedure was longer, the postoperative pain and swelling were less in the piezosurgery group [16].

### 40.5.2 Dental Implant Surgery

#### 40.5.2.1 Sinus Floor Elevation

Perforation of the Schneiderian membrane during lateral wall osteotomy, and/or while raising the maxillary sinus floor manually, is a common complication, which can affect the bone grafting procedure. Use of piezosurgery in sinus lift procedures not only minimizes the chance of perforation during osteotomy but also eases the separation of the membrane as well (Fig. 40.2a–c). In the commonly used lateral approach technique for sinus lift, piezoelectric devices have a superior action in each technique or step compared to traditional instruments. The chance of membrane perforation with conventional techniques is reported to be 14–56%, while studies on the use of piezosurgery devices report it to be 5–7% [8, 17, 18].

- Thinning buccal wall: With traditional instruments, it is difficult to thin the buccal wall with good control. Piezoelectric device makes precise osteoplasty easy and the bone fragments produced during osteoplasty can be used as grafting material.
- Bony window/osteotomy: Piezosurgery makes the frame of the bony window optimal with respect to the sinus

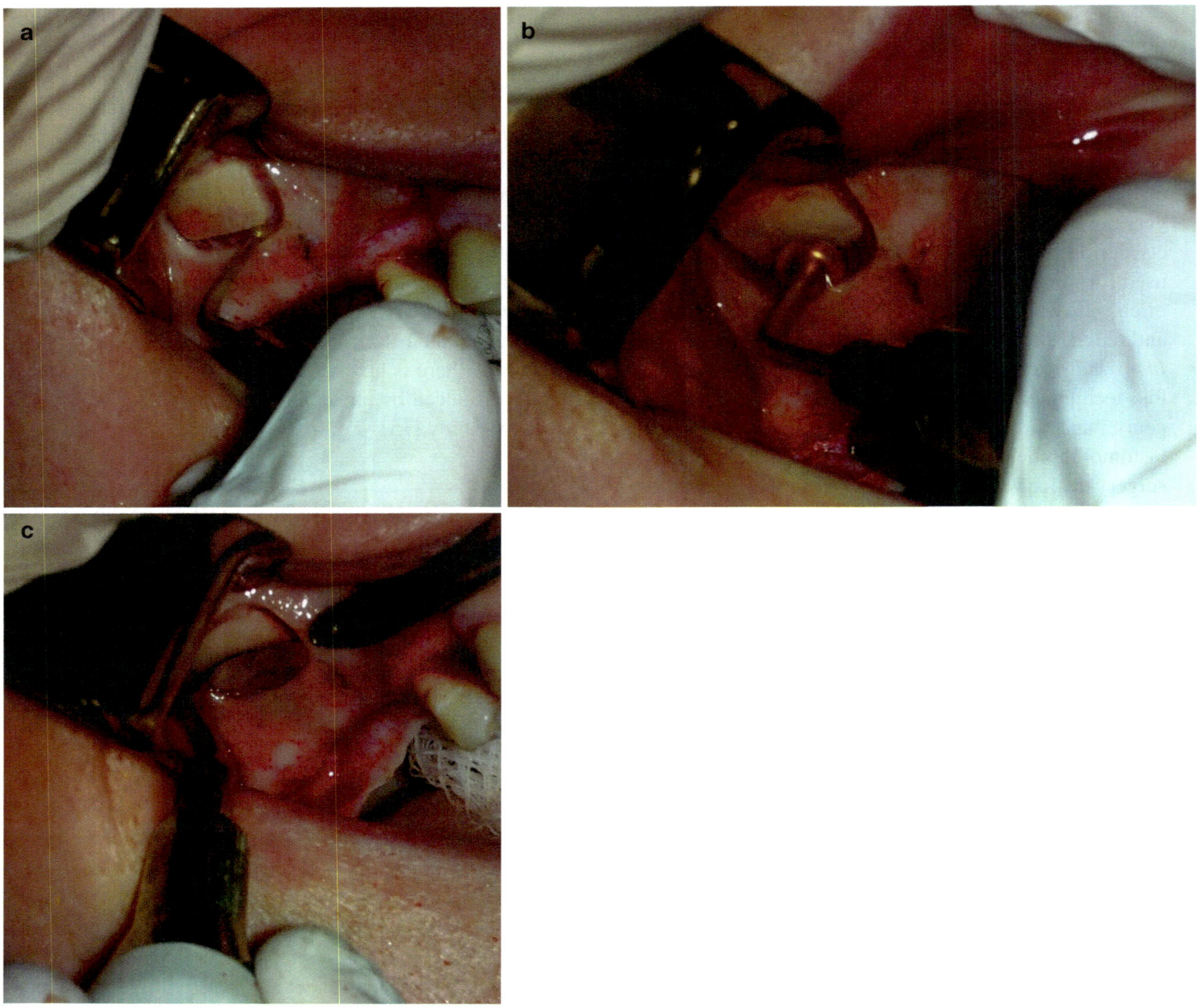




Fig. 40.2 (a) Piezosurgery insert used to perform outline of the lateral wall osteotomy to thin the wall. (b) Blunt piezosurgery insert used to infracture the window wall and initiate the separation of the schneiderian membrane from the sinus wall. (c) After the lateral sinus wall osteotomy completed, membrane separation initiated a third insert shaped as an elevator used to continue the separation of the membrane to create required space for the bone graft for augmentation

anatomy with decreased chance of membrane perforation.

- Sinus membrane separation: Most commercially available piezosurgery devices have special inserts that make the separation around the perimeter of bony window easier and decrease chance of tear or perforation during the manual lifting process.

#### 40.5.2.2 Implant Site Preparation

Implant site healing and ultimate osseointegration of implants is negatively influenced by the high temperatures created during site preparation. Results of an in vitro study done by Heinemann et al. in 2012 on porcine jaws comparing piezosurgery, Sonicflex®, and rotary instruments showed the highest temperature rise with use of piezosurgery, although the trabecular bone and osteocytes were still intact [19]. On the contrary, a recent randomized, controlled clinical trial by Da Silva Neto et al. in 2014 compared implant stability at various times postoperatively in osteotomies performed by conventional rotary instruments versus piezosurgery devices, and found implant stability to be higher with Piezosurgery [20]. The use of piezoelectric devices facilitates the use of selective enlargement of only one socket wall and Vercellotti called this: "differential ultrasonic socket preparation." [4].

#### 40.5.2.3 Alveolar Ridge Splitting

Ridge-splitting techniques for alveolar augmentation is indicated when there is adequate height of bone for implant placement but inadequate ridge thickness. The conventional ridge-splitting procedure uses chisels, rotary instruments, or saws, all of which have a high risk for damage to soft tissue, undesired propagation of the osteotomy and bone fracture, as well as prolonging treatment time due to the need for second-stage surgery to place the implants. (Fig. 40.3a, b) With use of piezosurgery, one can decrease the chance of the damage to adjacent structures during the osteotomy as well as reduce the risk of bone thermonecrosis, while simultaneously providing better control of propagation of the ridge split osteotomy. Although ridge splitting was traditionally used in the maxillary arch, piezoelectric bone surgery allows ridge expansion even in highly mineralized tissues like the mandible with ease [21, 22]. Blus et al. conducted a study on ridge splitting for more than 200 implants placed in 57 patients and reported 96.5% success rate with a 36-month follow up [23].

#### 40.5.2.4 Lateralization of the Inferior Alveolar Nerve

In order to place implants in atrophic edentulous mandibles, IAN lateralization can be used as an alternative to bone augmentation procedures (Fig. 40.4a–c). Bovi, in 2005, first reported a technique for IAN mobilization with simultaneous implant placement utilizing a piezoelectric device. He reported that IAN mobilization with a piezoelectric device minimizes the risk of irreversible damage to the IAN and enables the surgeon to make a smaller bony window, which, in turn, decreases overstretching of the mental nerve [24]. In an in vitro study, Metzger compared transposition of the IAN with use of a piezoelectric device versus conventional burs. His study also supported the lower rate of nerve injury from use of piezosurgery [25].

### 40.5.3 Bone Graft Harvesting

For bone augmentation, bone grafts in the form of chips or blocks can be used. Bone chips are primarily indicated in guided bone regeneration where the stabilization of the graft is not an issue, such as multiwalled defects. On the other hand, when the bony defect is large or stabilization is diffi-

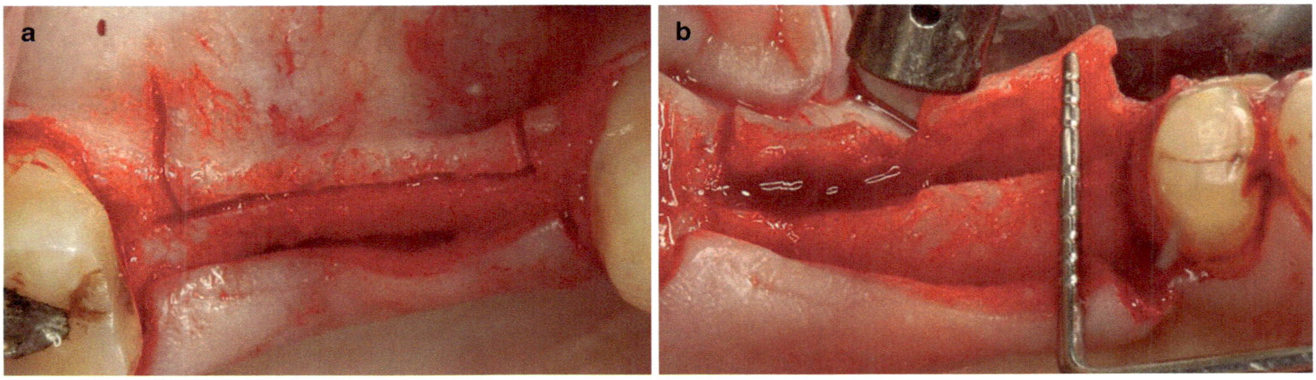




**Fig. 40.3** (**a**, **b**) Ridge split technique with piezo surgery. Bony osteotomies performed with piezoelectric device then ridge expanded to desired dimensions. From: Tarun Kumar, A., Triveni, B., Priyadharshini, M., & Mehta, G. (2016). Staged Ridge Split Procedure in the Management of Horizontal Ridge Deficiency Utilizing Piezosurgery. *Journal of Maxillofacial and Oral Surgery, 15*(4), 542–546 (Springer)

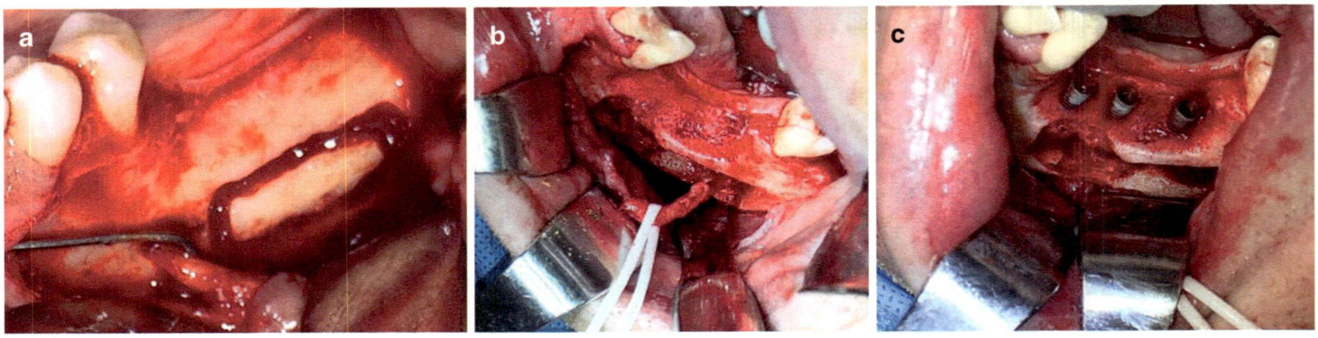




**Fig. 40.4** (**a–c**) Inferior alveolar nerve (IAN) lateralization for placement of implant

cult, block grafts must be utilized to augment vertical or horizontal dimension. Piezosurgery is used for harvesting all types of bone grafts, including autologous free block grafts, microvascular free flaps, and bone chips.

For example, piezosurgery is commonly used to harvest mandibular ramus block grafts. This requires use of two types of piezosurgery inserts. One is the standard saw-shaped right angle insert, which is used in an area, which can be viewed directly to make the depth cut and vertical cuts, while a second, dual-angled, insert is used specifically to make the inferior horizontal bone cut. In bone graft harvesting, piezosurgery allows better visibility, precise cuts, and good adaptation of the grafts along with better survival of bone cells. In a study by Happe in 2007 on 40 patients, bone grafts harvested from the mandibular ramus by piezosurgery resulted in 93% uneventfully healed donor sites and 96% uneventfully healed graft sites [26]. There was also minimal resorption of the graft. Shaping of block grafts can be better controlled with piezosurgery, although this can take longer than rotary instruments. In microvascular free bone flaps harvested with piezosurgery, the surgeon can decrease the chance of injury to the vascular bundle along the surface of bone. With the use of piezoelectric surgery, the clinician can cautiously osteotomize the fibula or other bone without any periosteal/pedicle dissection. In addition, the piezoelectric method also allows shaping and handling the pedicle while it is still attached to the donor site.

### 40.5.4 Orthognathic Surgery

Piezoelectric devices are increasingly being used in orthognathic surgery due to its precise cutting and lower risk of damage to adjacent teeth and nerves. Landes et al. performed a large study on 90 patients in whom orthognathic surgery was performed with piezosurgery. This study demonstrated decreased blood loss compared to conventional surgery but no significant difference in surgical times. Lefort I osteotomy only required the use of chisels in about 33% of cases [5, 27, 28]. In the same study, among patients who underwent bilateral sagittal split osteotomy (BSSO), inferior alveolar nerve sensitivity at 3-month follow up was retained in 98% of the cases, compared with 84% after conventional BSSO (Fig. 40.5). When performing surgically assisted rapid maxillary expansion (SARME), the advantage of using piezoelectric surgery is that it minimizes potential damage to the descending palatine artery while separating the pterygomaxillary junction, the nasopalatine artery while making the midline maxillary cut, and it lowers indirect thermal damage to the bony surfaces and adjacent structures, including teeth [29].

### 40.5.5 Aesthetic Facial Surgery

Conventionally, chisels are used for osteotomy of the lateral nasal bone during rhinoplasty, which transmit significant force to the surrounding soft tissues in a blind manner, and increases the risk for bleeding from injury to the adjacent vasculature. A study done by Robiony et al. assessed use of chisels versus piezosurgery and found a decreased risk of injury to adjacent soft tissues with use of piezosurgery. Use of chisels also may create inaccuracy due to blind use and the unguarded nature of the instrument. On the other hand, use of piezo will not incur this issue and gives the operator more control and accuracy [30].

### 40.5.6 Distraction Osteogenesis

Distraction osteogenesis (DO) is indicated when there is a need for significant amounts of bone augmentation or lengthening, or when the soft tissues that cover the bone will not

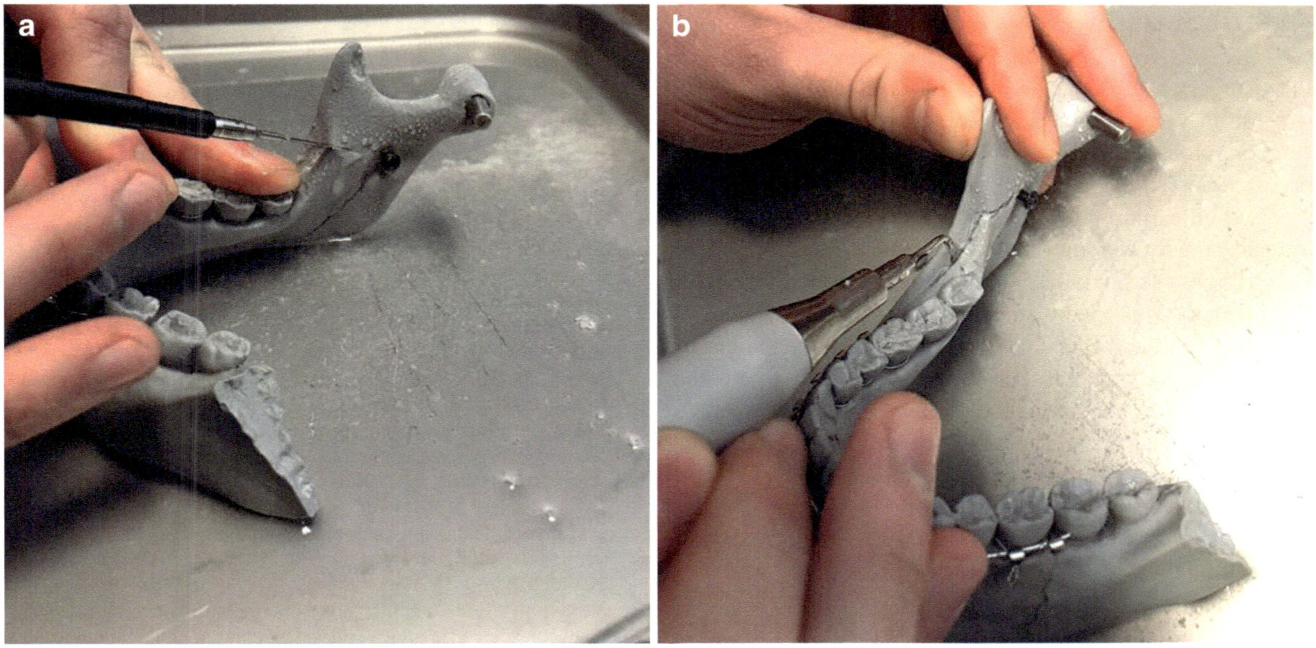

©Association of Oral and Maxillofacial Surgeons of India

**Fig. 40.5** (**a**, **b**) Orthognathic surgery using Piezo. Figure shows steps in a BSSO. Variations in the blade design can be used based on desired osteotomy

allow for osseous augmentation. The use of piezosurgery permits the initial osteotomy to be made delicately and accurately while minimizing injury to the soft-tissue flap and surrounding hard tissue, allowing maintenance of the vascularity needed for successful new bone formation [31]. Distraction Osteogenesis (DO) can be used for distraction of either the alveolar bone or the basal jawbone. DO with a piezoelectric device ensures the preservation of original bone structures, specifically the cancellous bone, which favors the healing process due to its high healing potential. In a recent article, DO with microdistractors using a piezoelectric device has shown favorable results in patients with Pierre Robin Sequence [32].

### 40.5.7 Temporomandibular Joint Surgeries

Osteotomies and osteoplasty in the temporomandibular joint (TMJ) region involves risk to the facial nerve as well as major vessels such as the internal maxillary artery and the masseteric artery. Due to anatomical complexity, the use of conventional bone-cutting tools such as burs and saws may put these vital structures at risk of injury or permanent damage. Given the advantages of piezosurgery as discussed previously in the chapter, its use in this specialized surgery is reasonable and advisable. In 2014, Anson Jose observed less bleeding along with minimal postoperative complications while treating TMJ ankylosis with piezosurgery [33].

### 40.5.8 Inferior Alveolar Nerve Preservation

The IAN is at risk whenever there is the need to extract impacted mandibular molars, enucleate large cysts, or remove benign mandibular tumors. In 2009, Dr. Kagan Degerliyurt presented an article describing a procedure called the "bone lid technique," which is performed by using a piezosurgery device when there is a definitive risk of damage to IAN [34, 35].

### 40.5.9 Trauma

Piezoelectric devices can be used for reconstruction in multiple trauma cases, such as comminuted frontal bar fractures, to cut and shape the inner table of a calvarial bone graft, to osteotomize a healing fracture while reducing the chance of adjacent tissue injury. Using piezosurgery in post-traumatic cases can help preserve bone, protect adjacent soft tissues, decrease blood loss, improve visibility, and ensure a better overall outcome [36].

## 40.6 Conclusion

Piezosurgery is a promising surgical tool for safe and effective use in various surgeries. For an oral and maxillofacial surgeon, piezosurgery allows safer and effective osteotomy or osteoplasty compared to conventional rotating instruments such as burs and saw blades, even in complex anatomical areas. Over the past decade, it has not only been increasingly used in OMFS but has been adapted for use in neurosurgery, orthopedic surgery, and otorhinolaryngology. In addition to the surgical advantages, it helps the patient by reducing procedural stress, postoperative swelling, pain and overall improves the surgical experience. The major drawback of piezosurgery is the lack of efficiency or cutting speed, which can be balanced by improved clinical outcomes. Future generations of ultrasonic devices may bring about better efficiency and ultimately replace all conventional cutting tools.

## References


1. Curie J, Curie P. Contractions et dilatations produites par des tensions dans les cristaux hémièdres à faces inclinées. C R Acad Sci Gen. 1880;93:1137–40.
2. Vercellotti T. Technological characteristics and clinical indications of piezoelectric bone surgery. Minerva Stomatol. 2004;53:207–14.
3. Aly L. Piezoelectric surgery: applications in oral & maxillofacial surgery. Future Dent J. 2018;4(2):105–11.
4. Vercellotti T. Essentials in piezosurgery: clinical advantages in dentistry. Milan: Quintessence; 2009.
5. Berengo M, Bacci C, Sartori M, et al. Histomorphometric evaluation of bone grafts harvested by different methods. Minerva Stomatol. 2006;55(4):189.
6. Leclercq P, Zenati C, Amr S, Dohan D. Ultrasonic bone cut. Part 1: State-of-the-art technologies and common applications. J Oral Maxillofac Surg. 2008;66(1):177–82.
7. Labanca M, Azzola F, Vinci R, Rodella LF. Piezoelectric surgery: twenty years of use. Br J Oral Maxillofac Surg. 2008;46(4):265–9.
8. Schlee M, Steigmann M, Bratu E, Garg A. Piezosurgery: basics and possibilities. Implant Dent. 2006;15(4):334–40.
9. Claire S, Lea SC, Walmsley AD. Characterisation of bone following ultrasonic cutting. Clin Oral Invest. 2013;17(3):905–12.
10. Schaeren S, Jaquiery C, Heberer M, Tolnay M, Vercellotti T, Martin I. Assessment of nerve damage using a novel ultrasonic device for bone cutting. J Oral Maxillofac Surg. 2008;66:593–6.
11. Preti G, Martinasso G, Peirone B, et al. Cytokines and growth factors involved in the osseointegration of oral titanium implants positioned using piezoelectric bone surgery versus a drill technique: a pilot study in minipigs. J Periodontol. 2007;78:716–22.
12. Leclercq P, Charlotte Z, Dohan DM. ultrasonic bone cut. Part 2: State-of-the-art specific clinical applications. J Oral Maxillofac Surg. 2008;66(1):183–8.
13. Beziat JL, Bera JC, Lavandier B, Gleizal A. Ultrasonic osteotomy as a new technique in craniomaxillofacial surgery. Int J Oral Maxillofac Surg. 2007;36:493–500.
14. Sivolella B, Bressan DF, Stellini E. Osteotomy for lower third molar germectomy: randomized prospective crossover clinical study comparing piezosurgery and conventional rotatory osteotomy. J Oral Maxillofac Surg. 2011;69(6):E15–23.
15. Gómez J, Sánchez R, Ferrer R, Duran-Sindreu F. Safety concerns of piezoelectric units in implantable cardioverter defibrillator. J Oral Maxillofac Surg. 2017;76(2):273–7.
16. Mantovani A, Schierano F, Gallesio M, Russo S, Carossa S. A split-mouth randomized clinical trial to evaluate the performance of piezosurgery compared with traditional technique in lower wisdom tooth removal. J Oral Maxillofac Surg. 2014;72(10):1890–7.
17. Pavlíková G, Foltán R, Horká M, Hanzelka T, Borunská H, Šedý J. Piezosurgery in oral and maxillofacial surgery. Int J Oral Maxillofac Surg. 2011;40(5):451–7.
18. Wallace SS, Mazor Z, Froum SJ, Cho SC, Tarnow DP. Schneiderian membrane perforation rate during sinus elevation using piezosurgery: clinical results of 100 consecutive cases. Int J Periodontics Rest Dent. 2007;27:413–9.
19. Heinemann F, Hasan I, Kunert-Keil C, Götz W, Gedrange T, Spassov A, Schweppe J, Gredes T. Experimental and histological investigations of the bone using two different oscillating osteotomy techniques compared with conventional rotary osteotomy. Ann Anat. 2012;194(2):165–70.
20. Da Silva Neto UT, Joly JC, Gehrke SA. Clinical analysis of the stability of dental implants after preparation of the site by conventional drilling or piezosurgery. Br J Oral Maxillofac Surg. 2014;52(2):149–53.
21. Vercellotti T. Piezoelectric surgery in implantology: a case report—a new piezoelectric ridge expansion technique. Int J Periodont Rest Dent. 2000;20:358–65.
22. Enislidis G, Wittwer G, Ewers R. Preliminary report on a staged ridge splitting technique for implant placement in the mandible: a technical notbovie. Int J Oral Maxillofac Impl. 2006;21:445–9.
23. Blus C, Szmukler-Moncler S. Split-crest and immediate implant placement with ultra-sonic bone surgery: a 3-year life-table analysis with 230 treated sites. Clin Oral Impl Res. 2006;17:700–7.
24. Bovi M. Mobilization of the inferior alveolar nerve with simultaneous implant insertion: a new technique. Case report. Int J Periodont Rest Dent. 2005;25(4):375–83.
25. Metzger M, Bormann K, Schoen R, Gellrich N, Schmelzeisen R. Inferior alveolar nerve transposition--an in vitro comparison between piezosurgery and conventional bur use. J Oral Implantol. 2006;32(1):19–25.
26. Happe A. Use of a piezoelectric surgical device to harvest bone grafts from the mandibular ramus: report of 40 cases. Int J Periodont Rest Dent. 2007;27:241–9.
27. Landes CA, Stubinger S, Ballon A, Sader R. Piezoosteotomy in orthognathic surgery versus conventional saw and chisel osteotomy. J Oral Maxillofac Surg. 2008;12:139–47.
28. Spinelli G, Lazzeri D, Conti M, Agostini T, Mannelli G. Comparison of piezosurgery and traditional saw in bimaxillary orthognathic surgery. J Craniomaxillofac Surg. 2014.
29. Olate S, Pozzer L, Unibazo A, Huentequeo-Molina C, Martinez F, De Moraes M. LeFort I segmented osteotomy experience with piezosurgery in orthognathic surgery. Int J Clin Experiment Med. 2014;7(8):2092–5.
30. RobionyM PF, Costa F, Toro C, Politi M. Ultrasound piezoelectric vibrations to perform osteotomies in rhinoplasty. J Oral Maxillofac Surg. 2007;65:1035–8.
31. Deepa D, Jain G, Bansal T. Piezosurgery in dentistry. J Oral Res Rev. 2016;8(1):27–31.
32. Galié M, Candotto V, Elia G, Clauser L. Piezosurgery: a new and safe technique for distraction osteogenesis in Pierre Robin sequence review of the literature and case report. Int J Surg Case Rep. 2015;6C(1):269–72.
33. Jose A, Nagori S, Virkhare A, Bhatt K, Bhutia O, Roychoudhury A. Piezoelectric osteoarthrectomy for management of ankylosis of the temporomandibular joint. Br J Oral Maxillofac Surg. 2014;52(7):624–8.

34. LaBanc JP. Inferior alveolar nerve repair after treatment of benign cysts and tumors of the mandible. Oral Maxillofac Surg Clin N Am. 1991;3:209–22.
35. Degerliyurt K, Akar V, Denizci S, Yucel E. Bone lid technique with piezosurgery to preserve inferior alveolar nerve. Oral Surg Oral Med Oral Path Oral Rad Endodontol. 2009;108(6):E1–5.
36. Kane S, Balasundaram I, Rahim I, Kanzaria A, Bridle C, Holmes S. Indications of Piezoelectric surgery in trauma oral and maxillofacial surgery. Brit J Oral Maxillofac Surg. 2014;52(8):E54–5.

# Computer-Assisted Navigation Surgery in Oral and Maxillofacial Surgery

# 41

Shintaro Sukegawa and Takahiro Kanno

## 41.1 Introduction

The anatomy of the oral and facial region is complex, having many vital organs and structures, including an intricate network of blood vessels and nerves as well as the brain, eyes, nose, and vital teeth. Plain radiography can be used for screening because of its simplicity, but it cannot characterize detailed anatomical relationships. Currently, imaging diagnosis must be performed with computed tomography (CT) and/or magnetic resonance imaging (MRI) before surgery to characterize the surgical area and surrounding anatomical structures. Recent developments in imaging technology have allowed for rapid processing and visualization of significant amounts of data yielded from a variety of digital imaging modalities. Prerequisites have been established for three-dimensional (3D) visualization as well as programs for the computer-assisted 3D planning of surgical procedures, and these image sources are now available to assist the surgeon in the operating room [1].

Today, surgeons can use computer-aided design and computer-aided modeling (CAD/CAM) software to assist with the planning and implementation of complex maxillofacial surgical procedures [2]. CAD/CAM software allows the clinician to import two-dimensional (2D) CT data in DICOM format (Digital Imaging and Communications in Medicine) to a computer workstation and create accurate 3D representations of the facial skeleton and related soft tissues. The data can then be used either to print a stereolithographic (STL) model or for virtual manipulation of the generated 3D model by segmentation, reflection (mirroring), insertion, or repositioning of 3D objects for treatment planning [3].

S. Sukegawa
Division of Oral and Maxillofacial Surgery, Kagawa Prefectural Central Hospital, Takamatsu, Kagawa, Japan

T. Kanno (✉)
Department of Oral and Maxillofacial Surgery, Shimane University Faculty of Medicine, Izumo, Shimane, Japan
e-mail: tkanno@med.shimane-u.ac.jp

Stereolithographic 3D models are useful for maxillo-mandibular reconstruction indicators such as

1. A guide for plate adaptation.
2. Planning bony osteotomies.
3. Planning for graft or flap placements.
4. Surgeries involving jaw repositioning.
5. Construction of patient-specific custom implants (PSI).

Not only are they useful in visualizing and planning, but also for providing haptic support to the surgeon for perceived excellent tactile feedback during virtual surgery. They also prove to be very useful in creating a more predictable workflow for the intended surgical intervention. Unfortunately, there is no single prediction method where the surgical plan as performed on the model can be directly transferred to the patient.

Computer-assisted surgery (CAS) uses data from image processing, and can be divided into two major categories:

1. Computer-assisted presurgical planning.
2. Intraoperative navigation.

Computer-assisted presurgical planning involves preoperative surgical simulation using physical or virtual 3D images or models, and helps the surgeon to appreciate the underlying skeletal anatomy in a more precise manner. The application of preoperative surgical simulations is being used in the field of dental implantology for determining the appropriate positions and sizes of implants as well as evalu-


K. Bonanthaya et al. (eds.), *Oral and Maxillofacial Surgery for the Clinician*, https://doi.org/10.1007/978-981-15-1346-6_41

ating and planning for bone augmentation when needed, and in the field orthognathic surgery for assessing the amount and direction of movement of the jaws.

The process of intraoperative navigation was developed to improve the sequence of "diagnosis-surgical planning-surgery," allowing surgeons to accurately visualize the positions of surgical instruments and guides in real time on a display of patient CT and/or MRI data. Intraoperative navigation systems integrate diagnostic imaging with the actual surgical field, allowing simultaneous visualization of the surgical site and the analogous image counterpart with the help of a sensor that enables more precise access and manipulation for areas with sensitive anatomy. These navigation systems have now evolved greatly to minimize invasiveness while improving accuracy. The development of intraoperative navigation surgery has enabled improvement in execution and predictability for greater precision during oral-maxillofacial surgery.

This section presents an overview of currently available navigation systems and their applications, focusing on clinical utility and solutions they offer for problems and challenges in the field of oral and maxillofacial surgery.

## 41.2 Medical Navigation Technology

"Navigation-assisted surgery" is a broad term and can be interpreted in various ways.

> This is most usefully represented by three questions: "Where is the anatomical target in our patient?", "How can we reach our target safely for our patient?", and "What is our current anatomical location?".

Besides these questions, navigation-assisted surgery may also be used as an "information center" to provide surgeons with accurate and efficiently retrievable information. Navigation systems used for surgery are very similar to a global positioning system (GPS), as is commonly found in automobiles.

> It comprises three principal components: (1) a localizer, which is analogous to a satellite; (2) a "hand-held" probe, which corresponds to the track waves emitted by the GPS unit; and (3) the CT scan data of the patient, which is analogous to a road map.

Intraoperative navigation systems were initially developed for use in neurosurgery, but they are now commonly used in surgery of the craniomaxillofacial region due to their high accuracy and reliability [1, 4] (Fig. 41.1).

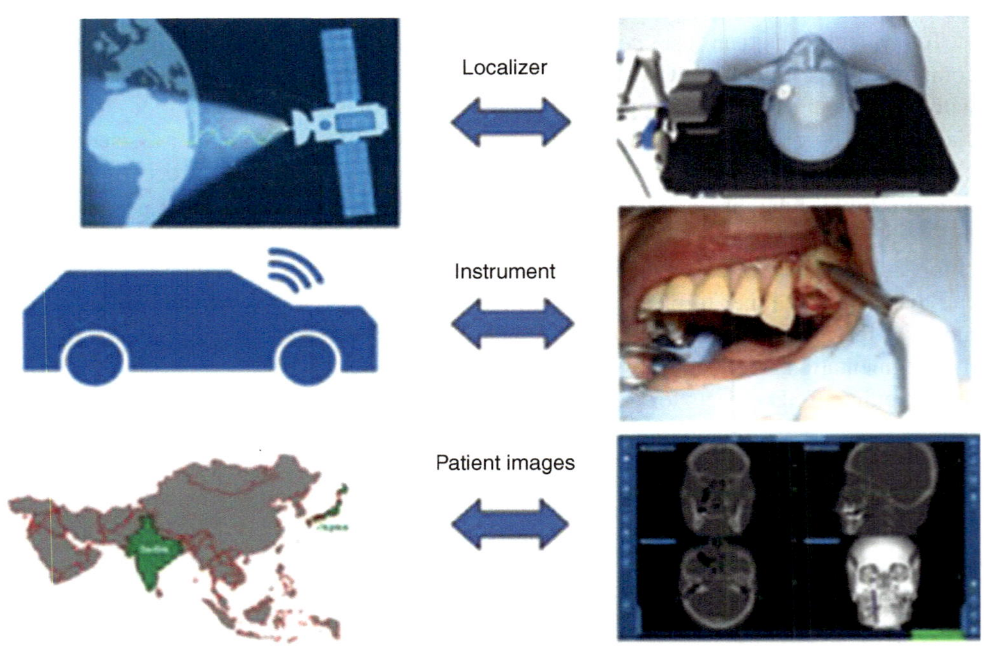




**Fig. 41.1** Components of a surgical navigation system. A surgical navigation system is comparable to a global positioning system (GPS) as is commonly used in automobiles, and is composed of three primary components: a localizer, which is analogous to a satellite in space; an instrument or surgical probe, which represents the track waves emitted by the GPS unit in the vehicle; and a CT scan data set, which is analogous to a road map

### 41.2.1 Differences Between Optical and Electromagnetic Tracking Systems

Two main technologies are currently available for intraoperative navigation, including optical and electromagnetic (Fig. 41.2), and they share the same function. However, they use very different technologies to relay position information to the surgeon. Two major components of the optical navigation system are measured using an infrared camera. These include the position of the reference frame, which is the optical point of reference for navigation and is also called the patient tracker, and a surgical probe with light reflectors. This enables the position of the surgical probe to be displayed on the CT or MRI image in real time. Care should be taken to ensure that both the tracker and the probe are detected by the infrared camera of the navigation system to track the instrument position within the surgical field [5]. By contrast, the electromagnetic system utilizes electromagnetic fields and reference points on a patient borne device, along with a wired instrument for the surgeon to manipulate within the surgical field. The system functions by creating a magnetic field of known intensity and then using microsensors in key instruments to allow the system to determine where the instrument is located relative to the patient's anatomy [6]. In contrast to an optical system, an electromagnetic system does not require a clear line of vision between the IR camera and the sensors, allowing equipment and objects to be placed between the sensors and the IR camera. However, the accuracy of this system is compromised when using ferromagnetic instruments.

### 41.2.2 Registration Techniques

Registration is the task of obtaining the mutual transformation matrix by calculating the relationship between the coordinates of the actual patient space and the coordinates of the medical image. In other words, this procedure involves the alignment of the patient and the image, and it is the most important process when performing surgical navigation.

Registration techniques are categorized into two major types: (1) marker-based [7] and (2) marker-free [8] (Fig. 41.3).

In the marker-based technique, registration requires identifiable markers to be placed within preoperative images that can be easily detected on the patient during the surgery. These markers include dental splints [9], skin adhesive reference markers, and bone-implanted screws [10]. In contrast, the marker-free technique is based on the patient's regional anatomy. This can be performed by registering easily identifiable soft tissue or bony structures on the patient's preoperative scans. Another technique for marker-free registration is laser surface scanning, which is used to match random points on the surface of facial skin to corresponding points on CT or MRI images. More recently, hybrid registration combining methods have been used that combine point registration and surface registration [11].

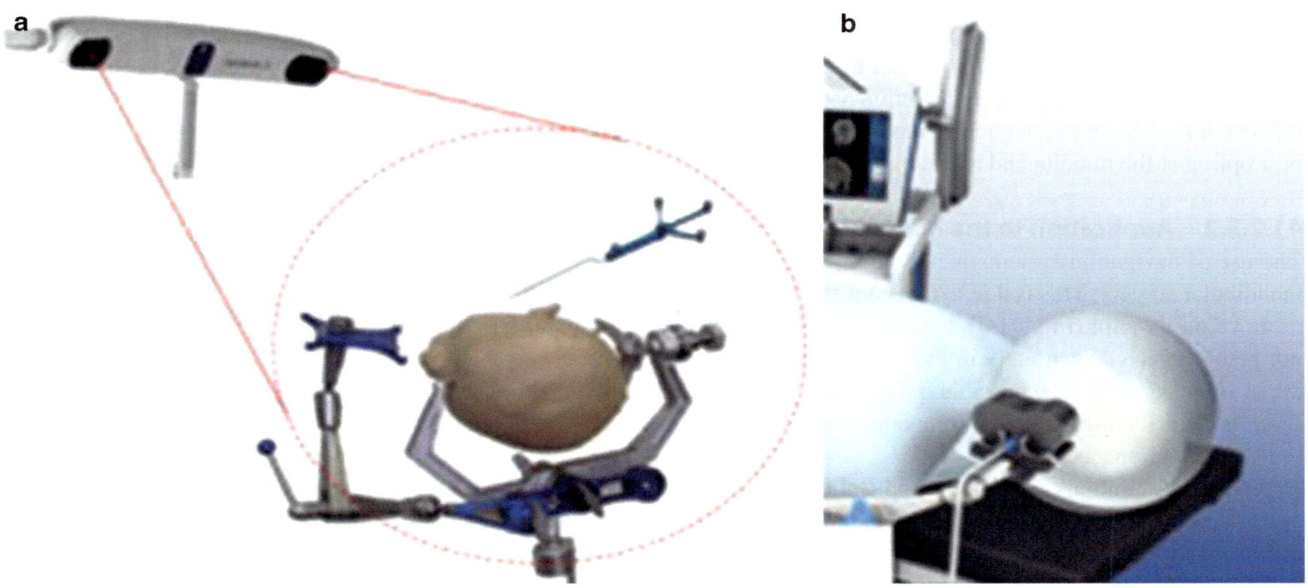




**Fig. 41.2** There are two main types of navigation systems currently available: (**a**) optical and (**b**) electromagnetic systems

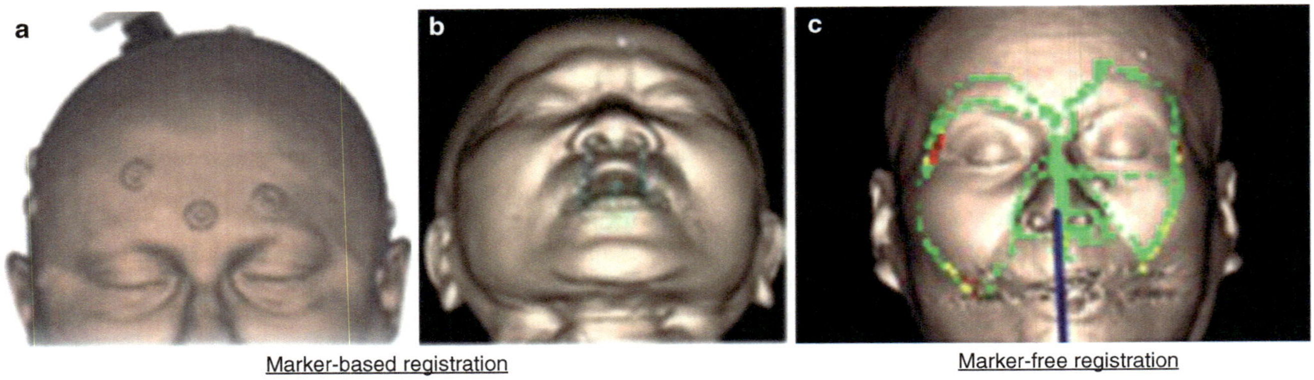


**Fig. 41.3** Registration techniques for navigation preparation can be categorized into two main groups: marker-based and marker-free. Marker-based registration requires markers that are apparent on preoperative images and that are easily detectable on the patient during the procedure, such as (**a**) skin adhesive reference markers or (**b**) a referencing dental splint (**c**) Marker-free registration relies on the patient's craniomaxillofacial anatomy. Laser surface scanning is applied in a distinct marker-free registration technique, where random points on the facial skin surface are matched to corresponding points on the soft tissues in preoperative computed tomography/magnetic resonance imaging (CT/MRI) images

### 41.2.3 Application to Oral-Maxillofacial Surgery

#### 41.2.3.1 Application to the Maxilla and Midface

The use of navigation systems significantly improves the degree of intraoperative precision and accuracy that can be predictably transferred from the planning stages to the actual surgery. However, navigational accuracy is limited by the type of system used, the method of procuring imaging data, and the intraoperative synchronization of the imaging data with the patient's actual position. The systems currently in use for maxillary and midface surgery are relatively reliable, as most have been modified from their neurosurgical counterparts [12]. Because the maxilla and midface are immovable, unlike the mandible, the position of the skull relative to the reference is stable, and the registration procedure directly reflects this. Therefore, navigation-assisted surgery is the best option at the maxilla and midface.

#### 41.2.3.2 Application to the Mandible

The use of navigation systems is not currently approved for mandibular surgery. This is due to the nature of the mandible to move on its joint (Fig. 41.4), resulting in the registration not being reflected accurately in the navigation of the mandible. However, it may be possible if the position of the mandible is held identical to its intraoperative position during image acquisition.

At present, solutions exist for the application of navigation systems to mandibular surgery. One such option is the use of a dynamic reference frame mounted to the mandible that enables the continuous tracking of mandibular movement during surgery [13]. This method utilizes a sensor frame and mandible/teeth supported markers for the direct tracking of the mandible during surgery. This permits free intraoperative movement of the mandible. The second option is to maintain an immobile intercuspation position, such as using a maxilla-mandibular fixation to maintain intraoperative synchronization [14]. Unfortunately, this is impossible to achieve in most intraoral procedures. Therefore, a third strategy has been developed in which the mandible is placed in a reproducible position against the maxilla using an occlusal splint. This method appears to produce no additional error.

## 41.3 Clinical Significance in Oral and Maxillofacial Surgery

There are numerous clinical applications for CAS and intraoperative navigation in oral and maxillofacial surgery. This is reiterated by literature support available over the last decade supporting its use.

### 41.3.1 Application for Oral-Maxillofacial Trauma

Computer-based surgery is a rapidly emerging approach used in some surgical disciplines, and can be used both as a research tool and to improve healthcare. Computer-based surgery, in combination with the use of a navigation system, has been shown to reduce overall operation time in complex anatomic areas, such as maxillofacial trauma surgery (e.g., orbital trauma reconstruction surgery), making surgery more reliable. Using 3D models based on CAS is suitable for preoperative preparation of reconstruction material for bone defects caused by trauma. On the other hand, navigation surgery is most suitable for intraoperative anatomical evaluation [15]. By combining these techniques, safer and minimally

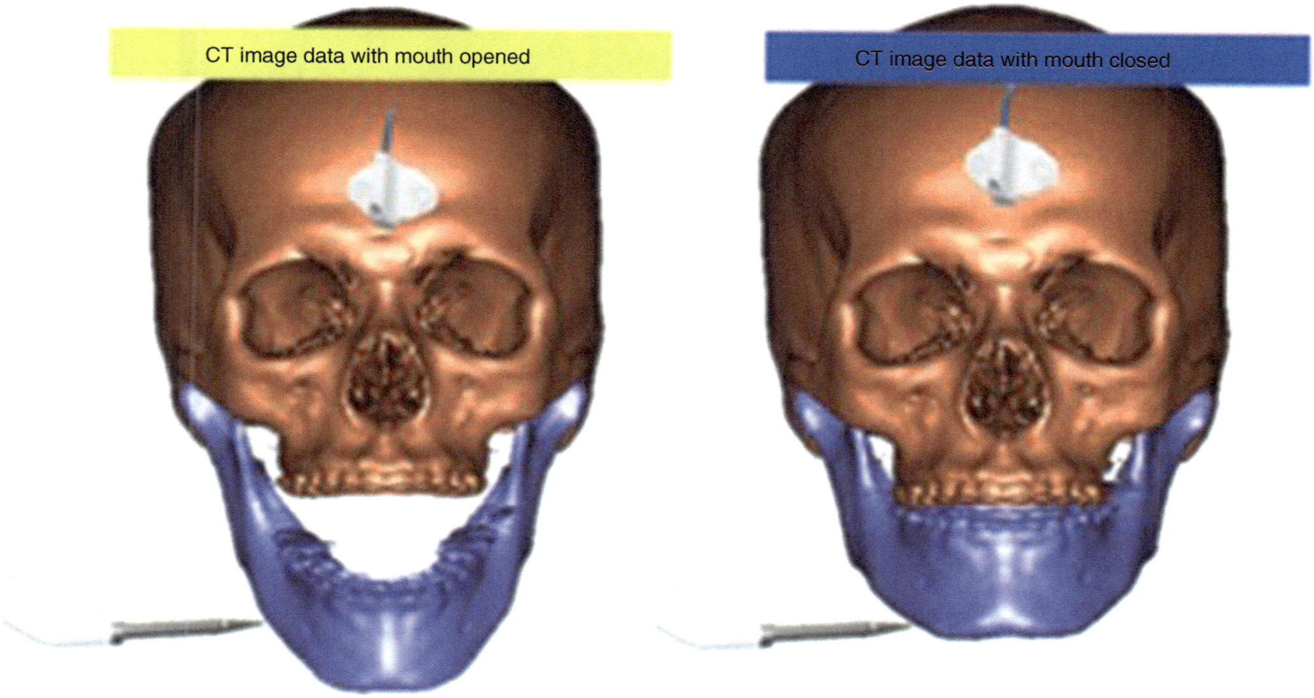


**Fig. 41.4** The positional relationship between the reference and the target becomes unstable due to the free mobility of the mandible. If the mandible were maintained in an identical position during image acquisition and the surgical procedure, then all structures within the image could be fixed in an identical position, thereby ensuring the accuracy of the navigation surgery

invasive surgery is possible. Maxillofacial trauma may be an important indicator suggesting the use of navigation systems (Figs. 41.5, 41.6, 41.7 and 41.8). Unilateral midfacial and orbital trauma surgery may also be indicators, and are normally treated with open reduction and fixation with navigation assistance.

The largest sample sizes for navigation surgery were found in the field of craniomaxillofacial trauma, offering significant positive results for orbital fracture treatment through navigation-assisted surgery. Midfacial trauma, and particularly unilateral midfacial trauma, was most common example of maxillofacial trauma available in the literature. Some of these reports described the treatment of patients with delayed zygomatic fractures requiring osteotomies to reposition the abnormally healed bones. This results in added complexity for the surgeon due to the lack of known anatomical landmarks. He et al. presented a protocol for the creation of artificial landmarks on the surface of the zygoma [16]. The technique involved the registration being performed with rigidly fixed, light-reflecting spheres placed on the patient's skull. Subsequent soft tissue surface scanning was performed using a laser pointer to complete the process.

Another challenging facet of oral and maxillofacial surgery is the management of orbital fractures. This can prove to be demanding even for the most experienced of surgeons. Literature indicates that intraoperative navigation is a very useful tool in post-traumatic orbital reconstruction. Another rising trend is the use of patient-specific implants (PSIs). A recently published literature also discusses the use of PSIs with navigation guidance [17]. A control group was treated with navigation using prebent titanium mesh. Several significant factors were reported favoring the study group. PSIs are poised to make a significant change in the management of orbital trauma.

Innovations such as intraoperative navigation and computer-assisted surgical planning have been shown to improve the efficacy, accuracy, and predictability of surgical procedures. The 3D reconstruction abilities of software could be used to virtually display the patient's anatomy throughout the case, allowing for stereotactic navigation. During the surgery, the intraoperative navigation system helps surgeons to control the positions of implants or of repositioned bone, and assists in verifying the final location. A navigation system enhances the surgeon's ability to measure the extent of resection and to confirm the orientation of bone grafts used for reconstruction. Using this approach, it is possible to minimize the human error factor by increasing the adherence to a pre-

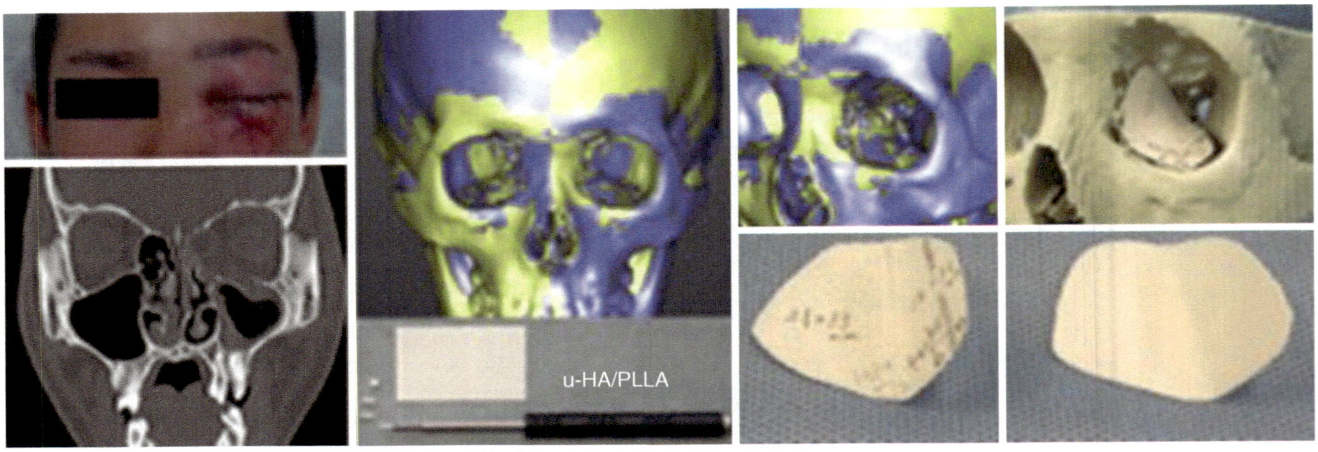




**Fig. 41.5** A 17-year-old male undergoing a large orbital floor to medial orbital fracture reconstruction. Surgeons first created a three-dimensional model that was mirrored by CAS, and determined the angle and form of reconstruction material using third-generation bioactive/bioresorbable materials, the SuperFIXORB-MX® (OsteotransMS®) system; TEIJIN Medical Technologies Co., Ltd, Osaka, Japan, according to the shape of the orbits to be reconstructed

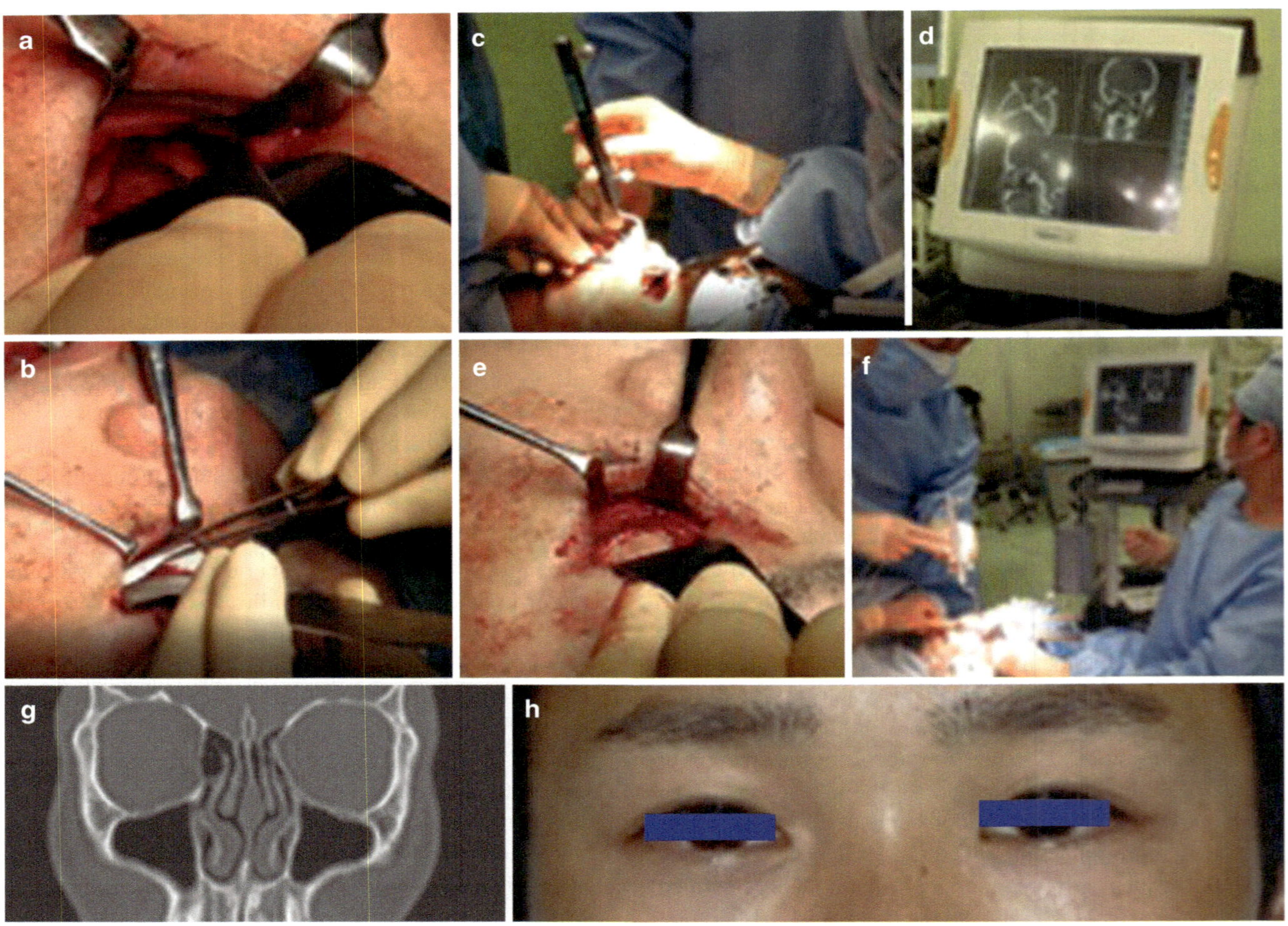




**Fig. 41.6** (**a–h**) A 17-year-old male undergoing a large orbital floor to medial orbital fracture reconstruction. Navigation will determine the exact intraoperative anatomical form. Reconstruction material before CAS was positioned at the reconstruction site. We then confirmed the exact position of the reconstruction material and reconstructed the orbital shape using the navigation system

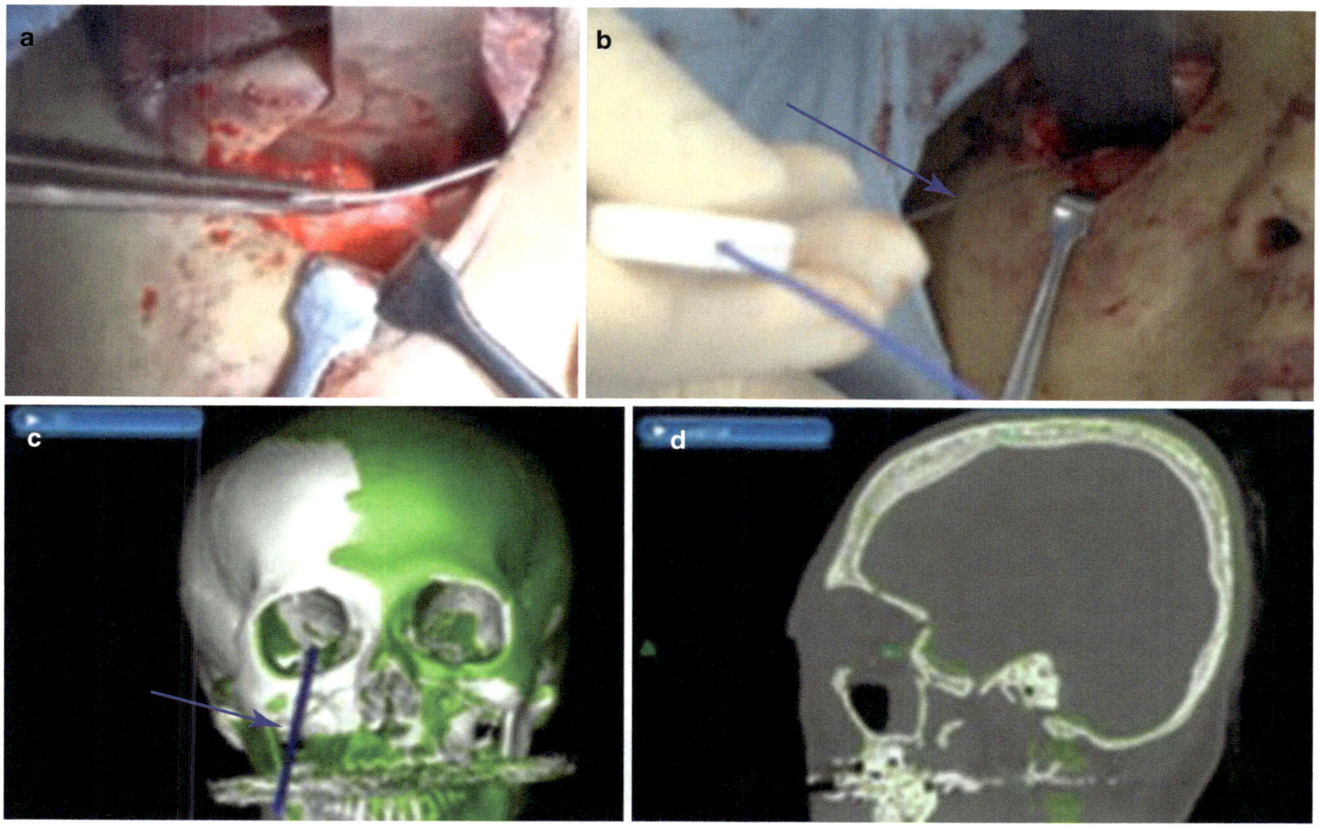




**Fig. 41.7** (**a**) The bioresorbable mesh plate was positioned to support the orbital globe. (**b**) The reconstructed site was confirmed to match the mirror image using a tip pointer with a navigation system. (**c**) Intraoperative navigation system screenshot showing a multiplane view of the position of the surgeon's navigation probe in relation to the orbital floor defect region at the time of localization. (**d**) Shows the reconstruction plan image, created using the mirroring technique

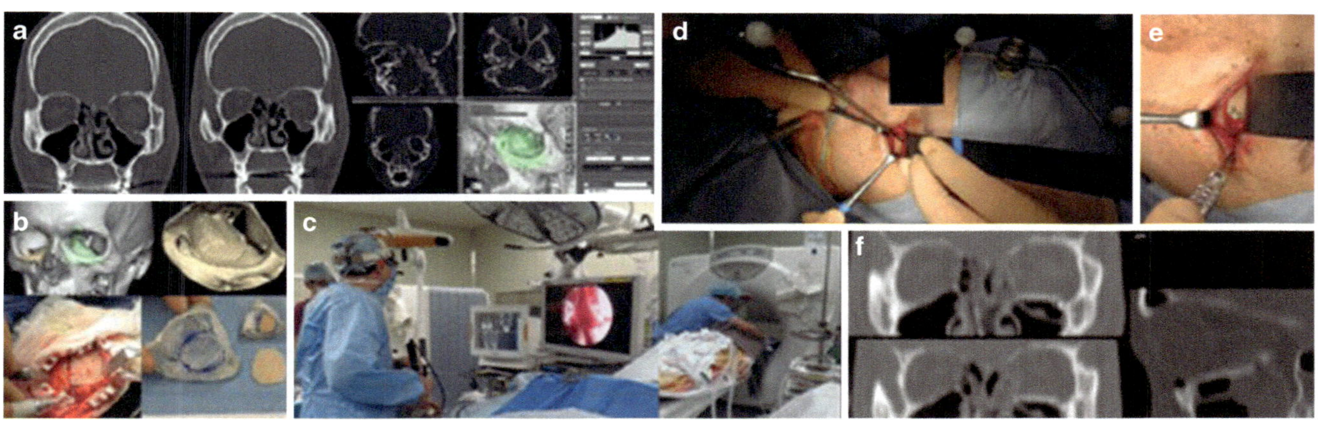




**Fig. 41.8** (**a, b**) A 33-year-old male undergoing a nasoorbitoethmoidal (NOE) and maxillary fractures open treatment, including a large orbital floor to medial orbital walls fractures reconstruction. We, maxillofacial surgeons, first created a three-dimensional (3D) precise preorbit to orbital groove model that was mirrored by computer-assisted simulation, and determined the anatomical form of reconstruction for autogenous bone harvested from calvaria using Piezosurgery® according to the 3D shape of the orbits to be reconstructed (produced by Yasojima Proceed Co., Ltd. Osaka, Japan). Navigation will determine the exact intraoperative 3D anatomical form. (**c**) The fractured deep medial orbital wall was precisely reduced under an endoscopic-assisted navigation-guided surgery by otorhinolaryngology-head and neck surgeons. (**d, e**) We then reconstructed the large orbital floor and confirmed the exact position of the autogenous calvarial bone for accurate reconstruction of the orbit using the navigation system, followed by fixation using titanium screws. (**f**) The use of intraoperative CT in the hybrid operation room can provide rapid CT data during surgery for the final 3D confirmation of complex orbital reconstruction cases

operative plan. Furthermore, this also helps in reducing the incidence of postoperative complications due to improperly positioned or oriented bone grafts, plates, or fixation screws. Virtual surgical planning (VSP) combined with 3D printing technology has improved surgical efficiency and precision through the generation of 3D surgical models, implants, and guides [18]. This increases the number of indicators suggesting the use of VSP by the surgeon, as it offers additional tools in preoperative planning and intraoperative decision making. Both VSP and 3D models may be used to plan the optimal reconstruction material in terms of the volume, shape, and dimensions required. They can also be used to produce templates for resective surgery to accurately demarcate the boundaries for resection and/or to plan more efficient and accurate reconstructive strategies. A further advantage of using 3D models is a reduction in total operative time and the elimination of potential complications from prolonged surgery.

### 41.3.2 Application for Oral-Maxillofacial Tumor/Cancer

Computer-assisted navigational surgery is a proven method for reducing operating time and increasing reliability in complex surgical procedures of the infratemporal fossa and the periorbital region [19] (Fig. 41.9). Navigation-assisted surgery was introduced in the field of oral, head, and neck tumors more than 20 years ago. The use of navigation in the management of benign and malignant lesions is discussed later.

Malignant lesions of the head and neck have a high rate of recurrence (25–48%). Tumor control essentially depends on the extent of the tumor, its location, and the margins of resection, with the latter being a very important prognostic factor in cancer surgery. Feichtinger et al. [20] used navigation systems to evaluate the resection margins in the treatment of six patients with carcinomas in the nasal cavity, maxillary sinus, and oral cavity. In four patients, further resection had to be performed after an assessment with a navigation system

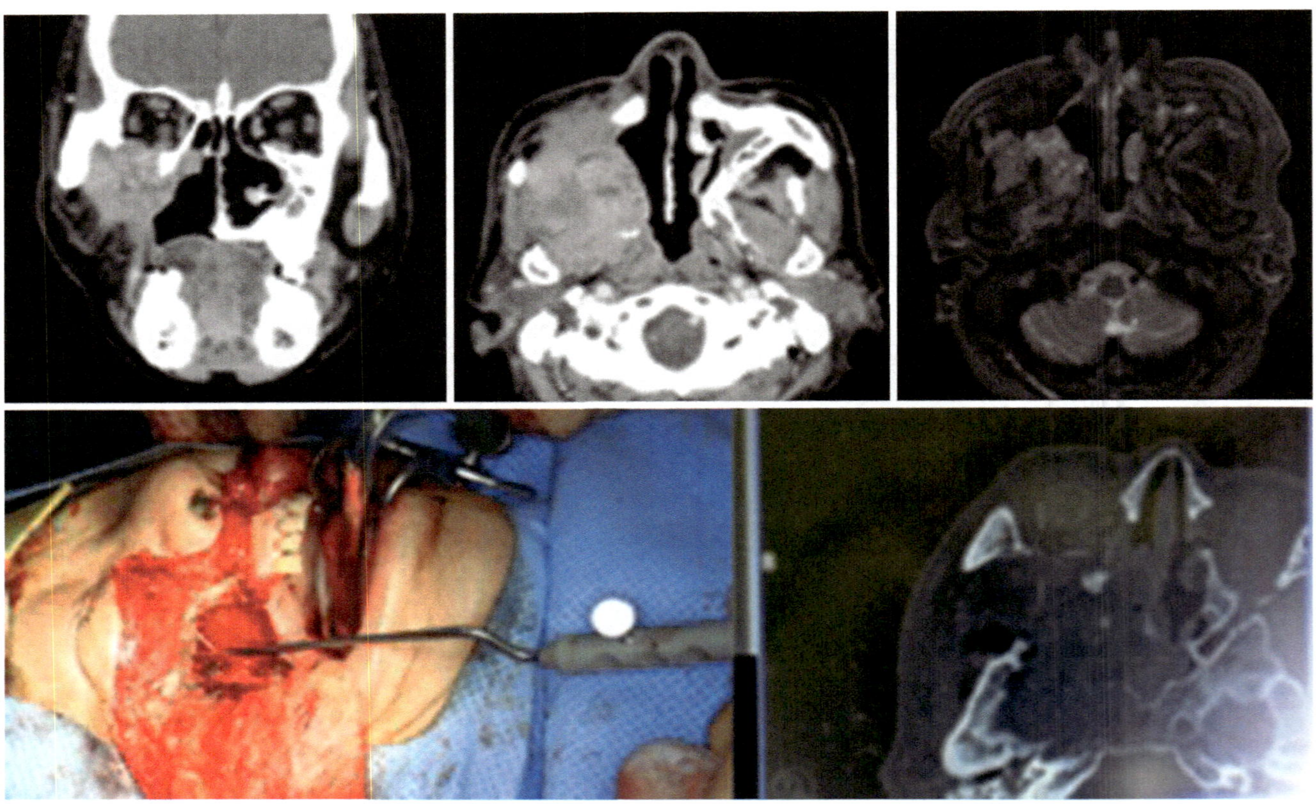



**Fig. 41.9** A 79-year-old male with recurrent ameloblastoma of maxilla-infratemporal fossa. Because of the complexity of the local anatomy, tumors in the infratemporal fossa present a challenge to oral and maxillofacial surgeons. Recurrent malignant tumors in this area are particularly difficult to resect because scars from previous operations may dislocate important structures. A navigation technique has been introduced to resect infratemporal fossa tumors and was successfully applied for the resection of recurrent malignant tumors. The visible navigation during surgery could increase the accuracy and safety of the operations and enhance surgeon confidence

using positron emission tomography (PET)-CT scans proved the initial resection to be unsatisfactory. This demonstrates that navigation surgery based on PET-CT image fusion is an excellent tool for improving the local control of advanced head and neck cancer.

Navigation-assisted surgery has also been successfully used in the management of benign tumors of the maxillofacial region [21]. This was performed with features such as mirroring and side-to-side comparisons, and was applied with successful results. Use of customized hydroxy-apatite prosthesis with pre-embedded titanium implants was used for reconstruction. Optimal positioning is secured using navigation. Some interesting techniques for reconstruction are discussed now.

It is important to remember that navigation is an excellent tool when it comes to its use in the skull base [22], the midface [23], and the neck [24]. However, its use in mandibular tumors is limited due to the possibility of changes in the spatial orientation of the lower jaw, as described earlier.

### 41.3.3 Application for Orthognathic Surgery

The primary determinants of success in orthognathic surgery include an accurate diagnosis, meticulous treatment planning, and the ability to transfer the plan precisely to the patient intraoperatively. In earlier years, this was performed by a process of model surgery in a laboratory using articulators on plaster casts, which were then transferred to the patient using acrylic splints during the surgical procedure (Figs. 41.10 and 41.11). The procedure was error prone at multiple levels within the sequence. Literature reports an error of up to 5 mm using this type of treatment sequence. With the advent and routine usage of CAD/CAM technology

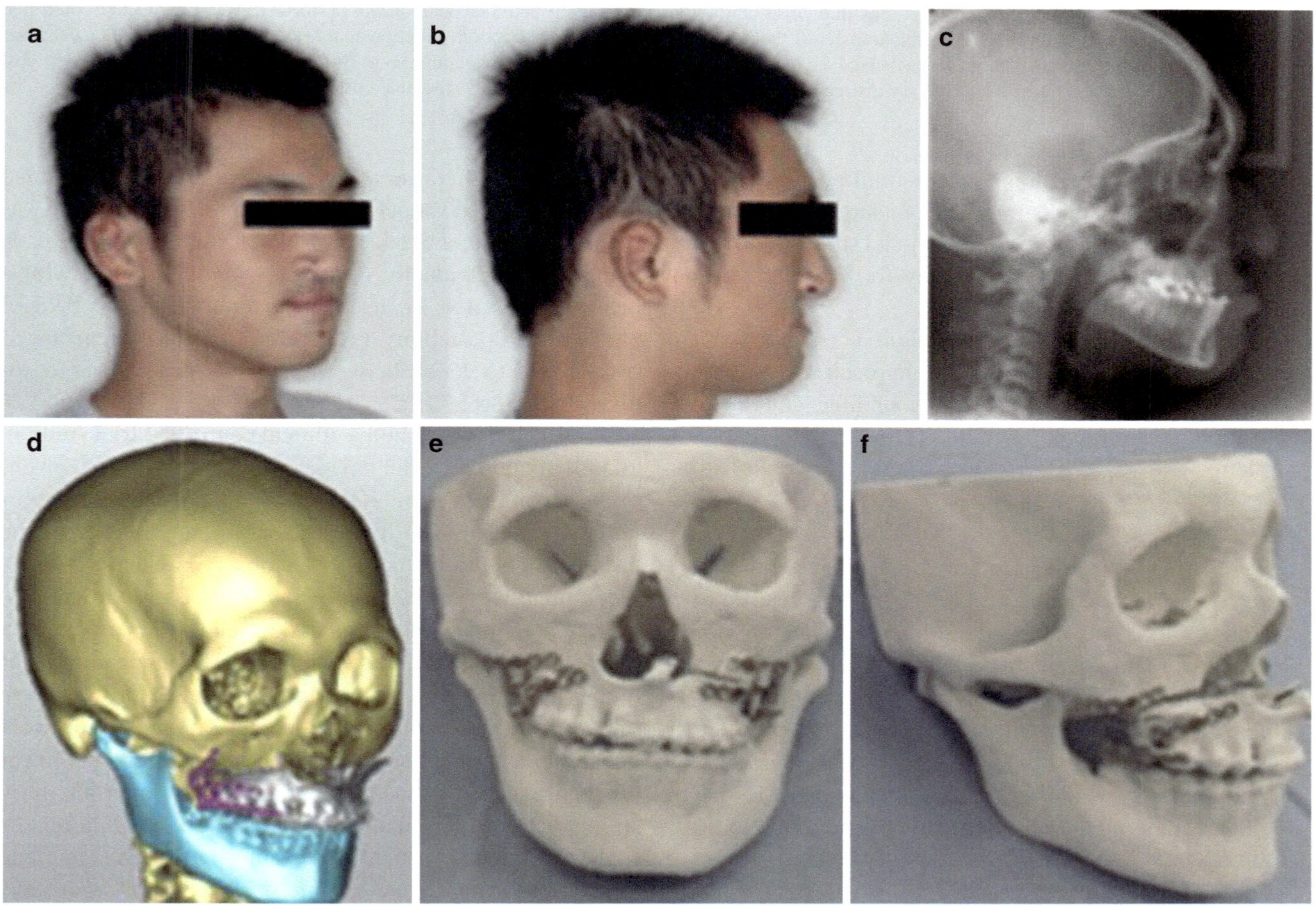




**Fig. 41.10** Optimal treatment planning and preparation using 3D models. CAS for cleft lip and palate-related severe maxillary hypoplasia deformity patients using maxillary distraction osteogenesis. (**a**–**c**) A 17 year old male undergoing maxillary distraction for cleft-related midfacial retrusion. (**d**) Detailed computer simulation for maxillary distraction surgery in a patient with severe maxillary hypoplasia deformity was used to determine the optimal treatment plan, such as the distraction direction and degree of advancement. (**e**, **f**) A 3D printed skeletal model was used to prepare for a maxillary semi-custom-made distractor setting with fabrication

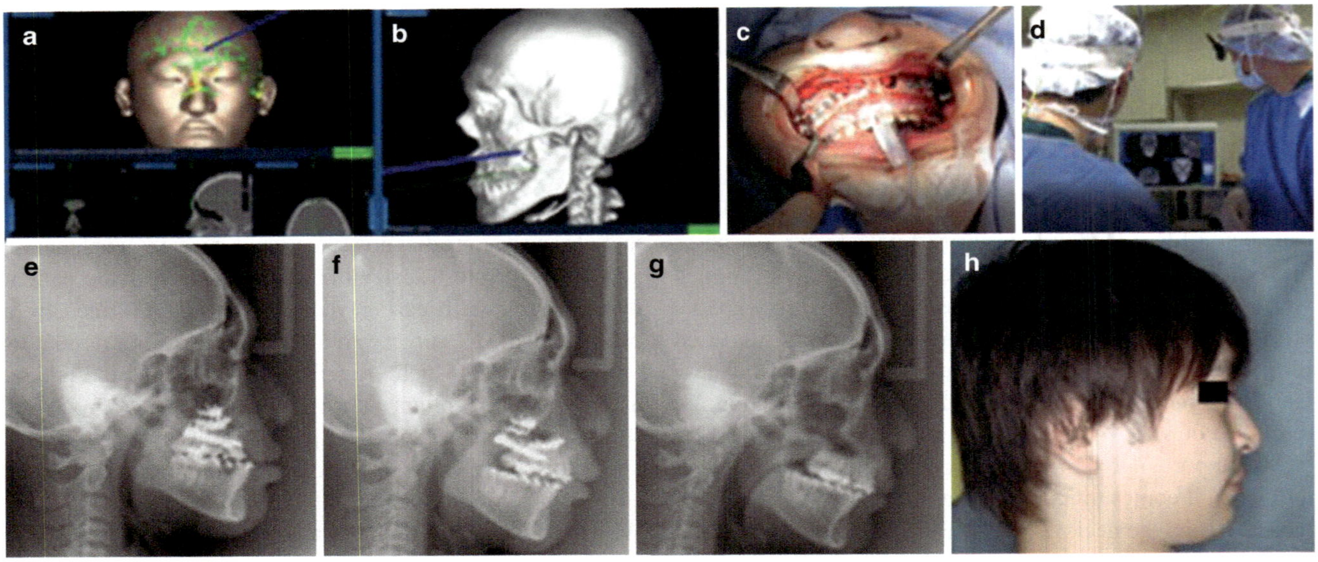



**Fig. 41.11** A 17-year-old male undergoing maxillary distraction for cleft-related midfacial retrusion. (**a–d**) Accurate transfer of the treatment plan to the patient in the operating room was acheived. Using the navigation system, precise placement of the maxillary distraction planned preoperatively at the set position was performed. The surgeon then confirmed the same distraction direction that was preoperatively planned by the intraoperative navigation. (**e–g**) Shows the radiographs during and post treatment. (**h**) Shows the final post surgical result of the patient

and virtual surgical planning, the workflow of treatment planning in orthognathic surgery has undergone a paradigm shift. The conventional workflow of model surgery and splint fabrications is slowly paving the way for VSP and custom printed 3D splints and guides.

Although the degree of inaccuracies associated with treatment planning is reduced using this approach, certain drawbacks such as autorotation of the mandible and lack of control on the vertical position of the maxilla are still prevalent.

There are three methods by which CAS is used in the practice of orthognathic surgery: (1) using real-time intraoperative guidance with surgical navigation for the repositioning of the maxilla and mandible; (2) use of 3D printed cutting guides for precise osteotomy and repositioning, with or without customized 3D printed osteosynthesis plates; and (3) the use of wafer-less surgical planning where the printed implant doubles as both a cutting guide for the osteotomy and as the fixation devices. Many clinical studies have evaluated the efficacy of these methods with promising results.

Mazzoni et al. were the first to report the use of intraoperative navigation in orthognathic surgery, in 2010 [25]. They calculated the overlap error to assess the accuracy of the technique after surface matching the virtually planned model and the postoperative CT scan. The accuracy was reported for the entire facial skeleton, rather than for each component individually (maxilla, mandible, chin), with a mean match error for each patient ranging from 0.28 to 1.99 mm. Repeatability (<2 mm) in the face area ranged from 77.5% to 96.2% between patients, with a mean reproducibility of 86.5%.

Zinser et al. published a clinical controlled trial study in 2013 that compared the navigation technique with conventional technique, using 3D surgical guides and intermaxillary splints [26]. The highest accuracy for transfer of the maxillary plan to the patient was observed when a 3D surgical guide was used, and no significant linear differences between the planned virtual model and the postoperative results were present in any direction. The navigation technique only showed a significant mean linear difference in the vertical dimension, and differences in angulation were not significant in either group. In contrast, significant linear differences were shown for the classic intermaxillary splints between the planning results and the actual results in the sagittal and vertical dimensions. Differences in plane angulations when using an interocclusal splint were also significant. The usefulness of navigation-assisted surgery for orthognathic surgery was supported based on previous reports.

Published literature demonstrates that all studies have met the 2-mm success criterion, which refers to a maximum difference of 2 mm between the virtual planning performed and the actual surgical outcome. Zinser et al. reported the only prospective controlled clinical trial comparing CAD-CAM splints, navigation surgery, and intermaxillary splints for the transfer of maxillary planning [26]. The CAD-CAM splints, patented by the authors, were used for maintaining the mandibular condyles (TMJ) in their centric relation. Mandibular positioning still poses a challenge during orthognathic surgery, with none of the solutions having attained "gold-standard" status.

An important clinical limitation for the use of navigation is the increase in operating time [27]. Though there is ample support for increased accuracy levels with the use of navigation, the prolonged operating time still remains a deterrent for the routine use of intraoperative navigation in orthognathic surgery. A recent study indicates that dynamic navigation systems have an entry error of approximately 0.4 mm [28] and an angular deviation error of approximately 4° [29]. Further technological developments can be expected in the field of orthognathic surgery, and an appropriate update for surgeons is required.

### 41.3.4 Application for Preimplant Bone Augmentation/Dental Implants

Loss of teeth and supporting structures is a common occurrence in the field of oral and maxillofacial surgery for patients who have suffered extensive alveolar bone defects caused by cysts, tumors, facial trauma, or severe periodontal disease [30]. Comprehensive reconstruction methods, including rehabilitation with multiple dental implants, are commonly required to restore function in these patients.

Issues like atrophic jaws, where dental implants cannot be placed due to the loss of bone corpus, are managed by regenerative procedures. Although bone augmentation at the mandibular posterior area is important for occlusion reconstruction using dental implants, it is difficult due to anatomical limitations arising from the inferior alveolar nerve (IAN) and the mandibular bone. However, bone augmentation at the mandibular posterior area can be performed safely and reliably using CAS with 3D modeling and navigation systems (Figs. 41.12 and 41.13).

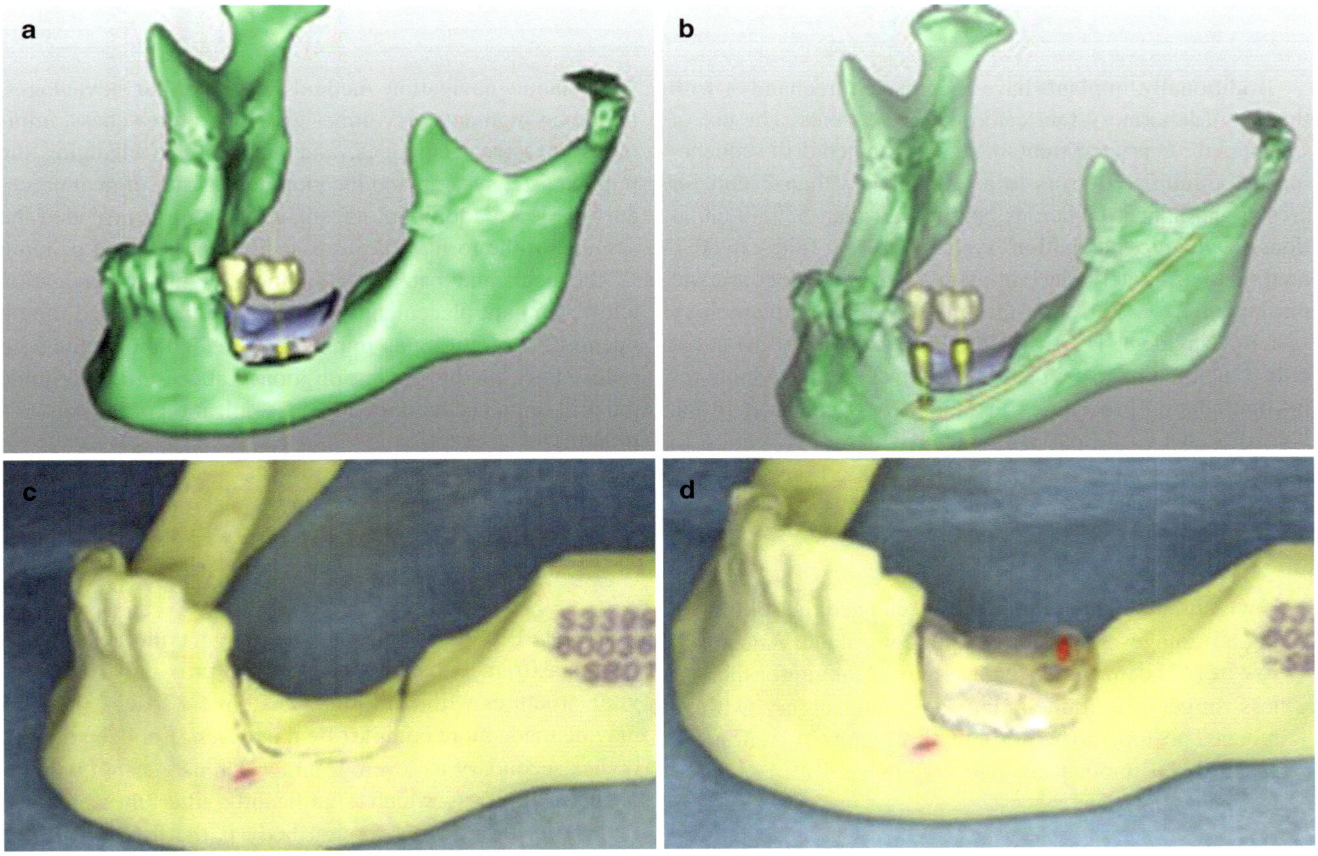




**Fig. 41.12** (**a–d**) Computer simulation based on preoperative CT data will determine the bone augmentation method for implantation. In this case, we chose bone augmentation using the sandwich technique. The necessary bone augmentation volume and position of the anatomically important inferior alveolar nerve (IAN) were confirmed using computer simulation. Based on this information, we will determine a safe bone cutting line. Surgeons then created a surgical guide using a 3D model based on simulation

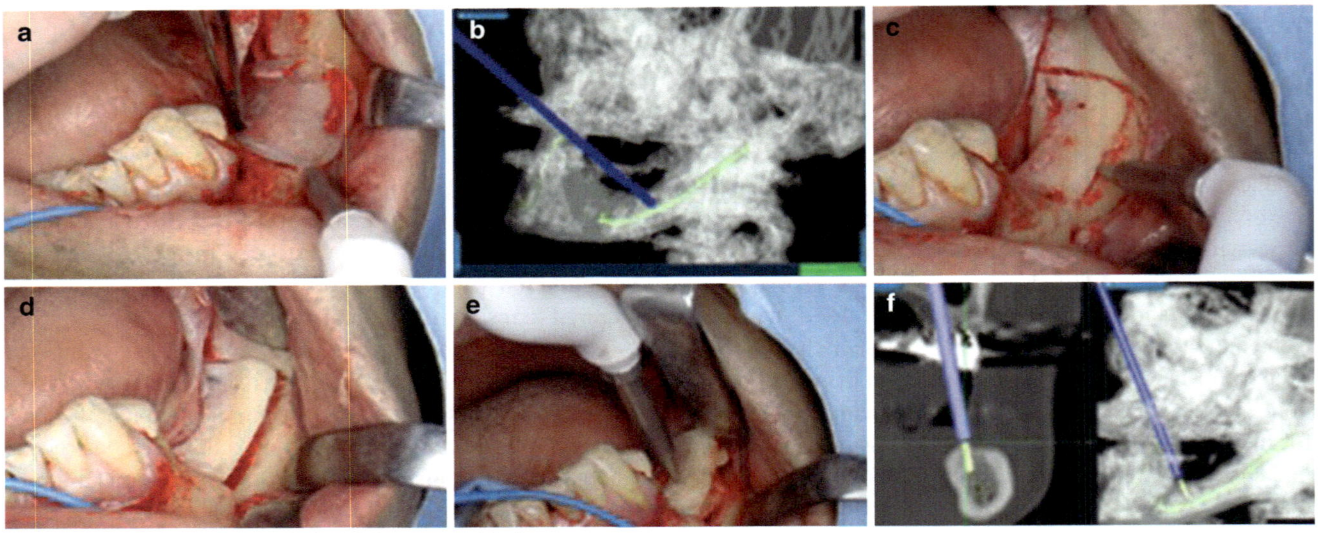




**Fig. 41.13** (**a–d**) This is a continuation of Fig. 41.12. While confirming the position of the IAN in real time based on intraoperative navigation, the surgeon cut the alveolar bone with reference to the surgical guide created before surgery. (**e**) The surgeon then inserted autologous bone taken from the donor and increased the alveolar bone vertically. The most important goal in this surgery is to acquire alveolar bone height as planned before surgery. (**f**) The bone height can be confirmed in real time based on intraoperative navigation

Traditionally, implants have been placed freehand or with the use of laboratory-fabricated guidance stents. The use of CT-guided 3D printed stents with coordinated drill sequencing has minimized errors to a level of less than 2 mm for crestal and apical deviations, and to less than 5° in angulations. Dynamic navigation systems use a time-effective method to accurately place implants with equivalent implant placement error. Currently the Image-Guided Implantology system (Navident; HERMANS Corp., Tokyo, Japan) is the only dynamic image navigation system (DINS) available for in-office dental procedures in Japan. Its counterpart in the United States is the passive optical dynamic navigation in implantology (X-Nav Technologies, Inc., Lansdale, PA, USA).

> Navigation in dental implantology can add the following advantages: (1) precise depth control and reduced risk of IAN damage [31]; (2) help in planning for flapless surgery or limited flap elevation surgery with reduced postoperative morbidity [32]; and (3) accurate spacing and implant angulation compared to using a freehand approach.

The use of virtual implant planning and intraoperative navigation allows for prosthodontic and surgical coordination due to its planning accuracy and implementation in actual surgical scenarios.

Dynamic navigation methods have similar advantages, including high accuracy, time- and cost-effectiveness, minimally invasive techniques, and flexibility in changing the implant size, system, and location during the surgical procedure [33]. An additional advantage is comfort provided the surgeon in the form of posture, facilitating reduced bending of the neck and back. For example, dynamic navigation allows implant placement for patients with a limited mouth opening, or requiring an implant at a second molar site with reduced access, by relying on a navigation screen to guide the drill sequence without direct visualization of the patient's mouth.

### 41.3.5 Clinical Applications for the Removal of Foreign Bodies

Retrieval of foreign bodies in the craniomaxillofacial region is often extremely dangerous due to the proximity to various vital structures within a limited anatomical space [34]. This may be made more complex by the presence of deep foreign bodies secondary to severe trauma such as gunshot wounds or blast injuries, which significantly alter the anatomy. Precise location of the foreign body is the first step in the retrieval process, and this may be accomplished with preoperative scans and 3D image rendering. The intraoperative step is next, and is more challenging, as the exact location of the foreign body within the surgical field must be ascertained. Traditional methods utilize a stereotactic "double needle" method with venipuncture needles for triangulation

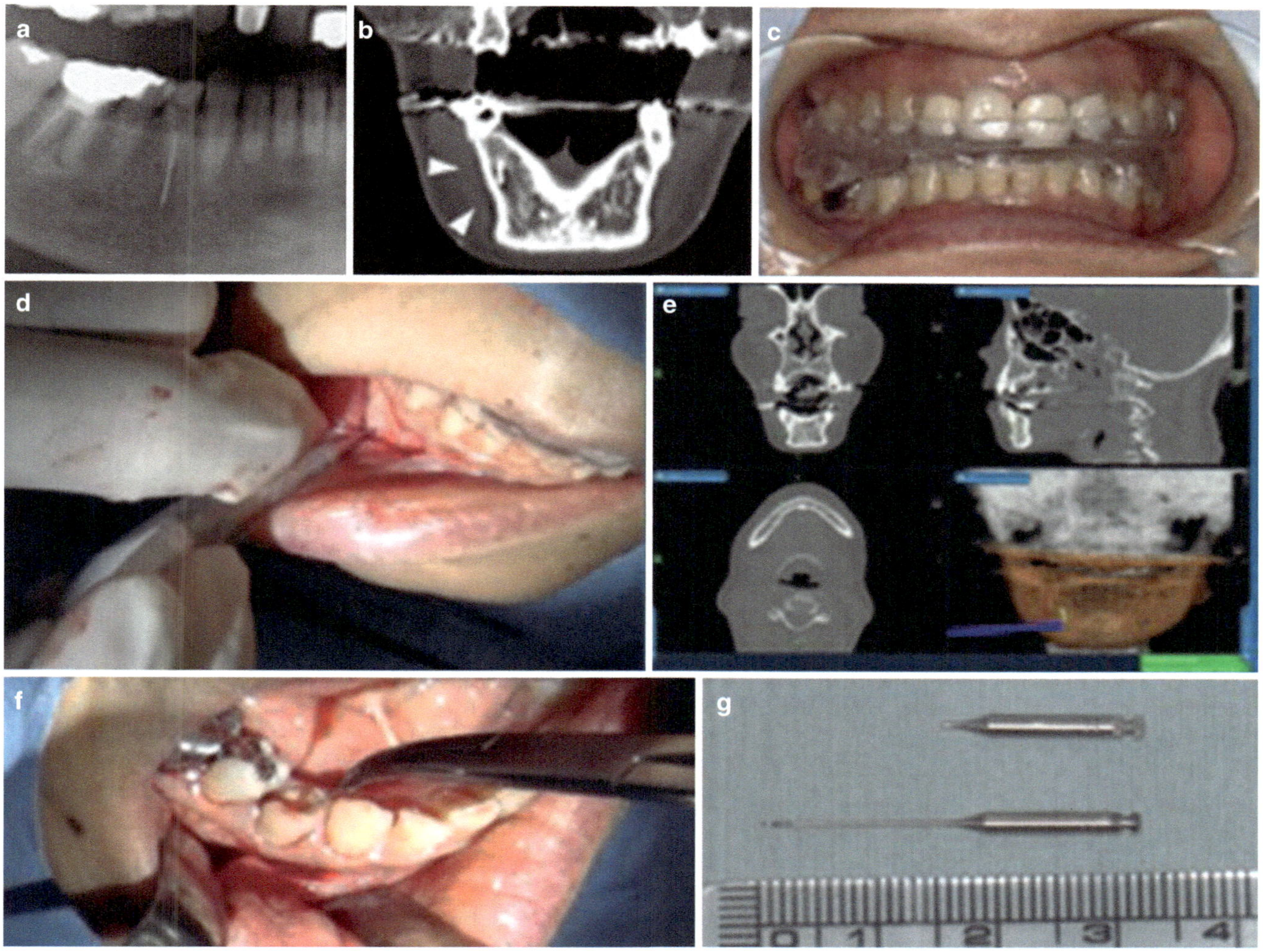




**Fig. 41.14** (**a–g**) A 65-year-old female with a foreign body due to dental instrument breakage in the mandible, occurring during an endodontic treatment for a restorative dental procedure. (**a**, **b**) Fracture of root canal instruments, with a fractured piece protruding beyond the apex, is a troublesome incident during endodontic treatment. Locating and retrieving these objects represents a challenge for maxillofacial surgeons because they are difficult to access due to the proximity between the foreign body and vital structures. Using the navigation system for mandible treatment is difficult as the mobile nature of the mandible complicates its synchronization with the preoperative imaging data during surgery. (**c**) The broken dental instrument was removed using a minimally invasive approach with a surgical navigation system and an interocclusal splint for stable, identically repeatable positioning of the mandible. (**d**, **e**) Based on the 3D position of the navigation probe, a location that best approximated and the most anterior extent of the fragment was selected. (**f**) A minimal vestibular incision was made at this location, a subperiosteal reflection was performed, and the foreign body location was confirmed using the navigation system. (**g**) The instrument was carefully visualized and extruded from the apical to the tooth crown side and was then removed using mosquito forceps through the medullary cavity of the crown side of the tooth

of the foreign body using plain radiographs [35]. This involved the two reference needles being sequentially placed until both met the foreign body on radiographs. Through blunt dissection, one of the needles is made to contact the foreign body and locate it. It is important to understand that it may be difficult to distinguish small changes in position on plain radiographs. The use of C-arm digital fluoroscopy was a significant advancement for this method, providing rapid radiography [36]. However, as with plain films, fluoroscopic images are 2D, which imposes limitations when locating objects in a 3D space. The use of intraoperative ultrasound imaging has also been proposed to localize foreign bodies. However, the precision involved in positioning may be questionable, and its use in the oral cavity may also be limited by the size of the instrument.

Intraoperative navigation systems could allow a foreign body to be accurately located in 3D space; these systems are very effective for removing a foreign body during facial surgery [37] (Figs. 41.14 and 41.15). One limitation of navigation is the incapability of the system to account for

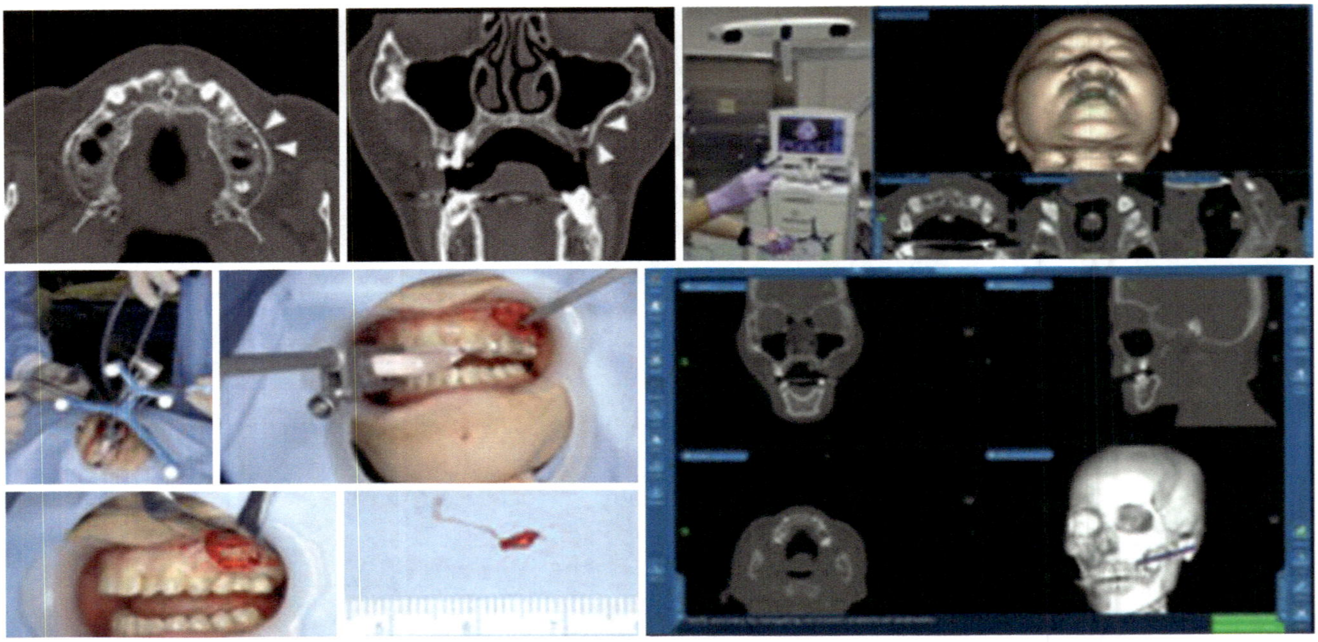


**Fig. 41.15** A 78-year-old female with a small foreign body in the maxilla. Accurate determination of the position of the foreign body in the maxillofacial region can be challenging. This may be due to a small-sized foreign body or a limited inflammatory response. Navigation systems are helpful in identifying the location of the foreign body, determining the optimal approach, and performing the surgical procedure using a minimally invasive surgical strategy. In this case, registration could be reliably performed before surgery using an optical navigation system that facilitates the process, utilizing splints with embedded reference points. This method can decrease the operation time

intraoperative soft-tissue changes. The use of navigation techniques superficial tissues or to minimize soft-tissue manipulation may help us overcome this to an extent.

### 41.3.6 Application for Dentoalveolar Surgery

Dynamic computer-based image navigation technology is a good method for increasing accuracy while minimizing the invasiveness of surgery. It has the additional advantage of real-time access to intraoperative radiographs, which enable us to perform complex dentoalveolar procedures with relative ease. Currently, the Image-Guided Implantology system (Navident; HERMANS Corp.) is the only dynamic image navigation system (DINS) available for in-office dental procedures in Japan. This is an ultraviolet-based optical system, which was approved by the US Food and Drug Administration for the placement of dental implants. However, its use for other dentoalveolar procedures is not approved. Its advantages in the field of dental implantology have already been discussed earlier. The use of dynamic navigation when applied to complex dentoalveolar procedures, such as the surgical removal of third molars, is similar to its use for dental implants, helping the surgeon prevent inadvertent damage to key structures like the IAN, roots of adjacent teeth, or the lingual plate of the mandible [38]. Common indications for the use of navigation in dentoalveolar surgery include third molar extractions and the location and extraction of supernumerary [39] or malposed teeth (Fig. 41.16), as well as teeth, which get iatrogenically displaced into the sinus, the sublingual pouch, or even the infra temporal fossa.

The use of CAS in oral and maxillofacial surgery has been enhanced with the increasing availability of CBCT. This in turn has promoted the use of Dynamic Image Navigation. As described earlier, the use of DINS during surgical extraction improves visualization of the regional anatomy, preventing or minimizing complications secondary to dentoalveolar surgery. In addition, improved instrument control allows for reduced bone removal, minimization of the surgical access size, and an overall reduction in the morbidity of the procedure. As discussed earlier, this technology also allows for improvement of the ergonomics involved during the surgery. Lastly, dynamic guidance can serve as an effective teaching tool for young surgeons by displaying the surgery and the locations of vital structures on screen.

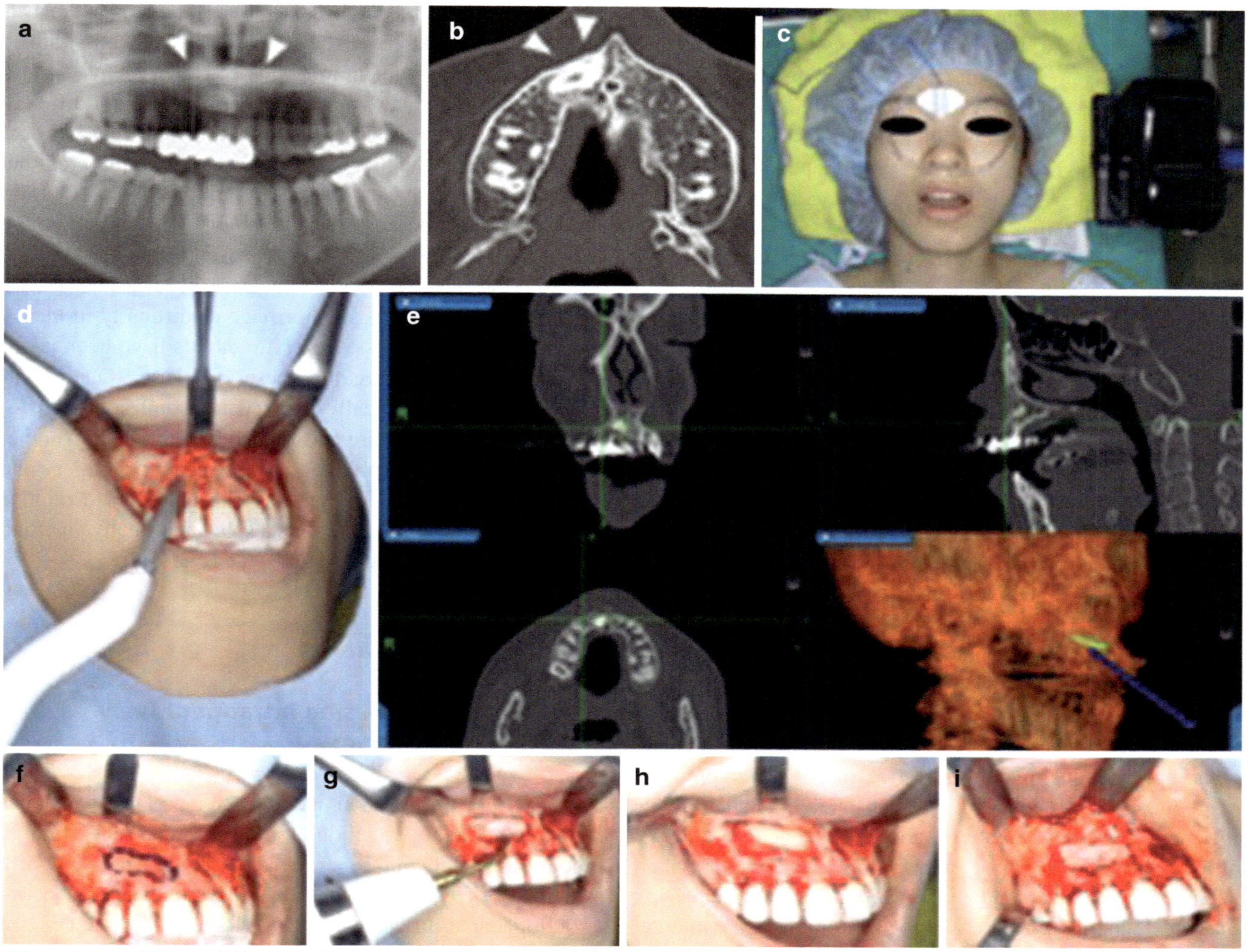




**Fig. 41.15** (**a**–**i**) A 24-year-old female with an impacted maxillary canine tooth. Bone lid surgery involves cutting a window into the cortical bone and removing a portion thereof; this portion is subsequently returned to its original position at the end of surgery. Bone lid surgery is a minimally invasive technique designed to avoid secondary large bone defects during osteotomies. However, because jaw bone lesions are completely covered with cortical bone, it can be difficult to accurately determine the position of the lesion from the outside. As a potential solution, we used navigation-assisted bone lid surgery. Using navigation, surgeons could confirm the state of the impacted tooth and surrounding tissue from above the covered bone. We were also able to establish a safe and reliable bone cutting line. In addition, the removed cortical bone was returned to the same (i.e., presurgical) position. Navigation-assisted bone lid surgery for the removal of impacted teeth increases surgical accuracy, minimizes invasion, and allows the bone to be returned to its original position (**a**, **b**)-pre operative OPG and CT (**c**–**e**)-shows intra operative navigation. (**f**) outline of canine marked (**g**, **h**) impacted canine being removed (**i**) the bone lid placed back in position

Wang reported the following advantages of surgical navigation in complicated extractions: (1) localization of teeth for accurate access planning and minimal bone removal; (2) differentiation of impacted teeth from erupting tooth germs; (3) ensured transfer of the preoperative plan to the surgical procedure; and (4) the marking of safety margins while preserving adjacent structures, to avoid complications [40].

### 41.3.7 Application for Temporomandibular Joint and Skull Base Surgery

The TMJ and surrounding anatomy, including the skull base, are extremely complex and require a cautious approach during surgery. Intraoperative navigation can play an important role for surgeries such as the removal of an ankylotic bony mass, tumor resection, and gap arthroplasty [41]. Successful treatment outcomes have been reported by studies for the use of navigation assistance in unilateral surgery for the TMJ. Other publications report that navigation is helpful and increases safety in TMJ surgery. A recent publication used navigation to compare prospectively treated groups of patients with recurrent malignant tumors of the infratemporal fossa. Although the results are not independently significant, they yielded a benefit to the navigation cohort. The authors concluded that surgeon confidence and safety during the operations improved, but the navigation system alone did not determine patient outcomes.

Management of tumors at the skull base or of end-stage degenerative TMJ disorders requires thorough knowledge of the regional anatomy and precise 3D planning of the resection margins with attention of vital structures in the immediate vicinity (Fig. 41.17). The location, invasion, and extent of the tumor are key determinants in deciding the surgical approach. In the past, malignant tumors that had infiltrated into the infratemporal fossa or the middle of the skull base were considered inoperable due to the compromised access and inability to achieve predictable tumor control or hemostasis.

The use of surgical navigation for skull base surgery offers the following advantages: (1) ensuring safer and quicker skull base access through a dynamic display of the precise operating site and the extent of bone drilling, thereby significantly reducing intraoperative risk; (2) mapping the anatomical structures and important landmarks such as the foramen ovale and rotundum; and (3) the incorporation of allied imaging modalities, such as 3D CT angiography and MRI, into the intraoperative navigation planning, increasing our understanding of the skull base anatomy and the internal carotid artery region.

As surgery of the skull base is not affected by the shifting brain, use of navigation in this field is more precise than in other neurosurgical procedures. The use of a navigation system for the resection of tumors of the skull base or of TMJ lesions increases surgical predictability while reducing the surgical duration.

### 41.3.8 Other Applications

Another application of intraoperative navigation is in surgery for the management of Eagle's syndrome, which may be due to the elongation of the styloid process of calcification of the stylomandibular ligament [42]. This condition involves a group of symptoms, including throat pain and foreign body sensation on the affected side, reflex otalgia, head and neck pain, and hypersalivation. Surgical treatment was indicated for patients with no symptomatic improvement following conservative treatment.

The surgery may be performed by two different approaches: (1) transcervical and (2) transoral. The cervical approach provides better surgical exposure of the area, but has the major disadvantage of an external incision. The transoral approach is cosmetically favorable, and is more commonly used. However, this approach offers very limited access. This may affect the management of intraoperative complications, including hemorrhage or difficulty in identifying the styloid process. Several methods have been advocated recently to overcome these problems. One report suggests an endoscopically assisted transoral approach for achieving better exposure and visibility of the field. Another method proposes a combination of piezoelectric surgery and surgical navigation for a transcervical approach to remove the styloid. This technique offers a safe and effective method for the treatment of Eagle's syndrome (Fig. 41.18).

## 41.4 Recent Advances

### 41.4.1 Navigation Using Intraoperatively Updated Images

The accuracy of surgical navigation in recent years has been augmented by the induction of intraoperative imaging modalities like the intraoperative CBCT, C-arm, and O-arm systems [43]. These offer intraoperative multiplanar reconstruction capabilities, which enable the improvement of surgical outcomes in demanding surgeries such as surgery of the orbital walls. Furthermore, the popularization of hybrid operating rooms (Fig. 41.19) equipped with both intraoperative imaging and navigation systems has revolutionized surgery of the maxillofacial region. It is now possible to continuously update intraoperative images to determine the best sequence to follow during surgeries (Fig. 41.20). The effectiveness of a navigation system using intraoperative CT images has been already demonstrated in orthopedic surgery and maxillofacial operations, which involve bone movement, such as trauma surgery and orthognathic surgery. Intraoperative CT images have allowed for rapid intraoperative evaluations, which when coupled with surgical navigation, may allow for performing more complicated maxillofacial surgery with increased accuracy.

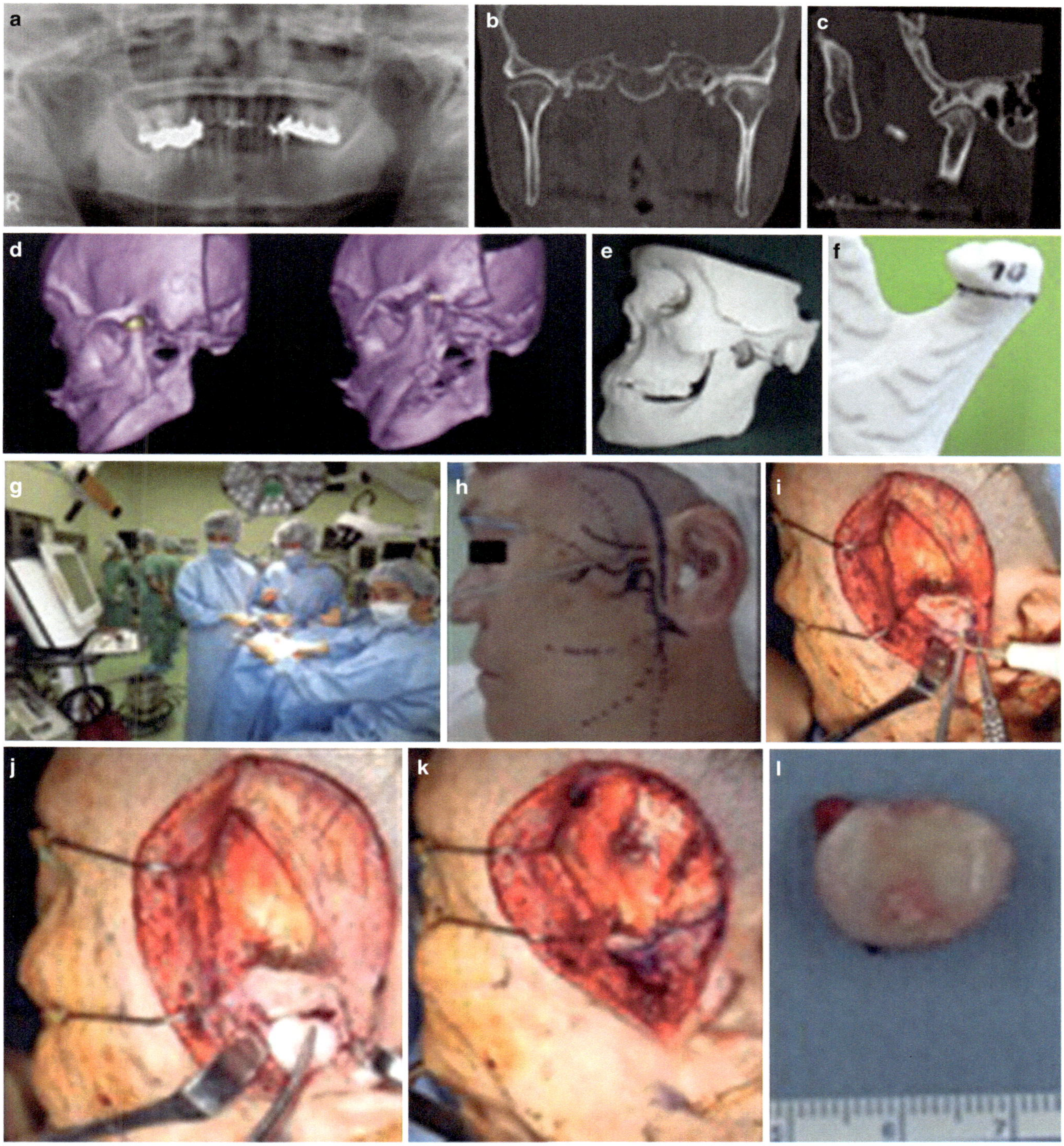




**Fig. 41.17** A 70-year-old female with temporomandibular joint (TMJ) ankylosis. Ankylosis surgery is used for gap arthroplasty and mobilization of the joints. (**a–c**) However, removal of the bony ankylosis and creation of a gap between the ramus of the mandible and the base of the skull can be difficult because of the size of the ankylosis and the anatomy on the inner aspect of the mandible. Virtual planning is useful in conjunction with surgical navigation to remove the ankylosis. (**d**) First, a computer simulation based on preoperative CT data was performed for the virtual surgery. (**e**, **f**) Once the virtual surgery was completed, templates were constructed using rapid prototyping techniques from the virtual plan and applied at the time of surgery to facilitate the bony cuts. (**g**, **h**) Using the intraoperative navigation system, the surgeon can see the medial aspect of the mandible on the navigation station CT and protect important structures on the medial side. (**i–l**) This visualization prevents significant bleeding from the vessels on the medial side of the mandible and prevents penetration into the middle cranial fossa during release of the ankylosis. The temporalis flap was used for prevention of reankylosis

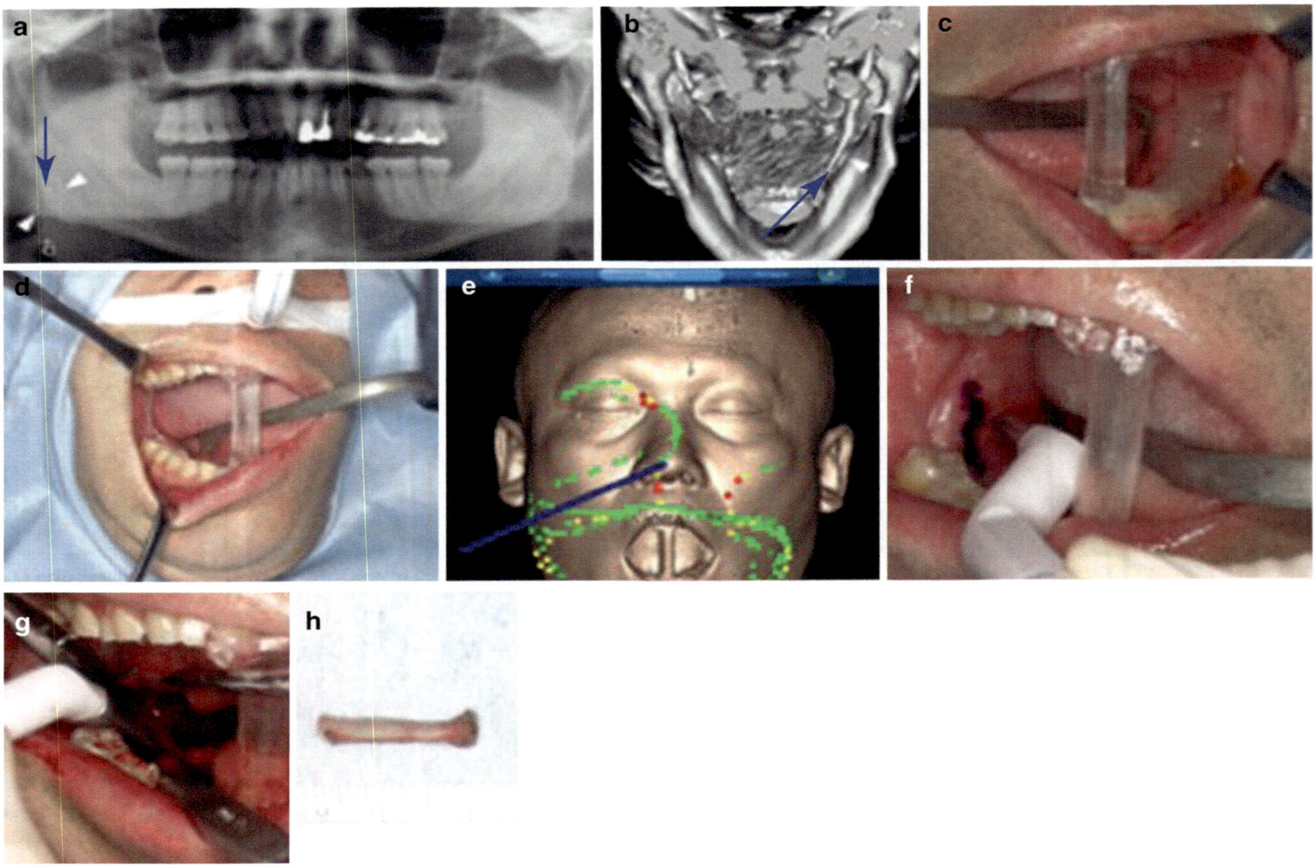




**Fig. 41.18** (**a**, **b**) A 45-year-old male with elongated styloid process syndrome (Eagle's syndrome). A minimally invasive approach with an intraoperative navigation system was used. (**c**) Preoperative preparation involved a custom interocclusal splint to produce the mouth opening conditions required during surgery. In this case, since the transoral approach was employed, it was important to reproduce the same mouth-opening conditions when obtaining the preoperative images required during surgery, because the position of the styloid process and the blood vessels may change depending on the position of the mandible during the mouth opening. Since it is difficult to implement the locational findings from the preoperative imaging data while performing surgery owing to the mobile nature of the mandible, a custom interocclusal splint for repeated maximum opening in the same mandibular position, while enabling surgical access, was used. (**d**) The patient was taken to the operating room, where the custom interocclusal splint was reinserted. (**e**) To perform patient-to-CT and MRI data registration, the instrumentation navigation probe was used to trace the reference array and soft tissue landmarks of the face. (**f**) Using the 3D position of the navigation probe, the location of the elongated styloid process was identified. (**g**, **h**) After confirmation of the resection location via the transoral approach, the styloid process was dissected using piezoelectric surgery. Follow-up examination showed an uneventful recovery with no associated complications. (The resection of the styloid process using an intraoperative navigation system and a custom interocclusal splint during a transoral approach, together with a piezoelectric cutting device, is safe and effective for the treatment of Eagle's syndrome)

### 41.4.2 Wearable Mount Display for Navigation-Assisted Surgery

Although intraoperative navigation yields helpful information on anatomical features, it is used in conjunction with a monitor. Generally, the direction of the monitor from the surgeon and operator is different from that the surgical field. Therefore, to see the navigation image, the surgeon and the operator must look up, which is stressful for the operator. It is important to minimize muscle tension and allow the surgeon to perform the operation in a

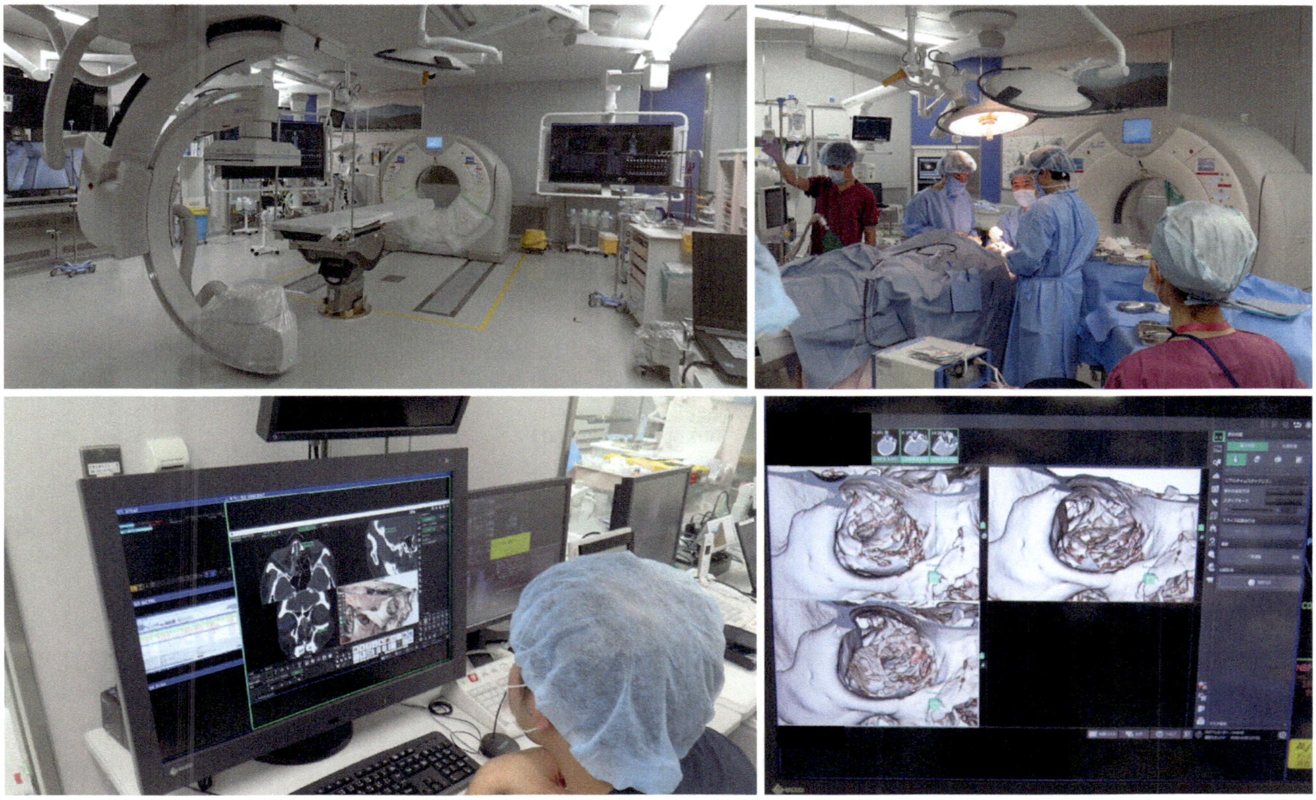



**Fig. 41.19** A hybrid operating room is a surgical theater equipped with advanced medical imaging devices, such as fixed C-arm and angiographic systems. Intraoperative CT imaging is convenient because the CT is installed in the hybrid operating room. Furthermore, recent advances in technology have made it possible to edit and use images simultaneously with intraoperative CT imaging

relaxed position. Moving the head to look at the monitor can result in considerable misalignment of the eye-hand-target axis during task execution, significantly affecting postural comfort and interventional safety. In recent years, head-mounted display monitors have been developed to address this problem. Such wearable displays can provide high-quality images [44]. Using a head-mounted display monitor, surgeons can finish the surgery without moving their head to check the navigation image. The head-mounted device also allows both the surgeon and the assistant to view both the navigation image and the surgical field without interrupting the flow of surgery. This contributes to rapid surgical operation, resulting in minimally invasive surgery. Navigation-assisted surgery with a head-mounted display is a revolutionary technique. In the future, head-mounted displays will be wearable devices that promote the use of navigation (Fig. 41.21).

## 41.5 Conclusions and Perspectives

CAS and navigation offers significant improvements in patient orientation and safety in every facet of maxillofacial surgery. Ranging from precisely planned orthognathic procedures to the removal of foreign bodies requiring

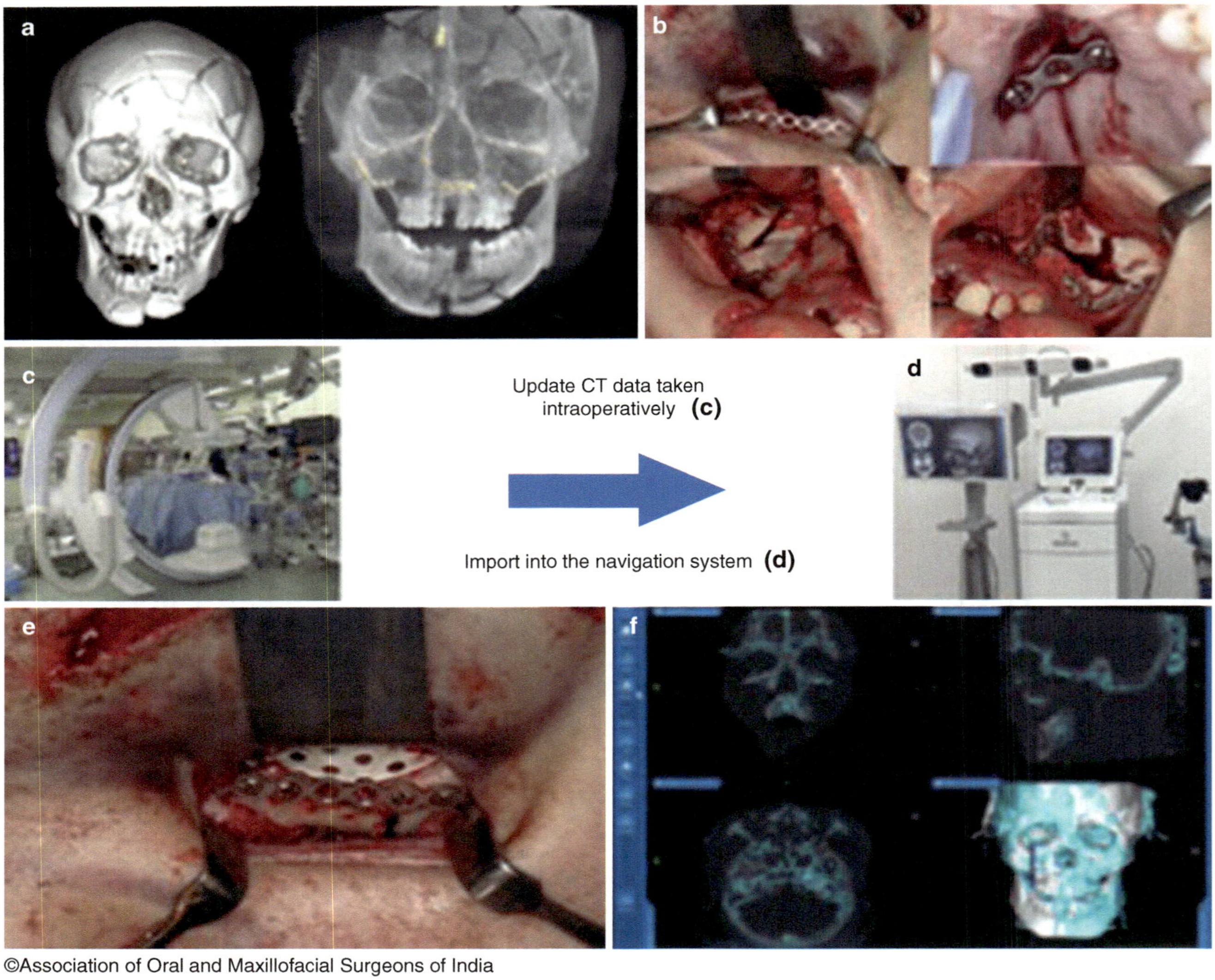


**Fig. 41.20** (**a**) A 19-year-old male with a complex facial fracture and orbital fracture. Navigation surgery is difficult to apply for treating a complex facial fracture with orbital fracture. (**b**) Since reconstruction of the buttress of the facial bone is performed prior to the treatment of the orbital fracture, preoperative CT data and the actual state of the facial bone are different. Therefore, a navigation system using preoperative CT data cannot be employed. (**c**) Using CT data obtained after facial fracture reduction, (**d**) it is possible to use a navigation system reflecting the updated patient condition. The use of CT in the hybrid room can provide rapid CT data during surgery. (**e**) The orbital floor defect has been repaired. (**f**) Post operative CT showing the accurate reduction of fractures

extremely flexible surgical options, and from minimally invasive dental implantology procedures to radical tumor resections of the skull base, they have made their mark improving procedure safety, predictability, and accuracy of surgery while also improving options for intraoperative adaptations. In the future, the application of CAS is expected to further reduce operative risks and surgery time, accompanied by a considerable decrease in patient stress.

Navigation systems are effective for delicate and accurate oral and maxillofacial surgery and neurosurgery, as well as for otolaryngology and orthopedic surgery. In the future, we expect to develop more convenient and reliable navigation systems using new technologies and devices.

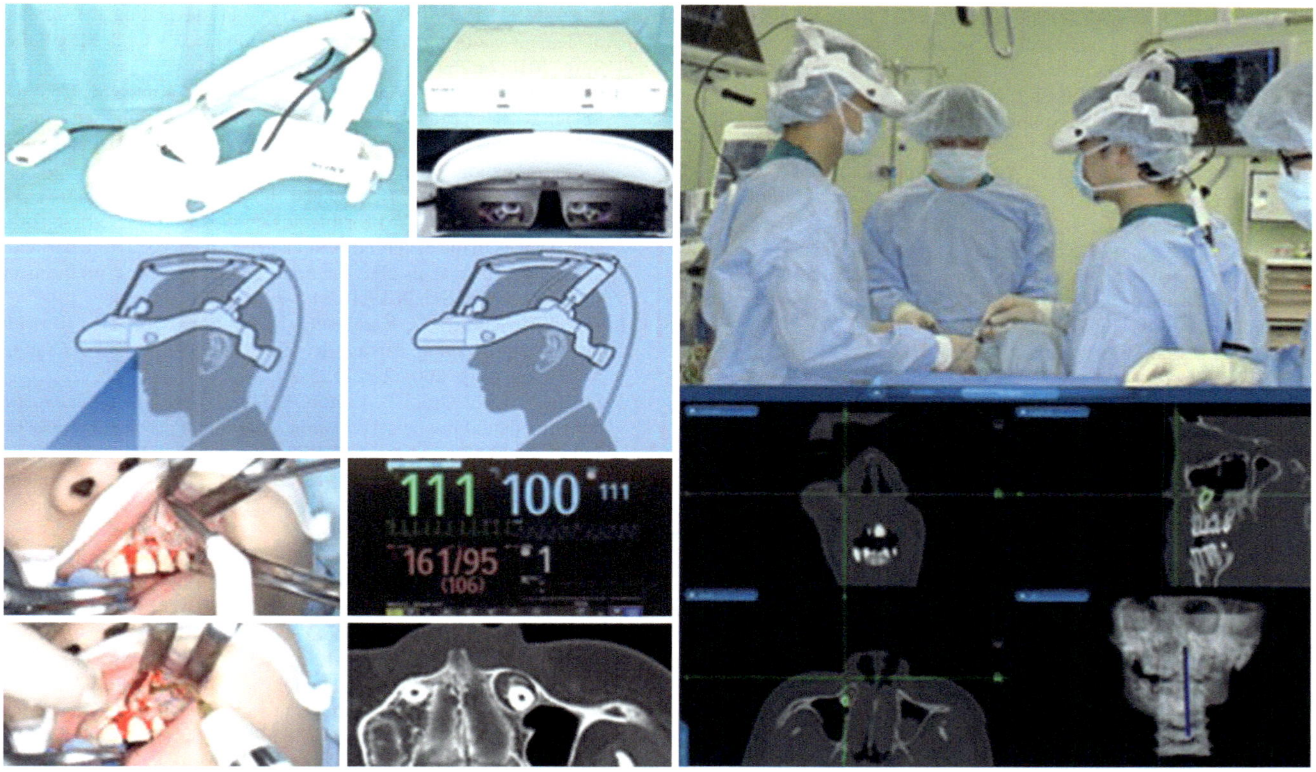



**Fig. 41.21** The head-mounted display can provide high-quality images with wearable technology. The head-mounted display unit was composed of a head-mount image processor unit (HMM-3000MT; Sony Corporation, Tokyo, Japan) and a head-mounted display monitor. Although the navigation system provides helpful information, it is used in conjunction with a monitor. Generally, the direction of the monitor differs from the surgical field. Therefore, to see the navigation image, the surgeon and the operator have to look up, which is stressful for the operator. Using a head-mounted display monitor, we could finish surgery without moving the head position. The surgeon must perform not only the surgery but also intraoperative systemic management. Multimodality patient information is important in such cases. Multimodality medical information fusion and processing have been developed in recent years. This head-mounted display system allows the integration of preoperative radiological findings with monitoring of navigation images and patient vital signs. Using the head-mounted display system, the surgeon can see multiple images in one view using a split screen, regardless of the head position. This technology facilitates safe surgical management with the navigation system

## References


1. Sukegawa S, Kanno T, Furuki Y. Application of computer-assisted navigation systems in oral and maxillofacial surgery. Jpn Dent Sci Rev. 2018;54:139–49.
2. Rodby KA, Turin S, Jacobs RJ, Cruz JF, Hassid VJ, Kolokythas A, Antony AK. Advances in oncologic head and neck reconstruction: systematic review and future considerations of virtual surgical planning and computer aided design/computer aided modeling. J Plast Reconstr Aesthet Surg. 2014;67:1171–85.
3. Bell RB. Computer planning and intraoperative navigation in cranio-maxillofacial surgery. Oral Maxillofac Surg Clin N Am. 2010;22:135–56.
4. Kanno T, Sukegawa S, Karino M, Furuki Y. Navigation-assisted orbital trauma reconstruction using a bioactive osteoconductive/bioresorbable u-HA/PLLA system. J Maxillofac Oral Surg. 2019;18:329–38.
5. Li L, Yang J, Chu Y, Wu W, Xue J, Liang P, Chen L. A novel augmented reality navigation system for endoscopic sinus and skull base surgery: a feasibility study. PLoS One. 2016;11:e0146996.
6. Samarakkody ZM, Abdullah B. The use of image guided navigational tracking systems for endoscopic sinus surgery and skull base surgery: a review. Egypt J Ear Nose Throat Allied Sci. 2016;17:133–7.
7. Hassfeld S, Mühling J, Zöller J. Intraoperative navigation in oral and maxillofacial surgery. Int J Oral Maxillofac Surg. 1995;24:111–9.
8. Marmulla R, Lüth T, Mühling J, Hassfeld S. Markerless laser registration in image-guided oral and maxillofacial surgery. J Oral Maxillofac Surg. 2004;62:845–51.
9. Bettschart C, Kruse A, Matthews F, Zemann W, Obwegeser JA, Grätz KW, Lübbers H-T. Point-to-point registration with mandibulo-maxillary splint in open and closed jaw position. Evaluation of registration accuracy for computer-aided surgery of the mandible. J Cranio-Maxillofac Surg. 2012;40:592–8.
10. Šiniković B, Kramer F-J, Swennen G, Lübbers H-T, Dempf R. Reconstruction of orbital wall defects with calcium phosphate cement: clinical and histological findings in a sheep model. Int J Oral Maxillofac Surg. 2007;36:54–61.
11. Jeon S, Park J, Chien J, Hong J. A hybrid method to improve target registration accuracy in surgical navigation. Minim Invasive Ther Allied Technol. 2015;24:356–63.

12. Gumprecht HK, Widenka DC, Lumenta CB. Brain lab vector vision neuronavigation system: technology and clinical experiences in 131 cases. Neurosurgery. 1999;44:97–104.
13. Casap N, Wexler A, Eliashar R. Computerized navigation for surgery of the lower jaw: comparison of 2 navigation systems. J Oral Maxillofac Surg. 2008;66:1467–75.
14. Li P, Li Z, Tian W, Tang W. A strategy for removal of foreign body in mandible with navigation system. Int J Oral Maxillofac Surg. 2015;44:885–8.
15. Dong QN, Karino M, Koike T, Ide T, Okuma S, Kaneko I, Osako R, Kanno T. Navigation-assisted isolated medial orbital wall fracture reconstruction using an U-HA/PLLA sheet via a transcaruncular approach. J Investig Surg. 2019:1–9.
16. He D, Li Z, Shi W, Sun Y, Zhu H, Lin M, Shen G, Fan X. Orbitozygomatic fractures with enophthalmos: analysis of 64 cases treated late. J Oral Maxillofac Surg. 2012;70:562–76.
17. Baumann A, Sinko K, Dorner G. Late reconstruction of the orbit with patient-specific implants using computer-aided planning and navigation. J Oral Maxillofac Surg. 2015;73:S101–6.
18. Azarmehr I, Stokbro K, Bell RB, Thygesen T. Surgical navigation: a systematic review of indications, treatments, and outcomes in oral and maxillofacial surgery. J Oral Maxillofac Surg. 2017;75:1987–2005.
19. Schmelzeisen R, Gellrich N-C, Schramm A, Schön R, Otten J-E. Navigation-guided resection of temporomandibular joint ankylosis promotes safety in skull base surgery. J Oral Maxillofac Surg. 2002;60:1275–83.
20. Zrnc TA, Wallner J, Zemann W, Pau M, Gstettner C, Brcic L, Assaf AT, Hassanzadeh H, Feichtinger M, Schwenzer-Zimmerer K. Assessment of tumor margins in head and neck cancer using a 3D-navigation system based on PET/CT image-fusion – a pilot study. J Cranio-Maxillofac Surg. 2018;46:617–23.
21. Sukegawa S, Kanno T, Shibata A, Matsumoto K, Sukegawa-Takahashi Y, Sakaida K, Furuki Y. Intraoperative navigation-assisted accurate bone lid surgery to remove a mandibular lesion: a case report. Oral Maxillofac Surg Cases. 2017;3:15–9.
22. Wei B, Sun G, Hu Q, Tang E. The safety and accuracy of surgical navigation technology in the treatment of lesions involving the skull base. J Craniofac Surg. 2017;28:1431–4.
23. Ricotta F, Cercenelli L, Battaglia S, Bortolani B, Savastio G, Marcelli E, Marchetti C, Tarsitano A. Navigation-guided resection of maxillary tumors: can a new volumetric virtual planning method improve outcomes in terms of control of resection margins? J Cranio-Maxillofac Surg. 2018;46:2240–7.
24. Luna-Ortiz K, Villa-Zepeda O, Carrillo JF, Molina-Frias E, Gómez-Pedraza A. Parapharyngeal space tumor: submandibular approach without mandibulotomy. J Maxillofac Oral Surg. 2018;17:616–24.
25. Mazzoni S, Badiali G, Lancellotti L, Babbi L, Bianchi A, Marchetti C. Simulation-guided navigation. J Craniofac Surg. 2010;21:1698–705.
26. Zinser MJ, Sailer HF, Ritter L, Braumann B, Maegele M, Zöller JE. A paradigm shift in orthognathic surgery? A comparison of navigation, computer-aided designed/computer-aided manufactured splints, and "classic" intermaxillary splints to surgical transfer of virtual orthognathic planning. J Oral Maxillofac Surg. 2013;71:2151.e1–2151.e21.
27. Holly LT, Foley KT. Intraoperative spinal navigation. Spine (Phila. Pa. 1976). 2003;28:S54–61.
28. Block MS, Emery RW. Static or dynamic navigation for implant placement-choosing the method of guidance. J Oral Maxillofac Surg. 2016;74:269–77.
29. Chao AH, Weimer K, Raczkowsky J, Zhang Y, Kunze M, Cody D, Selber JC, Hanasono MM, Skoracki RJ. Pre-programmed robotic osteotomies for fibula free flap mandible reconstruction: a preclinical investigation. Microsurgery. 2016;36:246–9.
30. Sukegawa S, Kawai H, Nakano K, Kanno T, Takabatake K, Nagatsuka H, Furuki Y. Feasible advantage of bioactive/bioresorbable devices made of forged composites of hydroxyapatite particles and poly-L-lactide in alveolar bone augmentation: a preliminary study. Int J Med Sci. 2019;16:311–7.
31. Gaggl A, Schultes G, Kärcher H. Navigational precision of drilling tools preventing damage to the mandibular canal. J Cranio-Maxillofac Surg. 2001;29:271–5.
32. Stefanelli L, DeGroot B, Lipton D, Mandelaris G. Accuracy of a dynamic dental implant navigation system in a private practice. Int J Oral Maxillofac Implants. 2019;34:205–13.
33. Emery RW, Merritt SA, Lank K, Gibbs JD. Accuracy of dynamic navigation for dental implant placement–model-based evaluation. J Oral Implantol. 2016;42:399–405.
34. Shuker ST, Sadda R. Craniomaxillofacial falling bullet injuries and management. J Oral Maxillofac Surg. 2010;68:1593–601.
35. Bedrock RD, Skigen A, Dolwick MF. Retrieval of a broken needle in the pterygomandibular space. J Am Dent Assoc. 1999;130:685–7.
36. Park S-S, Yang H-J, Lee U-L, Kwon M-S, Kim M-J, Lee J-H, Hwang S-J. The clinical application of the dental mini C-arm for the removal of broken instruments in soft and hard tissue in the oral and maxillofacial area. J Cranio-Maxillofac Surg. 2012;40:572–8.
37. Sukegawa S, Kanno T, Shibata A, Matsumoto K, Sukegawa-Takahashi Y, Sakaida K, Furuki Y. Use of an intraoperative navigation system for retrieving a broken dental instrument in the mandible: a case report. J Med Case Rep. 2017;11:14.
38. Emery RW, Korj O, Agarwal R. A review of in-office dynamic image navigation for extraction of complex mandibular third molars. J Oral Maxillofac Surg. 2017;75:1591–600.
39. Retana A, Emery RW, Keir V. Removal of impacted supernumerary teeth using a dynamic surgical navigation system: a case report. J Oral Maxillofac Surg. 2019;77:1130–4.
40. Wang H, Yang C-Y, Li Z. Traumatic displacement of teeth into maxillary sinus and the retrieval assisted by computer-assisted navigation. Medicine (Baltimore). 2018;97:e13865.
41. He Y, Huang T, Zhang Y, An J, He L. Application of a computer-assisted surgical navigation system in temporomandibular joint ankylosis surgery: a retrospective study. Int J Oral Maxillofac Surg. 2017;46:189–97.
42. Sukegawa S, Kanno T, Yoshimoto A, Matsumoto K, Sukegawa-Takahashi Y, Masui M, Furuki Y. Use of an intraoperative navigation system and piezoelectric surgery for styloidectomy in a patient with Eagle's syndrome: a case report. J Med Case Rep. 2017;11:322.
43. Wikner J, Riecke B, Gröbe A, Heiland M, Hanken H. Imaging of the midfacial and orbital trauma. Facial Plast Surg. 2014;30:528–36.
44. Matsuo A, Hamada H, Oba H, Shibata K. Virtual reality head-mounted display for endoscopically-assisted implant surgery. Br J Oral Maxillofac Surg. 2018;56:636–7.

# Part XIV

# Practice Management in Oral and Maxillofacial Surgery

# Human Factors Recognition to Enhance Team Working and Safer Patient Care

42

Peter A. Brennan and Rachel S. Oeppen

## 42.1 Introduction

Human error and organisational mistakes are a significant cause of morbidity for patients. It is important to recognise and address human factors (HF) in the context of our own performance optimisation, enhancing team working to improve patient safety, and better working lives for clinicians across surgery and medicine.

Medical errors are usually multi-factorial rather than the direct fault of any one individual. Organisational issues, poor team working and other HF are often at the root of many incidents and errors. The Surgical Checklist produced by the World Health Organization (WHO), and aviation-styled communication training initiatives have been advocated to optimise surgical performance by reducing human fallibility and misinterpretation between team members. Brief and debriefing processes and other performance improvement practices have been positively rated when incorporated into healthcare. Ergonomics and other factors such as stress and fatigue, emotional status, hunger, dehydration and situational awareness can all lead to human error, but these are often under-appreciated and in some cases even disregarded.

The aims of this chapter are to raise colleague awareness of both individual human factors and those relevant to organisations and to highlight relatively simple methods to actively reduce error in healthcare.

P. A. Brennan (✉)
Maxillofacial Unit, Queen Alexandria Hospital, Portsmouth, UK
e-mail: peter.brennan@porthosp.nhs.uk

R. S. Oeppen
Consultant Radiologist, University Hospital Southampton, Southampton, UK
e-mail: Rachel.oeppen@uhs.nhs.uk

## 42.2 The Scale of the Problem

Over 70% of plane crashes are due to a human mistake rather than a failure of the aircraft itself. Issues with communication can occur in up to 80% of air disasters. Recognition of factors leading to human error, including tiredness, stress, and repetitive tasks, and an acceptance that a certain degree of failure is almost inevitable, has improved air safety. These factors are being increasingly recognised by healthcare professionals [1]. The American Institute of Medicine report entitled "To Err Is Human" published in 1999 and subsequent work has found death from preventable medical errors, with those in surgery second only to medication errors as the most common reasons for death from medical error [2]. Recent estimates place avoidable patient deaths in USA hospitals at over 400,000 per year, with preventable harm in the top three causes of death [3].

While the authors were not able to source any statistics for the Indian sub-continent, death in UK hospitals from medical error is estimated to be about 4000 per year, with a disproportionate amount of harm caused by errors in surgery. To put this into context, this would be the equivalent of more than one A320 fatal airbus (Fig. 42.1) crashes occurring twice a month. Incidentally, the A320 is the aircraft involved in the widespread media coverage after an emergency landing on the River Hudson in January 2009 by Captain 'Sully' Sullenerger, subsequently dramatized in the well-known movie, Sully. Despite the WHO checklist, which is widely used throughout the modern world, the number of 'never events'—those that should never happen, including wrong site surgery and retained instruments or swabs—is increasing [4]. Although doctor-induced mistakes are quite rare, a near miss occurs far more commonly in the hospital environment. An investigation and detailed cause analysis following any incident can help organisations learn, prevent and reduce the chance of such errors occurring again in the future.


K. Bonanthaya et al. (eds.), *Oral and Maxillofacial Surgery for the Clinician*, https://doi.org/10.1007/978-981-15-1346-6_42

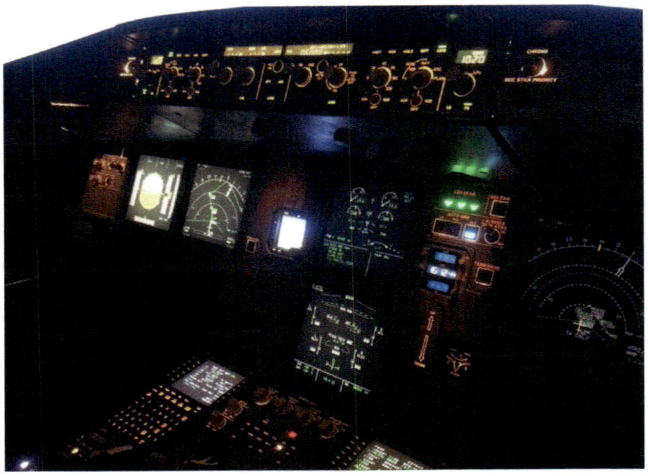

©Association of Oral and Maxillofacial Surgeons of India

Fig. 42.1 The flight deck of an Airbus A320 being configured for departure

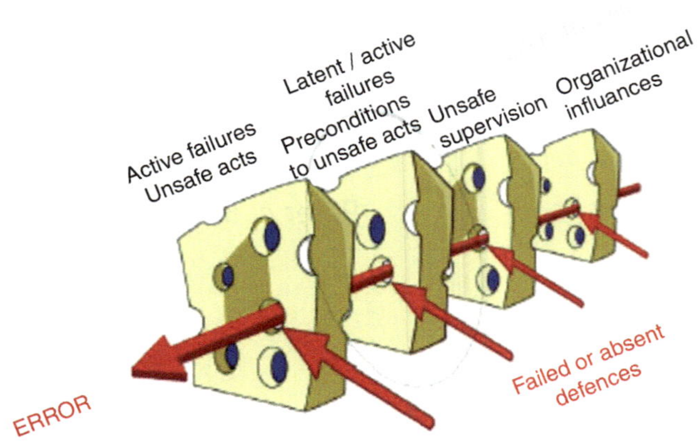


©Association of Oral and Maxillofacial Surgeons of India

Fig. 42.2 Schematic representation of the Swiss cheese model of human error. Each of the cheese slices acts as a barrier to an error occurring with the final chance for stopping the error being the elimination of the unsafe act itself. Error has its origin in organisation influences (latent failure) and those caused by individuals and teams (active failures)

## 42.3 How Do Human Errors Arise?

Recognition and understanding of those relevant HF involved in potential error is vital for improving patient safety. These factors include fatigue and tiredness, stress, communication style, effective team working, and good leadership. The well-known 'Swiss cheese model' of error (Reason [5]) is illustrated in Fig. 42.2. Organisational failures contributing to medical error could include pressures on individuals to meet hospital targets, having too many patients on an operating list than is deemed safe, too many patients in an outpatient clinic, working very long hours without taking a break or being expected to operate the following day after having being disturbed overnight with on-call emergencies.

Table 42.1 Avoiding human error traps

- Read out WHO Checklist with active participation of all team members. Engage with it as if your own life or limb depended on getting it right
- Ensure staff communicate well with each other
- Use briefing/debriefing to improve team working
- Limit avoidable distractions and any interruptions during essential parts of an operation (same as sterile cockpit in aviation).
- Promote use of positive two-way communication.
- Ensure 6–8 h of sleep, regular physical activity and adequate nutrition and hydration before starting surgery.
- Look out for each other as part of the team.
- Ensure you take regular breaks and eat and drink often during the day.
- Recognise when something doesn't seem right in yourself.
- Do not assume physically uncomfortable postures unless absolutely necessary. Adjust equipment, table for the comfort of you and your team.

### 42.3.1 Senior Management Support Is Essential in Helping to Reduce Medical Error

Senior management commitment is essential in ensuring safety across any organisation. An open culture has to be key in any hospital agenda and strategy. Poor leadership together with a 'blame culture' led to more than 35 deaths in the Bristol paediatric cardiac surgery service. As a result, a large number of changes were implemented to limit future preventable surgical incidents. Pilots, aircraft ground engineers and other aviation safety staff are encouraged to actively question any safety issues related to their aeroplane, and their employer must investigate concerns, even if this means stopping a flight from taking off. In healthcare, we should be following this safety model with higher hospital management and surgical team leaders creating a safe environment to report and action possible error. The surgical team has to endorse the use of evidence-based best practices, including use of the WHO Surgical Checklist, avoiding human error traps (Table 42.1) and early identification of those situations in which harm or error is more likely to occur (Table 42.2).

Table 42.2 Take special care—recognise situations in which error/harm is more likely

- Site- and side-specific procedures
- Staffing limitations high turnover rates
- Changes in physical environment
- Changes in staff/scheduling
- Staffing limitations
- High staff turnover
- Significant changes in life situation of team members—divorce, death in family
- Special patient factors, e.g. Jehovah witness unable to accept transfusion, obesity

While a surgeon's life or limb is not at stake during an operation (unlike an air disaster when a mistake made by an airline pilot might result in the death of all those on board, including the crew), the psychological effects of a major surgical incident or error can be devastating to both individuals and teams [6].

### 42.3.2 Human Factors That We Should Be Thinking About

There are many personal human factors that can cause error, including tiredness and fatigue, nutritional status, anger and stress, multitasking and loss of our own situational awareness. However, all too often as individuals we sometimes imagine that these factors do not apply to us, and therefore we might choose to ignore them (such as missing lunch, working for many hours without taking a break) significantly raising the risk of patient harm and potentially damaging our own health and well-being.

#### 42.3.2.1 Fatigue and Tiredness

These are known in aviation and other high-risk organisations (HROs) as significant factors that can cause human error. As a result, strict guidelines have been put in place in these HRO, with for example flight crews only being working a defined number of hours in any given month. Many airlines have a policy in place to make sure that one pilot is as refreshed as possible for the most dangerous aspects of flying such as the landing. Intense concentration can only be maintained for about 20–30 min. For example, one pilot will take over the actual landing when the other has done the first-stage descent. The effect of these personal factors in surgical performance is less understood than in aviation though tiredness will affect decision making, as well as doing complex tasks. Situational awareness will also be affected even if surgeons behave as if they are immune and operate for many hours without taking a break. The ability for sleep deprivation to degrade performance is dramatically under-estimated by healthcare providers [7].

With reference to the Swiss cheese analogy, tiredness, emotional factors and stressful surgery can all align together to raise the risk of serious error. Table 42.2 shows some of these high-risk situations. Good communication and team working and the ability to question decisions with a phrase such as 'can I check that I've got this correct' can be useful. Other phrases like 'I am not happy' and 'I am going to take over' can also be used in situations where an error might happen.

#### 42.3.2.2 Nutritional Status and Hydration

These factors significantly affect HF and our performance in a demanding operating room setting. Even modest levels of dehydration are known to impair cognitive function and performance [8]. Meals that contain protein, carbohydrates and fats such as those derived from olive oil, fish and avocado as well as certain nuts are considered to be best for optimal nutrition. Simple sugars (such as chocolate bars) and processed food do not readily support long-term concentration and the endurance that is needed in the operating theatre [8].

The authors recommend taking a short break of 10–15 min every 2–3 h when at work, especially if performing complex tasks or surgery. Of course, the procedure can continue if there is suitable expertise within the team, but each team member should plan to take a regular break, which can be staggered. Even a short time spent away from operating can help provide a fresh outlook, improve morale, and enable a toilet and food/water break. Recovery is aided through regular sleep, which is positively linked to healthy eating and drinking. Certain nutritional supplements may also support performance [9].

#### 42.3.2.3 Stress and Emotions While We Are Working

Emotional and psychological issues can affect performance. While these emotions can often be hidden, a trigger or so-called sentinel event that results in upset or even anger can occur, during times of high mental workload or in those stressful situations that we all will be familiar with. Many of us will have witnessed others (or ourselves) having an emotional outburst, including shouting at other team members. During these events, error is much more likely to occur. In these situations, visible anger usually results from additional hidden factors that others do not see in the so-called anger triangle (Fig. 42.3).

A simple thing to remember, **HALT** (Table 42.3), reminds us of sometimes overlooked personal issues and to ensure we stop to take a break. The importance of a short rest cannot be emphasised enough if it is safe, especially when these HALT

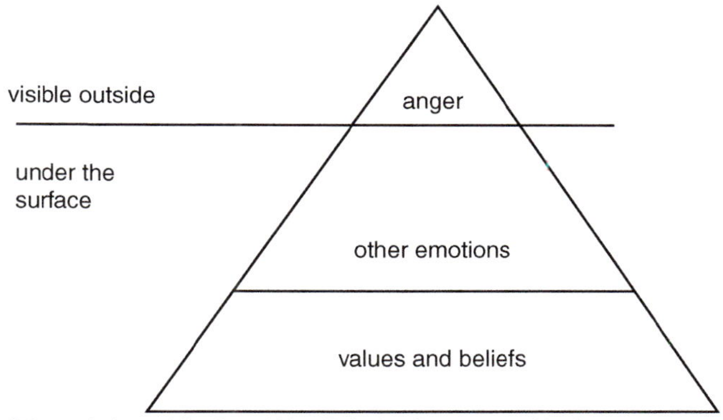




**Fig. 42.3** Anger triangle: many emotions may be hidden from others until a sentinel event causes an outburst of anger. During this time, error is much more likely

**Table 42.3** Try to stop or inform a member of the team when experiencing or witnessing these HALT factors

| | |
|---|---|
| H | Hungry |
| A | Angry or anxious |
| L | Lonely or late |
| T | Tired |

issues becomes apparent, and may prevent something serious from occurring.

Management strategies such as increasing our own emotional awareness and learning how to deal with personal stress may also be useful.

Effective communication with the rest of the team and questioning decisions where there might be some doubt by saying something like 'can I check that I have got this right?' is paramount. Other words such as 'I'm not happy' and 'I'm going to take over' can also be used in situations where potential errors are deemed more likely.

## 42.4 What About WHO and Other Checklists and Team Working Dynamics on Surgical Performance?

The WHO Surgical checklist has resulted in significant decreases to post-operative mortality and morbidity on a worldwide scale, yet errors persist and recur. While checklists, including WHO's, cannot address all aspects of medical and surgical practice, good team working with effective briefing can help to optimise team performance. There are many situations in surgery and other medical specialities when mental or physical workloads increase suddenly or dramatically (for example, during complex microvascular reconstruction) and these can have an adverse effect on performance. In such cases, team dynamics and an understanding of each individual's role within the wider team are crucial. Airlines enforce a 'sterile cockpit' policy in which noise is kept to only essential conversation below 10,000 ft (during high-risk procedures such as landing and take-off) and only essential conversation relating solely to procedure is permitted. The sterile flight deck concept is being advocated for reducing error in anaesthesia and surgery [10]. This should be discussed with all team members at the pre-operative briefing so that all know the need to stop non-essential communications at certain times. Poor team working has had tragic consequences on many occasions. In one well-known UK case (Elaine Bromiley), the airway was lost following induction of anaesthesia for a routine ENT procedure. The anaesthetists made repeated attempts to secure an airway, and had 'tunnel vision' about this rather than seeking assistance from surgeons or others for an emergency needle cricothyroidotomy.

Ancillary staff were well aware of the patient's prolonged hypoxic state but felt reluctant to assert themselves or state the need for alternative intervention. No individual took a leadership decision role and the team did not have designated roles during a difficult airway situation. As a result, the patient died when she could so easily have been saved. Lack of leadership, poor communication, inability to challenge hierarchy, and many other HF failings were to blame for this tragedy.

Effective team working is also valuable in promoting a sense of shared responsibility for patient safety. Team performance is often improved when front line staff actively monitor important performance criteria such as blood loss, regular swab counts, and needle and instrument checks.

The WHO checklist and other team tools have helped with theatre safety; however, never events still continue to occur [4]. Much more is needed around safer team interactions. The team brief, coupled to a debriefing after the day's operating, can enhance patient care, team working and feeling valued by all.

Airline pilots discuss the 'what if?' scenario in pre-flight briefings and know who will be doing what if something doesn't go well (Fig. 42.4). Some clinicians even go as far as to ask team members 'how could we kill this patient today?' Table 42.4 summarises items that could be included in a good briefing and debriefing. The nominated team leader can summarise what has been discussed and repeat back as necessary to confirm to everyone that there is shared understanding. We also suggest monitoring each other for signs of loss of situation awareness as well as looking for features of tiredness and fatigue.

An open culture and respect by all team members are crucial for better team working and enhancing patient safety. Even the most inexperienced pilot will question decisions of senior Captains without fear. While a hierarchal gradient between trainees and their boss is needed, this should be sufficiently flat to allow and encourage them to speak up when something does not seem right. At all times, this needs to be done in an environment where there is no fear of retribution for speaking up about something that may appear trivial.

This concept is important in the team brief so that students, trainees, and nurses all feel valued. We need to be aiming for a 'smooth and enjoyable flight' in our workplaces, even if the view isn't as exciting as from the flight deck.

## 42.5 Situational Awareness

An important HF principle is recognising and understanding how we relate and behave and how changes over time. Surgeons can sometimes develop tunnel vision during long procedures. This can be confounded by indicators that they recognise confirm their behaviour, and thus may need to rely

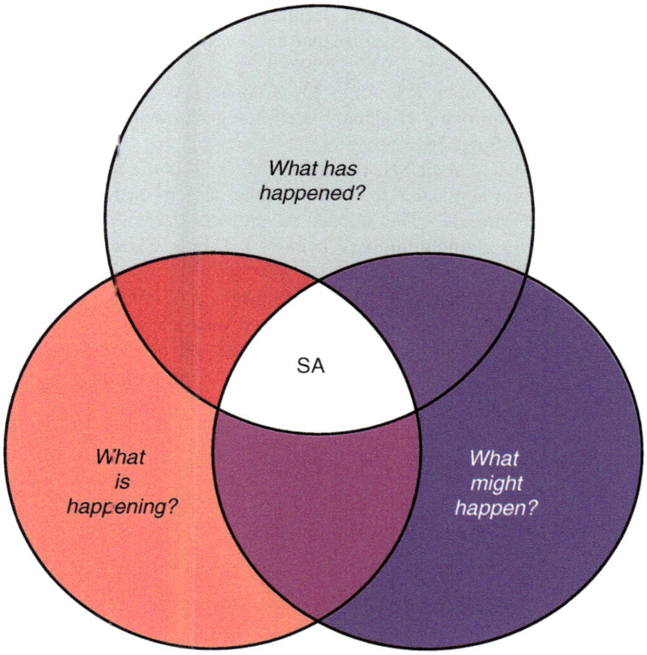


**Fig. 42.4** The three key elements that comprise situational awareness (SA)

**Table 42.4** Things to consider at a team brief

| |
|---|
| A well-prepared team knows their role, looks out for each other and helps all to feel valued. |
| *Briefing* |
| Introductions, transparent culture, 'anyone can speak if concerned' |
| Team working and leadership |
| Identify major parts of surgery and who is going to do what |
| Ask 'What am **I** going to do if something goes wrong?' |
| Situation awareness—how can I intervene when something doesn't seem quite right |
| Decision-making skills |
| *Debriefing* |
| • What went well today? |
| • One thing I (we) could do more of? |
| • One thing I (we) could do less of? |
| • What will I (we) do differently next time? |
| • Saying 'Thank you' to everyone |

on other team members to identify a problem. Losing track of time is one factor, which can lead to catastrophic consequences as highlighted by the Elaine Bromiley incident mentioned earlier. An otherwise competent team lost their situational awareness as critical minutes passed by during failed intubation attempts. Her husband Martin (airline pilot) knew about the same tunnel vision from a fatal plane crash, where a prolonged attempt to troubleshoot a landing light warning and a crew member's failure to assertively communicate led to the plane running out of fuel.

A lack of situation awareness causes many diving accidents. Recognising it for ourselves is important for developing surgical skill and where possible stopping what we are doing when things do not seem quite right. A well-briefed team will be able to recognise at a much earlier stage when something is not quite right [11].

A simple diagram showing the three key components of situational awareness is shown in Fig. 42.4.

## 42.6 HF Training When Not in the Operating Theatre

Technology developments have led surgeons to perform increasing minimally invasive procedures. Physicians also do more invasive procedures such as interventional radiology (IR), percutaneous coronary techniques and gastrointestinal endoscopic surgery. The lessons learnt from surgery and team briefs, WHO checklists and other HF training initiatives should be applied to other parts of the hospital.

Medicine is a challenging activity and patients are far more complex than aircraft. Greater control is needed wherever possible to minimise the risk of harm to others as a result of human error. HF training can readily be taught across medical practice leading to widespread improvements in safety. It is clear that any HF training includes important safety concepts, including better communication in teams, a culture of open reporting without blame, regular safety briefings and leadership skills. Aviation-based 'Crew Resource Management CRM' training has improved reduction in wrong site surgery. Hospitals need to recognise that they can influence attitudes, culture and values towards patient safety. HF training is simple, cost-effective and deliverable way of getting all staff members involved.

## 42.7 Conclusion

HF and better team working, as well as commitment towards continual performance improvement, are increasingly recognised as essential aspects of patient safety. Despite this, serious medical errors have not been abolished. Many errors can be prevented by recognising and using simple measures in our clinical practice. An appreciation of those factors that affect each of us as being potential contributors to error is a great step towards improving safety for our patients.

We believe and advocate that HF training is essential for medical staff as it is for airline employees. Since the introduction of compulsory HF training in the early 1990s, there has not been a single death on a UK-based airline due to human error in more than 3 billion passenger journeys. An individual would have to fly every day for 38,000 years before experiencing a human error–related aviation catastrophe. Surely we owe it to our patients to do everything we can to improve their safety too?

## References


1. O'Connor T, Papanikolaou V, Keogh I. Safe surgery, the human factors approach. Surgeon. 2010;8:93–5.
2. Leape LL, Berwick DM. Five years after To Err Is Human: what have we learned? JAMA. 2005;293:2384–9.
3. Makary MA, Daniel M. Medical error-the third leading cause of death in the US. BMJ. 2016;353:i2139.
4. Reid JH. Surgical never events should never happen. J Perioper Pract. 2011;21:373–8.
5. Reason J. A system approach to organizational error. Ergonomics. 2005;38:1708–21.
6. Abd Elwahab S, Doherty E. What about doctors? The impact of medical errors. Surgeon. 2014;12:297–300.
7. Parry DA, Oeppen RS, Amin MSA, Brennan PA. Sleep: its importance and the effects of deprivation on surgeons and other healthcare professionals. Br J Oral Maxillofac Surg. 2018;56:663–6.
8. Parry D, Oeppen RS, Gass H, Brennan PA. Impact of hydration and nutrition on personal performance in the clinical workplace. Br J Oral Maxillofac Surg. 2017;55:995–8.
9. Parry DA, Oeppen RS, Amin M, Brennan PA. Can dietary supplements improve a clinician's well-being and health? Br J Oral Maxillofac Surg. 2018;56:85–9.
10. Wadhera RK, Parker SH, Burkhart HM, et al. Is the "sterile cockpit" concept applicable to cardiovascular surgery critical intervals or critical events? The impact of protocol-driven communication during cardiopulmonary bypass. J Thorac Cardiovasc Surg. 2010;139:312–9.
11. Mishra A, Catchpole K, Dale T, McCulloch P. The influence of non-technical performance on technical outcome in laparoscopic cholecystectomy. Surg Endosc. 2008;22:68–73.

# 43 De Novo Practice of Oral and Maxillofacial Surgery

Srinivas Gosla Reddy and Avni Pandey Acharya

## 43.1 Introduction

The exhilarating and exciting emotion of starting your own practice can also be a daunting experience to a freshly passed out maxillofacial surgeon. Student loans taken during the course of one's studies also play a significant role in determining one's ability to take on any additional financial burden.

As oral and Maxillofacial surgery is a bridge between medicine and dentistry, there is a continual national debate regarding the need to pursue a dual degree. The option to pursue a condensed medical degree as part of the current syllabus is still not available in India. Thus, new residents should always strive to do additional training [residency, fellowship and diplomas] in their fields of interest to expand their expertise prior to starting their own set-ups [1]. It is a well-known fact that it is easier to gain knowledge and skills during the starting of one's career rather than later in life. The goal is to aim high by keeping one's feet grounded in the soil of academics.

The fire of determination and passion should always be kept alive in order to truly succeed and excel in our field. The truly successful surgeon is the one who has thrived against all the odds and taken advantage of every opportunity that has come his or her way. This chapter aims to guide the freshly passed out maxillofacial surgeon regarding further avenues of learning and about the establishment and expansion of one's surgical practice.

## 43.2 Professional Skill and Learning

For the freshly passed out maxillofacial surgeon, the option of acquiring financial stability always appears alluring. However, it is a well-known fact that enhanced surgical skills and strong academic knowledge cannot be traded for the financial gains obtained by prematurely starting one's surgical practice. Thus, it is always advisable to pursue additional training in the form of a fellowship, residency or diploma in one's area of interests [2, 3]. This trend will help the surgeon establish a niche practice where they specialize in a particular domain of oral and maxillofacial surgery, which eventually leads to improved surgical results and credibility for our profession. This kind of surgical practice will also help to create an edge over the plastic surgeon and the otolaryngologist and establish a distinguishable specialty offering an unequivocal service to patients. Despite the prevailing circumstances governing one's decision to enter practice immediately or continue training, everyone will eventually contribute to the OMFS field with their skills and knowledge.

Laskin [4] made an organized attempt to tackle this problem by dividing the scope of oral and maxillofacial surgery into three categories: areas of expertise, competence, and familiarity. To be addressed as an oral and maxillofacial surgeon, one needs to include the areas of expertise and competence in their work profile.

- Areas of expertise include oral pathology/oral medicine, dentoalveolar surgery, implantology, pre-prosthetic surgery, and maxillofacial traumatology.
- Areas of competence involve orthognathic surgery, temporomandibular joint surgery, and local reconstructive surgery.
- Areas of familiarity are cleft lip and palate surgery, regional reconstructive surgery, oncologic surgery, craniofacial surgery, and cosmetic surgery.

The first step in learning a skill is to know how a skill is learned. Educationists have constructed many models attempting to outline the learning process. The most widely accepted was first documented by Noel Bunch and was subsequently re-worked by Abraham Maslow (Figs. 43.1 and

S. G. Reddy (✉) · A. P. Acharya
GSR Institute of Cranio-maxillofacial & Facial Plastic Surgery, Hyderabad, Telangana, India


K. Bonanthaya et al. (eds.), *Oral and Maxillofacial Surgery for the Clinician*, https://doi.org/10.1007/978-981-15-1346-6_43

43.2). In the beginning, a student is in the 'unconsciously incompetent' phase. An undergraduate dental student in their third year would have no idea about administering local anaesthesia. After working on the skill for some time, they move on to the 'consciously incompetent' phase. Here, they have attempted different ways of anaesthetizing teeth and are now keenly aware of the various ways to give local anaesthesia along with their shortcomings in certain regional nerve blocks.

Most of our trainees will arrive somewhere between these two steps of knowing what they can and cannot perform. Educators must help them overcome their limitations. Once they are aware of their shortcomings, they can actively begin to correct them. With practice and appropriate teaching, they move to the third level of being 'consciously competent'. Here, the trainee can perform every step of local anaesthesia along with variations of different techniques. However, the steps require focus and assiduousness. Now, he or she would be considered as a competent surgeon who can practice independently although lacking in instinctiveness. As learning advances, with years of handwork and practice, they will reach to the concluding stage, 'unconsciously competent'. Now the local anaesthesia can be given while listening to music or talking to patients or colleagues [5].

The obstacle to a meticulous 'ability preparation' is that most of our instructors perform numerous components at an unknown and advanced skilled dimension, while the students are frequently unmindful of numerous components of what they have to learn. The individuals who have overlooked the subtleties of an expertise are entrusted with showing people who don't know about what abilities they are unequipped for performing. The initial step for an ace instructor is to perceive that the educator and understudy live at inverse finishes of the authority. Perception, readiness, practice and tolerance are the key components of learning in any skill [6].

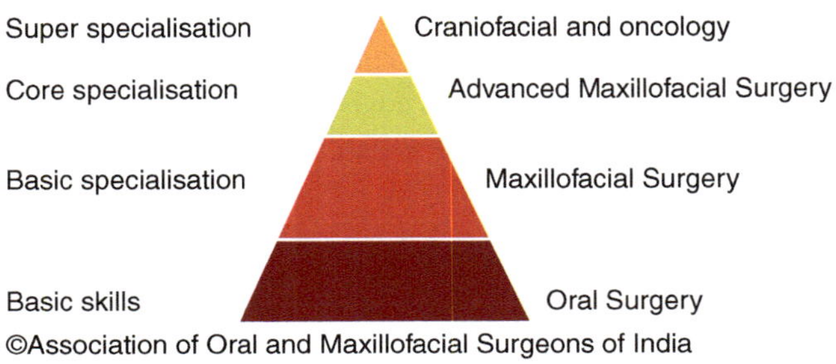


**Fig. 43.1** Gradation of maxillofacial surgery and importance of super specialization

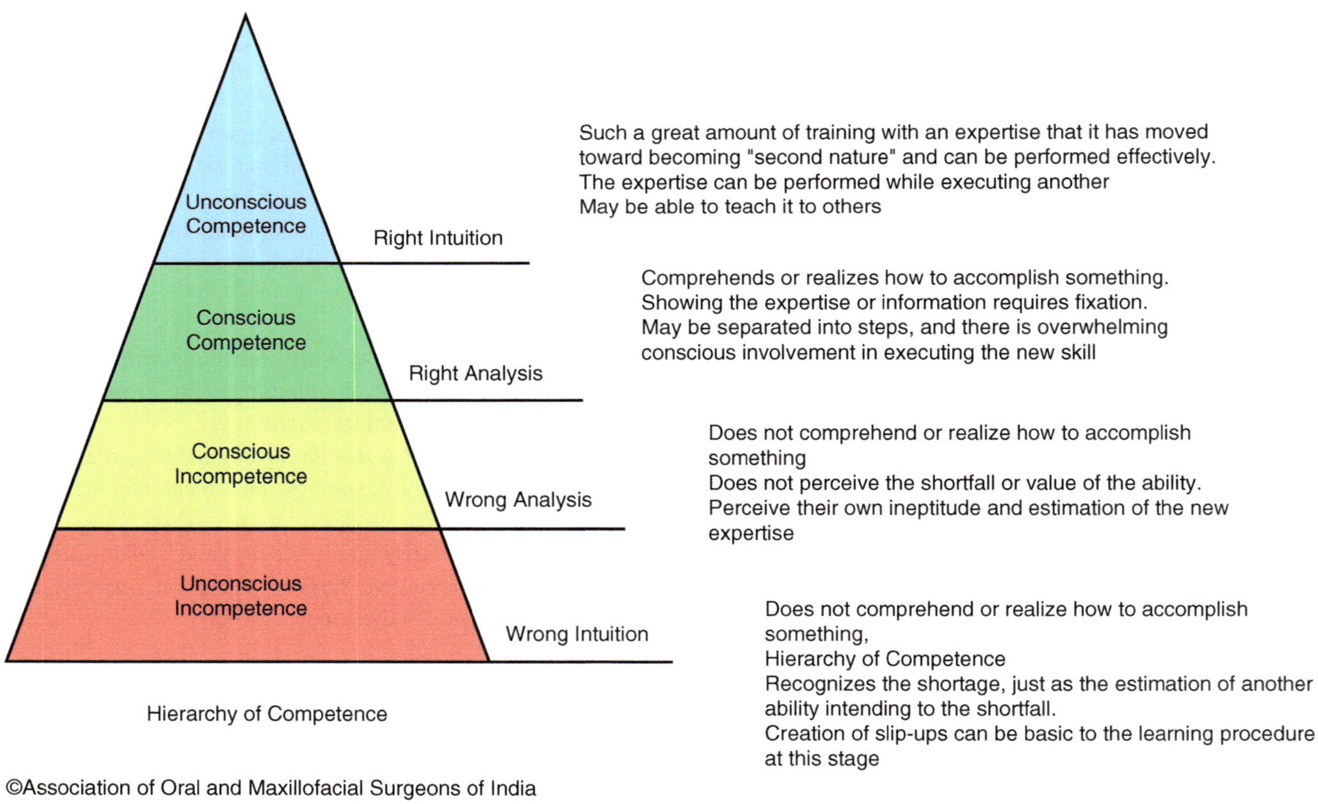


**Fig. 43.2** Competence hierarchy

### 43.2.1 Kolb's Learning Cycle [7]

David Kolb is renowned in educational circles for his Learning Style Inventory. In Kolb's speculation, the drive for the headway of new thoughts is given by new experiences. "Learning is the technique whereby data is made through the difference in comprehension" [7]. Kolb's experiential learning style theory is conventionally addressed by a four-stage learning cycle in which the understudy contacts all of the bases (Fig. 43.3). Along these lines, everyone responds to and needs the improvement of a wide scope of learning styles.

Here are brief depictions of the four Kolb learning styles:

- *Diverging (feeling and watching—CE/RO)*

These individuals can take a gander at things from alternate points of view. They are touchy. They want to observe as opposed to doing, tending to accumulate data and use creative ability to tackle issues. They are best at reviewing solid circumstances from unique perspectives.

Kolb called this style 'separating' in light of the fact that these individuals perform better in circumstances that require thoughts, for instance, conceptualizing. Individuals with a wandering learning style have wide social premiums and like to assemble data.

They are keen individuals, will in general be inventive and enthusiastic, and will be solid in expressions of the human experience. Individuals with the veering style like to work in gatherings, to tune in with a receptive outlook and to get individual criticism.

- *Assimilating (watching and thinking—AC/RO)*

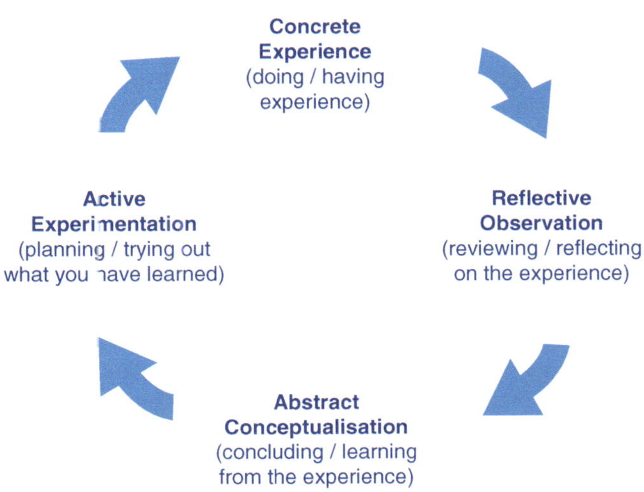




**Fig. 43.3** Kolb's Experiential learning cycle

The Assimilating learning inclination is for a compact, sensible methodology. These individuals require clear clarification as opposed to pragmatic chance. They exceed expectations at seeing wide-going data and sorting out it in a reasonable coherent configuration.

This learning style is essential for viability in data and science vocations. In formal learning circumstances, individuals with this style incline toward readings, addresses, investigating diagnostic models, and need room to thoroughly consider things.

- *Converging (doing and thinking—AC/AE)*

Individuals with this combining learning style can tackle issues and will utilize their figuring out ability to discover answers for reasonable issues. They lean toward specialized assignments and are less worried about individuals and relational angles.

Individuals with a combining learning style are more pulled into specialized errands and issues than social or relational issues. A meeting learning style empowers expert and innovation capacities. Individuals with a meeting style like to try different things with new thoughts, to recreate, and to work with handy applications.

- *Accommodating (doing and feeling—CE/AE)*

The Accommodating learning style is 'hands-on' and depends on instinct as opposed to rationale. These individuals utilize other individuals' examination and want to take a viable, experiential methodology. They are pulled in to new difficulties and encounters. They usually follow up on 'gut' nature as opposed to sensible examination.

Individuals with an obliging learning style will in general depend on others for data than complete their own examination. This learning style is common inside the all-inclusive community. To become familiar with specific, careful abilities, an understudy needs to go intensively through every one of the styles of learning. First, we have to observe, think and feel pursued by experimentation on models to learn the aptitude to do medical procedure on humans.

### 43.2.2 Transformative Learning Way

Transformative learning is the procedure by which we digest and decipher data based on our own encounters to date, to deal with ace Surgical aptitudes. This can be seen in a case of a boss helping a careful student with his or her first case. One of the key issues is for the chief to be accessible if for no other explanation other than to counsel, whenever required, and guarantee that things go easily. Grown-up students need to realize that they have the director's certainty and support and that they will be permitted to extend their range of abilities to attempt to take care of any issues they may experience, before the chief strides in.

The following enquiries of destinations and points can give understanding into the learner's self-appraisal capacity or trainee's self-assessment:

- Pre-employable appraisal or Pre-operative assessment
- Discourse of case, history, examination and examinations to date.
- Discourse of the means of the activity and who will attempt which part—the director ought not to set suddenly exclusive requirements, just what is sensible to accomplish for the dimension of the student.
- Conceivable complexities and their goals
- Armamentarium.
- Consent
- Break process

### 43.2.3 Intra-operative Educating

- The student endeavours to pursue the pre-operative plan and, if there is a deviation, guarantees to take assent from the supervisor.
- The supervisor controls through the central specialized advances and focuses on technical steps and gives assertion for leading following the next stage, simply after fruitful fulfilment of past advances.
- The teacher gives prompt input on what is being progressed admirably and what should be possible in an unexpected way.
- The chief considers enabling the student to accomplish more on the off chance that they are advancing admirably and exhorts them in like manner.

The teacher must attempt to 'dominate', if important to help the patient yet this positively doesn't imply that boss should hinder in each progression and make the student uncertain.

**Post-operative questioning**

This can begin to happen as the student is concluding the case; however, a few learners may discover this diverting, which may hamper their execution.

The chief should plan to question in a peaceful domain.

- Ask the student how they think they went, invigorate reflection and show general tenets; help them survey their execution; investigate ways they can set a few objectives to help address insufficiencies
- Provide explicit instances of how the student could have performed better. An administrator may figure the learner progressed nicely, yet on the off chance that they don't convey, the student may feel that some perspective was not progressed admirably. Strong correspondence is critical [8].

## 43.3 Career Goals

Oral and maxillofacial surgery gives a wide range of alternatives from a conventional private minor oral surgery practice to specialist maxillofacial surgery in trauma, temporomandibular surgeries, orthognathic surgeries, implantology, oncology, aesthetic surgery and cleft and craniofacial surgery [9]. The following are the alternatives, which can be taken by a newly passed oral and maxillofacial surgeon:

- *Associateship*—The possibility of associateship with an officially settled practice is by all accounts extremely appealing. By joining a specialist set-up, one stays away from the numerous costs and unpleasant circumstances involved in setting up one's own practice. However, one should make sure to join the right specialist practice. There is a lot of contrast between a specialist that genuinely needs a partner and a specialist that may need a partner for increasingly narrow-minded reasons. The practice may not have enough volume to support two specialists and the senior associate may. In this situation, the new specialist may be in charge of creating the new referrals. This can be a troublesome circumstance. In addition, one may anticipate that as the new associate one should take an excessive measure of call, see all patients with insurance formalities and not take an interest in the 'great cases'. Additionally, the desires of the senior associate might be farfetched and a lot of additional fault may be put on the new junior associate. Before getting engaged with any of the associateship, the term and conditions ought to be clear in the pre-legally binding stage [10].
- *Scholastics and Research*—Teaching is one of the alternatives for a specialist who has the enthusiasm to educate the new batch of upcoming surgeons. It is one of the best ways to remain connected with your field. There are many institutes looking for youthful surgeons with a keen interest in academics, research and administrations [11].
- *Organization*—Being a manager includes leading, managing, overseeing and supporting health care departments or associations to accomplish their pre-set goals. With the opening of a several corporate hospitals, administrators with a medical background are most desirable for such roles. The size, intricacy and mission of various healthcare organizations (hospital systems, academic medical centres, practice groups, insurance companies) require assistance from experienced specialists with fluctuating roles [12].

- *De novo Practice*—Opening one's own OMFS office from the ground up is an extremely tough task that is not for the weak hearted. It has been rightly said the war field ought not be entered without a weapon and thus one need to be confident in their surgical skills and also have a basic understanding of the administration involved with running one's own practice [10].

## 43.4 De Novo Practice

### 43.4.1 Requirements

- *Surgical Skills*: Never accept surgery as an easygoing endeavour and always keep the patient's prosperity over any of your own advantages. It is important to develop surgical skills early on in one's career as it is these skills that will carry you forward throughout life. However, one should also make an effort to get the right opportunity
- *Site or place of your practice*: Selection of the place where you will set up your centre is the first and most basic decision that one comes across. Choosing a location that has a geographic advantage [as in easily accessible via adequate public and private transport] and has an adequate population to support your practice is essential. Demand and supply also needs be considered when choosing your location. Too many competing specialists in the vicinity will definitely make attracting patients difficult. However, it must be said that the eventual fate of a practice depends on the surgical skills and services offered by the surgeon in charge. Lastly, the spot ought to be close to the living arrangement of the surgeon in case of a medical emergency [13].
- *Accounts or Finances*: It is prudent to begin a project of such magnitude with your financial capacity in mind. Very few specialists manage to acquire stipends during their residency programs and hence are not well acquainted with handling funds. One should avoid large and unnecessary expenses in the beginning. However, this does not mean that one should skip on the basic requirements for starting a well-equipped practice. Expansion, modernizing and incorporation of advanced technology into the practice must be kept as a long-term step wise plan. The computations of property expenses [rent/lease/loan], staff salaries, equipment costs, sterilization and biomedical waste management ought to be dependably considered in evaluating the finances [14].
- *Framework*: The rooms required in an OMFS workspace are as follows: reception room, business zone, financial zone, exams rooms, operatories, x-ray zones, research centre space, staff lounge, specialist's private office, restrooms, medicinal gas space, mechanical space, sterilization space, recovery space and storage space [10].
- *Marketing strategy*: Health care associations actualize business techniques through projects and administrations, and achievement relies upon program structure and execution. Beginning a business adventure without an arrangement is out and out welcoming a fiasco and human services is no exemption for this standard. Since we are specialist co-ops, we ought to dependably remember that this field is certifiably not a "high pay" creating field except if we are managing corporate divisions. That is the reason why practical objectives ought to be set to keep ourselves as well as other people away from the rat race of cash. This positively doesn't imply that you ought not dream about a sensible way of life.

### 43.4.2 Types of Practice

There are four different ways by which medical practices can be organized:

(a) *Sole Proprietor*—This is for the specialist who already has a foundation of maxillofacial surgical or other medical service organizations running in the family. The choice appears to be practical for the surgeon who has full control of his financial assets and is as of now experienced in the field [15].
(b) *Organization or associateship*—If you have fellow medicos who are of the same or diverse fields and are prepared to create a combined practice with you, then it is the most reasonable choice. Always scrutinize your colleagues before entering into such arrangements. The success of this arrangement relies upon mutual trust for each other. It is also necessary to discuss all the terms and conditions [expenses and division of profits] before entering such an arrangement.

Additionally, you can work under the umbrella of some settled specialist and eventually move toward becoming a partner in the not-so-distant future [15].

(c) *Corporate segment.* Joining corporate hospitals or chains is also an alternative. The hustles of marketing, equipment, and location can be obliterated. However, corporate hospitals today are keen on hiring well-settled specialists as patients are hesitant being treated by novice surgeons [15].
(d) *Trust or NGOs*—These organizations are created to help unaffording individuals for treatment. One cannot expect great monetary benefits from a trust or NGO. However, there is a feeling of fulfilment of helping other people. There are a few associations in and outside India, which raise funds for such organizations. A point worth noting is that there are numerous specialists who are working free of charge under such associations while simultaneously obtaining their standard pay elsewhere [15].

### 43.4.3 Qualities Needed

#### 43.4.3.1 Strategic Planning

Due to the contingent nature of the decision of essential structure be it sole owner or in affiliation, Strategic arranging is required. It is a definite methodical report demonstrating the manner in which it intends to advance from its present circumstance to the ideal future situation [16].

The SP procedure is isolated into progressive stages. The writing gives diverse names to unmistakable stages yet we are adopting established strategy, distinguishing five values simultaneously. The Mission, Vision and Values ought to be institutionalized amid the underlying stages.

- Mission
- This mission characterizes the general motivation behind the association, the objective customers, the administrations offered, its distinctive highlights, the geological territory in which the centre works, and occasionally the manner in which it works (quality, morals, productivity, and so forth.).
- Vision
- The vision displays the future picture. The substance of the vision ought to uncover what the human services association explicitly tries to be later on.
- Qualities
- Qualities are the arrangement of standards, rules and social viewpoints administering the Hospital Organization (HO) and deciding their institutional conduct. They comprise the association's moral code that gives it its 'spirit' and 'character'. These qualities foresee a particular reaction by the HO when a circumstance emerges that must be quickly settled.

#### 43.4.3.2 Technique Formulation

The accompanying five phases ought to be considered

- *First Stage: Analysing the External Environment*
- This examination generates data on those difficult to change external variables that can affect the association. This involves patients and contenders.
- Patients: The place that you will eventually set up should have a geographic advantage with the right patient demographic. All too often, a specialist will begin their facility in a distant, underdeveloped and immature zone due to the dread of rivalry. It is a well-known fact that a specialist practice survives on referrals and not only on walk-in patients.
- Contenders: Good work and identity are significant in keeping an edge over your rivals. Endeavour to build up your individual character, as far as work and morals are concerned, should be made.
- *Second Stage: Analysing the Internal Environment*
- This investigation generates data on everything pertinent that has/can and is happening inside the set-up. This investigation centres around three distinct angles:
  - Resources: It incorporates individuals, monetary spending plans, consumable and non-consumable supplies and their level of obsolescence.
  - Licensure—Legal parts of drug store, radiations, and different licenses with respect to specific region ought to be taken already relying upon the standards of the region.
  - Analysis of clinical and research work, action and spending plan ought to dependably be kept aside [16].
- *Third Stage: The SWOT matrix*
- When the outside and inside examinations have been finished and coordinated, the vital arrangement directing gathering will have an abundance of thoughts regarding conceivable vital activities that could be tended to in the arrangement. Then, the issues distinguished in the examination are characterized into four classifications to comprehend what to do and in what request. This is the SWOT investigation, an abbreviation framed from qualities (S), shortcomings (W), openings (O) and dangers (T), which orders the consequences of the examination.
- Every one of the outcomes, notwithstanding grouping them with SWOT criteria, can be weighted as far as significance or relative power (high, medium, and low; +, ++ or +++, and so on.). It permits the arranging group to build up a positioning, with the most vital components positioned in the principal position, situated to key priorities [17, 18].

**TOWS Matrix Analysis**

The TOWS Matrix is aimed at developing strategic options from an external-internal analysis. TOWS idea is firmly identified with SWOT investigation. Whereas SWOT Analysis starts with an internal analysis, the TOWS Matrix starts the other way around, with an external environment analysis; the threats and opportunities are examined first. As indicated by H. Weihrich (1982) [19], Dangers, Opportunities, Weaknesses, Strengths (of the association) ought to be examined in a specific order, as a critical thinking succession during the time spent on the procedure plan. To streamline, let's use TOWS examination in beginning an oral and maxillofacial medical procedure set-up:

Inner Strengths: The accompanying could be qualities of the endeavour:

- Proficient abilities of the head picked up by changed associations, confirmations and courses
- Focal Location of the set-up
- Access to demonstrated plan of action

- Relationship with other dental and restorative fields to give all administrations under one rooftop
- The individual variables of the specialist like family foundation, past experience, unique intrigue, administrative and specialized abilities, self-assurance, inventiveness, creativity and eagerness to go for broke

Inward Weaknesses

- less familiarity with the field of Oral and maxillofacial medical procedure
- Constrained patient base if there should arise an occurrence of elite oral and maxillofacial practice
- Understanding paying limit
- Issue of staff wear out

Individual shortcomings (inside negative factors or challenge) like deficient abilities, terrible work propensities or attributes like poor relational abilities, poor systems administration, ineffectual authority characteristics, absence of specialized mastery, absence of IT information, absence of comprehension of statistical surveying, absence of promoting skill and so on because of which wrong choices are generally taken.

The following stage is the planning of TOWS 'Matrix of key' choices, which empowers determination of supportable, open door, simpler, and quantifiable results. '*Inward*' are the shortcomings and qualities and '*outer*' are the dangers and shortcomings. Four quadrants with various vital circumstances are created as pursued:

*S-O*—How can the organization employ the expertise of its own professionals to respond to the needs of centres? By partnering up, the organization can convince the institutions that there is enough capacity, knowledge and experience to train young people to independent professionals at all levels of surgery.

- *SO circumstance—maxi-maxi system.* This circumstance compares to the maxi-maxi methodology whereby it is conceivable to have solid extension and broadened advancement. In such cases, if the cost is utilized as to prepare individuals and keep them on minimal effort at first to give complete consideration by the prime specialist will prompt bringing down of beginning costs. Along these lines, more income is produced amid starting days just to have the capacity to rise as market pioneer.

*S-T*—How can the organization use its skilled staff to compete with cheaper workers employed by competitors? A smart approach for the organization would be to communicate to the outside world that their staff has accredited diplomas and that it's important for health care centres to comply with legal requirements and safety standards.

- *ST circumstance—maxi-little system.* The wellspring of troubles in development and improvement are ominous outer conditions (predominance of dangers) like a lot of swarming of good oral specialists in the zone, or patients paying limit is low, and so on. The procedure should utilize vast interior qualities in endeavour to defeat dangers from environment. The technique of reaching and catching patient ought to be connected through free camps, minimal effort medications contrasted with encompassing zones and catching exchange out specialists. On the off chance that the ability of the prime specialist is awesome, settle on troublesome cases left by different specialists with the dread of disappointment. In addition more up-to-date methods and medical procedures ought to be aced by the specialist in such cases.

*W-O*—How can partnerships with other centres help the organization to improve itself and put more effort into patient acquisition? By presenting itself as an accredited apprenticeship provider, the organization will put itself on the market again and its shows that adapt to changing times and wants to offer different kinds of treatments.

- This circumstance has more vulnerabilities—shortcomings, yet its condition gives more open doors like less number of oral specialists in the town and so forth. The procedure ought to incorporate the utilization of these chances while decreasing or amending shortcomings inside. Executing the arrangement step by step is required in such cases. The emphasis ought to be on improving the patient experience by great work by prime specialist, less staff and nearly not all that extravagant set-up amid introductory stage. Along these lines, cost cutting should be possible successfully without settling on the treatment plan. As the patient information and OPD increments, further advances can be taken for extension.

*W-T*—How can the organization better position itself in the market and thus reduce the threat posed by competitors? By presenting itself as an accredited apprenticeship provider, the organization can claim that they are a serious competitor and can possibly offer healthcare services by apprentices at reduced rates, with the work still being done by the prime specialists.

- WT circumstance—smaller than usual little methodology. This circumstance is without any advancement openings. It works in antagonistic situations, and its potential for change is little. It doesn't have huge qualities, which could withstand dangers. Scaled-down smaller-than-expected technique comes down to a negative rendition of the shut down or in idealistic circumstance—to take a stab at survival keeping in mind the desire of restoration. Advertising is the key in such cases alongside advancement of uncommon careful just as relational abilities of the prime specialist. Additionally, creating specialty brands are of significance as the abilities are not present with basic maxillofacial specialists. These brands include clefts, oral oncology, all out TMJ substitution and so on [17].

- *Fourth Stage: Strategic Alternatives*
- Equipped with this arrangement of recommendations, the vital arrangement controlling gathering starts a procedure, which orders them into characterized territories of activity. These zones of activity are additionally at the same time distinguished and named relying upon the kind of recommendations they contain [16].
- *Fifth Stage: Strategic Areas and Objectives*
- Now, it is prudent to adjust the procedure definition created, to check whether in reality a methodology exists by asking the accompanying inquiries:
  - Does the plan give a key suggestion that will lead the setup to a truly remarkable position thinking about the challenge?
  - Does it offer an incentive in an alternate manner?
  - Are the key decisions that have been made substantial in the long haul?

On the off chance that there are negative answers, the detailing ought to be looked into to check whether, rather than shaping a key arrangement, an arrangement has been made with a progressively restricted scope [16].

#### 43.4.3.3 Operational Planning

The point of operational arranging is to make the arrangement totally explicit, viable and unmistakable. The Operation destinations unite the accompanying attributes:

- They must have a fixed length, in every case under 1 year. Middle-of-the road objectives can be built up to be completed in various stages after some time.
- They ought to be evaluated. To follow their level of consummation, pointers that measure this are oftentimes required.
- They ought to challenge and keep the association in a condition of alarm so as to accomplish them.
- As a capability to the previous, the Operational goals ought to be feasible.
- Each objective must have an assigned individual in control, who truly has the ability to change the execution of the unit or subunit.
- Each Objective must have a cost doled out to its usage, with the end goal that the all-out expense of all the goals is equivalent to the absolute expense of the key arrangement.
- Each Objective must have the financing and different assets (staff time, gear and so forth.) important to accomplish the goals.

When all the OOs are detailed, the execution has to be incorporated with that of the others inside a course of events of activities that incorporates every one of them and gives an outline of the connections, timing and succession of errands, just as the joined endeavours that the HO needs to perform at each stage.

#### 43.4.3.4 Assessment of Results

Auspicious evaluation of results ought to be done, which is dependent on development of number of patients, nature of administrations, nature of medical procedure, income age and work fulfilment. This should be possible by figuring the development charge. Arbitrary overviews on the web or discontent ought to be finished with the assistance of patients to keep up the pace of association and know the dimension of fulfilment of the patient with the health care providers, i.e. the head and the staffs. Likewise, number of patient waiting ought to dependably increase steadily for a feasible growth [16].

#### 43.4.3.5 Marketing Oral and Maxillofacial Surgery [20]

- It is a must that both the specialist and the staff also show consideration for the patient's needs and have a humble attitude. This will go a great length in gaining the good will of the patient and word-of-mouth referrals.
- Utilizing online marketing tools through advertisement and social networking are slowly becoming a must for every new practice.
- Showcasing your work in study clubs, get-togethers and association conferences will also make fellow medicos aware about your abilities.
- You can publish in the neighbourhood newsletters through knowledgeable articles with respect to your field.
- Conducting free camps for check-ups with the neighbourhood non-profit associations can also help showcase your aptitudes.

#### 43.4.3.6 Staff Hiring

The staff should be skilled in their work and maintain a humble and empathetic attitude. Always hire and maintain the correct staff

- Make clear what is expected of them through a detailed manual
- Train them to be focused in their specific roles and reward them for their endeavours

- Hold meetings at frequent intervals to address problems and figure out solutions
- Always be an instructor and a student [21]
- Know when to fire an employee

#### 43.4.3.7 Communication

Communication or Correspondence is most imperative for achieving the great name as an expert. Thinking from the patients' point of view and attempting to clarify in straightforward however non-phobic words about the method will help in building up the trust of patient for the specialist. This will likewise spare the legitimate ramifications if there should be an occurrence of adversity, which can emerge by not disclosing the intricacies appropriately to the patients. The way toward relieving a patient requires an all-encompassing methodology, which includes contemplations post treating a malady. It warrants a few aptitudes in a specialist along with the specialized ability. Studies have showed great correspondence ability in a specialist improves patient's consistence and general fulfilment. There are fundamental standards of rehearsing great correspondence. Persistent tuning in, compassion, and focusing on the para verbal and non-verbal parts of the correspondence are the essential steps that are often disregarded. Appropriate data about the nature, course and forecast of the infection are essential. Additionally, patients and orderlies ought to be clarified about the need and yield of costly examinations and dangers/benefits engaged with obtrusive strategies. One ought to be mindful while overseeing troublesome experiences and breaking awful news. Formal preparation of the specialists in improving relational abilities is vital and has demonstrated to improve outcomes. Furthermore, it is additionally helpful in overseeing difficult clinical experiences. This way diminishes the disappointment of both the specialist and the patient or chaperon in circumstances of enthusiastic upheavals. It has also appeared to diminish work pressure and increase work fulfillment [22].

#### 43.4.3.8 Record Keeping

Record keeping is vital to a successful practice especially in view of the legal implications that come along with a failure to maintain the same. One should maintain both a hard copy and a virtual copy of their records as backups are most essential. Informed consent forms should clearly record possible complications in a language understood by the patient. Photographic records at the preop, intraop, and postop phases need to be maintained and become especially important when a patient has unrealistic expectations. It is also important to maintain well-documented out-patient records and operative notes. Never forget the seventh principle of the Caldicott report, an NHS report on patient information, which says '*the duty to share information can be as important as the duty to protect patient confidentiality*' [23].

#### 43.4.3.9 Reformulating the Strategy

If at any point of time you come to realize that your practice is unable to achieve patient needs or financial goals, it is time to reconsider your strategy [16].

#### 43.4.3.10 Professional and Financial Growth in Career

Nothing is permanent in life and in one's career. You can run your profession for a particular timeframe to be trailed by slow decrease in the training with age. Wellbeing and prosperity play a vital depiction to build the life span of the training (Fig. 43.4a). Till 45 years, there is a tendency to achieve followed by continuous decrease in the field. The thought is to augment the achievement with slow decrease. A specialist can viably work till the age 55–60, which can be expanded till 65–70 with great wellbeing and consistent learning. It is the duty of old specialists to offer approach to novel specialists for the improvement of field. Supportable model can be made to prepare novice specialists followed by naming them as partners.

#### 43.4.3.11 Time Management (Fig. 43.4b)

Time is the most essential commodity that we have in our lives. Digitalization of many facets of hospital management has helped save time. This time can be re-invested in various other aspects of your clinical practice like discussion regarding treatment planning and discussion of various cases. Make sure you plan your day daily and weekly so that you are aware of the time that you have and be able to invest it wisely [24].

#### 43.4.3.12 Management of Finances (Fig. 43.4c)

One must learn how to handle finances appropriately; unnecessary and exorbitant spending at the earlier stages is not a wise idea and can lead to a sudden financial crisis, which can even lead to the premature end of one's career. As mentioned before, expansion and modernization of the practice should follow a well-thought-out long-term incremental approach. Similarly, it is wise to slowly create an alternate source of income to help tide over any financial crises that one may face throughout the course of their career [25].

## 43.5 Conclusion

Oral and maxillofacial surgery is gaining popularity as a field and general awareness is increasing in India. It is the responsibility of new surgeons to contribute their best to the field in order to get the maximum out of their careers

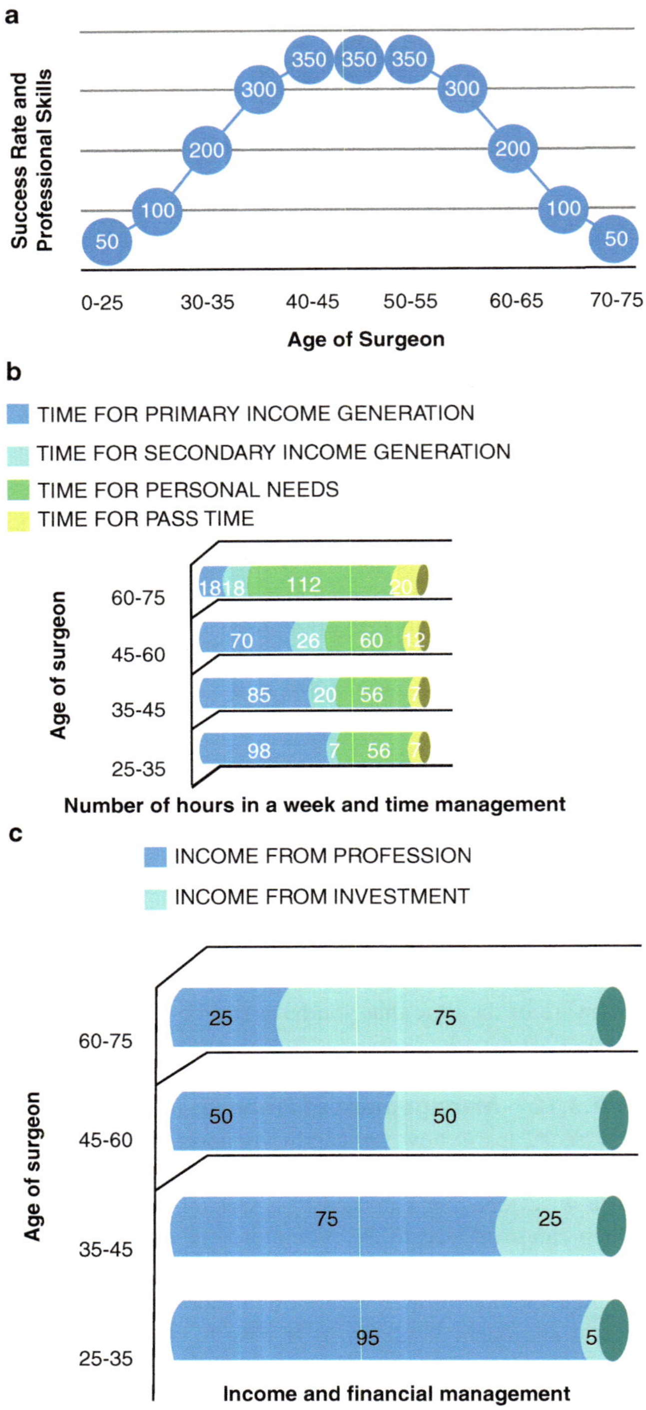


**Fig. 43.4** (**a**) Professional life cycle of oral and maxillofacial surgeon. (**b**) Time management in the life of a maxillofacial surgeon. (**c**) Finances management in the life of a maxillofacial surgeon

and life. As is said 'Do good and it will come back in unexpected ways to you'. Never lose your principles and ethics in this competitive world as it will only tarnish your reputation. Everyone has a specific purpose in this world. The aim is to find that purpose and work upon it with the help of the skills and knowledge you have gathered. These were my rules for success that I stumbled up on while achieving my goals. The newer generation is getting smarter and sharper and will surely contribute to a new set of rules and redefine success.

'Those are my principles, and if you don't like them, well, I have others'—Groucho Marx

**Disclosure** Authors have no financial conflicts to disclose.

## References


1. Samman N. The modern specialty of oral and maxillofacial surgery. 2009;14(6). Dental Bulletin, The Hong Kong Times.
2. Kumar S. Training pathways in oral and maxillofacial surgery across the globe—a mini review. J Maxillofac Oral Surg. 2017;16(3):269–76.
3. Clark PK, Markiewicz MR, Bell RB, Dierks EJ. Trends and attitudes regarding head and neck oncologic surgery: a survey of United States oral and maxillofacial surgery programs. J Oral Maxillofac Surg. 2012;70:717–29.
4. Laskin DM. The past, present, and future of oral and maxillofacial surgery. J Oral Maxillofac Surg. 2008;66:1037–40.
5. Smith M. Aristotle and education. 2001. http://infed.org/mobi/aristotle-and-education/
6. Sadideen H, et al. Surgical experts: born or made? Int J Surg. 2013;11:773–8.
7. Kolb DA. Experiential learning: experience as the source of learning and development, vol. 1. Englewood Cliffs, NJ: Prentice-Hall; 1984.
8. Knowles MS. The modern practice of adult education: Andragogy versus pedagogy (Revised edition). Prentice Hall/Cambridge: Englewood Cliffs; 1988.
9. Haider SM, et al. Oral & maxillofacial surgery; A historical review of the development of the surgical discipline. Int J Surg. 2018.
10. Niamtu J. Beginning a new oral and maxillofacial surgery practice.
11. Walker TW, et al. Educational paper: research in oral and maxillofacial surgery. Br J Oral Maxillofac Surg. 2010;48(8):629–32.
12. Ghosh R, et al. Management and leadership skills for doctors. BMJ. 2008;336
13. McDonald S, et al. Where to put an OMS practice, A supplement to the AAOMS. Today Newsletter. March/April 2007.
14. Pollock SL, et al. Financial arrangements in an oral and maxillofacial surgery practice, Part II, A supplement to the AAOMS. Today Newsletter. March/April 2009.
15. Miron-Shatz T, et al. Promoting business and entrepreneurial awareness in health care professionals: lessons from venture capital panels at Medicine 2.0 Conferences. J Med Internet Res. 2014;16(8):e184.

16. Rodríguez Perera Fde P, et al. Strategic planning in healthcare organizations. Rev Esp Cardiol (Engl Ed). 2012;65(8):749–54. Epub 2012 Jun 13.
17. Watkins M. From SWOT to TOWS: answering a reader's strategy question. Harv Bus Rev. 2007;27.
18. Wiley Encyclopedia of management, SWOT analysis.
19. Weihrich H. The TOWS Matrix: A tool for situational analysis, Long range planning. 1982;15(2):54–66. https://doi.org/10.1016/0024-6301(82)90120-0.
20. Bhangale V. Marketing of healthcare services in India: a study on factors influencing patients' decision making on choice of a hospital. J Manag Market Healthcare. 2011;4(4).
21. Mamoon Z, et al. Hiring the right people for your organization. Glob J Manag Bus Res Admin Manag. 2013;13(8).
22. Ranjan P, et al. How can doctors improve their communication skills? J Clin Diagn Res. 2015;9(3):JE01–4.
23. Mathioudakis A, et al. How to keep good clinical records. Breathe (Sheff). 2016;12(4):369–73.
24. Christie S, et al. How to improve your time management skills. BMJ. 2012;344
25. Halvorson GC. Healthcare tipping points. Healthcare Financ Manag. 2005;74:80.

# Medicolegal Issues in Maxillofacial Surgery

44

George Paul and Manjunath Rai

## 44.1 Introduction

In the modern world, human activity is governed by a set of rules and regulations collectively referred to as law. All professions must follow legal requirements and this is especially important while practising health care, including maxillofacial surgery. Doctors must be aware of their duties, rights and scope of practice within the framework of the laws governing their respective countries or states. This is especially important for maxillofacial surgeons, who straddle the line between medicine and dentistry. This chapter aims to outline the various legal issues that pertain to the maxillofacial surgeon. The laws referenced are mostly India centric, but the general principles are not very different from international laws.

## 44.2 What Are the Legal Issues That Must Concern the Maxillofacial Surgeon?

Since the role of a maxillofacial surgeon acts as a link between the medical and dental professions, the scope of practice has always been controversial. Maxillofacial surgeons have moved from beyond the oral cavity to the head and neck region, and even to distant body parts for procedures such as flap harvesting. All maxillofacial surgeons must be aware of what procedures they are allowed to practice under the law and what they must avoid.

During any procedure, legal documentation is of utmost importance. These include informed consent and filing medico-legal reports. Informed consent is a legal necessity to prove that a patient is willing to undergo a procedure. Medico-legal reports must be filed when one treats a case that could potentially become a legal issue. Maxillofacial surgeons may be called upon to testify as expert witnesses in legal cases such as assault and road traffic accidents. They should therefore be aware of procedures required to document evidence in these cases.

Finally, all medical professionals are vulnerable to malpractice suits. The surgeon must be aware of what actions could put them at risks for facing such suits and what procedure must be followed if one ever faces a malpractice litigation.

## 44.3 Scope of Practice of Maxillofacial Surgery as per the Indian Law

### 44.3.1 Historical Perspective

Oral and Maxillofacial Surgery has a unique place in the health care systems around the world. It is a stand-alone speciality in modern medicine that has its provenance in dentistry. However, when one realizes that modern medical systems are barely more than a century old, it is not long ago that the treatments of dental and oral diseases were a part of an integral system that encompassed holistic health care.

Dentistry as a separate autonomous specialty is an accident and an aberration in the history of modern medicine. In fact, the first dentists were medical doctors or surgeons like Pierre Fauchard in France who had a special interest in treating dental and oral conditions [1] and John Hunter [2] in England.

In the late nineteenth and early part of the twentieth centuries, dental schools and curriculums were established as courses separate from medical courses and the bifurcation became an established practice in different countries in almost all continents [3, 4].

It is through this prism that we need to view the speciality of OMFS and its future as a complex and distinct part of health care. In fact, training to become a maxillofacial

G. Paul (✉)
Kerala University of Health Sciences, Thrissur, Kerala, India

Dr MGR Medical University, Chennai, Tamil Nadu, India

M. Rai
Department of OMFS, A. J. Institute of Dental Sciences, Mangalore, Karnataka, India


K. Bonanthaya et al. (eds.), *Oral and Maxillofacial Surgery for the Clinician*, https://doi.org/10.1007/978-981-15-1346-6_44

surgeon through the route of dental surgery is unique when compared to other distinct regional specialties, which emerge as a post-medical qualification, e.g. ophthalmology, otolaryngology, or gastroenterology.

Realizing the need for adequate training in surgery, substantial additions were made to the dental and oral and maxillofacial surgery curricula by including several basic medical sciences and clinical medical subjects in the undergraduate and post-graduate level, to help meet the medical training requirements of a surgeon.

The impetus for the evolution of OMFS was provided by the two World Wars of the twentieth century and other armed conflicts, where dental and oral surgeons were found to be invaluable in the treatment of facial bone fractures. Thus, Oral and Maxillofacial Surgery was born as a speciality of dentistry and went on to encompass a wide range of surgical work, including pathologies of the mouth and jaws, TMJ surgeries, surgical corrections of dento-facial deformities and cosmetic surgery of the face.

In many countries, including those in Europe, this resulted in the concept of dual degrees (medical as well as dental degrees) to better address surgery in a complicated region of the body where one needed a clear understanding of surgical principles as well as sound dental concepts. Duality is often mistaken for an additional medical degree. In fact, duality includes the need for a dental degree for those with a medical background. In countries like USA, India and several Asian countries, oral and maxillofacial surgery continues to be a surgical speciality of dentistry, although some surgeons chose to do medicine as additional qualification to further their interests and knowledge [5]. Similarly, dentistry was offered as an additional degree for those with medical qualifications only. Dentistry was however an essential pre-qualification to become a maxillofacial surgeon. It must be remembered that 90% of the world population is still serviced by OMFS with a single dental qualification re-enforced by rigorous surgical training as part of their post-graduate curriculum. This includes the USA, Canada, Latin America and the Caribbean, Africa, China, Russia, Central Asia, South Asia, Middle East Asia, South West Asia, Japan, and Far East Asia [6–12]. Starting in the 1970s, several countries also offered integrated 6–7 year residencies leading to OMFS that provide an additional Medical or Dental degree depending on their original background.

The curriculum for Oral and Maxillofacial Surgery in India and several other countries has been suitably modified for patient safety and competence. In India, the speciality of OMFS is regulated by the Dentist Act of 1948 as more than 90% of OMFS are dental-qualified surgical specialists [13]. OMFS has been included as a recognized speciality with distinct privileges in the medical health care system and has been included in significant legislations at the national and state levels, including the Clinical Establishment Act of 2012.

### 44.3.2 Current Legal Privileges

Oral and Maxillofacial Surgery is a recognized department in most multi-specialty hospitals and they are given privileges such as admissions and autonomous departments within the surgical or dental services.

The Dentist Act has defined Oral and Maxillofacial Surgery as a surgical branch of dentistry dealing with diseases affecting the mouth, jaws, and face. The updated curriculum of OMFS is a focused training in surgical management of diseases, injuries and deformities of the face and gnathic system. Training includes interdisciplinary rotation with allied surgical specialities and standard competence in dealing with complex surgical situations in the mouth, jaws and face.

In an increasingly competitive surgical arena, different surgical specialities compete for ownership of procedures based on their diverse backgrounds. It is therefore expected that OMFS, as an emerging surgical specialty, is sometimes in conflict with other specialities.

The legal competence to perform procedures is dictated by the qualification and training received as part of the curriculum set up by the respective statutory bodies through due process of law.

The legal remit and privileges of OMFS in India are based on the training received as part of the curriculum of the master's degree in Oral and Maxillofacial Surgery as outlined by the Dental Council of India in its regulation issued from time to time. The current syllabus, curriculum and training equip the specialist to deal with a wide range of surgical procedures in the face, jaws, oral cavity and teeth. This includes comprehensive management of defects or deformities of dento-facial region caused by congenital anomalies, injuries or surgical ablation. However increased competence, like in any other surgical speciality, is achieved through experience and continuous training in the form of fellowships and structured courses.

Oral and Maxillofacial Surgery falls into a grey area, overlapped by several other surgical specialities. However, competence is defined by the scope offered by legally approved training within the framework set out by the statutory bodies in the respective countries. In India, OMFS is an advanced surgical specialty of dentistry and its remit is regulated by the Dental Council of India.

## 44.4 Legal Requirements to Be Followed When Dealing With a Patient

### 44.4.1 Informed Consent

Consent to medical treatment as an ethical and moral principle is probably as old as medical science. It is inconceivable that a medical practitioner at any point in history would have treated or operated on a patient without his or her permission. However, consent to treat as a legally binding entity is of recent origin. Today, it is validated by multiple principles drawn from social and behavioural sciences, moral philosophy, human rights, ethics and laws of a particular country. One of the main guiding principles of Informed consent involves the rights of patients to make clear assertions of what can or cannot be done to their bodies based on unbiased and full disclosure of the benefits and risks that will ensue from treatment. While most diagnostic treatment procedures are today performed only with a clear informed consent, there are some which attract particular attention in the matter of informed consent, e.g., HIV testing and high-dose radiation in vulnerable patients.

#### 44.4.1.1 Definition and Principles of Informed Consent

Farlex's free online dictionary [14] has a simple definition of Informed Consent. It is "Consent by a patient to a surgical or medical procedure or participation in a clinical study after achieving an understanding of the relevant medical facts and the risks involved." A more descriptive definition is sometimes employed to capture the nuances of informed consent. It may thus be defined as "Consent given by a patient after understanding his/her condition, procedure, risks and alternatives based on unbiased information by the medical professional in a language and manner which is unambiguous, lucid."

#### 44.4.1.2 History and Theory of Informed Consent [15]

The key historical signposts in the evolution of the Informed Consent as a valid legal document can be traced to cases from the US judicial system, though the basic principles find their roots in English Common law.

- While consent has been a well-known moral requirement before treatment, it gained legal sanctity only in 1914 with the case of Schloendorf Vs Society of New York Hospitals. It set the tone for a legally acceptable premise of self-determination [15]. Justice Benjamin Cardoza summarized the basic philosophy in his judgment thus "Every human being of adult years and sound mind has a right to determine what shall be done with his own body and a surgeon who performs an operation without his patients consent commits an assault for which he is liable."
- However, it was with a series of case in the 1960s and 1970s that self-determination came to be legally binding as a legal principle and more importantly the importance of full divulgence by the doctor based on which a consent can be made became a dictum. Important cases include the Salgo Vs Le Land Stanford Jr Case (1972) and the Canterbury Vs Spence Case (1972) [16]. Thereafter, not obtaining informed consent became legal violation, equivalent to assault or "battery".
- With the advent of new technology and emergence of new diseases like HIV, Informed Consent documents are constantly being upgraded to include new medical procedures.
- Informed Consent Document (ICD) in research was largely evolved due to the World War II atrocities in Nazi Concentration camps. ICDs in research have been formulated and reviewed by the Nuremburg conference and the Helsinki declaration. They are closely monitored for content by organizations such as the WHO, FDA, and the ICMR in India.

#### 44.4.1.3 Types of Informed Consent [17]

Informed consent may be of two types:

1. Implied and
2. Oral or written Consent
   - Implied Consent: It is given by the behaviour of the patient, such as entering the clinic and opening the mouth to be examined, etc.
   - Oral Consent: It is acceptable for inconsequential procedures such as examination, taking of impressions, or even routine low-exposure X Rays, etc.
   - Written Consent: While oral consent is an acceptable consent, it can often be challenged and the consent cannot often be proved or validated. It is therefore more binding to give a written informed consent.

#### 44.4.1.4 Informed Consent in Oral and Maxillofacial Surgery

Informed Consent for orthognathic surgery is particularly important because of the nature of the procedure. It is an elective procedure and the patient often seeks treatment for enhancement of aesthetics and function. The expectations are high and therefore the scope for disillusionment as well.

Orthognathic surgery is a highly skilled procedure in a complex anatomical area. Treatment often involves multiple specialists, including orthodontists, anaesthetists, general dentists, and other surgical specialists like neurosurgeons, otolaryngologists, or plastic surgeons. In addition to results falling below expectations, which are largely subjective, patients may also have morbidity in the form of neurological deficit, infections, occlusal discrepancy, TMJ problems, and in rare situations excessive exsanguinations and even death.

Maxillofacial Surgery is a unique speciality of dentistry and medicine and involves complex procedures and outcomes. Some of the procedures are cosmetic whereas others are ablative. Being a surgical procedure involving the mouth, jaws and face, there are several issues of deformity and disability.

The informed consent should include the following (Box 44.1):

**Box 44.1. Components of Informed consent for surgery**
1. the purpose of the proposed procedure;
2. a summary of the surgical approach;
3. expected benefits and limitations;
4. a description of postoperative recovery; possible complications and known side effects, including those that are rare.
5. risks associated with the procedure and/or medications should include alternatives, including the option of no treatment or surgery at all.

Irrespective of whether the surgery is a minor dento-alveolar extraction or major reconstructive procedure, it may be cautious to take an informed Consent, which includes chance of injury or consequences that have disutility for the patient. While operating as a team there are decisions that can be taken jointly by the other members in the treatment process, e.g., Neurosurgeons or orthodontists. For instance, in orthognathic surgery, the Informed Consent Document may have several distinct parts. Gasparini G, Boniello R et al. suggest a three-part informed consent to include pre-op orthodontics, orthognathic surgery and post-op orthodontic treatment [17].

The informed Consent document may need to include the following principles and the surgeon and his team can make appropriate changes to accommodate them. These have been enunciated by Lord Scarman in the case of Sidaway v Board of Governors of Bethlehem Royal Hospital [18].

1. The individual should be of adult years (18 years in India) and sound mind and should have the legal mental capacity to choose what happens to his body.
2. It should offer a choice that entails an opportunity to evaluate knowledgeably the options available and the risks attendant on each (including no surgery option)
3. The doctor should therefore disclose all material risks. The material risks are determined by the "prudent patient test," which determines what a "reasonable" patient in a position of a plaintiff (complainant) would attach significance to, in coming to a decision on the treatment given.

In addition to this, in the Indian context:

4. All informed consent must be in a language understood by the patient (vernacular languages like Tamil, Malayalam, Bhojpuri, Kannada, etc.)
5. In case of illiterates, the informed consent must be read to them in the presence of an independent witness who must sign on the space provided.
6. In children below 18, a parent or guardian can sign on behalf of the child.

Recent concerns have suggested that informed consent should also cover diagnostic tests. It is a common practice in some countries, including India, to do a routine HIV testing. These can be undertaken only with an informed consent, including pretesting counselling. Many countries also insist on informed consent for multiple high-dose radiation, especially with the use of CT scan.

**A standard Informed Consent form is attached and can be used as a template. Any change depending on local conditions can be added (addendum).

### 44.4.1.5 Informed Consent and Negligence in Oral and Maxillofacial Surgery

Informed consent regulations today are largely governed by the principles of medical negligence rather than the tort of battery as in the early days. Any injury, even expected, may be considered a negligent act if there is no informed consent, e.g., paresthesia following Impactions or BSSO. The situation can be defended if the patient was informed and consent obtained. The civil liability for the same will be similar to the liability for medical negligence.

Similarly, Informed consent does not absolve the surgeon from liability for negligence, if it is proved that it could have been avoided if the surgeon had exercised reasonable care.

In short, liability for negligence can be mitigated by an informed consent, but informed consent cannot totally absolve a surgeon for an obvious negligent act.

**Defence for non-information**

Sometimes, the surgeon may encounter a non-reported or rarely reported complication despite reasonable care. In these situations, they can take defence in the principle of "Act of God!!" These are complications or sequels that may not have been anticipated by a reasonable surgeon.

**Exceptions for the use of Informed consent**

- Life-threatening situations, e.g., Carotid Ligation, Tracheostomy, etc.
- Incapacity of patient by virtue of age or mental status (It is taken from the guardian/parent).

### 44.4.1.6 Informed Consent for Clinical Trials and New Techniques

Informed consent has to be obtained if the patient undergoing the surgery is the subject of a new device, implant, or technique which is not a standard one. In India, devices are not covered by the DCGI (Drug Controller General of India). New techniques on an experimental basis, particularly in teaching institutions, must be communicated to the patient and should be cleared by an Institutional Review Board (IRB) or

Independent Ethics Committee (IEC). The ICD requirements for research are clearly enunciated in India by the ICMR.

In conclusion, Informed Consent Documentation is an important and critical part of all treatment plans and often includes invasive or potentially harmful investigations. A proper informed consent that is realistic and involves full disclosure, if the patient is exposed to a chance of injury for which he has no utility, is a necessary part of all treatment protocols. Informed consent documents respect the right of patients to take a decision on how their body is treated based on all available information. It is a moral, ethical and legal obligation to obtain a consent based on credible information. It also provides a safety net for the surgeon when unexpected adverse complications occur.

### 44.4.2 Dentist/Maxillofacial Surgeons as Expert Witnesses

Dentists and maxillofacial Surgeons are often called upon to give evidence in case of civil or criminal cases. When surgeons are called upon to give evidence as part of forensic evidence, they need to have a grasp of the subject. Forensic medicine and odontology have been used in many sensational cases in India, the Rajiv Gandhi assassination being one of the better-known ones.

Surgeons are often called upon in other more common situations as well.

1. Evaluation of disability after dental or maxillofacial injuries.
2. For opinions regarding the procedures adopted by other doctors/dentists in cases of alleged negligence.

Expert witnesses are issued summons as discussed earlier in the chapter. The surgeon is obliged to present himself before the court at the appointed time. He may be questioned by the lawyers of the prosecution, defence or the insurance company, as to the nature of injury and the quantum of disability. The surgeon is to clearly state his/her opinion without ambiguity and should remain non-committal about subjects that they are not sure about. If the surgeon has issued a wound certificate, the copy of the same will be given to him for reference at the time of testifying. The witness is to merely state the facts. They are not expected to involve themselves with the law on the subject, e.g., Loss of teeth, fracture of jaw, etc. They may answer truthfully to any other question pertaining to the same.

Today, there are only a few quantified disability criteria for dental and maxillofacial impairment in India. They include "The Manual for Permanent Disability" brought out by the CGHS, WHO, and AIIMS in 1981. A compendium of suggested dental and maxillofacial deformities/disabilities has been suggested by Paul G and Thomas S in the published book *Medical Law for the Dental Surgeon* [19]. It has been extensively used in courts of law. If unsure, the surgeon may state if the injury is grievous or not. He may also elaborate on the actual disability that the defect might cause.

Examples of grievous injuries are:

1. Fractures and loss of teeth.
2. Fractures of jaw.
3. Extensive soft-tissue injuries and scarring
4. Neurosensory or motor disturbances
5. Restricted function, e.g. limited mouth opening

**Duties of Witness**

Failure to appear in court without valid reasons after warrant has been issued can invite contempt of court.

Exaggeration or false statements given under oath are not only unethical, but can invite punishment under sec.181, sec.193.

## 44.5 Medical Negligence in Maxillofacial Surgery

### 44.5.1 What Is Negligence?

Negligence is usually a civil wrong or tort. It is the single most important issue in medical law pertaining to litigation for damages.

By definition, negligent torts (civil wrongs) are not deliberate but rather a failure to act as a reasonable person should in the conduct of duties to someone whom he or she owes a duty to.

The liability for negligence can however also be criminal or statutory.

**Negligence as Tort (Civil liability)**

It has several formal definitions, but a convenient one by Alderson explains it rather lucidly as "the omission to do something which a reasonable man, guided upon those considerations which ordinarily regulate the conduct of human affairs, would do, or doing something which a prudent and reasonable man would not do."

For an act to be considered negligent, the following aspects must be present, in regard to a surgeon (Box 44.2).

**Box 44.2. Features of a Negligent act**

1. That the surgeon owed a certain standard of care.
2. That the doctor/surgeon did not maintain that standard.
3. That there was an injury resulting from the lack of care.
4. There should be a proximate or causal relationship between the negligent act and the resultant injury.

**Exceptions to negligence**

Normally, carelessness is neither culpable nor a ground for legal liability, as there is no wrongful intention. However, in medical negligence, the outcomes have serious implications on the patient in particular and the public in general. The consequences of negligence by a surgeon who owes a duty of care are enormous and the law has imposed a duty of carefulness on the doctor or health worker in the interest of safe practices. However, there are several situations, which do not conform to the strict definition of negligence. In India, several judicial orders have placed many actions by doctors outside the ambit of negligence.

A review of Consumer cases (Under the Consumer Protection Act) shows that some of the situations mentioned here do not come under medical negligence.

- Not providing an ambulance, due to non-availability of the service does not constitute a negligent act.
- Any adverse outcome for a procedure done in good faith, in an emergency, beyond the call of duty, is not considered a negligent act. It is also called the Good Samaritan Act in some countries.
- Mere patient dissatisfaction with progress of treatment or desired relief cannot be construed as negligence.
- Non-availability of beds in an ICU is not negligence.
- Giving precedence of one patient over the other based on clinical risks or emergencies is not negligence.
- A fee, being perceived as exorbitant by the patient, is not negligence.
- Non-availability of a doctor outside his or her working hours may not constitute negligence.

## 44.5.2 Duty of Care

**Minimum standard of care**

The degree of carelessness for a particular profession depends on the risk that it poses to the person who is exposed to it.

Professional standard of care is therefore that standard of care or skill that is laid down by a body of professionals on behalf of the medical profession and which a surgeon or physician is expected to bring to his duty.

If skill and knowledge fall below this established standard, it will be considered to be negligent. A body of professionals can establish this standard by publication in books, reports of scientific studies, or by protocols established by them, e.g., text books, journals and protocols created by professional associations. Today, evidence-based science is the hallmark of best practices and is defined by the quality of evidence established through Randomized Clinical Trials (RCT) and meta-analysis of peer-reviewed publications.

When there is a difference of opinion on technical matters, an alternate method recognized by another body of professionals will be acceptable as a valid procedure and will not be considered as negligence. This is ascertained by the application of Bolam's law [20], which recognizes reasonable difference of opinion based on credible evidence or experience among peer professional groups.

The Bolitho test uses a different legal parameter and has undermined the usual dependence on the Bolam test. The Bolitho test goes beyond dependence on just two opinions and looks at credible scientific evidence as more important than mere difference of opinions.

In this context, it is important to discuss the semantics of customary and acceptable.

A professional cannot adopt a procedure merely because it is customary. Customary standards have been looked at critically because it does not provide incentive to adopt better practices. Because a particular procedure has been done for many years does not make it an acceptable practice. An acceptable practice, on the other hand, is not only time tested but also scientifically sound. An acceptable practice is usually the product of evidence-based science as opposed to customary practice, which is either anecdotal or proven to be inadequate or irrelevant by scientific scrutiny.

An often-quoted legal principle is that "The skill, diligence, knowledge, means and methods are not those that are ordinarily or generally or customarily exercised or employed, but those that are reasonably exercised or applied, negligence cannot be excused on the ground that others practice the same kind of negligence."

It may therefore be said that a "health worker is under a duty to use that degree of skill which is expected of a reasonable competent practitioner in the same class to which he belongs, acting in the same or similar circumstances." The Supreme Court has defined this duty in the case of Indian Medical Association Vs V.P. Shanta [21] as "In general a professional man owes to his client a duty in tort (civil wrong) as well as in contract to exercise reasonable care in giving advice or performing services."

Importantly, the court held that this standard should be outlined by the medical profession and it is not the duty of the "lay courts" to decide on what constitutes "standard" care. Negligence, in these situations, may be dependent on the locality, availability of facilities, specialization of the doctor, proximity to specialists and advanced technology. However, it is important to remember the dictum "no man is bound in law to be a good surgeon, but all men are bound *not to act* as a surgeon until he is good and capable as such."

The foregoing dictum indicates that a physician or surgeon should not venture to do a procedure unless he is trained and competent in performing it. Merely admitting that he had inadequate experience is no legal remedy. In other words, it is not legally wrong to be ignorant, but it is legally wrong to act in ignorance.

### 44.5.3 The Test of Negligence

**The Bolam Test**

This is a classical test widely used in the United Kingdom. The Bolam test is an acceptable test used by the National Health Service of the U.K. when a situation of negligence presents itself as observed in the landmark case of *Bolam Vs Friern Hospital managing committee. (1957) 2 AIIER 118.*

The Bolam test establishes that standard procedures be the basis of treatment. Importantly, it provides for alternate management protocols. If there is more than one school of thought, both alternates will be acceptable as a standard.

**Bolitho Test**

In a minority judgment comments in Bolitho, it was emphasized that the word "responsible" in the traditional formulation of the Bolam test meant that responsible practice is that which withstands the scrutiny of "logical analysis" from a judicial perspective. Today, courts are increasingly scrutinizing risk analysis from a patient view point, which undermines the traditional view point of only the care giver.

**Negligence—Carelessness vs. Recklessness**

While both words have almost the same meaning, there is a small difference. A careless person may not think of the eventuality while being careless. On the other hand, the reckless person is fully cognizant of the injury that his act may cause, but still takes the risk of possible injury. The former is passive, whereas the latter is an active act. Both acts are however are *not intentional* and is therefore often used to describe negligence.

**Standards of Care in Hospitals**

Legal standards applicable to hospitals are somewhat similar to those required of doctors or other health workers.

The hospitals are bound to maintain standards in two ways.

1. The facilities of a hospital should be that of a reasonable hospital engaging in similar type of health care.
2. The Hospitals should maintain standards laid down by statutory provisions (if available). In India, there are now basic standards for all medical establishments, which are defined by a legislated statute called the Clinical Establishment Act. It provides for the basic requirements of different categories of hospitals and the role of personnel in providing standard care.

In addition, the hospitals may be answerable for the negligence of their doctors, nurses and other health workers through what is called vicarious liability.

### 44.5.4 Contributory Negligence

In some situations, negligence arises fully or in part due to the patients or the complainant's fault. As the patient, wholly or partly, contributes to the negligent act, it is called contributory negligence.

The standard to be adopted to assess contributory negligence is somewhat similar to the standard adopted for the doctor. It may be said that 'contributory negligence is when a competent adult (patient) may be negligent by contribution when his conduct falls short of the degree of care that society expects a reasonable person to do or not to do for his own safety'. This would obviously preclude children and mentally incapacitated adult.

Examples

1. When a patient refuses to take a prescribed medication resulting in postoperative infection.
2. A patient who removes inter-maxillary wiring on his own resulting in non-union.

### 44.5.5 Remedy for Negligence Under the Indian Legal Systems

Negligence can be

1. Tortious (Civil wrong)
2. Contractual (Breach of contract)
3. Criminal
4. Vicarious (Liability passed on to hospital or employer)

Negligence can be remedied depending on what legal provision the complainant wishes to seek remedy.

The punishment under the law of Tort (Tortious liability) is unliquidated damages, i.e. whatever damages the judge wishes to award depending on injury, circumstances and other considerations like age, earning potential, profession, etc.

If an implied agreement was made between doctor and patient, then the remedy would be as specified in the contract. The judge may order a specific performance to do or not do something he has agreed to. However, guarantees for treatment are against ethical guidelines for treatment and it is not applicable in medical law.

If the complainant seeks punitive action against the doctor, he may file a criminal case under the relevant statutes. The Indian Penal Code for example, has provisions to punish doctors for death or disability. The remedy under criminal law is always in the form of a punishment (Penal). It may involve imprisonment or fine or both. Rarely, the court can order compensation or specific performance as well. Criminal law sees negligence as a crime against the state and not just against the plaintiff.

Doctors may also be liable under professional statutory laws governing the practice of the profession. In India, statutory bodies such as the Medical Council of India or the Dental Council of India can prescribe punitive action in accordance with laid down laws. The laws can be initiated only against persons registered under the particular statutory body. The Medical Council of India, for instance, cannot take action against a dental-qualified maxillofacial surgeon.

In some instances, a doctor may not have to answer for his negligence directly. The hospital or establishment employing him may have to answer to the allegation to negligence. This is called vicarious liability and is usually relevant to salaried employees who work for a contract of services and not a contract for services.

However, in practice, for the sake of regularity, it may be said that all permanently or part-time employed doctors are only vicariously liable. However, if the patient is admitted by a doctor in his personal capacity, then the doctor will be personally liable.

**Contractual nature of liability**

In a doctor patient relationship, an implied contract is established when a doctor accepts a patient for treatment. A breach of any aspect of this implied contract may amount to negligence when the doctor is under duty to

1. Treat with care
2. Continue to treat and not terminate until patient is cured or the patient discontinues treatment.

This may be considered the contractual nature of medical liability. However, Medical ethics does not provide for a written contract, which can be violated as in the case of a commercial transaction. So any liability based on breach of an implied contract will essentially lie within the realm of tortious liability.

Written contracts with promise to cure, failing which a refund is assured is against the ethics of medical or dental practice. It is this author's view that such contracts can be technically void, considering the ethical and legal issues involved.

Tortious Liability is usually dealt with in Civil Courts. In India, medical negligence comes within the ambit of the Consumer Protection Laws established to provide speedy relief to plaintiffs seeking redressals for goods and services that fall short of standards. The Consumer Protection Act defines medical care as contract <u>for</u> services, which makes doctors and hospitals liable under the Consumer Protection Act of 1986. The Consumer Courts are quasi-judicial legal redressal forums established for speedy justice. They are tiered under the District, State and National Forums depending on the place of the cause of action and the pecuniary jurisdiction (amount claimed as damages).

**Criminal Liability**

This liability normally lies with an identifiable individual or groups of individuals. However, recent trends indicate that Hospitals also may be held vicariously liable just as in civil liabilities.

Criminal liability is penal and involves punishment in the form of imprisonment or fine or both. Criminal negligence is considered to be a crime against society and not just the aggrieved party and is in violation of penal codes of countries. In India, it is a violation of various sections of the Indian Penal Code 1868 (amended several times).

The important offences inviting criminal liability with regard to negligence are:

1. Sec 304 A (IPC)—negligent homicide. A rash or negligent act resulting in Death, e.g. death on the dental chair or hospital or operating room.
2. Sec 336 (IPC) An act endangering the life of a person (even if there is no injury), e.g. conscious sedation without essential monitors or oxygen, even if no harm is caused.
3. Sec (337) (IPC) A rash or negligent act causing a simple injury, e.g. mild reversible thermal burns caused by bone-sectioning equipment.
4. Sec (338) (IPC) A rash or negligent act resulting in grievous injury, e.g. fracture of jaw during extraction due to excessive or improper force or avascular necrosis following osteotomy.

While these are the common sections under which a doctor may be liable, other sections also apply. Any offence against the human body (Sec 299 to Sec 377) or offences against property (Sec 378–462) can be used against doctors, e.g. abetting suicide, causing miscarriage sec 312–316 (subject to exemption from the Medical Termination of pregnancy Act 1971), etc.

Sections 78, 80, 81, 87, 88 are directly or indirectly relevant to the medical practitioner. Some can be used in defence of the doctor accused of negligence. Section 88 for instance is an act done in good faith not intended to cause death. It is a good defence in emergency care. Sections 86 and 87 IPC are in respect to harm or death caused by an act not intended to cause harm or death and is done with consent in the best interest of patients. Section 499 deals with defamation. It can be used by doctors to counter malicious charges by patients intending to spoil the good name of the doctor by frivolous or vexatious charges. It can also be used by patients as a criminal violation of confidentiality statutes. For example, revealing HIV status when the patient is not likely to be a public health hazard.

It is important to understand some terms in connection with criminal liability (Box 44.3).

**Box 44.3. Terms related to criminal liability**

- *Cognizable Offence*: A police officer can arrest without a judicial warrant based on his investigation.
- *Non-Cognizable*: An arrest can only be made by a judicial warrant.
- *Bailable: the arresting officer can provide bail.* Bail is a matter of right and has to be given unless the officer apprehends that the accused may abscond or tamper with evidence.
- *Non-Bailable:* Bail can be secured only from a magistrate. Heinous and violent crimes fall in this category, e.g., if there is a significant risk that the offender may commit further crimes, abscond or tamper with evidence.
- *Compoundable:* A crime in which a compromise between the suspected offender and the victim or his attendant can be worked out it is said to be compoundable
- *Non-Compoundable*: If the crime is against society and is of a serious nature, no compromise can be made between the accused and the victim. These cases are said to be non-compoundable.
- *Sec 304 A* is cognizable, bailable and non-compoundable. It can be punished with imprisonment of either description for a term of 2 years or fine or both.
- *Sec 337 and 338* are cognizable, bailable and compoundable. Sec 337 may attract an imprisonment up to 3 months and a fine up to Rs 250/ or both. Sec 338 can involve imprisonment up to 2 years and a fine up to Rs 1000/ or both.

It is important for the surgeon to be aware of these liabilities. It is also important for him to understand his rights. For example, bail is a matter of right in the foregoing situations and it is to be given by the police officer attempting to arrest a medical professional. Bail is granted on the surety given by the doctor or a colleague. A doctor can give surety on his own reputation. The burden of providing reasons for refusing bail rests on the police officer and he will have to give convincing reasons for *not granting bail.*

**Representations to amend Criminal procedures for arresting Doctors**

Doctors cannot be arrested arbitrarily.

In a landmark case referred to as the Jacob Mathew Case (2002), the Supreme Court of India has prevented arbitrary arrest and detention of doctors even in case of death or serious disability, as a part of treatment. Criminal liability and arrest can only be made on the basis of a credible Medical Board opinion duly constituted or recognized by the Government.

**Statutory Liability**

A doctor or nursing home is liable if there is any infringement of Statutes (rules). They then become accountable to a statutory body. The liability depends on the kind of infringement and the provisions in the statute to deal with it. There are many statutes dealing with practice of Doctors and Dentists, as well as Hospitals. Recently, the newly legislated Clinical Establishment Act provides guidelines for the whole of India.

Doctors and dentists may also be liable to other statutory laws such as The Pollution Control Board and the Drugs and Cosmetics Act, etc.

### 44.5.6 Legal Procedure and Evidentiary Requirements

(With special reference to medical/dental Negligence)

Legal Procedure (Procedural Law) Relevant to Medical/Dental Negligence.

It is important for the doctor/dentist to know the legal procedure involved in medical negligence. The legal procedure is slightly different for civil negligence, criminal negligence, and negligence under the Consumer Protection Act.

To understand legal procedures, one must be familiar with some of the procedural laws. They are,

1. Civil Procedure Code.
2. Criminal Procedure Code
3. The Indian Evidence Act
4. The Limitation Act
5. The Court fees Act
6. Procedure under CPA.

**The Evidence Act**

It is a very important procedural law. There are three concepts in Evidentiary Law.

1. Facts
2. Facts in Issue
3. Relevant Facts.

The facts are the material evidence.

The "facts in issue" are those that have to be explicitly proved. The facts in issue are proved by bringing into evidence the relevant facts. Sections 6–55 deal with these relevant facts.

There are also other rules in Evidence Law.

- *Who needs to bring in Evidence?*

The person who has to legally bring in evidence to prove or disprove a fact is said to have the 'burden of proof'". When one has the burden of proof he has:

1. The burden of establishing a case
2. The burden of introducing evidence.

The general rule (with some exception) is that the onus of proving any particular fact lies with the party who alleges it and not with the party who denies it. In other words, the onus of proof lies with the complainant and not with the defendant.

Negligence can be proved by

1. Direct Evidence
2. Circumstantial Evidence
3. Res ipsa loquitor (The matter speaks for itself)
   - Another aspect of evidentiary law is *standard of proof*.

The standard of proof in civil cases can be based on probability and circumstantial evidence. However in a criminal case, the standard of proof is more stringent and should be beyond reasonable doubt as sanction in criminal law is more severe and penal in nature.

- The limitation act (1963)

It is the statute dealing with the time limit for various suits, appeals, bail application and other legal actions.

- *Cause of Action*:

This refers to the incident, which has necessitated a legal process. Limitation period begins as soon as the cause of action takes place. The period of time varies according to the suit and it is given in the schedule of limitations.

**Appeals/Application for leave of appeals**

For appeals, the day of judgment marks the beginning of limitation period after giving time for obtaining the copy of decree (Judgment Order). This will not include 'writs' as the limitation Act does not apply to them.

If a suit or appeal is made after the statutory limitation period, the court may reject the petition on grounds of being barred by limitation. The court may however accept a petition even if it is barred by limitation, if it is satisfied that the delay was unavoidable. However, in criminal cases, the Act does not provide a period of limitation. Criminal proceedings can be instituted at any time after the offence has been committed. However, as per the guidelines given in Section 468 of CrPC, the limitation periods run thus:

(a) 6 months for offences punishable with fine only.
(b) 1 year for offences punishable with imprisonment up to 1 year.
(c) 3 years for offences punishable with imprisonment up to 3 years (not less than 1 year).

If the limitation period ends on a day when the court is closed, then the next working day is included as the limitation period. It may therefore be said that a suit should be filed as soon as the cause of action occurs.

**Court Fees Act (Varies from State to State)**

Any party who wishes to approach a court with litigation has to pay a court fees with some exceptions like the Consumer Court. Each state may have a different court fee structure. In a suit for money, the fee is usually computed based on the amount claimed by the plaintiff. Court fees are paid in the form of Stamps, which may be adhesive or impressed or both.

## 44.6 Conclusion

This chapter is unique as most textbooks do not address issues pertaining to law and ethics in practice.

The maxillofacial surgeon is often confronted with questions on their remit and scope of work as it overlaps with several other specialties and is constantly in conflict with issues of qualification and areas of competence. The sections on these issues will throw light on their practice privileges in addition to dealing with litigation for medical negligence, which has become all pervasive.

**Disclosure** Authors have no financial conflicts to disclose.

## Annexures

### A.1 AOMSI—Informed Consent Forms for All Procedures https://www.aomsi.com/WebPages/downloads.aspx

1. **Health questionnaire**

AOMSI CONSENT FORM

For A Safer Tomorrow

**ORAL &MAXILLOFACIAL SURGERY**

**HEALTH QUESTIONNAIRE**

Patient's Name Age/Sex Date

---

**Please initial on each page after reading. If you have any questions, please ask your doctor BEFORE initialing.**

---

Have you had any of the following Problems? Please tick **YES** or **NO**

GENERAL PROBLEMS:

- Cold , cough ----------------------------------------Yes \ No
- Fever. ------------------------------------------------Yes \ No
- Sinusitis -----------------------------------------------Yes \ No

  **(If Yes, when was the last episode______________________)**

RESPIRATORY PROBLEMS:

- Nasal obstruction
- Asthma
- Shortness of breath
- Tuberculosis ( TB).
- Bronchitis.
- Emphysema
- Lung diseases.

  **(If Yes, when was the last episode______________________)**

HEART PROBLEMS:

- High blood pressure
- Chest pain

Signature ----------------

- Heart attack
- Heart murmur
- Pacemakers
- Rheumatic fever
- Irregular heart beat
- Infective endocarditis .
- Angioplasty / Angiogram.
- Bypass surgery.

  **(If Yes, mention the details of medication, Procedure date & last visit to the Physician____________________________________________**

  **____________________________________________________________)**

CNS PROBLEMS:

- Seizures/ epilepsy
- Stroke
- Paralysis
- Brain tumor
- Muscle weakness
- Neuralgia

**(If Yes, mention the details of medication, Procedure date & last visit to the Physician________________________________________________**

**____________________________________________________________)**

GIT PROBLEMS:

- Acidity
- Peptic ulcers
- Gall bladder stones
- Colitis
- Appendicitis

- Piles
- Fistula and fissure

Signature ---------------------

**(If Yes, mention the details of medication, Procedure date & last visit to the Physician_______________________________________________ )**

LIVER AND KIDNEY PROBLEMS:

- Cirrhosis
- Liver failure
- Kidney stones
- Kidney failure
- Prostate obstruction
- Urinary obstruction

**(If Yes, mention the details of medication, Procedure date & last visit to the Physician_______________________________________________**

**______________________________________________________)**

BLEEDING PROBLEMS:

- Anemia
- Clotting and bleeding time
- Platelet count
- Haemophilia

**(If Yes, mention the details of medication, Procedure date & last visit to the Physician_______________________________________________**

**______________________________________________________)**

ENDOCRINE PROBLEMS:

- Diabetes

- Thyroid
- Steroids.

Signature -----------------

**(If Yes, mention the details of medication, Procedure date & last visit to the Physician______________________________________________**

**______________________________________________________)**

PSYCHAITRIC PROBLEMS & COUNCILLING

**(If Yes, mention the details of medication, Procedure date & last visit to the Physician______________________________________________**

**______________________________________________________)**

ARTHRITIS:

**(If Yes, mention the details of medication, Procedure date & last visit to the Physician______________________________________________**

**______________________________________________________)**

RADIOTHERAPY:

**(If Yes, mention the details of Procedure date & last visit to the Physician______________________________________________**

**______________________________________________________)**

PREVIOUS SURGERIES:

**(If Yes, mention the details of medication, Procedure date & last visit to the Physician______________________________________________**

**______________________________________________________)**

ACQUIRED DISEASES:

- AIDS
- HEPATITIS – B & C

**(If Yes, mention the details of medication, Procedure date & last visit to the Physician________________________________________________**

**________________________________________________________________)**

Date of last physical exam: Date of last ECG:

Signature -----------------

Are you pregnant: YES/ NO**(If yes specify the trimester_____________)**

Are you breast feeding: YES/ NO**(If Yes, since how long______________)**

Have you been under the care of physician during last 2 years?

**(If yes, why & when_______________________________)**

Have you undergone general anesthesia for an operation?

**(If Yes,Operation details &any anesthesia complications noted____________________________________________)**

Are you taking medicine of any kind: YES/NO

**(If Yes, For what & since how long____________________________)**

Do you smoke YES/NO **(If yes, How long _________ how many________)**

Do you consume alcohol YES/NO **(If yes,How long ________how much_______)**

Do you chew Tobacco/ Areca nutYES/NO **(If yes,How long _____how much________)**

Are you allergic to any drugs: YES / NO

Pencillin... YES/NO Codeine...YES/NO

Local anesthetic...YES/NO Aspirin....YES/NO

General anesthetic....YES/NO Barbiturates....YES/NO

Any other allergies in specific ________________________

Do you wear dentures...YES/NO

Do you wear lenses...YES/NO

Any other medicines....YES/NO

**( If yes specify the medicine________________________________________)**

PATIENT SIGNATURE \ DATE ____________________________________

WITNESS SIGNATURE \ DATE ____________________________________

**2. Medication questionnaire**

# AOMSI CONSENT FORM

For A Safer Tomorrow

**HEALTH QUESTIONNAIRE**

Patient Name:_____________ Date____________

Primary care Physician __________ Primary care dentist

Phone______________ Phone__________________

Address_______________________________ Address_________________

Have you had any of the following ? Please check **YES** or **NO**

**Yes No**

Recurrent illness(Within one year)
Cough, cold , flu(Within 2 months)
Nose obstruction
Shortness of breath
Lung disease
Asthma
Bronchitis
Emphysema
Heart trouble
Chest pain
Heart attack
Irregular heart heat

Yes No

Heart murmur
Rheumatic fever
Scarlet fever
Arthritis
Artificial joints
Cortisone

High blood pressure
Pacemaker
Heart Surgery
Excessive bleeding
Anemia
Treatment of Tumor

Yes No
seizures/ epilepsy
psychiatric disorder
liver disease
stroke
hepatitis
Stomach ulcer
Diabetes
Kidney disease
HIV
AIDS
Others serious illness

Date of last physical exam____________________ Date of last ECG
_____________________

Yes___ No____ Are you pregnant?

Yes___ No____Have you been under the care of physician during the last two years?

Yes___ No____Have you been made unconscious for an operation?

List anesthesia complications_________________________________

Yes___ No____ Are you taking medicine of any kind? List___________________--

Yes___ No____ Do you smoke?___________ How long?________How much?_______

Are you allergic to any drugs : if Yes______________________

Yes___ No____Pencillin.Yes___ No____Codeine

Yes___ No____Novocain Local Anesthetic.Yes___ No____Aspirin

Yes___ No____General Anesthetics Yes___ No____Barbiturates

Yes___ No____ Do you wear dentures?
Yes___ No____Do you wear contact lenses
Yes___ No____Other medicines.

Signature of persons completing this form

______________________________________

Age________Weight____________-BP______________________

Reviewed by ____________________-______________Date Reviewed__________

### 3. Consent for Minor oral surgery

# AOMSI CONSENT FORM

For A Safer Tomorrow

---

## CONSENT FOR MINOR ORAL &MAXILLOFACIAL SURGERY

PATIENT 'S NAME : ………………………………………………
DATE : ………………………………………………
PLACE : ………………………………………………
DIAGNOSIS : ………………………………………………
TREATMENT PLAN : ………………………………………………

---

- My doctor has explained to me that there are certain inherent and potential risks and side effects associated with my proposed treatment and in this specific instance they include, but are not limited to :

1. Post-operative swelling and discomfort that may require several days of recovery.
2. Prolonged or heavy bleeding that may require additional treatment.
3. Injury or loosening of adjacent teeth or fillings.
4. Post-operative infection that may require additional treatment.
5. Stretching of the corners of the mouth that may cause cracking or bruising and may heal slowly.
6. Restricted mouth opening during healing sometimes related to swelling and muscle soreness and sometimes related to stress on the jaw joints(TMJ),especially when TMJ problem already exists.
7. A decision to leave a small piece of root in the jaw when its removal would require extensive surgery or risk of other complications.
8. Fracture of the jaw (usually only in more complicated extraction or surgery)
9. Injury to the nerve adjacent to teeth, resulting in pain numbness tingling or sensory disturbances on the chin, lip, cheek, gums or tongue and which may persist for several weeks, months, or in rare instances permanently.
10. It has been explained that during the course of treatment unforeseen conditions may result that may require change in the procedure, I authorize my Doctor to use professional judgement to perform such additional procedures that are necessary to complete my surgery.

The Anaesthetic I have chosen for my surgery is

- ☐ Local anaesthesia
- ☐ Local with oral premedication
- ☐ Local with intravenous sedation
- ☐ General anaesthesia

It has been explained to me and I fully understand that a perfect result is not or cannot be guaranteed.

I have read and fully understood the above and discussed this operation and alternative treatment with __________________. He has given me ample opportunity to ask questions about specific points and has answered those questions to my satisfaction.

PLEASE ASK YOUR DOCTOR IF U HAVE QUESTIONS CONCERNING THIS CONSENT FORM

_______________________________________________

PATIENTS (OR LEGAL GUARDIANS) SIGNATURE DATE

SURGEON's NAME:

_______________________________________________

**4. Consent for Implant**

# AOMSI CONSENT FORM

For A Safer Tomorrow

**ORAL & MAXILLOFACIAL SURGERY**

**CONSENT FOR DENTAL IMPLANT SURGERY**

Patients Name Age/Sex Date

______________________________________________________________

**Please initial on each page after reading. If you have any questions, please ask your doctor BEFORE initialing.**

______________________________________________________________

1. I hereby authorize Dr. ____________________________ and assistants to treat the condition described as ____________________________________________
______________________________________________________________.

2. The procedure offered to treat the condition has been explained to me and I understand the nature of the procedure to be: ______________________________
______________________________________________________________.

3. I understand that incisions will be made in my mouth for the purpose of placing one or more endosteal root form structures (implants) in my jaw to serve as anchors for a missing tooth or teeth replacement or to stabilize a crown (cap), bridge, or denture. I acknowledge that the doctor has explained to me the procedure, including the number and location of the incisions and the type of implant to be used. I understand that the crown, bridge or denture that will be attached to this implant(s) will be made and attached by Dr.______________________ and that a separate charge will be made by the office.

4. I understand that the implant(s) may need to remain covered by gum tissue for at least three months before being used and that a second surgical procedure may be needed to uncover the top of the implant. No guarantee can be or has been given that the implant(s) will last for a specific time period. It has been explained to me that once the implant is inserted, the entire treatment plan must be followed and completed on schedule.If the planned schedule is not carried out , the implant(s) may fail.

5. I have been informed of possible alternative methods of treatment (if any), including
______________________________________________________________
______________________________________________________________
I understand that other forms of treatment or no treatment at all are choices that I have and the risks of those choices have been presented to me.

6. My doctor has explained to me that there are certain inherent and potential risks and side effects of any surgical procedure and in this specific instance such risks include but are not limited to:

A. Post-operative discomfort , Pain and swelling that may require several days of at- home recuperation.
B. Prolonged or heavy bleeding that may require additional treatment.
C. Injury or damage to adjacent teeth and soft tissue.

Signature -----------------

D. Post-Operative infection and inflammation of soft tissues around the implant that may require additional treatment.

E. Stretching of the corners of the mouth that may cause cracking and bruising and may heal slowly.
F. Restricted mouth opening for several days; sometimes related to swelling and muscle soreness and sometimes related to stress on the jaw joints (TMJ).
G. Injury to nerve branches in the lower jaw resulting in numbness, pain or tingling of the chin, lips, cheek, gums or tongue on the operated side(s). These symptoms may persist for several weeks, months or, in rare instances may be permanent.
H. Opening into the sinus (a normal bony chamber above the upper back teeth) requiring additional treatment. If the sinus is intentionally entered (sinus-lift procedure with grafting), there may be several weeks of sinusitis symptoms requiring certain medications and additional recovery time.
I. Fracture of the jaw or perforation of thin bony plates.
J. use of other materials which may have to be removed at a later date: ______________
K. Bone loss around implants and loosening of implants.
L. implant or prosthesis fracture, or loss of the implant due to rejection by the body.
M. Allergic or adverse reactions to any medications.
N. Accidental swallowing of foreign material.
O.other ____________________________________________________________

7. It has been explained to me that during the course of surgery unforeseen conditions may be revealed which will necessitate extension of the original procedure or a different procedure from that set forth in paragraph 2 above. I authorize my doctor and his staff to perform such additional procedures as are necessary and desirable in the exercise of professional judgment.

8. I understand smoking is extremely detrimental to the success of my implant surgery. I agree to cease all forms of use of tobacco for 2-3 weeks after surgery, including the later uncovering procedure (when necessary), and to make a strong efforts to give up smoking entirely.

9. I consent to the administration of anesthesia I have chosen, which is:
☒ Local
☒ Local with Nitrous Oxide / Oxygen Analgesia
☒ Local with oral Premedication
☒ Local with Intravenous Sedation
☒ General Anesthesia

10.**ANESTHETIC RISKS** include: discomfort, swelling, bruising, infection, prolonged numbness and allergic reactions. There may be inflammation at the site of an intravenous injection (phlebitis which may cause prolonged discomfort and / or disability, and may require special care. Nausea and vomiting, although are rare, may be unfortunate side effects of IV anesthesia. Intravenous anesthesia is a serious medical procedure and, although considered safe, carries with it the risk of heart irregularities, heart attack, stroke, brain damage or death.

Signature -----------------

10. **YOUR OBLIGATIONS IF IV ANESTHESIA IS USED**

A. Because anesthetic medications cause prolonged drowsiness, you MUST be accompanied by a responsible adult to drive you home and stay with you until you are recovered sufficiently to care for yourself. This may be up to 24 hours.
B. During recovery time (24 hours) you should not drive, operate complicated machinery or devices or make important decisions such as signing documents, etc.
C. you must have a completely empty stomach. It is vital that you have nothing to eat or drink for eight (8) hours prior to your anesthetic. To do otherwise may be life-threatening.
D. However, it is important that you take any regular medications (high blood pressure, antibiotics, etc.) Or any other medications provided by this office, using only a small sip of water.

11. I understand that no guarantee can be promised and I give free and voluntary consent for treatment.

My signature below signifies that all questions have been answered to my satisfaction regarding this consent and I fully understand the risks involved of the proposed surgery and anesthesia. I certify that I speak, read, and write English.

**BEFORE SIGNING, PLEASE ASK YOUR DOCTOR IF YOU HAVE ANY QUESTIONS CONCERNING THIS CONSENT FORM.**

Patient's (or Guardian's) Signature &Date

WitnessSignature

1)

2)

Doctor`s Signature

**5. Consent for Orthognathic surgery**

AOMSI CONSENT FORM

For A Safer Tomorrow

## ORAL AND MAXILLOFACIAL SURGERY

### CONSENT FOR ORTHOGNATHIC SURGERY

Patient's Name ______________________ Age /sex __________ Date __________

**Please initial on each page after reading. If you have any questions, please ask your doctor BEFORE initialing.**

---

Orthognathic surgery is being planned for you, and it is important that you understand the benefits and risks of such surgery. This is NOT minor surgery and you have the right to be fully informed about your condition and the recommended treatment plan. The disclosures in this consent are not meant to alarm you, but rather to provide information you need in order to give or withhold your consent to the planned surgery.

1. I hereby authorize Dr.__________________________and staff to treat the condition described as:______________________________________________________________
______________________________________________________________

2. The surgical procedure planned to treat the above condition has been explained to me and I understand the nature of the treatment to be:___________________________________
______________________________________________________________

3. I have been informed of possible alternative forms of treatment (if any), including:_______
______________________________________________________________

4. My doctor has explained to me that there are certain potential risks and side effects of the surgery planned, some of which may be serious. They include, but are not limited to:

   A. Facial and jaw swelling after surgery, usually lasting several days.
   B. Bleeding, both during and after surgery, which may sometimes be severe enough to require blood transfusion. I have been informed about the opportunity for blood donation before surgery so that, my own blood may be transfused back to me (auto transfusion) if necessary.
   C. Allergic reaction to any of the medications given during or after surgery.
   D. Delayed healing of the bony segments; rarely requiring a second surgery and/or bone graft to repair.

E. Relapse: the tendency for the repositioned bone segments to return to their original position, which may require additional treatment, including surgery and/or bone grafting.

F. Bruising and discoloration of the skin around the jaws, eyes and nose. Possible Hematoma at injection site .

G. Diminished sense of smell (anosmia) in the upper jaw surgery.

H. A change in cosmetic appearance. Although this is primarily a procedure to restore jaw function, I am aware of some expected change in my appearance. I understand that certain cosmetic changes may not be totally predictable. There may also be changes in speech patterns which may require additional treatment.

I. Loss of feeling, pain or a tingling numbness in my chin, lips, tongue, gums, or teeth which occurs in a significant number of patients. Loss of taste sensation in tongue and palate . These symptoms may last for several days, weeks or months. I have been told that there is some chance that it may be permanent.

J. Possible decreased function of muscles of facial expression.

K. Scarring from external skin incisions if certain rigid fixation methods are used.

L. Malfunctioning or breakage of hard ware. Possible need for additional procedures to remove fixation devices, pins, screws, plates or splints.

M. In certain cases where bone cuts may be made in the marrow space between teeth, there is the possibility of devitalization of those teeth which may require later root canal procedures, and may result in the loss of these teeth.

N Fracture of the maxilla and mandible due to improper mobilization or incomplete osteotomies

O. In upper jaw surgery, the sinus will be affected for several weeks, and there may bleeding from nose in postoperative period. There may be a need for further sinus surgery to remedy any lingering problems.

P. Post-operative infection which may cause loss of adjacent bone and/or teeth and which may require additional treatment for a prolonged period of time.

Q Change in position of the jaw joints (TMJ) which may cause post-operative discomfort, bite change and chewing difficulties. If TMJ symptoms existed before surgery, there may be no improvement and even some worsening of these symptoms after surgery.

R. Stretching of the corners of the mouth with resulting discomfort and slow healing.

S. Inflammation of veins (phlebitis) that are used for IV fluids and medications, sometimes resulting in pain, swelling, discoloration and restriction of arm or hand movement for some time after surgery.

T. Hypernasality of voice due to swelling of nasal mucosa in immediate post operative period. Diffculty in swallowing and speech in cases of cleft patients due to velopharyngeal incompetence.

U I consent to being photographed (head and neck region only) before and After surgery and during the operation to be performed. .

These photographs may be used for medical, scientific or educational purposes, provided my name is not revealed by the pictures

**V** Airway compromise and fall back of tongue in cases of set back surgeries of mandible.

5. **General anesthesia** will be used for this surgery and I have been told of the risks, including bronchitis, pneumonia, hoarseness or voice changes, cardiac irregularities, heart attack or death. I am aware of the importance of not having anything by mouth (including clear liquids unless specifically authorized by my doctor or anesthesiologist) FOR EIGHT (8) HOURS PRIOR TO AND (8) HOURS AFTER SURGERY . **TO DO OTHERWISE MAY BE LIFE-THREATENING!**

6. I realize the importance of providing true and accurate information about my health, especially concerning possible pregnancy, allergies, medications and history of drug or alcohol use. If I misinform my doctor I understand the consequences may be life-threatening or otherwise adversely affect the results of my surgery.

**ABOUT WIRING OF TEETH**

If my teeth are wired together after this surgery, I understand there are certain associated risks and complications: oral hygiene will be diminished, there may be resulting gum disease, my teeth will feel slightly loose for some time after the wiring, compromised nutrition and there is always some concern about airway obstruction. I agree to carry wire cutters with me at all times when my jaws are wired and to avoid the use of alcohol and other activities that may cause nausea or airway problems.

Signature -----------------

**INFORMATION FOR FEMALE PATIENTS**

I have informed my doctor about my use of birth control pills. I have been advised that certain antibiotics and other medications may neutralize the preventive effect of birth control pills, allowing for conception and pregnancy. I agree to consult with my personal physician to initiate additional forms of birth control during the period of my treatment, and to continue those methods until advised by my personal physician that I can return to the use of oral birth control pills.

Signature -----------------

By signing this consent form, I acknowledge that I have read it completely and understand the procedure to be performed, the risks, and the alternatives to surgery. I have had all my questions answered to my satisfaction. I was under no pressure to sign this form and have made a voluntary choice to proceed with surgery. The fee for services has been explained to me and is satisfactory and I understand there is no warranty or guarantee as to the result and/or cure and that my condition may return or become worse. I certify that I speak, read and write English.

Patients (or guardian`s) signature & Date

Witness signature:

1.

2.

Doctor`s signature

**6. Consent for TMJ**

AOMSI CONSENT FORM

For A Safer Tomorrow

**ORAL AND MAXILLOFACIAL SURGERY**

**CONSENT FOR TREATMENT FOR REPAIR OF TEMPORO-MANDIBULAR JOINT**

Patient's Name Age/Sex Date

---

**Please initial on each page after reading. If you have any questions, please ask your doctor BEFORE initialing.**

---

Dr. ________________________________ has explained to me about the pathology (disease) that exists in my right and/or left temporomandibular joints (lower jaw joint).

I understand that my condition of limited or compromised function and/or pain may be secondary to a number of possible processes including, but not limited to

| | **Mark the symptoms** |
|---|---|
| 1. Traumatic injury | ☐ |
| 2. Malocclusion | ☐ |
| 3. Articular displacement (cartilage dislocation) | ☐ |
| 4. Degenerative joint disease, inflammation | ☐ |
| 5. Infection | ☐ |
| 6. Arthritis | ☐ |
| 7. Vascular injuries( hematoma formation) | ☐ |

8. Instrument breakage during arthroscopy ☐

9. Ankylosis( fibrous union / bony union of joint) ☐

10. Chronic pain ☐

11. Material failure ( foreign body reaction) ☐

12. Frey`s syndrome (sweating over temporal region on operated side) ☐

13. Neruosensory disturbances (numbness over skin and adjacent area of operated site) ☐

14. Otology complications ( ear related) ☐

15. Intracranial injuries ( Dural tear, cerebrospinal fluid leak) ☐

16. Post operative maxilla-mandibular fixation ☐

17. Objectionable scar formation. ☐

18 Facial swelling lasting for longer period of time ☐

I understand that the surgery to be performed is an exploratory procedure and the treatment rendered at that time will be based on the findings during surgery.

Surgical treatment may includes **mark the procedure**

1. Meniscus repair ☐

2. Meniscectomy (removal of cartilage) ☐

3. Placement of an implant ☐

4. Eminectomy ☐

5. Condylectomy. ☐

6. Arthroscopy ☐

7. Arthrocentisis ☐

8. Gap arthroplasty( release of ankylotic mass) ☐

9.Ligament Plication ☐

10.Interpositional Arthroplasty ☐

11.TMJ Reconstruction ☐

I (we) understand that my surgeon may discover other or different conditions which require additional or different procedures than those planned.

I (we) understand that no warranty or guarantee has been made to me as to a result or cure. I (we) also realize that the following risks and hazards may occur in connection with this particular procedure:

1. Facial nerve paralysis with inability to close eyelid on the affected side.

2. Inability to wrinkle the forehead.

3. Inability to blow air from mouth

4. burning sensation of eye due to inability to close eyelids

5. drooling of saliva from corner of mouth

6. Infection.

7. Resultant malocclusion (incorrect bite) and limited opening of jaw.

8. Lack of improvement or worsening of pain and jaw dysfunction.

9. Further degenerative changes with the temporomandibular joint (TMJ).

Patients (or guardian`s) signature & Date

Witness signature:

1.

2.

Doctor`s signature

**7. Consent for Trauma**

AOMSI CONSENT FORM

For A Safer Tomorrow

**ORAL &MAXILLOFACIAL SURGERY**

**CONSENT FOR TREATMENT FOR REPAIR OF FACIALBONE FRACTURES**

Patient's Name Age/Sex Date

**Please initial on each page after reading. If you have any questions, please ask your doctor BEFORE initialing.**

My doctor has explained to me that there are inherent and potential risk and side effects associated with my proposed treatment and in this specific instance, but they are not limited to

1. Damage to or loss of teeth in the area of trauma or fracture, loss of vitality of those teeth with requirement for future root canal therapy, loss of dental restoration, accidental swallowing or aspiration of tooth or foreign object, devitalization of bone and soft tissue in the area of trauma which may result in some loss of tissue.
2. Unusual procedures required during surgery such as incomplete removal of tooth, which endanger adjacent vital structures.
3. Post operative swelling, discomfort, bruising, bleeding, hematoma (blood clot), wound infection or dehiscence, sinusitis and limitations of function, any of which require further care.
4. Adverse or allergic reactions to medications or anesthesia causing multiple side effects, some of which may be serious and require additional care or hospitalization.
5. Reaction to foreign material which may have been introduced into the wound by the trauma, or "tattooing" of the skin or mucosa from particles of foreign material
6. Change in occlusion (bite) and jaw function after treatment; secondary problems of the jaw joint (TMJ) which may be prolonged, or even permanent, and which may require future treatment.
7. Possibility of otologic (ear related) complications such as perforation, infections, decrease in function of parotid gland( one of the gland responsible for saliva secretion),formation of fistula over preauricular& retromandibular region(areas of lateral

surface of face), mandibular hypomobility in long term experience, ankylosis of TMJ during surgeries of TMJ joint.

8. Scarring either inside or outside of the mouth, depending on the nature and force of the trauma and the locations of certain incisions required in treatment.
9. Facial muscle weakness particularly of the lip, eyelid or other muscles of expression caused by injury to motor nerves in the area of the trauma. Such weakness may be partial or total and may be temporary or permanent.

10. Sensory nerve injury causing pain, numbness, or other sensory alterations anywhere in the mouth, tongue, cheek, lip, and areas of facial skin which may be temporary or permanent.
11. Wiring the teeth together during the time required for healing of bone fractures will significantly reduce oral hygiene effectiveness, which may then lead to or worsen periodontal (gum) disease, bleeding gums, discomfort and loosening of teeth. Following treatment for facial injury, any such conditions must be treated. Jaw wiring will decrease normal diet and cause temporary weight loss.
12. Certain wires, screws, plates, splints or other fixation devices may be introduced, and some may require later removal.
13. Unusual effects related to hardware used such as metal sensitivity, Infection ,screw fracture, plate fracture or plate exposure.
14. Non-union or malunion of bony fractures, possibly requiring re-treatment. Some cosmetic or functional deformity may occur in areas adjacent to the trauma or repair

I understand that additional injury may be discovered during treatment that might necessitate a change in approach or a different procedure from those explained above and I authorize my doctor to perform such procedures that are necessary and advisable in the exercise of professional judgment.

I understand that this is complex treatment and there can be no guarantee of complete resolution of my present symptoms or jaw/teeth/facial bone injury. Occasionally there may be increased symptoms post-operatively (for example, numbness). I also understand that additional treatment may be necessary post-operatively, including (but not restricted to) physical therapy, reconstructive dentistry, orthodontics, retreatment of bone fractures including bone grafting, removal of certain fixation devices, or TMJ treatment. I agree to cooperate with my doctor's recommendations during treatment, realizing that lack of cooperation will result in a less-than-optimal result.

I have discussed my past medical history with my doctor and have disclosed all diseases and medications, including alcohol and drug use (past and present).

Signature ------------------------

I have had an opportunity to have all my questions answered by my doctor that all blanks on this form were filled in prior to my signing, and I certify that I understand English. My signature below signifies that I understand the surgery and anesthetic that is proposed for me, together with the known risks and complications associated. I hereby give my consent for such surgery and anesthesia I have chosen.

Patients(or guardian`s) signature &Date

Witness signature:

1.

2.

Doctor`s signature

**8. Requisites for translation of "informed consent" to vernacular languages**

AOMSI CONSENT FORM

For A Safer Tomorrow

Here is the Consent for informed consent and illiterates. This as per the standard requirement. You can dilute it or modify it.

1. All consent forms should be in the language of the majority of the population. Therefore it must be in the Vernacular of that region plus English or any other popular language. The English Consent form should be translated to the local language. There are two ways of doing it so that the essence and meaning are not lost.

A. Ethical committee approved consent forms in order to remain valid will need ' back translation'. The suggested or approved consent form must be translated into the vernacular. The thus translated matter must then be translated back to the original English by another person. Then the original and the 'back translated versions are compared. If the meaning remains unchanged then the translation is accepted. Please note that this is required only in approved consent forms in research etc. In the clinical setting the AOMSI consent for is only a template and such rigorous measures may not be necessary.

B. Alternately the approved consent in English can be translated by a Government approved translator ( usually a University translation department). E.g. The Tamil University in Tanjore does approved translations.

2. For obtaining Informed Consent of illiterate persons the Consent form can be read out to the person giving consent in the language he/ she understands in the presence of an independent third party or relative of patient who should be literate. The consent form is then signed and attested by the independent witness in addition to signature or thumb impression of the consenting person.

3. In case of children below 18 years, the parent or legal guardian can sign on behalf of the children. However, child rights activists and the new law in several countries may require a consent (particularly in older children who can comprehend issues). Technically, in India, children below 18 are considered to be 'not legally competent'.

4. In mentally retarded or persons incapable of consenting due to mental incapacity, the parent or legal guardian (if unavailable -institutional heads of organizations taking care of them can sign on their behalf).
5. In hearing impaired illiterates the consent must be explained by sign language or any means that is used for communication to translate the document. It needs third party attestation. Similarly, in visually impaired persons the consent can be obtained through Braille or by oral communication with third party attestation.

Today, in many countries video recorded informed consent procedures are utilised. It may become mandatory in India too.

Caveat: informed consent, however carefully taken can be challenged on the grounds of being an unequal contract influenced by fiduciary relationship in doctor- patient relationship.

The above is my personal opinions based on experience and the use of consent approved by Ethiconsult Services of which Dr George Paul was a member secretary. It can be modified as per personal perception of what constitutes adequate consent.

**9. Informed refusal of treatment**

AOMSI CONSENT FORM

For A Safer Tomorrow

**Informed refusal of treatment.**

This form is primarily used when any recommended treatment is refused by a patient. (It may also be used for patients with TMJ implants who remain both asymptomatic and without imaging changes in joints and who, contrary to FDA and AAOMS guidelines, do NOT wish to have TMJ implants removed)

I have been informed by DRof my condition and the recommended treatment consisting of :

______________________________________________________________________
______________________________________________________________________
______________________________________________________________________
________________________________________________

I have also been offered alternative treatment which include:

______________________________________________________________________
______________________________________________________________________
________________________________

Afterconsideringthetreatment possibilities offered, and having the benefits and risks of each explained to my satisfaction, I have voluntary chosen to :-

______________________________________________________________________
______________________________________________________________________
______________________________________________________________________
________________________________________________

I understand that my decision is contrary to my doctor's recommendation and that my condition may significantly worsen as a result, may require additional therapy additional therapy/ or hospitalization, and in rare circumstances may be life threatening. I AGREE TO RETURN TO THIS OFFICE FOR PERIODIC MONITORING OF MY CONDITION AS scheduled by my doctor.

I realize that I may consider my decision at any time by notifying my doctor.

Patient 's(or Guardian) signature Date

Witness's Signature Date

Doctor's Signature Date

## A.2 Quantification of Disability

### A.2.1 Quantification of Dento-facial Disability/ Deformity: A Proposal [19]

Form and function are the quintessence of human life. Disability and deformity are interruptions to this harmony. Disability/deformity may be congenital or acquired. Governments have a social responsibility to mitigate such afflictions by creating an environment for re integrating them into normal social life. Most welfare states provide benefits for persons with disability.

Disability can also be caused by accidents, interpersonal violence and iatrogenic causes. These situations have legal overtones and often require compensation in some form. Benefits and compensation can only be calculated if the disability is quantified. Orthopedic disabilities in Civil and Military life have been calibrated and quantified. Similarly other disabilities involving loco motor, neurological, visual and hearing deficit have also been quantified. Unfortunately the maxillofacial region has not been adequately addressed in any of these quantification charts.

Quantification of the maxillofacial region is unique on account of the fact that there are two criteria to be evaluated—Disability and Deformity. While disability is more readily calculated, deformity is highly subjective and therefore any award for the latter is bound to be arbitrary. However it is not possible to ignore the importance of deformity to the face, and an attempt is made to establish a broad parameter in which it can be assessed.

#### Review of Quantification Criteria

Quantification of orthopedic disability is well established and has been in use for social benefits, rehabilitation, assistance and percentage reservations in labour market placement of disabled people. It has also been in use for legal and insurance compensations due to accidents, interpersonal violence and occupational diseases. The Phulhems profile by the Canadian Army was established as early as 1943. The McBrides criteria was the established reference in India till 1980. It did cover some aspects of the maxillofacial region and was generally accepted for dental injuries and dental loss. The McBrides criteria (1955) was replaced in India by the "Manual for Doctors to Evaluate Permanent Physical Impairment" (1981). Unfortunately the impairment and disability of the face is covered rather incomprehensively and inadequately, relegating the whole area of the face to one half of a chapter, with hardly 30 points being allocated to the face. Not one maxillofacial surgeon sat on the expert committee of 45 advisors. In the realm of physical rehabilitation and orthopedics, numerous references are available. Kessler (1970) covered various aspects of upper and lower extremity disabilities. The American Academy of Orthopedic Surgeons Manual (1966) discusses the concept of permanent impairment through a series of questions that reveal the permanency of the deficit. The Govt. of India notification (1986) covers visual disabilities, locomotor disabilities and hearing and speech disabilities. It recommends that Kessler's formula can be taken as a general guideline.

Significantly the only other Indian guideline for Maxillofacial region comes through a Government of Tamilnadu notification (1974) where complete facial disfigurement is dealt with. It simply awards a 50% for total facial disfigurement. No break up figures is given for type or severity of disfigurement.

The American Association of Oral and maxillofacial Surgeons and American Medical Association have given guidelines for assessment of maxillofacial injuries and disabilities. They however need modification to suit our population and needs.

The authors have depended on two major sources while making this evaluation.

1. Objective Evaluation of Impairment and Ability in Locomotor Handicapped by Sabapathyvinayagam Ramar. An excellent reference book on Physical Medicine and Rehabilitation.
2. Guidelines to the Evaluation of Impairment of The Oral and Maxillofacial Region—issued by the American Association of Oral and Maxillofacial Region.

The authors have modified the guidelines of the above sources to arrive at the recommendations.

The general aim of the exercise was to evolve quantification criteria for disabilities and deformities of the Maxillofacial region taking into account the special features of the problems encountered in India. It also endeavours to simplify the percentages awarded by eliminating complex variables. **The evaluation adopts a position of awarding a 100% to the face to be divided between deformity (50%) and disability (50%). It does not try to evaluate facial impairment as a part of the total body as it would significantly reduce the quantum of impairment and thus defeat the purpose of this exercise.** Consider a situation where 100% has to be divided between cardiovascular, alimentary, central nervous and locomotor systems in addition to sexual dysfunction, liver dysfunction, renal, endocrine and metabolic dysfunctions. Further distribution amongst visual, hearing, etc. will certainly minimize any help of giving value to the face.

The evaluation has also eliminated the need to go into variables like age, sex and occupation, which will modify the award percentages. These will rest within the realm of the government agencies, judiciary or insurance agents.

The criteria formulated shall simply make a statement of disability/deformity based on standards established within the purview of the 100% for the face—equally divided amongst the various structures and functions. **The total of these shall remain within hundred utilizing the formula**

$$A + \frac{B(100 - A)}{100}$$

**where, A = higher value and**
**B = lower value.**

### Definitions

Based on Govt. of India Gazette Part I section 1 No. 4-2/83—HW III Ministry of Welfare, 1986.8

- *Impairment:* is defined as any loss (or) abnormality of psychological, physiological (or) anatomical structure (or) function.
- *Disability:* WHO defines disability in the context of health experience as any restriction or lack (resulting from an impairment) of ability to perform an activity in the manner (or) within the range considered normal for a human being.
- *Deformity:* facial disfigurement involving soft and hard tissues arising from multiple genetic factors, environment influences, acquired defects, neoplastic processes and trauma.

### Recommended Quantification for the Dento-facial Region

#### Areas of Deformity Evaluation—Hard Tissues:

A. **Loss of Teeth:**

| *Anteriors* | *Deformity/Disability* |
|---|---|
| All anteriors (upper and lower) | : 25% |
| Between 8 and 11 | : 20% |
| Between 4 and 7 | : 15% |
| Between 2 and 3 | : 10% |
| One tooth | : 05% |

Though these are disabilities and deformities that can be replaced, it deserves the above percentile as the strength and function of false teeth are not considered equal to natural teeth. Orthopedic deformities are evaluated even if prosthesis is given.

<u>Posteriors</u> <u>Disability</u>

– Excluding third molars and including premolars.

| | |
|---|---|
| All posteriors (16) | : 25% |
| Between 10 and 14 | : 20% |
| Between 6 and 9 | : 15% |
| Between 2 and 5 | : 10% |
| Occlusal discrepancy | : 10–20% |
| One tooth | : 05% |

**Loss of teeth due to progressive dental pathology (e.g. Periodontitis, caries) are not considered.** The dental surgeon will have to make an assessment based on the condition of remaining teeth or preexisting records.

B. **Loss of Bone** (Disability/Deformity)

Significant loss of bone causing
Deformity/Disability : 10–25%
Small bony fragment : 5%

C. **Mal-united Facial Bones: (Depending on extent of Disability/Deformity)**

Malunited facial bones 10–20%
– Occlusion to be combined whenever affected.

This is an incomplete quantification and will have to be assessed by the surgeon on the basis of the degree of disability/deformity caused by the malunion.

D. **Orbital Deformity (excluding visual field assessment)**

Subjective evaluation based on:
Bony orbit : 5–10%
Soft tissue e.g.) etropian, scar etc : 5–10%
Composite deformities including
Telecanthus etc : 15–25%

#### Areas of Deformity Evaluation—Soft Tissue

A. **Soft Tissue—Non-reversible**
Single linear scar : 5%
Multiple or deforming scars
Including Keloids : 10–30%
Significant loss of soft tissue
E.g. Loss of nose, ear, lips etc : 20–50%

B. **Facial Sensory Impairment (Ramar)**
Face has 34% sensory innervations of whole body.
Ophthalmic : 8%
Maxillary : 8%
Mandibular : 8%
Tongue : 10%

C. **Impairment Rate for Mouth Opening (Ramar)**
Impairment rate for interincisor distance of 4 cm : 0%
Impairment rate for interincisor distance of 3 cm : 10%
Impairment rate for interincisor distance of 2 cm : 20%
Impairment rate for interincisor distance of 1 cm : 30%
Impairment rate for interincisor distance of 0 cm : 50%

D. **Motor Disability (RAMAR)**
Jaw muscles (masticatory) : 5% right side, 5% left side
Tongue muscles : 15% either side.

E. **Facial Nerve Impairment**
Single branch : 05%
Five branches : 25%
Zygomaticotemporal : 10%

Bilateral problems are not addressed.

F. **Disfigurement criteria (AAOMS and AMA guidelines 1997 and 2002)**

- Class 1—(0–5%) Disorder of cutaneous structure e.g. visible scars
- Class 2—(5–10%) Loss of supporting structure with or without cutaneous disorder e.g. Depressed cheek and nose.
- Class 3—(10–15%) Absence of normal anatomical area of face. E.g. Loss of eye or part of nose. Visual or hearing loss will have to be separately evaluated.
- Class 4—(15–35%) Impairment of whole person. Facial disfigurement is so severe that it precludes social acceptance.

This criteria appears logical and it significantly simplifies an otherwise complex quantification of facial disfigurement. However we would encourage its use with the other mentioned parameters. The multiple percentages can be resolved with the Kessler's formula.

In multiple disabilities and deformities or when there is a combination of the two the Kessler's Formula $A+\frac{B(100-A)}{100}$ can be used, where A= the higher and B= lower value

Another formula has also been used by Ramar as per the Government of India notification: $A+\frac{B(90-A)}{90}$ again A being the higher value and B being the lower value.

The formula can be used in a few mock situations.

1. X has an injury resulting in the fracture of the mandible and loss of four incisors. He also develops a pareisis of the marginal mandibular nerve following surgery. His total percentile may be calculated thus: A = 15% and B = 5%.
   $15+\frac{5(100-15)}{100}=19.25$, whereas the sum of both would have been 20%.
2. Y has an injury resulting in the fracture of both condyles causing subsequent total bony ankylosis. He also has a large scar with keloid on his right cheek. His percentage is calculated thus:
   $50+\frac{20(100-50)}{100}=60$ whereas the sum of two injuries would have been 70. Please note that the value adjusts itself as the percentiles go up.

## Discussion

Quantifying all kinds of disabilities/deformities is an enormous task. This paper attempts to deal with only those disabilities resulting from accidents. Congenital disabilities/deformities such as those found in cleft—craniofacial anomalies will require a more extensive analysis. Similarly disabilities and deformities caused by aggressive tumours and cancers of the head and neck comprise a wide range of problems, which are not necessarily regional. Cancer in particular may have numerous associated problems ranging from donor site morbidity to psychological impact affecting quality of life and mental depression.

Dental injuries and their resultant disability/deformity are closely linked to aesthetics and mastication. For the purpose of awarding percentiles, the anterior teeth were considered for aesthetics and the posterior teeth for masticatory function. The awards are arbitrary and based on the relative dysfunction caused by the absence of teeth in the masticatory apparatus. The American Association of Oral and Maxillofacial Surgery (AAOMS) guidelines award percentages for the complete masticatory apparatus. It awards 24% for a person who is restricted to liquid diet (40–60% if tube feeding is necessary) and 5–19% if person is restricted to semisolids (includes those with ability to wear dentures). We have taken the liberty of awarding points for individual teeth. However if the whole masticatory apparatus is to be evaluated, one may separately evaluate absence of teeth, occlusal disharmony, TMJ movement (craniomandibular articulation), muscle power etc and arrive at a figure by using the Kessler's formula of $A+\frac{B(100-A)}{100}$.

This appears as a reasonable formula, which accounts for individual disabilities within the framework of the masticatory apparatus.

Further the AAOMS guidelines classifies the percentiles into two categories (1) Percentage of normal. (2) Percentage impairment of whole person. The dichotomy does not seem reasonable and is likely to cause further confusion. Finer details such as lateral excursion etc which, have been dealt with in the AAOMS guidelines have been ignored.

Similarly the concept of deformity and disfigurement has been dealt with differently in the AAOMS and the AMA guidelines. The matter of disfigurement is complicated by issues such as personality crisis and the impact of social acceptance. As suggested earlier this criteria can be incorporated into Kessler's formula, thus resolving the issue of multiple disabilities and deformities.

Finally the question of who can give a disability certificate. The Indian sources are silent in the matter of maxillofacial injuries. However the law in many American states clearly provides for the role of a Board qualified Oral Surgeon or maxillofacial Surgeon to issue disability certification for the maxillofacial region.

Contrary to general perception, it is not necessary that these criteria need to be made by statutory bodies. General usage can give legal legitimacy. It would of course be in the best interest of the Surgeon, patient and the public if these suggestions can be scrutinized, amended and enlarged to accommodate a larger spectrum of disabilities and deformities.

#### A.2.1.2 Duties of Witness

Failure to appear in court without valid reasons after warrant has been issued can invite contempt of court.

Exaggeration or false statements given under oath is not only unethical, but can invite punishment under sec. 181, Sec. 193.

## References


1. Bernhard Wolf Weinberger. Pierre Fauchard, Surgeon-dentist: a brief account of the beginning of modern dentistry, the first dental textbook, and professional life two hundred years ago. 1941.
2. Moore W. The knife man. Transworld; 2010. pp. 223–4. ISBN 978-1409044628. Retrieved 8 Mar 2012.
3. https://www.dental.upenn.edu/admissions-academics/graduate-dental-education-programs/oral-maxillofacial-surgery-residency-m-d/
4. http://dental.nyu.edu/academicprograms/advanced-education-programs/oms6.html
5. Martin-Granizo R. Double degree in oral and maxillofacial surgery — is it necessary? IJOMS. 2017;02:126.
6. Amin M, Ahmed B. Dental education in Pakistan: current trends and practice. J Coll Physicians Surg Pak. 2010;20(8):497–8.
7. Mawatha NK. Prospectus, MD oral and maxillofacial surgery and board certification. Postgraduate Institute of Medicine, University of Colombo. 2011.
8. Zheng J, Fang B, Zhang S, Yang C, Shen G, Qiu W, et al. Oral and maxillofacial surgery in China: past, present and future. Open J Stomatol. 2013;03:354–8.
9. Fiehn N-E. Perspectives on dental education in the Nordic Countries. J Dent Educ. 2002;66(12):1374–80.
10. EACMFS. White book. Russia. 1st ed. 2017. http://beta.jointogethergroup.com/Society/members/whitebook/export.asp?wb=31
11. Kumar S. Training programmes in oral and maxillofacial surgery across the globe – a mini review. J Maxillofac Oral Surg. 2017;16(3):269–76.
12. Revised Dentists (Code of Ethics) Regulations – 2014, Part II, Section 3, Sub-sec (1) of the Gazette of India.
13. http://www.thefreedictionary.com/informed+consent
14. Faden RR, Beauchamp TL. A history and theory of informed consent. Oxford University Press; 1986. p. 28, 123.
15. Faden RR, Beauchamp TL. A history and theory of informed consent. Oxford University Press; 1986.
16. Gasparini G, Boniello R, Moro A, Di Nardo F, Pelo S. Orthognathic surgery: a new preoperative informed consent model. J Craniofac Surg. 2009;20(1):90–2.
17. Krishnan NR, Kasthuri AS. Informed Consent MFAJI. 2007;63:164-166.
18. http://www.surgery.org/press/news-release.php?iid=125
19. Paul G. Medical law for the dental surgeon. Jaypee Publishers; 2004. p. 30.
20. Bolam Vs Friern Hospital managing committee. (1957) 2 AIIER 118.
21. IMA v VP Shantha and Oths 111 (1995) CPJ (SC).

# Research and Publishing in Oral and Maxillofacial Surgery

# 45

George Dimitroulis

## 45.1 Introduction

We have all been too quick to make up our minds and too slow to change them. In Oral and Maxillofacial Surgery, our opinions are slaves to our prior experience. Ignorant confidence is what defined early Surgery as there was a distinct lack of interest in proving and promoting what was effective. The "God complex" among early Surgeons meant that what they thought was true did not need scientific evidence. It is only in more recent times that Surgical practice has embraced evidence to guard against rumour, bias, misconceptions and misunderstandings. Indeed, just in the last few decades we have witnessed the gradual evolution of Surgery from eminence-based practice, the idea that senior experienced Surgeons held all the knowledge, to evidence-based practice, where fair tests are employed to compare one treatment against the other in order to find what works best. History has taught us that clinical research leads to reforms in the practice of Surgery while basic research leads to revolutions in Medicine.

Like in most other scientific disciplines, Surgical research is used to confirm facts, reaffirm the results of previous work, solve existing problems and ultimately develop new ideas of practical value. If you can understand more, you can make better decisions rather than blind guesses which is the hallmark of successful clinical practice. Judgements, predictions and plans are based on the latest available information and should be constantly updated in the light of new information derived from good research. The late British Economist John Maynard Keynes once said "when the facts change, I change my mind". So too, a good Surgeon must be open to new ideas and techniques which are essential to the progress and evolution of each surgical specialty, as change is only possible when key opinion leaders lead the charge.

G. Dimitroulis (✉)
Maxillofacial Unit, St. Vincent's Hospital – University of Melbourne, Melbourne, Australia

Essentially, the greatest discoveries in Surgery are those that force us to rethink our beliefs about human disorders and our role in managing it. Research builds our core knowledge, and the most useful knowledge is one that changes the behaviour and practice of Surgeons. The simple idea of washing your hands before handling patients met with immense resistance from the established medical community in the nineteenth century until the scientific evidence supporting microbial infection became too overwhelming to ignore. Knowledge increases your ability to predict the outcomes, and the knowledge of bacterial infections was one of the greatest breakthroughs in modern medicine that significantly reduced the mortality and morbidity of even the simplest of surgical procedures. Research has been pivotal to the success of surgery over the last two centuries and will continue to be an integral part of all future progress, especially in the rapidly expanding field of Oral and Maxillofacial Surgery.

Progress doesn't occur in a vacuum; it almost always builds on existing ideas with a series of incremental improvements. That is why most research is used to develop further knowledge on a topic by reaffirming the results, theories and problems of past work in the field. Occasionally, when trying to solve an existing problem, research may lead to the discovery of new problems, ideas and theories which makes the science of Surgery a dynamic process of knowledge acquisition that has no endpoint.

## 45.2 The Science of Research

The word Science comes from the Latin "scienta" which means knowledge or skill. Science is about new ideas and testing these in the most transparent way. What launched the Scientific revolution was the realization that we do not have the answers to their most important questions. To find the answers, experiments are what people devised when they weren't sure of the truth. Ignorance is the starting point of all


K. Bonanthaya et al. (eds.), *Oral and Maxillofacial Surgery for the Clinician*, https://doi.org/10.1007/978-981-15-1346-6_45

science, and curiosity about the world around us is what drives science. The more that is unknown, the greater the opportunity to discover, and that is how research has become an essential tool of discovery.

The word Research is derived from an old French term referring to seeking or searching. Research is all about the ability to test, reproduce, quantify and falsify an idea before it can be fully accepted as scientific fact. In research we learn more from the unexpected results than from those we anticipate. Understanding the research process helps generate new research questions. The trick is to ensure the right methods are used to answer the right questions. For example, when we are seeking verification, we must ask ourselves "Did I build the system right?", while if we want to validate something, we then ask "Did I build the right system?".

Scientific research is a systematic way of explaining things by collecting evidence which make practical applications possible. The goal of research is not only to yield new knowledge but also to make us better understand existing issues or topics. There are three main forms of Research; Exploratory research helps to identify a problem, while Constructive research proposes solutions to the problem. The third is Empirical research which tests the feasibility of the solution using either qualitative or quantitative methods. Qualitative research collects data in the form of words, images and video which is largely confined to the social sciences but may also have applications in Surgical techniques. The difference between quantitative (numbers) and qualitative (descriptions) research is well summarized by the famous scientist, Albert Einstein, who once said that "Not everything that matters can be measured, and not everything that can be measured matters". The world cannot be understood without numbers, and equally, it cannot be understood with numbers alone.

In Surgery, quantitative research is most often used to establish the existence of causal relationships between variables by collecting and analysing numerical data. By relying on random sampling, the quantitative research method allows for experimental, correlational and descriptive (i.e. survey) results that are easy to summarize, compare and generalize using statistics to determine the relationship between variables. For example, if the research question is about best mandibular reconstruction following tumour resection, the patients may be randomly assigned to different groups, each representing a different mode of reconstruction. If this is not feasible, the researcher may collect data related to the patient's demographics and situational characteristics to statistically control for their influence on the degree of morbidity following their particular mandibular reconstruction. Often the intent of the surgical research is to generalize from the study participants to a larger population which will require the researcher to employ probability sampling to select the study participants.

**Table 45.1** The scientific research method

| |
|---|
| a. Identifying problem through observation |
| b. Review the literature—look for gaps in knowledge |
| c. Specify aims/purpose of research |
| d. Determine specific question or hypothesis |
| e. Define the variables being measured |
| f. Choose method of data collection—avoid bias |
| g. Data analysis—choose your statistical method |
| h Data interpretation—keep an open mind |
| i. Test/revision of hypothesis |
| j. Conclusion/recommendations for surgical practice |
| k. Reporting/communicating/publishing findings |

## 45.3 The Scientific Research Method (Table 45.1)

Scientific research follows a structured process. Successful research is only possible when asking the right questions, engaging in the right observations, running the right experiments and networking with the right people to elicit ideas and feedback. The core principle of science and research are precision and transparency—being clear about your methods and honest with your results. Transparency is what gives science credibility. World-changing ideas and technology were built from a protracted process of trial and error. Experiments are designed to show what does work and what doesn't. It is by testing that we gain access to the feedback that drives progress. Formal research has a well-established pathway that follows the basic steps set out below.

### 45.3.1 Observation

Many people simply watch the world around them (on autopilot). Few people observe. An astute observer will see the problem only when they're not vested in the way things have been. Their ability to imagine how things should be is what drives change and progress. The hardest part of solving a problem is seeing it, and many surgeons blindly follow procedures that do more harm than good for the patient because they have failed to question the surgical technique they have been taught. In surgery, very few surgeons have ever asked the pivotal question—"Is there a better way?" Curiosity and an open mind is what drives progress, and unfortunately, most surgeons have achieved their chosen profession by not rocking the boat and adhering to conventional practices.

Many of the things we accept as objective truths are themselves assumptions based on uncertainty, even in the world of Surgery. No surgical concept or technique has an absolute and permanent value. Time, experience and better experimental tools give rise to new ideas that supplant the old ideas. In other words, all existing surgical ideas and techniques are sooner or later supplanted by new ideas and techniques which means surgery is a never ending marvel of evolution.

Before embarking on any kind of research, the first step is to look for any idea or technique that has not been adequately explained or supported by evidence. When looking to a topic or issue as a potential subject for research, the hierarchy of deliberation begins with (1) "Where is the evidence?", (2) "How sound is the evidence?" and (3) "Has the evidence been properly interpreted?". Once you have selected the appropriate subject or topic you would like to explore, the next step is to find out what the literature has to say and look for gaps in the existing knowledge.

### 45.3.2 Literature Review

All the world's information is now at our fingertips, and to access scientific publications is a matter of a few keystrokes. Search engines like Google Scholar and PubMed have opened up a whole new digital world of scientific literature that even the largest University libraries could never hope to subscribe to. Access to the world's scientific literature has never been simpler than it is today, and subscriptions to University libraries also allow students digital access to a wide range of local and international journals.

Once the research topic has been selected, a thorough review of the literature is required to establish what is already known. It is best to begin with the most recent peer-reviewed articles on the topic which will often summarize the existing body of knowledge. Meta-analysis papers, especially those that follow the PRISMA guidelines, are becoming more common, and these papers can form the foundation of your research topic. Good journal papers will commonly highlight the gaps in our knowledge, the weakness in the current evidence available, and what further research is required that will conveniently point you in the right direction.

### 45.3.3 Purpose of Research

Once you have gathered all the pertinent information from the literature review, the next step is to crystalize in your own mind why you are embarking on this research. The flaws or holes in previous research are identified so that the gaps in the literature will provide justification for the new research being proposed. Look for clues in the literature where there may be a deficiency in the evidence surrounding published statements, particularly those that make generalizations that are not adequately backed by evidence. Indeed, many Cochrane reviews have consistently concluded that the vast majority of clinical papers fail to provide the level of evidence required to make any firm conclusions. The aim or purpose of the research is pivotal to the whole project as it dictates the methodology required to adequately address the aims. It is also the main driver in funding applications and recruiting study participants.

### 45.3.4 Hypothesis

Science grows with every new piece of evidence with the hypothesis as the compass that directs the inquiries. Scientific theories have to make testable predictions that can be validated in experiments. Science is not just about confirmation; it is also about falsification. If a theory cannot be tested, then it's logically impossible to ever falsify it. Karl Popper said "if it is not falsifiable, it's not scientific". If a theory cannot be tested with experiments, then it falls in the realm of religion or philosophy or pure speculation. Questions that generate the greatest emotional response are a great indicator of challenging the way things are.

The gap in the literature creates a research question which is otherwise referred to as the Hypothesis. The Hypothesis is a prediction which is set out as a statement that defines the relationship between two or more variables. In research, it is the hypothesis that is being tested as to whether it is true or false. If the hypothesis turns out to be consistent with the observations, then it is said to be supported rather than proven as it is still subject to further scrutiny. But if it is rejected, then support is claimed for an alternative hypothesis. The Null hypothesis is when there is no relationship between the variables being investigated.

### 45.3.5 Define the Variables

In the hypothesis statement, there will be two or more variables that will be the focus of the study. The study is designed to establish the relationship between the variables. However, before commencing the study, the variables must be clearly defined so that there is no doubt as to what each variable represents. Without clear definitions of the variables, studies cannot be repeated and hence impossible to validate.

### 45.3.6 Data Collection

What isn't measured can't be managed. Without data, we cannot make informed decisions. We gather data to collect information that becomes knowledge which is finally displayed as wisdom. Data has to be collected, processed and analysed for it to become information which can be used to make better decisions. Ultimately, the answer is only as good as the quality of the data fed into it.

Apart from field studies such as surveys and clinical audits, OMF Surgeons also conduct experiments that involve laboratory controlled conditions, often by recruiting the resources of other medical specialities such as pathology, microbiology, radiology, biochemistry, pharmacology and haematology. Data collection is easiest when data points can be quantified or represented with numerical figures. Even descriptive surveys can be quantified provided the responses can be listed on a sliding scale ranging from good to bad, high to low or positive to negative. A typical example is the visual analogue scale used by OMF Surgery researchers to quantify pain scales, chewing ability and quality of life outcomes before and after jaw surgery.

In Medicine, randomized trials where the patients and experimenters are blinded are least vulnerable to bias than observational studies, which are most prone to bias. Unfortunately, randomized trials are more expensive than observational studies and require a lot more manpower and resources to properly execute. In surgery, we most commonly rely on observational studies as the best evidence we have to go on for two reasons. Firstly, control groups with which to compare treatment outcomes, unlike a placebo sugar drug, are rare as it is ethically impossible to undertake sham operations. And secondly, it is practically impossible to blind surgeons and patients when it comes to evaluating surgical procedures. Evidence in the field of Oral and Maxillofacial Surgery therefore relies largely on observational studies derived from surveys and clinical audits of case series.

### 45.3.7 Data Analysis

Data science is about understanding the world by spotting patterns and predicting how one variable will affect another. While our instincts may give us a reasonable sense of how the world works, we need data to sharpen the picture as we can be easily blinded by our own experiences and prejudices.

Data shows us there is more to OMF Surgery than we think we see. Good data science can often demonstrate counterintuitive results—what you least expected to see. Selection biases are distortions of the results introduced either by the data collecting tools or by the method of data accumulation.

Statistics is a valuable tool that helps determine whether the results you have found are likely to be due to a chance rather than a true finding. Make sure the data is collected on an Excel spreadsheet, and work out what level of confidence you will accept as statistically significant which, in clinical research, is often the 95% confidence level (i.e. $P$ value $<0.05$). In statistics, the smaller the sample, the lower the likelihood that it would mirror the broader population. Large samples yield more precise results, while small samples are more susceptible to extreme results. As sample sizes get larger, the statistical calculations from that sample get more precise. Small differences (1%) between two populations being measured require bigger sample numbers than large differences (25%) for the true value to emerge. This is called the power calculation which is an important measure to consider before embarking on any study. Statistics is a complex affair and beyond the scope of this chapter, so the services of an expert statistician may well be useful when it comes to crunching the data.

### 45.3.8 Data Interpretation

Information is interpreted by different people in different ways. People can look at the same set of facts and disagree. Data can be manipulated to support any argument. You don't always need a ton of data to find important insights. What you need is the right data. Numbers can be seductive. We can grow fixated with them, and in doing so, we can lose sight of more important considerations. When looking at data, it is not the raw crunching power you have that matters most, but what you do with it that is most important. Behind every statistic there is a certain set of assumptions and prejudices. Minds crave certainty, and when they don't find it, they impose it so we must keep an open mind when the data does not yield the results we expected to see.

### 45.3.9 Test or Revision of Hypothesis

Your judgement call about how the results support your hypothesis is essential to your conclusions. If the data does not support your hypothesis, then it is essential to state an alternate hypothesis that fits with what has been observed. The scientific method is tailor-made for cherry picking because of its hypotheses and caveats and refusal to embrace certainty. Even in Science, certainty still relies on the assumptions, interpretations and theories of researchers based on what they see. Nothing is definite, for doubt is an essential operating principle of science. This means that doubt still has a place in all scientific proofs, so that all evidence is provisional and not final. In other words, what you have ascertained in your research is not definite proof but rather tacit support for an idea.

### 45.3.10 Conclusions and Recommendations

The conclusion is a summary of the entire experiment or study that simply states the outcomes observed which must be clear, concise and to the point. Any ambiguity should be highlighted and recommendations made as to how future studies should be conducted to minimize the uncertainty. It may simply be a numbers game where more patients are required, or additional groups such as control patients which may provide a clearer outcome. For example, the effectiveness of Botox in Myofascial Pain (TMD) can never be properly evaluated if there are no control groups (i.e. that have normal saline injected) with which to compare.

The conclusion is the most sought after piece of information that others will first look at when reviewing your research. Although it sounds rather obvious, the conclusion(s) must be supported by the data; otherwise, the research makes no sense. The onus is on the researcher to make sure the conclusions also fulfil the goals and aims of the study. Recommendations based on the conclusions are essential in providing a practical guide to surgical practice. Research is what drives clinical advances in Surgery, and the change in behaviour of Surgeons can only be achieved with evidence.

### 45.3.11 Reporting/Communicating/Publishing Findings

Research is useless if it is not shared with the outside world. All humanity is now connected by digital technology which has rendered distance, time and costs irrelevant to the distribution and exchange of ideas. The digital world has made recording, storage and dissemination of information, research and ideas virtually free with costless reproduction and instantaneous global distribution. Reporting and publishing research findings is described in detail in Sect. 5.

## 45.4 Constraints in Surgical Research

Cultures that fail to encourage questioning also fail to come up with new ideas. Great institutions should teach us how to ask hard questions and where to look for answers. Knowing all the answers does not distinguish someone's intelligence—rather, the ability to ask the right questions and linking the unconnected is the mark of a true genius. Generally, it is considered a weakness and a sign of vulnerability for clinicians to appear unsure. Confidence in medicine is valued over uncertainty, but science is all about uncertainty which drives progress. If we knew it all, there would not be a need for research.

Nothing is as powerful as an idea whose time has come. New ideas are what drive behavioural change and innovation. A new behaviour needs social approval before others are likely to pick up the habit as their own. Only the curious, who are open to learning, have a much greater chance of creating a truly novel solution. Unfortunately, originality is not always embraced by the surgical profession who are generally conservative by nature.

It is much easier for Surgeons to accept familiar ideas than totally original ones because if the ideas are too original, then it may be too hard for the Surgeon to accept or understand. The goal is to push the envelope, not to tear the envelope. Radical ideas are best presented in a way that is less shocking and more appealing to mainstream surgical practice by planting the seeds of a simple idea before revealing the larger idea. If you want your ideas to be accepted by your peers, make your ideas more appealing by connecting it with other ideas that are already understood by your colleagues. Other constraints related to research involve ethics, funding and bias which are discussed below.

### 45.4.1 Ethics

There has been a push in recent years by institutions and clinical journals to have all animal and human research activities sanctioned by appropriate ethics review boards or panels attached to hospitals or Universities. Without ethics approval or clearance, it may be impossible to conduct even the simplest of clinical studies, including basic surveys. Some Journals now request a copy of the ethics clearance letter before the paper can even be put out to review.

Unlike pharmaceutical research, the level of evidence in clinical surgery is hampered by the fact that control subjects are often missing because you cannot ethically perform sham operations in humans. Therefore, when designing surgical experiments, consider whether animal, laboratory or cadaver studies may be useful instead. Otherwise, you are limited to clinical audits which provide useful information which may not be scientifically valid. For example, a hospital which boasts 100% survival of its patients achieves this by turning away the sickest patients. Or a hospital which has the worst outcomes may well be a tertiary referral centre that only treats the most complex of cases that other hospitals turn away. So, while clinical audits provide a snapshot of the Hospital Unit's activities, it tells us very little else as far as science, progress and innovation is concerned.

We must be suspicious of therapeutic claims that have not been properly tested. Equally, we must be even more suspicious of research results that cannot be replicated. Many people are driven by a deep human desire for recognition and affirmation of work well done. Sometimes it is possible to build an academic career by sounding clever, rather than being clever. Most academics chase large numbers of trivial publications instead of investing their energies in new frontiers. In other words, why search for something new when you can collect rents on everything that has already been done. Sadly, there are small numbers of academics and researchers who have built their careers on falsification and plagiarism. The desire for recognition and the need for promotion when combined with the pressure to publish can tip some academics, clinicians and scientists towards fraudulent activities where data is made up and text is plagiarized in order to churn out the maximum number of "scientific" papers. In science and surgery, reputation takes many years of hard dedication to build up and an instant to destroy when you're suspected of scientific fraud.

### 45.4.2 Funding

Scientists have an innate desire to innovate, share, collaborate and be recognized for it regardless of the financial incentives. Hence, good research requires funding from external sources. Unfortunately, the spirit of open scientific enquiry can sometimes be hijacked by the combination of self-interest and money, especially when industry offer to bankroll the study. Industry rely on profitable enterprises which grow shareholder value. Scientific support behind a product is perhaps the ultimate value-adding marketing tool, so industry are always looking out for research that shows positive outcomes related to their products. Furthermore, industry never leave anything to chance so they want control of scientific research through financial rewards to various research institutions. By directly funding research, industry have control over what is published (i.e. the positive results) and what stays buried in a locked cupboard (i.e. the negative results).

Therefore, the most respectable research is that which is funded by government or not-for-profit organizations such as Medical Societies and disease interest groups like the Heart Foundation or the Cancer Council and so on. Funding from non-industry groups are much more competitive as there is always a limited amount of money available for research so applications must be of high quality. Furthermore, the non-industry funding bodies give free reign to the scientists on how the data is used and published. Industry funding, on the other hand, have simpler applications but more control of the data which remains their property. Most importantly, industry insist on the final veto on whether or not the results are published.

### 45.4.3 Confirmation Bias

Confirmation bias is one of the shortcomings of science because the human mind is bad at seeing things it did not expect to see and a bit too eager to see what it expected to see. It is basically seeing what you want to see and ignoring everything else. In essence, confirmation bias is when you filter reality through biases by eagerly accepting evidence that confirms what you believe and ignoring evidence that refutes or challenges what you believe. Once we adopt a particular hypothesis or interpretation, we find it difficult to see things any other way. People will accept any explanation as long as it fits with their own understanding of the facts.

### 45.4.4 Cognitive Dissonance

Cognitive dissonance is another impediment to scientific progress that affects many people. It is simply a feeling of discomfort that people experience when presented with information that is inconsistent with their beliefs. When we are confronted with evidence that challenges our deeply held beliefs, we are more likely to reframe the evidence than we are to alter our beliefs. In most cases, instead of acknowledging an error in judgement, people tend to reformulate their views in a way that justifies their old opinions. We simply invent new reasons, new justifications, or new explanations or ignore it altogether. Some people go to absurd lengths to justify their beliefs or judgement even when confronted with clear contrary evidence. The more committed we are to a certain opinion, the less likely we are to relinquish it, even when confronted with massive or overwhelming contradictory evidence. As an example, the introduction of microvascular venous couplers in microsurgery was developed by those who could see the obvious benefits of speed and patency of the anastomosis, and yet was resisted by those who felt the skill of micro-suturing tiny veins would be lost, regardless of the benefits of reduced thrombosis and improved flap survival.

## 45.5 Publishing

Research cannot thrive without publishing. All research projects are conceived with publication as the end game. The excessively competitive field of research creates a tendency to rush to conclusions and publish results that have not been properly validated. Valid conclusions can only be drawn from reproducible data sets because results that initially look promising aren't always repeatable. It is little wonder that remarkably few published breakthroughs have ever led to any useful treatments.

There are numerous media that researchers can use to propagate their experimental findings which are discussed below.

### 45.5.1 Electronic Media

Digital technology has not only transformed but has revolutionized the way we live. The merger of the personal computer and the Internet allowed networking to blossom on a massive scale, and so surgeons and scientist are not wholly reliant on print media to propagate their ideas. Websites like ResearchGate encourage scientists and clinicians to upload their research, both published and unpublished, onto a digital platform for all to see and to foster collaboration between research groups across the world.

Digital media platforms like YouTube are fast becoming a quick, easy and virtually cost-free way of publishing your novel ideas and surgical techniques on the Internet for all to see. More and more Surgeons are bypassing the heavily fortified realm of print media for the highly accessible digital media which not only offers a global audience but also facilitates immediate upload of content with virtually no delay. The disadvantage is of course the lack of scrutiny which suggests the content has not been vetted by experts. Hence, the scientific value of the video post is virtually zero. While you may have a wide audience, it may not necessarily be the people you want to impress.

### 45.5.2 Magazines

Glossy magazines that specifically target general medical/dental practitioners are supported by lots of industry advertising which is interspersed with clinical articles that have not been peer-reviewed, but rather submitted on the invitation of the magazine editor. The articles, which often have more clinical pictures than text, are written by clinicians and academics as a general interest piece that provides the reader with an update of what is current clinical practice that is aimed at the non-specialist practicing clinician. Authors are generally paid for their contributions. These articles are of little value to the specialist trainee or clinician wanting to find out more about their own specialty.

### 45.5.3 Textbooks

Textbooks contain information that is current practice and accepted by the profession. Unfortunately, by the time a textbook is commissioned, written, published and finally released, the information is often about 2 years out of date. Therefore, the strength of textbooks is in the basic principle of surgical practice, and the weakness lies in the distinct lack of new information. Digital technology is gradually changing the need for printed textbooks as students are gravitating to knowledge that is presented in discrete digital packages with hyperlinks that cross-reference important concepts similar to "Wikipedia". While university and hospital libraries still purchase textbooks for student consumption, today's students are finding the expense of textbooks prohibitive and so seek other means of accessing surgical information and knowledge through the Internet, which is often up to date as long as they know what to look for and are able to critically evaluate the credibility of the information source.

### 45.5.4 Peer-Reviewed Journals

There are over 1 million academic papers published every year in over 24,000 academic journals where gaps in our knowledge are discussed and new experiments are conducted that might resolve these gaps. Unfortunately, published scientific papers tend to be biased towards reporting positive results. Negative results do not make headlines so they are rarely published. Publication in a journal is not a mark of truth but merely that the research has passed a certain standard that warrants entering the formal literature and further discussion.

Scientific journals sell scholarship back to the same universities whose scientists had produced, written, peer reviewed and edited largely for free. Hence the cost of producing scientific journals is kept as low as possible in order to facilitate as wide a distribution as possible. Unlike magazines, peer-reviewed journals with few exceptions keep industry advertising to a minimum as they are supposed to be impartial to avoid conflict of interest when reporting studies that may conflict with the interests of a big advertiser.

Peer-reviewed journals are the platform we use to announce new discoveries, to comment on or criticize the discovery of others and to synthesize and seek to build consensus about what is known. In Oral and Maxillofacial Surgery, case reports and technical notes account for about one-third of journal publications, while less than one in ten are randomized control (Level 2 evidence) or non-randomized control (Level 3 evidence) studies (Table 45.2). Because of the difficulty in performing high-level randomized control trials in surgery, Surgeons are more accepting of lower-level evidence which is based on observation. Indeed, it is unlikely to extract any high-level evidence research from surgical departments who rely on surgical trainees for their research output.

**Table 45.2** Levels of evidence (Oxford Centre for Evidence-Based Medicine)

| |
|---|
| *Level 1: Randomized control trials (RCT)* |
| High-quality, properly powered and conducted studies with reduced bias when double blinded and multicentred |
| *Level 2: Cohort clinical studies* |
| Prospective, comparative clinical study without randomization |
| *Level 3: Case-controlled studies* |
| Retrospective clinical study |
| *Level 4: Case series studies* |
| Cross-sectional study (clinical audit) with or without intervention |
| *Level 5: Case-based reasoning* |
| Includes case reports, expert opinions and bench research |

*Note*: The strength of systematic reviews and meta-analysis depends on the evidence levels of the papers being reviewed. If all the papers are Level 3 evidence, the systematic review will also be Level 3 evidence

**Table 45.3** Factors to consider in the design of a clinical study

1. Where is the study being conducted? (field, hospital, clinic, laboratory, etc.)
2. Are there ethical issues? (animal or human studies)
3. Define your study groups or variables being investigated
4. Selection criteria (inclusion/exclusion)
5. Are there matched controls?
6. Describe the surgical or technical details
7. Method of data collection (randomized or blinded)
8. Method of data handling (statistical method)

**Table 45.4** Criteria for a good surgical manuscript

1. Short, succinct title
2. Original ideas with practical or pragmatic applications
3. Clear purpose/aim(s)
4. Good grammar—clear and concise wording/short sentences
5. Methods described in adequate detail to allow independent verification
6. Results set out in clearly labelled tables, graphs, figures, photos, diagrams
7. Focused discussion with balanced literature that both support and refute results
8. The most recent references that adequately support discussion
9. Conclusion supported by the results of the study

**Table 45.5** Anatomy of a poor surgical manuscript

1. Long, convoluted and ambiguous title
2. Wild, unusual, unethical or dangerous ideas of little practical value
3. No clear aims or purpose stated
4. Plagiarism and duplication (study previously published elsewhere under different title)
5. Poor grammar—incorrect wording/long convoluted sentences/ emotive language
6. Methods inadequately or poorly described that cannot be repeated
7. No data, tables, figures, graphs, photos or diagrams provided
8. Convoluted discussion without clear direction and biased to supportive literature
9. Old or antiquated references
10. Conclusion not supported by the results of the study

All journals subscribe to the IMRD layout which means all submissions must have an Introduction, Methods, Results and Discussion sections. The introduction builds the case for why you pursued the line of research and the final sentence is always the statement of the aim(s) of your study. The Methods section describes how the study was performed in terms of setting (e.g. Hospital or Laboratory), subjects (i.e. animals or humans), recruitment (e.g. inclusion/exclusion criteria), data collection (e.g. Surveys, measurements), variables being compared (experimental vs. control) and data analysis (statistics used) (Table 45.3). The Results section simply states the summary of the outcomes as depicted in the tables and graphs, while the Discussion critically analyses and compares the results in light of what has already been previously published on the topic. The discussion must include references that both agree and disagree with your findings so that a balanced argument can be presented which will add weight to the study.

**Table 45.6** Guidelines for formatting papers for publication

| | | |
|---|---|---|
| 1. | Randomized control studies: | www.consort-statement.org |
| 2. | Observational studies: | www.strobe-statement.org |
| 3. | Systematic reviews: | www.prisma-statement.org |
| 4. | Case series: | www.processguideline.com |
| 5. | Case reports: | www.scareguideline.com |

The final paragraph in the discussion is a summary of the research results with mention of any practical clinical applications that may arise from the study.

Authors must keep in mind that originality and a clear message are essential in getting their papers published in the highly competitive world of scientific journal publishing (Table 45.4). The high impact factor journals generally attract articles with high evidence levels so it is imperative to select a journal that caters to the subject and evidence levels of your particular study to avoid rejection and delays in publication of your paper. Original contributions that add new information to the existing body of knowledge are more likely to be considered for publication. However, wild or fanciful ideas are unlikely to garner support from journal editors who are looking for papers that lend respectability to their journal.

Unlike works of fiction, good scientific communication is based on clear and concise wording with short titles and tightly controlled sentences that describe complex ideas in the simplest language possible. Poor grammar, emotive language and long-winded descriptive wording must be avoided so that the ideas being conveyed are not buried in a convoluted tangle of discourse (Table 45.5). When evaluating the importance and relevance of published articles, surgeons and scientists look for the facts, not fancy prose.

To improve the acceptability of your paper for publication in a peer-reviewed journal, there are general guidelines available online that help you set out your paper in a format that is recognized and accepted throughout the world (Table 45.6). By following the guidelines, you improve the chances of your paper being accepted for publication. For instance, if you want to submit an observational case cohort study, then the "STROBE" statement will guide you in how to properly format your paper. If it is a case report then it is worth checking out the "SCARE" guidelines. Alternatively, if you want to undertake a systematic review of a topic, the "PRISMA" statement is essential.

## 45.6 Conclusion

In Surgery there is no greater accomplishment than being the first to successfully implement a successful treatment that changes the history of medicine. However, the person with the first idea is usually not the one recognized by history. Credit often goes to the person who convinces the world, not to the one with the original idea, because the credibility of all new ideas requires convincing evidence. If you make a claim about something, you provide the evidence, or at least a reference to the evidence that backs your claim. Research is the essential tool that builds the evidence which provides a better understanding of how and why things worked or failed. Good surgical practice must be based on evidence.

Surgical innovation is a constant work in progress because any new ideas or techniques are quickly supplanted by an even better ideas and techniques. Gaps in the literature are what fuel research, and the journey of discovery is paved with potholes that need to be filled. To paraphrase the great scientist Sir Isaac Newton, if you want to see further than anyone else has seen before, you need to stand on the shoulders of giants. Your voyage of discovery begins once you have secured your footing on the shoulders of the surgeons and scientists who have gone before you, so you can see the path they have built for you to follow.

## Further Reading

Dimitroulis G. EDITORIAL – Getting published in peer-reviewed journals. Int J Oral Maxillofac Surg. 2011;40:1342–5.

Dimitroulis G. EDITORIAL – Research – why bother? Int J Oral Maxillofac Surg. 2011;40:1346.

Hardicre J. An overview of research ethics and learning from the past. Br J Nurs. 2014;23:483–6.

Knottnerus JA, Tugwell P. EDITORIAL – Evidence-based medicine: achievements and prospects. J Clin Epidemiol. 2017;84:1–2.

Lau SL, Samman N. Levels of evidence and journal impact factor in Oral & Maxillofacial Surgery. Int J Oral Maxillofac Surg. 2007;36:1–5.

Mohan M, Shetty D, Shetty T, Pandyak K. Rising from plagiarising. J Maxillofac Oral Surg. 2015;14:538–40.

Sollaci LB, Pereira MG. The introduction, methods, results, discussion (IMRAD) structure: a fifty year survey. J Med Libr Assoc. 2004;92:364–7.

Szklo M. Impact factor: good reasons for concern. Epidemiology. 2008;19:369.

GPSR Compliance

*The European Union's (EU) General Product Safety Regulation (GPSR) is a set of rules that requires consumer products to be safe and our obligations to ensure this.*

*If you have any concerns about our products, you can contact us on ProductSafety@springernature.com*

In case Publisher is established outside the EU, the EU authorized representative is:

Springer Nature Customer Service Center GmbH
Europaplatz 3
69115 Heidelberg, Germany

**Batch number: 10683583**

Printed by Printforce, the Netherlands